Formulas for drug calculations

Surface area rule:

$$\text{Child dose} = \frac{\text{Surface area (m}^2)}{1.73\text{m}^2} \times \text{Adult dose}$$

Calculating strength of a solution:

Solution Strength: *Desired Solution:*

$$\frac{x}{100} = \frac{\text{Amount of drug desired}}{\text{Amount of finished solution}}$$

Calculating flow rate for IV:

$$\text{Rate of Flow} = \frac{\text{Amount of fluid} \times \text{Administration set calibration}}{\text{Running time}}$$

$$\frac{x}{1} = \frac{\text{(ml) (gtt/min)}}{\text{min}}$$

Calculation of medication dosages:

Formula method:

$$\frac{\text{Amount ordered}}{\text{Amount on hand}} \times \text{Vehicle}$$

$$= \text{Number of tablets, capsules, or amount of liquid}$$

Vehicle is the drug form or amount of liquid containing the dosage. Amounts used in calculation by formula must be in the same system.

Ratio—proportion method:

1 tablet: tablet in mg on hand:: x tablet order in mg
         Know or have:: Want to know or order

Multiply means and extremes, divide both sides by known amount to get X. Amounts used in equation must be in same system.

Dimensional analysis method:

$$\text{Order in mg} \times \frac{1 \text{ tablet or capsule}}{\text{What 1 tablet or capsule is in mg}}$$

$$= \text{Tablets or capsules to be given}$$

If amounts are in different systems:

$$\text{Order in mg} \times \frac{1 \text{ tablet or capsule}}{\text{What 1 tablet or capsule is in g}} \times \frac{1}{1000 \text{ mg}}$$

$$= \text{Tablets or capsules to be given}$$

Mosby's
1992
Nursing
Drug
Reference

Linda Skidmore-Roth, R.N., M.S.N., N.P.

Formerly, New Mexico State University,
Nursing Faculty, Las Cruces, New Mexico;
El Paso Community College, El Paso, Texas

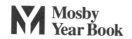

Mosby
Year Book

St. Louis   Baltimore   Boston   Chicago   London   Philadelphia   Sydney   Toronto

**Mosby
Year Book**

Dedicated to Publishing Excellence

Executive Editor: Don Ladig
Managing Editor: Robin Carter
Project Manager: Gayle May Morris
Production Editor: Mary Cusick Drone
Design: Elizabeth Fett

A NOTE TO THE READER:

The author and publisher have made every attempt to check dosages and nursing content for accuracy. Because the science of pharmacology is continually advancing, our knowledge base continues to expand. Therefore, we recommend that the reader always check product information for changes in dosage or administration before administering any medication. This is particularly important with new or rarely used drugs.

Mosby–Year Book, Inc.
11830 Westline Industrial Drive, St. Louis, Missouri 63146

ISSN 1044-8478
ISBN 0-8016-6198-6

GW/D   9   8   7   6   5   4   3   2

Clinical nursing consultants

Marie B. Andrews, R.N., B.S.N., M.S.N.
Lecturer, Texas Woman's University, Houston, Texas

Jean Krajicek Bartek, R.N., Ph.D.
Assistant Professor, University of Nebraska, Omaha, Nebraska

Nicki J. Beeler, R.N., M.S.N.
Instructor, Paris Junior College, Paris, Texas

Alice Bledig, R.N., Ph.D.
Professor, Southeastern Illinois Community College, Harrisburg, Illinois

Donnie F. Booth, R.N., Ph.D.
Director, School of Nursing, Southeastern Louisiana University, Hammond, Louisiana

Ruth Bowen, R.N., M.S.
Lecturer, Texas Woman's University, Denton, Texas

June Chandler, R.N., Ed.D.
Instructor, Florida Community College, Jacksonville, Florida

Mary Lou Cheatham, R.N., B.S.N., M.S.N.
Associate Professor, Ball State University, Muncie, Indiana

Leah M. Cleveland, R.N., Ed.D.
Professor, Saddleback College, Mission Viejo, California

Marilyn Edmunds, R.N., Ph.D.
Associate Professor, School of Nursing, University of Maryland, Baltimore, Maryland

Mary B. Gardner, R.N., M.S.
Lecturer, Assumption College, Worcester, Massachusetts

Barbara H. Goodkin, R.N., M.S.
Instructor, Washtenaw Community College, Ann Arbor, Michigan

Kathy Gutierrez, R.N., M.S.N.
Assistant Professor, Loretto Heights College, Denver, Colorado

Milly Gutkoski, R.N.C., M.N.
Assistant Professor, Montana State University, Bozeman, Montana

Patricia Hong, R.N., M.A.
Instructor, Anchorage Community College, Anchorage, Alaska

Joan M. Jenks, R.N., M.S.N.
Assistant Professor, Thomas Jefferson University, Philadelphia, Pennsylvania

Barbara Johnston, R.N., M.S.
Assistant Professor, Molloy College, Rockville Centre, New York

Linda L. Lilley, R.N., M.S.
Assistant Professor, Old Dominion University, Norfolk, Virginia

Suzanne E. Malloy, R.N., M.S.N.
Assistant Professor, San Jose State University, San Jose, California

Marylou Medlin, R.N., B.S.N., M.N.
Instructor, Charity Hospital School of Nursing, New Orleans, Louisiana

Clinical pharmacology consultants

Carmen Aceves-Blumenthal, M.S., R.Ph.
Assistant Professor, Southeastern College of Pharmaceutical Sciences, North Miami Beach, Florida

Richard H. Alper, Ph.D.
Assistant Professor, University of Kansas Medical Center, Kansas City, Kansas

Danial E. Baker, Pharm.D.
Assistant Professor, Washington State University, Pullman, Washington

R. Keith Campbell, Pharm.D.
Professor, Washington State University, Pullman, Washington

Catherine Celestin, Pharm.D.
Assistant Professor, Southeastern College of Pharmaceutical Sciences, North Miami Beach, Florida

Bruce D. Clayton, Pharm.D.
Professor, University of Arkansas, Little Rock, Arkansas

Edward H. Clouse, Ph.D.
Associate Professor, Southeastern College of Pharmaceutical Sciences, North Miami Beach, Florida

Jackson Como, Pharm.D.
Supervisor, Drug Information Service, University of Alabama, Birmingham, Alabama

David E. Domann, M.S., F.A.S.C.P.
Professional Services Manager, E.R. Squibb and Sons, Princeton, New Jersey

William Gerthoffer, Ph.D.
Associate Professor, University of Nevada School of Medicine, Reno, Nevada

Patricia A. Howard, B.S., R.Ph.
Clinical Instructor, University of Kansas Medical Center, Kansas City, Kansas

Norman Keltner, R.N., Ed.D.
Associate Professor, California State University, Bakersfield, California

James Lipp, Ph.D.
Associate Professor, Grand Valley State University, Allendale, Michigan

Lori A. Mangels, B.S.
Pharmacologist, The University of Michigan Medical School, Ann Arbor, Michigan

Judith K. Marquis, Ph.D.
Assistant Professor, Boston University School of Medicine, Boston, Massachusetts

Bozena B. Michniak, Ph.D., M.P.S.
Assistant Professor, University of South Carolina, Columbia, South Carolina

John Murski, B.S., R.Ph.
Pharmacology Consultant, Newtown, Pennsylvania

Keith M. Olsen, Pharm.D.
Assistant Professor, University of Arkansas, Little Rock, Arkansas

Canadian consultants

Linda Albert, R.N., B.N.
Instructor, Prince Edward Island
School of Nursing, Charlottetown,
Prince Edward Island

**Susanne Guy Alcolado, R.N.,
B.N., M.Ed.**
Assistant Director, Halifax
Infirmary Hospital School of
Nursing, Halifax, Nova Scotia

Linda M. Cameron, R.N., B.N.
Instructor, Foothills Hospital School
of Nursing, Calgary, Alberta

Margaret Chad, B.S.N.
Instructor, Diploma Nursing
Program, Saskatchewan Institute of
Applied Science and Technology,
Saskatoon, Saskatchewan

Edythe Ann Fleming, B.Sc.N.
Professor, Fanshawe College,
London, Ontario

Jacqueline Murphy, R.N., M.Sc.
Instructor and Staff Nurse, Foothills
Hospital School of Nursing,
Calgary, Alberta

Maureen J. Osis, R.N., M.N.
Clinical Nurse Specialist,
Calgary, Alberta

Kenneth W. Renton, Ph.D.
Professor and Head, Dalhousie
University Department of
Pharmacology, Halifax, Nova Scotia

**Roberta Ronayne, R.N., B.Sc.N.,
M.Sc.**
Assistant Professor, University of
Ottawa, Ottawa, Ontario

Shiela M. Stanton, R.N., M.S.N.
Associate Professor Emerita
Nursing, University of British
Columbia,
Vancouver, British Columbia

Linda Strand, Ph.D
Executive Director, Saskatchewan
Health, Regina, Saskatchewan

Sheila Rankin Zerr, R.N., M.Ed.
Assistant Professor, University of
Victoria, Victoria, British Columbia

Preface

Mosby's 1992 Nursing Drug Reference has been completely revised and updated with the addition of over 2000 new drug facts, 19 new drugs recently approved by the FDA, and—completely new to this edition—monographs on 23 major drug categories, which are printed on screened pages for easy access. The category monographs follow those of the individual drugs as closely as possible to facilitate comparison. Included in this new section are possible nursing diagnoses, categorized by uses or adverse effects, and lists of common generic drugs in each category with page references. New drugs include colfosceril palmitate (Exosurf Neonatal), a synthetic lung surfactant used for respiratory distress syndrome in premature infants; isradipine (DynaCirc) and bepridil HCl (Vascor), calcium channel blockers; hexamethylmelamine (Hexalen), an alkylating agent; dezocine (Dalgan), a synthetic opioid; and estazolam (ProSom) a benzodiazepine derivative. Over 125 new trade names have been added; obsolete trade names have been deleted. Another major addition is expanded content on IV drugs; over 185 IV-related facts have been incorporated. In addition, many new side effects, interactions, indications, and patient-teaching measures have been added, making this the most up-to-date nursing drug reference available.

Although drug references abound, few are available that are truly portable and geared specifically for clinical use by the practicing nurse or student. The guiding principle of this reference remains to provide the user with a book that allows easy access to drug information and nursing considerations that specifically tell the nurse what to do in terms consistent with the nursing process. Every detail—down to the choice of paper, typeface, cover, binding, use of color, and appendixes—has been carefully chosen with the user in mind.

Over 1000 generic and 4000 trade medications, alphabetized by generic name, are included. Trade names are given for all medications commonly used in the United States and Canada. Drugs available only in Canada are identified by an asterisk. The following information is provided, whenever possible, for safe and effective administration of each drug:

Pronunciations: Pronunciations are provided to help the nursing student master the more complex generic names.

Functional and chemical classifications: All known broad functional and chemical classifications are given. These classifications allow the nurse to see similarities and dissimilarities among drugs in the same functional but different chemical classes.

Controlled-substance schedule: Schedules are included for the United States (I, II, III, IV, V) and Canada (F, G).

Action: Pharmacologic properties are described in concise terms. Action is discussed to the cellular level when known.

Side effects and adverse reactions: Grouped by body system, common side effects are *italicized,* and life-threatening reactions are in ***bold italic type.*** This feature allows the nurse to instantly identify common and life-threatening reactions.

Dosages and routes: All available and approved dosages and routes are given for adult, pediatric, and geriatric patients.

Available forms: All available forms—including tablets, capsules, extended-release, injectables (IV, IM, SC), solutions, creams, ointments, lotions, gels, shampoos, elixirs, suspensions, suppositories, sprays, aerosols, and lozenges—are provided.

Contraindications: Contraindications are instances in which a medication should absolutely not be given. When the FDA has assigned pregnancy safety category D or X, it appears here.

Precautions: Special precautionary steps are given here, including FDA pregnancy safety categories A, B, and C.

Pharmacokinetics: Metabolism, distribution, and elimination are provided for all dosage forms, if known.

Interactions/incompatibilities: This section includes confirmed drug, food, and smoking interactions. The reaction is listed first, followed by the drug or nutrient causing that interaction, when applicable.

Nursing considerations: Highlighted nursing considerations are organized to foster use of the nursing process: Assess, Administer, Perform/provide, Evaluate, and Teach patient/family. Nursing considerations are consistently grouped under these headings to help the nurse group interventions that can be used for planning nursing care.

Laboratory test interferences: When known, laboratory test interferences are provided.

Treatment of overdose: Drugs and treatment for overdoses are provided for appropriate drugs.

The following appendixes are included to further enhance the usability of this reference: abbreviations, commonly used antibiotics in adults and children, nomogram, how to prepare a medication card, controlled substances, FDA pregnancy categories, bibliography, and combination products. Weights and measurements and formulas for drug calculations have been printed on the inside front cover, and a compatibility chart has been printed on the inside back cover for quick access.

I am indebted to the nursing and pharmacology consultants who reviewed the manuscript and galley pages and thank them for their criticism and encouragement. I would also like to thank Don Ladig and Robin Carter, my editors, whose active encouragement and enthusiasm have made this book better than it might otherwise have been. I am likewise grateful to Gayle May Morris, Mary Drone, and Elizabeth Fett. I also wish to thank the many users who have offered comments and suggestions concerning previous editions. I, along with the publisher, welcome comments from users of *Mosby's Nursing Drug Reference* so that we may continue to provide current and useful information in future editions.

Linda Skidmore-Roth

Contents

Drug categories, 1

Individual drugs, 39

Appendixes

Generic and trade index, 996

ALPHA-ADRENERGIC BLOCKERS

Action: Acts by binding to α-adrenergic receptors, causing dilation of peripheral blood vessels. Lowers peripheral resistance, resulting in decreased blood pressure.

Uses: Used for pheochromocytoma.

Side effects/adverse reactions: The most common side effects are: hypotension, tachycardia, nasal stuffiness, nausea, vomiting, and diarrhea.

Contraindications: Hypersensitive reactions may occur, and allergies should be identified before these products are given. Patients with myocardial infarction, coronary insufficiency, angina, or other evidence of coronary artery disease should not use these products.

Pharmacokinetics: Onset, peak, and duration vary between products.

Interactions/incompatibilities: Vasoconstrictive and hypertensive effects of epinephrine are antagonized by α-adrenergic blockers.

Possible nursing diagnoses:
• Altered tissue perfusion *[uses]*
• High risk for injury *[adverse reactions]*
• Sleep pattern disturbance *[adverse reactions]*

NURSING CONSIDERATIONS

Assess:
• Electrolytes: K, Na, Cl, CO_2
• Weight daily, I&O
• B/P lying, standing before starting treatment, q4h thereafter

Administer:
• Starting with low dose, gradually increasing to prevent side effects
• With food or milk for GI symptoms

Evaluate:
• Therapeutic response: decreased B/P, increased peripheral pulses
• Nausea, vomiting, diarrhea
• Skin turgor, dryness of mucous membranes for hydration status

Teach patient/family:
• To avoid alcoholic beverages
• To report dizziness, palpitations, fainting
• To change position slowly or fainting may occur
• To take drug exactly as prescribed
• To avoid all OTC products (cough, cold, allergy) unless directed by physician

---

Generic names:

phenoxybenzamine (p. 744)   phentolamine (p. 748)

ANTACIDS

Action: Antacids are basic compounds that neutralize gastric acidity and decrease the rate of gastric emptying. Products are divided into those containing aluminum, magnesium, calcium, or a combination of these.

Uses: Hyperacidity is decreased by antacids in conditions such as peptic ulcer disease, reflux esophagitis, gastritis, or hiatal hernia.

Side effects/adverse reactions: The most common side effect caused by aluminum-containing antacids is constipation, which may lead to fecal impaction and bowel obstruction. Diarrhea occurs often when magnesium products are given. Alkalosis may occur when systemic products are used. Constipation occurs more frequently than laxation with calcium carbonate. The release of CO_2 from carbonate-containing antacids causes belching, abdominal distention, and flatulence. Sodium bicarbonate may act as a systemic antacid and produce systemic electrolyte disturbances and alkalosis. Calcium carbonate and sodium bicarbonate may cause rebound hyperacidity and milk-alkali syndrome. Alkaluria may occur when products are used on a long-term basis, particularly in persons with abnormal renal function.

Contraindications: Sensitivity to aluminum or magnesium products may cause hypersensitive reactions. Aluminum products should not be used by persons sensitive to aluminum; magnesium products should not be used by persons sensitive to magnesium. Check for sensitivity before administering.

Precautions: Magnesium products should be given cautiously to patients with renal insufficiency and during pregnancy and lactation. Sodium content of antacids may be significant; use with caution for patients with hypertension, CHF, or those on a low-sodium diet.

Pharmacokinetics: Duration is 20-40 min. If ingested 1 hr after meals, acidity is reduced for at least 3 hr.

Interactions/incompatibilities: Drugs whose effects may be increased by some antacids: quinidine, amphetamines, pseudoephedrine, levodopa, valproic acid, dicumarol. Drugs whose effects may be decreased by some antacids: cimetidine, corticosteroids, ranitidine, iron salts, phenothiazines, phenytoin, digoxin, tetracyclines, ketoconazole, salicylates, isoniazid.

Possible nursing diagnoses:
- Pain *[uses]*
- Constipation *[adverse reactions]*
- Diarrhea *[adverse reactions]*

NURSING CONSIDERATIONS

Assess:

• Aggravating and alleviating factors of epigastric pain or hyperacidity; identify the location, duration, and characteristics of epigastric pain

• GI symptoms, including constipation, diarrhea, abdominal pain; if severe abdominal pain with fever occurs, these drugs should not be given

• Renal symptoms, including increasing urinary pH, electrolytes

Administer:

• All products with an 8-oz glass of water to ensure absorption in the stomach

• Another antacid if constipation occurs with aluminum products

Evaluate:

• The therapeutic effectiveness of the drug; absence of epigastric pain and decreased acidity should occur

Teach patient/family: Not to take other drugs within 1-2 hr of antacid administration, since antacids may impair absorption of other drugs

---

Generic names:

aluminum carbonate gel (p. 59)
aluminum hydroxide (p. 60)
aluminum phosphate (p. 61)
bismuth subsalicylate (p. 140)
calcium carbonate (p. 162)

dihydroxyaluminum (p. 342)
magaldrate (p. 563)
magnesium carbonate (p. 563)
magnesium oxide (p. 564)
magnesium trisilicate (p. 568)
sodium bicarbonate (p. 842)

ANTICONVULSANTS

Action: Anticonvulsants are divided into the barbiturates (p. 18), benzodiazepines (p. 19), hydantoins, succinimides, and miscellaneous products. Barbiturates and benzodiazepines are discussed in separate sections. Hydantoins act by inhibiting the spread of seizure activity in the motor cortex. Succinimides act by inhibiting spike and wave formation; they also decrease amplitude, frequency, duration, and spread of discharge in seizures.

Uses: Hydantoins are used in generalized tonic-clonic seizures, status epilepticus, and psychomotor seizures. Succinimides are used for absence (petit mal) seizures. Barbiturates are used in generalized tonic-clonic and cortical focal seizures.

Side effects/adverse reactions: Bone marrow depression is the most life-threatening adverse reaction associated with hydantoins or succinimides. The most common side effects are GI symptoms. Other common side effects for hydantoins are gingival hyperplasia and CNS effects such as nystagmus, ataxia, slurred speech, and mental confusion.

Contraindications: Hypersensitive reactions may occur, and allergies should be identified before these products are given.

Precautions: Persons with renal or hepatic disease should be watched closely.

Pharmacokinetics: Onset, peak, and duration vary widely among products. Most products are metabolized in the liver and excreted in urine, bile, and feces.

Interactions/incompatibilities: Decreased effects of estrogens, oral contraceptives (hydantoins).

Possible nursing diagnoses:
- High risk for injury *[uses]*
- Noncompliance
- Sleep pattern disturbance *[adverse reactions]*

NURSING CONSIDERATIONS
Assess:
- Renal function studies, including BUN, creatinine, serum uric acid, urine creatinine clearance before and during therapy
- Blood studies: RBC, Hct, Hgb, reticulocyte counts q wk for 4 wk then q mo
- Hepatic studies: AST, ALT, bilirubin, creatinine

Administer:
- With food, milk to decrease GI symptoms

Perform/provide:
- Good oral hygiene is important for hydantoins

Evaluate:
- Therapeutic response, including decreased seizure activity; document on patient's chart
- Mental status, including mood, sensorium, affect, behavorial changes; if mental status changes, notify physician
- Eye problems, including need for ophthalmic examinations before, during, and after treatment (slit lamp, funduscopy, tonometry)
- Allergic reaction, including red raised rash; if this occurs, drug should be discontinued
- Blood dyscrasia, including fever, sore throat, bruising, rash, jaundice
- Toxicity, including bone marrow depression, nausea, vomiting, ataxia, diplopia, cardiovascular collapse, Stevens-Johnson syndrome

Teach patient/family:
• To carry ID card or Medic-Alert bracelet stating drugs taken, condition, physician's name, phone number
• To avoid driving, other activities that require alertness

Generic names:

Hydantoins: ethotoin (p. 403)
mephenytoin (p. 589)
phenytoin (p. 752)
phensuximide (p. 745)

Succinimides: ethosuximide (p. 402)
methsuximide (p. 615)
phensuximide (p. 745)

Miscellaneous: acetazolamide (p. 42)

carbamazepine (p. 168)
clonazepam (p. 255)
diazepam (p. 322)
magnesium sulfate (p. 567)
paraldehyde (p. 714)
paramethadione (p. 715)
phenacemide (p. 737)
primidone (p. 784)
trimethadione (p. 937)
valproate acid (p. 954)

ANTIDIABETICS

Action: Antidiabetics are divided into the insulins that decrease blood sugar, phosphate, and potassium and increase blood pyruvate and lactate; and oral antidiabetics that cause functioning beta cells in the pancreas to release insulin.

Uses: Insulins are used for ketoacidosis and diabetes mellitus types I (IDDM) and II (NIDDM); oral antidiabetics are used for stable adult-onset diabetes mellitus type II (NIDDM).

Side effects/adverse reactions: The most common side effect of insulin and oral antidiabetics is hypoglycemia. Other adverse reactions for oral antidiabetics include blood dyscrasias, hepatotoxicity, and, rarely, cholestatic jaundice. Adverse reactions for insulin products include allergic responses and, more rarely, anaphylaxis.

Contraindications: Hypersensitive reactions may occur, and allergies should be identified before these products are given. Oral antidiabetics should not be used in juvenile or brittle diabetes, diabetic ketoacidosis, severe renal disease, or severe hepatic disease.

Precautions: Oral antidiabetics should be used with caution in the elderly, in cardiac disease, pregnancy, lactation, and in the presence of alcohol.

Pharmacokinetics: Onset, peak, and duration vary widely among products. Oral antidiabetics are metabolized in the liver, with metabolites excreted in urine, bile, and feces.

Interactions/incompatibilities: Interactions vary widely among products. Check individual monograph for specific information.

Possible nursing diagnosis:

• Altered nutrition: more than body requirements [uses]

NURSING CONSIDERATIONS
Assess:

• Blood, urine glucose levels during treatment to determine diabetes control (oral products)

• Fasting blood glucose, 2 hr PP (60-100 mg/dl normal fasting level) (70-130 mg/dl—normal 2-hr level)

Administer:

• Insulin, after warming to room temperature by rotating in palms to prevent lipodystrophy from injecting cold insulin

• Human insulin to those allergic to beef or pork

• Oral antidiabetic 30 min before meals

Perform/provide:

• Rotation of injection sites when giving insulin; use abdomen, upper back, thighs, upper arm, buttocks; keep a record of sites

Evaluate:

• Therapeutic response, including decrease in polyuria, polydipsia, polyphagia, clear sensorium, absence of dizziness, stable gait

• Hypoglycemic reaction that can occur during peak time

Teach patient/family:

• To avoid alcohol and salicylates except on advice of physician

• Symptoms of ketoacidosis: nausea, thirst, polyuria, dry mouth, decreased B/P, dry, flushed skin, acetone breath, drowsiness, Kussmaul respiration

• Symptoms of hypoglycemia: headache, tremors, fatigue, weakness; and that candy or sugar should be carried to treat hypoglycemia

• To test urine for glucose/ketones tid if this drug is replacing insulin

• To continue weight control, dietary restrictions, exercise, hygiene

---

Generic names:

Oral antidiabetics: acetohexamide (p. 44)
chlorpropamide (p. 229)
insulin, protamine zinc (p. 508)
insulin, regular (p. 823)
insulin, regular concentrated (p. 825)

insulin, zinc suspension (extended) (p. 511)
insulin, zinc suspension (prompt) (p. 512)
insulin, zinc suspension (intermediate) (p. 509)

ANTIDYSRHYTHMICS

Action: Antidysrhythmics are divided into four classes and miscellaneous antidysrhythmics:

• Miscellaneous antidysrhythmics are antidysrhythmics such as adenosine, which slows conduction through the AV node, and digoxin, which decreases conduction velocity and prolongs the effective refractory period in the AV node

• Class I increases the action potential duration and the effective refractory period and reduces disparity in the refractory period between a normal and infarcted myocardium

• Class II decreases the rate of SA node discharge, increases recovery time, slows conduction through the AV node, and decreases heart rate, which decreases O_2 consumption in the myocardium

• Class III increases the action potential duration and the effective refractory period

• Class IV inhibits calcium ion influx across the cell membrane during cardiac depolarization; decreases SA node discharge, decreases conduction velocity through the AV node

Uses: These products are used for PVCs, tachycardia, hypertension, angina pectoris.

Side effects/adverse reactions: Side effects and adverse reactions vary widely among products.

Contraindications: Contraindications vary widely among products.

Precautions: Precautions vary widely among products.

Pharmacokinetics: Onset, peak, and duration vary widely among products.

Interactions/incompatibilities: Interactions vary widely among products; check individual monograph for specific information.

Possible nursing diagnoses:
• Altered tissue perfusion: cardiopulmonary *[uses]*
• Decreased cardiac output *[uses]*
• Diarrhea *[adverse reactions]*
• Impaired gas exchange *[adverse reactions]*

NURSING CONSIDERATIONS
Assess:
• ECG continuously to determine drug effectiveness, PVCs or other dysrhythmias
• IV infusion rate to avoid causing nausea, vomiting
• For dehydration or hypovolemia
• B/P continuously for hypotension, hypertension
• I&O ratio

Evaluate:
• Therapeutic response, including decrease in B/P in hypertension, decreased B/P, edema moist rales in CHF
• Edema in feet and legs daily

Teach patient/family:
• Stress patient compliance with dosage schedule, even if feeling better
• To report bradycardia, dizziness, confusion, depression, fever

Generic names:

Class I: disyopyramide (p. 351)
encainide (p. 374)
flecainide (p. 422)
lidocaine (p. 546)
mexiletine (p. 634)
moricizine (p. 649)
phenytoin (p. 752)
procainamide (p. 787)
propafenone (p. 798)
quinidine (p. 819)
tocainide (p. 913)

Class II: acebutolol (p. 39)

esmolol (p. 386)
propranolol (p. 802)

Class III: amiodarone HCl (p. 74)
bretylium (p. 143)

Class IV: verapamil HCl (p. 958)

Miscellaneous: adenosine (p. 51)
digoxin (p. 337)

ANTIHISTAMINES

Action: Antihistamines compete with histamines for H_1 receptor sites. They antagonize in varying degrees most of the pharmacological effects of histamines.

Uses: Products are used to control the symptoms of allergies, rhinitis, and pruritus.

Side effects/adverse reactions: Most products cause drowsiness; however, two of the newer products, astemizole and terfenadine, produce little, if any, drowsiness. Other common side effects are headache and thickening of bronchial secretions. Serious blood dyscrasias may occur, but are rare. Urinary retention occurs with many of these products.

Contraindications: Hypersensitivity to H_1 receptor antagonists occurs rarely. Patients with acute asthma and lower respiratory tract disease should not use these products, since thick secretions may result. Other contraindications include narrow-angle glaucoma, bladder neck obstruction, stenosing peptic ulcer, symptomatic prostatic hypertrophy, newborn, lactation.

Precautions: These products must be used cautiously in conjunction with intraocular pressure, since they increase intraocular pressure. Caution should also be used in patients with renal and cardiac disease, hypertension, and seizure disorders and in the elderly.

Pharmacokinetics: Onset varies from 20-60 min, with duration lasting 4-12 hr. In general pharmacokinetics vary widely among products.

Drug interactions/incompatibilities: Barbiturates, narcotics, hypnotics, tricyclic antidepressants, or alcohol can increase CNS depression when taken with antihistamines.

Possible nursing diagnoses:
• Ineffective airway clearance *[uses]*

NURSING CONSIDERATIONS
Assess:
• I&O ratio; be alert for urinary retention, frequency, dysuria; drug should be discontinued if these occur
• CBC during long-term therapy, since hemolytic anemia may occur, but is rare

Administer:
• With food or milk to decrease GI symptoms; absorption may be decreased slightly

Perform/provide:
• Hard candy, gum, frequent rinsing of mouth for dryness

Evaluate:
• Therapeutic response, including absence of allergy symptoms, itching
• Blood dyscrasias: thrombocytopenia, agranulocytosis (rare)
• Respiratory status, including rate rhythm, increase in bronchial secretions, wheezing, chest tightness
• Cardiac status, including palpitations, increased pulse, hypotension

Teach patient/family:
• To notify physician if confusion, sedation, hypotension occurs
• To avoid driving or other hazardous activity if drowsiness occurs
• To avoid concurrent use of alcohol or other CNS depressants

---

Generic names:

astemizole (p. 105)
azatadine maleate (p. 113)
brompheniramine maleate (p. 145)
carbinoxamine maleate (p. 172)
chlorpheniramine maleate (p. 226)
diphenhydramine HCl (p. 346)
promethazine HCl (p. 796)
terfenadine (p. 877)
trimeprazine tartrate (p. 936)
tripelennamine HCl (p. 942)

clemastine fumarate (p. 246)
cyproheptadine HCl
(p. 288)
dexchlorpheniramine maleate
(p. 312)

triprolidine HCl
(p. 944)

ANTIHYPERTENSIVES

Action: Antihypertensives are divided into angiotensin-converting enzyme (ACE) inhibitors, β-adrenergic blockers, calcium channel blockers, centrally acting adrenergics, diuretics, peripherally acting antiadrenergics, and vasodilators. Beta blockers, calcium channel blockers, and diuretics are discussed in separate sections. Angiotensin-converting enzyme inhibitors act by selectively suppressing renin-angiotensin I to angiotensin II; dilation of arterial and venous vessels occurs. Centrally acting adrenergics act by inhibiting the sympathetic vasomotor center in the CNS that reduces impulses in the sympathetic nervous system; blood pressure, pulse rate, and cardiac output decrease. Peripherally acting antiadrenergics inhibit sympathetic vasoconstriction by inhibiting release of norepinephrine and/or depleting norepinephrine stores in adrenergic nerve endings. Vasodilators act on arteriolar smooth muscle by producing direct relaxation or vasodilation; a reduction in blood pressure, with concomitant increases in heart rate and cardiac output, occurs.

Uses: Used for hypertension and for heart failure not responsive to conventional therapy. Some products are used in hypertensive crisis, angina, and for some cardiac dysrhythmias.

Side effects/adverse reactions: The most common side effects are marked hypotension, bradycardia, tachycardia, headache, nausea, and vomiting. Side effects and adverse reactions may vary widely between classes and specific products.

Contraindications: Hypersensitive reactions may occur, and allergies should be identified before these products are given. Antihypertensives should not be used in patients with heart block or children.

Precautions: Antihypertensives should be used with caution in the elderly, in dialysis patients, and in the presence of hypovolemia, leukemia, and electrolyte imbalances.

Pharmacokinetics: Onset, peak, and duration vary widely among products. Most products are metabolized in the liver, with metabolites excreted in urine, bile, and feces.

Interactions/incompatibilities: Interactions vary widely among products; check individual monograph for specific information.

Possible nursing diagnoses:
• Altered tissue perfusion *[uses]*
• Decreased cardiac output *[uses]*
• Diarrhea *[adverse reactions]*
• Impaired gas exchange *[adverse reactions]*

NURSING CONSIDERATIONS

Assess:
• Blood studies: neutrophil; decreased platelets occur with many of the products
• Renal studies: protein, BUN, creatinine; watch for increased levels that may indicate nephrotic syndrome; obtain baselines in renal and liver function studies before beginning treatment

Perform/provide:
• Supine or Trendelenburg position for severe hypotension

Evaluate:
• Therapeutic response, including decrease in B/P in hypotension; decreased B/P, edema, moist rales in CHF
• Edema in feet and legs daily
• Allergic reaction, including rash, fever, pruritus, urticaria: drug should be discontinued if antihistamines fail to help
• Symptoms of CHF: edema, dyspnea, wet rales, B/P
• Renal symptoms: polyuria, oliguria, frequency

Teach patient/family:
• Stress patient compliance with dosage schedule, even if feeling better
• To rise slowly to sitting or standing position to minimize orthostatic hypotension

---

Generic names:

Angiotensin-converting enzyme inhibitor: enalapril (p. 372)

Centrally acting adrenergics:
clonidine HCl (p. 257)
guanabenz (p. 462)
guanfacine (p. 465)
methyldopa (p. 617)

Peripherally acting antiadrenergics: guanadrel (p. 463)

guanethidine (p. 464)
prazosin (p. 779)
reserpine (p. 826)
terazosin (p. 875)

Vasodilators: diazoxide (p. 323)
hydralazine (p. 479)
minoxidil (p. 642)
nitroprusside (p. 679)

Antiadrenergic: combined alpha/beta blocker—labetalol (p. 534)

ANTIINFECTIVES

Action: Antiifectives are divided into several groups, which include but are not limited to penicillins, cephalosporins, aminoglycosides, sulfonamides, tetracyclines, monobactam, erythromycins, and quinolones. These drugs act by inhibiting the growth and replication of susceptible bacterial organisms.

Uses: Used for infections of susceptible organisms. These products are effective against bacterial, rickettsial, and spirochete infections.

Side effects/adverse reactions: The most common side effects are nausea, vomiting, and diarrhea. Adverse reactions include bone marrow depression and anaphylaxis.

Contraindications: Hypersensitive reactions may occur, and allergies should be identified before these products are given. Cross-sensitivity can occur between products of different classes (penicillins or cephalosporins). Often persons allergic to penicillins will also be allergic to cephalosporins.

Precautions: Antiinfectives should be used with caution in persons with renal and liver disease.

Pharmacokinetics: Onset, peak, and duration vary widely among products. Most products are metabolized in the liver, and metabolites are excreted in urine, bile, and feces.

Interactions/incompatibilities: Interactions vary widely among products; check individual monograph for specific information.

Possible nursing diagnoses:
• High risk for infection *[uses]*
• Diarrhea *[adverse reactions]*

NURSING CONSIDERATIONS

Assess:
• Nephrotoxicity, including increased BUN, creatinine
• Blood studies: AST, ALT, CBC, Hct, bilirubin; test monthly if patient is on long-term therapy
• Bowel pattern q d; if severe diarrhea occurs, drug should be discontinued

Administer:
• For 10-14 days to ensure organism death, prevention of superimposed infection
• After C&S completed, drug may be taken as soon as culture is taken

Evaluate:
• Therapeutic response, including absence of fever, fatigue, malaise, draining wounds
• Urine output; if decreasing, notify physician; may indicate nephrotoxicity

• Allergic reaction, including rash, fever, pruritus, urticaria; drug should be discontinued
• Bleeding: ecchymosis, bleeding gums, hematuria, stool guaiac daily
• Overgrowth of infection: perineal itching, fever, malaise, redness, pain, swelling, drainage, rash, diarrhea, change in cough, sputum

Teach patient/family:
• Stress patient compliance with dosage schedule, even if feeling better
• To report sore throat, bruising, bleeding, joint pain; may indicate blood dyscrasias (rare)

Generic names:

Aminoglycosides: amikacin sulfate (p. 66)
gentamicin (p. 448)
kanamycin (p. 528)
neomycin (p. 666)
netilmicin (p. 670)
streptomycin (p. 854)
tobramycin (p. 911)

Cephalosporins: cefaclor (p. 181)
cefadroxil (p. 182)
cefamandole (p. 183)
cefazolin (p. 185)
cefixime (p. 186)
cefmetazole (p. 187)
cefonicid (p. 189)
cefoperazone (p. 190)
ceforanide (p. 192)
cefotaxime (p. 193)
cefuroxime axetil (p. 202)
cefuroxime sodium (p. 203)
cephalexin (p. 205)
cephalothin (p. 207)
cephapirin (p. 208)
cephradine (p. 210)
moxalactam disodium (p. 651)

Penicillins: amdinocillin (p. 64)
amoxicillin/clavulanate (p. 82)
ampicillin/sulbactam (p. 90)

azlocillin (p. 115)
bacampicillin (p. 118)
cloxacillin (p. 261)
cyclacillin (p. 280)
dicloxacillin (p. 327)
methicillin (p. 605)
mezlocillin (p. 635)
nafcillin (p. 656)
oxacillin (p. 695)
penicillin G benzathine (p. 720)
penicillin G potassium (p. 722)
penicillin G procaine (p. 724)
penicillin G sodium (p. 725)
penicillin V (p. 727)
piperacillin (p. 761)
ticarcillin (p. 904)
ticarcillin/clavulanate (p. 906)

Sulfonamides: sulfacytine (p. 860)
sulfasalazine (p. 866)
sulfisoxazole (p. 868)

Tetracyclines: demeclocycline HCl (p. 301)
doxycycline (p. 361)
minocycline (p. 640)
oxytetracycline (p. 707)
tetracycline (p. 885)

ANTINEOPLASTICS

Action: Antineoplastics are divided into alkylating agents, antimetabolites, antibiotic agents, hormonal agents, and miscellaneous agents. Alkylating agents act by cross-linking strands of DNA. Antimetabolites act by inhibiting DNA synthesis. Antibiotic agents act by inhibiting RNA synthesis and by delaying or inhibiting mitosis. Hormones alter the effect of androgens, luteinizing hormone, follicle-stimulating hormone, or estrogen by changing the hormonal environment.

Uses: Uses vary widely among products and classes of drugs. They are used to treat leukemia, Hodgkin's disease, lymphomas, and other tumors throughout the body.

Side effects/adverse reactions: Most products cause thrombocytopenia, leukopenia, and anemia, and, if these reactions occur, the drug may need to be stopped until the problem is corrected. Other side effects include nausea, vomiting, glossitis, and hair loss. Some products also cause hepatotoxicity, nephrotoxicity, and cardiotoxicity.

Contraindications: Hypersensitive reactions may occur, and allergies should be identified before these products are given. Also, persons with severe liver and kidney disease should not use these products unless the benefits outweigh the risks.

Precautions: Persons with bleeding, severe bone marrow depression, or renal or hepatic disease should be watched closely.

Pharmacokinetics: Onset, peak, and duration vary widely among products. Most products cross the placenta and are excreted in breast milk and in urine.

Interactions/incompatibilities: Toxicity may occur when used with other antineoplastics or radiation.

Possible nursing diagnoses:
- High risk for infection [adverse reactions]
- Altered nutrition: less than body requirements [adverse reactions]
- Altered oral mucous membrane [adverse reactions]

NURSING CONSIDERATIONS

Assess:
- CBC, differential, platelet count weekly; withhold drug if WBC is <4000 or platelet count is <75,000; notify physician of results
- Renal function studies, including BUN, creatinine, serum uric acid, and urine creatinine clearance before and during therapy
- I&O ratio; report fall in urine output of 30 ml/hr
- Monitor temperature q4h (may indicate beginning infection)
- Liver function tests before and during therapy (bilirubin, AST, ALT, LDH) as needed or monthly

Administer:
- Checking IV site for irritation; phlebitis

• Hydrate patient with 1-2 L of fluids over 8-12 hr before treatment
• Epinephrine for hypersensitivity reaction
• Antibiotics for prophylaxis of infection

Perform/provide:

• Strict medical asepsis, protective isolation if WBC levels are low
• Comprehensive oral hygiene, using careful technique and soft-bristle brush

Evaluate:

• Therapeutic response, including decreased tumor size
• Bleeding, including hematuria, guaiac, bruising or petechiae, mucosa, or orifices q8h; obtain prescription for viscous xylocaine
• Yellowing of skin, sclera, dark urine, clay-colored stools, itchy skin, abdominal pain, fever, diarrhea
• Edema in feet, joint pain, stomach pain, shaking
• Inflammation of mucosa, breaks in skin

Teach patient/family:

• To report signs of infection, including increased temperature, sore throat, malaise
• To report signs of anemia, including fatigue, headache, faintness, shortness of breath, irritability
• To report bleeding and avoid use of razors or commercial mouthwash

---

Generic names:

Alkylating agents: busulfan p. 153)
carboplatin (p. 173)
carmustine (p. 178)
chlorambucil (p. 213)
cisplatin (p. 244)
cyclophosphamide (p. 285)
dacarbazine (p. 292)
lomustine (p. 555)
mechlorethamine (p. 575)
melphalan (p. 583)
streptozocin (p. 855)
thiotepa (p. 897)
uracil mustard (p. 948)

Antimetabolites: cytarabine (p. 290)
fluorouracil (p. 431)
mercaptopurine (p. 594)
methotrexate (p. 609)

doxorubicin (p. 360)
mitomycin (p. 643)
mitoxantrone (p. 646)
plicamycin (p. 767)

Hormonal agents:
aminoglutethimide (p. 72)
estramustine (p. 392)
flutamide (p. 441)
goserelin acetate (p. 459)
leuprolide (p. 538)
megestrol (p. 582)
mitotane (p. 645)
tamoxifen (p. 873)
testolactone (p. 878)
trilostane (p. 935)

Miscellaneous agents:
asparaginase (p. 102)
etoposide (p. 409)

thioguanine (p. 893)

Antibiotic agents: bleomycin
(p. 142)
dactinomycin (p. 293)
daunorubicin HCl (p. 298)

interferon alfa-2A (p. 513)
interferon alfa-2B (p. 513)
procarbazine (p. 789)
vinblastine (p. 960)
vincristine (p. 962)

ANTIPSYCHOTICS

Action: Antipsychotics/neuroleptics are divided into several subgroups: phenothiazines, thioxanthenes, butyrophenones, dibenzoxazepines, dibenzodiazepines, and indolones and other heterocyclic compounds. Although chemically different, these subgroups share many pharmacological and clinical properties. All antipsychotics work to block postsynaptic dopamine receptors in the brain that are responsible for psychotic behavior, including hallucinations, delusions, and paranoia.

Uses: Antipsychotic behavior is decreased in conditions such as schizophrenia, paranoia, and mania. These agents are also effective for severe anxiety, intractable hiccups, nausea, vomiting, behavioral problems in children, and before surgery for relaxation.

Side effects/adverse reactions: The most common side effects include extrapyramidal symptoms such as pseudoparkinsonism, akathisia, dystonia, and tardive dyskinesia, which may be controlled by use of antiparkinsonian agents. Serious adverse reactions such as hypotension, agranulocytosis, cardiac arrest, and laryngospasm have occurred.

Contraindications: Persons with liver damage, severe hypertension or coronary disease, cerebral arteriosclerosis, blood dyscrasias, bone marrow depression, children <12 yr, or persons withdrawing from alcohol or barbiturates should not use antipsychotics until these conditions are corrected.

Precautions: Caution must be used when antipsychotics are given to the elderly, since metabolism is slowed and adverse reactions can occur rapidly. Hepatic and renal disease may cause poor metabolism and excretion of the drug. Seizure threshold is decreased with these products; increases in the dose of anticonvulsants may be required.

Pharmacokinetics: Onset, peak, and duration vary widely with different products and routes. Products are metabolized by the liver, are excreted in urine as metabolites, are highly bound to plasma proteins, cross the placenta, and enter breast milk. Half-life can be extended over 3 days.

Interactions/incompatibilities: Because other CNS depressants can cause oversedation, these combinations should be used carefully. Anticholinergics may decrease the therapeutic actions of phenothiazines and also cause increased anticholinergic effects.

Possible nursing diagnoses:

• Altered thought processes *[uses]*
• Sensory-perceptual alterations *[uses]*

NURSING CONSIDERATIONS

Assess:

• Bilirubin, CBC, liver function studies monthly, since these drugs are metabolized in the liver and excreted in urine
• I&O ratio: palpate bladder if low urinary output occurs, since urinary retention occurs with many of these products
• Affect, orientation, LOC, reflexes, gait, coordination, sleep pattern disturbances
• Dizziness, faintness, palpitations, tachycardia on rising

Administer:

• Antiparkinsonian agent if extrapyramidal symptoms occur
• Liquid concentrates mixed in glass of juice or cola, since taste is unpleasant

Perform/provide:

• Supervised ambulation until stabilized on medication; do not involve in strenuous exercise program because fainting is possible; patient should not stand still for long periods of time
• Increased fluids to prevent constipation
• Sips of water, candy, gum for dry mouth

Evaluate:

• The therapeutic effectiveness of the drug: decrease in excitement, hallucinations, delusions, paranoia, reorganization of thought patterns, speech
• B/P lying and standing; wide fluctuations between lying and standing B/P may require dosage or product change since orthostatic hypotension is occurring
• Extrapyramidal symptoms, including akathisia, tardive dyskinesia, pseudoparkinsonism

Teach patient/family:

• To rise from sitting or lying position gradually, since fainting may occur
• To remain lying down for at least 30 minutes after IM injections
• To avoid hot tubs, hot showers, or tub baths, since hypotension may occur
• To wear a sunscreen or protective clothing to prevent burns
• To take extra precautions during hot weather to stay cool; heat stroke can occur

Generic names:

Phenothiazines: chlorpromazine
HCl (p. 227)
fluphenazine (p. 436)
mesoridazine (p. 596)
perphenazine (p. 735)
prochlorperazine (p. 791)
promazine (p. 794)
thioridazine (p. 895)

thiothixene (p. 899)
trifluoperazine (p. 929)

Butyrophenone: haloperidol
(p. 469)

Miscellaneous: loxapine (p. 560)
molindone (p. 647)

BARBITURATES

Action: Barbiturates act by decreasing impulse transmission to the cerebral cortex.

Uses: All forms of epilepsy can be controlled, since the seizure threshold is increased. Uses also include febrile seizures in children, sedation, insomnia, hyperbilirubinemia, chronic cholestasis with some of these products. Ultra-short acting barbiturates are used as anesthetics.

Side effects/adverse reactions: The most common side effects are drowsiness and nausea. Serious adverse reactions such as Stevens-Johnson syndrome and blood dyscrasias may occur with high doses and long-term treatment.

Contraindications: Hypersensitivity may occur, and allergies should be identified before administering. Barbiturates are identified as pregnancy category (D) and should not be used in pregnancy. Other contraindications include porphyria and marked impairment of liver function.

Precautions: Caution must be used when these products are given to the elderly or debilitated; usually smaller doses are needed, since metabolism is slowed. Persons with renal and hepatic disease may show delayed excretion. Barbiturates may produce excitability in children.

Pharmacokinetics: Onset of action can be slow up to 1 hr, with a peak of 8 hr and a duration of 3-10 hr. These drugs are metabolized by the liver, excreted by the kidneys, cross the placenta, and enter breast milk.

Drug interactions/incompatibilities: Increased CNS depressant effect may occur with alcohol, MAO inhibitors, sedatives, or narcotics. These products should be used together cautiously. Oral anticoagulants, corticosteroids, griseofulvin, quinidine, oral contraceptives, and theophylline may show a decreased effect when used with barbiturates.

Possible nursing diagnoses:
- Sleep pattern disturbance *[uses]*
- High risk for injury *[adverse reactions]*

NURSING CONSIDERATIONS
Assess:

• Hepatic and renal studies: AST, ALT, bilirubin, creatinine, LDH, alkaline phosphatase, BUN if patient is on long-term therapy, since these products are metabolized and excreted by the liver and kidney

• Blood studies: CBC, hematocrit, hemoglobin, and prothrombin time if patient is on long-term therapy, since these products increase the possibility of bleeding and blood dyscrasias

Evaluate:

• Barbiturate toxicity: hypotension, pulmonary constriction; cold, clammy skin; cyanosis of lips; insomnia; nausea; vomiting, hallucinations, delirium, weakness

Teach patient/family:

• That physical dependency may result when used for extended periods of time (45-90 days, depending on dose)

• To avoid driving and activities that require alertness, since drowsiness and dizziness may occur

• To abstain from alcohol or other psychotropic medications unless prescribed by physician

• Not to discontinue medication abruptly after long-term use; withdrawal symptoms will occur

---

Generic names:

amobarbital (p. 79)
aprobarbital (p. 99)
butabarbital (p. 154)
mephobarbital (p. 590)
pentobarbital (p. 731)

phenobarbital (p. 742)
secobarbital (p. 835)
talbutal (p. 871)
thiopental (p. 894)

BENZODIAZEPINES

Action: Benzodiazepines potentiate the effects of γ-aminobutyrate (GABA), including any other inhibitory transmitters in the CNS, resulting in decreased anxiety.

Uses: Anxiety is relieved in conditions such as phobic disorders. Benzodiazepines are also used for acute alcohol withdrawal to relieve the possibility of delirium tremens, and some products are used before surgery for relaxation.

Side effects/adverse reactions: The most common side effects are dizziness, drowsiness, blurred vision, and orthostatic hypotension.

Contraindications: Hypersensitivity, acute narrow-angle glaucoma, children <6 months, liver disease (clonazepam), lactation (diazepam).

Precautions: Caution must be used when these products are given to the elderly or debilitated; usually smaller doses are needed, since metabolism is slowed. Persons with renal and hepatic disease may show delayed excretion. Clonazepam may increase incidence of seizures.

Pharmacokinetics: Onset of action is ½-1 hr, with a peak of 1-2 hr and a duration of 4-6 hr. These drugs are metabolized by the liver, excreted by the kidneys, cross the placenta, and enter breast milk.

Drug interactions/incompatibilities: Increased CNS depressant effect may occur with other CNS depressants. These products should be used together cautiously. Alcohol should not be used; fatal reactions can occur. The serum concentration and toxicity of digoxin may be increased.

Possible nursing diagnoses:

• Anxiety *[uses]*
• High risk for injury *[adverse reactions]*

NURSING CONSIDERATIONS
Assess:
• B/P (lying, standing), pulse; if systolic B/P drops 20 mm Hg, hold drug, notify physician; orthostatic hypotension is severe
• Hepatic and renal studies: AST, ALT, bilirubin, creatinine, LDH, alkaline phosphatase
Administer:
• With food or milk for GI symptoms; may give crushed if patient is unable to swallow medication whole
Evaluate:
• Physical dependency, withdrawal symptoms, including headache, nausea, vomiting, muscle pain, weakness after long-term use
Teach patient/family:
• That drug should not be used for everyday stress or long-term; not to take more than prescribed amount, since drug is habit forming
• To avoid driving and activities that require alertness, since drowsiness and dizziness occur
• To abstain from alcohol or other psychotropic medications unless prescribed by physician
• Not to discontinue medication abruptly after long-term use; withdrawal symptoms will occur

---

Generic names:

alprazolam (p. 55)   midazolam (p. 638)

BETA-ADRENERGIC BLOCKERS

Action: Beta blockers are divided into selective and nonselective blockers. Nonselective beta blockers produce a fall in blood pressure without reflex tachycardia or reduction in heart rate through a mixture of beta blocking effects; elevated plasma renins are reduced. Selective beta blockers competitively block stimulation of β-1 receptors in cardiac smooth muscle; these drugs produce chronotropic and inotropic effects.

Uses: Beta blockers are used for hypertension, ventricular dysrhythmias, and prophylaxis of angina pectoris.

Side effects/adverse reactions: The most common side effects are orthostatic hypotension, bradycardia, diarrhea, nausea, vomiting. Serious adverse reactions include blood dyscrasias, bronchospasm, and CHF.

Contraindications: Hypersensitive reactions may occur, and allergies should be identified before these products are given. β-adrenergic blockers should not be used in heart block, CHF, or cardiogenic shock.

Precautions: Beta blockers should be used with caution in the elderly or in renal and thyroid disease, COPD, CAD, diabetes mellitus, or pregnancy.

Pharmacokinetics: Onset, peak, and duration vary widely among products. Most products are metabolized in the liver, with metabolites excreted in urine, bile, and feces.

Interactions/incompatibilities: Interactions vary widely among products; check individual monograph for specific information.

Possible nursing diagnoses:
• Altered tissue perfusion *[uses]*
• Decreased cardiac output *[uses]*
• Diarrhea *[adverse reactions]*
• Impaired gas exchange *[adverse reactions]*

NURSING CONSIDERATIONS
Assess:
• Renal studies, including protein, BUN, creatinine; watch for increased levels that may indicate nephrotic syndrome; obtain baselines in renal and liver function studies before beginning treatment

- I&O, weight daily
- B/P during beginning treatment and periodically thereafter, pulse q4h, note rate, rhythm, quality
- Apical/radial pulse before administration; notify physician of significant changes

Administer:
- PO ac, hs, tablets may be crushed or swallowed whole
- Reduced dosage in renal dysfunction

Evaluate:
- Therapeutic response, including decrease in B/P in hypertension, decreased B/P, edema, moist rales in CHF
- Edema in feet and legs daily

Teach patient/family:
- Stress patient compliance with dosage schedule, even if feeling better
- To rise slowly to sitting or standing position to minimize orthostatic hypotension
- To report bradycardia, dizziness, confusion, depression, fever
- To take pulse at home; advise when to notify physician
- To comply with weight control, dietary adjustment, modified exercise program
- To wear support hose to minimize effects of orthostatic hypotension
- Not to discontinue drug abruptly; taper over 2 wk; may precipitate angina

---

Generic names:

Selective β-1 receptor blockers:
acebutolol (p. 39)
atenolol (p. 106)
esmolol (p. 386)
metoprolol (p. 630)

Nonselective β-1 and β-2 blockers: careolol (p. 175)

nadolol (p. 654)
pindolol (p. 759)
propranolol (p. 802)
timolol (p. 907)

Combined α-1, β-1, and β-2 receptor blocker: labetalol (p. 534)

CALCIUM CHANNEL BLOCKERS

Action: These products act by inhibiting calcium ion influx across the cell membrane in cardiac and vascular smooth muscle. This action produces relaxation of coronary vascular smooth muscle, dilates coronary arteries, decreases SA/AV node conduction, and dilates peripheral arteries.

Uses: These products are used for chronic stable angina pectoris, vasospastic angina, dysrhythmias, hypertension, and unstable angina.

Side effects/adverse reactions: The most common side effects are dysrhythmias and edema. Also common are headache, fatigue, drowsiness, and flushing.

Contraindications: Persons with 2nd or 3rd degree heart block, sick sinus syndrome, hypotension of <90 mm Hg systolic, Wolff-Parkinson-White syndrome or cardiogenic shock should not use these products, since worsening of those conditions may occur.

Precautions: CHF may worsen, since edema may be increased. Hypotension may worsen, since B/P is decreased. Patients with renal and liver disease should use these products cautiously, since they are metabolized in the liver and excreted by the kidneys.

Pharmacokinetics: Onset, peak, and duration vary widely with route of administration. Drugs are metabolized by the liver and excreted in the urine primarily as metabolites.

Interactions/incompatibilities: Increased levels of digoxin and theophylline may occur when used with these products. Increased effects of beta blockers and antihypertensives may occur with calcium channel blockers.

Possible nursing diagnoses:
• Altered tissue perfusion: cardiopulmonary *[uses]*
• Decreased cardiac output *[adverse reactions]*

NURSING CONSIDERATIONS

Assess:
• Cardiac system, including B/P, pulse, respirations, ECG intervals (PR, QRS, QT)

Administer:
• PO before meals and hs

Evaluate:
• Therapeutic response, including decreased anginal pain, decreased B/P, dysrhythmias

Teach patient/family:
• How to take pulse before taking drug; patient should record or graph pulses to identify changes
• To avoid hazardous activities until stabilized on this drug, since dizziness occurs frequently
• Need for compliance to all areas of medical regimen, including diet, exercise, stress reduction, drug therapy

Generic names:

diltiazem (p. 342)   nifedipine (p. 676)
nicardipine (p. 673)   verapamil HCl (p. 958)

CARDIAC GLYCOSIDES

Action: Products act by inhibiting sodium and potassium ATPase and then making more calcium available to activate contracted proteins. Cardiac contractility and cardiac output are increased.

Uses: These products are used for congestive heart failure, atrial fibrillation, atrial flutter, atrial tachycardia, and rapid digitalization in these disorders.

Side effects/adverse reactions: The most common side effects are cardiac disturbances, headache, hypotension, GI symptoms. Also common are blurred vision and yellow-green halos.

Contraindications: Hypersensitive reactions may occur, and allergies should be identified before these products are given. Also, persons with ventricular tachycardia, ventricular fibrillation, and carotid sinus syndrome should not use these products.

Precautions: Persons with acute MI and those who have or may develop serum potassium, calcium, or magnesium imbalances should use these products cautiously. Also, persons with AV block, severe respiratory disease, hypothyroidism, renal and liver disease, and the elderly should exercise caution when these drugs are prescribed.

Pharmacokinetics: Onset, peak, and duration vary widely with the route of administration. Digitoxin is inactivated by the liver, and inactive metabolites are excreted in urine. Digoxin is excreted in urine mainly as the parent drug and metabolites.

Interactions/incompatibilities: Toxicity may occur when used with diuretics, succinylcholine, quinidine, and thioamines. Increased blood levels may occur with propantheline bromide, spironolactone, quinidine, verapamil, aminoglycosides (PO), amiodarone, anticholinergics, and quinine. Diuretics may increase toxicity.

Possible nursing diagnoses:

• Altered tissue perfusion: cardiopulmonary *[uses]*
• Decreased cardiac output *[adverse reactions]*

NURSING CONSIDERATIONS

Assess:

• Cardiac system, including B/P, pulse, respirations, and increased urine output

• Apical pulse for 1 min before giving drug; if pulse <60, take again in 1 hr; if <60 notify physician
• Electrolytes, including potassium, sodium, chloride, calcium, magnesium; renal function studies, including BUN and creatinine; and blood studies, including AST, ALT, bilirubin
• I&O ratio, daily weights
• Monitor therapeutic drug levels

Administer:
• Potassium supplements if ordered for potassium levels <3.0

Evaluate:
• Therapeutic response, including decreased weight, edema, pulse, respiration, and increased urine output

Teach patient/family:
• How to take pulse before taking drug; patient should record or graph pulse to identify changes
• To avoid hazardous activities until stabilized on this drug, since dizziness occurs frequently
• Need for compliance to all areas of medical regimen, including diet, exercise, stress reduction, drug therapy

---

Generic names:

digitoxin (p. 336)   digoxin (p. 337)

CHOLINERGIC BLOCKERS

Action: Cholinergic blockers inhibit or block acetylcholine at receptor sites in the autonomic nervous system.

Uses: Many products are used to decrease secretions before surgery, to reverse neuromuscular blockade, and to decrease motility of GI, biliary, urinary tracts. Other products are used for Parkinson symptoms, including dystonia associated with neuroleptic drugs.

Side effect/adverse reactions: The most common side effects are dryness of the mouth and constipation, which can be prevented by frequent rinsing of the mouth and increasing water and bulk in the diet.

Contraindications: Hypersensitivity can occur, and allergies should be identified before administering these products. Persons with GI and GU obstruction should not use these products, since constipation and urinary retention may occur. They are also contraindicated in angle-closure glaucoma and myasthenia gravis.

Precautions: Caution must be used when these products are given to the elderly, since metabolism is slowed. Also, persons with tachycardia or prostatic hypertrophy should use these products with caution.

Pharmacokinetics: Onset, peak, and duration vary with route.

Drug interactions/incompatibilities: Increase in anticholinergic effect occurs when used with narcotics, barbiturates, antihistamines, MAO inhibitors, phenothiazines, amantadine.

Possible nursing diagnoses:

• Impaired physical mobility *[uses]*

• Pain *[uses]*

NURSING CONSIDERATIONS

Assess:

• I&O ratio; be alert for urinary retention, frequency, dysuria; drug should be discontinued if these occur

Administer:

• With food or milk to decrease GI symptoms

• Parenteral dose with patient recumbent to prevent postural hypotension; give parenteral dose slowly, monitoring vital signs

Perform/provide:

• Hard candy, gum, frequent rinsing of mouth for dryness

Evaluate:

• Therapeutic response, including absence of cramps, absence of extrapyramidal symptoms

• Urinary hesitancy, retention; palpate bladder if retention occurs

• Constipation; increase fluids, bulk, exercise

• For tolerance over long-term therapy, dose may need to be increased or changed

• Mental status: affect, mood, CNS depression, worsening of mental symptoms during early therapy

Teach patient/family:

• To avoid driving or other hazardous activity if drowsiness occurs

• To avoid concurrent use of cough, cold preparations with alcohol, antihistamines unless directed by physician

• To use with caution in hot weather, since medication may increase susceptibility to heat stroke

---

Generic names:

atropine sulfate (p. 109)
benztropine mesylate (p. 132)
biperiden HCl (p. 138)
glycopyrrolate (p. 457)

procyclidine HCl (p. 792)
scopolamine hydrobromide
(p. 834)
trihexyphenidyl HCl (p. 934)

CORTICOSTEROIDS

Action: Corticosteroids are divided into glucocorticoids and mineralocorticoids. Glucocorticoids decrease inflammation by the suppression of migration of polymorphonuclear leukocytes, fibroblasts, increased capillary permeability, and lysosomal stabilization. They also have varied metabolic effects and modify the body's immune responses to many different stimuli. Mineralocorticoids act by increasing resorption of sodium by increasing hydrogen and potassium excretion in the distal tubule.

Uses: Glucocorticoids are used to decrease inflammation and for immunosuppression. In addition, some products may be given for allergy, adrenal insufficiency, or cerebral edema. The mineralocorticoids are given for adrenal insufficiency or adrenogenital syndrome.

Side effects/adverse reactions: The most common side effects include change in behavior, including insomnia and euphoria; GI irritation, including peptic ulcer; metabolic reactions, including hypokalemia, hyperglycemia, and carbohydrate intolerance; and sodium and fluid retention. Most adverse reactions are dose dependent.

Contraindications: Hypersensitivity may occur and should be identified before administering. Since these products mask infection, they should not be used in systemic fungal infections or amebiasis. Mothers taking pharmacologic doses of corticosteroids should not nurse.

Precautions: Caution must be used when these products are prescribed for diabetic patients, since hyperglycemia may occur. Also, patients with glaucoma, seizure disorders, peptic ulcer, impaired renal function, CHF, hypertension, ulcerative colitis, or myasthenia gravis should be monitored closely if corticosteroids are given. Use with caution in children and the elderly and during pregnancy.

Pharmacokinetics: For oral preparations the onset of action occurs between 1-2 hr, and duration can be up to 2 days, with a half-life of 2-4 days. Pharmacokinetics vary widely among products. These products cross the placenta and appear in breast milk.

Drug interactions/incompatibilities: Decreased corticosteroid effect may occur with barbiturates, rifampin, phenytoin; corticosteroid dose may need to be increased. There is a possibility of GI bleeding when used with salicylates, indomethacin. Steroids may reduce salicylate levels. When using with digitalis glycosides, potassium-depleting diuretics, and amphotericin, serum potassium levels should be monitored.

Possible nursing diagnoses:
- High risk for infection *[adverse reactions]*
- Body-image disturbance *[adverse reactions]*
- High risk for violence: self-directed (suicide) *[adverse reactions]*

NURSING CONSIDERATIONS

Assess:
- Potassium, blood sugar, urine glucose while on long-term therapy; hypokalemia and hyperglycemia are common
- Weight daily; notify physician if weekly gain of >5 lb, since these products alter fluid and electrolyte balance
- I&O ratio; be alert for decreasing urinary output and increasing edema
- Plasma cortisol levels during long-term therapy (normal level is 138-635 nmol/L SI U when drawn at 8 A.M.
- Infection, including increased temperature, WBC, even after withdrawal of medication; drug masks symptoms of infection
- Adrenal insufficiency: nausea, anorexia, fatigue, dizziness, dyspnea, weakness, joint pain

Administer:
- With food or milk to decrease GI symptoms

Evaluate:
- Therapeutic response, including decreased inflammation
- Potassium depletion, including paresthesias, fatigue, nausea, vomiting, depression, polyuria, dysrhythmias, weakness
- Mental status, including affect, mood, behavioral changes, aggression; if severe personality changes occur, including depression, drug may need to be tapered and then discontinued

Teach patient/family:
- That ID as steroid user should be carried
- Not to discontinue this medication abruptly or adrenal crisis can result
- Teach patient all aspects of drug use, including cushingoid symptoms
- That single daily or alternate-day doses should be taken in the morning before 9 A.M.
- To take with meals or a snack

Generic names:

Glucocorticoids: beclomethasone dipropionate (p. 123)
betamethasone (p. 134)
betamethasone benzoate (p. 135)
betamethasone disodium phosphate (p. 134)
betamethasone sodium phosphate (p. 134)
cortisone acetate (p. 272)
dexamethasone (p. 308)
dexamethasone acetate (p. 308)
methylprednisolone acetate (p. 621)
methylprednisolone sodium succinate (p. 621)
paramethasone acetate (p. 716)
prednisolone (p. 780)
prednisolone acetate (p. 780)
prednisolone phosphate (p. 780)
prednisolone sodium phosphate (p. 781)
prednisolone tebutate (p. 780)

dexamethasone sodium phosphate
(p. 308)
flunisolide (p. 427)
hydrocortisone (p. 482)
hydrocortisone acetate (p. 882)
hydrocortisone sodium phosphate
(p. 484)
hydrocortisone sodium succinate
(p. 484)
methylprednisolone (p. 621)

prednisone (p. 782)
triamcinolone (p. 923)
triamcinolone acetonide (p. 926)
triamcinolone diacetate (p. 923)
triamcinolone hexacetonide
(p. 923)

Mineralocorticoid: fludrocortisone
acetate (p. 426)

DIURETICS

Action: Diuretics are divided into subgroups: thiazides and thiazide-like
diuretics, loop diuretics, carbonic anhydrase inhibitors, osmotic diuretics,
and potassium-sparing diuretics. Each one of these subgroups differs in
its mechanism of action. Thiazides and thiazide-like diuretics increase
excretion of water and sodium by inhibiting resorption in the early distal
tubule. Loop diuretics inhibit resorption of sodium and chloride in the
thick ascending limb of the loop of Henle. Carbonic anhydrase inhibitors
increase sodium excretion by decreasing sodium–hydrogen ion exchange
throughout the renal tubule. Carbonic anhydrase inhibitors also decrease
secretion of aqueous humor in the eye and thus decrease intraocular
pressure. Osmotic diuretics increase the osmotic pressure of glomerular
filtrate, thus decreasing net absorption of sodium. The potassium-sparing
diuretics interfere with sodium resorption at the distal tubule, thus decreasing potassium excretion.

Uses: Blood pressure is reduced in hypertension; edema is reduced in
CHF; intraocular pressure is decreased in glaucoma.

Side effects/adverse reactions: Hypokalemia, hyperuricemia, and hyperglycemia occur most frequently with thiazide diuretics. Aplastic anemia, blood dyscrasias, volume depletion, and dehydration may occur
when thiazide-like diuretics, loop diuretics, or carbonic anhydrase inhibitors are given. Side effects and adverse reactions vary widely for the
miscellaneous products.

Contraindications: Persons with electrolyte imbalances (sodium, chloride, potassium), dehydration, or anuria should not be given these products until the problem is corrected.

Precautions: Caution must be used when diuretics are given to the elderly,
since electrolyte disturbances and dehydration can occur rapidly. Hepatic
and renal disease may cause poor metabolism and excretion of the drug.

Pharmacokinetics: Onset, peak, and duration vary widely among the different subgroups of these drugs.

Interactions/incompatibilities: Cholestyramine and colestipol will decrease the absorption of thiazide diuretics. Concurrent use of thiazides with diazoxide may increase hyperuricemia, hyperglycemia, and antihypertensive effects of thiazides. Ototoxicity may occur when loop diuretics are used with aminoglycosides. Thiazide and loop diuretics may increase therapeutic and toxic effects of lithium.

Possible nursing diagnoses:
- Fluid volume excess *[uses]*
- Decreased cardiac output *[adverse reactions]*

NURSING CONSIDERATIONS

Assess:
- Weight, I&O daily to determine fluid loss; check skin turgor for dehydration
- Electrolytes: potassium, sodium, chloride: include BUN, blood sugar, CBC, serum creatinine, blood pH, ABGs, uric acid, calcium; electrolyte imbalances may occur quickly
- B/P lying, standing; postural hypotension may occur, since fluid loss occurs from intravascular spaces first

Administer:
- In A.M. to avoid interference with sleep if using drug as a diuretic
- Potassium replacement if potassium is less than 3.0

Evaluate:
- The therapeutic effectiveness of the drug: improvement in edema of feet, legs, sacral area daily if medication is being used in CHF; improvement in B/P if medication is being used as a diuretic; improvement in intraocular pressure if medication is being used to decrease aqueous humor in the eye
- Signs of metabolic alkalosis, including drowsiness and restlessness
- Signs of hypokalemia with some products, including postural hypotension, malaise, fatigue, tachycardia, leg cramps, weakness

Teach patient/family:
- To take drug early in the day (diuretic) to prevent nocturia

---

Generic names:

Thiazides: chlorothiazide (p. 222) hydrochlorothiazide (p. 480)

Thiazide-like: chlorthalidone (p. 231)

Carbonic anhydrase inhibitors: acetazolamide (p. 42) acetazolamide sodium (p. 42) methazolamide (p. 602)

indapamide (p. 501)
metolazone (p. 628)

Loop: bumetanide (p. 147)
ethacrynate acid (p. 396)
ethacrynate sodium
(p. 396)
furosemide (p. 444)

Potassium-sparing: amiloride
(p. 67)
spironolactone (p. 849)
triamterene (p. 926)

Osmotic: mannitol (p. 568)
urea (p. 950)

NARCOTICS

Action: Narcotics act by depressing pain impulse transmission at the spinal cord level by interacting with opioid receptors. Products are divided into opiates and nonopiates.

Uses: Most products are used to control moderate-to-severe pain and are used before and after surgery.

Side effects/adverse reactions: GI symptoms, including nausea, vomiting, anorexia, constipation, and cramps are the most common side effects. Other common side effects include lightheadedness, dizziness, sedation. Serious adverse reactions such as respiratory depression, respiratory arrest, circulatory depression, and increased intracranial pressure may result, but are less common and usually dose dependent.

Contraindications: Hypersensitive reactions occur frequently. Check for sensitivity before administering. These drugs should not be used if narcotic addiction is suspected, and they are also contraindicated in acute bronchial asthma and upper airway obstruction.

Precautions: Caution must be used when these products are given to persons with an addictive personality, since the possibility of addiction is so great. Also, persons with increased intracranial pressure may experience an even greater increase in intracranial pressure. Persons with severe heart disease, hepatic or renal disease, respiratory conditions, and seizure disorders should be monitored closely for worsening condition.

Pharmacokinetics: Onset of action is immediate by IV route and rapid by IM and PO routes. Peak occurs from 1-2 hr, depending on route, with a duration of 2-8 hr, depending on route. These agents cross the placenta and appear in breast milk.

Drug interactions/incompatibilities: Barbiturates, other narcotics, hypnotics, antipsychotics, or alcohol can increase CNS depression when taken with narcotics.

Possible nursing diagnoses:
• Pain *[uses]*
• Impaired gas exchange *[adverse reactions]*

NURSING CONSIDERATIONS

Assess:
• I&O ratio; be alert for urinary retention, frequency, dysuria; drug should be discontinued if these occur

Administer:
• With antiemetic if nausea or vomiting occurs
• When pain is beginning to return; determine dosage interval by patient response

Perform/provide:
• Assistance with ambulation; patient should not be ambulating during drug peak

Evaluate:
• Therapeutic response, including decrease in pain
• Respiratory dysfunction, including respiratory depression, rate, rhythm, character; notify physician if respirations are <12 per minute
• CNS changes: dizziness, drowsiness, hallucinations, euphoria, LOC, pupil reaction
• Allergic reactions: rash, urticaria
• Need for pain medication, physical dependence

Teach patient/family:
• To report any symptoms of CNS changes, allergic reactions, or shortness of breath
• That physical dependency may result when used for extended periods of time
• That withdrawal symptoms may occur, including nausea, vomiting, cramps, fever, faintness, anorexia
• To avoid alcohol and other CNS depressants

Generic names:

alfentanil HCl (p. 53)
buprenorphine HCl (p. 149)
butorphanol tartrate (p. 156)
codeine phosphate (p. 264)
codeine sulfate (p. 264)
dezocine (p. 320)
fentanyl citrate (p. 417)
pentazocine lactate (p. 730)
propoxyphene HCl (p. 801)
morphine sulfate (p. 650)
nalbuphine HCl (p. 658)
oxycodone HCl (p. 702)
oxymorphone HCl (p. 705)
pentazocine HCl (p. 730)

levorphanol tartrate (p. 541)
meperidine HCl (p. 587)
methadone HCl (p. 599)

fentanyl transdermal (p. 418)
hydromorphone HCl (p. 487)
propoxyphene napsylate (p. 801)

NONSTEROIDAL ANTIINFLAMMATORIES

Action: These products act by inhibition of prostaglandin synthesis. Products have analgesic, antiinflammatory, antipyretic properties.

Uses: Products are used to control pain, inflammation associated with acute, chronic rheumatoid arthritis, osteoarthritis, and ankylosing spondylitis. Some products may be used for relief of mild-to-moderate pain, tendinitis, bursitis, fever, sunburn, migraine, dysmenorrhea.

Side effects/adverse reactions: GI symptoms, including nausea, vomiting, anorexia, are the most common side effects. May cause dizziness, drowsiness, or blurred vision. Serious adverse reactions include nephrotoxicity and blood dyscrasias.

Contraindications: Hypersensitive reactions occur frequently. Check for sensitivity before administering. Patients sensitive to aspirin or iodides should not use these agents.

Precautions: Patients with bleeding disorders should use cautiously, since bleeding tendencies may increase. GI disorders may be intensified, since these products are irritating to the GI system. Use with caution in lactation and in impaired renal or hepatic function.

Pharmacokinetics: Peak occurs from 0.5-4 hr after oral ingestion, and elimination half-life may be as long as 5 hr. They are highly bound to plasma proteins and metabolized in the liver, with metabolites excreted in the urine.

Interactions/incompatibilities: Increased anticoagulant effect may occur with coumarin. Increased toxicity may occur when used with phenytoin, sulfonamide, or sulfonylureas. Aspirin may decrease activity of nonsteroidals.

Possible nursing diagnoses:
• Pain [uses]
• Impaired physical mobility [uses]
• Activity intolerance [uses]
• Sensory/perceptual alteration: auditory [adverse reactions]

NURSING CONSIDERATIONS
Assess:
• Hepatic and renal studies: AST, ALT, bilirubin, creatinine, LDH, al-

kaline phosphatase, BUN if patient is on long-term therapy, since these products are metabolized and excreted by the liver and kidney

• Blood studies: CBC, hematocrit, hemoglobin, and prothrombin time if patient is on long-term therapy, since these products increase the possibility of bleeding and blood dyscrasias

Administer:

• With food or milk to decrease gastric irritation; give 30 min before or 1 hr after meals with a full glass of water

Evaluate:

• Hepatotoxicity: dark urine, clay-colored stools, yellowing of skin, sclera, itching, abdominal pain, fever, diarrhea, which may occur with long-term use

Teach patient/family:

• Not to exceed recommended dosage; acute poisoning may result

• That therapeutic response takes 2 wk in arthritis

• To avoid use of alcohol, since GI bleeding may result

• To avoid taking with aspirin while on nonsteroidal therapy

Generic names:

diclofenac (p. 326)
fenoprofen calcium (p. 415)
ibuprofen (p. 496)
indomethacin (p. 503)
ketoprofen (p. 533)
ketorolac tromethamine (p. 534)
meclofenamate (p. 578)

mefenamic acid (p. 580)
naproxen (p. 664)
naproxen sodium (p. 664)
piroxicam (p. 765)
sulindac (p. 869)
tolmetin sodium (p. 917)

SALICYLATES

Action: Salicylates have analgesic, antipyretic, and antiinflammatory effects. The antiinflammatory and analgesic activities may be mediated through the inhibition of prostaglandin synthesis. Antipyretic action results from inhibition of the hypothalamic heat-regulating center.

Uses: The primary uses of salicylates are relief of mild-to-moderate pain and fever and in inflammatory conditions such as arthritis, thromboembolic disorders, and rheumatic fever.

Side effects/adverse reactions: The most common side effects are GI symptoms and rash. Serious blood dyscrasias and hepatotoxicity may result when used for long periods of time at high doses. Tinnitus or impaired hearing may indicate that blood salicylate levels are reaching or exceeding the upper limit of the therapeutic range.

Contraindications: Hypersensitivity to salicylates is common. Check for sensitivity before administering. Persons with bleeding disorders, GI bleeding, and vitamin K deficiency should not use these products, since salicylates increase prothrombin time. Children should not use these products, since salicylates have been associated with Reye's syndrome.

Precautions: Caution is needed when salicylates are given to patients with anemia, hepatic or renal disease, or Hodgkin's disease. Caution should also be exercised in pregnancy and lactation.

Pharmacokinetics: Onset of action occurs in 15-30 min, with a peak of 1-2 hr and a duration up to 6 hr. These drugs are metabolized by the liver and excreted by the kidneys.

Drug interactions/imcompatibilities: Increased effects of anticoagulants, insulin, methotrexate, heparin, valproic acid, and oral sulfonylureas may occur when used with salicylates. Aspirin may decrease serum concentrations of nonsteroidal antiinflammatory agents.

Possible nursing diagnoses:
- Pain *[uses]*
- Impaired physical mobility *[uses]*
- Activity intolerance *[uses]*
- Sensory/perceptual alteration: auditory *[adverse reactions]*

NURSING CONSIDERATIONS
Assess:
- Hepatic and renal studies: AST, ALT, bilirubin, creatinine, LDH, alkaline phosphatase, BUN if patient is on long-term therapy, since these products are metabolized and excreted by the liver and kidney
- Blood studies: CBC, hematocrit, hemoglobin, and prothrombin time if patient is on long-term therapy, since these products increase the possibility of bleeding and blood dyscrasias

Administer:
- With food or milk to decrease gastric irritation; give 30 min before or 1 hr after meals with a full glass of water

Evaluate:
- Hepatotoxicity: dark urine, clay-colored stools, yellowing of skin, sclera, itching, abdominal pain, fever, diarrhea, which may occur with long-term use
- Ototoxicity: tinnitus, ringing, roaring in ears; audiometric testing is needed before and after long-term therapy

Teach patient/family:
- That blood sugar levels should be monitored closely, if patient is diabetic
- Not to exceed recommended dosage; acute poisoning may result
- That therapeutic response takes 2 wk in arthritis

- To avoid use of alcohol, since GI bleeding may result
- To notify physician if ringing in the ears or persistent GI pain occurs
- To take with full glass of H_2O to reduce risk of lodging in esophagus

Generic names:

aspirin (p. 103)
choline magnesium trisalicylate
(p. 235)
choline salicylate (p. 237)

magnesium salicylate (p. 565)
salsalate (p. 831)
sodium thiosalicylate (p. 847)

THYROID HORMONES

Action: Acts by increasing metabolic rates, resulting in increased cardiac output, O_2 consumption, body temperature, blood volume, growth, development at cellular level, respiratory rate, enzyme system activity.

Uses: Products are used for thyroid replacement.

Side effects/adverse reactions: The most common side effects include insomnia, tremors, tachycardia, palpitations, angina, dysrhythmias, weight loss, and changes in appetite. Serious adverse reactions include thyroid storm.

Contraindications: Persons with adrenal insufficiency, myocardial infarction, or thyrotoxicosis should not use these products.

Precautions: The elderly and patients with angina pectoris, hypertension, ischemia, cardiac disease, or diabetes mellitus or insipidus should be watched closely when using these products. Caution should be used in pregnancy (A) and lactation.

Pharmacokinetics: Pharmacokinetics vary widely among products; check specific monographs.

Interactions/incompatibilities:
- Impaired absorption of thyroid products may occur when administered with cholestyramine (separate by 4-5 hr)
- Increased effects of anticoagulants, sympathomimetics, tricyclic antidepressants, catecholamines may occur
- Decreased effects of digitalis, glycosides, insulin, hypoglycemics may occur
- Decreased effects of thyroid products may occur with estrogens

Possible nursing diagnoses:
- Knowledge deficit
- Noncompliance
- Body image disturbance

NURSING CONSIDERATIONS
Assess:
• B/P, pulse before each dose
• I&O ratio
• Weight q d in same clothing, using same scale, at same time of day
• Height, growth rate if given to a child
• T3, T4, which are decreased; radioimmunoassay of TSH, which is increased; ratio uptake, which is decreased if patient is on too low a dosage of medication

Administer:
• At same time each day to maintain drug level
• Only for hormone imbalances, not to be used for obesity, male infertility, menstrual conditions, lethargy

Perform/provide:
• Removal of medication 4 wk before RAIU test

Evaluate:
• Therapeutic response: absence of depression; increased weight loss; diuresis; pulse; appetite; absence of constipation; peripheral edema; cold intolerance; pale, cool, dry skin; brittle nails; alopecia; coarse hair; menorrhagia; night blindness; paresthesias; syncope; stupor; coma; rosy cheeks
• Increased nervousness, excitability, irritability; may indicate too high doses of medication usually after 1-3 wk of treatment
• Cardiac status: angina, palpitation, chest pain, change in VS

Teach patient/family:
• That hair loss will occur in child and is temporary
• To report excitability, irritability, anxiety; indicates overdose
• Not to switch brands unless directed by physician
• That hypothyroid child will show almost immediate behavior/personality change
• That treatment drug is not to be taken to reduce weight
• To avoid OTC preparations with iodine; read labels
• To avoid iodine food, salt-iodinized, soy beans, tofu, turnips, some seafood, some bread

---

Generic names:

levothyroxine sodium (T4) (p. 542)
liothyronine sodium (T3) (p. 550)
liotrix (p. 551)

thyroglobulin (p. 901)
thyroid USP (p. 902)
thyrotropin (TSH) (p. 904)

VITAMINS

Action: Action varies widely among products and classes; check specific monographs.

Uses: Vitamins are used to correct and prevent vitamin deficiencies.

Side effects/adverse reactions: There is an absence of side effects or adverse reactions with the water-soluble vitamins (C, B). However, fat-soluble vitamins (A, D, E, K) may accumulate in the body and cause adverse reactions (refer to specific monographs).

Contraindications: Hypersensitive reactions may occur, and allergies should be identified before these products are given.

Pharmacokinetics: Onset, peak, and duration vary widely among products; check individual monograph for specific information.

Possible nursing diagnosis:
• Nutrition, less than body requirements *[uses]*

NURSING CONSIDERATIONS
Administer:
• PO with food for better absorption
Perform/provide:
• Storage in tight, light-resistant container
Evaluate:
• Therapeutic response
Teach patient/family:
• Not to take more than prescribed amount

Generic names:

Fat-soluble: phytonadione (p. 756)
vitamin A (p. 964)
vitamin D (p. 965)
vitamin E (p. 966)
vitamin K-menadiol (p. 584)

Water-soluble: ascorbic acid (C) (p. 100)

cyanocobalamin hydroxocobalimin (B_{12}) (p. 278)
pyridoxine (B_6) (p. 813)
riboflavin (B_2) (p. 828)
thiamine (B_1) (p. 891)

Miscellaneous: multiple vitamins (p. 652)

absorbable gelatin

Gelfoam

Func. class.: Hemostatic
Chem. class.: Purified gelatin solution

Action: Absorbs blood, provides area for clot formation, healthy tissue growth
Uses: Hemostasis during surgery, decubitus ulcers
Dosage and routes:
• *Adult:* TOP hold in place for 15 sec after saturating with isotonic NaCL injection
Decubitus ulcer
• *Adult:* TOP place into ulcer, may add more as needed, not to be removed
Available forms include: Sponge, pack, cone, powder
Side effects/adverse reactions: None reported
Contraindications: Hypersensitivity, frank infection, abnormal bleeding, postpartum bleeding
Pharmacokinetics:
IMPLANT: Absorbed in 4-6 wk
NURSING CONSIDERATIONS
Administer:
• By lightly packing, do not overpack foam
• Dry, hold for 10-15 sec, remove
• Moist, place in sterile saline or thrombin solution, squeeze after removing, blot before applying
• After debridement of decubiti unless dressing change qd; do not remove sponge, may add more sponges over top of old ones
Perform/provide:
• Discard unused portion; do not resterilize
Evaluate:
• Infection: fever, redness, inflammation

Teach patient/family:
• That foam is absorbed in 4-6 wk, does not need to be removed

---

acebutolol

(ase-bute′-oh-lole)
Monitan,* Sectral
Func. class.: Antihypertensive
Chem. class.: Nonselective β-blocker

Action: Competitively blocks stimulation of β-adrenergic receptor within vascular smooth muscle; produces chronotropic, inotropic activity (decreases rate of SA node discharge, increases recovery time), slows conduction of AV node, decreases heart rate, which decreases O_2 consumption in myocardium; also, decreases renin-aldosterone-angiotensin system at high doses, inhibits β-2 receptors in bronchial system (high doses)
Uses: Mild to moderate hypertension, sinus tachycardia, persistent atrial extrasystoles, tachydysrhythmias, prophylaxis of angina pectoris
Dosage and routes:
Hypertension
• *Adult:* PO 400 mg qd or in 2 divided doses, may be increased to desired response
Ventricular dysrhythmia
• *Adult:* PO until dose 200 mg bid, may increase gradually, usual range 600-1200 mg daily
Available forms include: Caps 200, 400 mg, tabs 100, 200, 400 mg (Canada only)
Side effects/adverse reactions:
*CV: **Profound hypotension, bradycardia, CHF,** cold extremities, postural hypotension, **2nd or 3rd degree heart block***
CNS: Insomnia, fatigue, dizziness,

---

italics = common side effects   ***bold italic*** = life threatening reactions

mental changes, memory loss, hallucinations, depression, lethargy, drowsiness, strange dreams, catatonia

GI: Nausea, diarrhea, vomiting, ***mesenteric arterial thrombosis, ischemic colitis***

INTEG: Rash, fever, alopecia

HEMA: Agranulocytosis, thrombocytopenia, purpura

EENT: Sore throat, dry burning eyes

GU: Impotence

ENDO: Increased hypoglycemic response to insulin

*RESP: **Bronchospasm,*** dyspnea, wheezing

Contraindications: Hypersensitivity to β-blockers, cardiogenic shock, heart block (2nd, 3rd degree), sinus bradycardia, CHF, cardiac failure

Precautions: Major surgery, pregnancy (B), lactation, diabetes mellitus, renal disease, thyroid disease, COPD, asthma, well compensated heart failure, aortic, mitral valve disease

Pharmacokinetics:

PO: Peak 2-4 hr; half-life 6-7 hr, excreted unchanged in urine, protein binding 5%-15%

Interactions/incompatibilities:

• Increased hypotension, bradycardia: reserpine, hydralazine, methyldopa, prazosin, anticholinergics

• Decreased antihypertensive effects: indomethacin

• Increased hypoglycemic effect: insulin

• Decreased bronchodilation: theophyllines

NURSING CONSIDERATIONS
Assess:

• B/P during beginning treatment, periodically thereafter; pulse q4h; note rate, rhythm, quality

• Apical/radial pulse before administration; notify physician of any significant changes (pulse <60 bpm)

• Baselines in renal, liver function tests before therapy begins

Administer:

• PO ac, hs, tablet may be crushed or swallowed whole

• Reduced dosage in renal dysfunction

Perform/provide:

• Storage protected from light, moisture; placed in cool environment

Evaluate:

• Therapeutic response: decreased B/P after 1-2 wk

• Edema in feet, legs daily

• Skin turgor, dryness of mucous membranes for hydration status

Teach patient/family:

• Not to discontinue drug abruptly, taper over 2 wk, may cause precipitate angina

• Not to use OTC products containing α-adrenergic stimulants (such as nasal decongestants, OTC cold preparations) unless directed by physician

• To report bradycardia, dizziness, confusion, depression, fever

• To take pulse at home, advise when to notify physician

• To avoid alcohol, smoking, sodium intake

• To comply with weight control, dietary adjustments, modified exercise program

• To carry Medic Alert ID to identify drug that you are taking, allergies

• To avoid hazardous activities if dizziness is present

• To report symptoms of CHF: difficult breathing, especially on exertion or when lying down, night cough, swelling of extremities

Lab test interferences:

Interference: Glucose/insulin tolerance tests

---

* Available in Canada only

Treatment of overdose: Lavage, IV atropine for bradycardia, IV theophylline for bronchospasm, digitalis, O$_2$, diuretic for cardiac failure, hemodialysis, IV glucose for hyperglycemia, IV diazepam (or phenytoin) for seizures

---

acetaminophen

(a-seat-a-mee'noe-fen)

Anapap, Atasol,* Campain,* Dapa, Datril, Liquiprin, Panadol, Parten, Pedric, Robigesic,* Rounax,* Tempra, Tylenol, Valadol, Valcrin

Func. class.: Nonnarcotic analgesic

Chem. class.: Nonsalicylate, para aminophenol derivative

Action: Blocks pain impulses in CNS that occur in response to inhibition of prostaglandin synthesis; antipyretic action results from inhibition of hypothalamic heat-regulating center.

Uses: Mild to moderate pain or fever

Dosage and routes:
• *Adult and child >10 yr:* PO 325-650 mg q4h prn, not to exceed 4 g/day; REC: 325-650 mg q4h prn, not to exceed 4 g/day
• *Child 0-3 mo:* 40 mg/dose
• *Child 4-11 mo:* 80 mg/dose
• *Child <1 yr:* PO/REC 15-60 mg/dose all q4-6h, not to exceed 65 mg/kg/day
• *Child 1-2 yr:* PO/REC 60 mg/dose
• *Child 2-3 yr:* PO/REC 120 mg/dose
• *Child 3-4 yr:* PO/REC 180 mg/dose
• *Child 4-5 yr:* PO/REC 240 mg/dose

• *Child 5-10 yr:* PO/REC 325 mg/dose

Available forms include: Rectal supp 120, 125, 325, 600, 650 mg; chewable tab 80 mg; caps 325, 500, 650 mg; elix 120, 160, 325 mg/5 ml; liq 160 mg/5 ml, 500mg/15ml; sol 100 mg/1 ml, 120 mg/2.5 ml

Side effects/adverse reactions:
SYST: **Anaphylaxis**
HEMA: **Leukopenia, neutropenia, hemolytic anemia** (long-term use), **thrombocytopenia, pancytopenia**
CNS: Stimulation, drowsiness
GI: Nausea, vomiting, abdominal pain, **hepatotoxicity**
INTEG: Rash, urticaria, **angioedema**
TOXICITY: **Cyanosis, anemia, neutropenia, jaundice, pancytopenia, CNS stimulation, delirium then vascular collapse, convulsions, coma, death**

Contraindications: Hypersensitivity

Precautions: Anemia, hepatic disease, renal disease, chronic alcoholism, pregnancy (B)

Pharmacokinetics:
PO: Onset 10-30 min, peak ½-2 hr, duration 4-6 hr
REC: Onset slow, duration 4-6 hr
Metabolized by liver, excreted by kidneys, crosses placenta, excreted in breast milk, half-life 1-4 hr

Interactions/incompatibilities:
• Increased effects of: chloramphenicol
• Decreased effects of acetaminophen: cholestyramine, oral contraceptives, anticholinergics
• Increased effect of acetaminophen: diflunisal, caffeine

NURSING CONSIDERATIONS
Assess:
• Liver function studies: AST, ALT, bilirubin, creatinine if patient is on long-term therapy

---

italics = common side effects   **bold italic** = life threatening reactions

• Renal function studies: BUN, urine creatinine if patient is on long-term therapy
• Blood studies: CBC, pro-time if patient is on long-term therapy
• I&O ratio; decreasing output may indicate renal failure (long-term therapy)

Administer:
• To patient crushed or whole; chewable tablets may be chewed
• With food or milk to decrease gastric symptoms

Evaluate:
• Therapeutic response: absence of pain, fever
• Hepatotoxicity: dark urine, clay-colored stools, yellowing of skin, sclera, itching, abdominal pain, fever, diarrhea if patient is on long-term therapy
• Allergic reactions: rash, urticaria; if these occur, drug may need to be discontinued
• Renal dysfunction: decreased urine output

Teach patient/family:
• Not to exceed recommend dosage; acute poisoning may result
• To read label on other OTC drugs; many contain acetaminophen

Treatment of overdose: Drug level q4h, gastric lavage, administer acetylcysteine

---

acetazolamide/ acetazolamide sodium

(a-set-a-zole′a-mide)
Cetazol, Diamox, Hydrazol/Diamox Parenteral

Func. class.: Diuretic; carbonic anhydrase inhibitor
Chem. class.: Sulfonamide derivative

Action: Inhibits carbonic anhydrase activity in proximal renal tubules to decrease reabsorption of water, sodium, potassium, bicarbonate; decreases carbonic anhydrase in CNS, increasing seizure threshold; able to decrease aqueous humor in eye, which lowers intraocular pressure

Uses: Open-angle glaucoma, narrow-angle glaucoma (preoperatively, if surgery delayed), epilepsy (petit mal, grand mal, mixed), edema in CHF, drug-induced edema, acute mountain sickness

Dosage and routes:
Closed-angle glaucoma
• *Adult:* PO/IM/IV 250 mg q4h, or 250 mg bid, to be used for short-term therapy
Open-angle glaucoma
• *Adult:* PO/IM/IV 250 mg-1g/day in divided doses for amounts over 250 mg
Edema
• *Adult:* IM/IV 250-375 mg/day in AM
• *Child:* IM/IV 5 mg/kg/day in AM
Seizures
• *Adult:* PO/IM/IV 8-30 mg/kg/day, usual range 375-1000 mg/day
• *Child:* PO/IM/IV 8-30 mg/kg/day in divided doses tid or qid, or 300-900 mg/m²/day, not to exceed 1.5 g/day
Mountain sickness
• *Adult:* PO 250 mg q8-12h
Available forms include: Tabs 125, 250 mg; caps sust rel 500 mg; inj IM/IV 500 mg

Side effects/adverse reactions:
*GU: Frequency, hypokalemia, polyuria, **uremia,** glucosuria, hematuria, dysuria*
CNS: Drowsiness, paresthesia, anxiety, depression, headache, dizziness, confusion, stimulation, fa-

tigue, *convulsions,* sedation, nervousness

GI: Nausea, vomiting, anorexia, constipation, diarrhea, melena, weight loss, *hepatic insufficiency*

EENT: Myopia, tinnitus

INTEG: Rash, pruritus, urticaria, fever, *Stevens-Johnson syndrome,* photosensitivity

ENDO: Hyperglycemia

HEMA: Aplastic anemia, hemolytic anemia, leukopenia, agranulocytosis, thrombocytopenia, purpura, pancytopenia

Contraindications: Hypersensitivity to sulfonamides, severe renal disease, severe hepatic disease, electrolyte imbalances (hyponatremia, hypokalemia), hyperchloremic acidosis, Addison's disease, long-term use in narrow-angle glaucoma, COPD

Precautions: Hypercalciuria, pregnancy (C)

Pharmacokinetics:

PO: Onset 1-1½ hr, peak 2-4 hr, duration 6-12 hr

PO—SUS REL: Onset 2 hr, peak 8-12 hr, duration 18-24 hr

IV: Onset 2 min, peak 15 min, duration 4-5 hr

65% absorbed if fasting (oral), 75% absorbed if given with food; half-life 2½-5½ hr; excreted unchanged by kidneys (80% within 24 hr), crosses placenta

Interactions/incompatibilities:

• Increased action of: amphetamines, procainamide, quinidine, tricyclics, flecainide, ephedrine, pseudoephedrine

• Toxicity: salicylates

• Hypokalemia: with other diuretics, corticosteroids, amphotericin B

• IV compatibility: cimetidine, D_5W, $D_{10}W$, NaCl, LR

NURSING CONSIDERATIONS
Assess:

• Weight daily, I&O daily to determine fluid loss; effect of drug may be decreased if used qd

• Rate, depth, rhythm of respiration, effect of exertion

• B/P lying, standing; postural hypotension may occur

• Electrolytes: potassium, sodium, chloride; include BUN, blood sugar, CBC, serum creatinine, blood pH, ABGs, liver function tests

Administer:

• PO or IV if possible, IM administration is painful

• In AM to avoid interference with sleep if using drug as diuretic

• Potassium replacement if potassium is less than 3.0

• With food if nausea occurs; absorption may be decreased slightly

Perform/provide:

• Storage in dark, cool area; use reconstituted solution within 24 hr

• Dilute 500 mg in >5 ml sterile H_2O for injection; direct IV—give at 100-500 mg/min; may be diluted further in compatible IV solutions and infused over 4-8 hr

Evaluate:

• Therapeutic response: improvement in edema of feet, legs, sacral area daily if medication is being used in CHF; or decrease in aqueous humor if medication is being used in glaucoma

• Improvement in CVP q8h

• Signs of metabolic acidosis: drowsiness, restlessness

• Signs of hypokalemia: postural hypotension, malaise, fatigue, tachycardia, leg cramps, weakness

• Rashes, temperature elevation qd

• Confusion, especially in elderly; take safety precautions if needed

---

italics = common side effects   *bold italic* = life threatening reactions

Teach patient / family:
• To increase fluid intake 2-3 L/day unless contraindicated; to rise slowly from lying or sitting position
• To notify physician if sore throat, unusual bleeding, bruising, paresthesias, tremors, flank pain, or skin rash occurs
• To avoid hazardous activities if drowsiness occurs

Lab test interferences:
False positive: Urinary protein

Treatment of overdose: Lavage if taken orally, monitor electrolytes, administer dextrose in saline, monitor hydration, CV, renal status

---

acetohexamide

(a-seat-oh-hex′a-mide)
Dimelor,* Dymelor
Func. class.: Antidiabetic
Chem. class.: Sulfonylurea (1st generation)

Action: Causes functioning β-cells in pancreas to release insulin, leading to drop in blood glucose levels; may improve binding between insulin and insulin receptors or increase number of insulin receptors; not effective if patient lacks functioning β-cells

Uses: Stable adult-onset diabetes mellitus (type II), NIDDM

Dosage and routes:
• *Adult:* PO 250 mg-1.5 g/day; usually given before breakfast, unless large dose is required, then dose is divided in two

Available forms include: Tabs 250, 500 mg scored

Side effects / adverse reactions:
CNS: Headache, weakness, tinnitus, fatigue, dizziness, vertigo
GI: Nausea, vomiting, diarrhea, *hepatotoxicity, jaundice,* heartburn
HEMA: Leukopenia, thrombocytopenia, agranulocytosis, aplastic anemia, increased AST, ALT, alk phosphatase
INTEG: Rash, allergic reactions, pruritus, urticaria, eczema, photosensitivity, erythema
ENDO: Hypoglycemia

Contraindications: Hypersensitivity to sulfonylureas, juvenile or brittle diabetes

Precautions: Pregnancy (C), elderly, cardiac disease, renal disease, hepatic disease, thyroid disease, severe hypoglycemic reactions

Pharmacokinetics:
PO: Completely absorbed by GI route, onset 1 hr, peak 2-4 hr, duration 12-24 hr, half-life 6-8 hr, metabolized in liver, excreted in urine (metabolites, unchanged drug)

Interactions / incompatibilities:
• Increased hypoglycemic effects: oral anticoagulants, salicylates, sulfonamides, nonsteroidal antiinflammatories, guanethidine, methyldopa, MAOIs, chloramphenicol, insulin, cimetidine
• Decreased action of acetohexamide: calcium channel blockers, corticosteroids, oral contraceptives, thiazide diuretics, thyroid preparations, estrogens, phenobarbital, phenothiazines, phenytoin, rifampin, sympathomimetics
• Decreased effect of both drugs: diazoxide

NURSING CONSIDERATIONS
Administer:
• Drug 30 min before meals

Perform / provide:
• Storage in tight container in cool environment

Evaluate:
• Therapeutic response: decrease in polyuria, polydipsia, polyphagia,

---

clear sensorium, absence of dizziness, stable gait

• Hypoglycemic/hyperglycemic reaction that can occur soon after meals

Teach patient/family:

• To check for symptoms of cholestatic jaundice: dark urine, pruritus, yellow sclera; if these occur physician should be notified

• To use capillary blood glucose test while on this drug

• To test urine glucose levels with Chemstrip 3 ×/day

• Symptoms of hypo/hyperglycemia, what to do about each

• Drug must be continued on daily basis; explain consequence of discontinuing drug abruptly

• To take drug in morning to prevent hypoglycemic reactions at night

• Not to drink alcohol

• To avoid OTC medications unless prescribed by physician

• That diabetes is life-long illness; that this drug is not a cure

• That all food included in diet plan must be eaten in order to prevent hypoglycemia

• To carry Medic-Alert ID for emergency purposes

Treatment of overdose: 10%-50% glucose solution or 1 mg glucagon

---

acetohydroxamic acid

(a-set-oh-hye-drox-am′ic)

Lithostat

Func. class.: Ammonia detoxicant, reversible urease inhibitor

Chem. class.: Hydroxylamine, ethyl acetate compound

Action: Inhibits bacterial enzyme urease, which decreases conversion of urea to ammonia; the reduced ammonia levels and decreased pH increase the effectiveness of antimicrobial agents

Uses: Adjunctive treatment in chronic urea-splitting urinary infection

Dosage and routes:

• *Adult:* PO 250 mg tid-qid q6-8h when stomach is empty, not to exceed 1.5 g/day

• *Child:* PO 10 mg/kg/day in 2-3 divided doses

Available forms include: Tabs 250 mg

Side effects/adverse reactions:

*HEMA: **Hemolytic anemia, reticulocytosis, thrombocytopenia, bone marrow depression***

CNS: Headache, depression, restlessness, anxiety, nervousness

GI: Nausea, vomiting, anorexia, malaise

INTEG: Rash on face, arms, alopecia

CV: Phlebitis, ***deep vein thrombosis, pulmonary embolism,*** palpitation

Contraindications: Hypersensitivity, severe renal disease, nonurease-producing organisms, pregnancy (X)

Precautions: Deep vein thrombosis, hepatic disease, renal disease, lactation

Pharmacokinetics:

PO: Peak 15-60 min, half-life 3½-10 hr, metabolized, excreted in urine as unchanged drug (15%-60%)

Interactions/incompatibilities:

• Decreased absorption of both drugs: iron preparations

• Rash: alcohol

NURSING CONSIDERATIONS
Assess:

• I&O ratio; observe for decrease in urinary output

• CBC, platelets, reticulocytes before, during therapy (q3 mo)

---

italics = common side effects   ***bold italic*** = life threatening reactions

Administer:
• On empty stomach only, to facilitate absorption

Perform/provide:
• Storage in tight container at room temperature

Evaluate:
• Therapeutic response: decrease in stone formation on x-ray, decreased pain in kidney region, absence of hematuria, signs of anemia

Teach patient/family:
• To avoid alcohol, OTC preparations that contain alcohol; skin rashes have occurred
• To report any pain, redness, or hard area, usually in legs, may indicate phlebitis
• Stress patient compliance with medical regimen; bone marrow depression may occur
• To increase fluids to 3-4 L/day
• To use contraception during treatment

---

acetylcholine chloride

(a-se-teel-koe'leen)
Miochol direct-acting

Func. class.: Miotic, cholinergic
Chem. class.: Quaternary ammonium compound

Action: Intense, immediate miosis (pupil constriction) by causing contraction of sphincter muscle of iris

Uses: Anterior segment surgery; cataract removal keratoplasty, peripheral iridectomy or cyclodialysis

Dosage and routes:
• *Adult and child:* INSTILL 0.5-2 ml of a 1% sol in anterior chamber of eye (instillation by physician)

Available forms include: Sol 1:100

Side effects/adverse reactions:
CV: Hypotension, bradycardia

EENT: Blurred vision, lens opacities

Contraindications: Hypersensitivity, when miosis is undesirable

Precautions: Acute cardiac failure, bronchial asthma

Pharmacokinetics:
INSTILL: Miosis occurs immediately, duration 10 min

NURSING CONSIDERATIONS
Administer:
• Check vial for percentage of solution
• Check label for expiration date
• After shaking vial to mix drug to clear solution, push stopper to mix solvent with powder; do not use if stopper cannot be forced down
• After cleaning stopper with alcohol or other germicidal
• IV atropine 0.6-0.8 mg for systemic reactions

Perform/provide:
• Used reconstituted solution immediately; discard unused portion

Teach patient/family:
• To report change in vision, blurring or loss of sight, trouble breathing, sweating, flushing

---

acetylcysteine

(a-se-til-sis'tay-een)
Airbron,* Mucomyst, Parvolex

Func. class.: Mucolytic
Chem. class.: Amino acid L-cysteine

Action: Decreases viscosity of secretions by breaking disulfide links of mucoproteins; increases hepatic glutathione, which is necessary to inactivate toxic metabolites in acetaminophen overdose

Uses: Acetaminophen toxicity, bronchitis, pneumonia, cystic fibrosis, emphysema, atelectasis, tuberculosis, complications of thoracic, cardiovascular surgery, diagnosis in bronchial lab tests

Dosage and routes:
• *Adult and child:* INSTILL 1-2 ml (10%-20% sol) q1-4h prn or 3-5 ml (20% sol) or 6-10 ml (10% sol) tid or qid

Acetaminophen toxicity
• *Adult and child:* PO 140 mg/kg, then 70 mg/kg q4h × 17 doses to total of 1330 mg/kg

Available forms include: Sol 10%, 20%

Side effects/adverse reactions:
CNS: Dizziness, drowsiness, headache, fever, chills
GI: Nausea, stomatitis, constipation, vomiting, anorexia, *hepatotoxicity*
EENT: Rhinorrhea, tooth damage
CV: Hypotension
INTEG: Urticaria, rash, fever, clamminess
RESP: Bronchospasm, burning, hemoptysis, chest tightness

Contraindications: Hypersensitivity, increased intracranial pressure, status asthmaticus

Precautions: Hypothyroidism, Addison's disease, CNS depression, brain tumor, asthma, hepatic disease, renal disease, COPD, psychosis, alcoholism, convulsive disorders, lactation, pregnancy (B)

Pharmacokinetics:
INH/INSTILL: Onset 1 min, duration 5-10 min, metabolized by liver, excreted in urine

Interactions/incompatibilities:
• Do not use with iron, copper, rubber
• Do not mix with antibiotics: tetracycline, chlortetracycline, oxytetracycline, erythromycin, lactobionate, amphotericin-B, sodium ampicillin; iodized oil, chymotrypsin, trypsin, hydrogen peroxide

NURSING CONSIDERATIONS
Assess:
• VS, cardiac status including checking for dysrhythmias, increased rate, palpitations
• ABGs for increased CO_2 retention in asthma patients
• Antidotal use: liver function tests, acetaminophen levels; inform physician if dose is vomited or vomiting is persistent

Administer:
• Store in refrigerator: use within 96 hr of opening
• Before meals ½-1 hr for better absorption, to decrease nausea
• 20% solutions diluted with NS over water for injection; may give 10% solution undiluted
• Only after patient clears airway by deep breathing, coughing
• Antidotal use: give within 24 hr; give with cola or soft drink to disguise taste; can be given with H_2O through tubes; use within 1 hr
• By syringe 2-3 doses of 1-2 ml of 20% or 2-4 ml of 10% solution
• Decreased dose to elderly patients; their metabolism may be slowed
• Gum, hard candy, frequent rinsing of mouth for dryness of oral cavity
• Only if suction machine is available

Perform/provide:
• Storage in refrigerator after opening
• Assistance with inhaled dose: bronchodilator if bronchospasm occurs
• Mechanical suction if cough insufficient to remove excess bronchial secretions

Evaluate:
• Therapeutic response: absence of purulent secretions when coughing

italics = common side effects   ***bold italic*** = life threatening reactions

• Cough: type, frequency, character including sputum
• Rate, rhythm of respirations, increased dyspnea; discontinue if bronchospasm occurs
• Antidotal use: decrease in hepatic encephalopathy

Teach patient/family:
• Avoid driving or other hazardous activities until patient is stabilized on this medication
• Avoid alcohol, other CNS depressants; will enhance sedating properties of this drug
• That unpleasant odor will decrease after repeated use
• That discoloration of solution after bottle is opened does not impair its effectiveness
• Avoid smoking, smoke-filled rooms, perfume, dust, environmental pollutants, cleaners

---

activated charcoal

Arm-a-char, Charcoaide, Charcocaps, Charcodote, Charcotabs, Digestalin

Func. class.: Antiflatulent/antidote

Action: Binds poisons, toxins, irritants; increases adsorption in GI tract; inactivates toxins and binds until excreted

Uses: Flatulence, poisoning, dyspepsia, distention, deodorant in wounds, diarrhea

Dosage and routes:
Poisoning
• *Adult and child:* PO 5-10 × weight of substance ingested, minimum dose 30 g/250 ml of water
Flatulence/dyspepsia
• *Adult:* PO 600 mg-5 g tid-qid
Available forms include: Powder; liq 12.5, 25, 40 g; caps 260 mg; tabs 325, 650 mg

Side effects/adverse reactions:
GI: Nausea, black stools, vomiting, constipation, diarrhea

Contraindications: Hypersensitivity to this drug, unconsciousness/semiconsciousness, poisoning of cyanide, mineral acids, alkalies

Pharmacokinetics:
PO: Not metabolized, excreted in feces

Interactions/incompatibilities:
• Decreased effectiveness of both drugs: ipecac, laxatives
• Do not mix with dairy products

NURSING CONSIDERATIONS
Assess:
• Respiration, pulse, B/P to determine charcoal effectiveness if taken for barbiturate/narcotic poisoning

Administer:
• After inducing vomiting first unless contraindicated (i.e., cyanide or alkalies)
• After mixing with water or fruit juice to form thick syrup; do not use dairy products to mix charcoal
• Repeat dose if vomiting occurs soon after dose
• After spacing at least 1 hr before or after other drugs, or absorption will be decreased
• With a laxative to promote elimination
• Alone; do not administer with ipecac
• Through a nasogastric tube if patient unable to swallow
• Keeping container tightly closed to prevent absorption of gases

Evaluate:
• Therapeutic response: LOC, alert (poisoning)

Teach patient/family:
• That stools will be black

---

acyclovir (topical)

(ay-sye'kloe-ver)
Zovirax

Func. class.: Local antiinfective
Chem. class.: Antiviral

Action: Interferes with viral DNA replication

Uses: Simple mucocutaneous herpes simplex, in immunocompromised clients with initial herpes genitalis

Dosage and routes:
• *Adult and child:* TOP apply to all lesions q3h while awake, 6 times/day × 1 wk

Available forms include: Top oint 5% (50 mg/g)

Side effects/adverse reactions:
INTEG: Rash, urticaria, stinging, burning, pruritus, vulvitis

Contraindications: Hypersensitivity

Precautions: Pregnancy (C), lactation

NURSING CONSIDERATIONS
Administer:
• Using finger cot or rubber glove to prevent further infection
• Enough medication to completely cover lesions
• After cleansing with soap, water before each application, dry well

Perform/provide:
• Storage at room temperature in dry place

Evaluate:
• Allergic reaction: burning, stinging, swelling, redness
• Therapeutic response: decrease in size, number of lesions

Teach patient/family:
• Not to use in eyes, or use when there is not evidence of infection
• To apply with glove to prevent further infection
• To avoid use of OTC creams, ointments, lotions unless directed by physician
• To use medical asepsis (hand washing) before, after each application and avoid contact with eyes
• Strict adherence to prescribed regimen to maximize successful treatment outcome
• Begin taking drug when symptoms arise

acyclovir sodium

(ay-sye-kloe-ver)
Zovirax

Func. class.: Antiviral
Chem. class.: Acylic purine nucleoside analog

Action: Interferes with DNA synthesis needed for viral replication

Uses: Mucocutaneous herpes simplex virus, herpes genitalis (HSV-1, HSV-2)

Dosage and routes:
Herpes simplex
• *Adult and child >12 yr:* IV INF 5 mg/kg over 1 hr q8h × 5 days
• *Child <12 yr:* IV INF 250 mg/m² over 1 hr q8h × 5 days

Genital herpes
• *Adult:* PO 200 mg q4h 5×/day while awake for 5 days to 6 mo depending whether initial, recurrent, or chronic

Available forms include: Caps 200 mg; inj IV 500 mg, oint (see topical listings)

Side effects/adverse reactions:
CNS: Tremors, confusion, lethargy, hallucinations, *convulsions,* dizziness, *headache*

HEMA: Anemia, increased bleeding time, *bone marrow depression, granulocytopenia, thrombocytopenia, leukopenia, megaloblastic anemia*

GI: Nausea, vomiting, diarrhea, increased ALT, AST, abdominal pain, glossitis, colitis

GU: Oliguria, proteinuria, hematuria, *vaginitis, moniliasis, glomerulonephritis, acute renal failure*, changes in menses

INTEG: Rash, urticaria, pruritus, phelebitis at IV site

Contraindications: Hypersensitivity, herpes zoster in immunosuppressed individual

Precautions: Lactation, hepatic disease, renal disease, electrolyte imbalance, dehydration, pregnancy (C)

Pharmacokinetics:

IV: Peak 1 hr, half-life 20 min-3 hr, (terminal), metabolized by liver, excreted by kidneys as unchanged drug (95%), crosses placenta

Interactions/incompatibilities:

• Increased neurotoxicity, nephrotoxicity: aminoglycosides, amphotericin, interferon, probenecid, methotrexate

• IV incompatibility: dobutamine, dopamine, all protein products

• IV-compatible solutions: D_5W, LR, or NaCl solutions

NURSING CONSIDERATIONS

Assess:

• Signs of infection, anemia

• I&O ratio; report hematuria, oliguria, fatigue, weakness; may indicate nephrotoxicity; check for protein in urine during treatment

• Any patient with compromised renal system, since drug is excreted slowly in poor renal system function; toxicity may occur rapidly

• Liver studies: AST, ALT

• Blood studies: WBC, RBC, Hct, Hgb, bleeding time; blood dyscrasias may occur; drug should be discontinued

• Renal studies: urinalysis, protein, BUN, creatinine, CrCl

• C&S before drug therapy; drug may be taken as soon as culture is taken; repeat C&S after treatment

Administer:

• Increased fluids to 3 L/day to decrease crystalluria when given IV

• After reconstituting with 10 ml compatible solution/500 mg of drug, concentration of 50 mg/ml, shake, use within 12 hr; give over at least 1 hr by infusion pump to prevent nephrotoxicity

Perform/provide:

• Storage at room temperature for up to 12 hr after reconstitution

• Adequate intake of fluids (2000 ml) to prevent deposit in kidneys

Evaluate:

• Therapeutic response: absence of itching, painful lesions

• Bowel pattern before, during treatment; if severe abdominal pain with bleeding occurs, drug should be discontinued

• Skin eruptions: rash, urticaria, itching

• Allergies before treatment, reaction of each medication; place allergies on chart, Kardex in bright red letters; notify all people giving drugs

Teach patient/family:

• That drug may be taken orally before infection occurs; drug should be taken when itching or pain occurs, usually before eruptions

• That partners need to be told that patient has herpes; they could become infected

• That drug does not cure infection, just controls symptoms

• To report sore throat, fever, fatigue; could indicate superimposed infection

• That drug must be taken in equal intervals around the clock to maintain blood levels for duration of therapy

• To notify physician of side effects of bruising, bleeding, fatigue, malaise; may indicate blood dyscrasias

---

adenosine
Adenocard

Func. class.: Antidysrhythmic
Chem. class.: Endogenous nucleoside

Action: Slows conduction through the AV node, can interrupt reentry pathways through AV node, and can restore normal sinus rhythm in patients with paroxysmal supraventricular tachycardia (PSVT)
Uses: Paroxysmal supraventricular tachycardia
Dosage and routes:
• *Adult:* IV BOL 6 mg; if conversion to normal sinus rhythm does not occur within 1-2 min, give 12 mg by rapid IV BOL; may repeat 12 mg dose again
Available forms include: Inj 3 mg/ml
Side effects/adverse reactions:
GI: Nausea, metallic taste, throat tightness, groin pressure
RESP: Dyspnea, chest pressure, hyperventilation
CNS: Lightheadedness, dizziness, arm tingling, numbness, apprehension, blurred vision, headache
CV: Chest pain, ***atrial tachydysrhythmias,*** sweating, palpitations, hypotension, *facial flushing*
Contraindications: Hypersensitivity, 2nd or 3rd degree heart block, AV block, sick sinus syndrome, atrial flutter, atrial fibrillation, ventricular tachycardia
Precautions: Pregnancy (C), lactation, children, asthma
Pharmacokinetics: Cleared from plasma in <30 sec, half-life 10 sec

Interactions/incompatibilities:
• Increased effects of adenosine: dipyridamole
• Decreased activity of adenosine; theophylline or other methylxanthines (caffeine)
• Higher degree of heart block: carbamazepine
NURSING CONSIDERATIONS
Assess:
• Cardiac status continually
Evaluate:
• Therapeutic response: decreased anginal pain, decreased B/P, dysrhythmias
• Cardiac status: B/P, pulse, respiration, ECG intervals (PR, QRS, QT)
Lab test interferences:
Increase: Liver function tests
Treatment of overdose: Defibrillation, vasopressor for hypotension

---

albumin, normal serum 5%/25%
(al-byoo'min)
Albuminar 5%, Albutein 5%, Buminate 5%, Plasbumin 5%, Albuminar 25%, Albumisol 25%, Buminate 25%, Plasbumin 25%

Func. class.: Blood derivative
Chem. class.: Placental human plasma

Action: Exerts oncotic pressure, which expands volume of circulating blood
Uses: Restores plasma volume in burns, hyperbilirubinemia, shock, hypoproteinemia, varicella zoster infections (supportive treatment)
Dosage and routes:
Burns
• *Adult:* IV dose to maintain plasma albumin at 30-50 g/L, use 5% sol initially, then 25% sol after 24 hr

---

italics = common side effects   ***bold italic*** = life threatening reactions

Shock
• *Adult:* IV 500 ml of 5% sol q30 min, as needed
• *Child:* ¼-½ adult dose in non-emergencies

Hypoproteinemia
• *Adult:* IV 1000-2000 ml of 5% sol qd, not to exceed 5-10 ml/min or 25-100 g of 25% sol qd, not to exceed 3 ml/min, titrated to patient response

Hyperbilirubinemia/erythoblastosis fetalis
• *Infant:* IV 1 g of 25% sol/kg before transfusion

Available forms include: Inj IV 50, 250 mg/ml

Side effects/adverse reactions:
GI: Nausea, vomiting, increased salivation
INTEG: Rash, urticaria
CNS: Fever, chills, flushing, headache
RESP: Altered respirations, pulmonary edema
CV: Fluid overload, hypotension, erratic pulse, tachycardia

Contraindications: Hypersensitivity, congestive heart failure, severe anemia

Precautions: Decreased salt intake, decreased cardiac reserve, lack of albumin deficiency, hepatic disease, renal disease, pregnancy (C)

Pharmacokinetics: In hyponutrition states metabolized as protein/energy source.

NURSING CONSIDERATIONS
Assess:
• Blood studies Hct, Hgb; if serum protein declines, dyspnea, hypoxemia can result
• Decreased B/P, erratic pulse, respiration
• I&O ratio: urinary output may decrease

• CVP, pulmonary wedge pressure will increase if overload occurs
Administer:
• IV slowly, to prevent fluid overload; dilute with NS for injection or D₅W; may be given undiluted; use infusion pump
• Within 4 hr of opening
Perform/provide:
• Adequate hydration before, during administration
• Check type of albumin, some stored at room temperature, some need to be refrigerated
Evaluate:
• Therapeutic response: increased B/P, decreased edema, increased serum albumin
• Allergy: fever, rash, itching, chills, flushing, urticaria, nausea, vomiting, hypotension, requires discontinuation of infusion, use of new lot if therapy reinstituted
• CVP reading: distended neck veins indicate circulatory overload; shortness of breath, anxiety, insomnia, expiratory rales, frothy blood-tinged cough, cyanosis indicate pulmonary overload
Lab test interferences:
False increase: Alk phosphatase

---

albuterol

(al-byoo'ter-ole)
Proventil, Salbutamol,* Ventolin
Func. class.: Adrenergic β-2 agonist

Action: Causes bronchodilation by action on β₂ receptors by increasing levels of cAMP, which relaxes smooth muscle with very little effect on heart rate
Uses: Prevention of exercise-induced asthma, bronchospasm
Dosage and routes:
Asthma

---

* Available in Canada only

• *Adult:* INH 2 puffs 15 min before exercising
Bronchospasm
• *Adult:* INH 1-2 puffs q4-6h PO 2-4 mg tid-qid, not to exceed 8 mg
Available forms include: Aerosol 90 µg/actuation; tabs 2, 4 mg; syr 2 mg/5 ml

Side effects/adverse reactions:
CNS: Tremors, anxiety, insomnia, headache, dizziness, stimulation, restlessness, hallucinations, flushing, irritability
EENT: Dry nose, irritation of nose and throat
CV: Palpitations, tachycardia, hypertension, angina, hypotension, dysrhythmias
GI: Heartburn, nausea, vomiting
MS: Muscle cramps
RESP: **Bronchospasm**
GU: Difficulty in urination
Contraindications: Hypersensitivity to sympathomimetics, tachydysrhythmias, severe cardiac disease
Precautions: Lactation, pregnancy (C), cardiac disorders, hyperthyroidism, diabetes mellitus, hypertension, prostatic hypertrophy, narrow angle glaucoma, seizures
Pharmacokinetics:
PO: Onset ½ hr, peak 2½ hr, duration 4-6 hr, half-life 2½ hr
INH: Onset 5-15 min, peak ½-2 hr, duration 3-6 hr, half-life 4 hr
Metabolized in the liver, excreted in urine, crosses placenta, breast milk, blood-brain barrier
Interactions/incompatibilities:
• Increased action of: aerosol bronchodilators
• Increased action of albuterol: tricyclic antidepressants, MAOIs
• May inhibit action of albuterol: other β-blockers
NURSING CONSIDERATIONS
Assess:
• Respiratory function: vital capacity, forced expiratory volume, ABGs, lung sounds, heart rate and rhythm
Administer:
• After shaking, exhale, place mouthpiece in mouth, inhale slowly, hold breath, remove, exhale slowly
• Gum, sips of water for dry mouth
• PO with meals to decrease gastric irritation
Perform/provide:
• Storage in light-resistant container, do not expose to temperatures over 86° F
Evaluate:
• Therapeutic response: absence of dyspnea, wheezing after 1 hr
Teach patient/family:
• Not to use OTC medications, extra stimulation may occur
• Use of inhaler, review package insert with patient
• To avoid getting aerosol in eyes
• To wash inhaler in warm water qd and dry
• To avoid smoking, smoke-filled rooms, persons with respiratory infections
Treatment of overdose: Administer a β₂-adrenergic blocker

---

alfentanil HCl

(al-fen′ta-nil)
Alfenta
Func. class.: Narcotic analgesic
Chem. class.: Opiate, synthetic

Action: Inhibits ascending pain pathways in limbic system, thalamus, midbrain, hypothalamus
Uses: In combination with other drugs in general anesthesia, as a primary anesthetic in general surgery
Dosage and routes:
Combination

---

italics = common side effects   ***bold italic*** = life threatening reactions

- *Adult:* IV 8-50 μg/kg, may increase by 3-15 μg/kg

Anesthetic induction
- *Adult:* IV 130-245 μg/kg, then 0.5-1.5 μg/kg/min

Available forms include: Inj 500 μg/ml

Side effects/adverse reactions:

CNS: Drowsiness, dizziness, confusion, headache, sedation, euphoria, delirium, agitation, anxiety
GI: Nausea, vomiting, anorexia, constipation, cramps, dry mouth
GU: Urinary retention, dysuria
INTEG: Rash, urticaria, bruising, flushing, diaphoresis, pruritus
EENT: Tinnitus, blurred vision, miosis, diplopia
CV: Palpitation, bradycardia, change in B/P, facial flushing, syncope, asystole
RESP: Respiratory depression, apnea
MS: Rigidity

Contraindications: Child <12 yr, hypersensitivity

Precautions: Pregnancy (C), lactation, increased intracranial pressure, acute MI, severe heart disease, renal disease, hepatic disease, asthma, respiratory conditions, convulsive disorders

Pharmacokinetics: Half-life 1-2 hr, 90% bound to plasma proteins, duration 30 min

Interactions/incompatibilities:

- Respiratory depression, hypotension, profound sedation: alcohol, sedative hypnotics, or other CNS depressants, antihistamines, phenothiazines
- Compatible IV solution: LR, 0.9% NaCl, D_5W, D_5/0.9% NaCl

NURSING CONSIDERATIONS

Assess:
- I&O ratio, check for decreasing output; may indicate urinary retention

- CNS changes: dizziness, drowsiness, hallucinations, euphoria, LOC, pupil reaction

Administer:
- Direct IV over 1½-3 min
- Cont. IV by diluting 20 ml of drug in 230 ml of diluent (40 μg/ml)

Perform/provide:
- Storage in light-resistant area at room temperature

Evaluate:
- Therapeutic response: maintenance of anesthesia
- Allergic reactions: rash, urticaria
- Respiratory dysfunction: respiratory depression, character, rate, rhythm: notify physician if respirations are <12/min

Lab test interferences:
Increase: Amylase

Treatment of overdose: Narcan 0.2-0.8 IV, O_2, IV fluids, vasopressors

---

allopurinol

(al-oh-pure'i-nole)
Apoallopurinol,* Novapurol,* Purimol,* Lopurin, Zyloprim, Zurinol
Func. class.: Antigout drug
Chem. class.: Enzyme inhibitor

Action: Inhibits the enzyme xanthine oxidase, reducing uric acid synthesis

Uses: Chronic gout, hyperuricemia associated with malignancies, recurrent calcium oxalate calculi

Dosage and routes:

Gout/hyperuricemia
- *Adult:* PO 200-600 mg qd depending on severity
- *Child 6-10 yr:* 300 mg qd
- *Child <6 yr:* 150 mg qd

Impaired renal function
- *Adult:* PO 200 mg qd when CrCl is 20 to 10 ml/min

---

*Available in Canada only

Recurrent calculi
• *Adult:* PO 200-300 mg qd
Uric acid nephropathy prevention
• *Adult:* PO 600-800 mg qd × 2-3 days
Available forms include: Tabs 100, 300 mg
Side effects/adverse reactions:
*HEMA: **Agranulocytosis, thrombocytopenia, aplastic anemia, pancytopenia, leukopenia, bone marrow depression***
CNS: Headache, drowsiness, neuritis, paresthesia
GI: Nausea, vomiting, anorexia, malaise, metallic taste, cramps, peptic ulcer, diarrhea, stomatitis
MISC: Myopathy, arthralgia, hepatomegaly, hyperbilirubinemia, cholestatic jaundice, renal failure
EENT: Retinopathy, cataracts, epistaxis
INTEG: Fever, chills, dermatitis, pruritus, purpura, erythema, ecchymosis
Contraindications: Hypersensitivity
Precautions: Pregnancy (B), lactation, renal disease, hepatic disease
Pharmacokinetics:
PO: Peak 2-4 hr; excreted in feces, urine, half-life 2-3 hr, terminal half-life 18-30 hr
Interactions/incompatibilities:
• Increased action of: oral anticoagulants, chlorpropamide, cyclophosphamide, hydantoin, theophylline, vidarabine, thiazide diuretics
• Decreased effects of: probenecid
• Rash: ampicillin, amoxicillin
NURSING CONSIDERATIONS
Assess:
• Uric acid levels q2 wk; uric acid levels should be 6 mg/dl
• CBC, AST, BUN, creatinine before starting treatment, monthly

• I&O ratio; increase fluids to prevent stone formation
Administer:
• With meals, to prevent GI symptoms
• A few days before antineoplastic therapy
Evaluate:
• Therapeutic response: decreased pain in joints, decreased stone formation in kidney
• Nutritional status: discourage organ meat, sardines, salmon, legumes, gravies (high purine foods)
Teach patient/family:
• To increase fluid intake to 3-4 L/day
• To report skin rash, stomatitis, malaise, fever, aching; drug should be discontinued
• To avoid hazardous activities if drowsiness or dizziness occurs
• To avoid alcohol, caffeine; will increase uric acid levels
• Avoid large doses of vitamin C; kidney stone formation may occur
Lab test interferences:
Increase: AST/ALT, alk phosphatase
Decrease: Hct/Hgb, leukocytes, serum glucose

---

alprazolam
(al-pray′zoe-lam)
Xanax
Func. class.: Antianxiety
Chem. class.: Benzodiazepine

Controlled Substance Schedule IV
Action: Depresses subcortical levels of CNS, including limbic system, reticular formation
Uses: Anxiety, panic disorders, anxiety with depressive symptoms
Dosage and routes:
• *Adult:* PO 0.25-0.5 mg tid, not

---

italics = common side effects   ***bold italic*** = life threatening reactions

to exceed 4 mg in divided doses/day
• *Geriatric:* PO 0.25 mg bid-tid
Available forms include: Tab 0.25, 0.5, 1 mg
Side effects/adverse reactions:
CNS: Dizziness, drowsiness, confusion, headache, anxiety, tremors, stimulation, fatigue, depression, insomnia, hallucinations
GI: Constipation, dry mouth, nausea, vomiting, anorexia, diarrhea
INTEG: Rash, dermatitis, itching
*CV: Orthostatic hypotension, **ECG changes, tachycardia,*** hypotension
EENT: Blurred vision, tinnitus, mydriasis
Contraindications: Hypersensitivity to benzodiazepines, narrow-angle glaucoma, psychosis, pregnancy (D), child <18 yr
Precautions: Elderly, debilitated, hepatic disease, renal disease
Pharmacokinetics:
PO: Onset 30 min, peak 1-2 hr, duration 4-6 hr, therapeutic response 2-3 days, metabolized by liver, excreted by kidneys, crosses placenta, breast milk, half-life 12-15 hr
Interactions/incompatibilities:
• Increased CNS depression: anticonvulsants, alcohol, antihistamines, sedative/hypnotics
• Decreased action of alprazolam: disulfiram, cimetidine
• Decreased action of: levodopa
NURSING CONSIDERATIONS
Assess:
• B/P (lying, standing), pulse; if systolic B/P drops 20 mm Hg, hold drug, notify physician
• Blood studies: CBC during long-term therapy; blood dyscrasias have occurred rarely
• Hepatic studies: AST, ALT, bilirubin, creatinine, LDH, alk phosphatase
• I&O; may indicate renal dysfunction
• For indications of increasing tolerance and abuse
Administer:
• With food or milk for GI symptoms
• Crushed if patient is unable to swallow medication whole
• Sugarless gum, hard candy, frequent sips of water for dry mouth
Perform/provide:
• Assistance with ambulation during beginning therapy; drowsiness/dizziness occurs
• Safety measures, including siderails
• Check to see PO medication has been swallowed
Evaluate:
• Therapeutic response: decreased anxiety, restlessness, sleeplessness
• Mental status: mood, sensorium, affect, sleeping pattern, drowsiness, dizziness
• Physical dependency, withdrawal symptoms: anxiety, panic attacks, agitation, convulsions, headache, nausea, vomiting, muscle pain, weakness
• Suicidal tendencies
Teach patient/family:
• That drug may be taken with food
• Not to be used for everyday stress or longer than 3 mo, unless directed by physician; not to take more than prescribed amount, may be habit forming
• Avoid OTC preparations unless approved by physician
• To avoid driving, activities that require alertness, since drowsiness may occur
• To avoid alcohol ingestion or other psychotropic medications, unless prescribed by physician

• Not to discontinue medication abruptly after long-term use
• To rise slowly or fainting may occur
• That drowsiness might worsen at beginning of treatment

Lab test interferences:
Increase: AST/ALT, serum bilirubin
False increase: 17-OHCS
Decrease: RAIU

Treatment of overdose: Lavage, VS, supportive care

---

alprostadil

(al-pros′ta-dil)
Prostin VR Pediatric
Func. class.: Hormone
Chem. class.: Prostaglandin

Action: Relaxes smooth muscles of ductus arteriosus; results in increased O_2 content throughout body
Uses: Patent ductus arteriosus (temporary treatment)
Dosage and routes:
• *Infants:* IV INF 0.1 μg/kg/min, until desired response, then reduce to lowest effective amount, not to exceed 0.4 μg/kg/min
Available forms include: Inj IV 500 μg/ml
Side effects/adverse reactions:
MISC: Sepsis, hypokalemia, peritonitis, hypoglycemia, hyperkalemia
RESP: Apnea
HEMA: DIC (disseminated intravascular coagulation), *thrombocytopenia*
CNS: Fever, *convulsions,* lethargy, cerebral bleeding, hypothermia, stiffness
GI: Diarrhea, regurgitation
GU: Oliguria, hematuria, *anuria*
CV: Bradycardia, tachycardia, hypotension, *CHF, ventricular fibrillation, shock,* flushing, *cardiac arrest*

Contraindications: *Hypersensitivity,* respiratory distress syndrome (RDS)
Precautions: Bleeding disorders
Pharmacokinetics:
PO: 15-30 min, metabolized in lungs, up to 80%, excreted in urine (metabolites)

NURSING CONSIDERATIONS
Assess:
• ABGs, arterial pH, arterial pressure, continuous ECG; if arterial pressure decreases, reduce or stop drug
Administer:
• Only with emergency equipment available by trained clinicians
• After diluting with NS or D_5W injection to a concentration of 500 mcg/ml, dilute further with 0.9% NaCl, D_5W; 500 μg of drug/250 mg of dilute = 2 μg/ml
Perform/provide:
• Arterial pressure measurement during infusion
• Refrigeration for drug; discard all mixed unused portion
Evaluate:
• Apnea and bradycardia; if these occur, discontinue drug
• Therapeutic response: increased PO_2 (cyanotic heart disease)
• Increased pH, B/P, output, decreased ratio of PA to AP (restricted systemic blood flow)
Teach patient/family:
• Regarding diagnosis, prognosis, treatment

---

alteplase

(al-teep′lase)
Activase
Func. class.: Antithrombotic
Chem. class.: Tissue plasminogen activator (TPA)

Action: Produces fibrin conversion

italics = common side effects   ***bold italic*** = life threatening reactions

of plasminogen to plasmin; able to bind to fibrin, convert plasminogen in thrombus to plasmin, which leads to local fibrinolysis, limited systemic proteolysis

Uses: Lysis of obstructing thrombi-associated with acute MI

Dosage and routes:
• *Adult:* IV a total of 100 mg; 6-10 mg given IV Bol over 1-2 min, 60 mg given over first hour, 20 mg given over second hour, 20 mg given over third hour; or 1.25 mg/kg given over 3 hr for smaller patients

Available forms include: Powder for inj 20 mg (11.6 million IU)/vial, 50 mg (29 million IU)/vial

Side effects/adverse reactions:
SYST: **GI, GU, intracranial, retroperitoneal bleeding,** *surface bleeding*
CV: **Sinus bradycardia, ventricular tachycardia, accelerated idioventricular rhythm**
INTEG: Urticaria, rash

Contraindications: Hypersensitivity, active internal bleeding, recent CVA, severe uncontrolled hypertension, intracranial/intraspinal surgery/trauma, aneurysm

Precautions: Pregnancy (C), lactation, children

Pharmacokinetics: Cleared by liver, 80% cleared within 10 min of drug termination

Interactions/incompatibilities:
• Increased bleeding: heparin, acetylsalicylic acid, dipyridamole
• Do not add other drugs to IV solution

NURSING CONSIDERATIONS
Assess:
• VS, B/P, pulse, respirations, neurologic signs, temperature at least q4h; temperature >104° F is indicator of internal bleeding; monitor rhythm closely; ventricular

dysrhythmias may occur with hyperfusion
• For bleeding during first hr of treatment: hematuria, hematemesis, bleeding from mucous membranes, epistaxis, ecchymosis

Administer:
• After reconstituting with provided diluent, add appropriate amount of sterile water for injection (no preservatives) to 1 mg/ml, mix by slow inversion or dilute with NaCl, D_5W to a concentration of 0.5 mg/ml; flush line with NaCl after administration
• Heparin therapy after thrombolytic therapy is discontinued, TT, ACT, or APTT less than 2 X control (about 3-4 hr)
• Reconstituted IV solution within 8 hr
• Within 6 hr of coronary occlusion for best results

Perform/provide:
• Avoidance of invasive procedures, injection, rectal temperature
• Pressure for 30 sec to minor bleeding sites; inform physician if this does not attain hemostasis, apply pressure dressing
• Storage of powder at room temperature or refrigerate, protect from excessive light

Evaluate:
• Allergy: fever, rash, itching, chills; mild reaction may be treated with antihistamines
• Blood studies (Hct, platelets, PTT, PT, TT, APTT) before starting therapy; PT or APTT must be less than 2 X control before starting therapy TT or PT q3-4h during treatment

Lab test interferences:
Increase: PT, APTT, TT

---

aluminum acetate

Acid Mantle, Burow's Solution, Buro-Sol, modified Burow's solution, Bluboro, Domeboro

Func. class.: Astringent
Chem. class.: Aluminum product

Action: Maintains skin acidity, which is protective to skin surface
Uses: Skin irritation, inflammation, athlete's foot, insect bites, poison ivy, eczema, acne, rash, bruises, pruritus (anal)
Dosage and routes:
• *Adult and child:* TOP apply for 15-30 min, q4-8h (1:10-40); Gargle use 1:10 sol prn
Available forms include: Solution, cream (Canada only)
Side effects/adverse reactions:
INTEG: Irritation, increasing inflammation
Contraindications: Tight, occlusive dressing
Interactions/incompatibilities:
• Inhibits action of: topical collagenase ointment
• Decreased action of aluminum acetate: soap
NURSING CONSIDERATIONS
Administer:
• 1 pk/1 pt water (1:10-40 water)
Perform/provide:
• Wet dressings using only loose fitting dressing
Evaluate:
• Area of body to receive topical application, irritation, rash, breaks, dryness
Teach patient/family:
• To discontinue use if irritation occurs
• To avoid using near eye area
• To retain otic preparation for 2-3 min

aluminum carbonate gel

Basaljel

Func. class.: Antacid
Chem. class.: Aluminum product

Action: Neutralizes gastric acidity, binds phosphates in GI tract, these phosphates are excreted
Uses: Antacid, phosphate stones (prevention), phosphate binder in chronic renal failure
Dosage and routes:
Urinary phosphate stones
• *Adult:* SUSP 5-10 ml as needed; EXTRA STREN SUSP 2.5-5 ml as needed; PO 1-2 as needed
Antacid
• *Adult:* SUSP 15-45 ml in water or juice 1 hr pc, hs; EXTRA STREN SUSP 5-15 ml in water or juice 1 hr pc, hs; PO 2-6 1 hr pc, hs
Available forms include: Caps 500, 608 mg; tabs 500, 608 mg; susp 400mg/5 ml; extra stren susp 1000 mg/ml
Side effects/adverse reactions:
GI: Constipation, anorexia, obstruction, fecal impaction
META: Hypophosphatemia, hypercalciuria
Contraindications: Hypersensitivity to this drug or aluminum products, appendicitis
Precautions: Elderly, fluid restriction, decreased GI motility, GI obstruction, dehydration, renal disease, sodium-restricted diets, pregnancy (C)
Pharmacokinetics:
PO: Excreted in feces
Interactions/incompatibilities:
• Decreased effectiveness of: tetracyclines, ketoconazole
• Decreased absorption of: anticholinergics, chlordiazepoxide, cimetidine, corticosteroids, iron salts,

---

italics = common side effects   ***bold italic*** = life threatening reactions

phenothiazines, phenytoin, digitalis
• Enteric-coated drugs: separate by 1 hr

NURSING CONSIDERATIONS
Administer:
• Laxatives, or stool softeners if constipation occurs
• After shaking

Perform/provide:
• I&O, strain urine if using for urinary calculi

Evaluate:
• Therapeutic response: absence of pain, decreased acidity
• Hypophosphatemia: anorexia, weakness, fatigue, bone pain, hyporeflexia
• Constipation, if product is being used as an antacid, may need to switch to magnesium antacid
• Phosphate levels, urinary pH, Ca^{++}, electrolytes

Teach patient/family:
• Increase fluids to 2000 ml/day unless contraindicated
• Avoid phosphate foods (most dairy products, eggs, fruits, carbonated beverages) during drug therapy
• Add cheese, corn, pasta, plums, prunes, lentils after drug is discontinued
• Limit sodium intake

---

aluminum hydroxide

Alternagel, Alu-Cap, Al-U-Creme, Aluminett, Amphojel, Basaljel,* Dialume, Hydroxal, Nephrox, No-Co-Gel, Nutrajel
Func. class.: Antacid
Chem. class.: Aluminum product

Action: Neutralizes gastric acidity, binds phosphates in GI tract, these phosphates are excreted

Uses: Antacid, hyperphosphatemia in chronic renal failure

Dosage and routes:
• *Adult:* SUSP 5-10 ml 1 hr pc, hs; PO 600 mg 1 hr pc, hs, chewed with milk or water

Hyperphosphatemia in renal failure
• *Adult:* SUSP 500 mg-2 g bid-qid

Available forms include: Caps 475, 500 mg; tabs 300, 500 mg; chewable tabs 600 mg; susp (4%) 600 mg/5 ml; liq 320 mg/5ml, 600 mg/5 ml

Side effects/adverse reactions:
GI: Constipation, anorexia, *obstruction,* fecal impaction
META: Hypophosphatemia, hypercalciuria

Contraindications: Hypersensitivity to this drug or aluminum products

Precautions: Elderly, fluid restriction, decreased GI motility, GI obstruction, dehydration, renal disease, sodium-restricted diets, pregnancy (C)

Pharmacokinetics:
PO: Onset 20-40 min, excreted in feces

Interactions/incompatibilities:
• Decreased effectiveness of: tetracyclines, anticholinergics, phenothiazines, isoniazid, quinidine, phenytoin, digitalis, iron salts, warfarin, ketoconazole; separate by at least 2 hr

NURSING CONSIDERATIONS
Assess:
• Phosphate levels since drug is bound in GI system

Administer:
• Laxatives, or stool softeners if constipation occurs
• After shaking liquid
• By nasogastric tube if patient unable to swallow

*Available in Canada only

- With small amount of water or milk

Evaluate:
- Therapeutic response: absence of pain, decreased acidity
- Hypophosphatemia: anorexia, weakness, fatigue, bone pain, hyporeflexia
- Constipation, increase bulk in diet if needed
- Phosphate levels, urinary pH, Ca^{++}, electrolytes

Teach patient/family:
- Increase fluids to 2000 ml/day unless contraindicated
- Avoid phosphate foods (most dairy products, eggs, fruits, carbonated beverages) during drug therapy
- Add cheese, corn, pasta, plums, prunes, lentils after drug is discontinued
- Stools may appear white or speckled
- To check with MD after 2 wks of self-prescribed antacid use

---

aluminum phosphate

Phosphaljel

Func. class.: Antacid
Chem. class.: Aluminum products

Action: Neutralizes gastric acidity, binds phosphates in GI tract, these phosphates are excreted
Uses: Antacid
Dosage and routes:
- *Adult:* SUSP 15-30 ml 1 hr pc, hs
- *Adult:* Intragastric dilute 1:3 or 1:4

Available forms include: Susp 233 mg/5 ml
Side effects/adverse reactions:
GI: Constipation, anorexia, ***obstruction,*** fecal impaction
META: Hyperphosphatemia

Contraindications: Hypersensitivity to this drug or aluminum products
Precautions: Elderly, fluid restriction, decreased GI motility, GI obstruction, dehydration, renal disease, sodium-restricted diets, pregnancy (C)
Pharmacokinetics:
PO: Onset 20-40 min, excreted in feces
Interactions/incompatibilities:
- Decreased effectiveness of: tetracyclines, ketoconazole, isoniazid, phenothiazines, iron salts, digitalis

NURSING CONSIDERATIONS
Administer:
- Laxatives, or stool softeners if constipation occurs
- After shaking solution
Evaluate:
- Therapeutic response: absence of pain, decreased acidity
- Constipation, increase bulk in diet if needed or alternate with magnesium antacids
- Phosphate levels, urinary pH, Ca^{++}, electrolytes
Teach patient/family:
- Increase fluids to 2000 ml unless contraindicated
- Not to switch antacids unless directed by physician
- To use PO meds 1-2 hrs after antacid
- That antacid may cause premature dissolution of enteric-coated tablets

---

amantadine HCl

(a-man'ta-deen)
Symmetrel

Func. class.: Antiviral, antiparkinsonian agent
Chem. class.: Tricyclic amine

Action: Prevents uncoating of nu-

---

italics = common side effects   ***bold italic*** = life threatening reactions

cleic acid in viral cell, preventing penetration of virus to host; causes release of dopamine from neurons
Uses: Prophylaxis or treatment of influenza type A, extrapyramidal reactions, parkinsonism, respiratory tract infections
Dosage and routes:
Influenza type A
• *Adult and child >9 yr:* PO 200 mg/day in single dose or divided bid
• *Child 1-9 yr:* PO 4.4-8.8 mg/kg/day divided bid-tid, not to exceed 200 mg/day
Extrapyramidal reaction/parkinsonism
• *Adult:* PO 100 mg bid, up to 400 mg/day in EPS; give for 1 wk then 100 mg as needed in parkinsonism
Available forms include: Caps 100 mg; syr 50 mg/5 ml
Side effects/adverse reactions:
CNS: Headache, dizziness, drowsiness, fatigue, anxiety, psychosis, depression, hallucinations, tremors, *convulsions*
CV: Orthostatic hypotension, *CHF*
INTEG: Photosensitivity, dermatitis
EENT: Blurred vision
HEMA: Leukopenia
GI: Nausea, vomiting, constipation, dry mouth
GU: Frequency, retention
Contraindications: Hypersensitivity, lactation, child <1 yr, pregnancy (C)
Precautions: Epilepsy, CHF, orthostatic hypotension, psychiatric disorders, hepatic disease, renal disease
Pharmacokinetics:
PO: Onset 48 hr, half-life 24 hr, not metabolized, excreted in urine (90%) unchanged, crosses placenta, excreted in breast milk
Interactions/incompatibilities:
• Increased anticholinergic re-

sponse: atropine, other anticholinergics
• Increased CNS stimulation: CNS stimulants
NURSING CONSIDERATIONS
Assess:
• I&O ratio; report frequency, hesitancy
• CHF, confusion, mottling of skin
Administer:
• Before exposure to influenza; continue for 10 days after contact
• At least 4 hr before hs to prevent insomnia
• After meals for better absorption, to decrease GI symptoms
• In divided doses to prevent CNS disturbances: headache, dizziness, fatigue, drowsiness
Perform/provide:
• Storage in tight, dry container
Evaluate:
• Therapeutic response: absence of temperature, malaise, cough, dyspnea in infection; tremors, shuffling, gait in Parkinson's disease
• Bowel pattern before, during treatment
• Skin eruptions, photosensitivity after administration of drug
• Respiratory status: rate, character, wheezing, tightness in chest
• Allergies before initiation of treatment, reaction of each medication; place allergies on chart, Kardex in bright red letters; notify all people giving drugs
• Signs of infection
Teach patient/family:
• Change body position slowly to prevent orthostatic hypotension
• Aspects of drug therapy: need to report dyspnea, weight gain, dizziness, poor concentration, dysuria, behavioral changes
• To avoid hazardous activities if dizziness occurs
• To take drug exactly as pre-

scribed; parkinsonian crisis may occur if drug is discontinued abruptly
• To avoid alcohol

Treatment of overdose: Withdraw drug, maintain airway, administer epinephrine, aminophylline, O_2, IV corticosteroids, physostigmine

---

ambenonium chloride

(am-be-noe′nee-um)
Mytelase caplets
Func. class.: Cholinergics
Chem. class.: Synthetic quaternary ammonium compound

Action: Inhibits destruction of acetylcholine, which increases concentration at sites where acetylcholine is released; this facilitates transmission of impulses across myoneural junction

Uses: Myasthenia gravis when other drugs cannot be used

Dosage and routes:
• *Adult:* PO 5 mg q3-4h, then gradually increased q1-2 days, usually 5-40 mg is sufficient

Available forms include: Tabs 10 mg

Side effects/adverse reactions:
INTEG: Rash, urticaria
CNS: Dizziness, headache, sweating, confusion, weakness, *convulsions,* incoordination, *paralysis*
GI: Nausea, diarrhea, vomiting, cramps, increased salivary, gastric secretions, dysphagia
CV: Tachycardia, dysrhythmias, bradycardia, hypotension, AV block, ECG changes, cardiac arrest
GU: Frequency, incontinence
*RESP: **Respiratory depression, bronchospasm, constriction, laryngospasm, respiratory arrest***
EENT: Miosis, blurred vision, lacrimation

Contraindications: Obstruction of intestine, renal system, hypersensitivity
Precautions: Seizure disorders, bronchial asthma, coronary occlusion, hyperthyroidism, dysrhythmias, peptic ulcer, megacolon, poor GI motility, pregnancy (C), bradycardia, hypotension, lactation, children

Pharmacokinetics:
PO: Onset 2-30 min, duration 3-8 hr

Interactions/incompatibilities:
• Decreased action of ambenonium: aminoglycosides, anesthetics, antidysrhythmics, mecamylamine, polymyxin, quinidine, magnesium, corticosteroids
• Increased action of: neuromuscular blockers

NURSING CONSIDERATIONS
Assess:
• VS, respiration q2h
• I&O ratio; check for urinary retention or incontinence
Administer:
• Only with atropine sulfate available for cholinergic crisis
• Only after all other cholinergics have been discontinued
• Increased doses if tolerance occurs
• With food or milk to decrease GI symptoms; may decrease action of this drug
• Larger doses after exercise or fatigue
• On empty stomach for better absorption
Perform/provide:
• Storage at room temperature
Evaluate:
• Therapeutic response: increased muscle strength, improved gait, absence of labored breathing (if severe)
• Bradycardia, hypotension, bron-

---

italics = common side effects **bold italic** = life threatening reactions

chospasm, headache, dizziness, convulsions, respiratory depression; drug should be discontinued if toxicity occurs
• Muscle strength: hand grasp
Teach patient/family:
• To take drug exactly as prescribed
• That drug is not a cure, it only relieves symptoms
• To wear Medic Alert ID specifying myasthenia gravis, drugs taken
Treatment of overdose: Discontinue med, respiratory support, atropine 1-4 mg

---

amcinonide

(am-sin'oh-nide)
Cyclocort
Func. class.: Topical corticosteroid
Chem. class.: Synthetic fluorinated agent, group II potency

Action: Possesses antipruritic, antiinflammatory actions
Uses: Psoriasis, eczema, contact dermatitis, pruritus
Dosage and routes:
• *Adult and child:* Apply to affected area bid-tid, rub completely into skin
Available forms include: Cream 0.1%; oint 0.1%
Side effects/adverse reactions:
INTEG: Burning, dryness, itching, irritation, acne, folliculitis, hypertrichosis, perioral dermatitis, hypopigmentation, atrophy, striae, miliaria, allergic contact dermatitis, secondary infection
Contraindications: Hypersensitivity to corticosteroids, fungal infections
Precautions: Pregnancy (C), lactation, viral infections, bacterial infections

NURSING CONSIDERATIONS
Assess:
• Temperature, worsening of rash; if fever develops drug should be discontinued
Administer:
• Only to affected areas; do not get in eyes
• Medication, then cover with occlusive dressing (only if prescribed), seal to normal skin, change q12h, systemic absorption may occur
• Only to dermatoses; do not use on weeping, denuded, or infected area
Perform/provide:
• Cleansing before application of drug
• Treatment for a few days after area has cleared
• Storage at room temperature
Evaluate:
• Therapeutic response: absence of severe itching, patches on skin, flaking
• For systemic absorption: increased temperature, inflammation, irritation
Teach patient/family:
• To avoid sunlight on affected area; burns may occur
• If local irritation or fever develops, discontinue drug, notify physician

---

amdinocillin

(am-din-oh-sill'in)
Coactin
Func. class.: Broad spectrum antibiotic
Chem. class.: Penicillin-Misc. B-Lactam

Action: Interferes with cell wall replication of susceptible organisms; the cell wall, rendered os-

---

motically unstable, swells, bursts from increased osmotic pressure
Uses: Urinary tract infections caused by *E. coli*
Dosage and routes:
• *Adult:* IM/IV 10 mg/kg q4-6h
Available forms include: Powder for inj IM, IV 500 mg, 1 g
Side effects/adverse reactions:
*HEMA: **Eosinophilia, thrombocytosis, anemia, neutropenia, leukopenia***
GI: Nausea, vomiting, diarrhea
CNS: Lethargy, dizziness
Contraindications: Hypersensitivity to penicillins; neonates
Precautions: Hypersensitivity to cephalosporins, allergies, renal disease, hepatic disease, pregnancy (B)
Pharmacokinetics:
IV: Peak 24-45 min
IM: Peak 2-3 hr
Interactions/incompatibilities:
• Decreased antimicrobial effectiveness of amdinocillin: tetracyclines, erythromycins
• Increased penicillin concentrations when used with: aspirin, probenecid
• Incompatible with all other drugs in solution

NURSING CONSIDERATIONS
Assess:
• I&O ratio; report hematuria, oliguria since penicillin in high doses is nephrotoxic, monitor BUN, creatinine
• Any patient with a compromised renal system since drug is excreted slowly in poor renal system function; toxicity may occur rapidly
• Liver studies: AST, ALT
• Blood studies: WBC, RBC, Hct/Hgb, bleeding time
• Renal studies: urinalysis, protein, blood
• Culture, sensitivity before drug

therapy; drug may be taken as soon as culture is taken
Administer:
• IM after reconstituting with 2.2 ml of sterile H₂O, 0.9% NaCl/500 mg of drug (200 mg/ml), shaken, given deeply into large muscle
• IV after reconstituting with 4.8 ml of sterile H₂O/500 mg of drug (100 mg/ml) shake; must be further diluted in 50 ml of compatible solutions and given over 15 min; check site for inflammation, extravasation
• Drug after C&S completed
Perform/provide:
• Adrenaline, suction, tracheostomy set, endotracheal intubation equipment on the unit
• Adequate intake of fluids (2000 ml) during diarrhea episodes
• Scratch test to assess allergy after securing order from physician; usually done when penicillin is only drug of choice
• Storage of reconstituted solution at room temperature for 16 hr or 24 hr refrigerated
Evaluate:
• Therapeutic effectiveness: absence of temperature, draining wounds, C&S negative
• Bowel pattern before, during treatment
• Skin eruptions after administration of penicillin to 1 wk after discontinuing drug
• Respiratory status: rate, character, wheezing, tightness in chest
• Allergies before initiation of treatment, reaction of each medication; place allergies on chart, Kardex in bright red
Teach patient/family:
• Aspects of drug therapy: need to complete entire course of medication to ensure organism death (7-14 days); culture may be taken after

italics = common side effects   ***bold italic*** = life threatening reactions

completed course of medication
• To report sore throat, fever, fatigue (could indicate a superimposed infection)
• To wear or carry a Medic Alert ID if allergic to penicillins
• To notify nurse of diarrhea

Lab test interferences:
False positive: Urine glucose, urine protein
Decrease: Uric acid

Treatment of overdose: Withdraw drug, maintain airway, administer epinephrine, aminophylline, O_2, IV corticosteroids for anaphylaxis

---

amikacin sulfate

(am-i-kay′sin)
Amikin
Func. class.: Antibiotic
Chem. class.: Aminoglycoside

Action: Interferes with protein synthesis in bacterial cell by binding to ribosomal subunit, which causes misreading of genetic code; inaccurate peptide sequence forms in protein chain, causing bacterial death

Uses: Severe systemic infections of CNS, respiratory, GI, urinary tract, bone, skin, soft tissues caused by *P. aeruginosa, E. coli, Enterobacter, Acinetobacter, Providencia, Citrobacter, Staphylococcus, Serratia, Proteus*

Dosage and routes:
Severe systemic infections
• *Adult and child:* IV INF 15 mg/kg/day in 2-3 divided doses q8-12h in 100-200 ml D_5W over 30-60 min, not to exceed 1.5 g; decreased doses are needed in poor renal function as determined by blood levels, renal function studies; IM 15 mg/kg/day in divided doses q8-12h
• *Neonates:* IV INF 10 mg/kg initially, then 7.5 mg/kg q12h in D_5W over 1-2 hr
Severe urinary tract infections
• *Adults:* IM 250 mg bid
• *Adults with poor renal function:* 7.5 mg/kg initially, then increased as determined by blood levels, renal function studies

Available forms include: Inj IM, IV 50, 250 mg/ml

Side effects/adverse reactions:
*GU: **Oliguria, hematuria, renal damage, azotemia, failure, nephrotoxicity***
CNS: Confusion, depression, numbness, tremors, ***convulsions***, muscle twitching, ***neurotoxicity***
*EENT: **Ototoxicity**,* deafness, visual disturbances
*HEMA: **Agranulocytosis, thrombocytopenia, leukopenia, eosinophilia, anemia***
GI: Nausea, vomiting, anorexia, increased ALT, AST, bilirubin, hepatomegaly, ***hepatic necrosis***, splenomegaly, diarrhea, steatorrhea
CV: Hypotension
INTEG: Rash, burning, urticaria, photosensitivity, dermatitis

Contraindications: Mild to moderate infections, severe renal disease, hypersensitivity to aminoglycosides

Precautions: Neonates, mild renal disease, pregnancy (D), lactation, myasthenia gravis, hearing deficits, Parkinson's disease, elderly

Pharmacokinetics:
IM: Onset rapid, peak 1-2 hr
IV: Onset immediate, peak 1-2 hr
Plasma half-life 2-3 hr; not metabolized, excreted unchanged in urine, crosses placental barrier

Interactions/incompatibilities:
• Increased ototoxicity, neurotoxicity, nephrotoxicity: other aminoglycosides, amphotericin B, poly-

myxin, vancomycin, ethacrynic acid, furosemide, mannitol, methoxyflurane, cisplatin, cephalosporins
• Decreased effects of: parenteral penicillins, digoxin, vitamin B_{12}
• Do not mix in solution or syringe: carbenicillin, ticarcillin, amphotericin B, cephalothin, erythromycin, heparin

NURSING CONSIDERATIONS
Assess:
• Weight before treatment; calculation of dosage is usually done based on ideal body weight, but may be calculated on actual body weight
• I&O ratio, urinalysis daily for proteinuria, cells, casts; report sudden change in urine output
• VS during infusion, watch for hypotension, change in pulse
• IV site for thrombophlebitis including pain, redness, swelling q30 min, change site if needed; apply warm compresses to discontinued site
• Serum peak, drawn at 30-60 min after IV infusion or 60 min after IM injection, trough level drawn just before next dose; blood level should be 2-4 times bacteriostatic level
• Urine pH if drug is used for UTI; urine should be kept alkaline

Administer:
• IV, dilute 500 mg of drug/100-200 ml of compatible solutions and give over ½-1hr; flush after administration with D_5W or 0.9% NaCl
• IM injection in large muscle mass, rotate injection sites
• Drug in evenly spaced doses to maintain blood level
• Bicarbonate to alkalinize urine if ordered for UTI, as drug is most active in alkaline environment

Perform/provide:
• Adequate fluids of 2-3 L/day unless contraindicated to prevent irritation of tubules
• Flush of IV line with NS or D_5W after infusion
• Supervised ambulation, other safety measures with vestibular dysfunction

Evaluate:
• Therapeutic effect: absence of fever, draining wounds, negative C&S after treatment
• Renal impairment by securing urine for CrCl testing, BUN, serum creatinine; lower dosage should be given in renal impairment (CrCl <80 ml/min)
• Deafness by audiometric testing, ringing, roaring in ears, vertigo; assess hearing before, during, after treatment
• Dehydration: high sp gr, decrease in skin turgor, dry mucous membranes, dark urine
• Overgrowth of infection including increased temperature, malaise, redness, pain, swelling, perineal itching, diarrhea, stomatitis, change in cough, sputum
• C&S before starting treatment to identify organism
• Vestibular dysfunction: nausea, vomiting, dizziness, headache; drug should be discontinued if severe
• Injection sites for redness, swelling, abscesses; use warm compresses at site

Teach patient/family:
• To report headache, dizziness, symptoms for overgrowth of infection, renal impairment
• To report loss of hearing, ringing, roaring in ears or feeling of fullness in head

Treatment of overdose: Hemodialysis, monitor serum levels of drug

---

italics = common side effects   ***bold italic*** = life threatening reactions

amiloride HCl

(a-mill'oh-ride)

Midamor

Func. class.: Potassium-sparing diuretic

Chem. class.: Pyrazine

Action: Acts primarily on distal tubule, secondarily by inhibiting reabsorption of sodium, and increasing potassium retention

Uses: Edema in CHF in combination with other diuretics, for hypertension, adjunct with other diuretics to maintain potassium

Dosage and routes:

• *Adult:* PO 5 mg qd, may be increased to 10-20 mg qd if needed

Available forms include: Tab 5 mg

Side effects/adverse reactions:

GU: Polyuria, dysuria, frequency

ELECT: Acidosis, hyponatremia, hyperkalemia, hypochloremia

CNS: Headache, dizziness, fatigue, weakness, headache, paresthesias

GI: Nausea, diarrhea, dry mouth, vomiting, anorexia, cramps, constipation, dry mouth, abdominal pain, jaundice, bleeding, anorexia

EENT: Loss of hearing, tinnitus, blurred vision, nasal congestion, increased intraocular pressure

INTEG: Rash, pruritus, alopecia, urticaria

MS: Cramps, joint pain

CV: Orthostatic hypotension

HEMA: Aplastic anemia, agranulocytopenia, leukopenia, thrombocytopenia (rare)

Contraindications: Anuria, hypersensitivity, hyperkalemia, impaired renal function

Precautions: Dehydration, pregnancy (B), diabetes, acidosis, lactation

Pharmacokinetics:

PO: Onset 2 hr, peak 6-10 hr, duration 24 hr; excreted in urine, feces, half-life 6-9 hr

Interactions/incompatibilities:

• Enhanced action of: antihypertensives, lithium toxicity may be provoked

• Hyperkalemia: other potassium-sparing diuretics, potassium products, ACE inhibitors, salt substitutes

NURSING CONSIDERATIONS

Assess:

• Weight, I&O daily to determine fluid loss; effect of drug may be decreased if used qd

• Rate, depth, rhythm of respiration, effect of exertion

• B/P lying, standing; postural hypotension may occur

• Electrolytes: potassium, sodium, chloride; include BUN, CBC, serum creatinine, blood pH, ABGs

Administer:

• In AM to avoid interference with sleep if using drug as a diuretic

• With food, if nausea occurs, absorption may be decreased slightly

Evaluate:

• Improvement in edema of feet, legs, sacral area daily if medication is being used in CHF

• Improvement in CVP q8h

• Signs of drowsiness, restlessness

• Rashes, temperature elevation qd

• Confusion especially in elderly; take safety precautions if needed

Teach patient/family:

• Adverse reactions: muscle cramps, weakness, nausea, dizziness

• Take with food or milk for GI symptoms

• Take early in day to prevent nocturia

• Avoid potassium-rich foods: oranges, bananas; salt substitutes

Lab test interferences:

Interfere: GTT

---

* Available in Canada only

Treatment of overdose: Lavage if taken orally, monitor electrolytes, administer sodium bicarbonate for K^+ >6.5 mEq/L, monitor hydration, CV, renal status

---

amino acid injection

(a-mee'noe)
FreAmine HBC, HepatAmine
Func. class.: Nitrogen product

Action: Needed for anabolism to maintain structure, decrease catabolism, promote healing
Uses: Hepatic encephalopathy, cirrhosis, hepatitis, nutritional support in cancer
Dosage and routes:
• *Adult:* IV 80-120 g/day; 500 ml of amino acids/500 ml $D_{50}W$ given over 24 hr
Available forms include: Inj IV many strengths, types
Side effects/adverse reactions:
CNS: Dizziness, headache, confusion, *loss of consciousness*
CV: Hypertension, *CHF, pulmonary edema*
GI: Nausea, vomiting, liver fat deposits, abdominal pain
GU: Glycosuria, osmotic diuresis
ENDO: Hyperglycemia, rebound hypoglycemia, electrolyte imbalances, hyperosmolar syndrome, hyperosmolar hyperglycemic non-ketotic syndrome, alkalosis, acidosis, hypophosphatemia, hyperammonemia, dehydration, hypocalcemia
INTEG: Chills, flushing, warm feeling, rash, urticaria, extravasation necrosis, phlebitis at injection site
Contraindications: Hypersensitivity, severe electrolyte imbalances, anuria, severe liver damage, maple syrup urine disease, PKU
Precautions: Renal disease, pregnancy (C), children, diabetes mellitus, CHF

NURSING CONSIDERATIONS
Assess:
• Electrolytes (K, Na, Ca, Cl, Mg), blood glucose, ammonia, phosphate
• Renal, liver function studies: BUN, creatinine, ALT, AST, bilirubin
• Injection site for extravasation: redness along vein, edema at site, necrosis, pain, hard tender area; site should be changed immediately
• Monitor respiratory function q4h: auscultate lung fields bilaterally for rales, respirations, quality, rate, rhythm
• Monitor temperature q4h for increased fever, indicating infection; if infection suspected, infusion is discontinued, tubing bottle cultured
• Monitor for impending hepatic coma: asterixis, confusion, fetor, lethargy
• Urine glucose q6h using Chemstrips, which are not affected by infusion substances
Administer:
• Total parenteral nutrition only mixed with dextrose to promote protein synthesis
• Immediately after mixing in pharmacy under strict aseptic technique using laminar flowhood, use infusion pump, in-line filter
• Using careful monitoring technique; do not speed up infusion; pulmonary edema, glucose overload will result
Perform/provide
• Storage depends on type of solution; consult manufacturer
• Changing dressing and IV tubing to prevent infection q24-48h or q5-7 days if transparent dressing is used

---

italics = common side effects   ***bold italic*** = life threatening reactions

Evaluate:

• Hyperammonemia: nausea, vomiting, malaise, tremors, anorexia, convulsions

• Therapeutic response: weight gain, decrease in jaundice in liver disorders, increased LOC

Teach patient/family

• Reason for use of TPN

• If chills, sweating are experienced, they should be reported at once

---

amino acid solution

Aminosyn, FreAmine III, Novamine, Travasol

Func. class.: Nitrogen product

Action: Needed for anabolism to maintain structure, decrease catabolism, promote healing

Uses: Nutritional support in cancer, trauma, intestinal obstruction, short bowel syndrome, severe malabsorption

Dosage and routes:

• *Adult:* IV 1-1.5 g/kg/day titrated to patient's needs

• *Child:* IV 2-3 g/kg/day titrated to patient's needs

Available forms include: Inj IV many types, strengths

Side effects/adverse reactions:

CNS: Dizziness, headache, confusion, *loss of consciousness*

CV: Hypertension, *CHF, pulmonary edema*

GI: Nausea, vomiting, liver fat deposits, abdominal pain, jaundice

GU: Glycosuria, osmotic diuresis

ENDO: Hyperglycemia, rebound hypoglycemia, electrolyte imbalances, hyperosmolar syndrome, hyperosmolar hyperglycemic non-ketotic syndrome, alkalosis, acidosis, hypophosphatemia, hyper-

ammonemia, dehydration, hypocalcemia

INTEG: Chills, flushing, warm feeling, rash, urticaria, extravasation necrosis, phlebitis at injection site

Contraindications: Hypersensitivity, severe electrolyte imbalances, anuria, severe liver damage, maple syrup urine disease, PKU

Precautions: Renal disease, pregnancy (C), children, diabetes mellitus, CHF

NURSING CONSIDERATIONS

Assess:

• Electrolytes (K, Na, Ca, Cl, Mg), blood glucose, ammonia, phosphate

• Renal, liver function studies: BUN, creatinine, ALT, AST, bilirubin

• Injection site for extravasation: redness along vein, edema at site, necrosis, pain, hard tender area; site should be changed immediately

• Monitor respiratory function q4h: auscultate lung fields bilaterally for rales, respirations, quality, rate, rhythm

• Monitor temperature q4h for increased fever, indicating infection; if infection suspected, infusion is discontinued, tubing, bottle cultured

• Urine glucose q6h using Tes-Tape, Clinistix, Keto-Diastix, which are not affected by infusion substances, blood glucose is preferred testing method

Administer:

• Total parenteral nutrition only mixed with dextrose to promote protein synthesis

• Immediately after mixing in pharmacy under strict aseptic technique using laminar flowhood, use infusion pump, in-line filter

• Using careful monitoring technique; do not speed up infusion;

pulmonary edema, glucose overload will result

Perform/provide

• Storage depends on type of solution; consult manufacturer

• Changing dressing and IV tubing to prevent infection q24-48h

Evaluate:

• Hyperammonemia: nausea, vomiting, malaise, tremors, anorexia, convulsions

• Therapeutic response: weight gain, decrease in jaundice in liver disorders, increased serum albumin

Teach patient/family

• Reason for use of TPN

• If chills, sweating are experienced, they should be reported at once

---

aminocaproic acid

(a-mee-noe-ka-proe′ik)

Amicar, (EACA)

Func. class.: Hemostatic

Chem. class.: Synthetic monoaminocarboxylic acid

Action: Inhibits fibrinolysis by inhibiting plasminogen activator substances

Uses: Hemorrhage from hyperfibrinolysis, adjunctive therapy in hemophilia

Dosage and routes:

• *Adult:* PO/IV 5 g loading dose, then 1-1.25 g q1h if needed, not to exceed 30 g/day

Available forms include: Inj IV 250 mg/ml; tab 500 mg; syr 250 mg/ml

Side effects/adverse reactions:

GU: Dysuria, frequency, oliguria, **renal failure,** *ejaculatory failure, menstrual irregularities*

GI: Nausea, vomiting, abdominal cramps, diarrhea

INTEG: Rash

CNS:Headache, dizziness, malaise, fatigue, hallucinations, delirium, psychosis, **convulsions,** weakness

HEMA: **Thrombosis**

CV: **Dysrhythmias,** orthostatic hypotension, bradycardia

EENT: Tinnitus, nasal congestion, conjunctival suffusion

Contraindications: Hypersensitivity, abnormal bleeding, postpartum bleeding, DIC, upper urinary tract bleeding, new burns

Precautions: Neonates/infants, mild or moderate renal disease, hepatic disease, thrombosis, cardiac disease, pregnancy (C)

Pharmacokinetics:

PO/IV: Peak 2 hr, excreted by kidneys as unmetabolized drug rapidly absorbed

Interactions/incompatibilities:

Increased coagulation: estrogens, oral contraceptives

NURSING CONSIDERATIONS

Assess:

• I&O, if urinary output decreases, notify physician and stop drug

• Blood studies: coagulation factors, platelets, protamine coagulation test for extravascular clotting, thrombopheblitis

• B/P, pulse for increase

• Drug level: 0.13 mg/ml is required to decrease fibrinolysis

• Creatine phosphokinase, urinalysis

Administer:

• Give IV loading dose over 30 min to avoid hypotension

• IV push slowly, with plastic syringe only

• IV after dilution with 4-5 g/250 ml NS, D₅W, LR, give over 1 hr; may give by continuous infusion after loading dose(s) of 1 g/hr diluted in 50-100 ml of compatible solutions; use infusion pump

---

italics = common side effects   **bold italic** = life threatening reactions

Perform/provide:
• Storage in tight container in cool environment, do not freeze
Evaluate:
• Allergy: fever, rash, itching, jaundice
• Myopathy: if weakness, fever, myoglobinemia, or oliguria; discontinue drug
• Bleeding: mucous membrane, epistaxis, ecchymosis, petechiae, hematuria, hematemesis
Teach patient/family:
• To report any signs of bleeding (gums, under skin, urine, stools, emesis) or myopathy
• To change position slowly to decrease orthostatic hypotension
• Proper administration for 8-10 days following dental procedure in hemophilia
Lab test interferences:
Increased: K^+, CPK

---

aminoglutethimide

(a-meen-noe-gloo-te-th'i-mide)
Cytadren
Func. class.: Antineoplastic, adrenal steroid inhibitor
Chem. class.: Hormone

Action: Acts by inhibiting DNA, RNA, protein synthesis; is derived from *Streptomyces verticillus;* replication is decreased by binding to DNA, which causes strand splitting; phase specific in G_2 and M phases; blocks biosynthesis of all steroid hormones (cortisol, androgens, progestins)
Uses: Suppression of adrenal function in Cushing's syndrome, metastatic breast cancer, adrenal cancer
Dosage and routes:
• *Adult:* PO 250 mg qid at 6 hr intervals, may increase by 250 mg/day q1-2 wk, not to exceed 2 g/day
Available forms include: Tabs 250 mg
Side effects/adverse reactions:
GI: Nausea, vomiting, anorexia, ***hepatotoxicity***
INTEG: Rash, pruritus, hirsutism
CV: ***Hypotension,*** tachycardia
CNS: Drowsiness, morbilliform skin rash, dizziness, headache, lethargy
Contraindications: Hypersensitivity, hypothyroidism, pregnancy (D)
Precautions: Renal disease, hepatic disease, respiratory disease
Pharmacokinetics: Half-life 13 hr, metabolized in liver, excreted in urine, crosses placenta
Interactions/incompatibilities:
• Accelerated metabolism of: dexamethasone
NURSING CONSIDERATIONS
Assess:
• Renal function studies: BUN, serum uric acid, urine CrCl, electrolytes before, during therapy
• I&O ratio; report fall in urine output of 30 ml/hr
• Monitor temperature q4h; may indicate beginning infection
• Liver function tests before, during therapy (bilirubin, AST, ALT, LDH) as needed or monthly
• RBC, Hct, Hgb, since these may be decreased
Administer:
• Antacid before oral agent; give last dose of the day after evening meal before bedtime
• Local or systemic drugs for infection if indicated
Perform/provide:
• Special skin care
• Liquid diet, including cola, Jell-O; dry toast or crackers as ordered may be added if patient is not nauseated or vomiting

---

• Nutritious diet with iron and vitamin supplements as ordered
Evaluate:
• Food preferences; list likes, dislikes
• Inflammation of mucosa, breaks in skin
• Yellowing of skin, sclera, dark urine, clay-colored stools, itchy skin, abdominal pain, fever, diarrhea
• Symptoms indicating severe allergic reaction: rash, pruritus, urticaria, purpuric skin lesions, itching, flushing
Teach patient/family:
• To report any complaints, side effects to nurse or physician
• That masculinization can occur, is reversible after discontinuing treatment
• Correct self-administration of adjuvant corticosteroids

---

aminophylline (theophylline ethylenediamine)
(am-in-off'i-lin)
Amoline, Corophyllin,* Lixaminol, Phyllocontin, Somophyllin-DF, Truphylline
Func. class.: Spasmolytic
Chem. class.: Xanthine, ethylenediamide

Action: Relaxes smooth muscle of respiratory system by blocking phosphodiesterase, which increases cyclic AMP
Uses: Bronchial asthma, bronchospasm, Cheyne-Stokes respirations
Dosage and routes:
• *Adult:* PO 500 mg, then 250-500 mg q6-8h; CONT IV 0.3-0.9 mg/kg/hr (maintenance); RECT 500 mg q6-8h
• *Child:* PO 7.5 mg/kg, then 3-6 mg/kg q6-8h; IV 7.5 mg/kg, then 3-6 mg/kg q6-8h injected over 5 min, do not exceed 25 mg/min; may give loading dose of 5.6 mg/kg over ½ hr; CONT IV 1 mg/kg/hr (maintenance)
• *Neonates:* IV/PO 1 mg/kg initially for plasma increases of each 2 μg/ml, then 1 mg/kg q6h
Available forms include: Inj IV, IM, rectal supp 250, 500 mg; rectal sol 300 mg/5 ml; elix 250 mg/5 ml; oral liq 105 mg/5 ml; tabs 100, 200 mg, tabs con-rel 225 mg; tabs sust-rel 300 mg
Side effects/adverse reactions:
CNS: Anxiety, restlessness, insomnia, dizziness, **convulsions,** headache, light-headedness, muscle twitching
CV: Palpitations, sinus tachycardia, hypotension, flushing, dysrhythmias
GI: Nausea, vomiting, anorexia, diarrhea, bitter taste, dyspepsia, anal irritation (suppositories), epigastric pain
RESP: Increased rate
INTEG: Flushing, urticaria
GU: Urinary frequency
Contraindications: Hypersensitivity to xanthines, tachydysrhythmias
Precautions: Elderly, CHF, cor pulmonale, hepatic disease, active peptic ulcer disease, diabetes mellitus, hyperthyroidism, hypertension, children, pregnancy (C), glaucoma, prostatic hypertrophy
Pharmacokinetics:
IV: Peak 30 min
Interactions/incompatibilities:
• Do not mix in syringe with other drugs
• Increased action of aminophylline: cimetidine, propranolol, erythromycin, troleandomycin
• May increase effects of: anticoagulants
• Cardiotoxicity: β-blockade

---

italics = common side effects   ***bold italic*** = life threatening reactions

- Increased elimination: smoking
- Decreased effects of: lithium

NURSING CONSIDERATIONS
Assess:
- Theophylline blood levels (therapeutic level is 10-20 μg/ml); toxicity may occur with small increase above 20 μg/ml
- Monitor I&O; diuresis occurs, dehydration may result in elderly or children
- Whether theophylline was given recently

Administer:
- PO after meals to decrease GI symptoms; absorption may be affected
- IV after diluting in 5% dextrose to decrease burning sensation at injection site; only clear solutions
- May be diluted for IV INF in 100-200 ml compatible solution
- Avoid IM injection; pain occurs
- Rectal dose if patient is unable to take PO

Perform/provide:
- Storage of diluted solution for 24 hr if refrigerated

Evaluate:
- Therapeutic response: decreased dyspnea, respiratory rate, rhythm
- Respiratory rate, rhythm, depth; auscultate lung fields bilaterally; notify physician of abnormalities
- Allergic reactions: rash, urticaria; if these occur, drug should be discontinued

Teach patient/family
- To check OTC medications, current prescription medications for ephedrine; will increase CNS stimulation
- To avoid hazardous activities; dizziness may occur
- If GI upset occurs, to take drug with 8 oz water; avoid food, since absorption may be decreased
- To remain in bed 15-20 min after

rectal suppository is inserted to avoid removal
- To notify physician of toxicity: insomnia, anxiety, nausea, vomiting, rapid pulse, convulsions
- To notify physician of change in smoking habit; a change in dose may be required

---

amiodarone HCl

(a-mee'-oh-da-rone)
Cordarone

Func. class.: Antidysrhythmic (Class III)
Chem. class.: Iodinated benzofuran derivative

Action: Increases action potential duration and effective refractory period, noncompetitive α- and β-adrenergic inhibition
Uses: Severe ventricular tachycardia, ventricular fibrillation
Dosage and routes:
- *Adult:* Loading dose 800-1600 mg/day 1-3 wk; then 600-800 mg/day 1 mo; maintenance 200-600 mg/day
Available forms include: Tabs 200 mg
Side effects/adverse reactions:
CNS: Headache, dizziness, involuntary movement, tremors, peripheral neuropathy, malaise, fatigue, ataxia, paresthesias, insomnia
GI: Nausea, vomiting, diarrhea, abdominal pain, anorexia, constipation, *hepatotoxicity*
CV: Hypotension, bradycardia, *sinus arrest, CHF,* dysrhythmias, *SA node dysfunction*
INTEG: Rash, photosensitivity, blue-gray skin discoloration, rash, alopecia, spontaneous ecchymosis
EENT: Blurred vision, halos, photophobia, *corneal microdeposits,* dry eyes

---

ENDO: Hyperthyroidism or hypothyroidism
MS: Weakness, pain in extremities
RESP: **Pulmonary fibrosis**, pulmonary inflammation
MISC: Flushing, abnormal taste or smell, edema, abnormal salivation, coagulation abnormalities

Precautions: Goiter, Hashimoto's thyroiditis, sinus node dysfunction, 2nd, 3rd degree AV block, electrolyte imbalances, pregnancy (C), bradycardia, lactation

Pharmacokinetics:
PO: Onset 1-3 wk, peak 2-10 hr; half-life 53 days; metabolized by liver, excreted by kidneys

Interactions/incompatibilities:
• Bradycardia: β-blockers, calcium channel blockers
• Increased levels of: digitalis, quinidine, procainamide, flecainide, disopyramide, phenytoin
• Increased anticoagulant effects: warfarin
• Bradycardia, arrest: lidocaine

NURSING CONSIDERATIONS
Assess:
• I&O ratio; electrolytes: K, Na, Cl
• Liver function studies: AST, ALT, bilirubin, alk phosphatase
• ECG continuously to determine drug effectiveness, measure PR, QRS, QT intervals, check for PVCs, other dysrhythmias
• For dehydration or hypovolemia
• B/P continuously for hypotension, hypertension

Administer:
• Reduced dosage slowly with ECG monitoring

Evaluate:
• For rebound hypertension after 1-2 hr
• CNS symptoms: confusion, psychosis, numbness, depression, involuntary movements; if these occur drug should be discontinued

• Hypothyroidism: lethargy, dizziness, constipation, enlarged thyroid gland, edema of extremities, cool, pale skin
• Hyperthyroidism: restlessness, tachycardia, eyelid puffiness, weight loss, frequent urination, menstrual irregularities, dyspnea, warm, moist skin
• Pulmonary toxicity: dyspnea, fatigue, cough, fever, chest pain; drug should be discontinued
• Cardiac rate, respiration: rate, rhythm, character, chest pain

Teach patient/family:
• To use sunscreen or stay out of sun to prevent burns
• To report side effects immediately
• That skin discoloration is usually reversible
• That dark glasses may be needed for photophobia

Treatment of overdose: O₂, artificial ventilation, ECG, administer dopamine for circulatory depression, administer diazepam or thiopental for convulsions, isoproterenol

amitriptyline HCl
(a-mee-trip'ti-leen)
Amitril, Apo-Amitriptyline,* Elavil, Emitrip, Endep, Enovil, Levate,* Meravil,* Novotriptyn,* Rolavil*
Func. class.: Antidepressant—tricyclic
Chem. class.: Tertiary amine

Action: Blocks reuptake of norepinephrine, serotonin into nerve endings, increasing action of norepinephrine, serotonin in nerve cells
Uses: Major depression
Dosage and routes:
• *Adult:* PO 50-100 mg hs, may in-

crease to 200 mg qd, not to exceed 300 mg/day; IM 20-30 mg qid, or 80-120 mg hs
• *Adolescent/geriatric:* PO 30 mg/day in divided doses, may be increased to 150 mg/day

Available forms include: Tabs 10, 25, 50, 75, 100, 150 mg; inj IM 10 mg/ml

Side effects/adverse reactions:
*HEMA: **Agranulocytosis, thrombocytopenia, eosinophilia, leukopenia***
CNS: Dizziness, drowsiness, confusion, headache, anxiety, tremors, stimulation, weakness, insomnia, nightmares, EPS (elderly), increased psychiatric symptoms
GI: Diarrhea, dry mouth, nausea, vomiting, ***paralytic ileus,*** increased appetite, cramps, epigastric distress, jaundice, ***hepatitis,*** stomatitis
GU: Retention
INTEG: Rash, urticaria, sweating, pruritus, photosensitivity
*CV: Orthostatic hypotension, **ECG changes, tachycardia, hypertension,*** palpations
EENT: Blurred vision, tinnitus, mydriasis, ophthalmoplegia

Contraindications: Hypersensitivity to tricyclic antidepressants, recovery phase of myocardial infarction

Precautions: Suicidal patients, convulsive disorders, prostatic hypertrophy, schizophrenia, psychotic, severe depression, increased intraocular pressure, narrow-angle glaucoma, urinary retention, cardiac disease, hepatic disease/renal disease, hyperthyroidism, electroshock therapy, elective surgery, child <12 yr, pregnancy (C)

Pharmacokinetics:
PO/IM: Onset 45 min, peak 2-12 hr, therapeutic response 2-3 wk;

metabolized by liver, excreted in urine/feces, crosses placenta, excreted in breast milk, half-life 10-50 hr

Interactions/incompatibilities:
• Decreased effects of: guanethidine, clonidine, indirect acting sympathomimetics (ephedrine)
• Increased effects of: direct acting sympathomimetics (epinephrine), alcohol, barbiturates, benzodiazepines, CNS depressants
• Hyperpyretic crisis, convulsions, hypertensive episode: MAOI (pargyline [Eutonyl])

NURSING CONSIDERATIONS
Assess:
• B/P (lying, standing), pulse q4h; if systolic B/P drops 20 mm Hg hold drug, notify physician; take vital signs q4h in patients with cardiovascular disease
• Blood studies: CBC, leukocytes, differential, cardiac enzymes if patient is receiving long-term therapy
• Hepatic studies: AST, ALT, bilirubin, creatinine
• Weight qwk, appetite may increase with drug
• ECG for flattening of T wave, bundle branch block, AV block, dysrhythmias in cardiac patients

Administer:
• Increased fluids, bulk in diet if constipation, urinary retention occur
• With food or milk for GI symptoms
• Crushed if patient is unable to swallow medication whole
• Dosage hs if over-sedation occurs during day; may take entire dose hs; elderly may not tolerate once/day dosing
• Gum, hard sugarless candy, or frequent sips of water for dry mouth

Perform/provide:
• Storage at room temperature, do not freeze

• Assistance with ambulation during beginning therapy since drowsiness/dizziness occurs
• Safety measure including siderails primarily in elderly
• Checking to see PO medication swallowed

Evaluate:
• EPS primarily in elderly: rigidity, dystonia, akathisia
• Mental status: mood, sensorium, affect, suicidal tendencies; increase in psychiatric symptoms: depression, panic
• Urinary retention, constipation; constipation is more likely to occur in children
• Withdrawal symptoms: headache, nausea, vomiting, muscle pain, weakness; do not usually occur unless drug was discontinued abruptly
• Alcohol consumption; if alcohol is consumed, hold dose until morning

Teach patient/family:
• That therapeutic effects may take 2-3 wk
• Use caution in driving or other activities requiring alertness because of drowsiness, dizziness, blurred vision
• To avoid alcohol ingestion, other CNS depressants
• Not to discontinue medication quickly after long-term use, may cause nausea, headache, malaise
• To wear sunscreen or large hat since photosensitivity occurs

Lab test interferences:
Increase: Serum bilirubin, blood glucose, alk phosphatase
Decrease: VMA, 5-HIAA
False increase: Urinary catecholamines

Treatment of overdose: ECG monitoring, induce emesis, lavage, activated charcoal, administer anticonvulsant

ammonia, aromatic spirit

Func. class.: Respiratory stimulants
Chem. class.: Aromatic hydroalcoholic solution of ammonia

Action: Stimulates medulla (respiratory, vasomotor areas) by irritation of sensory receptors in mucosa of nasal passages, esophagus, stomach
Uses: To treat, prevent fainting
Dosage and routes:
• *Adult and child:* INH prn; PO 2-4 ml diluted in water
Available forms include: Inh 0.33, 0.4 ml; sol
Side effects/adverse reactions:
None known

NURSING CONSIDERATIONS
Assess:
• Vital signs, B/P after administration of inhalant
Administer:
• By inhalation, do not place packets in pockets, may open, cause caustic burns
• Orally by diluting 2-4 ml in >30 ml of water
Perform/provide:
• Storage protected from light at room temperature
Evaluate:
• Cause of fainting

ammonium chloride

Func. class.: Acidifier
Chem. class.: Ammonium

Action: Lowers urinary pH, liberates hydrogen and chloride ions in blood and extracellular fluid with

---

italics = common side effects　　　***bold italic*** = life threatening reactions

decreased pH and correction of alkalosis

Uses: Alkalosis (metabolic), systemic and urinary acidifer, expectorant, diuretic

Dosage and routes:

Alkalosis

• *Adult and child:* IV INF 0.9-1.3 ml/min of a 2.14% sol, not to exceed 2 ml/min

Acidifier

• *Adult:* PO 4-12 g/day in divided doses

• *Child:* PO 75 mg/kg/day in divided doses

Expectorant

• *Adult:* PO 250-500 mg q2-4h as needed

Available forms include: Tabs 500 mg, 1 g; inj IV 0.4, 5 mEq/ml

Side effects/adverse reactions:

CNS: Drowsiness, headache, confusion, stimulation, tremors, *twitching, hyperreflexia, tetany, EEG changes*

CV: Bradycardia, dysrhythmias, bounding pulse

GU: Glycosuria, thirst

GI: Gastric irritation, nausea, vomiting, anorexia, diarrhea

INTEG: Rash, pain at infusion site

META: Acidosis, hypokalemia, hyperchloremia, hyperglycemia

RESP: Apnea, irregular respirations, hyperventilation

Contraindications: Hypersensitivity, severe hepatic disease, severe renal disease

Precautions: Severe respiratory disease, cardiac edema, infants, pregnancy (C), children

Pharmacokinetics:

PO: Absorbed in 3-6 hr; metabolized in liver, excreted in urine and feces

Interactions/incompatibilities:

• Increased toxicity: PAS

• Decreased effects of: amphetamines, tricyclic antidepressants, salicylates, sulfonylureas

• Increased risk of systemic acidosis: spironolactone

NURSING CONSIDERATIONS

Assess:

• Respiratory rate, rhythm, depth, notify physician of abnormalities that may indicate acidosis

• Electrolytes and CO_2, chloride before and during treatment

• Urine pH, urinary output, urine glucose, specific gravity during beginning treatment

• I&O ratio, report large increases or decreases

Administer:

• PO with meals if GI symptoms occur

• IV slowly to avoid pain at infusion site and toxicity

• After diluting solutions to 2.14% (IV); each 20-ml vial must be further diluted by adding 1-2 vials/500-1000 ml of compatible solution and given at a rate of 5 ml/min or less

• With water for expectorant not compatible with milk or other alkaline solutions

Evaluate:

• For CNS symptoms: confusion, twitching, hyperreflexia, stimulation, headache that may indicate ammonia toxicity

• For cardiac dysrhythmias

• For respiratory symptoms: hyperventilation

Teach patient/family:

• To increase potassium in diet: bananas, oranges, cantelope, honeydew, spinach, potatoes, dry fruit

Lab test interferences:

Increase: Blood ammonia, AST/ALT

Decrease: Serum magnesium, urine urobilinogen

---

amobarbital/amobarbital sodium

(am-oh-bar'bi-tal)

Amytal, Isobec/Amytal sodium

Func. class.: Sedative/hypnotic-barbiturate (intermediate acting)

Chem. class.: Amylobarbitone

Controlled Substance Schedule II (USA), Schedule G (Canada)

Action: Depresses activity in brain cells primarily in reticular activating system in brainstem, also selectively depresses neurons in posterior hypothalamus, limbic structures; able to decrease seizure activity by inhibition of impulses in CNS

Uses: Sedation, preanesthetic sedation, insomnia, anticonvulsant, adjunct in psychiatry, hypnotic

Dosage and routes:

Preanesthetic sedation

• *Adult and child:* PO/IM 200 mg 1-2 hr preoperatively

Sedation

• *Adult:* PO 30-50 mg bid or tid, may be from 15-120 mg bid-qid

• *Child:* PO 2 mg/kg/day in 4 divided doses

Anticonvulsant/psychiatry

• *Adult:* IV 65-500 mg given over several min, not to exceed 100 mg/min; not to exceed 1 g

• *Child <6 yr:* IV/IM 3-5 mg/kg over several min

Insomnia

• *Adult:* PO/IM 65-200 mg hs, not to exceed 5 ml in one site

• *Child:* IM 3-5 mg/kg at hs, not to exceed 5 ml in one site

Available forms include: Tabs 30, 50, 100 mg; caps 65, 200 mg; powder for inj IM, IV 250, 500 mg/vial

Side effects/adverse reactions:

CNS: Lethargy, drowsiness, hang-over, dizziness, stimulation in the elderly and children, *lightheadedness,* physical dependence, CNS depression, mental depression, slurred speech

GI: Nausea, vomiting, diarrhea, constipation

INTEG: Rash, urticaria, pain, abscesses at injection site, *angioedema,* thrombophlebitis, *Stevens-Johnson syndrome*

CV: Hypotension, bradycardia

RESP: Depression, apnea, laryngospasm, bronchospasm

HEMA: Agranulocytosis, thrombocytopenia, megaloblastic anemia (long-term treatment)

Contraindications: Hypersensitivity to barbiturates, respiratory depression, addiction to barbiturates, severe liver impairment, porphyria

Precautions: Anemia, pregnancy (B), lactation, hepatic disease, renal disease, hypertension, elderly, acute/chronic pain

Pharmacokinetics:

PO: Onset 45-60 min, duration 6-8 hr

IV: Onset 5 min, duration 3-6 hr

Metabolized by liver, excreted by kidneys (inactive metabolites), crosses placenta, highly protein bound, excreted in breast milk, half-life 16-40 hr

Interactions/incompatibilities:

• Increased CNS depression: alcohol, MAOIs, sedative, narcotics

• Decreased effect of: oral anticoagulants, corticosteroids, griseofulvin, quinidine, oral contraceptives, estrogens

• Increased half-life of: doxycycline

NURSING CONSIDERATIONS

Assess:

• VS q30 min after parenteral route for 2 hr

• Blood studies: Hct, Hgb, RBCs, serum folate, vitamin D (if on long-term therapy); pro-time in patients receiving anticoagulants

• Hepatic studies: AST, ALT, bilirubin; if increased, drug is usually discontinued

Administer:

• After removal of cigarettes, to prevent fires

• Deep IM injection in large muscle mass to prevent tissue sloughing, abscesses, no more than 5 ml/site

• After trying conservative measures for insomnia

• After mixing with sterile water for injection to a concentration of 100 mg/ml, may dilute further with compatible solution; inject within 30 min of preparation; don't shake solution or use cloudy solution

• IV only with resuscitative equipment available, administer at <100 mg/min (only by qualified personnel)

• ½-1 hr before hs for expected sleeplessness

• On empty stomach for best absorption

Perform/provide:

• Assistance with ambulation after receiving dose

• Safety measures: siderails, nightlight, callbell within easy reach

• Checking to see PO medication swallowed

Evaluate:

• Therapeutic response: ability to sleep at night, decreased amount of early morning awakening if taking drug for insomnia, or decrease in number, severity of seizures if taking drug for seizure disorder

• Mental status: mood, sensorium, affect, memory (long, short)

• Physical dependency: more frequent requests for medication, shakes, anxiety

• Barbiturate toxicity: hypotension; pulmonary constriction; cold, clammy skin; cyanosis of lips; insomnia; nausea; vomiting; hallucinations; delirium; weakness; coma, pupillary constriction, mild symptoms may occur in 8-12 hr without drug

• Respiratory dysfunction: respiratory depression, character, rate, rhythm; hold drug if respirations are <10/min or if pupils are dilated

• Blood dyscrasias: fever, sore throat, bruising, rash, jaundice, epistaxis

Teach patient/family:

• That hangover is common

• Drug is indicated only for short-term treatment of insomnia and is probably ineffective after 2 wk

• That physical dependency may result when used for extended periods of time (45-90 days depending on dose)

• To avoid driving or other activities requiring alertness

• To avoid alcohol ingestion or CNS depressants; serious CNS depression may result

• Not to discontinue medication quickly after long-term use; drug should be tapered over 1 wk

• To tell all prescribers that a barbiturate is being taken

• That withdrawal insomnia may occur after short-term use; do not start using drug again, insomnia will improve in 1-3 nights, may experience increased dreaming

• That effects may take 2 nights for benefits to be noticed

• Alternate measures to improve sleep: reading, exercise several hours before hs, warm bath, warm milk, TV, self-hypnosis, deep breathing

Lab test interferences:
False increase: Sulfobromophthalein

Treatment of overdose: Lavage, activated charcoal, warming blanket, vital signs, hemodialysis, alkalinize urine

---

amoxapine

(a-mox′a-peen)
Asendin

Func. class.: Antidepressant—tricyclic
Chem. class.: Dibenzoxazepine derivative—secondary amine

Action: Blocks reuptake of norepinephrine, serotonin into nerve endings, increasing action of norepinephrine, serotonin in nerve cells

Uses: Depression

Dosage and routes:
• *Adult:* PO 50 mg tid, may increase to 100 mg tid on 3rd day of therapy; not to exceed 300 mg/day unless lower doses have been given for at least 2 wk, may be given daily dose hs, not to exceed 600 mg/day in hospitalized patients

Available forms include: Tabs 10, 25, 50, 75, 100, 150 mg

Side effects/adverse reactions:
HEMA: Agranulocytosis, thrombocytopenia, eosinophilia, leukopenia
CNS: Dizziness, drowsiness, confusion, headache, anxiety, tremors, stimulation, weakness, insomnia, nightmares, EPS (elderly), increased psychiatric symptoms, paresthesia
GI: Diarrhea, dry mouth, nausea, vomiting, *paralytic ileus,* increased appetite, cramps, epigastric distress, jaundice, *hepatitis,* stomatitis
GU: Retention, *acute renal failure*
INTEG: Rash, urticaria, sweating, pruritus, photosensitivity
CV: Orthostatic hypotension, ECG changes, tachycardia, *hypertension,* palpitations
EENT: Blurred vision, tinnitus, mydriasis, ophthalmoplegia

Contraindications: Hypersensitivity to tricyclic antidepressants, recovery phase of myocardial infarction, convulsive disorders, prostatic hypertrophy

Precautions: Suicidal patients, severe depression, increased intraocular pressure, narrow-angle glaucoma, urinary retention, cardiac disease, hepatic disease, hyperthyroidism, electroshock therapy, elective surgery, elderly, pregnancy (C)

Pharmacokinetics:
PO: Steady state 7 days; metabolized by liver, excreted by kidneys, crosses placenta, half-life 8 hr

Interactions/incompatibilities:
• Decreased effects of: guanethidine, clonidine, indirect-acting sympathomimetics (ephedrine)
• Increased effects of: direct-acting sympathomimetics (epinephrine), alcohol, barbiturates, benzodiazepines, CNS depressants
• Hyperpyretic crisis, convulsions, hypertensive episode: MAOI (pargyline [Eutonyl])

NURSING CONSIDERATIONS
Assess:
• B/P (lying, standing), pulse q4h; if systolic B/P drops 20 mm Hg hold drug, notify physician; take vital signs q4h in patients with cardiovascular disease
• Blood studies: CBC, leukocytes, differential, cardiac enzymes if patient is receiving long-term therapy

---

italics = common side effects   ***bold italic*** = life threatening reactions

- Hepatic studies: AST, ALT, bilirubin, creatinine
- Weight qwk, appetite may increase with drug
- ECG for flattening of T wave, bundle branch block, AV block, dysrhythmias in cardiac patients

Administer:
- Increased fluids, bulk in diet if constipation, urinary retention occur
- With food or milk for GI symptoms
- Crushed if patient is unable to swallow medication whole
- Dosage hs if over-sedation occurs during day; may take entire dose hs; elderly may not tolerate once/day dosing
- Gum, hard candy, or frequent sips of water for dry mouth

Perform/provide:
- Storage at room temperature, do not freeze
- Assistance with ambulation during beginning therapy since drowsiness/dizziness occurs
- Safety measures including siderails primarily in elderly
- Checking to see PO medication swallowed

Evaluate:
- EPS primarily in elderly: rigidity, dystonia, akathisia
- Mental status: mood, sensorium, affect, suicidal tendencies, increase in psychiatric symptoms: depression, panic
- Urinary retention, constipation; constipation is more likely to occur in children
- Withdrawal symptoms: headache, nausea, vomiting, muscle pain, weakness; do not usually occur unless drug was discontinued abruptly
- Alcohol consumption; if alcohol is consumed, hold dose until morning

Teach patient/family:
- That therapeutic effects may take 2-3 wk
- Use caution in driving or other activities requiring alertness because of drowsiness, dizziness, blurred vision
- To avoid alcohol ingestion, other CNS depressants
- Not to discontinue medication quickly after long-term use, may cause nausea, headache, malaise
- To wear sunscreen or large hat since photosensitivity occurs

Lab test interferences:
Increase: Serum bilirubin, blood glucose, alk phosphatase
False increase: Urinary catecholamines
Decrease: VMA, 5-HIAA

Treatment of overdose: ECG monitoring, induce emesis, lavage, activated charcoal, administer anticonvulsant

---

amoxicillin/clavulanate potassium
(a-mox-i-sill'in)
Augmentin, Clavulin*

Func. class.: Broad spectrum antibiotic
Chem. class.: Aminopenicillin-B lactamase inhibitor

Action: Interferes with cell wall replication of susceptible organisms; the cell wall, rendered osmotically unstable, swells, and bursts from osmotic pressure
Uses: Sinus infections, pneumonia, otitis media, skin, urinary tract infections; effective for strains of *E. coli, P. mirabilis, H. influenzae, S. faecalis, S. pneumoniae,* and β-lactamase-producing organisms

Dosage and routes:
- *Adult:* PO 250-500 mg q8h depending on severity of infection
- *Child:* PO 20-40 mg/kg/day in divided doses q8h

Available forms include: Tabs 250, 500 mg; chew tabs 125, 250 mg; powder for oral susp 125, 250 mg/5 ml

Side effects/adverse reactions:

HEMA: Anemia, ***bone marrow depression, granulocytopenia, leukopenia, eosinophilia,*** thrombocytopenic purpura

GI: Nausea, diarrhea, vomiting, increased AST, ALT, abdominal pain, glossitis, colitis, black tongue

GU: Oliguria, proteinuria, hematuria, *vaginitis, moniliasis, **glomerulonephritis***

CNS: Headache

META: Hyperkalemia, hypokalemia, alkalosis, hypernatremia

Contraindications: Hypersensitivity to penicillins; neonates

Precautions: Pregnancy (B), hypersensitivity to cephalosporins

Interactions/incompatibilities:
- Decreased antimicrobial effectiveness of amoxicillin: tetracyclines, erythromycins
- Increased amoxicillin concentrations: aspirin, probenecid

Pharmacokinetics:

PO: Peak 2 hr, duration 6-8 hr; half-life 1-1⅓ hr, metabolized in liver, excreted in urine, crosses placenta, enters breast milk

NURSING CONSIDERATIONS
Assess:
- I&O ratio; report hematuria, oliguria since penicillin in high doses is nephrotoxic
- Any patient with a compromised renal system, since drug is excreted slowly in poor renal system function; toxicity may occur rapidly
- Liver studies: AST, ALT

- Blood studies: WBC, RBC, H&H, bleeding time
- Renal studies: urinalysis, protein, blood
- Culture, sensitivity before drug therapy; drug may be taken as soon as culture is taken

Administer:
- After C&S completed

Perform/provide:
- Adrenaline, suction, tracheostomy set, endotracheal intubation equipment on unit
- Adequate intake of fluids (2000 ml) during diarrhea episodes
- Scratch test to assess allergy after securing order from physician; usually done when penicillin is only drug of choice
- Storage refrigerated for 2 wk, or room temperature for 1 wk

Evaluate:
- For therapeutic effectiveness: absence of temperature, draining wounds
- Bowel pattern before, during treatment
- Skin eruptions after administration of penicillin to 1 wk after discontinuing drug
- Respiratory status: rate, character, wheezing, tightness in chest
- Allergies before initiation of treatment, reaction of each medication; place allergies on chart, Kardex in bright red

Teach patient/family:
- Aspects of drug therapy: need to complete entire course of medication to ensure organism death (10-14 days); culture may be taken after completed course of medication
- To report sore throat, fever, fatigue (could indicate a superimposed infection)
- That drug must be taken in equal intervals around the clock to maintain blood levels, take on empty

---

italics = common side effects   ***bold italic*** = life threatening reactions

stomach with full glass of water
• To wear or carry a Medic Alert ID if allergic to penicillins
• To notify nurse of diarrhea

Lab test interferences:
False positive: Urine glucose, urine protein

Treatment of overdose: Withdraw drug, maintain airway, administer epinephrine, aminophylline, O_2, IV corticosteroids for anaphylaxis

---

amoxicillin trihydrate

(a-mox-i-sill'in)
Amoxican,* Amoxil, Apo-Amoxi,* Larotid, Novamoxin,* Polymox, Robamox, Sumox, Trimox, Utimox, Wymox

Func. class.: Broad-spectrum antibiotic
Chem. class.: Aminopenicillin

Action: Interferes with cell wall replication of susceptible organisms; the cell wall, rendered osmotically unstable, swells, and bursts from osmotic pressure

Uses: Effective for gram-positive cocci *(S. aureus, S. pyogenes, S. faecalis, S. pneumoniae)*, gram-negative cocci *(N. gonorrhoeae, N. meningitidis, E. coli)*, gram-positive bacilli *(C. diphtheriae, L. monocytogenes)*, gram-negative bacilli *(H. influenzae, P. mirabilis, Salmonella)*

Dosage and routes:
Systemic infections
• *Adult:* PO 750 mg-1.5 g qd in divided doses q8h
• *Child:* PO 20-40 mg/kg/day in divided doses q8h
Gonorrhea/urinary tract infections
• *Adult:* PO 3 g given with 1 g probenecid as a single dose
Available forms include: Caps 250,

500 mg; chew tabs 125, 250 mg; powder for oral susp 50, 125, 250 mg/5 ml

Side effects/adverse reactions:
HEMA: Anemia, increased bleeding time, *bone marrow depression, granulocytopenia*
GI: Nausea, vomiting, diarrhea, increased AST, ALT, abdominal pain, glossitis, colitis
CNS: Headache
SYST: **Anaphylaxis, respiratory distress**

Contraindications: Hypersensitivity to penicillins; neonates

Precautions: Pregnancy (B), hypersensitivity to cephalosporins

Interactions/incompatibilities:
• Decreased antimicrobial effectiveness of amoxicillin: tetracyclines, erythromycins
• Increased amoxicillin concentrations: aspirin, probenecid

Pharmacokinetics:
PO: Peak 2 hr, duration 6-8 hr; half-life 1-1⅓ hr, metabolized in liver, excreted in urine, crosses placenta, enters breast milk

NURSING CONSIDERATIONS
Assess:
• I&O ratio; report hematuria, oliguria since penicillin in high doses is nephrotoxic
• Any patient with a compromised renal system, since drug is excreted slowly in poor renal system function; toxicity may occur rapidly
• Liver studies: AST, ALT
• Blood studies: WBC, RBC, H&H, bleeding time
• Renal studies: urinalysis, protein, blood
• Culture, sensitivity before drug therapy; drug may be taken as soon as culture is taken

Administer:
• After C&S completed

---

* Available in Canada only

Perform/provide:

• Adrenaline, suction, tracheostomy set, endotracheal intubation equipment on unit

• Adequate intake of fluids (2000 ml) during diarrhea episodes

• Scratch test to assess allergy after securing order from physician; usually done when penicillin is only drug of choice

• Storage in tight container; after reconstituting, oral suspension refrigerated for 2 wk or stored at room temperature for 1 wk

Evaluate:

• Therapeutic effectiveness: absence of temperature, draining wounds

• Bowel pattern before, during treatment

• Skin eruptions after administration of penicillin to 1 wk after discontinuing drug

• Respiratory status: rate, character, wheezing, tightness in the chest

• Allergies before initiation of treatment, reaction of each medication; place allergies on chart, Kardex in bright red

Teach patient/family:

• Aspects of drug therapy: need to complete entire course of medication to ensure organism death (10-14 days); culture may be taken after completed course of medication

• To report sore throat, fever, fatigue, diarrhea (could indicate a superimposed infection)

• That drug must be taken in equal intervals around the clock to maintain blood levels, take on empty stomach with a full glass of water

• To wear or carry a Medic Alert ID if allergic to penicillins

Lab test interferences:

False positive: Urine glucose, urine protein

Treatment of overdose: Withdraw

drug, maintain airway, administer epinephrine, aminophylline, O₂, IV corticosteroids for anaphylaxis

---

amphetamine sulfate

(am-fet′a-meen)

Racemic Amphetamine Sulfate

Func. class.: Cerebral stimulant

Chem. class.: Amphetamine

Controlled Substance Schedule II

Action: Increases release of norepinephrine, dopamine in cerebral cortex to reticular activating system

Uses: Narcolepsy, exogenous obesity, attention deficit disorder

Dosage and routes:

Narcolepsy

• *Adult:* PO 5-60 mg qd in divided doses

• *Child >12 yr:* PO 10 mg qd increasing by 10 mg/day at weekly intervals

• *Child 6-12 yr:* PO 5 mg qd increasing by 5 mg/wk, max 60 mg/day

Attention deficit disorder

• *Child >6 yr:* PO 5 mg qd-bid increasing by 5 mg/day at weekly intervals

• *Child 3-6 yr:* PO 2.5 mg qd increasing by 2.5 mg/day at weekly intervals

Obesity

• *Adult:* PO 5-30 mg in divided doses 30-60 min before meals

Available forms include: Tabs 5, 10 mg; sus rel caps 15 mg

Side effects/adverse reactions:

CNS: Hyperactivity, insomnia, restlessness, talkativeness, dizziness, headache, chills, stimulation, dysphoria, irritability, aggressiveness, tremor

GI: Nausea, vomiting, anorexia, dry mouth, diarrhea, constipation, weight loss, metallic taste, cramps

---

italics = common side effects   ***bold italic*** = life threatening reactions

GU: Impotence, change in libido
CV: Palpitations, tachycardia, hypertension, dysrhythmias, decreased heart rate
INTEG: Urticaria
Contraindications: Hypersensitivity to sympathomimetic amines, hyperthyroidism, hypertension, glaucoma hypertrophy, severe arteriosclerosis, drug abuse, cardiovascular disease, anxiety
Precautions: Gilles de la Tourette's disorder, pregnancy (X), lactation, child <3 yr
Pharmacokinetics:
PO: Onset 30 min, peak 1-3 hr, duration 4-20 hr, metabolized by liver, excreted by kidneys, crosses placenta, breast milk, half-life 10-30 hr
Interactions/incompatibilities:
• Hypertensive crisis: MAOIs or within 14 days of MAOIs
• Increased effect of amphetamine: acetazolamide, antacids, sodium bicarbonate
• Decreased effect of amphetamine: barbiturates, tricyclics
• Decreased effect of: guanethidine
NURSING CONSIDERATIONS
Assess:
• VS, B/P since this drug may reverse antihypertensives; check patients with cardiac disease more often
• CBC, urinalysis, in diabetes: blood sugar, urine sugar; insulin changes may need to be made since eating will decrease
• Height, growth rate in children, growth rate may be decreased
Administer:
• At least 6 hr before hs to avoid sleeplessness
• For obesity only if patient is on weight reduction program that includes dietary changes, exercise; patient will develop tolerance, and

weight loss won't occur without additional methods; give 30-60 min before meals
• Gum, hard candy, frequent sips of water for dry mouth
Evaluate:
• Mental status: mood, sensorium, affect, stimulation, insomnia; aggressiveness may occur
• Physical dependency; should not be used for extended time; dose should be discontinued gradually
• Withdrawal symptoms: headache, nausea, vomiting, muscle pain, weakness
• Drug tolerance will develop after long-term use
• Dosage should not be increased if tolerance develops
Teach patient/family:
• To decrease caffeine consumption (coffee, tea, cola, chocolate) which may increase irritability, stimulation
• Avoid OTC preparations unless approved by physician
• To taper off drug over several weeks, or depression, increased sleeping, lethargy may occur
• To avoid alcohol ingestion
• To avoid hazardous activities until patient is stabilized on medication
• To get needed rest, patients will feel more tired at end of day
Treatment of overdose: Administer fluids, hemodialysis, peritoneal dialysis, antihypertensives for increased B/P; ammonium Cl for increased excretion

---

amphotericin B
(am-foe-ter′i-sin)
Fungizone
Func. class.: Antifungal
Chem. class.: Amphoteric polyene

Action: Increases cell membrane

permeability in susceptible organisms by binding sterols; decreases K, Na, and nutrients in cell

Uses: Histoplasmosis, blastomycosis, coccidioidomycosis, cryptococcosis, aspergillosis, phycomycosis, candidiasis, sporotrichosis causing severe meningitis, septicemia, skin infections

Dosage and routes:
• *Adult and child:* IV INF 1 mg/ 250 ml D_5W (0.1 mg/ml) over 2-4 hr or 0.25 mg/kg/day over 6 hr; may be increased gradually up to 1 mg/kg/day, not to exceed 1.5 mg/ kg; INTRATHECAL 0.1 mg, gradually increased to 0.5 mg q48-72 hr

Available forms include: Powder for inj 50 mg

Side effects/adverse reactions:
EENT: Tinnitus, deafness, diplopia, blurred vision

INTEG: Burning, irritation, necrosis at injection site, flushing, dermatitis, skin rash (topical route)

CNS: Headache, fever, chills, peripheral nerve pain, paresthesias, peripheral neuropathy, ***convulsions,*** dizziness

GU: Hypokalemia, axotemia, hyposthenuria, ***renal tubular acidosis,*** nephrocalcinosis, ***permanent renal impairment, anuria, oliguria***

GI: Nausea, vomiting, anorexia, diarrhea, cramps, ***hemorrhagic gastroenteritis, acute liver failure***

*MS: **Arthralgia, myalgia,*** generalized pain, weakness

HEMA: Normochromic, normocytic anemia, ***thrombocytopenia, agranulocytosis, leukopenia, eosinophilia,*** hypokalemia, hyponatremia, hypomagnesemia

Contraindications: Hypersensitivity, severe bone marrow depression

Precautions: Renal disease, pregnancy (B)

Pharmacokinetics:
IV: Peak 1-2 hr, initial half-life 24 hr, metabolized in liver, excreted in urine (metabolites), breast milk, highly bound to plasma proteins; penetrates poorly CSF, bronchial secretions, aqueous humor, muscle, bone

Interactions/incompatibilities:
• Increased nephrotoxicity: other nephrotoxic antibiotics (aminoglycosides, cisplatin, vancomycin, cyclosporine, polymixin B)
• Increased hypokalemia: corticosteroids, digitalis, skeletal muscle relaxants
• Antagonism: miconazole
• Do not mix in sodium solutions or diluent with preservatives

NURSING CONSIDERATIONS
Assess:
• VS q15-30 min during first infusion; note changes in pulse, B/P
• I&O ratio; watch for decreasing urinary output, change in sp gr; discontinue drug to prevent permanent damage to renal tubules
• Blood studies: CBC, K, Na, Ca, Mg q2 wk
• Weight weekly; if weight increases over 2 lb/wk, edema is present, renal damage should be considered

Administer:
• After diluting with 10 ml sterile water (no preservatives), then dilute with 500 ml of solution to concentration of 0.1 mg/ml
• Test dose of 1 mg/20 ml D_5W; give over 10-30 min
• IV using in-line filter (mean pore diameter >1 μm) using distal veins, check for extravasation, necrosis q8h
• Drug only after C&S confirms organism, drug needed to treat con-

---

italics = common side effects   ***bold italic*** = life threatening reactions

dition; make sure drug is used in life-threatening infections

Perform/provide:

• Protection from light during infusion, cover with foil

• Symptomatic treatment as ordered for adverse reactions: aspirin, antihistamines, antiemetics, antispasmodics

• Storage, protected from moisture and light; diluted solution is stable for 24 hr

Evaluate:

• Therapeutic response: decreased fever, malaise, rash, negative C&S for infecting organism

• For renal toxicity: increasing BUN, serum creatinine; if BUN is >40 mg/dl or if serum creatinine >3 mg/dl, drug may be discontinued or dosage reduced

• For hepatotoxicity: increasing AST, ALT, alk phosphatase, bilirubin

• For allergic reaction: dermatitis, rash; drug should be discontinued, antihistamines (mild reaction) or epinephrine (severe reaction) administered

• For hypokalemia: anorexia, drowsiness, weakness, decreased reflexes, dizziness, increased urinary output, increased thirst, paresthesias

• For ototoxicity: tinnitus (ringing, roaring in ears) vertigo, loss of hearing (rare)

Teach patient/family:

• That long-term therapy may be needed to clear infection (2 wk-3 mo depending on type of infection)

---

amphotericin B (topical)

(am-foe-ter′i-sin)

Fungizone

Func. class.: Local antiinfective
Chem. class.: Antifungal (polyene)

Action: Increases cell membrane permeability in susceptible organisms by binding sterols

Uses: Cutaneous, mucocutaneous infections caused by *Candida*

Dosage and routes:

• *Adult and child:* TOP bid-qid for 7-21 days or longer if needed

Available forms include: Cream, lotion, oint 3%

Side effects/adverse reactions:

INTEG: Urticaria, stinging, burning, dry skin, pruritus, contact dermatitis, erythema, staining of nail lesions

Contraindications: Hypersensitivity

Precautions: Pregnancy (B), lactation

NURSING CONSIDERATIONS

Administer:

• Enough medication to completely cover lesions, apply liberally and rub thoroughly into affected area

• After cleansing with soap, water before each application, dry well (as ordered)

Perform/provide:

• Storage at room temperature in dry place

Evaluate:

• Allergic reaction: burning, stinging, swelling, redness

• Therapeutic response: decrease in size, number of lesions

Teach patient/family:

• That skin and clothing may become discolored

• To apply with glove to prevent further infection

• To avoid use of OTC creams, ointments, lotions unless directed by physician

• To use medical asepsis (hand washing) before, after each application to prevent further infection

• Not to cover with occlusive dressing

- To continue even if condition improves
- That clothing may stain

---

ampicillin/ampicillin sodium/ampicillin trihydrate
(am-pi-sill'in)

Amcap, Amcill, Ampicin, Ampilean,* Ampicin-PRB,* Apo-Ampi,* D-Amp, NovoAmpicillin,* Omnipen, Penbritin,* Pfizerpen A, Principen, Roampicillin, Supen, Omnipen-N, Pen A/N, Polycillin-N, Totacillin-N

Func. class.: Broad-spectrum antibiotic
Chem. class.: Aminopenicillin

Action: Interferes with cell wall replication of susceptible organisms; the cell wall, rendered osmotically unstable, swells, bursts from osmotic pressure

Uses: Effective for gram-positive cocci *(S. aureus, S. pyogenes, S. faecalis, S. pneumoniae)*, gram-negative cocci *(N. gonorrhoeae, N. meningitidis)*, gram-negative bacilli *(H. influenzae, P. mirabilis, Salmonella, Shigella, L. monocytogenes)*, gram-positive bacilli

Dosage and routes:
Systemic infections
- *Adult:* PO 1-2 g qd in divided doses q6h; IV/IM 2-8 g qd in divided doses q4-6h
- *Child:* PO 50-100 mg/kg/day in divided doses q6h; IV/IM 100-200 mg/kg/day in divided doses q6h

Meningitis
- *Adult:* IV 8-14 g/day in divided doses q3-4h × 3 days
- *Child:* IV 200-300 mg/kg/day in divided doses q3-4h × 3 days

Gonorrhea
- *Adult:* PO 3.5 g given with 1 g probenecid as a single dose

Available forms include: Powder for inj IV, IM 125, 250, 500 mg, 1, 2, 10 g; IV inf 500 mg, 1, 2 g; caps 250, 500 mg; powder for oral susp 100, 125, 250, 500 mg/5 ml

Side effects/adverse reactions:
INTEG: Rash, urticaria
HEMA: Anemia, increased bleeding time, **bone marrow depression, granulocytopenia**
GI: Nausea, vomiting, diarrhea
GU: Oliguria, proteinuria, hematuria, *vaginitis, moniliasis, **glomerulonephritis***
CNS: Lethargy, hallucinations, anxiety, depression, twitching, **coma, convulsions**

Contraindications: Hypersensitivity to penicillins

Precautions: Pregnancy (B); hypersensitivity to cephalosporins; neonates

Pharmacokinetics:
PO: Peak 2 hr
IV: Peak 5 min
IM: Peak 1 hr
Half-life 50-110 min; metabolized in liver, excreted in urine, bile, breast milk, crosses placenta

Interactions/incompatibilities:
- Possible increased bleeding: oral anticoagulants
- Decreased antimicrobial effectiveness of ampicillin: tetracyclines, erythromycins
- Increased ampicillin concentrations: aspirin, probenecid
- Decreased effectiveness of: oral contraceptives
- Increased ampicillin-induced skin rash: allopurinol

NURSING CONSIDERATIONS
Assess:
- I&O ratio; report hematuria, oliguria since penicillin in high doses is nephrotoxic

---

italics = common side effects   ***bold italic*** = life threatening reactions

• Any patient with compromised renal system, since drug is excreted slowly in poor renal system function; toxicity may occur rapidly
• Liver studies: AST, ALT
• Blood studies: WBC, RBC, H&H, bleeding time
• Renal studies: urinalysis, protein, blood
• Culture, sensitivity before drug therapy; drug may be taken as soon as culture is taken
• Sodium levels when high doses of injectables are given to cardiac patients

Administer:
• After diluting with sterile H_2O 0.9-1.2 ml/125 mg drug, administer over 3-5 min (up to 500 mg), 10-15 min, (>500 mg) by direct IV; may be diluted in 50 ml or more of compatible solutions to a concentration of 30 mg/ml or less
• After C&S completed
• On empty stomach for best absorption

Perform/provide:
• Adrenaline, suction, tracheostomy set, endotracheal intubation equipment on unit
• Adequate intake of fluids (2000 ml) during diarrhea episodes
• Scratch test to assess allergy after securing order from physician; usually done when penicillin is only drug of choice
• Storage in tight container; after reconstituting oral suspension refrigerated for 2 wk or stored at room temperature for 1 wk

Evaluate:
• Therapeutic effectiveness: absence of temperature, draining wounds
• Bowel pattern before, during treatment
• Skin eruptions after administra-

tion of penicillin to 1 wk after discontinuing drug
• Respiratory status: rate, character, wheezing, tightness in chest
• Allergies before initiation of treatment; reaction of each medication; place allergies on chart, Kardex in bright red

Teach patient/family:
• To take oral penicillin on empty stomach with full glass of water
• Aspects of drug therapy: need to complete entire course of medication to ensure organism death (10-14 days); culture may be taken after completed course of medication
• To report sore throat, fever, fatigue, diarrhea (could indicate superimposed infection)
• That drug must be taken in equal intervals around the clock to maintain blood levels
• To wear or carry a Medic Alert ID if allergic to penicillins

Lab test interferences:
False positive: Urine glucose, urine protein

Treatment of overdose: Withdraw drug, maintain airway, administer epinephrine, aminophylline, O_2, IV corticosteroids for anaphylaxis

---

ampicillin sodium, sulbactam sodium

Unasyn

Func. class.: Broad-spectrum antibiotic
Chem. class.: Aminopenicillin

Action: Interferes with cell wall replication of susceptible organisms; the cell wall, rendered osmotically unstable, swells, bursts from osmotic pressure
Uses: Skin infections (*S. aureus, E. coli, K.* sp, *P. mirabilis, B. fra-*

gilis, *Enterobacter* sp., *A. calcoaceticus*), intraabdominal infections (*Enterobacter*, *K*. sp., *B*. sp., *E. coli*) gynecologic infections (*E. coli*, *Bacteroides* sp.)

Dosage and routes:
• *Adult:* IV 1 g ampicillin, 0.5 g sulbactam to 2 g ampicillin and 1 g sulbactam q6h, not to exceed 4 g/day sulbactam

Available forms include: Powder for inj 1.5 g (1 g ampicillin, 0.5 g sulbactam), 3.0 g (2 g ampicillin, 1 g sulbactam)

Side effects/adverse reactions:
HEMA: Anemia, increased bleeding time, *bone marrow depression, granulocytopenia*
GI: Nausea, vomiting, diarrhea, increased AST, ALT, abdominal pain, glossitis, colitis
GU: Oliguria, proteinuria, hematuria, *vaginitis, moniliasis, glomerulonephritis*
CNS: Lethargy, hallucinations, anxiety, depression, twitching, *coma, convulsions*

Contraindications: Hypersensitivity to penicillins

Precautions: Pregnancy, hypersensitivity to cephalosporins, neonates

Pharmacokinetics:
IV: Peak 5 min; half-life 50-110 min; little metabolized in liver, 75% to 85% of both drugs excreted in urine, diffuses to breast milk, crosses placenta

Interactions/incompatibilities:
• Decreased antimicrobial effectiveness of ampicillin: tetracyclines, erythromycins
• Increased ampicillin concentration: aspirin, probenecid

NURSING CONSIDERATIONS
Assess:
• Bowel pattern before, during treatment

• Respiratory status: rate, character, wheezing, tightness in chest
• I&O ratio; report hematuria, oliguria, since penicillin in high doses is nephrotoxic
• Any patient with compromised renal system, since drug is excreted slowly in poor renal system function; toxicity may occur rapidly
• Liver studies: AST, ALT
• Blood studies: WBC, RBC, Hct/Hgb, bleeding time
• Renal studies: urinalysis, protein, blood
• C&S before drug therapy; drug may be taken as soon as culture is taken

Administer:
• IV after diluting 1.5 g/4 ml or more sterile H_2O for inj; may be given over 15 min directly or diluted in 50 ml or more of compatible solution
• After C&S completed; on empty stomach

Perform/provide:
• Adrenaline, suction, tracheostomy set, endotracheal intubation equipment on unit for possible anaphylaxis
• Adequate intake of fluids (2000 ml) during diarrhea episode
• Scratch test to assess allergy after securing order from physician; usually done when penicillin is only drug choice
• Storage in tight container, out of light

Evaluate:
• Therapeutic response: absence of temperature, draining wounds, negative C&S
• Skin eruptions after administration of ampicillin 1 wk after discontinuing drug
• Allergies before initiation of treatment; reaction of each medication; place allergies on chart

---

italics = common side effects   ***bold italic*** = life threatening reactions

Teach patient/family:
• To report sore throat, fever, fatigue (could indicate superimposed infection)
• To wear or carry Medic Alert ID if allergic to penicillin products

Lab test interferences:
False positive: Urine glucose, urine protein

Treatment of overdose: Withdraw drug, maintain airway, administer epinephrine, aminophylline, O_2, IV corticosteroids for anaphylaxis

---

amrinone lactate

(am'ri-none)
Inocor

Func. class.: Cardiac inotropic agent
Chem. class.: Bipyrimidine derivative

Action: Positive inotropic agent with vasodilator properties; reduces preload and afterload by direct relaxation on vascular smooth muscle

Uses: Short-term management of CHF that has not responded to other medication; can be used with digitalis

Dosage and routes:
• *Adult:* IV BOL 0.75 mg/kg given over 2-3 min; start infusion of 5-10 µg/kg/min; may give another bolus ½ hr after start of therapy, not to exceed 10 mg/kg total daily dose

Available forms include: Inj 5 mg/ml

Side effects/adverse reactions:
*HEMA: **Thrombocytopenia***
CV: Dysrhythmias, hypotension, headache, chest pain
GI: Nausea, vomiting, anorexia, abdominal pain, ***hepatotoxicity, ascites,*** jaundice, hiccups

INTEG: Allergic reactions, burning at injection site
RESP: Pleuritis, ***pulmonary densities, hypoxemia***

Contraindications: Hypersensitivity to this drug or bisulfites, severe aortic disease, severe pulmonic valvular disease, acute myocardial infarction

Precautions: Lactation, pregnancy (C), children, renal disease, hepatic disease, atrial flutter/fibrillation

Pharmacokinetics:
IV: Onset 2-5 min, peak 10 min, duration variable; half-life 4-6 hr, metabolized in liver, excreted in urine as drug and metabolites 60%-90%

Interactions/incompatibilities:
• Excessive hypotension: antihypertensives

NURSING CONSIDERATIONS
Assess:
• B/P and pulse q5 min during infusion; if B/P drops 30 mm Hg, stop infusion and call physician
• Electrolytes: potassium, sodium, chloride, calcium; renal function studies: BUN, creatinine; blood studies: platelet count
• ALT, AST, bilirubin daily
• I&O ratio and weight qd, diuresis should increase with continuing therapy
• If platelets are $<150,000/mm^3$ drug is usually discontinued and another drug started

Administer:
• Do not mix with glucose solutions directly, chemical reaction occurs over 24 hr; precipitate forms if amrinone and furosemide come in contact
• Into running dextrose infusion through Y connector or directly into tubing; dilute with normal saline to concentration of 1-3 mg/ml,

---

*Available in Canada only

do not mix with glucose for long-term infusion
• By infusion pump for doses other than bolus
• Potassium supplements if ordered for potassium levels <3.0
Evaluate:
• Extravasation, change site q48h
• Therapeutic response: increased cardiac output, decreased PCWP, adequate CVP, decreased dyspnea, fatigue, edema
Treatment of overdose: Discontinue drug, support circulation

---

amyl nitrate

(am′il)
Amyl Nitrate Aspirols, Amyl Nitrate Vaporole

Func. class.: Coronary vasodilator
Chem. class.: Nitrate

Action: Relaxes vascular smooth muscle, may dilate coronary blood vessels, resulting in reduced venous return, decreased cardiac output; reduces preload, afterload, which decreases left ventricular end diastolic pressure, systemic vascular resistance
Uses: Acute angina pectoris
Dosage and routes:
Angina
• *Adult:* INH 0.18-0.3 ml as needed, 1-6 inhalations from 1 cap, may repeat in 3-5 min
Cyanide poisoning
• *Adult:* INH 0.3 ml ampule inhaled 15 sec until preparation of sodium nitrite infusion is ready
Available forms include: Inh pearls 0.18, 0.3 ml
Side effects/adverse reactions:
*CV: Postural hypotension, **tachycardia, cardiovascular collapse,** palpitations

CNS: Headache, dizziness, weakness, syncope
GI: Nausea, vomiting, abdominal pain
INTEG: Flushing, pallor, sweating
MISC: Muscle twitching, ***hemolytic anemia, methemoglobinemia***
Contraindications: Hypersensitivity to nitrites, severe anemia, acute myocardial infarction, increased intracranial pressure, hypertension
Precautions: Lactation, children, drug abuse, head injury, cerebral hemorrhage, hypotension, pregnancy (C)
Pharmacokinetics:
INH: Onset 30 sec, duration 3-5 min; metabolized by liver, ⅓ excreted in urine, half-life 1-4 min
Interactions/incompatibilities:
• Increased hypotension: alcohol, β-blockers, antihypertensive
NURSING CONSIDERATIONS
Assess:
• B/P, supine and sitting, pulse during treatment until stable
Administer:
• After wrapping, crushing ampule to avoid cuts
• Ordered analgesic if headache develops
• To patient who is sitting or lying down during treatment; keep head low, use deep breaths, which will decrease dizziness
• Drug, and have patient rest for 15 min
Perform/provide:
• Storage in light-resistant area in cool environment
Evaluate:
• Therapeutic response: relief of chest pain (angina)
• For drug tolerance: the need for more medication for each attack
• For postural hypotension, headache during treatment, which are

---

common side effects because of vasodilation

Teach patient/family:
• To keep a record of angina attacks, and what aggravates condition; prolonged chest pain may indicate MI, seek emergency treatment
• That medication may explode in presence of flame
• To take several deep breaths despite foul odor
• To make position changes slowly to prevent orthostatic hypotension
• To keep drug out of reach of children and in secure place, as there is high abuse potential

---

anistreplase (APSAC)

Eminase

Func. class.: Thrombolytic enzyme
Chem. class.: Anisolated plasminogen streptokinase activator complex

---

Action: Promotes thrombolysis by promoting conversion of plasminogen to plasmin
Uses: Management of acute myocardial infarction
Dosage and routes:
• *Adult:* IV 30 U over 4-5 min as soon as possible after onset of symptoms
Available forms include: Powder, lyophilized 30 U/vial
Side effects/adverse reactions:
HEMA: Decreased Hct, *GI, GU, intracranial, retroperitoneal,* surface bleeding, *thrombocytopenia*
INTEG: Rash, urticaria, phlebitis at site, itching, flushing
CNS: Headache, fever, sweating, agitation, dizziness, paresthesia, tremor, vertigo
GI: Nausea, vomiting

RESP: Altered respirations, dyspnea, *bronchospasm,* lung edema
MS: Low back pain, arthralgia
CV: Hypotension, dysrhythmias, conduction disorders
SYST: Anaphylaxis
Contraindications: Hypersensitivity, active internal bleeding, intraspinal or intracranial surgery, neoplasms of CNS, severe hypertension, cerebral embolism/thrombosis/hemorrhage
Precautions: Arterial emboli from left side of heart, pregnancy (B), ulcerative colitis/enteritis, renal disease, hepatic disease, hypocoagulation, COPD, subacute bacterial endocarditis, rheumatic valvular disease, intraarterial diagnostic procedure or surgery (10 days), recent major surgery
Pharmacokinetics: Half-life 105 min
Interactions/incompatibilities:
• Increased bleeding potential: aspirin, indomethacin, phenylbutazone, anticoagulants
NURSING CONSIDERATIONS
Assess:
• VS, B/P, pulse, respirations, neurologic signs, temperature at least q4h, temp >104° F or indicators of internal bleeding, cardiac rhythm after intracoronary administration
Administer:
• Reconstitute only with sterile water for injection (not bacteriostatic water), and roll (not shake) to enhance reconstitution
• As soon as thrombi are identified; not useful for thrombi more than 1 wk old
• Cryoprecipitate or fresh, frozen plasma if bleeding occurs
• Heparin therapy after thrombolytic therapy is discontinued, TT or

---

APTT less than 2 times control (about 3-4 hr)
• About 10% of patients have high streptococcal antibody titers, requiring increased loading doses
Perform/provide:
• Bed rest during entire course of treatment
• Storage of powder in refrigerator; use within 30 min after reconstitution
• Avoid invasive procedures: inj, rectal temperature
• Treat fever with acetaminophen
• Pressure of 30 sec to minor bleeding sites; inform physician if hemostasis not attained, apply pressure dressing
Evaluate:
• Allergy: fever, rash, itching, chills; mild reaction may be treated with antihistamines
• Bleeding during 1st hr of treatment (hematuria, hematemesis, bleeding from mucous membranes, epistaxis, ecchymosis)
• Blood studies (Hct, platelets, PTT, PT, TT, APTT) before starting therapy; PT or APTT must be less than 2 times control before starting therapy; TT or PT q3-4h during treatment
Lab test interferences:
Increase: PT, APTT, TT

---

anthralin

(an'thra-lin)
Anthra-Derm, Lasan, Drithocreme
Func. class.: Antipsoriatic/antieczema medication
Chem. class.:

Action: Inhibits epidermal cell replication by decreasing mitosis by inhibiting nucleic protein synthesis
Uses: Psoriasis, eczema, chronic dermatitis

Dosage and routes:
• *Adult and child:* TOP apply to affected area qd or bid
Available forms include: Top cream 0.1%, 0.2%, 0.25%, 0.4%, 0.5%, 1%; top oint 0.1%, 0.25%, 0.4%, 0.5%, 1%
Side effects/adverse reactions:
INTEG: Rash on normal skin, folliculitis, discoloration of nails, hair, skin
GU: Renal irritation, *toxicity*
Contraindications: Hypersensitivity, renal disease, inflamed skin, child, lactation
Precautions: Erythema, pregnancy (C)
Pharmacokinetics:
TOP: Absorption poor, absorbed amount excreted in urine
NURSING CONSIDERATIONS
Assess:
• Urinalysis qwk, for albumin, casts
Administer:
• Cover with dressing or paper tape to avoid staining clothing
• After putting on gloves to protect healthy skin, wash after application
• After covering healthy skin with a protectant such as petrolatum or zinc oxide to prevent damage to adjacent tissues
• For 2-4 wk as needed
• To scalp after olive oil or mineral oil is applied to head, remove scales using comb
• At hs, leave on required time (10 min-12 hr)
Perform/provide:
• Removal of gauze bandage, cream by applying mineral oil before cleaning area; if area is not cleaned, maceration may occur
• Storage in tight covered container at room temperature
Evaluate:
• Therapeutic response: decreased itching, redness, dry scaly area

---

italics = common side effects   ***bold italic*** = life threatening reactions

• Area of the body involved, including time involved, what helps or aggravates condition

Teach patient/family:

• To avoid application on normal skin or getting cream in eyes or mucous membranes

• That skin, nails, hair may turn brown-yellow color if applied to these areas

• To discontinue use if rash, irritation, folliculitis develops

---

antihemophilic factor (AHF)

(an-tee-hee-moe-fill'ik)

Hemofil M, Koate H.P., Koate H.S., Kryobulin VH,* Monoclate

Func. class.: Hemostatic
Chem. class.: Factor VIII

Action: Necessary for clotting, activates factor X in conjunction with activated factor IX, transformation of prothrombin to thrombin

Uses: Hemophilia A, patients with acquired circulating factor VIII inhibitors, factor VIII deficiency

Dosage and routes: Depends on severity of deficiency

• *Adult and child:* IV 10-20 U/kg q8-24 h; INF 10-20 ml/3 min

Available forms include: Inj IV (number of units noted on label)

Side effects/adverse reactions:

GI: Nausea, vomiting, abdominal cramps, jaundice, *viral hepatitis*

INTEG: Rash, flushing, *urticaria*

CNS: Headache, *lethargy, chills, fever, flushing*

HEMA: Thrombosis, hemolysis, AIDS

CV: Hypotension, tachycardia

RESP: Bronchospasm

Contraindications: Hypersensitivity, monoclonal antibody-derived factor VIII

Precautions: Neonates/infants, hepatic disease, blood types A, B, AB, pregnancy (C), factor VIII inhibitor

Pharmacokinetics:

IV: Half-life 4 hr, terminal 15 hr

NURSING CONSIDERATIONS

Assess:

• Blood studies (coagulation factors assay by % normal: 5% prevents spontaneous hemorrhage, 30%-50% for surgery, 80%-100% for severe hemorrhage)

• Pulse: discontinue infusion if significant increase

• Hct, Coombs' with blood types A, B, AB

• Test for factor VIII inhibitors before starting treatment, may require concomitant antiinhibitor coagulant complex therapy

Administer:

• After rotating gently to mix

• IV slowly, plastic syringe to reconstitute, administer; adheres to glass; use another needle as a vent when reconstituting

• After dilution with warm NS, D_5W, LR, give within 3 hr

• IV INF: give at ≤2 ml/min if concentration exceeds 34 U/ml or over 3 min if concentration is less than 34 U/ml

Perform/provide:

• Storage in refrigerator, do not freeze, after reconstitution, do not refrigerate

Evaluate:

• Therapeutic response

• Allergy: fever, rash, itching, jaundice; give Benadryl, continue therapy if reaction is mild

• Blood group of patient, donors (if applicable; most factor VIII not from specific blood group donors)

• Bleeding: ankles, knees, elbows, other joints

---

*Available in Canada only

Teach patient/family:
• To report any signs of bleeding: gums, under skin, urine, stools, emesis
• To avoid salicylates (increase bleeding tendencies)
• To prepare, administer factor VIII concentrates at first sign of danger
• Signs of viral hepatitis, AIDS
• That immunization for hepatitis B may be given first
• To report hives, urticaria, chest tightness, hypotension; may be monoclonal antibody-derived factor VIII
• To be checked q2-3 mo for HIV screen

---

antithrombin III, human
ATnativ

Func. class.: Antithrombin
Chem. class.: Pooled human plasma

Action: Inactivates thrombin and the activated forms of factors IX, X, XI, XII, resulting in inhibition of coagulation
Uses: Hereditary antithrombin III deficiency in connection with surgical or obstetrical procedures or for thromboembolism
Dosage and routes: Dosage is individualized. After first dose, antithrombin III level should increase to about 120% of normal; thereafter maintain at levels >80%; this is usually achieved by administering maintenance doses once every 24 hr
Available forms include: Lyophilized powder, 50 ml infusion bottles containing 500 IU antithrombin III with 10 ml sterile water for injection

Side effects/adverse reactions:
SYST: Bleeding, surface bleeding, ***anaphylaxis,*** vasodilatory effects
Precautions: Pregnancy (C), children
Pharmacokinetics: Unknown
NURSING CONSIDERATIONS
Assess:
• VS, B/P, pulse, respirations, neurologic signs, temperature at least q4h, temperature 104° F or indicators of internal bleeding, cardiac rhythm
• For neurologic changes that may indicate intracranial bleeding
• Retroperitoneal bleeding: back pain, leg weakness, diminished pulses
• Heparin after fibrinogen level is over 100 mg/dl; heparin infusion to increase PTT to 1.5-2 × baseline for 3-7 days
• After reconstituting with 10 ml of NS or D₅W; do not shake
• IV therapy using 0.22 or 0.45 micro filter
Perform/provide:
• Bed rest during entire course of treatment
• Avoidance of venous or arterial puncture, inj, rectal temperature
• Treatment of fever with acetaminophen or aspirin

---

apomorphine HCl
(a-poe-mor'feen)

Func. class.: Emetic, dopamine agonist
Chem. class.: Morphine, hydrochloric acid

Controlled Substance Schedule II
Action: Acts centrally by stimulating chemoreceptor trigger zone, which in turn acts on vomiting center
Uses: In poisoning/drug overdose

---

italics = common side effects   ***bold italic*** = life threatening reactions

to induce vomiting promptly (10-15 min); is almost 100% effective

Dosage and routes:
• *Adult:* IM/SC 2-10 mg then 200-300 ml evaporated milk or water, do not repeat
• *Child >1 yr:* IM/SC 0.07 mg/kg then 16 oz evaporated milk or water, do not repeat
• *Child <1 yr:* IM/SC 0.07 mg/kg then 8 oz evaporated milk or water, do not repeat

Available forms include: Soluble tabs (parenteral) 6 mg

Side effects/adverse reactions:
CNS: Euphoria, depression, restlessness, tremor, muscle weakness
GI: Nausea, anorexia, dry mouth, diarrhea, constipation, weight loss, metallic taste, cramps, salivation
CV: Circulatory failure, tachycardia, irregular rapid pulse, decreased B/P
RESP: Respiratory depression

Contraindications: Hypersensitivity to narcotics, respiratory depression, corrosive poisoning, coma, shock, narcosis from CNS depressants

Precautions: Children, cardiac decompensation, elderly, pregnancy (C)

Pharmacokinetics:
PO: Onset 10-15 min
SC: Onset 1-2 min, metabolized by liver, excreted by kidneys

Interactions/incompatibilities:
• Incompatible with iodides, iron preparations, tannins, oxidizing agents

NURSING CONSIDERATIONS
Assess:
• Vital signs, B/P; check patients with cardiac disease more often, administer to conscious patients only

Administer:
• Dopamine antagonists to reverse emetic effect of this drug

• Activated charcoal if this drug doesn't work; may begin lavage after 10-15 min

Perform/provide:
• Only clear solutions; do not expose to light or air

Evaluate:
• Type of poisoning; do not administer if petroleum products or caustic substances have been ingested: kerosene, gasoline, lye, Drano
• Respiratory status before, during, after administration of emetic, check rate, rhythm, character; respiratory depression can occur rapidly with elderly or debilitated patients; record B/P, pulse; check for odor of alcohol on breath, clothes

---

apraclonidine HCl
(ap-raa-kloe'ni-deen)
Iopidine

Func. class.: Topical ophthalmic agent
Chem. class.: Selective α-adrenergic agonist

Action: Reduces intraocular pressure by reducing aqueous formation; exact mechanism of action unknown

Uses: Control elevations of intraocular pressure after laser iridotomy or trabeculoplasty

Dosage and routes
• *Adult:* Instill 1 gtt 1 hr before laser surgery, second gtt at completion of surgery

Available forms include: Sol 1% apraclonidine HCl, 0.01% benzalkonium chloride

Side effects/adverse reactions:
EENT: Upper lid elevation, conjunctival blanching, mydriasis, burning, dryness, itching, blurred vision, conjunctival microhemorrhage, foreign body sensation, dry

mouth, taste abnormalities, nasal dryness/burning
GI: Abdominal pain, diarrhea, cramps, emesis
CV: Bradycardia, palpitations, vasovagal attack, orthostatic episode
CNS: Insomnia, irritability, restlessness, headache, dream disturbances
OTHER: Shortness of breath, head cold sensation, sweaty palms, fatigue, paresthesia, pruritus
Contraindications: Hypersensitivity to this drug or clonidine, severe cardiovascular disease
Precautions: Pregnancy (C), lactation, children

NURSING CONSIDERATIONS
Assess:
• Cardiac status; watch for bradycardia, palpitations, especially in cardiac disease (including hypertension)
• Vasovagal attack during laser surgery primarily in individuals with history of such episodes
Administer:
• 1 hr before surgery and at completion of surgery; do not press on lacrimal sac
Perform/provide:
• Storage at room temperature, away from light
Teach patient/family
• Drug may cause burning, itching, blurring, dryness of eye area

---

aprobarbital

(a-proe-bar'bi-tal)
Alurate
Func. class.: Sedative/hypnotic-barbiturate
Chem. class.: Barbitone (intermediate acting)

Controlled Substance Schedule III (USA), Schedule G (Canada)

Action: Depresses activity in brain cells primarily in reticular activating system in brainstem, also selectively depresses neurons in posterior hypothalamus, limbic structures
Uses: Sedation, insomnia
Dosage and routes:
Sedation
• *Adult:* PO 15-40 mg tid or qid; use reduced dose in geriatrics
Insomnia
• *Adult:* PO 40-160 mg qhs, use reduced dose in geriatrics
Available forms include: Elix 40 mg/5 ml
Side effects/adverse reactions:
CNS: Lethargy, drowsiness, hangover, dizziness, confusion, *convulsion,* stimulation in elderly, lightheadedness
GI: Nausea, vomiting
INTEG: Rash, urticaria, *angioedema, Stevens-Johnson syndrome*
Contraindications: Hypersensitivity to barbiturates, respiratory disease, porphyria, addiction to barbiturates
Precautions: Hypertension, hepatic disease, renal disease, pregnancy (D)
Pharmacokinetics:
PO: Onset 1 hr, peak 3 hr, duration 6-8 hr; metabolized by liver, excreted by kidneys (up to 50% in unchanged form); half-life 27 hr
Interactions/incompatibilities:
• Increased CNS depression: alcohol, MAOIs, sedative, narcotics
• Decreased effect of: oral anticoagulants, corticosteroids, griseofulvin, quinidine, oral contraceptives, estrogens
• Decreased half-life of: doxycycline

NURSING CONSIDERATIONS
Assess:
• Blood studies: Hct, Hgb, RBCs,

---

serum folate (if on long-term therapy); pro-time in patients receiving anticoagulants

• Hepatic studies: AST, ALT, bilirubin; if increased, the drug is usually discontinued

Administer:

• After removal of cigarettes, to prevent fires

• After trying conservative measures for insomnia

• ½-1 hr before hs for sleeplessness

• On empty stomach for best absorption

Perform/provide:

• Assistance with ambulation after receiving dose

• Safety measures: siderails, nightlight, callbell within easy reach

Evaluate:

• Therapeutic response: ability to sleep at night, decreased amount of early morning awakening if taking drug for insomnia

• Mental status: mood, sensorium, affect, memory (long, short)

• Physical dependency: more frequent requests for medication, shakes, anxiety

• Barbiturate toxicity: hypotension; pulmonary constriction; cold, clammy skin; cyanosis of the lips; insomnia; nausea; vomiting; hallucinations; delirium; weakness; coma, pupillary constriction; mild symptoms may occur in 8-12 hr without drug

• Respiratory dysfunction: respiratory depression, character, rate, rhythm; hold drug if respirations are <12 /min or if pupils are dilated

• Blood dyscrasias: fever, sore throat, bruising, rash, jaundice, epistaxis

Teach patient/family:

• That hangover is common

• That drug is indicated only for short-term treatment of insomnia; is probably ineffective after 2 wk

• That physical dependency may result when used for extended periods of time (45-90 days depending on dose)

• To avoid driving or other activities requiring alertness

• To avoid alcohol ingestion or CNS depressants; serious CNS depression may result

• Not to discontinue medication quickly after long-term use; drug should be tapered over 1-2 wk

• To tell all prescribers that barbiturate is being taken

• That withdrawal insomnia may occur after short-term use; do not start using drug again, insomnia will improve in 1-3 nights, may experience increased dreaming

• That effects may take 2 nights for benefits to be noticed

• Alternate measures to improve sleep: reading, exercise several hours before hs, warm bath, warm milk, TV, self-hypnosis, deep breathing

Lab test interferences:

False increase: Sulfobromophthalein

Treatment of overdose: Lavage, activated charcoal, warming blanket, vital signs, hemodialysis, alkalinize urine

---

ascorbic acid (vitamin C)
(a-skor'bic)

Ascorbicap, Ascorbineed, Best-C, Cecon, Cemill, C-Long, C-Syrup 500, Cenolate, Cetane, Cevalin, Cevi-Bid, Ce-Vi-Sol, Cevita, Redoxon,* Solucap C, Vitacee, Viterra C

Func. class.: Vitamin C, water-soluble vitamin

Action: Needed for wound healing,

collagen synthesis, antioxidant, carbohydrate metabolism

Uses: Vitamin C deficiency, scurvy, delayed wound and bone healing, chronic disease, urine acidification, before gastrectomy

Dosage and routes:

Scurvy

• *Adult:* PO/SC/IM/IV 100 mg-500 mg qd, then 50 mg or more qd
• *Child:* PO/SC/IM/IV 100-300 mg qd, then 35 mg or more qd

Wound healing/chronic disease/ fracture

• *Adult:* SC/IM/IV/PO 200-500 mg qd
• *Child:* SC/IM/IV/PO 100-200 mg added doses

Urine acidification

• *Adult:* 4-12 g qd in divided doses

Available forms include: Tabs 25, 50, 100, 250, 500, 1000, 1500 mg; tabs effervescent 1000 mg; tabs chewable 100, 250, 500 mg; tabs timed release 500, 750, 1000, 1500 mg; caps timed release 500 mg; crys 4 g/tsp; powd 4 g/tsp; liq 35 mg/0.6 ml; sol 100 mg/ml; syr 20 mg/ml, 500 mg/5 ml; inj SC, IM, IV 100, 250, 500 mg/ml

Side effects/adverse reactions:

CNS: Headache, insomnia, dizziness, fatigue, flushing

GI: Nausea, vomiting, diarrhea, anorexia, heartburn, cramps

GU: Polyuria, urine acidification, oxalate or urate renal stones

HEMA: **Hemolytic anemia in patients with G-6-PD**

Contraindications: None significant

Precautions: Gout, pregnancy (A)

Pharmacokinetics:

PO, INJ: Metabolized in liver, unused amounts excreted in urine (unchanged) and metabolites, crosses placenta, breast milk

Interactions/incompatibilities:

• Increased effects of: salicylates, oral contraceptives
• Increased side effects of: PAS, digitalis, sulfonamides
• Decreased effects of: phenothiazines, disulfiram, amphetamines, heparin, coumarin (massive doses)

NURSING CONSIDERATIONS

Assess:

• I&O ratio
• Ascorbic acid levels throughout treatment if continued deficiency is suspected

Administer:

• By direct IV 100 mg over at least 1 min
• By IV INF diluted with compatible solutions and given over 15 min

Evaluate:

• Therapeutic response: absence of anorexia, irritability, pallor, joint pain, hyperkeratosis, petechiae, poor wound healing
• Nutritional status: citrus fruits, vegetables
• Injection sites for inflammation

Teach patient/family

• Necessary foods to be included in diet
• That if oral contraceptives are taken, increased levels of vitamin C are needed
• That smoking decreases vitamin C levels, not to exceed prescribed dose; increases will be excreted in urine, except time release

Lab test interferences:

• False positive, negatives in glucose tests
• False negative occult blood

---

italics = common side effects   ***bold italic*** = life threatening reactions

asparaginase (L-aspara-ginase)

(a-spar'a-gin-ase)
Elspar, Kidrolase
Func. class.: Antineoplastic
Chem. class.: E. coli enzyme

Action: Indirectly inhibits protein synthesis in tumor cells; without amino acid, DNA, RNA synthesis is halted; a nonvesicant

Uses: Acute lymphocytic leukemia in combination with other antineoplastics

Dosage and routes:
In combination
• *Adult:* IV 1000 IU/kg/day × 10 days given over 30 min; IM 6000 IU/m²/day
Sole induction
• *Adult:* IV 200 IU/kg/day × 28 days
Available forms include: Inj 10,000 IU

Side effects/adverse reactions:
SYST: Anaphylaxis, hypersensitivity
HEMA: Thrombocytopenia, leukopenia, myelosuppression, anemia, decreased clotting factors
GI: Nausea, vomiting, anorexia, cramps, stomatitis, hepatotoxicity, pancreatitis
GU: Urinary retention, *renal failure,* glycosuria, polyuria, azotemia, uric acid neuropathy
INTEG: Rash, urticaria, chills, fever
ENDO: Hyperglycemia
RESP: Fibrosis, pulmonary infiltrate
CV: Chest pain
CNS: Neuritis, dizziness, headache, *coma,* depression, fatigue, confusion, hallucinations

Contraindications: Hypersensitivity, infants, pregnancy (D), lactation, pancreatitis

Precautions: Renal disease, hepatic disease

Pharmacokinetics: Half-life 4-9 hr, terminal 1.4-1.8 hr

Interactions/incompatibilities:
• Decreased action of: methotrexate
• Do not use with radiation
• Increased toxicity: vincristine, prednisone
• Synergism: in combination with cytarabine, azauridine

NURSING CONSIDERATIONS
Assess:
• For signs and symptoms of pancreatitis (nausea, vomiting, severe abdominal pain), anaphylaxis (bronchospasm, dyspnea), cyanosis
• CBC, differential, platelet count weekly; withhold drug if WBC is <4000 or platelet count is <75,000; notify physician of these results
• Pulmonary function tests, chest X-ray studies before, during therapy; chest X-ray film should be obtained q2 wk during treatment
• Renal function studies: BUN, serum uric acid, ammonia urine CrCl, electrolytes before, during therapy
• I&O ratio; report fall in urine output of 30/ml/hr
• Monitor temperature q4h; may indicate beginning infection
• Liver function tests before, during therapy (bilirubin, AST, ALT, LDH) as needed or monthly
• RBC, Hct, Hgb since these may be decreased
• Serum, urine glucose levels

Administer:
• Allopurinol or sodium bicarbonate to reduce uric acid levels, alkalinization of urine
• IV infusion using 21-, 23-, 25-gauge needle; administer by slow

IV infusion after diluting 10,000 IU/5 ml of sterile H₂0 or 0.9% NaCl (no preservatives); use of filter may be necessary if fibers are present
• After intradermal skin testing and desensitization, give 0.1 ml (2 IU) intradermally after reconstituting with 5 ml sterile H₂O or 0.9% NaCl for injection; then add 0.1 ml of reconstituted drug to 9.9 ml diluent (20 IU/ml); observe for 1 hr, check for wheal
• Transfusion for anemia
• Antispasmodic

Perform/provide:
• Deep-breathing exercises with patient 3-4 × day; place in semi-Fowler's position
• Increase fluid intake to 2-3 L/day to prevent urate deposits, calculi formation
• Diet low in purines: absence of organ meats (kidney, liver), dried beans, peas to maintain alkaline urine
• Rinsing of mouth 3-4 × day with water, club soda
• Brushing of teeth 2-3 × day with soft brush or cotton-tipped applicators for stomatitis; use unwaxed dental floss
• Warm compresses at injection site for inflammation
• Nutritious diet with iron, vitamin supplements
• HOB increased to facilitate breathing

Evaluate:
• Bleeding: hematuria, guaiac, bruising or petechiae, mucosa or orifices q8h
• Dyspnea, rales, nonproductive cough, chest pain, tachypnea fatigue, increased pulse, pallor, lethargy, or swelling around eyes or lips, anaphylaxis may occur

• Food preferences; list likes, dislikes
• Yellowing of skin and sclera, dark urine, clay-colored stools, itchy skin, abdominal pain, fever, diarrhea
• Local irritation, pain, burning, discoloration at injection site
• Symptoms indicating severe allergic reaction: rash, pruritus, urticaria, purpuric skin lesions, itching, flushing, dyspnea
• Frequency of stools, characteristics: cramping, acidosis; signs of dehydration: rapid respirations, poor skin turgor, decreased urine output, dry skin, restlessness, weakness

Teach patient/family:
• To report any complaints or side effects to nurse or physician
• To report any changes in breathing or coughing

Lab test interferences:
Decrease: Thyroid function tests

---

aspirin

(as'pir-in)
Ancasal,* ASA, Aspirin,* Ecotrin, Empirin, Entrophen,* Novasen,* Sal-Adult,* Sal-Infant,* Supasa*
Func. class.: Nonnarcotic analgesic
Chem. class.: Salicylate

Action: Acts by blocking pain impulses in CNS that occur in response to inhibition of prostaglandin synthesis; antipyretic action results from inhibition of hypothalamic heat-regulating center
Uses: Mild to moderate pain or fever including arthritis, thromboembolic disorders, transient ischemic attacks in men, rheumatic fever, postmyocardial infarction

---

italics = common side effects   ***bold italic*** = life threatening reactions

Dosage and routes:
Arthritis
• *Adult:* PO 2.6-5.2 g/day in divided doses q4-6h
• *Child:* PO 90-130 mg/kg/day in divided doses q4-6h
Pain/fever
• *Adult:* PO/REC 325-650 mg q4h prn, not to exceed 4 g/day
• *Child:* PO/REC 40-100 mg/kg/day in divided doses q4-6h prn
Thromboembolic disorders
• *Adult:* PO 325-650 mg/day or bid
Transient ischemic attacks in men
• *Adult:* PO 650 mg bid or 325 mg qid
Available forms include: Tabs 65, 81, 325, 500, 650, 975 mg; chewable tabs 81 mg; caps 325, 500 mg; tabs controlled-release 800 mg; tabs time-release 650 mg; supp 60, 120, 125, 130, 195, 200, 300, 325, 600, 650 mg, 1.2 g; cream; gum 227.5 mg
Side effects/adverse reactions:
*HEMA: **Thrombocytopenia, agranulocytosis, leukopenia, neutropenia, hemolytic anemia,*** increased pro-time, PT, bleeding time
CNS: Stimulation, drowsiness, dizziness, confusion, ***convulsion,*** headache, flushing, hallucinations, ***coma***
*GI: Nausea, vomiting, **GI bleeding,*** diarrhea, heartburn, anorexia, ***hepatitis***
INTEG: Rash, urticaria, bruising
EENT: Tinnitus, hearing loss
CV: Rapid pulse, pulmonary edema
RESP: Wheezing, hyperpnea
ENDO: Hypoglycemia, hyponatremia, hypokalemia
Contraindications: Hypersensitivity to salicylates, GI bleeding, bleeding disorders, children < 3 yr, children with flu-like symptoms,

pregnancy (C), lactation, vitamin K deficiency, peptic ulcer
Precautions: Anemia, hepatic disease, renal disease, Hodgkin's disease, pre/post operatively
Pharmacokinetics:
PO: Onset 15-30 min, peak 1-2 hr, duration 4-6 hr
REC: Onset slow, duration 4-6 hr Metabolized by liver, excreted by kidneys, crosses placenta, excreted in breast milk, half-life 1-3½ hr
Interactions/incompatibilities:
• Decreased effects of aspirin: antacids, steroids, urinary alkalizers
• Increased blood loss: alcohol, heparin
• Increased effects of: anticoagulants, insulin, methotrexate
• Decreased effects of: probenecid, spironolactone, sulfinpyrazone, sulfonylamides
• Toxic effects: PABA, furosemide, carbonic anhydrase inhibitors
• Decreased blood sugar levels: salicylates
• Gastric ulcer: steroids, antiinflammatories
NURSING CONSIDERATIONS
Assess:
• Liver function studies: AST, ALT, bilirubin, creatinine if patient is on long-term therapy
• Renal function studies: BUN, urine creatinine if patient is on long-term therapy
• Blood studies: CBC, Hct, Hgb, pro-time if patient is on long-term therapy
• I&O ratio; decreasing output may indicate renal failure (long-term therapy)
Administer:
• To patient crushed or whole; chewable tablets may be chewed
• With food or milk to decrease

gastric symptoms; give 30 min before or 2 hr after meals

Evaluate:

• Hepatotoxicity: dark urine, clay-colored stools, yellowing of skin, sclera, itching, abdominal pain, fever, diarrhea if patient is on long-term therapy

• Allergic reactions: rash, urticaria; if these occur, drug may need to be discontinued

• Renal dysfunction: decreased urine output

• Ototoxicity: tinnitus, ringing, roaring in ears; audiometric testing needed before, after long-term therapy

• Visual changes: blurring, halos, corneal, retinal damage

• Edema in feet, ankles, legs

• Prior drug history; there are many drug interactions

Teach patient/family:

• To report any symptoms of hepatotoxicity, renal toxicity, visual changes, ototoxicity, allergic reactions (long-term therapy)

• Not to exceed recommended dosage; acute poisoning may result

• To read label on other OTC drugs; many contain aspirin

• That the therapeutic response takes 2 wk (arthritis)

• To avoid alcohol ingestion; GI bleeding may occur

Lab test interferences:

Increase: Coagulation studies, liver function studies, serum uric acid, amylase, CO_2, urinary protein

Decrease: Serum potassium, PBI, cholesterol

Interfere: Urine catecholamines, pregnancy test

Treatment of overdose: Lavage, activated charcoal, monitor electrolytes, VS

astemizole
(a-stem´-mi-zole)

Hismanal

Func. class.: Antihistamine

Chem. class.: H_1-histamine antagonist

Action: Acts on blood vessels, GI, respiratory system by competing with histamine for H_1-receptor site; decreases allergic response by blocking pharmacologic effects of histamine

Uses: Rhinitis, allergy symptoms

Dosage and routes:

• *Adult and child > 12 yr:* PO 10 mg qd, to reduce time to steady state may take 30 mg day 1, 20 mg day 2, followed by 10 mg daily

Available forms include: Tabs 10 mg

Side effects/adverse reactions:

GU: Frequency, dysuria, urinary retention, impotence

HEMA: **Hemolytic anemia, thrombocytopenia, leukopenia, agranulocytosis, pancytopenia**

RESP: Thickening of bronchial secretions, dry nose, throat

GI: Nausea, diarrhea, abdominal pain, vomiting, constipation

CNS: Headache, stimulation, drowsiness, sedation, fatigue, confusion, blurred vision, tinnitus, restlessness, tremors, paradoxical excitation in children or elderly

INTEG: Rash, eczema, photosensitivity, urticaria

CV: Hypotension, palpitations, bradycardia, tachycardia

Contraindications: Hypersensitivity, newborn or premature infants, lactation

Precautions: Pregnancy (C), elderly, children, respiratory disease, narrow-angle glaucoma, prostatic

hypertrophy, bladder neck obstruction, asthma
Pharmacokinetics:
PO: Peak 1-2 hr, 97% bound to plasma proteins; half-life is biphasic 3½ hr, 16-23 hr
Interactions/incompatibilities:
• Increased CNS depression: alcohol, other CNS depressants, procarbazine
• Increased anticholinergic effects: MAOIs
• Decreased action of: oral anticoagulants
NURSING CONSIDERATIONS
Assess:
• I&O ratio: be alert for urinary retention, frequency, dysuria; drug should be discontinued if these occur
• CBC during long-term therapy
Administer:
• On empty stomach, 1 hr before or 2 hr after meals
Perform/provide:
• Hard candy, gum, frequent rinsing of mouth for dryness
• Storage in tight, light-resistant container
Evaluate:
• Therapeutic reponse: absence of running or congested nose or rashes
• Respiratory status: rate, rhythm, increase in bronchial secretions, wheezing, chest tightness
Teach patient/family:
• All aspects of drug use; to notify physician if confusion, sedation, hypotension occurs
• To avoid driving or other hazardous activity if drowsiness occurs
• To avoid alcohol or other CNS depressants
Lab test interferences:
False negative: Skin allergy tests
Treatment of overdose: Administer ipecac syrup or lavage, diaz-epam, vasopressors, barbiturates (short-acting)

---

atenolol

(a-ten'oh-lole)
Apo-Atenol* Tenormin
Func. class.: Antihypertensive
Chem. class.: β-Blocker, β-1, 2 blocker (high doses)

Action: Competitively blocks stimulation of β-adrenergic receptor within vascular smooth muscle; produces negative chronotropic activity, positive inotropic activity (decreases rate of SA node discharge, increases recovery time), slows conduction of AV node, decreases heart rate, decreases O_2 consumption in myocardium; also, decreases renin-aldosterone-angiotensin system at high doses, inhibits β-2 receptors in bronchial system
Uses: Mild to moderate hypertension, prophylaxis of angina pectoris
Dosage and routes:
• *Adult:* PO 50 mg qd, increasing q1-2 wk to 100 mg qd; may increase to 200 mg qd for angina
Available forms include: Tabs 50, 100 mg
Side effects/adverse reactions:
*CV: **Profound hypotension, bradycardia, CHF,** cold extremities, postural hypotension, 2nd or 3rd degree heart block*
CNS: Insomnia, fatigue, dizziness, mental changes, memory loss, hallucinations, depression, lethargy, drowsiness, strange dreams, catatonia
*GI: Nausea, diarrhea, vomiting, **mesenteric arterial thrombosis, ischemic colitis***
INTEG: Rash, fever, alopecia

HEMA: Agranulocytosis, thrombocytopenia, purpura
EENT: Sore throat, dry burning eyes
GU: Impotence
ENDO: Increased hypoglycemic response to insulin
RESP: Bronchospasm, dyspnea, wheezing
Contraindications: Hypersensitivity to β-blockers, cardiogenic shock, heart block (2nd, 3rd degree), sinus bradycardia, CHF, cardiac failure
Precautions: Major surgery, pregnancy (C), lactation, diabetes mellitus, renal disease, thyroid disease, COPD, asthma, well compensated heart failure
Pharmacokinetics:
PO: Peak 2-4 hr; half-life 6-7 hr, excreted unchanged in urine, protein binding 5%-15%
Interactions/incompatibilities:
• Increased hypotension, bradycardia: reserpine, hydralazine, methyldopa, prazosin, anticholinergics, digoxin
• Decreased antihypertensive effects: indomethacin
• Increased hypoglycemic effect: insulin
• Mutual inhibition: sympathomimetics (cough, cold preparations)
• Decreased bronchodilation: theophyllines
• Paradoxical hypertension: clonidine

NURSING CONSIDERATIONS
Assess:
• I&O, weight daily
• B/P, pulse q4h; note rate, rhythm, quality
• Apical/radial pulse before administration; notify physician of any significant changes
• Baselines in renal, liver function tests before therapy begins

Administer:
• PO ac, hs, tablet may be crushed or swallowed whole
• Reduced dosage in renal dysfunction
Perform/provide:
• Storage protected from light, moisture; placed in cool environment
Evaluate:
• Therapeutic response: decreased B/P after 1-2 wk
• Edema in feet, legs daily
• Skin turgor, dryness of mucous membranes for hydration status
Teach patient/family:
• Not to discontinue drug abruptly, taper over 2 wk
• Not to use OTC products unless directed by physician
• To report bradycardia, dizziness, confusion, depression, fever
• To take pulse at home, advise when to notify physician
• To avoid alcohol, smoking, sodium intake
• To comply with weight control, dietary adjustments, modified exercise program
• To carry Medic Alert ID to identify drug that you are taking, allergies
• To avoid hazardous activities if dizziness is present
Lab test interferences:
Interference: Glucose/insulin tolerance tests
Treatment of overdose: Lavage, IV atropine for bradycardia, IV theophylline for bronchospasm, digitalis, O_2, diuretic for cardiac failure, hemodialysis

---

italics = common side effects   ***bold italic*** = life threatening reactions

atracurium besylate

(a-tra-cyoor'ee-um)

Tracrium

Func. class.: Neuromuscular blocker (nondepolarizing)

Chem. class.: Biquaternary ammonium ester

Action: Inhibits transmission of nerve impulses by binding with cholinergic receptor sites, antagonizing action of acetylcholine

Uses: Facilitation of endotracheal intubation, skeletal muscle relaxation during mechanical ventilation, surgery, or general anesthesia

Dosage and routes:

• *Adult:* IV BOL 0.4-0.5 mg/kg, then 0.08-0.10 mg/kg 20-45 min after 1st dose if needed for prolonged procedures

Available forms include: Inj IV 10 mg/ml

Side effects/adverse reactions:

CV: Bradycardia, tachycardia, increase, decrease B/P

*RESP: **Prolonged apnea, bronchospasm, cyanosis, respiratory depression***

EENT: Increased secretions

INTEG: Rash, flushing, pruritus, urticaria

Contraindications: Hypersensitivity

Precautions: Pregnancy (C), cardiac disease, lactation, children <2 yr, electrolyte imbalances, dehydration, neuromuscular disease, respiratory disease

Pharmacokinetics:

IV: Onset 2 min, duration 20-60 min; half-life 2 min, 29 min (terminal), excreted in urine, feces (metabolites), crosses placenta

Interactions/incompatibilities:

• Increased neuromuscular blockade: aminoglycosides, clindamycin, lincomycin, quinidine, local anesthetics, polymyxin antibiotics, lithium, narcotic analgesics, thiazides, enflurane, isoflurane

• Dysrhythmias: theophylline

• Do not mix with barbiturates in solution or syringe

NURSING CONSIDERATIONS

Assess:

• For electrolyte imbalances (K, Mg), may lead to increased action of this drug

• Vital signs (B/P, pulse, respirations, airway) until fully recovered; rate, depth, pattern of respirations, strength of hand grip

• I&O ratio; check for urinary retention, frequency, hesitancy

Administer:

• Using nerve stimulator by anesthesiologist to determine neuromuscular blockade

• Anticholinesterase to reverse neuromuscular blockade

• By slow IV over 1-2 min (only by qualified person, usually an anesthesiologist), do not administer IM

• Only slightly discolored solution

Perform/provide:

• Storage in light-resistant area

• Reassurance if communication is difficult during recovery from neuromuscular blockade

Evaluate:

• Therapeutic response: paralysis of jaw, eyelid, head, neck, rest of body

• Recovery: decreased paralysis of face, diaphragm, leg, arm, rest of body

• Allergic reactions: rash, fever, respiratory distress, pruritus; drug should be discontinued

Treatment of overdose: Edrophonium or neostigmine, atropine, monitor VS; may require mechanical ventilation

---

atropine sulfate

(a′troe-peen)

Func. class.: Anticholinergic-para sympatholytic

Chem. class.: Belladonna alkaloid

Action: Blocks acetylcholine at parasympathetic neuroeffector sites; increases cardiac output, heart rate by blocking vagal stimulation in heart; dries secretions by blocking vagus

Uses: Bradycardia, bradydysrhythmia, anticholinesterase insecticide poisoning, blocking cardiac vagal reflexes, decreasing secretions before surgery, antispasmodic with GU, biliary surgery

Dosage and routes:

Bradycardia/bradydysrhythmias

• *Adult:* IV BOL 0.5-1 mg given q1-2 hr, not to exceed 2 mg

• *Child:* IV BOL 0.01-0.03 mg/kg up to 0.4 mg or 0.3 mg/m², may repeat q4-6h

Insecticide poisoning

• *Adult and child:* IM/IV 2 mg qh until muscarinic symptoms disappear, may need 6 mg qh

Presurgery

• *Adult:* SC/IM/IV 0.4-0.5 mg before anesthesia

• *Child:* SC 0.1-0.6 mg 30 min before surgery

Available forms include: Inj 0.05, 0.1, 0.3, 0.4, 0.5, 0.8, 1 mg/ml; tabs 0.4 mg; tabs sol 0.4, 0.6 mg

Side effects/adverse reactions:

GU: Retention, hesitancy, impotence, dysuria

CNS: Headache, dizziness, involuntary movement, confusion, psychosis, anxiety, *coma,* flushing, drowsiness, insomnia

GI: Dry mouth, nausea, vomiting, abdominal pain, anorexia, constipation, *paralytic ileus,* abdominal distention

CV: Hypotension, paradoxical bradycardia, angina, PVCs, hypertension, tachycardia, ectopic ventricular beats

INTEG: Rash, urticaria, contact dermatitis, dry skin, flushing

EENT: Blurred vision, photophobia, glaucoma, eye pain, pupil dilation, nasal congestion

MISC: Suppression of lactation, decreased sweating

Contraindications: Hypersensitivity to belladonna alkaloids, angleclosure glaucoma, GI obstructions, myasthenia gravis, thyrotoxicosis, ulcerative colitis, prostatic hypertrophy, tachycardia/tachydysrhythmias, asthma

Precautions: Pregnancy (C), renal disease, lactation, CHF, tachydysrhythmias, hyperthyroidism, COPD, hepatic disease, child <6 yr, hypertension

Pharmacokinetics:

IV: Peak 2-4 min

IM: Peak 30 min

Half-life 2-3 hr, excreted unchanged by kidneys (70%-90% in 24 hr); metabolized in liver, crosses placenta, excreted in breast milk

Interactions/incompatibilities:

• Decreased effects of: phenothiazines

• Increased anticholinergics, effects of: anticholinergics, antidepressants, amantadine, MAOIs

• Incompatible with all drugs in solution or syringe (except analgesics)

NURSING CONSIDERATIONS

Assess:

• I&O ratio; check for urinary retention, daily output

• ECG for hypertension, ectopic

---

italics = common side effects   ***bold italic*** = life threatening reactions

ventricular beats, PVC, tachycardia

• For bowel sounds, check for constipation

Administer:

• IV undiluted or diluted with 10 ml sterile H_2O, give at a rate of 0.6 mg/min

• Increased bulk, water in diet if constipation occurs

• Frequent mouth rinsing, gum or candy for dry mouth

Perform/provide:

• Sugarless hard candy, gum, frequent rinsing of mouth for dryness

Evaluate:

• Respiratory status: rate, rhythm, cyanosis, wheezing, dyspnea, engorged neck veins

• Increased intraocular pressure: eye pain, nausea, vomiting, blurred vision, increased tearing

• Cardiac rate: rhythm, character, B/P continuously

• Allergic reaction: rash, urticaria

Teach patient/family:

• To report blurred vision, chest pain, allergic reactions

Treatment of overdose: O_2, artificial ventilation, ECG, administer dopamine for circulatory depression, administer diazepam or thiopental for convulsions; assess need for antidysrhythmics

---

atropine sulfate (optic)

(a′troe-peen)

Atropisol, BufOpto Atropine, Isopto Atropine

Func. class.: Mydriatic

Chem. class.: Belladonna alkaloid

Action: Blocks response of iris sphincter muscle, muscle of accommodation of ciliary body to cholinergic stimulation, resulting in dilation, paralysis of accommodation

Uses: Iritis, cycloplegic refraction

Dosage and routes:

• *Adult:* INSTILL SOL 1-2 gtts of a 1% sol qd-tid for iritis or 1 hr before refracting (cycloplegic refraction); INSTILL OINT 2-3 ×/day

• *Child:* INSTILL SOL 1-2 gtts of a 0.5% sol qd-tid for iritis or bid × 1-3 days before exam (cycloplegic refraction); INSTILL OINT qd-bid 2-3 days before exam

Available forms include: Oint 0.5%, 1%; sol 0.5%, 1%, 2%, 3%

Side effects/adverse reactions:

SYST: Tachycardia, confusion, fever, flushing, dry skin, dry mouth, abdominal discomfort (infants: bladder distention, irregular pulse, respiratory depression)

Contraindications: Hypersensitivity, infants <3 mo, open or narrow angle glaucoma, conjunctivitis, Down's Syndrome

Pharmacokinetics:

INSTILL: Peak 30-40 min (mydriasis), 60-180 min (cycloplegia), duration 6-12 days

NURSING CONSIDERATIONS

Evaluate:

• Therapeutic response: decrease in inflammation (iritis) or cycloplegic refraction

• Eye pain, discontinue use if pain occurs

Teach patient/family:

• To report change in vision, blurring or loss of sight, trouble breathing, sweating, flushing

• Method of instillation: pressure on lacrimal sac for 1 min, do not touch dropper to eye

• That blurred vision will decrease with repeated use of drug

• Not to do hazardous things until able to see

---

*Available in Canada only

- To omit next instillation if side effects are present
- Wait 5 min to use other drops
- Do not blink more than usual

---

auranofin

(aur-an-oo-fin)
Ridaura
Func. class.: Gold salt
Chem. class.: Active gold compound (2%)

Action: Antiinflammatory action unknown, may decrease phagocytosis, lysosomal activity or decrease prostaglandin synthesis; decreases concentration of rheumatoid factor, immunoglobulins
Uses: Rheumatoid arthritis
Dosage and routes:
- *Adult:* PO 6 mg qd or 3 mg bid, may increase to 9 mg/day after 3 mo
Available forms include: Caps 3 mg
Side effects/adverse reactions:
*HEMA: **Thrombocytopenia, agranulocytosis, aplastic anemia, leukopenia, eosinophilia***
*INTEG: Rash, pruritus, dermatitis, **exfoliative dermatitis,** urticaria, alopecia, photosensitivity*
CNS: Dizziness, syncope
GI: Diarrhea, abdominal cramping, stomatitis, nausea, vomiting, enterocolitis, anorexia, flatulence, metallic taste, dyspepsia, jaundice, increased AST, ALT, glossitis, gingivitis, melena, constipation
*GU: **Proteinuria, hematuria,** increased BUN, creatinine, vaginitis*
*RESP: **Interstitial pneumonitis, fibrosis,** cough, dyspnea*
Contraindications: Hypersensitivity to gold, necrotizing enterocolitis, bone marrow aplasia, child <6 yr, lactation, pulmonary fibrosis,
exfoliative dermatitis, blood dyscrasias, recent radiation therapy
Precautions: Elderly, CHF, diabetes mellitus, allergic conditions, ulcerative colitis, renal disease, liver disease, pregnancy (C)
Pharmacokinetics:
PO: Absorbed by GI tract, peak 2 hr, steady state 8-16 wk, excreted in urine, feces

NURSING CONSIDERATIONS
Assess:
- Respiratory status: dyspnea, wheezing; if respiratory problems occur, drug should be discontinued
- I&O ratio
- Urine: hematuria, proteinuria, increased BUN, creatinine, may require decrease in dosage
- Platelet counts q mo, drug should be discontinued if <100,000/mm³
- Hepatic test: ALT, AST, alk phosphatase, HCL as ordered for diarrhea
Administer:
- bid or may give as single dose q am with food or drink
Evaluate:
- Therapeutic response: ability to move joints with less pain
- Diarrhea stools; if severe, drug should be discontinued
- Allergy: rash, dermatitis, pruritus; drug should be discontinued if any of these occur
- Gold toxicity: decreased Hgb, WBC <4000/mm³, granulocytes <1500/mm³, platelets <150,000/mm³, severe diarrhea, stomatitis, hematuria, rash, itching, proteinuria
Teach patient/family
- That drug must be taken as prescribed to be useful, to obtain lab work monthly
- That diarrhea is common, but if blood appears in stools or urine notify physician at once, that patient

italics = common side effects   ***bold italic*** = life threatening reactions

should check for bruising, petechiae, bleeding gums
• To report skin conditions, stomatitis, fatigue, jaundice; may indicate blood dyscrasias
• To avoid exposure to sunlight or ultraviolet light
• That therapeutic effect may take 3-4 mo
• To use dilute hydrogen peroxide for mild stomatitis, avoid hot spicy foods, food with high acidic content; use soft toothbrush, rinse more frequently, floss daily
• That contraception should be used during treatment
• To use sunscreen to prevent burns
Lab test interferences:
False positive: TB test

---

aurothioglucose/gold sodium thiomalate

(aur-oh-thye-oh-gloo'kose)
Solganal/Myochrysine
Func. class.: Gold salts
Chem. class.: Active gold compound

Action: Antiinflammatory action unknown; may decrease phagocytosis, lysosomal activity, prostaglandin synthesis
Uses: Rheumatoid arthritis, psoriatic arthritis
Dosage and routes:
• *Adult:* IM 10 mg, then 25 mg q wk × 2-3 wk, then 50 mg/wk until total of 1 g is administered, then 25-50 mg q3-4 wk if there is improvement without toxicity (aurothioglucose) total of 800 mg-1 g
• *Adult:* IM 10 mg, then 25 mg after 1 wk, then 50 mg q wk for total of 14-20 doses, then 50 mg q2 wk × 4, then 50 mg q3 wk × 4, then 50 mg q mo for maintenance (gold sodium thiomalate)

• *Child 6-12 yr:* IM 1 mg/kg/wk × 20 wk, or ¼ of adult dose (aurothioglucose)
• *Child:* IM 1 mg/kg/wk × 20 wk, then q3-4 wk if improvement without toxicity (gold sodium thiomalate) not to exceed 2.5 mg
Available forms include: IM inj 50 mg/ml
Side effects/adverse reactions:
EENT: Iritis, corneal ulcers
HEMA: **Thrombocytopenia, agranulocytosis, aplastic anemia, leukopenia, eosinophilia**
INTEG: Rash, pruritus, dermatitis, urticaria, alopecia, photosensitivity, *exfoliative dermatitis, angioedema*
GI: Stomatitis, nausea, vomiting, metallic taste, jaundice, *hepatitis,* diarrhea
GU: Proteinuria, hematuria, *nephrosis, tubular necrosis*
RESP: Interstitial pneumonitis, pharyngitis, *pulmonary fibrosis*
CNS: Dizziness, syncope, EEG abnormalities, *encephalitis*
CV: Bradycardia, rapid pulse
SYST: **Anaphylaxis**
Contraindications: Hypersensitivity to gold, systemic lupus erythematosus, uncontrolled diabetes mellitus, marked hypertension, recent radiation therapy, CHF, lactation, renal disease, liver disease
Precautions: Decrease tolerance in elderly, children, blood dyscrasias, pregnancy (C)
Pharmacokinetics:
IM: Peak 4-6 hr; half-life 3-27 days, excreted in urine, feces
Interactions/incompatibilities:
• Increased blood dyscrasias: antimalarials, cytotoxic agents, immunosuppressants, oxyphenbutazone, phenylbutazone, penicillamine

---

NURSING CONSIDERATIONS
Assess:

• Respiratory status: dyspnea, wheezing; if respiratory problems occur, drug should be discontinued
• I&O ratio
• For pregnancy before administration; do not give in pregnancy
• Urine: hematuria, proteinuria, increased BUN, creatinine, may require decrease in dosage
• Platelet counts q mo, drug should be discontinued if <100,000/mm³
• Hepatic test: ALT, AST, alk phosphatase

Administer:

• bid or may give as single dose q AM
• Deep IM, never IV
• Slowly, keep recumbent for 10 min after injection, monitor for transient reaction

Evaluate:

• Therapeutic response: ability to move joints with less pain
• Diarrhea stools; if severe, drug should be discontinued
• Allergy: rash, dermatitis, pruritus; drug should be discontinued if any of these occur
• Gold toxicity: decreased Hgb, WBC <4000/mm³, granulocytes <1500/mm³, platelets <150,000/mm³, severe diarrhea, stomatitis, hematuria, rash, itching, proteinuria

Teach patient/family

• That drug must be taken as prescribed to be useful, to obtain lab work monthly
• That diarrhea is common, but if blood appears in stools or urine, notify physician at once, that patient should check for bruising, petechiae, bleeding gums
• To report skin conditions, stomatitis, fatigue, jaundice, which may indicate blood dyscrasias; report fever, chills, which may indicate infection
• That therapeutic effect may take 3-4 months
• To use dilute hydrogen peroxide for mild stomatitis, avoid hot spicy foods or food with high acidic content; use soft toothbrush, rinse more frequently
• That contraception should be used during treatment
• To use sunscreen to prevent burns

Lab test interferences:

False positive: TB test

---

azatadine maleate
(a-za'ta-deen)
Optimine

Func. class.: Antihistamine
Chem. class.: Piperidine H_1-receptor antagonist

Action: Acts on blood vessels, GI, respiratory system by competing with histamine for H_1-receptor site; decreases allergic response by blocking histamine

Uses: Allergy symptoms, rhinitis, chronic urticaria

Dosage and routes:

• *Adult:* PO 1-2 mg bid, not to exceed 4 mg/day

Available forms include: Tabs 1 mg

Side effects/adverse reactions:

CNS: Dizziness, drowsiness, poor coordination, fatigue, anxiety, euphoria, confusion, paresthesia, neuritis, sweating, chills

CV: Hypotension, palpitations, tachycardia

RESP: Increased thick secretions, wheezing, chest tightness

HEMA: **Thrombocytopenia, agranulocytosis, hemolytic anemia**

GI: Constipation, dry mouth, nausea, vomiting, anorexia, diarrhea

---

italics = common side effects   ***bold italic*** = life threatening reactions

INTEG: Rash, urticaria, photosensitivity

GU: Retention, dysuria, frequency, impotence

EENT: Blurred vision, dilated pupils, tinnitus, nasal stuffiness, dry nose, throat, mouth

Contraindications: Hypersensitivity to H_1-receptor antagonist, acute asthma attack, lower respiratory tract disease, child <12 yr

Precautions: Increased intraocular pressure, renal disease, cardiac disease, bronchial asthma, seizure disorder, stenosed peptic ulcers, hyperthyroidism, prostatic hypertrophy, bladder neck obstruction, pregnancy (B)

Pharmacokinetics:

PO: Peak 4 hr; metabolized in liver, excreted by kidneys, crosses placenta, crosses blood-brain barrier, minimally bound to plasma proteins, half-life 9-12 hr

Interactions/incompatibilities:

• Increased CNS depression: barbiturates, narcotics, hypnotics, tricyclic antidepressants, alcohol
• Decreased effect of: oral anticoagulants, heparin
• Increased effect of azatadine: MAOIs

NURSING CONSIDERATIONS
Assess:

• I&O ratio; be alert for urinary retention, frequency, dysuria; drug should be discontinued if these occur
• CBC during long-term therapy

Administer:

• With meals if GI symptoms occur; absorption may slightly decrease

Perform/provide:

• Hard candy, gum, frequent rinsing of mouth for dryness
• Storage in tight container at room temperature

Evaluate:

• Therapeutic response: absence of running or congested nose, or rashes
• Blood dyscrasias: thrombocytopenia, agranulocytosis; these occur rarely
• Respiratory status: rate, rhythm, increase in bronchial secretions, wheezing, chest tightness

Teach patient/family:

• All aspects of drug use; to notify physician if confusion, sedation, or hypotension occurs
• To avoid driving or other hazardous activities if drowsiness occurs
• To avoid concurrent use of alcohol or other CNS depressants

Lab test interferences:

False negative: Skin allergy tests

Treatment of overdose: Administer ipecac syrup or lavage, diazepam, vasopressors, barbiturates (short-acting)

---

azathioprine

(ay-za-thye'oh-preen)
Imuran

Func. class.: Immunosuppressant
Chem. class.: Purine analog

Action: Produces immunosuppression by inhibiting purine synthesis in cells

Uses: Renal transplants to prevent graft rejection, refractory rheumatoid arthritis, refractory ITP, glomerulonephritis, nephrotic syndrome, bone marrow transplant

Dosage and routes:

Prevention of rejection

• *Adult and child:* PO 3-5 mg/kg/ day, then maintenance of at least 1-2 mg/kg/day

Refractory rheumatoid arthritis

• *Adult:* PO 1/mg/kg/day, may increase dose after 2 mo by 0.5 mg/

kg/day, not to exceed 2.5 mg/kg/ day

Available forms include: Tabs 50 mg; inj IV 100 mg

Side effects/adverse reactions:

GI: Nausea, vomiting, stomatitis, esophagitis, *pancreatitis, hepatotoxicity, jaundice*

HEMA: Leukopenia, thrombocytopenia, anemia, pancytopenia

INTEG: Rash

MS: Arthralgia, muscle wasting

Contraindications: Hypersensitivity, pregnancy (D)

Precautions: Severe renal disease, severe hepatic disease

Pharmacokinetics: Metabolized in liver, excreted in urine (active metabolite), crosses placenta

Interactions/incompatibilities:

• Increased action of azathioprine: allopurinol

NURSING CONSIDERATIONS

Assess:

• Blood studies: Hgb, WBC, platelets during treatment monthly; if leukocytes are <3000/mm³ drug should be discontinued

• Liver function studies: alk phosphatase, AST, ALT, bilirubin

Administer:

• For several days before transplant surgery

• All medications PO if possible, avoiding IM injections since bleeding may occur

• With meals to reduce GI upset

Evaluate:

• Hepatotoxicity: dark urine, jaundice, itching, light-colored stools; drug should be discontinued

Teach patient/family:

• That therapeutic response may take 3-4 mo in rheumatoid arthritis

• To report fever, rash, severe diarrhea, chills, sore throat, fatigue since serious infections may occur

• To use contraceptive measures

during treatment, for 12 wk after ending therapy

• To avoid crowds

---

azlocillin sodium

(az-loe-sill′in)

Azlin

Func. class.: Broad spectrum antibiotic

Chem. class.: Extended spectrum penicillin

Action: Interferes with cell wall replication of susceptible organisms; the cell wall, rendered osmotically unstable, swells, bursts from osmotic pressure

Uses: Lower respiratory infections, skin, bone, bacterial septicemia, urinary tract infections, yaws; effective for gram-positive cocci *(S. aureus, S. pyogenes, S. faecalis)*, gram-positive bacilli *(C. perfringens, C. tetani)*, gram-negative bacilli *(Bacteroides, P. aeruginosa, E. coli)*, *H. influenzae, P. mirabilis*

Dosage and routes:

• *Adult:* IV 100-350 mg/kg/day in 4-6 divided doses, max 24 g

Cystic fibrosis

• *Child:* IV 75 mg/kg q4h max 24 g

Available forms include: Powder for inj 2, 3, 4 g

Side effects/adverse reactions:

HEMA: Anemia, increased bleeding time, *bone marrow depression, granulocytopenia*

GI: Nausea, vomiting, diarrhea, increased AST, ALT, abdominal pain, glossitis, colitis

GU: Oliguria, proteinuria, hematuria, *vaginitis, moniliasis, glomerulonephritis*

CNS: Lethargy, hallucinations, anx-

---

iety, depression, twitching, ***coma, convulsions***
META: Hypokalemia, alkalosis, hypernatremia
Contraindications: Hypersensitivity to penicillins
Precautions: Pregnancy (B), hypersensitivity to cephalosporins, neonates
Pharmacokinetics: Half-life 55-70 min, metabolized in liver, excreted in urine, bile, breast milk (small amount), crosses placenta
Interactions/incompatibilities:
• Decreased antimicrobial effectiveness of azlocillin: tetracyclines, erythromycins
• Increased azlocillin concentrations: aspirin, probenecid
NURSING CONSIDERATIONS
Assess:
• I&O ratio; report hematuria, oliguria since penicillin in high doses is nephrotoxic
• Any patient with compromised renal system, since drug is excreted slowly in poor renal system function; toxicity may occur rapidly
• Liver studies: AST, ALT
• Blood studies: WBC, RBC, H&H, bleeding time
• Renal studies: urinalysis, protein, blood
• Culture, sensitivity before drug therapy; drug may be taken as soon as culture is taken
Administer:
• IV after reconstituting 1 g/10 ml of compatible solution, shake
• After C&S completed
• Slowly (direct IV) over 5 min to prevent chest discomfort
• After further dilution in 50-100 ml of compatible solution, give over 30 min; change IV site q48h
Perform/provide:
• Adrenaline, suction, tracheostomy set, endotracheal intubation equipment on unit
• Adequate intake of fluids (2000 ml) during diarrhea episodes
• Scratch test to assess allergy after securing order from physician; usually done when penicillin is only drug of choice
• Storage in cool environment; solution is stable for 24 hr at room temperature
Evaluate:
• For therapeutic effectiveness: absence of temperature, draining wounds
• Bowel pattern before, during treatment
• Skin eruptions after administration of penicillin to 1 wk after discontinuing drug
• Respiratory status: rate, character, wheezing, tightness in chest
• Allergies before initiation of treatment; reaction of each medication; place allergies on chart, Kardex in bright red
Teach patient/family:
• Culture may be taken after completed course of medication
• To report sore throat, fever, fatigue (could indicate superimposed infection)
• To wear or carry a Medic Alert ID if allergic to penicillins
• To notify nurse of diarrhea
Lab test interferences:
False positive: Urine glucose, urine protein
Decrease: Uric acid
Treatment of overdose: Withdraw drug, maintain airway, administer epinephrine, aminophylline, O_2, IV corticosteroids for anaphylaxis

aztreonam

(az-tree'oo nam)

Azactam

Func. class.: Misc antibiotic
Chem. class.: Monobactam

Action: Inhibits organisms by inhibiting bacterial cell wall synthesis, which causes death of organism (bactericidal)

Uses: Urinary tract infection; septicemia; skin, muscle, bone infection; and other infections caused by gram-negative organisms

Dosage and routes:

Urinary tract infections

• *Adult:* IV/IM 500 mg − 1 g q8-12h

Systemic infections

Adult: IV/IM 1-2 g q8-12h

Severe systemic infections

Adult: IV/IM 2 g q6-8h, do not exceed 8 g/day

Continue treatment for 48 hr after negative culture or until patient is asymptomatic

Available forms include: Powder for inj 500 mg, 1, 2 g

Side effects/adverse reactions:

HEMA: Anemia, increased bleeding time, ***bone marrow depression, granulocytopenia***

GI: *Nausea, vomiting, diarrhea,* increased AST, ALT, abdominal pain, glossitis, colitis

CNS: Lethargy, hallucinations, anxiety, depression, twitching, ***coma, convulsions,*** malaise

EENT: Tinnitus, diplopia, nasal congestion

GU: Vaginal candidiasis, vaginitis, breast tenderness

Contraindications: Hypersensitivity

Precautions: Pregnancy (B), lactation, children, impaired renal, hepatic function

Pharmacokinetics:

IV: Peak immediate, trough 8 hr

IM: Peak 1 hr

Half-life: 1.7 hr, half-life prolonged in renal disease; protein binding 56%; metabolized by liver, excreted in urine, small amounts appear in breast milk, placenta

Interactions/incompatibilities:

• Decreased effect of both drugs: β-lactamase antibiotics (cefoxitin, imipenem)

• Incompatible with nafcillin, metronidazole, cephradine

NURSING CONSIDERATIONS

Assess:

• Signs of bruising, bleeding, anemia

• Bowel pattern before, during treatment

• Respiratory status: rate, character, wheezing, tightness in chest

• I&O ratio; report hematuria, oliguria, since this drug in high doses is nephrotoxic

• Any patient with compromised renal system, since drug is excreted slowly in poor renal system function; toxicity may occur rapidly

• Liver studies: AST, ALT

• Blood studies: WBC, RBC, Hgb & Hct, bleeding time

• Renal studies: urinalysis, protein, blood

Administer:

• Direct IV after diluting with 6-10 ml sterile H_2O/15 ml drug; give over 3-5 min

• IV INF after diluting with 3 ml or more sterile H_2O/1 g drug; then dilute with 50-100 ml of compatible solution; give over ½-1 hr

• IM; dilute each g with at least 3 ml of 0.9% NaCl; give into large muscle

• Drug after C&S completed

Perform/provide:

- Adequate fluid intake (2000/ml) during diarrhea episodes
- Storage in refrigerator

Evaluate:
- Therapeutic response: absence of fever, purulent drainage, redness, inflammation
- Skin eruptions after administration of drug to 1 wk after discontinuing drug
- Allergies before initiation of treatment, reaction of medication; highlight allergies on chart

Teach patient/family:
- Culture may be taken after completed course of medication
- To report sore throat, fever, fatigue; could indicate superimposed infection

---

bacampicillin HCl

(ba-kam-pi-sill'in)
Penglobe,* Spectrobid
Func. class.: Broad spectrum antibiotic
Chem. class.: Aminopenicillin

Action: Interferes with cell wall replication of susceptible organisms; the cell wall, rendered osmotically unstable, swells, bursts from osmotic pressure

Uses: Respiratory tract infections, skin urinary tract infections; effective for gram-positive cocci *(S. faecalis, S. pneumoniae),* gram-negative cocci *(N. gonorrhoeae),* gram-negative bacilli *(E. coli, H. influenzae, P. mirabilis)*

Dosage and routes:
- *Adult:* PO 400-800 mg q12h
- *Child:* PO 25-50 mg/kg/day in divided doses q12h

Available forms include: Tabs 400 mg; powder for oral susp 125 mg/ 5 ml

Side effects/adverse reactions:
HEMA: Anemia, increased bleeding time, **bone marrow depression, granulocytopenia**
GI: Nausea, vomiting, diarrhea, increased AST, ALT, abdominal pain, glossitis, colitis
GU: Oliguria, proteinuria, hematuria, *vaginitis, moniliasis, glomerulonephritis*
CNS: Lethargy, hallucinations, anxiety, depression, twitching, **coma, convulsions**

Contraindications: Hypersensitivity to penicillins; neonates

Precautions: Pregnancy (B), hypersensitivity to cephalosporins

Pharmacokinetics:
PO: Peak 30-60 min, duration 5-6 hr, half-life ½-1 hr, metabolized in liver, excreted in urine

Interactions/incompatibilities:
- Decreased antimicrobial effectiveness of bacampicillin: tetracyclines, erythromycins
- Increased bacampicillin concentrations: aspirin, probenecid
- Do not give with disulfiram

NURSING CONSIDERATIONS
Assess:
- I&O ratio; report hematuria, oliguria since penicillin in high doses is nephrotoxic
- Any patient with compromised renal system, since drug is excreted slowly in poor renal system function; toxicity may occur rapidly
- Liver studies: AST, ALT
- Blood studies: WBC, RBC, H&H, bleeding time
- Renal studies: urinalysis, protein, blood
- Culture, sensitivity before drug therapy; drug may be taken as soon as culture is taken

Administer:
- After C&S completed

---

* Available in Canada only

Perform/provide:
• Adrenaline, suction, tracheostomy set, endotracheal intubation equipment on unit
• Adequate intake of fluids (2000 ml) during diarrhea episodes
• Scratch test to assess allergy after securing order from physician; usually done when penicillin is only drug of choice
• Storage in dry tight container, oral suspension refrigerated for 2 wk or at room temperature for 1 wk

Evaluate:
• For therapeutic effectiveness: absence of temperature, draining wounds
• Bowel pattern before, during treatment
• Skin eruptions after administration of penicillin to 1 wk after discontinuing drug
• Respiratory status: rate, character, wheezing, tightness in chest
• Allergies before initiation of treatment; reaction of each medication; place allergies on chart, Kardex in bright red

Teach patient/family:
• Aspects of drug therapy: culture may be taken after completed course of medication
• To report sore throat, fever, fatigue (could indicate superimposed infection)
• To wear or carry a Medic Alert ID if allergic to penicillins
• To notify nurse of diarrhea
• That drug should be taken on an empty stomach, with a full glass of water

Lab test interferences:
False positive: Urine glucose, urine protein
Decrease: Uric acid
Treatment of overdose: Withdraw drug, maintain airway, administer epinephrine, aminophylline, O_2, IV corticosteroids for anaphylaxis

---

bacitracin
(bass-i-tray′sin)
Baci-IM
Func. class.: Antibacterial
Chem. class.: Bacillus subtilis derivative

Action: Inhibits bacterial cell wall synthesis, thereby interfering with osmotic pressure within cell
Uses: Staphylococcal pneumonia, empyema
Dosage and routes:
• *Infants >2.5 kg:* IM 1,000 U/kg/day in divided doses q8-12h
• *Infants <2.5 kg:* IM 900 U/kg/day in divided doses q8-12h
Available forms include: Inj IM 10,000, 50,000 U
Side effects/adverse reactions:
INTEG: Rash, pain at injection site
GI: Nausea, vomiting
*GU: **Proteinuria, casts, azotemia***
Contraindications: Hypersensitivity, severe renal disease
Precautions: Pregnancy (C)
Pharmacokinetics: Peak 1-2 hr, duration >12 hr, metabolized in liver, excreted in urine
Interactions/incompatibilities:
• Increased nephrotoxicity, neurotoxicity: aminoglycosides, polymyxin
• Increased neuromuscular blockage: nondepolarizing skeletal muscle relaxants, anesthetics

NURSING CONSIDERATIONS
Assess:
• I&O ratio; report oliguria, change in urinary output; high doses are nephrotoxic
• Any patient with compromised renal system; drug is excreted slowly in poor renal system func-

---

tion; toxicity may occur rapidly
• Renal studies: urinalysis, protein, blood, BUN, creatinine, urine pH (keep at 6.0)
• C&S before drug therapy; drug may be taken as soon as culture is taken; repeat C&S after treatment

Administer:
• After reconstituting with NS
• IM in deep muscle mass; rotate injection site; do not give IV/SC

Perform/provide:
• Storage in refrigerator; protect from direct sunlight
• Adrenalin, suction, tracheostomy set, endotracheal intubation equipment on unit
• Adequate intake of fluids (2000 ml) during diarrhea episodes

Evaluate:
• Therapeutic response: absence of fever, cough, dyspnea, malaise
• Bowel pattern before, during treatment; if severe diarrhea occurs, drug should be discontinued
• Skin eruptions, itching: rash, urticaria, erythema
• Respiratory status: rate, character, wheezing, tightness in chest, dyspnea on exertion
• Allergies before treatment, reaction of each medication; place allergies on chart, Kardex in bright red; notify all people giving drugs

Teach patient/family:
• To report sore throat, fever, fatigue; could indicate superimposed infection

Dosage and routes:
• *Adult and child:* Apply to conjunctival sac bid-qid until desired response
Available forms include: Oint 500 U/g

Side effects/adverse reactions:
EENT: Poor corneal wound healing, visual haze (temporary), overgrowth of nonsusceptible organisms

Contraindications: Hypersensitivity

Precautions: Antibiotic hypersensitivity, pregnancy (C)

NURSING CONSIDERATIONS
Administer:
• After washing hands, cleanse crusts or discharge from eye before application

Perform/provide:
• Storage at room temperature

Evaluate:
• Therapeutic response: absence of redness, inflammation, tearing
• Allergy: itching, lacrimation, redness, swelling

Teach patient/family:
• To use drug exactly as prescribed
• Not to use eye makeup, towels, washcloths, eye medication of others; reinfection may occur
• That drug container tip should not be touched to eye
• To report itching, increased redness, burning, stinging, swelling; drug should be discontinued
• That drug may cause blurred vision when ointment is applied

---

bacitracin (ophthalmic)
(bass-i-tray'sin)

Func. class.: Antiinfective

Action: Inhibits cell wall synthesis in bacteria
Uses: Infection of eye

---

bacitracin (topical)
(bass-i-tray'sin)
Baciguent, Bacitin*

Func. class.: Local antiinfective
Chem. class.: Antibacterial

Action: Interferes with bacterial

cell wall function by inhibiting protein synthesis

Uses: Topical staphylococci, streptococci

Dosage and routes:
• *Adult and child:* TOP bid-qid or more often if needed

Available forms include: Oint 500 U/g

Side effects/adverse reactions:
INTEG: Rash, urticaria, stinging, burning, contact dermatitis

Contraindications: Hypersensitivity

Precautions: Pregnancy (C), lactation

NURSING CONSIDERATIONS
Administer:
• After C&S is obtained, if lesion is weeping
• Enough medication to completely cover lesions
• After cleansing with soap, water before each application, dry well (as ordered)

Perform/provide:
• Storage at room temperature in dry place

Evaluate:
• Allergic reaction: burning, stinging, swelling, redness
• Therapeutic response: decrease in size, number of lesions
• For systemic effects and superimposed infections

Teach patient/family:
• To apply with glove to prevent further infection
• To avoid use of OTC creams, ointments, lotions unless directed by physician
• To use medical asepsis (hand washing) before, after each application to prevent further infection
• To watch for superimposed infections with long-term use

baclofen

(bak'loe-fen)
Lioresal, Lioresal DS
Func. class.: Skeletal muscle relaxant, central acting
Chem. class.: GABA chlorophenyl derivative

Action: Inhibits synaptic responses in CNS by decreasing GABA, which decreases neurotransmitter function; decreases frequency, severity of muscle spasms

Uses: Spinal cord injury, spasticity in multiple sclerosis

Dosage and routes:
• *Adult:* PO 5 mg tid × 3 days, then 10 mg tid × 3 days, then 15 mg tid × 3 days, then 20 mg tid × 3 days, then titrated to response, not to exceed 80 mg/day

Available forms include: Tabs 10, 20 mg

Side effects/adverse reactions:
CNS: Dizziness, weakness, fatigue, drowsiness, headache, disorientation, insomnia, paresthesias, tremors

EENT: Nasal congestion, blurred vision, mydriasis, tinnitus

CV: Hypotension, chest pain, palpitations, edema

GI: Nausea, constipation, vomiting, increased AST, alk phosphatase, abdominal pain, dry mouth, anorexia

GU: Urinary frequency

INTEG: Rash, pruritus

Contraindications: Hypersensitivity

Precautions: Peptic ulcer disease, renal disease, hepatic disease, stroke, seizure disorder, diabetes mellitus, pregnancy (C), elderly

Pharmacokinetics:
PO: Peak 2-3 hr, duration >8 hr,

---

half-life 2½-4 hr, partially metabolized in liver, excreted in urine (unchanged)

Interactions/incompatibilities:

• Increased CNS depression: alcohol, tricyclic antidepressants, narcotics, barbiturates, sedatives, hypnotics

NURSING CONSIDERATIONS

Assess:

• B/P, weight, blood sugar, and hepatic function periodically

• For increased seizure activity in epilepsy patient; this drug decreases seizure threshold

• I&O ratio; check for urinary retention, frequency, hesitancy

• ECG in epileptic patients; poor seizure control has occurred in patients taking this drug

Administer:

• With meals for GI symptoms

• Gum, frequent sips of water for dry mouth

Perform/provide:

• Storage in tight container at room temperature

• Assistance with ambulation if dizziness or drowsiness occurs

Evaluate:

• Therapeutic response: decreased pain, spasticity

• Allergic reactions: rash, fever, respiratory distress

• Severe weakness, numbness in extremities

• Psychologic dependency: increased need for medication, more frequent requests for medication, increased pain

• CNS depression: dizziness, drowsiness, psychiatric symptoms

• Dosage, as individual titration is required

Teach patient/family:

• Not to discontinue medication quickly; hallucinations, spasticity,

tachycardia will occur; drug should be tapered off over 1-2 wk

• Not to take with alcohol, other CNS depressants

• To avoid altering activities while taking this drug

• To avoid hazardous activities if drowsiness or dizziness occurs

• To avoid using OTC medication: cough preparations, antihistamines, unless directed by physician

• To increase fluid intake >2L/day

Lab test interferences:

Increase: AST, alk phosphatase, blood glucose

Treatment of overdose: Induce emesis of conscious patient, lavage, dialysis

---

beclomethasone dipropionate

(be-kloe-meth'a-sone)
Beclovent, Vancenase, Vanceril, Beconase

Func. class.: Corticosteroid, synthetic

Chem. class.: Glucocorticoid

Action: Prevents inflammation by depression of migration of polymorphonuclear leukocytes, fibroblasts, reversal of increased capillary permeability and lysosomal stabilization; does not suppress hypothalamus and pituitary function

Uses: Chronic asthma, rhinitis

Dosage and routes:

• *Adult:* INH 2-4 puffs tid-qid, not to exceed 20 inhalations/day

• *Child:* 6-12 yr: INH 1-2 puffs tid-qid, not to exceed 10 inhalations/day

Available forms include: Aerosol 42 μg/actuation

Side effects/adverse reactions:

RESP: **Bronchospasm**

GI: Dry mouth

EENT: Hoarseness, candidal infections of oral cavity, sore throat

Contraindications: Hypersensitivity, status asthmaticus (primary treatment), nonasthmatic bronchial disease, bacterial, fungal, or viral infections of mouth, throat, or lungs, children < 3 yr

Precautions: Nasal disease/surgery, pregnancy (C)

Pharmacokinetics:

INH: Onset 10 min, excreted in feces (metabolites), half-life 3-15 hr, crosses placenta, metabolized in lungs, liver, GI system

NURSING CONSIDERATIONS
Assess:
• Adrenal function periodically for HPA axis suppression

Administer:
• INH with water to decrease possibility of fungal infections
• Titrated dose, use lowest effective dose

Perform/provide:
• Gum, rinsing of mouth for dry mouth

Evaluate:
• Therapeutic response: decreased dyspnea, wheezing, dry rales on auscultation

Teach patient/family:
• That ID as steroid user should be carried
• To notify physician if therapeutic response decreases; dosage adjustment may be needed
• Proper administration technique
• Wash inhaler with warm water and dry after each use
• Teach patient all aspects of drug usage including Cushingoid symptoms
• Symptoms of adrenal insufficiency: nausea, anorexia, fatigue, dizziness, dyspnea, weakness, joint pain, depression
• To keep out of children's reach

beclomethasone dipropionate (nasal)

(be-kloe-meth'a-sone)
Beconase Nasal Inhaler, Vancenase Nasal Inhaler, Beclovent, Vanceril

Func. class.: Synthetic corticosteroid

Chem. class.: Beclomethasone diester

Action: Antiinflammatory, vasoconstrictive properties in nasal passages

Uses: Seasonal or perennial rhinitis

Dosage and routes:
• *Adult and child >12 yr:* INSTILL 1-2 sprays in each nostril bid-qid

Available forms include: Aero 42 µg/spray

Side effects/adverse reactions:

EENT: Dryness, nasal irritation, burning, sneezing, secretions with blood, nasal ulcerations, ***perforation of nasal septum,*** candida infection, earache

*ENDO: **Adrenal suppression***

INTEG: Rash, urticaria, pruritus

CNS: Headache, paresthesia

*RESP: **Acute status asthmaticus***

Contraindications: Hypersensitivity, systemic corticosteroid therapy

Precautions: Pregnancy (C), lactation, children <12, nasal ulcers, recurrent epistaxis respiration

Pharmacokinetics:

INSTILL: Readily absorbed; peak, concentration, other data have not been determined

NURSING CONSIDERATIONS
Assess:
• Adrenal function periodically for HPA axis suppression

Administer:
• After cleaning aerosol top daily with warm water, dry thoroughly

---

italics = common side effects   ***bold italic*** = life threatening reactions

Perform/provide:
• Storage in cool environment, do not puncture or incinerate container
Evaluate:
• Adrenal suppression: 17-KS, plasma cortisol for decreased levels
• Nasal passages during long-term treatment for changes in mucus
Teach patient/family:
• To clear nasal passages if sneezing attack occurs, repeat dose
• To continue using product even if mild nasal bleeding occurs, is usually transient
• Method of installation after providing written instructions from manufacturer
• To clear nasal passages before administration, use decongestant if needed, shake inhaler, invert, tilt head backward, insert nozzle into nostril, away from septum, hold other nostril closed and depress activator, inhale through nose, exhale through mouth

---

belladonna alkaloids

(bell-a-don′a)
Bellafoline
Func. class.: Gastrointestinal anticholinergic
Chem. class.: Belladonna alkaloid

Action: Inhibits muscarinic actions of acetylcholine at postganglionic parasympathetic neurone effector sites
Uses: Treatment of peptic ulcer disease, irritable bowel syndrome in combination with other drugs; for other GI disorders
Dosage and routes:
• *Adult:* PO 0.25-0.5 mg tid; SC 0.125-0.5 mg qd or bid
• *Child >6 yr:* PO 0.125-0.25 mg tid

Available forms include: Tabs 0.25 mg; inj SC 0.5 mg/ml
Side effects/adverse reactions:
CNS: Confusion, stimulation in elderly, headache, insomnia, dizziness, drowsiness, anxiety, weakness, hallucination
GI: Dry mouth, constipation, paralytic ileus, heartburn, nausea, vomiting, dysphagia, absence of taste
GU: Hesitancy, retention, impotence
CV: Palpitations, tachycardia
EENT: Blurred vision, photophobia, mydriasis, cycloplegia, increased ocular tension
INTEG: Urticaria, rash, pruritus, anhidrosis, fever, allergic reactions, flushing
Contraindications: Hypersensitivity to anticholinergics, narrow-angle glaucoma, GI obstruction, myasthenia gravis, paralytic ileus, GI atony, toxic megacolon
Precautions: Hyperthyroidism, coronary artery disease, dysrhythmias, CHF, ulcerative colitis, hypertension, hiatal hernia, hepatic disease, renal disease, pregnancy (C), urinary obstruction
Pharmacokinetics:
PO: Duration 4-6 hr; metabolized by liver, excreted in urine, half-life 13-38 hr
Interactions/incompatibilities:
• Increased anticholinergic effect: amantadine, tricyclic antidepressants, MAOIs
• Increased effect of: nitrofurantoin
• Decreased effect of: phenothiazines, levodopa
NURSING CONSIDERATIONS
Assess:
• VS, cardiac status: checking for dysrhythmias, increased rate, palpitations, flushing

• I&O ratio; check for urinary retention or hesitancy

Administer:

• ½-1 hr ac for better absorption

• Decreased dose to elderly patients; their metabolism may be slowed

• Gum, hard candy, frequent rinsing of mouth for dryness of oral cavity

Perform/provide:

• Storage in tight container protected from light

• Increased fluids, bulk, exercise to patient's lifestyle to decrease constipation

Evaluate:

• Therapeutic response: absence of epigastric pain, bleeding, nausea, vomiting

• GI complaints: pain, bleeding (frank or occult), nausea, vomiting, anorexia, constipation

Teach patient/family:

• Avoid driving or other hazardous activities until stabilized on medication

• Avoid alcohol or other CNS depressants; will enhance sedating properties of this drug

• To avoid hot environments, stroke may occur, drug suppresses perspiration

• Use sunglasses when outside to prevent photophobia

---

bentiromide

(ben-teer'oh-mide)
Chymex
Func. class.: Digestant
Chem. class.: Synthetic peptide with PABA

Action: A peptide that carries a PABA marker that can be detected
Uses: Pancreatic exocrine insufficiency screening, to assess pan-

creatic enzyme replacement therapy

Dosage and routes:

• *Adult and child >12 yr:* PO 500 mg with 8 oz water

• *Child <12 yr:* PO 14 mg/kg with 8 oz water

Available forms include: Sol 500 mg/7.5 ml

Side effects/adverse reactions:

CNS: Headache, dizziness, drowsiness, weakness

GI: Nausea, vomiting, *diarrhea,* abdominal pain, flatulence, increased liver enzymes

RESP: Acute respiratory distress, stridor

Contraindications: Hypersensitivity

Precautions: Pregnancy (B), lactation, children, diabetes

Pharmacokinetics:

Peak 2-3 hr, metabolized in liver, excreted in urine (metabolites)

Interactions/incompatibilities:

• Decreased action of: sulfonamides

• Increased therapeutic and toxic effects of: salicylates

NURSING CONSIDERATIONS
Administer:

• After 8 hr NPO

• Whole, not to be crushed or chewed

• With water, give 16 oz of water 2 hr after dose, another 16 oz 4-6 hr after dose

Perform/provide:

• Storage at room temperature

• Collection of urine specimens (10-20 ml) for testing at hours 1-6 after drug administration

Evaluate:

• Bowel pattern before, during treatment: diarrhea may occur

Teach patient/family:

• To drink water 2-3 L for 24 hr

---

italics = common side effects   ***bold italic*** = life threatening reactions

following test to promote elimination of drug
• Retest can be done 1 wk after initial test
• To void before taking drug

Lab test interferences:
False increase: PABA drugs, arylamines

---

benzalkonium chloride

(benz-al-koe′nee-um)
Benasept, Benzachlor-50,* Bena-All, Ionax Scrub,* Sabol Shampoo,* Zalkon, Zalkonium Chloride, Zephiran, Zephiran Chloride,* Mercurochrome II, Benza, Dermo-Sterol
Func. class.: Disinfectant
Chem. class.: Quaternary ammonium cationic surfactant

Action: Inhibits and destroys organisms by enzyme inactivation (bactericidal/bacteriostatic)
Uses: Irrigate eye, vagina, body cavities, disinfection of skin before surgery

Dosage and routes:
• *Adult and child:* TOP 1:750 for minor wounds, disinfection before surgery; 1:3000-20,000 deep infected wounds; 1:2000-5000 vaginal irrigation; 1:5000-10,000 denuded skin, eye, mucous membrane irrigation; 1:5,000-20,000 bladder, urethral irrigation
Available forms include: Top sol 0.1%, 0.13%, 17%, 17.5%, 50%; tinct 0.13%

Side effects/adverse reactions:
CNS: Confusion, restlessness
INTEG: Irritation, contact dermatitis, hypersensitivity, rash, burning
GI: Nausea, vomiting
RESP: Dyspnea, *respiratory paralysis, coma* (if ingested)
Contraindications: Hypersensitivity, occlusive dressing, casts/traction

Interactions/incompatibilities:
• Decreased action of benzalkonium: soap
• Not to be used with fluorescein, nitrates, lanolin, potassium permanganate, kaolin, zinc sulfate, zinc oxide, caramel, aluminum, iodine, peroxide, yellow oxide of mercury, citrates, sulfonamides

NURSING CONSIDERATIONS
Administer:
• After diluting with sterile water for injection for irrigating wounds
• To ⅓ of body or less to avoid chilling

Perform/provide:
• Rust tablets for cleaning metal objects, or instrument will rust
• Wet dressings using clear solution only; discontinue if necrosis occurs

Evaluate:
• Area of body involved: irritation, rash, breaks, dryness, scales, discharge

Teach patient/family:
• To store at room temperature no longer than 1 wk
• To use applicator, insert high into vagina, notify physician of itching, discharge, burning

Treatment of ingestion: Administer milk, soap solution, gastric lavage, supportive care

---

benzocaine (oral)

(ben-zoe-kane)
Orabase with Benzocaine, Oracin, Ora-Jel, Spec-T Anesthetic, Trocaine, Tyzomint, Solarcaine, Dermoplast, Chiggerex, Benzocal, Americaine
Func. class.: Topical local anesthetic
Chem. class.: Ester

Action: Inhibits conduction of

---

nerve impulses from sensory nerves

Uses: Oral irritation, sore throat, toothache, cold sore, canker sore, sunburn, minor cuts, insect bites, pain, itching

Dosage and routes:
• *Adult and child >12 yr:* TOP apply to affected area; LOZ suck as needed

Available forms include: Cream 1%, 5%; lotion 0.5%, 8%; oint 2%, 5%, 20%; sol 2.1%, 2.5%, 6.3%, 20%; lozenges 3, 5, 6.25, 10 mg; topical aerosol 20%; gel 6.3%, 7.5%, 10%, 20%

Side effects/adverse reactions:
EENT: Itching, irritation in ear
INTEG: Rash, urticaria

Contraindications: Hypersensitivity

Precautions: Pregnancy (C)

Pharmacokinetics:
TOP: Peak 1 min, duration ½-1 hr

NURSING CONSIDERATIONS
Administer:
• To gums as needed for teething pain
• Lozenges for temporary sore throat pain

Perform/provide:
• Storage in tight, light-resistant container; do not freeze, puncture, or incinerate aerosol container

Evaluate:
• Affected area for redness, swelling, pain

Teach patient/family:
• To avoid contact with eyes
• Not to use for prolonged periods of time <1 wk; if condition remains, physician should be contacted

benzocaine (otic)

(ben'zoe-caine)
Americaine-Otic, Auralgan, Eardro, Myringacaine, Tympagesic, Otocain

Func. class.: Otic
Chem. class.: Paraminobenzoic acid ethyl ester (PABA)

Action: Inhibits nerve impulse conduction in sensory nerves (surface anesthesia), decreases ear pain

Uses: Removal of cerumen, otitis media pain

Dosage and routes:
• *Adult and child:* INSTILL in ear canal tid × 2 days

Otitis media pain
• *Adult and child:* INSTILL in ear canal, plug with cotton, repeat q1-2h prn

Available forms include: Sol 1.4%, 5%, 20%

Side effects/adverse reactions:
EENT: Itching, irritation in ear
INTEG: Rash, urticaria

Contraindications: Hypersensitivity, perforated eardrum

Pharmacokinetics:
INSTILL: Peak 1 min, duration ½-1 hr

NURSING CONSIDERATIONS
Administer:
• After removing impacted cerumen by irrigation
• After cleaning stopper with alcohol
• After restraining child if necessary
• Warming solution to body temperature

Evaluate:
• Therapeutic response: decreased ear pain
• For redness, swelling, pain in ear, which indicates superimposed infection

---

italics = common side effects   ***bold italic*** = life threatening reactions

Teach patient/family:
• Method of instillation, using aseptic technique including not touching dropper to ear
• That dizziness may occur after instillation
• Report ear pain >48 hr

---

benzocaine (topical)

(ben'zoe-caine)

Americaine, Anbesol, Benzocol, Cloerex, Dermoplast, Hurricaine, Oracin, Ora-Jel, Rhulicream, Solarcaine, Spec T Anesthetic, Trocaine

Func. class.: Topical anesthetic
Chem. class.: PABA ethyl ester

Action: Inhibits nerve impulses from sensory nerves which produces anesthesia
Uses: Pruritus, sunburn, toothache, sore throat, cold sores, oral pain, rectal pain, irritation
Dosage and routes:
• *Adult and child:* Apply syr/gel to affected area; suck loz as needed; apply oint to affected area bid-tid
Available forms include: Aerosol 20%; gel 6.3%, 7.5%, 10%, 20%; sol 2.5%, 6.3%, 20%
Side effects/adverse reactions:
HEMA: Methemoglobinemia (infants)
INTEG: Rash, irritation, sensitization
Contraindications: Hypersensitivity to PABA or procaine, infants <1 yr, application to large areas
Precautions: Child <6 yr, sepsis, pregnancy (C), denuded skin
NURSING CONSIDERATIONS
Administer:
• After cleansing and drying of affected area
• Holding 6-12 in from affected area if using aerosol

Evaluate:
• Allergy: rash, irritation, reddening, swelling
• Therapeutic response: absence of pain, itching of affected area
• Infection: if affected area is infected, do not apply
Teach patient/family:
• To report rash, irritation, redness, swelling
• How to apply spray, ointment, jelly, and how to use syrup or lozenges
• Not to get aerosol in eyes or inhale spray

---

benzonatate

(ben-zoe'na-tate)

Tessalon

Func. class.: Antitussive, nonnarcotic
Chem. class.: Tetracaine derivative

Action: Inhibits cough reflex by anesthetizing stretch receptors in respiratory system, direct action on cough center in medulla
Uses: Nonproductive cough
Dosage and routes:
• *Adult and child:* PO 100 mg tid, not to exceed 600 mg/day
• *Child <10 yr:* PO 8 mg/kg in 3-6 divided doses
Available forms include: Perles 100 mg
Side effects/adverse reactions:
CNS: Dizziness, drowsiness, headache
GI: Nausea, constipation, upset stomach
EENT: Nasal congestion, burning eyes
CV: Increased B/P, chest tightness, numbness
INTEG: Urticaria, rash, pruritus
Contraindications: Hypersensitivity

Precautions: Pregnancy (C), lactation

Pharmacokinetics:

PO: Onset 15-20 min, duration 3-8 hr, metabolized by liver, excreted in urine

NURSING CONSIDERATIONS

Perform/provide:

• Storage in tight, light-resistant containers

• Increased fluids, bulk, exercise to patient's lifestyle to decrease constipation, liquefy sputum

• Chest percussion to bring up secretion if needed

Evaluate:

• Therapeutic response: absence of cough

• Cough: type, frequency, character including sputum

Teach patient/family:

• Avoid driving, other hazardous activities until patient is stabilized on this medication

• Not to chew or break capsules; will anesthetize mouth

• To avoid smoking, smoke-filled rooms, perfumes, dust, environmental pollutants, cleaners

---

benzoyl peroxide

(ben'zoe-ill per-ox'ide)

Benoxyl, Benzac, Benzagel, Desquam-X,* Oxy-5, Oxy-10, Persadox, Persa-Gel, Xerac BP, Pan Oxyl, Propa P.H. Acne

Func. class.: Antiacne medication

Action: Antibacterial activity especially against predominant bacteria causing acne

Uses: Mild-moderate acne

Dosage and routes:

• *Adult and child:* TOP apply to affected area qd or bid

Available forms include: Topical cleansers, lotions, creams, sticks, pads, gels, bars

Side effects/adverse reactions:

INTEG: Local skin irritation, stinging, warmth (dryness), scaling, erythema, edema, allergic, contact dermatitis

Contraindications: Hypersensitivity to benzoic acid derivatives

Precautions: Pregnancy (C), lactation, children <12 yr

Pharmacokinetics:

TOP: 50% absorbed through skin, metabolized to benzoic acid, excreted in urine

NURSING CONSIDERATIONS

Administer:

• Then wash hands immediately to avoid irritation

Perform/provide:

• Storage at room temperature

Evaluate:

• Therapeutic response: decreased amount of acne on body

• Area of body involved, including time involved, what helps or aggravates condition

• Allergic reaction: rash, irritation, scaling, dermatitis; discontinue use

Teach patient/family:

• To avoid application on normal skin or getting cream in eyes, nose, or other mucous membranes

• To discontinue use if rash or irritation develops

• May cause transitory warmth or stinging over area treated

• Expect dryness, peeling of area treated

• Avoid contact with hair or clothing; they may stain

• Cosmetics may be used over drug

• That dryness and peeling can be expected

---

italics = common side effects   ***bold italic*** = life threatening reactions

benzphetamine HCl

(benz-fet′a-neen)
Didrex
Func. class.: Anorexiant
Chem. class.: Amphetamine-like analog

Controlled Substance Schedule III

Action: Direct stimulation of satiety center in hypothalamic, limbic regions

Uses: Exogenous obesity

Dosage and routes:
• *Adult:* PO 25-50 mg qd-tid

Available forms include: Tabs 25, 50 mg

Side effects/adverse reactions:

CNS: Hyperactivity, insomnia, restlessness, talkativeness, dizziness, headache, chills, stimulation, dysphoria, irritability, aggressiveness, tremors, diaphoresis, fatigue, depression, confusion

GI: Nausea, vomiting, anorexia, dry mouth, diarrhea, constipation, weight loss, metallic taste, cramps

GU: Impotence, change in libido, dysuria, polyuria, menstrual changes

CV: Palpitations, tachycardia, hypertension, hypotension

INTEG: Urticaria

EENT: Mydriasis, eye irritation, blurred vision

HEMA: Bone marrow depression, leukopenia, agranulocytosis

Contraindications: Hypersensitivity to sympathomimetic amines, hyperthyroidism, hypertension, glaucoma, severe arteriosclerosis, drug abuse, cardiovascular disease, anxiety, pregnancy (X)

Precautions: Gilles de la Tourette's disorder, lactation, child <12 yr, elderly

Pharmacokinetics:
PO: Onset 30 min, peak 1-3 hr, duration 4-20 hr; metabolized by liver, excreted by kidneys, crosses placenta, breast milk, half-life 10-30 hr

Interactions/incompatibilities:
• Hypertensive crisis: MAOIs or within 14 days of MAOIs
• Increased effect of benzphetamine: acetazolamide, antacids, sodium bicarbonate, ascorbic acid, ammonium chloride
• Decreased effect of benzphetamine: tricyclics
• Decreased effect of: guanethidine, other antihypertensives

NURSING CONSIDERATIONS

Assess:
• VS, B/P since this drug may reverse antihypertensives; check patients with cardiac diseases more often
• CBC, urinalysis, in diabetes: blood sugar, urine sugar; insulin changes may need to be made since eating will decrease
• Height, growth rate in children; growth rate may be decreased

Administer:
• At least 6 hr before hs to avoid sleeplessness
• For obesity only if patient is on weight reduction program that includes dietary changes, exercise; patient will develop tolerance and weight loss won't occur without additional methods, give 1 hour before meals
• Gum, hard candy, frequent sips of water for dry mouth

Evaluate:
• Mental status: mood, sensorium, affect, stimulation, insomnia, aggressiveness may occur
• Physical dependency; should not be used for extended time; dose should be discontinued gradually

---

* Available in Canada only

• Withdrawal symptoms: headache, nausea, vomiting, muscle pain, weakness
• Drug tolerance will develop after long-term use
• Dosage should not be increased if tolerance develops

Teach patient/family:
• To decrease caffeine consumption (coffee, tea, cola, chocolate); may increase irritability, stimulation
• Avoid OTC preparations unless approved by physician
• To taper off drug over several weeks, or depression, increased sleeping, lethargy may occur
• To avoid alcohol ingestion
• To avoid hazardous activities until patient is stabilized on medication
• To get needed rest; patients will feel more tired at end of day

Treatment of overdose: Administer fluids, hemodialysis, peritoneal dialysis; antihypertensive for increased B/P; ammonium Cl for increased excretion

---

benzquinamide HCl

(benz-kwin'a-mide)
Emete-Con, Quantril

Func. class.: Antiemetic
Chem. class.: Benzoquinolize amide

Action: Acts centrally by blocking chemoreceptor trigger zone, which in turn acts on vomiting center
Uses: To inhibit nausea, vomiting associated with anesthetic, surgery
Dosage and routes:
• *Adult:* IM 50 mg or 0.5-1 mg/kg, may be repeated in 1 hr, then q3-4 hr prn; IV 25 mg or 0.2-0.4 mg/kg as a one-time dose

Available forms include: Inj 50 mg/vial
Side effects/adverse reactions:
CNS: Drowsiness, fatigue, restlessness, tremor, headache, stimulation, dizziness, insomnia, twitching, excitement, nervousness, extrapyramidal symptoms
GI: Nausea, anorexia
CV: Premature atrial or ventricular contractions, atrial fibrillation, hypertension, hypotension
INTEG: Rash, urticaria, fever, chills, flushing, hives, shivering, sweating, temperature
EENT: Dry mouth, blurred vision, hiccups, salivation
Contraindications: Hypersensitivity, hypertension
Precautions: Children, pregnancy (C), lactation, elderly
Pharmacokinetics:
IM/IV: Onset 15 min, duration 3-4 hr, metabolized by liver, excreted in urine, feces, half-life 40 min
NURSING CONSIDERATIONS
Assess:
• Vital signs, B/P; check patients with cardiac disease more often; hypotension, hypertension, dysrhythmias may occur
Administer:
• After reconstituting with 2.2 ml sterile water for injection to a concentration of 25 mg/ml; do not use sodium chloride
• Reduced dosage if patient is receiving pressor drugs
• Direct IV 25 mg over ½-1 min by Y tubing; incompatible with saline solutions
Perform/provide:
• Storage of injection before, after reconstitution in light-resistant container, single dose container
Evaluate:
• Therapeutic response: absence of nausea, vomiting

---

italics = common side effects   ***bold italic*** = life threatening reactions

• Observe for drowsiness; instruct patient not to drive, operate machinery
Treatment of overdose:
• Supportive care; atropine may be helpful

---

benztropine mesylate

(benz'troe-peen)
Apo-Benzotropine, Bensylate, Cogentin
Func. class.: Cholinergic blocker
Chem. class.: Tertiary amine

Action: Blockade of central acetylcholine receptors
Uses: Parkinson symptoms, extrapyramidal symptoms associated with neuroleptic drugs
Dosage and routes:
Drug-induced extrapyramidal symptoms
• *Adult:* IM/IV 1-2 mg 1-2 × day; give PO dose as soon as possible; PO 1-2 mg bid/tid, increase by 0.5 mg q 5-6 days
Parkinson symptoms
• *Adult:* PO 0.5-1 mg qd, increased 0.5 mg q5-6 days titrated to patient response
Available forms include: Tabs 0.5, 1, 2 mg; inj IM, IV 1 mg/ml
Side effects/adverse reactions:
MS: Muscular weakness, cramping
INTEG: Rash, urticaria, dermatoses
MISC: Increased temperature, flushing, decreased sweating, hyperthermia, heat stroke, numbness of fingers
CNS: Confusion, anxiety, restlessness, irritability, delusions, hallucinations, headache, sedation, depression, incoherence, dizziness, memory loss
EENT: Blurred vision, photophobia, dilated pupils, difficulty swallowing, dry eyes, mydriasis

CV: Palpitations, tachycardia, hypotension, bradycardia
GI: Dryness of mouth, constipation, nausea, vomiting, abdominal distress, *paralytic ileus,* epigastric distress
GU: Hesitancy, retention
Contraindications: Hypersensitivity, narrow-angle glaucoma, myasthenia gravis, GI/GU obstruction, child <3 yr, peptic ulcer, megacolon
Precautions: Pregnancy (C), elderly, lactation, tachycardia, prostatic hypertrophy, liver, kidney disease, drug abuse history, dysrhythmias, hypotension, hypertension, psychiatric patients
Pharmacokinetics:
IM/IV: Onset 15 min, duration 6-10 hr
PO: Onset 1 hr, duration 6-10 hr
Interactions/incompatibilities:
• Increased anticholinergic effect: antihistamines, phenothiazines, amantadine
• Decreased effect of: levodopa
• Increased schizophrenic symptoms: haloperidol
NURSING CONSIDERATIONS
Assess:
• I&O ratio; retention commonly causes decreased urinary output
Administer:
• With or after meals to prevent GI upset; may give with fluids other than water
• At hs to avoid daytime drowsiness in patient with parkinsonism
• Parenteral dose slowly; keep in bed for at least 1 hr after dose
Perform/provide:
• Storage at room temperature
• Hard candy, frequent drinks, gum to relieve dry mouth
Evaluate:
• Parkinsonism, extrapyramidal symptoms: shuffling gait, muscle

---

* Available in Canada only

rigidity, involuntary movements

• Urinary hesitancy, retention; palpate bladder if retention occurs

• Constipation; increase fluids, bulk, exercise if this occurs

• For tolerance over long-term therapy; dose may need to be increased or changed

• Mental status: affect, mood, CNS depression, worsening of mental symptoms during early therapy

Teach patient/family:

• Not to discontinue this drug abruptly; to taper off over 1 wk

• To avoid driving or other hazardous activities, drowsiness may occur

• To avoid OTC medication: cough, cold preparations with alcohol, antihistamines unless directed by physician

---

bepridil HCl

Vascor

Func. class.: Calcium channel blocker type 4

Action: Inhibits calcium ion influx across cell membrane during cardiac depolarization; produces relaxation of coronary vascular smooth muscle, dilates coronary arteries, decreases SA/AV node conduction, dilates peripheral arteries

Uses: Stable angina, used alone or in combination with propranolol

Dosage and routes:

Angina

Adult: 200-450 mg q d

Available forms include: Tabs, film-coated, 200, 300, 400 mg

Side effects/adverse reactions:

CV: Dysrhythmia, edema, CHF, bradycardia, hypotension, palpitations, AV block

GI: Nausea, vomiting, diarrhea, gastric upset, constipation, increased liver function studies

GU: Nocturia, polyuria

CNS: Headache, fatigue, drowsiness, dizziness, anxiety, depression, weakness, insomnia, confusion, lightheadedness, nervousness

Contraindications: Sick sinus syndrome, 2nd or 3rd degree heart block, Wolff-Parkinson-White syndrome, hypotension less than 90 mm Hg systolic, cardiogenic shock

Precautions: CHF, hypotension, hepatic injury, pregnancy (C), lactation, children, renal disease, concomitant β-blocker therapy

Pharmacokinetics: Peak 2-3 hr, 99% plasma protein bound, half-life 42 hr; completely metabolized in the liver and excreted in urine and feces

Interactions/incompatibilities:

• Increased effects: β-blockers

• Decreased effects of: lithium, rifampin

• Increased levels of: digoxin

NURSING CONSIDERATIONS

Administer:

• Before meals, hs

Evaluate:

• Therapeutic response: decreased anginal pain, decreased B/P

• Cardiac status: B/P, pulse, respiration, ECG intervals (PR, QRS, QT), dysrhythmias

Teach patient/family:

• How to take pulse before taking drug; record or graph should be kept

• To avoid hazardous activities until stabilized on drug, dizziness is no longer a problem

• To limit caffeine consumption

• To avoid OTC drugs unless directed by a physician

• Stress patient compliance to all areas of medical regimen: diet, exercise, stress reduction, drug therapy

Lab test interferences:
Increase: Liver function tests
Treatment of overdose: Defibrillation, atropine for AV block, vasopressor for hypotension

---

betamethasone/betamethasone sodium phosphate/betamethasone disodium phosphate/betamethasone acetate, betamethasone sodium phosphate

Betnelan, Celestone/Celestone Phosphate*/Betnesol/Celestone Soluspan

Func. class.: Corticosteroid, synthetic
Chem. class.: Glucocorticoid, long-acting

Action: Decreases inflammation by suppression of migration of polymorphonuclear leukocytes, fibroblasts, reversal of increased capillary permeability and lysosomal stabilization
Uses: Immunosupression, severe inflammation, prevention of neonatal respiratory distress syndrome (by administering to mothers)
Dosage and routes:
• *Adult:* PO 0.6-7.2 mg qd; IM/IV 0.6-7.2 mg qd in joint or soft tissue (sodium phosphate)
• *Pregnant adult:* IM 12 mg 36-48 hr, before premature delivery, then same dose in 24 hr (betamethasone acetate)
Available forms include: Tabs 0.6 mg; syr 0.6 mg/5 ml; inj 3, 4 mg/ml
Side effects/adverse reactions:
INTEG: Acne, poor wound healing,

ecchymosis, bruising, petechiae
CNS: Depression, flushing, sweating, headache, ecchymosis, bruising, mood changes
*CV: Hypertension, **circulatory collapse, thrombophlebitis, embolism,** tachycardia, **necrotizing angiitis, CHF***
*HEMA: **Thrombocytopenia***
MS: Fractures, osteoporosis, weakness
*GI: Diarrhea, nausea, abdominal distention, **GI hemorrhage**, increased appetite, **pancreatitis***
EENT: Fungal infections, increased intraocular pressure, blurred vision
Contraindications: Psychosis, hypersensitivity, idiopathic thrombocytopenia, acute glomerulonephritis, amebiasis, fungal infections, nonasthmatic bronchial disease, child <2 yr, AIDS, TB
Precautions: Pregnancy (C), diabetes mellitus, glaucoma, osteoporosis, seizure disorders, ulcerative colitis, CHF, myasthenia gravis, renal disease, esophagitis, peptic ulcer
Pharmacokinetics:
PO: Onset 1-2 hr, peak 1 hr, duration 3 days
IM/IV: Onset 10 min, peak 4-8 hr, duration 1-1½ days
Metabolized in liver, excreted in urine as steroids, crosses placenta
Interactions/incompatibilities:
• Decreased action of betamethasone: cholestyramine, colestipol, barbiturates, rifampin, ephedrine, phenytoin, theophylline
• Decreased effects of: anticoagulants, anticonvulsants, antidiabetics, ambenonium, neostigmine, isoniazid, toxoids, vaccines
• Increased side effects: alcohol, salicylates, indomethacin, amphotericin B, digitalis preparations
• Increased action of betametha-

sone: salicylates, estrogens, indomethacin

NURSING CONSIDERATIONS
Assess:
• Potassium, blood sugar, urine glucose while on long-term therapy; hypokalemia and hyperglycemia
• Weight daily, notify physician of weekly gain >5 lb
• B/P q4h, pulse, notify physician if chest pain occurs
• I&O ratio, be alert for decreasing urinary output and increasing edema
• Plasma cortisol levels during long-term therapy (normal level: 138-635 nmol/L SI units when drawn at 8 AM)

Administer:
• IV, only sodium phosphate product; give > 1 min; may be given by IV INF in compatible sol
• After shaking suspension (parenteral)
• Titrated dose, use lowest effective dose
• IM injection deeply in large mass, rotate sites, avoid deltoid, use 21G needle
• In one dose in AM to prevent adrenal suppression, avoid SC administration, damage may be done to tissue
• With food or milk to decrease GI symptoms

Perform/provide:
• Assistance with ambulation in patient with bone tissue disease to prevent fractures

Evaluate:
• Therapeutic response: ease of respirations, decreased inflammation
• Infection: increased temperature, WBC even after withdrawal of medication; drug masks infection symptoms
• Potassium depletion: paresthe-

sias, fatigue, nausea, vomiting, depression, polyuria, dysrhythmias, weakness
• Edema, hypertension, cardiac symptoms
• Mental status: affect, mood, behavioral changes, aggression

Teach patient/family:
• That ID as steroid user should be carried
• To notify physician if therapeutic response decreases; dosage adjustment may be needed
• Not to discontinue this medication abruptly or adrenal crisis can result
• To avoid OTC products: salicylates, alcohol in cough products, cold preparations unless directed by physician
• Teach patient all aspects of drug usage including Cushingoid symptoms
• Symptoms of adrenal insufficiency: nausea, anorexia, fatigue, dizziness, dyspnea, weakness, joint pain

Lab test interferences:
Increase: Cholesterol, sodium, blood glucose, uric acid, calcium, urine glucose
Decrease: Calcium, potassium, T_4, T_3, thyroid ^{131}I uptake test, urine 17-OHCS, 17-KS, PBI
False negative: Skin allergy tests

---

betamethasone benzoate
(bay-ta-meth'a-sone)
Beben, Benisone, Uticort

Func. class.: Topical corticosteroid
Chem. class.: Synthetic fluorinated agent, group III potency

Action: Possesses antipruritic, antiinflammatory actions

Uses: Psoriasis, eczema, contact dermatitis, pruritus

Dosage and routes:
• *Adult and child:* Apply to affected area qid

Available forms include: Oint 0.025%; cream 0.025%; lotion 0.025%; gel 0.025%

Side effects/adverse reactions:
INTEG: Burning, dryness, itching, irritation, acne, folliculitis, hypertrichosis, perioral dermatitis, hypopigmentation, atrophy, striae, miliaria, allergic contact dermatitis, secondary infection

Contraindications: Hypersensitivity to corticosteroids, fungal infections

Precautions: Pregnancy (C), lactation, viral infections, bacterial infections

NURSING CONSIDERATIONS
Assess:
• Temperature; if fever develops, drug should be discontinued

Administer:
• Only to affected areas; do not get in eyes
• Medication, then cover with occlusive dressing (only if prescribed), seal to normal skin, change q12h, systemic absorption may occur
• Only to dermatoses; do not use on weeping, denuded, or infected area

Perform/provide:
• Cleansing before application of drug
• Treatment for a few days after area has cleared
• Storage at room temperature

Evaluate:
• Therapeutic response: absence of severe itching, patches on skin, flaking
• For systemic absorption: increased temperature, inflammation, irritation

Teach patient/family:
• To avoid sunlight on affected area; burns may occur

---

betamethasone valerate
(bay-ta-meth′a-sone)
Beta Cort,* Betaderm,* Beta-Val, Betatrex, Valnac, Valisone

Func. class.: Topical corticosteroid
Chem. class.: Synthetic fluorinated agent

Action: Possesses antipruritic, antiinflammatory actions

Uses: Psoriasis, eczema, contact dermatitis, pruritus

Dosage and routes:
• *Adult and child:* Apply to affected area qid

Available forms include: Oint 0.1%; cream 0.01%, 0.1%; lotion 0.1%

Side effects/adverse reactions:
INTEG: Burning, dryness, itching, irritation, acne, folliculitis, hypertrichosis, perioral dermatitis, hypopigmentation, atrophy, striae, miliaria, allergic contact dermatitis, secondary infection

Contraindications: Hypersensitivity to corticosteroids, fungal infections

Precautions: Pregnancy (C), lactation, viral infections, bacterial infections

NURSING CONSIDERATIONS
Assess:
• Temperature; if fever develops, drug should be discontinued

Administer:
• Only to affected areas; do not get in eyes
• Medication, then cover with occlusive dressing (only if prescribed), seal to normal skin,

change q12h, systemic absorption may occur

• Only to dermatoses; do not use on weeping, denuded, or infected area

Perform/provide:

• Cleansing before applying drug
• Treatment for a few days after area has cleared
• Storage at room temperature

Evaluate:

• Therapeutic response: absence of severe itching, patches on skin, flaking
• For systemic absorption: increased temperature, inflammation, irritation

Teach patient/family:

• To avoid sunlight on affected area; burns may occur

---

bethanechol chloride

(be-than'e-kile)

Duvoid, Myotonachol, Urecholine, Urabeth

Func. class.: Cholinergic stimulant
Chem. class.: Synthetic choline ester

Action: Stimulates muscarinic ACh receptors directly; mimics effects of parasympathetic nervous system stimulation; stimulates gastric motility, stimulates ganglia

Uses: Urinary retention (postoperative, postpartum), neurogenic atony of bladder with retention

Dosage and routes:

• *Adult:* PO 10-50 mg bid-qid; SC 2.5-10 mg tid-qid prn

Test dose

• *Adult:* SC 2.5 mg repeated 15-30 min intervals × 4 doses to determine effective dose

Available forms include: Tabs 5, 10, 25, 50 mg; inj SC 5 mg/ml

Side effects/adverse reactions:

INTEG: Rash, urticaria, flushing, increased sweating, hypothermia
CNS: Dizziness, headache, confusion, weakness, ***convulsions***
GI: Nausea, bloody diarrhea, vomiting, cramps, fecal incontinence
CV: Hypotension, bradycardia, orthostatic hypotension, reflex tachycardia, ***cardiac arrest, circulatory collapse***
GU: Frequency, incontinence
*RESP: **Acute asthma, dyspnea***
EENT: Miosis, increased salivation, lacrimation, blurred vision

Contraindications: Hypersensitivity, severe bradycardia, asthma, severe hypotension, hyperthyroidism, peptic ulcer, parkinsonism, seizure disorders, CAD, coronary occlusion, mechanical obstruction

Precautions: Hypertension, pregnancy (C), lactation, child <8 yr, urinary retention

Pharmacokinetics:

PO: Onset 30-90 min, duration 6 hr
SC: Onset 5-15 min, duration 2 hr, excreted by kidneys

Interactions/incompatibilities:

• Increased action of bethanechol: other cholinergics
• Hypotension: ganglionic blockers
• Decreased action of bethanechol: procainamide, quinidine

NURSING CONSIDERATIONS

Assess:

• B/P, pulse; observe after parenteral dose for 1 hr
• I&O ratio; check for urinary retention or incontinence

Administer:

• Parenteral dose by SC route; use of IM, IV may result in cardiac arrest
• Only with atropine sulfate available for cholinergic crisis
• Only after all other cholinergics have been discontinued

---

italics = common side effects   ***bold italic*** = life threatening reactions

• Increased doses if tolerance occurs
• With food or milk to decrease GI symptoms (bilateral vagotomy), may decrease action of this drug
• On empty stomach for better absorption

Perform/provide:
• Storage at room temperature
• Bedpan/urinal if given for urinary retention
• Use of rectal tube if ordered to increase passage of gas when used for abdominal distention

Evaluate:
• Therapeutic response: absence of urinary retention, abdominal distention
• Bradycardia, hypotension, bronchospasm, headache, dizziness, convulsions, respiratory depression; drug should be discontinued if toxicity occurs

Teach patient/family:
• To take drug exactly as prescribed
• To make position changes slowly, orthostatic hypotension may occur

Treatment of overdose: Administer atropine 0.6-1.2 mg IV or IM (adult)

Lab test interferences:
Increase: AST, lipase/amylase, bilirubin, BSP

---

biperiden HCl, biperiden lactate

(bye-per'i-den)
Akineton
Func. class.: Cholinergic blocker

Action: Centrally acting competitive anticholinergic
Uses: Parkinson symptoms, extrapyramidal symptoms secondary to neuroleptic drug therapy

Dosage and routes:
Extrapyramidal symptoms
• *Adult:* PO 2-6 mg bid-tid; IM/IV 2 mg q30 min, if needed, not to exceed 8 mg/24 hr
Parkinson symptoms
• *Adult:* PO 2 mg tid-qid
Available forms include: Tabs 2 mg; inj IM/IV 5 mg/ml (lactate)

Side effects/adverse reactions:
CNS: Confusion, anxiety, restlessness, irritability, delusions, hallucinations, headache, sedation, depression, incoherence, dizziness, euphoria, tremors, memory loss
EENT: Blurred vision, photophobia, dilated pupils, difficulty swallowing, mydriasis
CV: Palpitations, tachycardia, postural hypotension, bradycardia
GI: Dryness of mouth, constipation, nausea, vomiting, abdominal distress, *paralytic ileus*
GU: Hesitancy, retention
MS: Weakness, cramping
INTEG: Rash, urticaria, dermatoses
MISC: Increased temperature, flushing, decreased sweating, hyperthermia, heat stroke, numbness of fingers

Contraindications: Hypersensitivity, narrow-angle glaucoma, myasthenia gravis, GI/GU obstruction, megacolon, stenosing peptic ulcers

Precautions: Pregnancy (C), elderly, lactation, tachycardia, prostatic hypertrophy, dysrhythmias, liver, kidney disease, drug abuse, hypotension, hypertension, psychiatric patients, children

Pharmacokinetics:
IM/IV: Onset 15 min, duration 6-10 hr
PO: Onset 1 hr, duration 6-10 hr

Interactions/incompatibilities:
• Increased levels of: digoxin, levodopa

• Increased schizophrenic symptoms: haloperidol
• Increased anticholinergic effect: antihistamines, phenothiazines, amantadine

NURSING CONSIDERATIONS
Assess:
• I&O ratio; retention commonly causes decreased urinary output
Administer:
• Parenteral dose with patient recumbent to prevent postural hypotension
• With or after meals to prevent GI upset; may give with fluids other than water
• At hs to avoid daytime drowsiness in patient with parkinsonism
• Parenteral dose slowly (>1 min); keep in bed for at least 1 hr after dose
Perform/provide:
• Storage at room temperature
• Hard candy, frequent drinks, gum to relieve dry mouth
Evaluate:
• Parkinsonism, extrapyramidal symptoms: shuffling gait, muscle rigidity, involuntary movements
• Urinary hesitancy, retention; palpate bladder if retention occurs
• Constipation; increase fluids, bulk, exercise if this occurs
• For tolerance over long-term therapy; dose may need to be increased or changed
• Mental status: affect, mood, CNS depression, worsening of mental symptoms during early therapy
Teach patient/family:
• Not to discontinue this drug abruptly, to taper off over 1 wk
• To avoid driving or other hazardous activities, drowsiness may occur
• To avoid OTC medication: cough, cold preparations with alcohol, antihistamines unless directed by physician

bisacodyl
(bis-a-koe′dill)
Apo-Bisacodyl,* Bisco-Lax, Dulcolax, Fleet Bisacodyl, Theralax, Dacodyl, Deficol
Func. class.: Laxative, stimulant
Chem. class.: Diphenylmethane

Action: Acts directly on intestine by increasing motor activity, thought to irritate colonic intramural plexus
Uses: Short-term treatment of constipation, bowel or rectal preparation for surgery, examination
Dosage and routes:
• *Adult:* PO 10-15 mg in PM or AM, may use up to 30 mg for bowel or rectal preparation; REC 10 mg; ENEMA 1.25 oz
• *Child >3 yr:* PO 5-10 mg
• *Child >2 yr:* REC 10 mg
• *Child <2 yr:* REC 5 mg
• *Child <6 yr:* ENEMA one-half contents of micro enema
Available forms include: Enteric coated tabs 5 mg; rec supp 10 mg
Side effects/adverse reactions:
CNS: Muscle weakness
GI: Nausea, *vomiting, anorexia, cramps,* diarrhea, rectal burning (suppositories)
META: Protein-losing enteropathy, alkalosis, hypokalemia, ***tetany,*** electrolyte, fluid imbalances
Contraindications: Hypersensitivity, rectal fissures, abdominal pain, nausea/vomiting, appendicitis, acute surgical abdomen, ulcerated hemorrhoids, acute hepatitis, fecal impaction, intestinal/biliary tract obstruction
Precautions: Pregnancy (C)

italics = common side effects   ***bold italic*** = life threatening reactions

Pharmacokinetics:
PO: Onset 6-10 min, acts within 6-12 hr
REC: Onset 15-16 min
Metabolized by liver, excreted in urine, bile, feces, breast milk

Interactions/incompatibilities:
• Gastric irritation: antacids, milk, H₂ Blockers

NURSING CONSIDERATIONS
Assess:
• Blood, urine electrolytes if drug is used often by patient
• I&O ratio to identify fluid loss

Administer:
• Alone only with water for better absorption; do not take within 1 hr of other drugs or within 1 hr of antacids, milk, or cimetidine
• In morning or evening (oral dose)

Evaluate:
• Therapeutic response: decrease in constipation
• Cause of constipation; identify whether fluids, bulk, or exercise is missing from lifestyle
• Cramping, rectal bleeding, nausea, vomiting; if these symptoms occur, drug should be discontinued

Teach patient/family:
• Swallow tabs whole; do not chew
• Not to use laxatives for long-term therapy; bowel tone will be lost
• That normal bowel movements do not always occur daily
• Do not use in presence of abdominal pain, nausea, vomiting
• Notify physician if constipation unrelieved or if symptoms of electrolyte imbalance occur: muscle cramps, pain, weakness, dizziness

---

bismuth subsalicylate
(bis-meth)
Pepto-Bismol
Func. class.: Antidiarrheal
Chem. class.: Salicylate

Action: Inhibits prostaglandin synthesis responsible for GI hypermotility, stimulates absorption of fluid and electrolytes

Uses: Diarrhea (cause undetermined), prevention of diarrhea when traveling

Dosage and routes:
• *Adult:* PO 1-2 tabs chewed or swallowed tid (subgallate), or 30 ml or 2 tabs q30-60 min, not to exceed 8 doses for >2 days (subsalicylate)
• *Child 10-14 yr:* PO 15 ml
• *Child 6-10 yr:* PO 10 ml
• *Child 3-6 yr:* PO 5 ml

Available forms include: Chewable tabs 262 mg; susp 262 mg/15 ml

Side effects/adverse reactions:
HEMA: Increased bleeding time
GI: Increased fecal impaction (high doses), dark stools
CNS: Confusion, twitching
EENT: Hearing loss, tinnitus, metallic taste, blue gums

Contraindications: Child <3 yr
Precautions: Salicylate or coumarin therapy

Pharmacokinetics:
PO: Onset 1 hr, peak 2 hr, duration 4 hr

Interactions/incompatibilities:
• Increased side effects: alcohol, aminosalicyclic acid, carbonic anhydrase inhibitors
• Increased action of bismuth: ammonium chloride
• Decreased action of bismuth: antacids, corticosteroids
• Decreased action of: uricosurics, indomethacin, antidiabetics, tetracyclines

NURSING CONSIDERATIONS
Assess:
• Skin turgor; shift if dehydration is suspected
• Electrolytes (K, Na, Cl) if diarrhea is severe or continues for a long term

---

Administer:
- But stop use if symptoms do not improve within 2 days or become worse, or if diarrhea is accompanied by high fever
- Increased fluids to rehydrate the patient

Evaluate:
- Therapeutic response: decreased diarrhea or absence of diarrhea when traveling
- Bowel pattern before drug therapy, after treatment

Teach patient/family:
- To chew or dissolve in mouth, do not swallow whole
- To avoid other salicylates unless directed by physician
- Stools may turn gray; tongue may darken

Lab test interferences:
Interfere: radiographic studies of GI system

---

bitolterol mesylate

(bye-tole′-ter-ol)
Tornalate
Func. class.: Adrenergic β₂-agonist
Chem. class.: Acid ester of colterol

Action: Causes bronchodilation by action on β₂ receptors with increased synthesis of cAMP, relaxes bronchial smooth muscle, inhibits mast cell degranulation, and stimulates cilia to remove secretions with very little effect on heart rate

Uses: Asthma, bronchospasm

Dosage and routes:
- *Adult and chiid >12 yr:* INH 2 puffs, wait 1-3 min before 3rd puff if needed, not to exceed 3 INH q6h or 2 INH q4h

Available forms include: Aerosol 0.37 mg/actuation

Side effects/adverse reactions:
CNS: Tremors, anxiety, insomnia, headache, dizziness, stimulation, restlessness, hallucinations
EENT: Dry nose, irritation of nose and throat
CV: Palpitations, tachycardia, hypertension, angina, hypotension
GI: Heartburn, nausea, vomiting, anorexia
MS: Muscle cramps
RESP: Bronchospasm, dyspnea

Contraindications: Hypersensitivity to sympathomimetics

Precautions: Lactation, pregnancy (C), cardiac disorders, hyperthyroidism, diabetes mellitus

Pharmacokinetics:
INH: Onset 3 min, peak ½-1 hr, duration 5-8 hr

Interactions/incompatibilities:
- Increased action of: aerosol bronchodilators
- Increased action of bitolterol: tricyclic antidepressants, MAOIs
- May inhibit action when used with other β-blockers

NURSING CONSIDERATIONS
Assess:
- Respiratory function: vital capacity, forced expiratory volume, ABGs

Administer:
- After shaking, exhale, place mouthpiece in mouth, inhale slowly, hold breath, remove, exhale slowly
- Gum, sips of water for dry mouth

Perform/provide:
- Storage in light-resistant container, do not expose to temperatures over 86° F

Evaluate:
- Therapeutic response: absence of dyspnea, wheezing over 1 hr

Teach patient/family:
- Not to use OTC medications; extra stimulation may occur

---

italics = common side effects   ***bold italic*** = life threatening reactions

• Use of inhaler, review package insert with patient
• To avoid getting aerosol in eyes
• To wash inhaler in warm water and dry qd
• On all aspects of drug; avoid smoking, smoke-filled rooms, persons with respiratory infections
Treatment of overdose: Administer a β_2 adrenergic blocker

---

bleomycin sulfate
(blee-oh-mye'sin)
Blenoxane
Func. class.: Antineoplastic, antibiotic
Chem. class.: Glycopeptide

Action: Inhibits synthesis of DNA, RNA, protein; this drug is derived from *Streptomyces verticillus;* replication is decreased by binding to DNA, which causes strand splitting; drug is phase specific in the G_2 and M phases; a nonvesicant
Uses: Cancer of head, neck, penis, cervix, vulva of squamous cell origin, Hodgkin's disease, lymphosarcoma, reticulum cell sarcoma, testicular carcinoma
Dosage and routes:
• *Adult:* SC/IV/IM 0.25-0.5 U/kg 1-2 × /wk or 10-20 U/m², then 1 U/day or 5 U/wk; may also be given intraarterially; do not exceed total dose, 400 µg in lifetime
Available forms include: Inj IV, SC, IM 5 units
Side effects/adverse reactions:
SYST: Anaphylaxis
GI: Nausea, vomiting, anorexia, stomatitis, weight loss
INTEG: Rash, hyperkeratosis, nail changes, alopecia, fever and chills
RESP: Fibrosis, pneumonitis, wheezing, *pulmonary toxicity*
CNS: Fever, chills

IDIOSYNCRATIC REACTION: Hypotension, confusion, fever, chills, wheezing
Contraindications: Hypersensitivity
Precautions: Renal, hepatic, respiratory disease, pregnancy (D)
Pharmacokinetics: Half-life 2 hr when CrCl >35 ml/min half-life is increased in lower clearance, metabolized in liver, 50% excreted in urine (unchanged)
Interactions/incompatibilities:
• Increased toxicity: other antineoplastics or radiation therapy
• Decreased serum digoxin levels: digoxin
NURSING CONSIDERATIONS
Assess:
• IM test dose
• Pulmonary function tests: chest x-ray before and during therapy; should be obtained q2 wk during treatment
• Temperature q4h; fever may indicate beginning infection
• Serum creatinine
Administer:
• IM/SC after reconstituting 5 U/ 1-5 ml sterile H_2O, D_5W, 0.9% NaCl, or bacteriostatic water for inj; do not use products containing benzyl alcohol when giving to neonates
• Direct IV after reconstituting 15 U/5 ml of D_5W or 0.9% NaCl; give over 10-15 min
• IV INF after further diluting with 50-100 ml D_5W or 0.9% NaCl
• Two test doses 2-5U before initial dose; monitor for anaphylaxis
• Antiemetic 30-60 min before giving drug to prevent vomiting, continue antiemetics 6-10 hr after treatment
• Topical or systemic analgesics for pain of stomatitis as ordered; anti-

histamines and antipyretics for fever and chills
• Intraarterial/IV injections over >10 min

Perform/provide:
• Deep breathing exercises with patient tid-qid; place in semi-Fowler's position
• Liquid diet: carbonated beverage, gelatin may be added if patient is not nauseated or vomiting
• Rinsing of mouth tid-qid with water, club soda; brushing of teeth with baking soda bid-tid with soft brush or cotton-tipped applicators for stomatitis; use unwaxed dental floss
• HOB increased to facilitate breathing

Evaluate:
• Dyspnea, rales, unproductive cough, chest pain, tachypnea, fatigue, increased pulse, pallor, lethargy
• Food preferences; list likes, dislikes
• Effects of alopecia and skin color on body image; discuss feelings about body changes
• Buccal cavity q8h for dryness, sores, ulceration, white patches, oral pain, bleeding, dysphagia
• Local irritation, pain, burning, discoloration at injection site
• Symptoms indicating severe allergic reaction: rash, pruritus, urticaria, purpuric skin lesions, itching, flushing
• Storage for 2 wk after reconstituting at room temperature; discard unused portions

Teach patient/family:
• To report any complaints, side effects to nurse or physician
• To report any changes in breathing, coughing, fever
• That hair may be lost during treatment and wig or hairpiece may make patient feel better; tell patient that new hair may be different in color, texture
• To avoid foods with citric acid, hot or rough texture
• To report any bleeding, white spots, ulcerations in mouth; to examine mouth qd and report symptoms

---

bretylium tosylate
(bre-til′ee-urn)
Bretylate,* Bretylol
Func. class.: Antidysrhythmic (Class III)
Chem. class.: Quaternary ammonium compound

Action: After a transient release of norepinephrine, inhibits further release by postganglionic nerve endings; increases action potential duration and effective refractory period

Uses: Serious ventricular tachycardia, cardioversion, ventricular fibrillation; for short-term use only

Dosage and routes:
Severe ventricular fibrillation
• *Adult:* IV BOL 5 mg/kg, increase to 10 mg/kg repeated q15 min; IV INF 1-2 mg/min or give 5-10 mg/kg over 10 min q6h (maintenance)

Ventricular dysrhythmias
• *Adult:* IV INF 500 mg diluted in 50 ml D₅W or NS, infuse over 10-30 min, may repeat in 1 hr, maintain with 1-2 mg/min or 5-10 mg/kg over 10-30 min q6h; IM 5-10 mg/kg undiluted; repeat in 1-2 hr if needed; maintain with same dose q6-8h

Available forms include: Inj IV 50 mg/ml

Side effects/adverse reactions:
CNS: Syncope, dizziness, confusion, psychosis, anxiety

---

italics = common side effects   ***bold italic*** = life threatening reactions

GI: Nausea, vomiting
CV: Hypotension, postural hypotension, bradycardia, angina, PVCs, substernal pressure, transient hypertension, precipitation of angina
RESP: Respiratory depression
Contraindications: Hypersensitivity, digitalis toxicity, aortic stenosis, pulmonary hypertension, children
Precautions: Renal disease, pregnancy (C), lactation
Pharmacokinetics:
IV: Onset 5 min
IM: Onset ½-2 hr, peak 6-9 hr
Half-life 4-17 hr, excreted unchanged by kidneys (70%-80% in 24 hr), not metabolized
Interactions/incompatibilities:
• Increased or decreased effects of bretylium: quinidine, procainamide, propranolol or other antidysrhythmics
• Hypotension: antihypertensives
• Toxicity: digitalis
• Incompatible with all medications in solution or syringe
NURSING CONSIDERATIONS
Assess:
• ECG continuously to determine drug effectiveness, PVCs or other dysrhythmias
• IV inf rate to avoid causing nausea, vomiting
• For dehydration or hypovolemia
• B/P continuously for hypotension, hypertension
• I&O ratio
Administer:
• IV INF by diluting 500 mg of drug/50 ml or more D₅/LR, D₅W, 0.9% NaCl, D₅/0.45% NaCl, D₅/0.9% NaCl; give over 15-30 min
• By continuous infusion using an infusion pump
• IM inj, rotate sites, inject <5 ml in any one site

• Reduced dosage slowly with ECG monitoring
Perform/provide:
• Place patient in supine position unless otherwise ordered
• Have suction equipment available
Evaluate:
• For rebound hypertension after 1-2 hr
• Cardiac status: rate, rhythm, character, continuously
Lab test interferences:
Decrease: Urinary epinephrine, urinary norepinephrine, urinary VMA epinephrine
Treatment of overdose: O₂, artificial ventilation, ECG, administer dopamine for circulatory depression, administer diazepam or thiopental for convulsions

---

bromocriptine mesylate
(broe-moe-krip'teen)
Parlodel
Func. class.: Dopamine receptor agonist; ovulation stimulant
Chem. class.: Ergot alkaloid derivative

Action: Inhibits prolactin release by activating postsynaptic dopamine receptors; activation of straital dopamine receptors could be reason for improvement in Parkinson's disease
Uses: Female infertility, Parkinson's disease, prevention of postpartum lactation, amenorrhea caused by hyperprolactinemia, acromegaly
Dosage and routes:
Hyperprolactinemic indications
• *Adult:* PO 1.25-2.5 mg with meals; may increase by 2.5 mg q3-7 days, usual 5-7.5 mg
Acromegaly

• *Adult:* PO 1.25-2.5 mg × 3 days hs, may increase by 1.25-2.5 mg q3-7 days, usual range 20-30 mg/day

Postpartum lactation
• *Adult:* PO 2.5 mg qid-tid with meal × 14 or 21 days

Parkinson's disease
• *Adult:* PO 1.25 mg bid with meals, may increase q2-4 wk by 2.5 mg/day, not to exceed 100 mg qd

Available forms include: Caps 5 mg; tabs 2.5 mg

Side effects/adverse reactions:
EENT: Blurred vision, diplopia, burning eyes, nasal congestion
CNS: Headache, depression, restlessness, anxiety, nervousness, confusion, *convulsions,* hallucinations, dizziness, fatigue, drowsiness, abnormal involuntary movements
GU: Frequency, retention, incontinence, diuresis
GI: Nausea, vomiting, anorexia, cramps, constipation, diarrhea, dry mouth, GI hemorrhage
INTEG: Rash on face, arms, alopecia
CV: Orthostatic hypotension, decreased B/P, palpitation, extra systole, *shock,* dysrhythmias, bradycardia

Contraindications: Hypersensitivity to ergot, severe ischemic disease, pregnancy (D)

Precautions: Lactation, hepatic disease, renal disease, children

Pharmacokinetics:
PO: Peak 1-3 hr, duration 4-8 hr, 90%-96% protein bound, half-life 3 hr, metabolized by liver (inactive metabolites), excreted in urine, feces

Interactions/incompatibilities:
• Decreased action of bromocriptine: phenothiazines, imipramine, haloperidol, droperidol, amitriptyline, oral contraceptives
• Increased action of: antihypertensives

NURSING CONSIDERATIONS
Assess:
• B/P; establish baseline, compare with other reading; this drug decreases B/P

Administer:
• With meal to prevent GI symptoms
• At hs so dizziness, orthostatic hypotension do not occur

Perform/provide:
• Storage at room temperature in tight container

Evaluate:
• Therapeutic response (Parkinson's disease): decreased dyskinesia, decreased slow movements, decreased drooling

Teach patient/family:
• To change position slowly, to prevent orthostatic hypotension
• To use contraceptives during treatment with this drug; pregnancy may occur; to use methods other than oral contraceptives
• That therapeutic effect may take 2 mo: galactorrhea, amenorrhea
• To avoid hazardous activity if dizziness occurs

Lab test interferences:
Increase: Growth hormone, AST/ALT, CPK, BUN, uric acid, alk phosphatase, GGTP

---

brompheniramine maleate

(brome-fen-ir'a-meen)
Brombay, Dimetane, Dimetane-Ten, Rolabromophen, Spentane, Veltane, and others
Func. class.: Antihistamine
Chem. class.: Alkylamine, H_1-receptor antagonist

Action: Acts on blood vessels, GI,

---

italics = common side effects   *bold italic* = life threatening reactions respiratory system by competing with histamine for H_1-receptor site; decreases allergic response by blocking histamine

Uses: Allergy symptoms, rhinitis

Dosage and routes:
• *Adult:* PO 4-8 mg tid-qid, not to exceed 36 mg/day; TIME REL 8-12 mg bid-tid, not to exceed 36 mg/day; IM/IV/SC 5-20 mg q6-12h, not to exceed 40 mg/day
• *Child >6 yr:* PO 2 mg tid-qid, not to exceed 12 mg/day; IM/IV/SC 0.5 mg/kg/day divided tid or qid
• *Child <6 yr:* Only as directed by physician

Available forms include: Tabs 4 mg; tabs, time rel 8, 12 mg; elix 2 mg/5 ml; inj IM/SC/IV 10, 100 mg/ml

Side effects/adverse reactions:
CNS: Dizziness, drowsiness, poor coordination, fatigue, anxiety, euphoria, confusion, paresthesia, neuritis
CV: Hypotension, palpitations, tachycardia
RESP: Increased thick secretions, wheezing, chest tightness
HEMA: Thrombocytopenia, agranulocytosis, hemolytic anemia
GI: Dry mouth, nausea, vomiting, anorexia, constipation, diarrhea
INTEG: Photosensitivity
GU: Retention, dysuria, frequency, impotence
EENT: Blurred vision, dilated pupils, tinnitus, nasal stuffiness, dry nose, throat, mouth

Contraindications: Hypersensitivity to H_1-receptor antagonists, acute asthma attack, lower respiratory tract disease, child <6 yr

Precautions: Increased intraocular pressure, renal disease, cardiac disease, hypertension, bronchial asthma, seizure disorder, stenosed peptic ulcers, hyperthyroidism, prostatic hypertrophy, bladder neck obstruction, pregnancy (C)

Pharmacokinetics:
PO: Peak 2-5 hr, duration to 48 hr; metabolized in liver, excreted by kidneys, excreted in breast milk, half-life 12-34 hr

Interactions/incompatibilities:
• Increased CNS depression: barbiturates, narcotics, hypnotics, tricyclic antidepressants, alcohol
• Decreased effect of: oral anticoagulants, heparin
• Increased drying effect: MAOIs

NURSING CONSIDERATIONS
Assess:
• I&O ratio; be alert for urinary retention, frequency, dysuria; drug should be discontinued if these occur
• CBC during long-term therapy

Administer:
• Direct IV undiluted or diluted with 10 ml 0.9% NaCl, given over 1 min or more
• IV INF by diluting in D_5W, 0.9% NaCl
• With meals if GI symptoms occur; absorption may slightly decrease

Perform/provide:
• Hard candy, gum, frequent rinsing of mouth for dryness
• Storage in tight container at room temperature

Evaluate:
• Therapeutic response: absence of running or congested nose or rashes
• Blood dyscrasias: thrombocytopenia, agranulocytosis (rare)
• Respiratory status: rate, rhythm, increase in bronchial secretions, wheezing, chest tightness

Teach patient/family:
• Not to crush or chew sustained release forms
• All aspects of drug use; to notify

---

*Available in Canada only

physician if confusion, sedation, hypotension occurs
• To avoid driving or other hazardous activities if drowsiness occurs
• To avoid use of alcohol or other CNS depressants while taking drug
Lab test interferences:
False negative: Skin allergy tests
Treatment of overdose: Administer ipecac syrup or lavage, diazepam, vasopressors, barbiturates (short-acting)

---

buclizine HCl
(byoo'kli-zeen)
Bucladin-S, Softran, Equivert, Vibazine
Func. class.: Antiemetic, antihistamine, anticholinergic
Chem. class.: H₁-receptor antagonist (piperazine)

Action: Acts centrally by blocking chemoreceptor trigger zone, which in turn acts on vomiting center
Uses: Motion sickness, dizziness, nausea, vomiting
Dosage and routes:
• *Adult:* PO 25-50 mg prn ½ hr before travel; may be repeated q4-6h prn
Available forms include: Tabs 50 mg
Side effects/adverse reactions:
CNS: Drowsiness, dizziness, fatigue, restlessness, headache, insomnia
GI: Nausea, anorexia, bitterness
EENT: Dry mouth, blurred vision
Contraindications: Hypersensitivity to cyclizines, shock
Precautions: Children, narrowangle glaucoma, lactation, prostatic hypertrophy, elderly, pregnancy (C)
Pharmacokinetics:
PO: Duration 4-6 hr, other pharmacokinetics not known

NURSING CONSIDERATIONS
Assess:
• VS, B/P
Administer:
• Tablets may be swallowed whole, chewed, or allowed to dissolve
Evaluate:
• Signs of toxicity of other drugs or masking of symptoms of disease: brain tumor, intestinal obstruction
• Drowsiness, dizziness
Teach patient/family:
• To avoid hazardous activities or activities requiring alertness; dizziness may occur; instruct patient to request assistance with ambulation
• To avoid alcohol, other depressants

---

bumetanide
(byoo-met'a-nide)
Bumex
Func. class.: Loop diuretic
Chem. class.: Sulfonamide derivative

Action: Acts on ascending loop of Henle by increasing excretion of chloride, sodium
Uses: Edema in CHF, liver disease, renal disease (nephrotic syndrome), pulmonary edema, ascites (nephrotic syndrome), hypertension
Dosage and routes:
• *Adult:* PO 0.5-2.0 mg qd, may give 2nd or 3rd dose at 4-5 hr intervals, not to exceed 20 mg/day, may be given on alternate days or intermittently; IV/IM 0.5-1.0 mg/day, may give 2nd or 3rd dose at 2-3 hr intervals, not to exceed 20 mg/day
Available forms include: Tabs 0.5, 1, 2 mg; inj IV, IM 0.25/ml

---

italics = common side effects   ***bold italic*** = life threatening reactions

Side effects/adverse reactions:

*GU: Polyuria, **renal failure,** glycosuria*

ELECT: Hypokalemia, hypochloremic alkalosis, hypomagnesemia, hyperuricemia, hypocalcemia, hyponatremia

CNS: Headache, fatigue, weakness, vertigo

*GI: Nausea, diarrhea, dry mouth, vomiting, anorexia, cramps, upset stomach, abdominal pain, **acute pancreatitis, jaundice***

*EENT: **Loss of hearing,** ear pain, tinnitus, blurred vision*

*INTEG: Rash, pruritus, purpura, **Stevens-Johnson syndrome,** sweating, photosensitivity*

MS: Cramps, arthritis, stiffness

ENDO: Hyperglycemia

*HEMA: **Thrombocytopenia, agranulocytosis, neutropenia***

*CV: Chest pain, hypotension, **circulatory collapse,** ECG changes*

Contraindications: Hypersensitivity to sulfonamides, anuria, hepatic coma, hypovolemia, lactation

Precautions: Dehydration, ascites, severe renal disease, pregnancy (C)

Pharmacokinetics:

PO: Onset ½-1 hr, duration 4 hr

IM: Onset 40 min, duration 4 hr

IV: Onset 5 min, duration 2-3 hr, Excreted by kidneys, crosses placenta, excreted by breast milk

Interactions/incompatibilities:

• Decreased diuretic effect: indomethacin

• Ototoxicity: cisplatin, aminoglycosides

• Increased effect: antihypertensives

• Increased toxicity: lithium, nondepolarizing skeletal muscle relaxants

• Decreased effects of: antidiabetics

NURSING CONSIDERATIONS

Assess:

• Hearing with high doses

• Weight, I&O daily to determine fluid loss; effect of drug may be decreased if used qd

• Rate, depth, rhythm of respiration, effect of exertion

• B/P lying, standing; postural hypotension may occur

• Electrolytes: potassium, sodium, chloride; include BUN, blood sugar, CBC, serum creatinine, blood pH, ABGs, uric acid, calcium, magnesium

• Glucose in urine if patient is diabetic

Administer:

• Direct IV over at least 1 min

• INT IV after dilution in LR, D_5W, 0.9% NaCl

• In AM to avoid interference with sleep if using drug as a diuretic

• Potassium replacement if potassium is less than 3.0

• With food if nausea occurs; absorption may be decreased slightly

Evaluate:

• Improvement in edema of feet, legs, sacral area daily if medication is being used in CHF

• Improvement in CVP q8h

• Signs of metabolic alkalosis: drowsiness, restlessness

• Signs of hypokalemia: postural hypotension, malaise, fatigue, tachycardia, leg cramps, weakness

• Rashes, temperature elevation qd

• Confusion, especially in elderly; take safety precautions if needed

Teach patient/family:

• To increase fluid intake 2-3 L/day unless contraindicated, to rise slowly from lying or sitting position

• Adverse reactions: muscle cramps, weakness, nausea, dizziness

---

*Available in Canada only

- Take with food or milk for GI symptoms
- Take early in day to prevent nocturia

Treatment of overdose: Lavage if taken orally, monitor electrolytes, administer dextrose in saline, monitor hydration, CV, renal status

---

bupivacaine HCl

(byoop-a-va'caine)
Marcaine, Sensorcaine
Func. class.: Local anesthetic
Chem. class.: Amide

Action: Competes with calcium for sites in nerve membrane that control sodium transport across cell membrane; decreases rise of depolarization phase of action potential

Uses: Epidural anesthesia, peripheral nerve block, caudal anesthesia

Dosage and routes:
Varies depending on route of anesthesia

Available forms include: Inj 0.25%, 0.5%, 0.75%; inj with epinephrine 0.25%, 0.5%, 0.75%

Side effects/adverse reactions:
CNS: Anxiety, restlessness, *convulsions, loss of consciousness,* drowsiness, disorientation, tremors, shivering
CV: Myocardial depression, cardiac arrest, dysrhythmias, bradycardia, hypotension, hypertension, fetal bradycardia
GI: Nausea, vomiting
EENT: Blurred vision, tinnitus, pupil constriction
INTEG: Rash, urticaria, allergic reactions, edema, burning, skin discoloration at injection site, tissue necrosis
RESP: Status asthmaticus, respiratory arrest, anaphylaxis

Contraindications: Hypersensitivity, child <12 yr, elderly, severe liver disease

Precautions: Elderly, severe drug allergies, pregnancy (C)

Pharmacokinetics:
Onset 4-17 min, duration 4-8 hr, excreted in urine (metabolites), metabolized by liver

Interactions/incompatibilities:
- Dysrhythmias: epinephrine, halothane, enflurane
- Hypertension: MAOIs, tricyclic antidepressants, phenothiazines
- Decreased action of bupivacaine: chloroprocaine

NURSING CONSIDERATIONS
Assess:
- B/P, pulse, respiration during treatment
- Fetal heart tones if drug is used during labor

Administer:
- Only with crash cart, resuscitative equipment nearby
- Only drugs without preservatives for epidural or caudal anesthesia

Perform/provide:
- Use of new solution, discard unused portions

Evaluate:
- Therapeutic response: anesthesia necessary for procedure
- Allergic reactions: rash, urticaria, itching
- Cardiac status: ECG for dysrhythmias, pulse, B/P during anesthesia

Treatment of overdose: Airway, O₂, vasopressor, IV fluids, anticonvulsants for seizures

---

buprenorphine HCl

(byoo-preen'or-feen)
Buprenex
Func. class.: Narcotic analgesics
Chem. class.: Opiate, thebaine derivative

Controlled Substance Schedule V

---

italics = common side effects | ***bold italic*** = life threatening reactions

Action: Depresses pain impulse transmission at the spinal cord level by interacting with opioid receptors

Uses: Moderate to severe pain

Dosage and routes:
• *Adult-* IM/IV 0.3-0.6 mg q6h prn, reduce dosage in elderly

Available forms include: Inj IM, IV 1, 2 mg/ml, 0.3 mg/ml (1ml vials)

Side effects/adverse reactions:
CNS: Drowsiness, dizziness, confusion, headache, sedation, euphoria

GI: Nausea, vomiting, anorexia, constipation, cramps

GU: Increased urinary output, dysuria

INTEG: Rash, urticaria, bruising, flushing, diaphoresis, pruritus

EENT: Tinnitus, blurred vision, miosis, diplopia

CV: Palpitations, bradycardia, change in B/P

RESP: Respiratory depression

Contraindications: Hypersensitivity, addiction (narcotic)

Precautions: Addictive personality, pregnancy (C), lactation, increased intracranial pressure, MI (acute), severe heart disease, respiratory depression, hepatic disease, renal disease

Pharmacokinetics:
IM: Onset 10-30 min, peak ½ hr, duration 3-4 hr

IV: Onset 1 min, peak 5 min, duration 2-5 hr

REC: Onset slow, duration 4-6 hr
Metabolized by liver, excreted by kidneys, crosses placenta, excreted in breast milk, half-life 2½-3½ hr, 96% bound to plasma proteins

Interactions/incompatibilities:
• Effects may be increased with other CNS depressants: alcohol, narcotics, sedative/hypnotics, antipsychotics, skeletal muscle relaxants

NURSING CONSIDERATIONS
Assess:
• I&O ratio; check for decreasing output; may indicate urinary retention

Administer:
• IV slowly over 2-3 min
• With antiemetic if nausea, vomiting occur
• When pain is beginning to return; determine dosage interval by patient response

Perform/provide:
• Assistance with ambulation
• Safety measures: siderails

Evaluate:
• CNS changes, dizziness, drowsiness, hallucinations, euphoria, LOC, pupil reaction
• Allergic reactions: rash, urticaria
• Respiratory dysfunction: respiratory depression, character, rate, rhythm; notify physician if respirations are <12/min
• Need for pain medication, physical dependence
• Therapeutic response: decrease in pain, absence of grimacing

Teach patient/family:
• To report any symptoms of CNS changes, allergic reactions
• That physical dependency may result when used for extended periods of time

Treatment of overdose: Narcan 0.2-0.8 mg IV, O₂, IV fluids, vasopressors

---

buproprione
(byoo-proe′ pee-on)
Wellbutrin

Func. class.: Misc. antidepressant

Action: Inhibits reuptake of dopa-

mine, serotonin, norepinephrine
Uses: Depression
Dosage and routes:
Adult: PO 100 mg bid initially, then increase after 3 day to 100 mg tid if needed; may increase after 1 month to 150 mg tid
Available forms: 75, 100 mg
Side effects/adverse reactions:
*CNS: Headache, agitation, confusion, **seizures,** akathisia,* delusions, insomnia, sedation, tremors
CV: Dysrhythmias, hypertension, palpitations, tachycardia, hypotension
GI: Nausea, vomiting, dry mouth, increased appetite, constipation
GU: Impotence, frequency, retention
INTEG: Rash, pruritus, sweating
EENT: Blurred vision, auditory disturbance
Contraindications: Hypersensitivity, seizure disorder, eating disorders
Precautions: Renal and hepatic disease, recent MI, cranial trauma, pregnancy (B), lactation, children
Pharmacokinetics: Onset 2-4 wk, half-life 12-14 hr, metabolized by liver
Interactions/incompatibilities:
• Increased adverse reactions: levodopa, MAO inhibitors, phenothiazines, tricyclic antidepressants, benzodiazepines, alcohol
NURSING CONSIDERATIONS
Assess:
• Blood studies: CBC, leukocytes, differential, cardiac enzymes if patient is on long-term therapy
• Liver function tests before, during therapy: bilirubin, AST, ALT, creatinine
• ECG: watch for flattening of T wave, bundle branch block, AV block, dysrhythmias in cardiac patients

Administer:
• Increased fluids, bulk in diet if constipation, urinary retention occur
• With food or milk for GI symptoms
• Gum, hard candy, or frequent sips of water for dry mouth
Perform/provide:
• Assistance with ambulation during beginning therapy, since sedation occurs
• Safety measures, including siderails, primarily in elderly
• Checking to see PO medication is swallowed
Evaluate:
• Therapeutic response: decreased depression, ability to function in daily activities, ability to sleep throughout the night
• Mental status: mood sensorium, affect, suicidal tendencies, increase in psychiatric symptoms
• EPS primarily in elderly: akathisia
• Withdrawal symptoms: headache, nausea, vomiting, muscle pain, weakness occurs if drug is discontinued abruptly
• Alcohol consumption: if alcohol is consumed, hold dose until morning
Teach patient/family:
• Therapeutic effects may take 2-4 wk
• Use caution in driving or other activities requiring alertness; sedation and blurred vision may occur
• To avoid alcohol ingestion, other CNS depressants
• Not to discontinue medication quickly after long-term use, may cause nausea, headache, malaise
Treatment of overdose: ECG monitoring; induce emesis, lavage,

---

italics = common side effects   ***bold italic*** = life threatening reactions

activated charcoal; administer anticonvulsant

---

buspirone HCl

(byoo-spear'-own)

Buspar

Func. class.: Antianxiety agent

Chem. class.: Azaspirodecane-dione

Action: Unknown; may act by inhibiting 5-HT, a receptor in brain tissue

Uses: Management and short-term relief of anxiety disorders

Dosage and routes:

• *Adult:* PO 5 mg tid, may increase by 5 mg/day q2-3 days, not to exceed 60 mg/day

Available forms include: Tabs 5, 10 mg

Side effects/adverse reactions:

CNS: Dizziness, headache, depression, stimulation, insomnia, nervousness, lightheadedness, numbness, paresthesia, incoordination, tremors, excitement, involuntary movements, confusion, akathisia

GI: Nausea, dry mouth, diarrhea, constipation, flatulence, increased appetite, rectal bleeding

CV: Tachycardia, palpitations, hypotension, hypertension, *CVA, CHF, MI*

EENT: Sore throat, tinnitus, blurred vision, nasal congestion, red, itching eyes, change in taste, smell

GU: Frequency, hesitancy, menstrual irregularity, change in libido

MS: Pain, weakness, muscle cramps, spasms

RESP: Hyperventilation, chest congestion, shortness of breath

INTEG: Rash, edema, pruritus, alopecia, dry skin

MISC: Sweating, fatigue, weight gain, fever

Contraindications: Hypersensitivity, child <18 yr

Precautions: Pregnancy (B), lactation, elderly, impaired hepatic/renal function

Interactions/incompatibilities:

• Increased B/P: MAOIs; do not use together

• Increased effects: psychotropic drugs, alcohol (avoid use)

• Increased ALT: trazodone

NURSING CONSIDERATIONS

Assess:

• B/P (lying, standing), pulse; if systolic B/P drops 20 mm Hg, hold drug, notify physician

• Blood studies: CBC during long-term therapy; blood dyscrasias have occurred rarely

• Hepatic studies: AST, ALT, bilirubin, creatinine, LDH, alk phosphatase

• I&O; may indicate renal dysfunction

• Mental status: mood, sensorium, affect, sleeping pattern, drowsiness, dizziness

Administer:

• With food or milk for GI symptoms

• Crushed if patient unable to swallow medication whole

• Sugarless gum, hard candy, frequent sips of water for dry mouth

Perform/provide:

• Assistance with ambulation during beginning therapy; drowsiness, dizziness occur

• Safety measures, including side-rails if drowsiness occurs

• Check to see PO medication swallowed

Evaluate:

• Therapeutic response: decreased anxiety, restlessness, sleeplessness

• Suicidal tendencies

Teach patient/family:

• That drug may be taken with food

---

* Available in Canada only

- Avoid OTC preparations unless approved by physician
- To avoid driving, activities requiring alertness, since drowsiness may occur
- To avoid alcohol ingestion or other psychotropic medications, unless prescribed by physician
- Not to discontinue medication abruptly after long-term use
- To rise slowly or fainting may occur
- That drowsiness might worsen at beginning of treatment
- 1-2 wk of therapy may be required before therapeutic effects occur

Treatment of overdose: Gastric lavage, VS, supportive care

busulfan

(byoo-sul'fan)
Myleran

Func. class.: Antineoplastic alkylating agent
Chem. class.: Nitrosurea

Action: Changes essential cellular ions to covalent bonding with resultant alkylation; this interferes with normal biologic function of DNA; activity is not phase specific, action is due to myelosuppression

Uses: Chronic myelocytic leukemia

Dosage and routes:
- *Adult:* PO 4-12 mg/day initially until WBC levels fall to 10,000/mm³, then drug is stopped until WBC levels raise over 50,000/mm³, then 1-3 mg/day
- *Child:* PO 0.06-0.12 mg/kg or 1.8-4.6 mg/m² day; dose is titrated to maintain WBC levels at 20,000/mm³

Available forms include: Tab 2 mg

Side effects/adverse reactions:
*HEMA: **Thrombocytopenia, leukopenia, pancytopenia, severe bone marrow depression***
GI: Nausea, vomiting, *diarrhea, weight loss*
GU: Impotence, sterility, amenorrhea, gynecomastia, *renal toxicity,* hyperuremia
INTEG: Dermatitis, hyperpigmentation
*RESP: **Fibrosis,** pneumonitis*
*OTHER: **Chromosomal aberrations***

Contraindications: Radiation, chemotherapy, lactation, pregnancy (3rd trimester) (D), "blastic" phase of chronic myelocytic leukemia, hypersensitivity

Precautions: Childbearing age men, women, leukopenia, thrombocytopenia, anemia, hepatotoxicity, renal toxicity

Pharmacokinetics:
Well absorbed orally, excreted in urine, crosses placenta, excreted in breast milk

Interactions/incompatibilities:
Increased toxicity: other antineoplastics or radiation

NURSING CONSIDERATIONS
Assess:
- CBC, differential, platelet count weekly; withhold drug if WBC is <4000 or platelet count is <75,000; notify physician of results
- Pulmonary function tests, chest x-ray films before, during therapy; chest film should be obtained q2wk during treatment
- Renal function studies: BUN, serum uric acid, urine CrCl before, during therapy
- I&O ratio; report fall in urine output of 30 ml/hr
- Monitor for cold, fever, sore throat (may indicate beginning infection)
- For decreased hyperuricemia

Administer:
• Antacid before oral agent, give drug after evening meal, before bedtime
• Antiemetic 30-60 min before giving drug to prevent vomiting
• Allopurinol or sodium bicarbonate to maintain uric acid levels, alkalinization of urine
• Antibiotics for prophylaxis of infection

Perform/provide:
• Comprehensive oral hygiene
• Strict medical asepsis, protective isolation if WBC levels are low
• Deep breathing exercises with patient tid-qid; place in semi-Fowler's position for pulmonary reactions
• Increase fluid intake to 2-3 L/day to prevent urate deposits, calculi formation
• Diet low in purines: organ meats (kidney, liver), dried beans, peas to maintain alkaline urine
• Storage in tight container

Evaluate:
• Bleeding: hematuria, guaiac, bruising or petechiae, mucosa or orifices q8h, no rectal temps
• Dyspnea, rales, unproductive cough, chest pain, tachypnea
• Food preferences; list likes, dislikes
• Edema in feet, joint, stomach pain, shaking
• Inflammation of mucosa, breaks in skin, use viscous xylocaine for oral pain

Teach patient/family:
• Of protective isolation precautions
• To avoid use of aspirin, or ibuprofen; razors, commercial mouthwash
• To report signs of anemia, (fatigue, headache, irritability, faintness, shortness of breath

• To report symptoms of bleeding (hematuria, tarry stools)
• That impotence or amenorrhea can occur, are reversible after discontinuing treatment
• To report any changes in breathing or coughing even several months after treatment

---

butabarbital/butabarbital sodium

(byoo-ta-bar'bi-tal)
Butisol, Medarsed, Butatran, Buticaps, Butisol Sodium
Func. class.: Sedative/hypnotic-barbiturate
Chem. class.: Barbitone (intermediate acting)

Controlled Substance Schedule III (USA), Schedule G (Canada)
Action: Depresses activity in brain cells primarily in reticular activating system in brainstem; also selectively depresses neurons in posterior hypothalamus and limbic structures
Uses: Sedation, insomnia, preoperatively

Dosage and routes:
Sedation
• *Adult:* PO 15-30 mg tid or qid
• *Child:* PO 6 mg/kg/day or 180 mg/m² in divided doses tid, range may vary from 7.5-30 mg tid
Insomnia
• *Adult:* PO 50-100 mg hs
Preoperatively
• *Adult:* PO 50-100 mg 1-2 hr preoperatively
Available forms include: Tabs 15, 30, 50, 100 mg; caps 15, 30 mg; elix 30, 33.3 mg/5 ml, powder
Side effects/adverse reactions:
CNS: Lethargy, drowsiness, hangover, dizziness, stimulation in elderly and children, lightheaded-

---

ness, physical dependence, CNS depression, mental depression, slurred speech

GI: Nausea, vomiting, diarrhea, constipation

INTEG: Rash, urticaria, pain, abscesses at injection site, *angioedema,* thrombophlebitis, *Stevens-Johnson syndrome*

CV: Hypotension, bradycardia

RESP: Depression, *apnea, laryngospasm, bronchospasm*

HEMA: Agranulocytosis, thrombocytopenia, megaloblastic anemia (long-term treatment)

Contraindications: Hypersensitivity to barbiturates, respiratory depression, addiction to barbiturates, severe liver impairment, porphyria

Precautions: Anemia, pregnancy (D), lactation, hepatic disease, renal disease, hypertension, elderly, acute/chronic pain

Pharmacokinetics:

PO: Onset 40-60 min, duration 6-8 hr; metabolized by liver, excreted by kidneys; half-life 66-140 hr

Interactions/incompatibilities:

• Increased CNS depression: alcohol, MAOIs, sedative, narcotics

• Decreased effect of: oral anticoagulants, corticosteroids, griseofulvin, quinidine, oral contraceptives, estrogens

• Decreased half-life of: doxycycline

NURSING CONSIDERATIONS

Assess:

• Blood studies: Hct, Hgb, RBCs, serum folate (if on long-term therapy); pro-time in patients receiving anticoagulants

• Hepatic studies: AST, ALT, bilirubin; if increased, the drug is usually discontinued

Administer:

• After removal of cigarettes, to prevent fires

• After trying conservative measures for insomnia

• ½-1 hr before hs for sleeplessness

• On empty stomach for best absorption

Perform/provide:

• Assistance with ambulation after receiving dose

• Safety measure: siderails, nightlight, callbell within easy reach

• Checking to see PO medication swallowed

Evaluate:

• Therapeutic response: ability to sleep at night, decreased amount of early morning awakening if taking drug for insomnia

• Mental status: mood, sensorium, affect, memory (long, short)

• Physical dependency: more frequent requests for medication, shakes, anxiety

• Barbiturate toxicity: hypotension; pulmonary constriction; cold, clammy skin; cyanosis of lips; insomnia; nausea; vomiting; hallucinations; delirium; weakness, coma, pupillary constriction; mild symptoms may occur in 8-12 hr without drug

• Respiratory dysfunction: respiratory depression, character, rate, rhythm; hold drug if respirations are <10/min or if pupils are dilated

• Blood dyscrasias: fever, sore throat, bruising, rash, jaundice, epistaxis

Teach patient/family:

• That hangover is common

• That drug is indicated only for short-term treatment of insomnia and is probably ineffective after 2 wk

• That physical dependency may result when used for extended periods of time (45-90 days depending on dose)

---

italics = common side effects   ***bold italic*** = life threatening reactions

• To avoid driving or other activities requiring alertness
• To avoid alcohol ingestion or CNS depressants; serious CNS depression may result
• Not to discontinue medication quickly after long-term use; drug should be tapered over 1-2 wk
• To tell all prescribers that a barbiturate is being taken
• That withdrawal insomnia may occur after short-term use; do not start using drug again, insomnia will improve in 1-3 nights
• That effects may take 2 nights for benefits to be noticed
• Alternate measures to improve sleep (reading, exercise several hours hs, warm bath, warm milk, TV, self-hypnosis, deep breathing)

Lab test interferences:
False increase: Sulfobromophthalein test

Treatment of overdose: Lavage, activated charcoal, warming blanket, vital signs, hemodialysis, alkalinize urine

---

butoconazole nitrate
(byoo'-toe-kone-a-zole)
Femstat

Func. class.: Local antiinfective
Chem. class.: Antifungal

Action: Binds sterols in fungal cell membrane, which increases permeability
Uses: Vaginal infections caused by *Candida*
Dosage and routes:
• *Adult:* INTRA VAG 1 applicatorful hs × 3 days (nonpregnant), 6 days (2nd/3rd trimester pregnancy)
Available forms include: Vaginal cream 2%
Side effects/adverse reactions:
GU: Rash, stinging, burning, vulvo vaginal itching, soreness, swelling

Contraindications: Hypersensitivity
Precautions: Pregnancy (C), lactation

NURSING CONSIDERATIONS
Administer:
• 1 applicatorful every night into vagina
Perform/provide:
• Storage at room temperature in dry place
Evaluate:
• Allergic reaction: burning, stinging, itching, discharge, soreness
• Therapeutic response: decrease in itching, or white discharge
Teach patient/family:
• May experience increased dreaming
• To apply with applicator only
• To avoid use of any other vaginal product unless directed by physician
• To use medical asepsis (hand washing) before, after each application
• To abstain from sexual intercourse until treatment is completed
• To notify physician if symptoms persist

---

butorphanol tartrate
(byoo-tor'fa-nole)
Stadol

Func. class.: Narcotic analgesics
Chem. class.: Opiate

Action: Depresses pain impulse transmission at the spinal cord level by interacting with opioid receptors
Uses: Moderate to severe pain
Dosage and routes:
• *Adult:* IM 1-4 mg q3-4h prn; IV 0.5-2 mg q3-4h prn

Available forms include: Inj IM, IV 1, 2 mg/ml

Side effects/adverse reactions:

CNS: Drowsiness, dizziness, confusion, headache, sedation, euphoria, weakness

GI: Nausea, vomiting, anorexia, constipation, cramps

GU: Increased urinary output, dysuria, urinary retention

INTEG: Rash, urticaria, bruising, flushing, diaphoresis, pruritus

EENT: Tinnitus, blurred vision, miosis, diplopia

CV: Palpitations, bradycardia, change in B/P

*RESP: **Respiratory depression,** pulmonary hypertension*

Contraindications: Hypersensitivity, addiction (narcotic), CHF, myocardial infarction

Precautions: Addictive personality, pregnancy (B), lactation, increased intracranial pressure, respiratory depression, hepatic disease, renal disease, child <18 yr

Pharmacokinetics:

IM: Onset 10-30 min, peak ½ hr, duration 3-4 hr

IV: Onset 1 min, peak 5 min, duration 2-4 hr

REC: Onset slow, duration 4-6 hr, metabolized by liver, excreted by kidneys, crosses placenta, excreted in breast milk, half-life 2½-3½ hr

Interactions/incompatibilities:

• Effects may be increased with other CNS depressants: alcohol, narcotics, sedative/hypnotics, antipsychotics, skeletal muscle relaxants

NURSING CONSIDERATIONS

Assess:

• I&O ratio; check for decreasing output; may indicate urinary retention

• For withdrawal symptoms in narcotic dependent patients: pulmonary embolus, vascular occlusion, abscesses, ulcerations

Administer:

• IV over 3-5 min

• IM deeply in large muscle mass

• With antiemetic if nausea, vomiting occur

• When pain is beginning to return; determine dosage interval by patient response

Perform/provide:

• Storage in light-resistant area at room temperature

• Assistance with ambulation

• Safety measures: siderails, night light, call bell within easy reach

Evaluate:

• Therapeutic response: decrease in pain

• CNS changes: dizziness, drowsiness, hallucinations, euphoria, LOC, pupil reaction

• Allergic reactions: rash, urticaria

• Respiratory dysfunction: respiratory depression, character, rate, rhythm; notify physician if respirations are <10/min

• Need for pain medication, physical dependence

Teach patient/family:

• To report any symptoms of CNS changes, allergic reactions

• That physical dependency may result when used for extended periods of time

• Withdrawal symptoms may occur: nausea, vomiting, cramps, fever, faintness, anorexia

Lab test interferences:

Increase: Amylase

Treatment of overdose: Narcan 0.2-0.8 mg IV, O₂, IV fluids, vasopressors

---

italics = common side effects   ***bold italic*** = life threatening reactions

caffeine

(kaf-een)

No-Doz, Tirend, Vivarin, Dexitac, Quick Pep

Func. class.: Analeptic
Chem. class.: Xanthine

Action: Increases calcium permeability in sarcoplasmic reticulum, promotes accumulation of cAMP, and competitively blocks adenosine receptors

Uses: Mild CNS stimulation, in combination with analgesics, diuretics for tension and fluid retention associated with menstruation

Dosage and routes:
• *Adult:* PO 100-200 mg q4h prn; IM 500 mg; timed rel 200-250 mg q4-6h
• *Infant and child:* 8 mg/kg, not to exceed 500 mg

Available forms include: Tabs 65, 150 mg; time rel caps 200, 250 mg; inj 850 mg/ml

Side effects/adverse reactions:

CNS: Hyperactivity, insomnia, restlessness, talkativeness, dizziness, headache, *stimulation,* irritability, aggressiveness, tremors, twitching, mild delirium, tinnitus

GI: Nausea, vomiting, anorexia, gastric irritation, diarrhea

GU: Diuresis

CV: Tachycardia, extrasystole, dysrhythmias, palpitations

INTEG: Hyperesthesia

Contraindications: Hypersensitivity

Precautions: Dysrhythmias, Gilles de la Tourette's disorder, pregnancy (B), lactation, renal, psychological disorders

Pharmacokinetics:

PO: Onset 15 min, peak ½-1 hr, metabolized by liver, excreted by kidneys, crosses placenta, breast milk, half-life 3-4 hr

Interactions/incompatibilities:
• Increased effect of caffeine: oral contraceptives, cimetidine

NURSING CONSIDERATIONS

Assess:
• VS, B/P

Evaluate:
• Therapeutic response: increased CNS stimulation, decreased drowsiness
• Mental status: mood, sensorium, affect, stimulation, insomnia, irritability
• Tolerance or dependency: an increased amount may be used to get same effect
• Overdose: pain, fever, dehydration, insomnia, hyperactivity

Teach patient/family:
• To decrease other caffeine consumption (coffee, tea, cola, chocolate), which may increase irritability, stimulation
• To taper off drug over several weeks if used long-term

Lab test interferences:

Increase: Urinary cathecholamines
False positive: Serum urate

Treatment of overdose: Lavage, activated charcoal, monitor electrolytes, VS, administer anticonvulsants if needed

---

calcifediol

(kal-si-fe-dye'ole)

Calderol

Func. class.: Vitamin D analog
Chem. class.: Sterol

Action: Increases intestinal absorption of calcium for bones; increases renal tubular absorption of phosphate, increases mobilization of

---

calcium from bones, bone resorption

Uses: Metabolic bone disease with chronic renal failure, osteopenia, osteomalacia, hypocalcemia

Dosage and routes:
• *Adult:* PO 300-350 μg qwk divided into qd or qod doses; may increase q4wk

Available forms include: Caps 20, 50 μg

Side effects/adverse reactions:
EENT: Tinnitus
CNS: Drowsiness, headache, vertigo, fever, lethargy
GI: Nausea, diarrhea, vomiting, jaundice, anorexia, dry mouth, constipation, cramps, metallic taste
MS: Myalgia, arthralgia, decreased bone development
GU: Polyuria, hypercalciuria, hyperphosphatemia, hematuria
CV: dysrhythmias

Contraindications: Hypersensitivity, hyperphosphatemia, hypercalcemia

Precautions: Pregnancy (C), renal calculi, lactation, CV disease

Pharmacokinetics:
PO: Peak 4 hr, duration 15-20 days; half-life 12-22 days

Interactions/incompatibilities:
• Decreased absorption of calcifediol: cholestyramine, colestipol HCl, mineral oil
• Hypercalcemia: thiazide diuretics
• Cardiac dysrhythmias: cardiac glycosides
• Decreased effect of this drug: corticosteroids

NURSING CONSIDERATIONS
Assess:
• BUN, urinary calcium, AST, ALT, cholesterol, creatinine, uric acid, chloride, magnesium, electrolytes, urine pH, phosphate; may increase, calcium should be kept at 9-10 mg/dl, vitamin D 50-135 IU/dl, phosphate 70 mg/dl
• Alk phosphatase; may be decreased
• For increased blood level since toxic reactions may occur rapidly

Administer:
• PO may be increased q4wk depending on blood level

Perform/provide:
• Storage in tight, light-resistant containers at room temperature
• Restriction of sodium, potassium if required
• Restriction of fluids if required for chronic renal failure

Evaluate:
• For dry mouth, metallic taste, polyuria, bone pain, muscle weakness, headache, fatigue, tinnitus, change in LOC, irregular pulse, dysrhythmias, increased respirations, anorexia, nausea, vomiting, cramps, diarrhea, constipation; may indicate hypercalcemia
• Renal status: decreased urinary output (oliguria, anuria), edema in extremities, weight gain 5 lb, periorbital edema
• Nutritional status, diet for sources of vitamin D (milk, some seafood), calcium (dairy products, dark green vegetables), phosphates (dairy products)

Teach patient/family:
• The symptoms of hypercalcemia
• Foods rich in calcium

Lab test interferences:
False increase: Cholesterol

---

calcitonin (human)
(kal-si-toe′nin)
Cibacalcin

Func. class.: Parathyroid agents (calcium regulator)
Chem. class.: Polypeptide hormone

Action: Decreases bone resorption,

---

blood calcium levels; increases deposits of calcium in bones

Uses: Paget's disease

Dosage and routes:

Paget's disease

• *Adult:* SC 0.5 mg/day initially; may require 0.5 mg bid × 6 mo, then decrease until symptoms reappear

Available forms include: Inj (SC) 0.5 mg/vial

Side effects/adverse reactions:

INTEG: Rash, flushing, pruritus of ear lobes, edema of feet

CNS: Headache, tetany, chills, weakness, dizziness

GU: Diuresis

GI: Nausea, diarrhea, vomiting, anorexia, abdominal pain, salty taste

MS: Swelling, tingling of hands

CV: Chest pressure

RESP: Dyspnea

Contraindications: Hypersensitivity

Precautions: Renal disease, children, lactation, osteogenic sarcoma, pregnancy (C)

Pharmacokinetics:

IM/SC: Onset 15 min, peak 4 hr, duration 8-24 hr; metabolized by kidneys, excreted as inactive metabolites

NURSING CONSIDERATIONS

Assess:

• GI symptoms, polyuria, flushing, head swelling, tingling, headache; may indicate hypercalcemia

• Nutritional status; diet for sources of vitamin D (milk, some seafood), calcium (dairy products, dark green vegetables), phosphates

Administer:

• By SC route only, rotate injection sites; use within 6 hr of reconstitution, give hs to minimize nausea, vomiting

Perform/provide:

• Store at <77° F, protect from light

Evaluate:

• BUN, creatinine, uric acid, chloride, electrolytes, urine pH, urinary calcium, magnesium, phosphate, urinalysis, (calcium should be kept at 9-10 mg/dl, vitamin D 50-135 IU/dl), alk phosphatase baseline and q3-6 mo

• Increased drug level since toxic reactions occur rapidly, have calcium chloride on hand if calcium level drops too low; check for tetany

• Urine for sediment

Teach patient/family:

• Method of injection if patient will be responsible for self-medication

---

calcitonin (salmon)

(kal-si-toe′nin)

Calcimar, Miacalcin

Func. class.: Parathyroid agents (calcium regulator)

Chem. class.: Polypeptide hormone

Action: Decreases bone resorption, blood calcium levels; increases deposits of calcium in bones

Uses: Hypercalcemia, postmenopausal osteoporosis, Paget's disease

Dosage and routes:

Osteoporosis/Paget's disease

• *Adult:* SC/IM 100 IU qd, maintenance for Paget's disease 50-100 IU qd or qod

Hypercalcemia

• *Adult:* IM 4-8 IU/kg q6-12h

Available forms include: Inj SC/IM 200 MRC units/ml, 100 IU/ml

Side effects/adverse reactions:

INTEG: Rash, pruritus of ear lobes, edema of feet

CNS: Headache, flushing, ***tetany,*** chills, weakness, dizziness
GU: Diuresis
GI: Nausea, diarrhea, vomiting, anorexia, abdominal pain, salty taste
MS: Swelling, tingling of hands
Contraindications: Hypersensitivity, children, lactation
Precautions: Renal disease, osteoporosis, pernicious anemia, Zollinger-Ellison syndrome, pregnancy (C)
Pharmacokinetics:
IM/SC: Onset 15 min, peak 4 hr, duration 8-24 hr; metabolized by kidneys, excreted as inactive metabolites

NURSING CONSIDERATIONS
Assess:
• BUN, creatinine, uric acid, chloride, electrolytes, urine pH, urinary calcium, magnesium, phosphatase, urinalysis, calcitonin antibody formation (calcium should be kept at 9-10 mg/dl, vitamin D 50-135 IU/dl), alk phosphatase
• Increased level since toxic reactions may occur rapidly
• Urine for sediment and casts
Administer:
• After test dose of 10 IU/ml, give 0.1 ml intradermally, watch 15 min; give only with epinephrine and emergency meds available
• IM injection in deep muscle mass slowly, rotate sites
Perform/provide:
• Storage in light-resistant area, refrigerate
• Restriction of sodium, potassium if required
Evaluate:
• GI symptoms, polyuria, flushing, head swelling, tingling, headache; may indicate hypercalcemia
• Nutritional status; diet for sources of vitamin D (milk, some seafood),

calcium (dairy products, dark green vegetables), phosphates
• Systemic allergic reaction to drug: skin test before 1st dose
Teach patient/family:
• Avoid OTC products
• To administer drug SC if patient will be responsible for self-medication

---

calcitriol (1,25-Dihydroxycholecalciferol)
(kal-si-tyre′ole)
Rocaltrol
Func. class.: Parathyroid agents (calcium regulator)
Chem. class.: Vitamin D hormone

Action: Increases intestinal absorption of calcium, provides calcium for bones, increases renal tubular resorption of phosphate
Uses: Hypocalcemia in chronic renal dialysis, hypoparathyroidism, pseudo-hypoparathyroidism
Dosage and routes:
Hypocalcemia
• *Adult:* PO 0.25 μg qd, may increase by 0.25 μg/day q4-8wk, maintenance 0.25 μg qod-1 μg qd
Hypoparathyroidism/pseudohypoparathyroidism
• *Adult and child >1 yr:* PO 0.25 μg qd, may be increased q2-4wk; maintenance 0.25-2 μg qd
Available forms include: Caps 0.25, 0.5 μg
Side effects/adverse reactions:
CNS: Drowsiness, headache, vertigo, fever, lethargy
GI: Nausea, diarrhea, vomiting, jaundice, anorexia, dry mouth, constipation, cramps, metallic taste
MS: Myalgia, arthralgia, decreased bone development
GU: Polyuria, hypercalciuria, hyperphosphatemia, hematuria

---

italics = common side effects   ***bold italic*** = life threatening reactions

Contraindications: Hypersensitivity, hyperphosphatemia, hypercalcemia

Precautions: Pregnancy (C), renal calculi, lactation, CV disease

Pharmacokinetics:
PO: Peak 4 hr, duration 15-20 days, half-life 3-6 hr

Interactions/incompatibilities:
• Decreased absorption of calcitriol: cholestyramine, mineral oil
• Hypercalcemia: thiazide diuretics, calcium supplement
• Cardiac dysrhythmias: cardiac glycosides, verapamil
• Decreased effect of calcifediol: barbiturates, phenytoin, corticosteroids

NURSING CONSIDERATIONS
Assess:
• BUN, urinary calcium, AST, ALT, cholesterol, creatinine, uric acid, chloride, magnesium, electrolytes, urine pH, phosphate; may increase calcium, should be kept at 9-10 mg/dl, vitamin D 50-135 IU/dl, phosphate 70 mg/dl
• Alk phosphatase; may be decreased
• For increased drug level since toxic reactions may occur rapidly

Perform/provide:
• Storage protected from light, heat, moisture
• Restriction of sodium, potassium if required
• Restriction of fluids if required for chronic renal failure

Evaluate:
• For dry mouth, metallic taste, polyuria, bone pain, muscle weakness, headache, fatigue, change in LOC, dysrhythmias, increased respirations, anorexia, nausea, vomiting, cramps, diarrhea, constipation; may indicate hypercalcemia
• Renal status: decreased urinary output (oliguria, anuria), edema in extremities, weight gain 75 lb, periorbital edema
• Nutritional status, diet for sources of vitamin D (milk, some seafood), calcium (dairy products, dark green vegetables), phosphates (dairy products) must be avoided

Teach patient/family:
• The symptoms of hypercalcemia
• Foods rich in calcium
• To avoid products with sodium: cured meats, dairy products, cold cuts, olives, beets, pickles, soups, meat tenderizers in chronic renal failure
• To avoid products with potassium: oranges, bananas, dried fruit, peas, dark green leafy vegetables, milk, melons, beans in chronic renal failure
• Avoid OTC products containing calcium, potassium, or sodium in chronic renal failure
• Avoid all preparations containing vitamin D

Lab test interferences:
False increase: Cholesterol

---

calcium carbonate

Alka-2, Amitone, Apo-Cal, Biocal Calcilac, Calglycine, Chooz, Dicarbosil, El-Da-Minte, Equilet, Gustalac, Mallamint, Os-Cal, P.H. Tablets, Titracid, Titralac, Trialea, Tums, Calsup, Caltrate

Func. class.: Antacid, calcium supplement

Chem. class.: Calcium product

Action: Neutralizes gastric acidity
Uses: Antacid, calcium supplement
Dosage and routes:
• *Adult:* PO 1 g 4-6 × /day, chewed with water; SUSP 1 g 1 hr pc, hs

Available forms include: Chewable

---

tabs 350, 420, 500, 750 mg; tabs 650 mg; gum 500 mg; susp 1 g/5 ml
Side effects/adverse reactions:
GI: Constipation, anorexia, ***obstruction,*** nausea, vomiting, flatulence, diarrhea, rebound hyperacidity, eructation
*CV: **Hemorrhage, rebound hypertension***
META: Hypercalcemia, metabolic alkalosis
GU: Renal dysfunction, renal stones, ***renal failure***
Contraindications: Hypersensitivity, hypercalcemia, hyperparathyroidism, bone tumors
Precautions: Elderly, fluid restriction, decreased GI motility, GI obstruction, dehydration, renal disease, pregnancy (C)
Pharmacokinetics:
PO: Onset 3 min, excreted in feces
Interactions/incompatibilities:
• Increased plasma levels of: quinidine, amphetamines
• Decreased levels of: salicylates, calcium channel blockers, ketoconazole, tetracyclines, iron salts
• Hypercalcemia: thiazide diuretics
NURSING CONSIDERATIONS
Assess:
• Ca⁺ (serum, urine), Ca⁺ should be 8.5-10.5 mg/dl, urine Ca⁺ should be 150 mg/day, monitor weekly
Administer:
• As antacid 1 hr pc and hs
• As supplement 1½ h pc and hs
• Only with regular tablets or capsules, do not give with enteric-coated tablets
• Laxatives, or stool softeners if constipation occurs
Evaluate:
• Therapeutic response: absence of pain, decreased acidity
• Milk-alkali syndrome: nausea, vomiting, disorientation, headache

• Constipation; increase bulk in the diet if needed
• Hypercalcemia: headache, nausea, vomiting, confusion
Teach patient/family:
• Increase fluids to 2000 ml unless contraindicated
• Not to switch antacids unless directed by physician

---

calcium chloride/calcium gluceptate/calcium gluconate/calcium lactate
Func. class.: Electrolyte replacements—calcium product

Action: Cation needed for maintenance of nervous, muscular, skeletal, enzyme reactions, normal cardiac contractility, coagulation of blood; affects secretory activity of endocrine, exocrine glands
Uses: Prevention and treatment of hypocalcemia, hypermagnesemia, hypoparathyroidism, neonatal tetany, cardiac toxicity caused by hyperkalemia, lead colic
Dosage and routes:
Calcium chloride
• *Adult:* IV 500 mg-1 g q1-3 days as indicated by serum calcium levels, give at <1 ml/min; IAV 200-800 mg injected in ventricle of heart
• *Child:* IV 25 mg/kg over several min
Calcium gluceptate
• *Adult:* IV 5-20 ml; IM 2-5 ml
• *Newborn:* 0.5 ml/100 ml of blood transfused
Calcium gluconate
• *Adult:* PO 0.5-2 g bid-qid; IV 0.5-2 g at 0.5 ml/min (10% solution)
• *Child:* PO/IV 500 mg/kg/day in divided doses
Calcium lactate

• *Adult:* PO 325 mg-1.3 g tid with meals
• *Child:* PO 500 mg/kg/day in divided doses
Available forms include: Many, check product listings
Side effects/adverse reactions:
Hypercalcemia: Drowsiness, lethargy, muscle weakness, headache, constipation, ***coma,*** anorexia, nausea, vomiting, polyuria, thirst
CV: Shortened Q-T, heart block
Contraindications: Hypercalcemia, digitalis toxicity, ventricular fibrillation, renal calculi
Precautions: Pregnancy (C), lactation, children, renal disease, respiratory disease, cor pulmonale, digitalized patient, respiratory failure
Interactions/incompatibilities:
• Increased dysrhythmias: digitalis glycosides
• Decreased action: calcium channel blockers
NURSING CONSIDERATIONS
Assess:
• ECG for decreased QT and T wave inversion: hypercalcemia, drug should be reduced or discontinued
• Calcium levels during treatment (8.5-1.5 g/dl is normal level)
Administer:
• Through small-bore needle into large vein, give over several min, if extravasation occurs, necrosis will result (IV); may be given directly or diluted in compatible IV sol; IM injection may cause severe burning, necrosis, and tissue sloughing
• In large vein, avoiding scalp
• PO with or following meals to enhance absorption
Perform/provide:
• Seizure precautions: padded side rails, decreased stimuli, (noise,

light); place airway suction equipment, padded mouth gag if Ca levels are low
• Store at room temperature
Evaluate:
• Cardiac status: rate, rhythm, CVP, (PWP, PAWP if being monitored directly)
• Therapeutic response: decreased twitching, paresthesias, muscle spasms, absence of tremors, convulsions, dysrhythmias, dyspnea, laryngospasm, negative Chvostek's sign, negative Trousseau's sign
Teach patient/family:
• To remain recumbent ½ hr after IV dose
• To add food high in vitamin D content
• To add calcium-rich foods to diet: dairy products, shellfish, dark green leafy vegetables; and decrease oxalate-rich and zinc-rich foods: nuts, legumes, chocolate, spinach, soy
Lab test interferences:
Increase: 11-OCHS
False decrease: Magnesium
Decrease: 17-OHCS

---

calcium polycarbophol
(pol-i-kar'boe-fol)
Mitrolan
Func. class.: Laxative
Chem. class.: Bulk-forming

Action: Attracts water, expands in intestine to increase peristalsis; also absorbs excess water in stool; decreases diarrhea
Uses: Constipation, irritable bowel syndrome (diarrhea), acute, nonspecific diarrhea
Dosage and routes:
• *Adult:* PO 1 g qid prn, not to exceed 6 g/24 hr

---

*Available in Canada only

• *Child 6-12 yr:* PO 500 mg bid prn, not to exceed 3 g/24 hr
• *Child 3-6 yr:* PO 500 mg bid prn, not to exceed 1.5 g/24 hr
Available forms include: Chew tab 500 mg
Side effects/adverse reactions:
*GI: **Obstruction,*** abdominal distention, laxative dependency, flatus
Contraindications: Hypersensitivity, GI obstruction
Precautions: Pregnancy (C)
Pharmacokinetics:
PO: Onset 12-24 min, peak 1-3 days
Interactions/incompatibilities:
• Gastric irritation: antacids, milk, H_2 blockers

NURSING CONSIDERATIONS
Assess:
• Blood, urine electrolytes if drug is used often by patient
• I&O ratio to identify fluid loss
Administer:
• Alone for better absorption; do not take within 1 hr of other drugs or within 1 hr of antacids, milk, or H_2 blockers
• In morning or evening (oral dose)
Evaluate:
• Therapeutic response: decrease in constipation
• Cause of constipation; identify whether fluids, bulk, or exercise is missing from lifestyle
• Cramping, rectal bleeding, nausea, vomiting; if these symptoms occur, drug should be discontinued
Teach patient/family:
• Not to use laxatives for long-term therapy; bowel tone will be lost
• That normal bowel movements do not always occur daily
• Do not use in presence of abdominal pain, nausea, vomiting
• Notify physician if constipation unrelieved or if symptoms of electrolyte imbalance occur: muscle

cramps, pain, weakness, dizziness
• Chew thoroughly and follow with water

---

capreomycin sulfate

(kap-ree-oh-mye'sin)
Capastat Sulfate
Func. class.: Antitubercular
Chem. class.: S. carpreolus polypeptide antibiotic

Action: Inhibits RNA synthesis, decreases tubercle bacilli replication
Uses: Pulmonary tuberculosis as adjunct
Dosage and routes:
• *Adult:* IM 15 mg/kg/day × 2-3 mo, then 1 g 2-3 ×/wk × 18-24 mo, not to exceed 20 mg/kg/day, must be given with another antitubercular medication
Available forms include: Powder for inj 1 mg/5 ml vial
Side effects/adverse reactions:
INTEG: Pain, irritation, sterile abscess at injection site, photosensitivity, rash, urticaria
CNS: Headache, vertigo, fever
EENT: Tinnitus, ***deafness, ototoxicity***
*GU: **Proteinuria,*** decreased CrCl, increased BUN, serum Cr, ***tubular necrosis,*** hypokalemia, alkalosis, ***hematuria, albuminuria, nephrotoxicity***
*HEMA: **Eosinophilia, leukocytosis, leukopenia***
Contraindications: Hypersensitivity
Precautions: Renal disease, hearing impairment, allergy history, hepatic disease, myasthenia gravis, parkinsonism, pregnancy (C)
Pharmacokinetics:
IM: Peak 1-2 hr, half-life 4-6 hr; excreted in urine unchanged

---

italics = common side effects   **bold italic** = life threatening reactions

Interactions/incompatibilities:
• Increased renal toxicity: aminoglycosides, polymyxin, colistin, vancomycin
• Increased neuroblocking action: phenothiazine, tubocurarine, neostigmine

NURSING CONSIDERATIONS
Assess:
• Liver studies q wk: ALT, AST, bilirubin; potassium
• Renal status: before; q wk: BUN, creatinine, output, sp gr, urinalysis
• Blood levels of drug
• Audiometric testing before, during, after treatment

Administer:
• After reconstituting with NS or sterile water for injection, wait 2-3 min before giving
• With other antituberculars
• IM in large muscle mass, rotate sites
• Reduced dosage in renal impairment, if BUN >20 mg/dl, drug should be decreased or discontinued

Evaluate:
• Therapeutic response: decreased dyspnea, fatigue
• Ototoxicity: tinnitus, vertigo, change in hearing
• Hepatic status: decreased appetite, jaundice, dark urine, fatigue

Teach patient/family:
• That compliance with dosage schedule, duration is necessary
• Side effects, adverse reactions: hearing loss, change in urine or urinary habits

---

captopril
(kap′toe-pril)
Capoten
Func. class.: Antihypertensive
Chem. class.: Renin-angiotensin antagonist

Action: Selectively suppresses renin-angiotensin-aldosterone system; inhibits ACE, prevents conversion of angiotensin I to angiotensin II, results in dilation of arterial, venous vessels

Uses: Hypertension, heart failure not responsive to conventional therapy

Dosage and routes:
Malignant hypertension
• *Adult:* PO 25 mg increasing q2h until desired response, not to exceed 450 mg/day
Hypertension
• *Initial dose:* 12.5 mg 2-3 × daily; may increase to 50 mg bid-tid at 1-2 wk intervals; usual range: 25-150 mg bid-tid; max 450 mg
CHF
• *Adult:* PO 12.5 mg 2-3 × daily given with a diuretic, digitalis; may increase to 50 mg bid-tid, after 14 days, may increase to 150 mg tid if needed

Available forms include: Tabs 12.5, 25, 37.5, 50, 100 mg

Side effects/adverse reactions:
CV: Hypotension
GU: Impotence, dysuria, nocturia, proteinuria, *nephrotic syndrome, acute reversible renal failure,* polyuria, oliguria, frequency
HEMA: Neutropenia
INT: Rash, *angioedema*
RESP: Bronchospasm, dyspnea, cough
META: Hyperkalemia
GI: Loss of taste
CNS: Fever, chills

Contraindications: Hypersensitivity, pregnancy (C), lactation, heart block, children, K-sparing diuretics

Precautions: Dialysis patients, hypovolemia, leukemia, scleroderma, lupus erythematosis, blood dyscrasias, CHF, diabetes mellitus, renal disease, thyroid disease, COPD, asthma

Pharmacokinetics:

PO: Peak 1 hr; duration 2-6 hr; half-life 6-7 hr, metabolized by liver (metabolites), excreted in urine, crosses placenta, excreted in breast milk

Interactions/incompatibilities:

• Increased hypotension: diuretics, other antihypertensives, ganglionic blockers, adrenergic blockers

• Do not use with vasodilators, hydralazine, prazosin, potassium-sparing diuretics, sympathomimetics

NURSING CONSIDERATIONS

Assess:

• Blood studies: neutrophils, decreased platelets

• B/P

• Renal studies: protein, BUN, creatinine, watch for increased levels that may indicate nephrotic syndrome

• Baselines in renal, liver function tests before therapy begins

• K levels, although hyperkalemia rarely occurs

• Dip-stick of urine for protein qd in first morning specimen, if protein is increased a 24 hr urinary protein should be collected

Administer:

• IV infusion of 0.9% NaCl (as ordered) to expand fluid volume if severe hypotension occurs

Perform/provide:

• Storage in tight container at 30° C or less

• Supine or Trendelenburg position for severe hypotension

Evaluate:

• Therapeutic response: decrease in B/P in hypertensives, decreased B/P, edema, moist rales (CHF)

• Edema in feet, legs daily

• Allergic reaction: rash, fever, pruritus, urticaria; drug should be discontinued if antihistamines fail to help

• Symptoms of CHF: edema, dyspnea, wet rales, B/P

• Renal symptoms: polyuria, oliguria, frequency

Teach patient/family:

• Administer 1 hr before meals

• Not to discontinue drug abruptly

• Not to use OTC (cough, cold, or allergy) products unless directed by physician

• Tell patient to avoid sunlight or wear sunscreen if in sunlight, photosensitivity may occur

• Stress patient compliance with dosage schedule, even if feeling better

• To rise slowly to sitting or standing position to minimize orthostatic hypotension

• Notify physician of: mouth sores, sore throat, fever, swelling of hands or feet, irregular heartbeat, chest pain, signs of angioedema

• Excessive perspiration, dehydration, vomiting; diarrhea may lead to fall in blood pressure—consult physician if these occur

• May cause dizziness, fainting; light-headedness may occur during 1st few days of therapy

• May cause skin rash or impaired perspiration

• How to take B/P

Lab test interferences:

False positive: Urine acetone

Treatment of overdose: 0.9% Na Ca IV/INF hemodialysis

---

carbachol

(kar'ba-kole)

Miostat, Carbacel, Isopto Carbachol, Carcholin, Doryl, Lentin, Mistura C, P.V. Carbachol, Muro-carb

Func. class.: Miotic, cholinergic

Action: Contracts spincther muscle

of iris, causes spasms of ciliary muscle, deepening of anterior chamber

Uses: Ocular surgery, glaucoma (open-angle, narrow-angle)

Dosage and routes:

Ocular surgery

• *Adult:* INSTILL 0.5 ml (intraocular) of 0.01% solution in anterior chamber of eye (done by physician) for miosis during surgery

Glaucoma

• *Adult:* INSTILL 1-2 gtt (topical) of 0.75%-3% solution into eye bid-tid; OINT apply bid

Available forms include: 0.75%, 1.5%, 2.25%, 3.0% sol for topical use; sol, powders for preparing sol for inj, oint

Side effects/adverse reactions:

CV: **Marked hypotension,** bradycardia, headache

GI: Nausea, vomiting, abdominal discomfort, diarrhea, salivation

EENT: Blurred vision, varying degrees of myopia, decreased visual acuity in dim light, slight conjunctival hyperemia, altered distance vision, decreased night vision, eye ache

RESP: Asthma attacks

Contraindications: Hypersensitivity, when miosis is undesirable, corneal abrasions

Precautions: Bradycardia, CAD, hyperthyroidism, asthma, pregnancy, obstruction of GI or urinary tract, peptic ulcer, parkinsonism, epilepsy, peritonitis

Pharmacokinetics:

INSTILL/OINT: Miosis onset 10-20 min, duration 4-8 hr; decreased IOP onset 4 hr duration 8 hr

NURSING CONSIDERATIONS

Assess:

• Heart, respiratory rate, B/P

Perform/provide:

• Use of reconstituted solution immediately, discard unused potion

Teach patient/family:

• To report change in vision, blurring or loss of sight, trouble breathing, sweating, flushing

• Method of instillation, including pressure on lacrimal sac for 1 min, and not to touch dropper to eye

• That long-term therapy may be required in glaucoma

• That blurred vision will decrease with repeated use of drug

• Not to drive during first few days of treatment

---

carbamazepine

(kar-ba-maz′e-peen)

Apo-Carbamazepine,* Epitol, Mazepine,* Tegretol

Func. class.: Anticonvulsant

Chem. class.: Iminostilbene derivative

Action: Inhibits nerve impulses by limiting influx of sodium ions across cell membrane in motor cortex

Uses: Tonic-clonic, complex-partial, mixed seizures; trigeminal neuralgia

Dosage and routes:

Seizures

• *Adult and child >12 yr:* PO 200 mg bid, may be increased by 200 mg/day in divided doses q6-8h; adjustment is needed to minimum dose to control seizures

• *Child <12 yr:* PO 10-20 mg/kg/day in 2-3 divided doses

Trigeminal neuralgia

• *Adult:* PO 100 mg bid, may increase 100 mg q12h until pain subsides, not to exceed 1.2 g/day;

maintenance is 200-400 mg bid
Available forms include: Tabs,
chewable 100 mg; tabs 200 mg
Side effects/adverse reactions:
*HEMA: **Thrombocytopenia, agranulocytosis, leukocytosis, neutropenia, aplastic anemia, eosinophilia,** increased pro-time*
CNS: Drowsiness, dizziness, confusion, fatigue, *paralysis,* headache, hallucinations
GI: Nausea, constipation,diarrhea,
anorexia, vomiting, abdominal
pain, stomatitis, glossitis, increased liver enzymes, *hepatitis*
*INTEG: Rash, **Stevens-Johnson
syndrome,** urticaria*
EENT: Tinnitus, dry mouth, blurred
vision, diplopia, nystagmus, conjunctivitis
*CV: **Hypertension, CHF,** hypoten-*
sion, aggravation of cardiac artery
disease
RESP: Pulmonary hypersensitivity
(fever, dyspnea, pneumonitis)
GU: Frequency, retention, albuminuria, glycosuria, impotence
Contraindications: Hypersensitivity to carbamazepine or tricyclic
antidepressants, bone marrow
depression, concomitant use of
MAOIs
Precautions: Glaucoma, hepatic
disease, renal disease, cardiac disease, psychosis, pregnancy (C),
lactation, child <6 yr
Pharmacokinetics:
PO: Onset slow, peak 4-8 hr, metabolized by liver, excreted in
urine, feces, crosses placenta, excreted in breast milk, half-life 14-
16 hr
Interactions/incompatibilities:
• Toxicity: troleandomycin, erythromycin, cimetidine, isoniazid,
propoxyphene, lithium
• Decreased effects of: phenobarbital, phenytoin, primidone

• Increased effects of: vasopressin,
lypressin, desmopressin
NURSING CONSIDERATIONS
Assess:
• Renal studies: urinalysis, BUN,
urine creatinine q3mo
• Blood studies: RBC, Hct, Hgb,
reticulocyte counts q wk for 4 wk
then q mo; if myelosupression oc-
curs, drug should be discontinued
• Hepatic studies: ALT, AST, bili-
rubin, creatinine
• Drug levels during initial treat-
ment; should remain at 3-9 µg/ml;
anorexia may indicate increased
blood levels
• Description of seizures
Administer:
• With food, milk to decrease GI
symptoms
• Chewable tablets; tell patient to
chew tablet, not swallow it whole
Perform/provide:
• Storage at room temperature
• Hard candy, frequent rinsing of
mouth, gum for dry mouth
• Assistance with ambulation during early part of treatment; dizziness occurs
Evaluate:
• Therapeutic response: decreased
seizure activity, document on patient's chart
• Mental status: mood, sensorium,
affect, behavioral changes; if mental status changes notify physician
• Eye problems: need for ophthalmic examinations before, during,
after treatment (slit lamp, fundoscopy, tonometry)
• Allergic reaction: purpura, red
raised rash, if these occur, drug
should be discontinued
• Blood dyscrasias: fever, sore
throat, bruising, rash, jaundice
• Toxicity: bone marrow depression, nausea, vomiting, ataxia, dip-

---

italics = common side effects   ***bold italic*** = life threatening reactions

lopia, cardiovascular collapse, Stevens-Johnson syndrome

Teach patient/family:
• To carry Medic-Alert ID stating drugs taken, condition, physician's name, phone number
• To avoid driving, other activities that require alertness
• To avoid alcohol ingestion; convulsions may result
• Not to discontinue medication quickly after long-term use
• Urine may turn pink to brown

Lab test interferences:
Decrease: Thyroid function tests
Treatment of overdose: Lavage, VS

---

carbamide peroxide (otic)

(kar'ba-mide per-ox'ide)
Debrox, Murine Ear Drops

Func. class.: Otic
Chem. class.: Urea compound, hydrogen peroxide

Action: Foaming action facilitates removal of impacted cerumen

Uses: Impacted cerumen, prevention of ceruminosis

Dosage and routes:
• *Adult and child:* INSTILL 5-10 gtts bid × 3-4 days
Available forms include: Sol 6.5%

Side effects/adverse reactions:
EENT: Itching, irritation in ear, redness

Contraindications: Hypersensitivity, otic surgery, perforated eardrum

Precautions: Pregnancy (C)

NURSING CONSIDERATIONS
Administer:
• Drug, then irrigate to remove cerumen
• By allowing drops to enter ear canal, do not touch dropper to ear

Evaluate:
• Therapeutic response: loosened cerumen, ability to hear better

Teach patient/family:
• Method of instillation, using aseptic technique

---

carbamide peroxide (urea peroxide)

(kar'ba-mide per-ox'ide)
Cank-aid, Clear Drops, Gly-Oxide Liquid, Orajel Brace-Aid Rinse, Proxigel

Func. class.: Topical antiinfective
Chem. class.: Equimolar compound of urea, hydrogen peroxide

Action: Releases oxygen on contact with mouth tissues, this provides cleansing effect; decreases inflammation, pain, mouth odors caused by bacteria

Uses: Oral and lip irritation, sore throat, toothache, cold sore, canker sore, aid to oral hygiene (when dental appliances are worn), cleansing of oral wounds/lesions

Dosage and routes:
• *Adult and child >3 yr:* TOP apply to affected area qid or prn; leave on 1-3 min
Available forms include: Sol 10%; gel 11%

Side effects/adverse reactions:
EENT: Itching, irritation in oral cavity
INTEG: Rash, urticaria

Contraindications: Hypersensitivity, child <3 yr

Precautions: Pregnancy (C)

NURSING CONSIDERATIONS
Administer:
• Gel by placing small amount directly on affected area, massage, do not expectorate or rinse mouth for at least 5 min
• Solution undiluted by placing

---

*Available in Canada only

several drops on affected area, on tongue, mix with saliva, swish 3 min, expectorate

Perform/provide:
• Storage in tight, light-resistant container at room temperature

Evaluate:
• Redness, swelling, pain in mouth or oral cavity

Teach patient/family:
• Not to use over 1 wk; notify physician if increased inflammation, redness, swelling, fever occur; drug should be discontinued
• That foaming will occur on contact with saliva
• Best to take after meals and hs

---

carbarsone

(kar-bar′sone)

Func. class.: Amebicide
Chem. class.: Pentavalent organic arsenic

Action: Organism death occurs in intestinal lumen by inhibition of sulfhydryl enzymes

Uses: Intestinal amebiasis

Dosage and routes:
• *Adult:* PO 250 mg bid-tid × 10 days; REC 2 g/200 ml warm 2% NaHCO₃ sol, qod × 5 doses
• *Child:* PO 75 mg/kg/day in 3 divided doses × 10 days

Available forms include: Caps 250 mg; powder

Side effects/adverse reactions:
RESP: Congestion
HEMA: **Agranulocytosis, aplastic anemia**
INTEG: Rash, pruritus, **exfoliative dermatitis**
CNS: Neuritis, **convulsion, hemorrhagic encephalitis, coma**
EENT: Blurred vision, sore throat, retinal edema
GI: Nausea, vomiting, diarrhea,

epigastric distress, anorexia, constipation, abdominal cramps, irritation, hepatomegaly, jaundice, **hepatitis, gastric necrosis,** weight decrease
GU: Polyuria, albuminuria, **nephrotoxicity**
CV: Tachycardia, hypotension, edema

Contraindications: Hypersensitivity to this drug or arsenic, renal disease, hepatic disease, contracted visual or color fields

Precautions: Pregnancy (D)

Pharmacokinetics:
PO: Slowly excreted by kidneys, accumulation may occur

NURSING CONSIDERATIONS
Assess:
• Stools during entire treatment; should be clear at end of therapy, stools must be clear for 1 yr before patient is considered cured
• ECG before, during, after therapy; be aware that inversion of T waves occurs
• Vision by ophthalmalogic exam during, after therapy; vision problems occur often
• I&O, stools for number, frequency, character
• Blood studies: CBC as dyscrasias occur

Administer:
• Dimercaprol for arsenic toxicity as ordered
• PO after meals to avoid GI symptoms

Perform/provide:
• Storage in tight container

Evaluate:
• Allergic reaction: fever, rash, itching, chills; drug should be discontinued if these occur
• Nephrotoxicity: polyuria, albuminuria, hematuria
• Arsenic toxicity: sore throat, edema, pruritus, nausea, vomiting,

---

italics = common side effects   **bold italic** = life threatening reactions

dizziness, anorexia, epigastric pain, weight decrease, gastritis, hepatitis, visual problems, convulsions, polyuria, agranulocytosis
• Superimposed infection: fever, monilial growth, fatigue, malaise
• Tachycardia, decreasing B/P, GI symptoms, weakness, neuromuscular symptoms
• Diarrhea for 2-3 days
Teach patient/family:
• To report any side effects
• Proper hygiene after BM: handwashing technique
• Avoid contact of drug with eyes, mouth, nose, other mucous membranes
• Need for compliance with dosage schedule, duration of treatment
Treatment of overdose: Administer dimercaprol, gastric lavage, O₂, IV fluids

---

carbinoxamine maleate
(kar-bi-nox′a-meen)
Clistin
Func. class.: Antihistamine
Chem. class.: Ethanolamine derivative, H₁-receptor antagonist

---

Action: Acts on blood vessels, GI system, respiratory system, by competing with histamine for H₁-receptor site; decreases allergic response by blocking histamine
Uses: Allergy symptoms, rhinitis
Dosage and routes:
• *Adult:* PO 4-8 mg tid-qid
• *Child >6 yr:* PO 4-6 mg tid-qid
• *Child 3-6 yr:* PO 2-4 mg tid-qid
• *Child 1-3 yr:* 2 mg tid-qid
Available forms include: Tabs 4 mg
Side effects/adverse reactions:
CNS: Dizziness, drowsiness, poor coordination, fatigue, anxiety, eu-

phoria, confusion, paresthesia, neuritis
CV: Hypotension, palpitations, tachycardia
RESP: Increased thick secretions, wheezing, chest tightness
*HEMA: **Thrombocytopenia, agranulocytosis, hemolytic anemia***
GI: Constipation, dry mouth, nausea, vomiting, anorexia, diarrhea
INTEG: Rash, urticaria, photosensitivity
GU: Retention, dysuria, frequency
EENT: Blurred vision, dilated pupils, tinnitus, nasal stuffiness, dry nose, throat, mouth
Contraindications: Hypersensitivity to H₁-receptor antagonists, acute asthma attack, lower respiratory tract disease
Precautions: Increased intraocular pressure, renal disease, cardiac disease, hypertension, bronchial asthma, seizure disorder, stenosed peptic ulcers, hyperthyroidism, prostatic hypertrophy, bladder neck obstruction, pregnancy (C)
Pharmacokinetics:
PO: Onset ½-1 hr, duration 4-6 hr; degraded in liver, excreted by kidneys (inactive)
Interactions/incompatibilities:
• Increased CNS depression: barbiturates, narcotics, hypnotics, tricyclic antidepressants, alcohol, antianxiety agents
• Decreased effect of: oral anticoagulants, heparin
• Increased effect of: MAOIs
NURSING CONSIDERATIONS
Assess:
• I&O ratio; be alert for urinary retention, frequency, dysuria; drug should be discontinued if these occur
• CBC during long-term therapy
Administer:
• With meals if GI symptoms oc-

---

cur; absorption may slightly decrease

Perform/provide:
• Hard candy, gum, frequent rinsing of mouth for dryness
• Storage in tight container at room temperature

Evaluate:
• Therapeutic response: absence of running or congested nose, rashes
• Blood dyscrasias: thrombocytopenia, agranulocytosis (rare)
• Respiratory status: rate, rhythm, increase in bronchial secretions, wheezing, chest tightness
• Cardiac status: palpitations, increased pulse, hypotension

Teach patient/family:
• All aspects of drug use; to notify physician if confusion, sedation, hypotension occurs
• To avoid driving or other hazardous activity if drowsiness occurs
• To avoid concurrent use of alcohol, other CNS depressants

Lab test interferences:
False negative: Skin allergy tests
Treatment of overdose: Administer ipecac syrup or lavage, diazepam, vasopressors, barbiturates (short-acting)

---

carboplatin
(kar-boe'-pla-tin)
Paraplatin
Func. class.: Antineoplastic-alkylating agent
Chem. class.: Platinum coordination compound

Action: Produces interstrand DNA cross-links and, to a lesser extent, DNA-protein cross-links
Uses: Palliative treatment of ovarian carcinoma recurrent after treatment with other antineoplastic agents, including cisplatin

Dosage and routes (single agent):
• *Adult:* IV INF 360 mg/m² given over >15 min on day 1 q4wk; do not repeat single intermittent courses until neutrophil count is >2,000/mm³ and platelet count is >100,000/mm³
Available forms: Inj 50, 150, 450 mg/vial

Side effects/adverse reactions:
EENT: Tinnitus, hearing loss, ***vestibular toxicity***
HEMA: ***Thrombocytopenia, leukopenia, pancytopenia, neutropenia,*** anemia, bleeding
CV: Cardiac abnormalities
GI: Severe nausea, vomiting, diarrhea, weight loss
GU: ***Renal tubular damage,*** renal insufficiency, impotence, sterility, amenorrhea, gynecomastia
INTEG: Alopecia, dermatitis, rash, erythema, pruritus, urticaria
CNS: ***Convulsions, central neurotoxicity,*** peripheral neuropathy
RESP: Mucositis
META: Hypomagnesemia, hypocalcemia, hypokalemia, hyponatremia, hyperuremia
Contraindications: Hypersensitivity to this drug, platinum products, mannitol, severe bone marrow depression, significant bleeding, pregnancy (D)
Precautions: Radiation therapy with 1 mo, chemotherapy within 1 mo, lactation, liver disease
Pharmacokinetics: Initial half-life 1-2 hr, postdistribution half-life 2½-6 hr, not bound to plasma proteins, excreted by the kidneys
Interactions/incompatibilities:
• Increased nephrotoxicity or ototoxicity: aminoglycosides
NURSING CONSIDERATIONS
Assess:
• CBC, differential, platelet count weekly; withhold drug if WBC

italics = common side effects   ***bold italic*** = life threatening reactions

count is <4000/mm³ or platelet count is <100,000/mm³; notify physician of results
• Renal function studies: BUN, creatinine, serum uric acid, urine CrCl before and during therapy
• I&O ratio; report fall in urine output of <30 ml/hr
• Monitor temperature q4h (may indicate beginning of infection)
• Liver function tests before and during therapy (bilirubin, AST, ALT, LDH) as needed or monthly

Administer:
• IV after reconstituting to a concentration of 10 mg/ml (INT INF) or 0.5 mg/ml (direct IV)
• IV INF over 5-6 hr; do not use needles or IV administration sets containing aluminum, may cause precipitate
• Antiemetic 30-60 min before giving drug to prevent vomiting, and PRN
• Allopurinol or sodium bicarbonate to maintain uric acid levels, alkalinization of urine
• Antibiotics for prophylaxis of infection
• Diuretic (furosemide 40 mg IV) after infusion

Perform/provide:
• Storage protected from light at room temperature; reconstituted solutions are stable for 8 hr at room temperature
• Deep breathing exercises with patient tid-qid; place in semi-Fowler's position
• Increase fluid intake 2-3 L/day to prevent urate deposits and calculi formation and to speed elimination of drug
• Diet low in purines: organ meats (kidney, liver), dried beans, peas to maintain alkaline urine

Evaluate:
• Bleeding: hematuria, stool guaiac, bruising or petechiae, mucosa or orifices q8h
• Dyspnea, rales, unproductive cough, chest pain, tachypnea
• Food preferences; list likes, dislikes
• Effects of alopecia on body image, discuss feelings about body changes
• Yellowing of skin, sclera, dark urine, clay-colored stools, itchy skin, abdominal pain, fever, diarrhea
• Edema in feet, joint pain, stomach pain, shaking
• Inflammation of mucosa, breaks in skin

Teach patient/family:
• To report any complaints or side effects to nurse or physician
• That impotence or amenorrhea can occur, reversible after treatment is discontinued
• To report any changes in breathing or coughing
• That hair may be lost during treatment; a wig or hairpiece may make patient feel better; new hair may be different in color, texture

carboprost tromethamine

(kar'boe-prost)
Prostin/M15
Func. class.: Oxytocic
Chem. class.: Prostaglandin

Action: Stimulates uterine contractions causing complete abortion in approximately 16 hr
Uses: Abortion between 13-20 wk gestation
Dosage and routes:
• *Adult:* IM 250 µg, then 250 µg q1½-3½ hr, may increase to 500 µg if no response, not to exceed 12 mg total dose

Available forms include: Inj IM 250 µg/ml carboprost, 83 µg/ml tromethamine

Side effects/adverse reactions:

CNS: Fever, chills, headache

GI: Nausea, vomiting, diarrhea

Contraindications: Hypersensitivity, severe hepatic disease, severe renal disease, pelvic inflammatory disease (PID), respiratory disease, cardiac disease

Precautions: Asthma, anemia, jaundice, diabetes mellitus, convulsive disorders, past uterine surgery

Pharmacokinetics: Onset: 15 min, peak 2 hr; metabolized in lungs, liver, excreted in urine (metabolites)

NURSING CONSIDERATIONS

Assess:

• B/P, pulse; watch for change that may indicate hemorrhage

• Respiratory rate, rhythm, depth; notify physician of abnormalities

Administer:

• IM in deep muscle mass, rotate injection sites if additional doses are given

• After having crash cart available on unit

Perform/provide:

• Emotional support before and after the abortion

Evaluate:

• For length, duration of contraction; notify physician of contractions lasting over 1 min or absence of contractions

• For incomplete abortion, pregnancy must be terminated by another method, drug is teratogenic

Teach patient/family:

• To report increased blood loss, abdominal cramps, increased temperature or foul-smelling lochia

• Methods of comfort control and pain control

careolol

(kar-ee'oe-lole)

Cartol

Func. class.: Antihypertensive

Chem. class.: Nonselective β-blocker

Action: Produces fall in B/P without reflex tachycardia or significant reduction in heart rate through mixture of α-blocking, β-blocking effects; elevated plasma renins are reduced

Uses: Mild to moderate hypertension

Dosage and routes:

• *Adult:* PO 2.5 mg tid initially, may gradually increase to desired response

Available forms include: Tabs 2.5, 5, 10 mg

Side effects/adverse reactions:

CV: Orthostatic hypotension, **bradycardia, CHF, chest pain, ventricular dysrhythmias, AV block, peripheral vascular insufficiency,** palpitations

CNS: Dizziness, mental changes, drowsiness, fatigue, headache, catatonia, depression, anxiety, nightmares, paresthesia, lethargy, insominia, decreased concentration

GI: Nausea, vomiting, diarrhea, dry mouth, flatulence, constipation, anorexia

INTEG: Rash, alopecia, urticaria, pruritus, fever

HEMA: **Agranulocytosis, thrombocytopenic purpura (rare)**

EENT: Tinnitus, visual changes, sore throat, double vision, dry burning eyes

GU: Impotence, dysuria, ejaculatory failure, urinary retention

RESP: **Bronchospasm,** dyspnea, wheezing, nasal stuffiness, pharyngitis

---

italics = common side effects **bold italic** = life threatening reactions

MS: Joint pain, arthralgia, muscle cramps, pain

OTHER: Facial swelling, decreased exercise tolerance, weight change, Raynaud's disease

Contraindications: Hypersensitivity to β-blockers, cardiogenic shock, heart block (2nd, 3rd degree), sinus bradycardia, CHF, bronchial asthma

Precautions: Major surgery, pregnancy (C), lactation, diabetes mellitus, renal disease, thyroid disease, COPD, well-compensated heart failure, CAD, nonallergic bronchospasm

Pharmacokinetics:

PO: Onset 1-2 hr, peak 2-4 hr, duration 8-12 hr, half-life 6-8 hr, metabolized by liver (metabolites inactive), excreted in urine, bile, crosses placenta, excreted in breast milk

Interactions/incompatibilities:

• Increased hypotension: diuretics, other antihypertensives, halothane, cimetidine, nitroglycerin, prazosin
• Decreased β-blocker effects: sympathomimetics, nonsteroidal antiinflammatory agents, salicylates
• Increased hypoglycemia effect: insulin
• Increased effects of: lidocaine
• Decreased bronchodilating effects of: theophylline

NURSING CONSIDERATIONS
Assess:
• I&O, weight daily
• B/P, pulse q4h; note rate, rhythm, quality
• Apical/radial pulse before administration; notify physician of any significant changes
• Baselines in renal, liver function tests before therapy begins

Administer:
• PO: ac, hs; tablet may be crushed or swallowed whole

• Reduced dosage in renal dysfunction

Perform/provide:
• Storage in dry area at room temperature, do not freeze

Evaluate:
• Therapeutic response: decreased B/P after 1-2 wk
• Edema in feet, legs daily
• Skin turgor, dryness of mucous membranes for hydration status

Teach patient/family:
• Not to discontinue drug abruptly; taper over 2 wk or may precipitate angina
• Not to use OTC products containing α-adrenergic stimulants (nasal decongestants, OTC cold preparations) unless directed by physician
• To report bradycardia, dizziness, confusion, depression, fever
• To take pulse at home, advise when to notify physician
• To avoid alcohol, smoking, sodium intake
• To comply with weight control, dietary adjustments, modified exercise program
• To carry Medic Alert ID to identify drug being taken, allergies
• To avoid hazardous activities if dizziness is present
• To report symptoms of CHF: difficult breathing, especially on exertion or when lying down, night cough, swelling of extremities
• Take medication hs to minimize orthostatic hypotension
• Wear support hose to minimize effects of orthostatic hypotension

Lab test interferences:

False increase: Urinary catecholamines

Interference: Glucose, insulin tolerance tests

Treatment of overdose: Lavage, IV atropine for bradycardia, IV the-

---

ophylline for bronchospasm, digitalis, O_2, diuretic for cardiac failure; hemodialysis is useful for removal; administer vasopressor (norepinephrine) for hypotension, isoproterenol for heart block

carisoprodol
(kar-eye-soe-proe'dole)
Rela, Soma
Func. class.: Skeletal muscle relaxant, central acting
Chem. class.: Meprobamate congener

Action: Depresses CNS by blocking interneuronal activity in descending reticular formation, spinal cord, producing sedation
Uses: Relieving pain, stiffness in musculoskeletal conditions
Dosage and routes:
• *Adult and child >12 yr:* PO 350 mg tid, hs
Available forms include: Tabs 350 mg
Side effects/adverse reactions:
CNS: Dizziness, weakness, drowsiness, headache, tremor, depression, insomnia, ataxia, irritability
EENT: Diplopia, temporary loss of vision
CV: Postural hypotension, tachycardia
GI: Nausea, vomiting, hiccups, epigastric discomfort
INTEG: Rash, pruritus, fever, facial flushing
Contraindications: Hypersensitivity, child <12 yr, intermittent porphyria
Precautions: Renal disease, hepatic disease, addictive personalities, pregnancy (C)
Pharmacokinetics:
PO: Onset ½ hr, duration 4-6 hr, metabolized by liver, excreted in

urine, crosses placenta, excreted in breast milk (large amounts), half-life 8 hr
Interactions/incompatibilities:
• Increased CNS depression: alcohol, tricylic antidepressants, narcotics, barbiturates, sedatives, hypnotics
NURSING CONSIDERATIONS
Assess:
• Blood studies: CBC, WBC, differential; blood dyscrasias may occur
• Liver function studies: AST, ALT, alk phosphatase; hepatitis may occur
• ECG in epileptic patients; poor seizure control has occurred with patients taking this drug
• Idiosyncratic reaction, anaphylaxis within a few min or hr of first to fourth dose
Administer:
• With meals for GI symptoms
Perform/provide:
• Storage in tight container at room temperature
• Assistance with ambulation if dizziness, drowsiness occurs
Evaluate:
• Therapeutic response: decreased pain, spasticity
• Allergic reactions: rash, fever, respiratory distress
• Severe weakness, numbness in extremities
• Psychologic dependency: increased need for medication, more frequent requests for medication, increased pain
• CNS depression: dizziness, drowsiness, psychiatric symptoms
Teach patient/family:
• Not to discontinue the medication quickly; insomnia, nausea, headache, spasticity, tachycardia will occur; drug should be tapered off over 1-2 wk

italics = common side effects   ***bold italic*** = life threatening reactions

• Not to take with alcohol, other CNS depressants
• To avoid altering activities while taking this drug
• To avoid hazardous activities if drowsiness, dizziness occurs
• To avoid using OTC medication: cough preparations, antihistamines, unless directed by physician
Treatment of overdose: Induce emesis of conscious patient, lavage, dialysis

---

carmustine (BCNU)

(kar-mus'teen)
BiCNU
Func. class.: Antineoplastic alkylating agent
Chem. class.: Nitrosourea

Action: Alkylates DNA, RNA; is able to inhibit enzymes that allow synthesis of amino acids in proteins
Uses: Brain tumors such as glioblastoma, medulloblastoma, astrocytoma; multiple myeloma, Hodgkin's disease, other lymphomas
Dosage and routes:
• *Adult:* IV 75-100 mg/m² over 1-2 hr × 2 days or 200 mg/m² × 1 dose q6-8wk; if leukocytes fall below 2000 or platelets below 25,000 only 50% of dose should be given
Available forms include: Inj IV 100 mg; powder
Side effects/adverse reactions:
HEMA: Thrombocytopenia, leukopenia, myelosuppression, anemia
GI: Nausea, vomiting, anorexia, stomatitis, hepatotoxicity
GU: Azotemia, renal failure
INTEG: Burning, hyperpigmentation at injection site
RESP: Fibrosis, pulmonary infiltrate
Contraindications: Hypersensitivity, leukopenia, thrombocytopenia
Precautions: Pregnancy (D)
Pharmacokinetics:
Degraded within 15 min, crosses blood-brain barrier; 70% excreted in urine within 96 hr, 10% excreted as CO_2, fate of 20% is unknown
Interactions/incompatibilities:
• Increased toxicity: other antineoplastics, or radiation
• Enhanced action: Vitamin A or caffeine
• Increased toxicity: cimetidine, other antineoplastics or radiation
NURSING CONSIDERATIONS
Assess:
• CBC, differential, platelet count weekly; withhold drug if WBC is <4000 or platelet count is <75,000; notify physician of results
• Liver function tests: AST, ALT, bilirubin
• Pulmonary function tests, chest x-ray films before, during therapy; chest film should be obtained q2wk during treatment
• Renal function studies: BUN, serum uric acid, urine CrCl before, during therapy
• I&O ratio; report fall in urine output of 30 ml/hr
• Monitor for cold, cough, fever (may indicate beginning infection)
Administer:
• IV after diluting 100 mg drug/3 ml ethyl alcohol (provided); then further dilute 27 ml sterile H_2O for INJ; then dilute with 500 ml 0.9% NaCl or D_5W
• Antiemetic 30-60 min before giving drug to prevent vomiting
• Antibiotics for prophylaxis of infection
Perform/provide:
• Storage in refrigerator
• Strict medical asepsis, protective isolation if WBC levels are low

---

• Special skin care
• Deep breathing exercises with patient tid-qid; place in semi-Fowler's position
• Increase fluid intake to 2-3 L/day to prevent urate deposits, calculi formation
• Rinsing of mouth tid-qid with water or club soda; brushing of teeth bid-tid with soft brush or cotton tipped applicators for stomatitis; use unwaxed dental floss, use viscous xylocaine
• Warm compresses at injection site for inflammation

Evaluate:
• Bleeding: hematuria, guaiac, bruising or petechiae, mucosa or orifices q8h
• Dyspnea, rales, unproductive cough, chest pain, tachypnea
• Food preferences; list likes, dislikes
• Inflammation of mucosa, breaks in skin

Teach patient/family:
• Of protective isolation precautions
• To report any changes in breathing or coughing
• To avoid foods with citric acid, hot or rough texture
• To report any bleeding; white spots, or ulceration in mouth to physician; tell patient to examine mouth qd
• To avoid use of aspirin, ibuprofen; razors, commercial mouthwash
• To report signs of anemia (fatigue, irritability, shortness of breath, faintness)
• To report signs of infection (sore throat, fever)

cascara sagrada/cascara sagrada aromatic fluid extract/cascara sagrada fluid extract

(kas-kar'a)

Func. class.: Laxative
Chem. class.: Anthraquinone

Action: Direct chemical irritation in colon; increases propulsion of stool
Uses: Constipation, bowel, or rectal preparation for surgery or examination

Dosage and routes:
• *Adult:* PO 325 mg hs; FLUID 1 ml qd; AROMATIC FLUID 5 ml qd
• *Child 2-12 yr:* PO/FLUID/AROMATIC FLUID ½ adult dose
• *Child <2 yr:* PO/FLUID/AROMATIC FLUID ¼ adult dose
Available forms include: Powder, tabs 325 mg; oral sol

Side effects/adverse reactions:
GI: Nausea, vomiting, anorexia, cramps, diarrhea
META: Hypocalcemia, enteropathy, alkalosis, hypokalemia, ***tetany***

Contraindications: Hypersensitivity, GI bleeding, obstruction, CHF, lactation, abdominal pain, nausea/vomiting, appendicitis, acute surgical abdomen, alcoholics (aromatic form)
Precautions: Pregnancy (C)
Pharmacokinetics:
PO: Peak 6-12 hr; metabolized by liver, excreted by kidneys, in feces
Interactions/incompatibilities:
• Decreased absorption: antibiotics, digitalis, nitrofurantoin, salicylates, tetracyclines, oral anticoagulants

NURSING CONSIDERATIONS
Assess:
• Blood, urine electrolytes if drug is used often by patient

---

italics = common side effects   ***bold italic*** = life threatening reactions

• I&O ratio to identify fluid loss
Administer:
• Alone for better absorption; do not take within 1 hr of other drugs or within 1 hr of antacids, milk, or H₂ blockers
• In morning or evening (oral dose)
Evaluate:
• Therapeutic response: decrease in constipation
• Cause of constipation; identify whether fluids, bulk, or exercise is missing from lifestyle
• Cramping, rectal bleeding, nausea, vomiting; if these symptoms occur, drug should be discontinued
Teach patient/family:
• Swallow tabs whole; do not chew
• Not to use laxatives for long-term therapy; bowel tone will be lost
• That normal bowel movements do not always occur daily
• Do not use in presence of abdominal pain, nausea, vomiting
• Notify physician if constipation unrelieved or if symptoms of electrolyte imbalance occur: muscle cramps, pain, weakness, dizziness

---

castor oil
Alphamul, Emulsoil, Fleet Castor Oil, Kelloff's Castor Oil, Neoloid, Purge

Func. class.: Laxative

Action: Directly acts on intestine by increasing motor activity, thought to irritate colonic intramural plexus
Uses: Bowel, rectal preparation for surgery or examination
Dosage and routes:
• *Adult:* PO 1.25-3.7 mg; LIQ 15-60 ml
• *Child >2 yr:* LIQ 5-15 ml
• *Child <2 yr:* LIQ 1.25-7.5 ml
• *Infants:* LIQ 1-4 ml

Available forms include: Liq 36.4%, 60%, 64%, 95%; caps 0.62 ml/cap
Side effects/adverse reactions:
GI: Nausea, vomiting, anorexia, cramps, diarrhea, rebound constipation, colon irritation, flatus
META: Alkalosis, hypokalemia, electrolytes, fluid imbalance
Contraindications: Hypersensitivity, fecal impaction, GI bleeding, pregnancy (X), lactation, abdominal pain, nausea/vomiting, appendicitis, acute surgical abdomen
Pharmacokinetics:
PO: Peak 2-3 hr; excreted in breast milk

NURSING CONSIDERATIONS
Assess:
• Blood, urine electrolytes if drug is used often by patient
• I&O ratio to identify fluid loss
Administer:
• Alone for better absorption; do not take within 1 hr of other drugs or within 1 hr of antacids, milk, or cimetidine
• In morning or evening (oral dose)
Perform/provide:
• Storage in cool environment, do not freeze
Evaluate:
• Therapeutic response: decrease in constipation
• Cause of constipation; identify whether fluids, bulk, or exercise is missing from lifestyle
• Cramping, rectal bleeding, nausea, vomiting; if these symptoms occur, drug should be discontinued
Teach patient/family:
• Swallow tabs whole; do not chew
• Not to use laxatives for long-term therapy; bowel tone will be lost
• That normal bowel movements do not always occur daily
• Do not use in presence of abdominal pain, nausea, vomiting

---

* Available in Canada only

• Notify physician if constipation unrelieved or if symptoms of electrolyte imbalance occur: muscle cramps, pain, weakness, dizziness, severe thirst
• Keep out of children's reach

---

cefaclor

(sef'a-klor)
Ceclor
Func. class.: Antibiotic
Chem. class.: Cephalosporin (2nd generation)

Action: Inhibits bacterial cell wall synthesis, which renders cell wall osmotically unstable

Uses: Gram-negative bacilli: *H. influenzae, E. coli, P. mirabilis, Klebsiella;* gram-positive organisms: *S. pneumoniae, S. pyogenes, S. aureus;* upper and lower respiratory tract, urinary tract, skin infections, otitis media

Dosage and routes:
• *Adult:* PO 250-500 mg q8h, not to exceed 4 g/day
• *Child >1 mo:* PO 20-40 mg/kg/qd in divided doses q8h, not to exceed 1 g/day
Available forms include: Caps 250, 500 mg; oral susp 125, 250 mg/5 ml

Side effects/adverse reactions:
CNS: Headache, dizziness, weakness, paresthesia, fever, chills
GI: Nausea, vomiting, *diarrhea, anorexia,* pain, glossitis, bleeding, increased AST, ALT, bilirubin, LDH, alk phosphatase, abdominal pain
GU: Proteinuria, vaginitis, pruritus, candidiasis, increased BUN, ***nephrotoxicity, renal failure***
HEMA: ***Leukopenia, thrombocytopenia, agranulocytosis,*** anemia, ***neutropenia, lymphocytosis, eo-***

sinophilia, pancytopenia, hemolytic anemia
INTEG: Rash, urticaria, dermatitis, ***anaphylaxis***
RESP: Dyspnea

Contraindications: Hypersensitivity to cephalosporins, infants <1 mo

Precautions: Hypersensitivity to penicillins, pregnancy (B), lactation, renal disease

Pharmacokinetics:
Peak ½-1 hr, half-life 36-54 min, 25% bound by plasma proteins, 60%-85% eliminated unchanged in urine in 8 hr, crosses placenta, excreted in breast milk

Interactions/incompatibilities:
• Decreased effects: tetracyclines, erythromycins
• Increased toxicity: aminoglycosides, furosemide, probenecid, sulfinpyrazone, colistin, ethacrynic acid, vancomycin

NURSING CONSIDERATIONS
Assess:
• Sensitivity to penicillins and other cephalosporins
  Nephrotoxicity: increased BUN, creatinine
• I&O daily
• Blood studies: AST, ALT, CBC, Hct, bilirubin, LDH, alk phosphatase, Coombs' test monthly if patient is on long-term therapy
• Electrolytes: potassium, sodium, chloride monthly if patient is on long-term therapy
• Bowel pattern qd; if severe diarrhea occurs, drug should be discontinued; may indicate pseudomembranous colitis

Administer:
• For 10-14 days to ensure organism death, prevent superimposed infection
• With food if needed for GI symptoms
• After C&S completed

---

italics = common side effects   ***bold italic*** = life threatening reactions

Evaluate:
- Therapeutic response: decreased fever, malaise, chills
- Urine output; if decreasing, notify physician (may indicate nephrotoxicity)
- Allergic reactions: rash, urticaria, pruritus, chills, fever, joint pain; angioedema may occur a few days after therapy begins
- Bleeding: ecchymosis, bleeding gums, hematuria, stool guaiac daily
- Overgrowth of infection: perineal itching, fever, malaise, redness, pain, swelling, drainage, rash, diarrhea, change in cough, sputum

Teach patient/family:
- If diabetic, to use Clinistix or Ketodiastix
- Not to drink alcohol or meds with alcohol or reaction may occur
- To use yogurt or buttermilk to maintain intestinal flora, decrease diarrhea
- Take all medication prescribed for length of time ordered
- To report sore throat, bruising, bleeding, joint pain; may indicate blood dyscrasias (rare)

Lab test interferences:
Increase (false): Creatinine (serum urine), urinary 17-KS
False positive: Urinary protein, direct Coombs', urine glucose
Interference: Cross-matching
Treatment of overdose: Epinephrine, antihistamines, resuscitate if needed (anaphylaxis)

---

cefadroxil

(sef-a-drox'ill)
Duricef, Ultracef
Func. class.: Antibiotic
Chem. class.: Cephalosporin (1st generation)

Action: Inhibits bacterial cell wall

synthesis, rendering cell wall osmotically unstable
Uses: Gram-negative bacilli: *E. coli, P. mirabilis, Klebsiella (UTI only);* gram-positive organisms: *S. pneumoniae, S. pyogenes, S. aureus;* upper, lower respiratory tract, urinary tract, skin infections, otitis media; tonsillitis; particularly for urinary tract infections

Dosage and routes:
- *Adult:* PO 1-2 g qd or q12h, give a loading dose of 1 g initially; dosage reduction indicated in renal impairment (CrCl < 50 ml/min)
- *Child:* 30 mg/kg/day

Available forms include: Caps 500 mg; tabs 1 g; oral susp 125, 250, 500 mg/5 ml

Side effects/adverse reactions:
CNS: Headache, dizziness, weakness, paresthesia, fever, chills
GI: Nausea, vomiting, *diarrhea, anorexia,* pain, glossitis, bleeding, increased AST, ALT, bilirubin, LDH, alk phosphatase, abdominal pain, ***pseudomembranous colitis***
GU: Proteinuria, vaginitis, pruritus, candidiasis, increased BUN, ***nephrotoxicity, renal failure***
HEMA: ***Leukopenia, thrombocytopenia, agranulocytosis,*** anemia, ***neutropenia, lymphocytosis, eosinophilia, pancytopenia, hemolytic anemia***
INTEG: Rash, urticaria, dermatitis, ***anaphylaxis***
RESP: Dyspnea

Contraindications: Hypersensitivity to cephalosporins, infants <1 mo
Precautions: Hypersensitivity to penicillins, pregnancy (B), lactation, renal disease

Pharmacokinetics:
Peak 1-1½ hr, half-life 1-2 hr, 20% bound by plasma proteins, crosses placenta, excreted in breast milk

---

Interactions/incompatibilities:
• Decreased effects: tetracyclines, erythromycins
• Increased toxicity: aminoglycosides, furosemide, probenecid, sulfinpyrazone, colistin, ethacrynic acid, vancomycin

NURSING CONSIDERATIONS

Assess:
• Sensitivity to penicillin and other cephalosporins
• Nephrotoxicity: increased BUN, creatinine
• I&O daily
• Blood studies: AST, ALT, CBC, Hct, bilirubin, LDH, alk phosphatase, Coombs' test monthly if patient is on long-term therapy
• Electrolytes: potassium, sodium, chloride monthly if patient is on long-term therapy
• Bowel pattern qd; if severe diarrhea occurs drug should be discontinued; may indicate pseudomembranous colitis

Administer:
• For 10-14 days to ensure organism death, prevent superimposed infection
• With food if needed for GI symptoms
• After C&S completed

Evaluate:
• Therapeutic response: decreased fever, malaise, chills
• Urine output; if decreasing, notify physician; may indicate nephrotoxicity
• Allergic reactions: rash, urticaria, pruritus, chills, fever, joint pain; angioedema; may occur few days after therapy begins
• Bleeding: ecchymosis, bleeding gums, hematuria, stool guaiac daily
• Overgrowth of infection: perineal itching, fever, malaise, redness, pain, swelling, drainage, rash, diarrhea, change in cough, sputum

Teach patient/family:
• If diabetic to use Clinistix or Ketodiastix
• Not to drink alcohol or use meds with alcohol or reaction may occur
• To use yogurt or buttermilk to maintain intestinal flora, decrease diarrhea
• Take all medication prescribed for length of time ordered
• To report sore throat, bruising, bleeding, joint pain; may indicate blood dyscrasias (rare)

Lab test interferences:
Increase (false): Creatinine (serum urine), urinary 17-KS
False positive: Urinary protein, direct Coombs', urine glucose
Interference: Cross-matching
Treatment of overdose: Epinephrine, antihistamines, resuscitate if needed (anaphylaxis)

---

cefamandole nafate
(sef-a-man′dole)
Mandol
Func. class.: Antibiotic
Chem. class.: Cephalosporin (2nd generation)

Action: Inhibits bacterial cell wall synthesis, rendering cell wall osmotically unstable
Uses: Gram-negative bacilli: *H. influenzae, E. coli, P. mirabilis, Klebsiella;* gram-positive organisms: *S. pneumoniae, S. pyogenes, S. aureus;* upper, lower respiratory tract, urinary tract, skin infections, peritonitis, septicemia, surgical prophylaxis

Dosage and routes:
• *Adult:* IM/IV 500 mg-1 g q4-8h; may give up to 2 g q4h for severe infections
• *Child >1 mo:* IM/IV 50-100 mg/

---

kg/day in divided doses q4-8h, not to exceed adult dose
• Dosage reduction indicated in renal impairment (CrCl < 5 ml/min)
Available forms include: Inj IM, IV 500 mg, 1, 2, 10 g; IV 1, 2 g
Side effects/adverse reactions:
CNS: Headache, dizziness, weakness, paresthesia, fever, chills
GI: Nausea, vomiting, diarrhea, anorexia, pain, glossitis, bleeding, increased AST, ALT, bilirubin, LDH, alk phosphatase, abdominal pain
GU: Proteinuria, vaginitis, pruritus, candidiasis, increased BUN, *nephrotoxicity, renal failure*
HEMA: Leukopenia, thrombocytopenia, agranulocytosis, anemia, *neutropenia, lymphocytosis, eosinophilia, pancytopenia, hemolytic anemia,* bleeding, *hypoprothrombinemia*
INTEG: Rash, urticaria, dermatitis, *anaphylaxis*
RESP: Dyspnea
Contraindications: Hypersensitivity to cephalosporins, infants <1 mo
Precautions: Hypersensitivity to penicillins, pregnancy, lactation, renal disease
Pharmacokinetics:
Peak 1-1½ hr, half-life ½-1 hr, 60%-75% bound by plasma proteins, crosses placenta, excreted in breast milk
Interactions/incompatibilities:
• Do not mix with tetracyclines, erythromycins, calcium chloride, magnesium salts, aminoglycosides, cimetidine in same parenteral fluid
• Decreased effects: tetracyclines, erythromycins
• Increased toxicity: aminoglycosides, furosemide, probenecid, sulfinpyrazone, colistin, ethacrynic acid, vancomycin
• Disulfiram reaction: disulfiram

NURSING CONSIDERATIONS
Assess:
• Sensitivity to penicillin or other cephalosporins
• Nephrotoxicity: increased BUN, creatinine
• I&O daily
• Blood studies: AST, ALT, CBC, Hct, bilirubin, LDH, alk phosphatase, Coombs' test, pro-time monthly if patient is on long-term therapy
• Electrolytes: potassium, sodium, chloride monthly if patient is on long-term therapy
• Bowel pattern qd, if severe diarrhea occurs drug should be discontinued; may indicate pseudomembranous colitis
• IV site for extravasation or phlebitis, change site q72h
Administer:
• IV, check for irritation, extravasation often, dilute 1 g of drug/10 ml normal saline or sterile H_2O for inj, run over 3-5 min; may be further diluted with 100 ml of compatible sol and run over 15-30 min; may also be diluted in 1000-ml compatible sol
• For 10-14 days to ensure organism death, prevent superimposed infection
• After C&S completed
Evaluate:
• Therapeutic response: decreased fever, malaise, chills
• Urine output, if decreasing, notify physician; may indicate nephrotoxicity
• Allergic reactions: rash, urticaria, pruritus, chills, fever, joint pain, angioedema; may occur few days after therapy begins
• Bleeding: ecchymosis, bleeding gums, hematuria, stool guaiac daily
• Overgrowth of infection: perineal itching, fever, malaise, redness,

---

*Available in Canada only

pain, swelling, drainage, rash, diarrhea, change in cough, sputum
Teach patient/family:
• If diabetic, to use Clinistix or Ketodiastix
• Not to drink alcohol or meds with alcohol or reaction may occur
• To report sore throat, bruising, bleeding, joint pain; may indicate blood dyscrasias (rare)
Lab test interferences:
Increase (false): Urinary 17-KS
False positive: Urinary protein, direct Coombs', urine glucose
Interference: Cross-matching
Treatment of overdose: Epinephrine, antihistamines, resuscitate if needed (anaphylaxis)

---

cefazolin sodium

(sef-a'zoe-lin)
Ancef, Kefzol
Func. class.: Antibiotic
Chem. class.: Cephalosporin (1st generation)

Action: Inhibits bacterial cell wall synthesis rendering cell wall osmotically unstable
Uses: Gram-negative bacilli: *H. influenzae, E. coli, P. mirabilis, Klebsiella;* gram-positive organisms: *S. pneumoniae, S. pyogenes, S. aureus;* upper, lower respiratory tract, urinary tract, skin infections, bone, joint, biliary, genital infections, endocarditis, surgical prophylaxis, septicemia
Dosage and routes:
Life-threatening infections
• *Adult:* IM/IV 1-1.5 g q6h
• *Child >1 mo:* IM/IV 100 mg/kg in 3-4 equal doses
Mild/moderate infections
• *Adult:* IM/IV 250-500 mg q8h
• *Child >1 mo:* IM/IV 25-50 mg/kg in 3-4 equal doses

• Dosage reduction indicated in renal impairment (CrCl < 54 ml/min)
Available forms include: Inj IM, IV, 250, 500 mg, 1, 5, 10 g
Side effects/adverse reactions:
CNS: Headache, dizziness, weakness, paresthesia, fever, chills
GI: Nausea, vomiting, *diarrhea, anorexia,* pain, glossitis, bleeding, increased AST, ALT, bilirubin, LDH, alk phosphatase, abdominal pain, oral candidiasis
GU: Proteinuria, vaginitis, pruritus, candidiasis, increased BUN, ***nephrotoxicity, renal failure***
*HEMA: **Leukopenia, thrombocytopenia, agranulocytosis,** anemia, **neutropenia, lymphocytosis, eosinophilia, pancytopenia, hemolytic anemia***
INTEG: Rash, urticaria, dermatitis, ***anaphylaxis***
Contraindications: Hypersensitivity to cephalosporins, infants <1 mo
Precautions: Hypersensitivity to penicillins, pregnancy (B), lactation, renal disease
Pharmacokinetics:
IM: Peak ½-2 hr, half-life 1½-2¼ hr
IV: Peak 10 min, eliminated unchanged in urine 70% to 86% protein bound
Interactions/incompatibilities:
• Do not mix with tetracyclines, erythromycins, calcium salts, magnesium salts, barbiturates, aminoglycosides in same parenteral fluid
• Decreased effects: tetracyclines, erythromycins
• Increased toxicity: aminoglycosides, furosemide, probenecid, sulfinpyrazone, colistin, ethacrynic acid

---

italics = common side effects   ***bold italic*** = life threatening reactions

NURSING CONSIDERATIONS
Assess:
• Sensitivity to penicillin or other cephalosporins
• Nephrotoxicity: increased BUN, creatinine
• I&O daily
• Blood studies: AST, ALT, CBC, Hct, alk phosphatase, bilirubin, LDH, Coombs' test monthly if patient is on long-term therapy
• Electrolytes: potassium, sodium, chloride monthly if patient is on long-term therapy
• Bowel pattern qd; if severe diarrhea occurs drug should be discontinued; may indicate pseudomembranous colitis
• IV site for extravasation or phlebitis, change site q72h

Administer:
• IV, check for irritation, extravasation often, dilute in 10 ml sterile H₂O for INJ and run over 3-5 min; may be further diluted with 50-100 ml of compatible sol and run over ½-1 hr
• For 10-14 days to ensure organism death, prevent superimposed infection
• After C&S completed

Evaluate:
• Therapeutic response: decreased fever, malaise, chills
• Urine output, if decreasing, notify physician; may indicate nephrotoxicity
• Allergic reactions: rash, urticaria, pruritus, chills, fever, joint pain, angioedema; may occur few days after therapy begins
• Bleeding: ecchymosis, bleeding gums, hematuria, stool guaiac daily
• Overgrowth of infection: perineal itching, fever, malaise, redness, pain, swelling, drainage, rash, diarrhea, change in cough, sputum

Teach patient/family:
• If diabetic, to use Clinistix or Ketodiastix
• Not to use alcohol or meds with alcohol or reaction may occur

Lab test interferences:
Increase (false): Urinary 17-KS
False positive: urinary protein, direct Coombs', urine glucose
Interference: Cross-matching

Treatment of overdose: Epinephrine, antihistamines, resuscitate if needed (anaphylaxis)

---

cefixime
(sef-ex'ime)
Suprex

Func. class.: Broad-spectrum antibiotic
Chem. class.: Cephalosporin (3rd generation)

Action: Inhibits bacterial cell wall synthesis, rendering cell wall osmotically unstable
Uses: Uncomplicated UTI *(E. coli, P. mirabilis)*, pharyngitis and tonsillitis *(S. pyogenes)*, otitis media *(H. influenzae)*, *M. catarrhalis*, acute bronchitis, and acute exacerbations of chronic bronchitis *(S. pneumoniae, H. influenzae)*

Dosage and routes:
• *Adult:* PO 400 mg qd as a single dose or 200 mg q12h
• *Child >50 kg or >12 yrs:* PO use adult dosage
• *Child: <50 kg or <12 years:* PO 8 mg/kg/day as a single dose or 4 mg/kg q12h
•*Available forms include:* Tabs 200, 400 g; powder for oral susp 100 mg/5 ml

Side effects/adverse reactions:
CNS: Headache, dizziness, paresthesia, fever, chills, lethargy, fatigue, confusion

GI: Nausea, vomiting, diarrhea, anorexia, pain, glossitis, bleeding, increased AST, ALT, bilirubin, LDH, alk phosphatase, heartburn, dysgeusia, flatulence

GU: Proteinuria, vaginitis, pruritus, increased BUN, *nephrotoxicity, renal failure,* pyuria, dysuria

HEMA: Leukopenia, thrombocytopenia, agranulocytosis, anemia, *neutropenia, lymphocytosis, eosinophilia, pancytopenia, hemolytic anemia*

INTEG: Rash, urticaria, *exfoliative dermatitis, anaphylaxis*

RESP: Bronchospasm, dyspnea, tight chest

Contraindications: Hypersensitivity to cephalosporins, infants <6 mo

Precautions: Hypersensitivity to penicillins, pregnancy (B), lactation, renal disease

Pharmacokinetics:
PO: Peak 1 hr
Half-life 3-4 hr, 65% bound by plasma proteins, 50% eliminated unchanged in urine; crosses placenta, excreted in breast milk

Interactions/incompatibilities:
• Decreased bactericidal effects: tetracyclines, erythromycins, chloramphenicol
• Increased renal toxicity: aminoglycosides, furosemide, colistin, ethacrynic acid, vancomycin

NURSING CONSIDERATIONS
Assess:
• Sensitivity to penicillin or other cephalosporins
• Nephrotoxicity: increased BUN, creatinine
• I&O daily
• Blood studies: AST, ALT, CBC, Hct, bilirubin, LDH, alk phosphatase; Coombs' test monthly if patient is on long-term therapy
• Bowel pattern qd; if severe diarrhea occurs, drug should be discontinued (may indicate pseudomembranous colitis)

Administer:
• For 10-14 days to ensure organism death, prevent superimposed infection
• After C&S completed

Evaluate:
• Therapeutic response: decreased fever, malaise, chills
• Urine output, if decreasing, notify physician (may indicate nephrotoxicity)
• Allergic reactions: rash, urticaria, pruritus, chills, fever, joint pain, angioedema; may occur a few days after therapy begins
• Bleeding: ecchymosis, bleeding, itching, fever, malaise, redness, pain, swelling, drainage, rash, diarrhea, change in cough, sputum

Teach patient/family:
• To report sore throat, bruising, bleeding, joint pain (may indicate blood dyscrasias [rare])
• If diabetic, to use Clinistix or Ketodiastix
• Not to use alcohol or meds with alcohol or reaction may occur

Lab test interferences:
Increase (false): Urinary 17-KS
False positive: Urinary protein, direct Coombs', urine glucose
Interference: Cross-matching

Treatment of overdose: Epinephrine, antihistamines, resuscitate if needed (anaphylaxis)

cefmetazole
(sef-met'a-zole)
Zefazone
Func. class.: Broad-spectrum antibiotic
Chem. class.: Cephalosporin (2nd generation)

Action: Inhibits bacterial cell wall

italics = common side effects   ***bold italic*** = life threatening reactions

synthesis, rendering cell wall osmotically unstable

Uses: Gram-negative bacilli: *H. influenzae, E. coli, Proteus, Klebsiella, B. fragilis;* gram-positive organisms: *S. pneumoniae, S. pyogenes, S. aureus;* anaerobes, including *Clostridium;* infections of lower respiratory tract, urinary tract, skin, bone; septicemia; intraabdominal infections

Dosage and routes:
• *Adult:* IV 1-8 g divided q6-12h × 5-14 days
• *Available forms include:* Powder for inj 1, 2 gm/vial

Side effects/adverse reactions:

CNS: Headache, dizziness, paresthesia, fever, chills, lethargy, fatigue, confusion

GI: Nausea, vomiting, diarrhea, anorexia, pain, glossitis, bleeding, increased AST, ALT, bilirubin, LDH, alk phosphatase, heartburn, flatulence

*GU: **Proteinuria,*** vaginitis, pruritus, candidiasis, increased BUN, ***nephrotoxicity, renal failure***

*HEMA: **Leukopenia, thrombocytopenia, agranulocytosis,*** anemia, ***neutropenia, lymphocytosis, eosinophilia, pancytopenia, hemolytic anemia***

INTEG: Rash, urticaria, ***exfoliative dermatitis,*** thrombophlebitis ***angioedema,*** erythema, pruritus

*SYST: **Anaphylaxis***

Contraindications: Hypersensitivity to cephalosporins, infants <1 mo

Precautions: Hypersensitivity to penicillins, pregnancy (B), lactation, renal disease

Pharmacokinetics:

IM: Peak 30-45 min, 68% bound by plasma proteins, excreted by kidneys, half-life 1-3 hr

Interactions/incompatibilities:
• Do not mix with aminoglycosides in same parenteral fluid
• Decreased bactericidal effects: tetracyclines, erythromycins, chloramphenicol
• Increased renal toxicity and ototoxicity: aminoglycosides, furosemide, colistin, ethacrynic acid, vancomycin
• Increased plasma level of cefmetazole

NURSING CONSIDERATIONS
Assess:
• Sensitivity to penicillin and other cephalosporins
• Nephrotoxicity: increased BUN, creatinine
• I&O daily
• Blood studies: AST, ALT, CBC, Hct, bilirubin, LDH, alk phosphatase, Coombs' test monthly if patient is on long-term therapy
• Electrolytes: potassium, sodium, chloride monthly if patient is on long-term therapy
• Bowel pattern qd, if severe diarrhea occurs drug should be discontinued (may indicate pseudomembranous colitis)
• IV site for extravasation or phlebitis, change site q72h

Administer:
• IV after reconstituting with diluent specified on package, give over 3-5 min
• For 10-14 days to ensure organism death, prevent superimposed infection
• After C&S completed

Evaluate:
• Therapeutic response: decreased fever, malaise, chills
• Urine output; if decreasing, notify physician (may indicate nephrotoxicity)
• Allergic reactions: rash, urticaria, pruritis, chills, fever, joint

pain, 7-10 days after therapy begins
• Bleeding: ecchymosis, bleeding gums, hematuria, stool guaiac daily
• Overgrowth of infection: perineal itching, fever, malaise, redness, pain, swelling, drainage, rash, diarrhea, change in cough, sputum

Teach patient/family:
• If diabetic, to use Clinistix or Ketodiastix
• Not to use alcohol or meds with alcohol or reaction may occur
• To report sore throat, bruising, bleeding, joint pain (may indicate blood dyscrasias [rare])

Lab test interferences:
Increase (false): Creatinine (serum urine), urinary 17-KS
False positive: Urinary protein, direct Coombs', urine glucose
Interference: Cross-matching

Treatment of overdose: Epinephrine, antihistamines, resuscitate if needed (anaphylaxis)

---

cefonicid sodium

(se-fon′i-sid)
Monocid
Func. class.: Antibiotic
Chem. class.: Cephalosporin (2nd generation)

Action: Inhibits bacterial cell wall synthesis rendering cell wall osmotically unstable

Uses: Gram-negative bacilli: *H. influenzae, E. coli, P. mirabilis, Klebsiella;* gram-positive organisms: *S. pneumoniae, S. pyogenes, S. aureus;* lower respiratory tract, urinary tract, skin infections, otitis media, peritonitis, septicemia

Dosage and routes:
Life-threatening infections
• *Adult:* IM/IV BOL or INF 1-2 g/24 hr; divide in two doses if giving 2 g

• Dosage reduction indicated in renal impairment

Available forms include: Inj IM, IV, 500 mg, 1, 10 g

Side effects/adverse reactions:
CNS: Headache, dizziness, weakness, paresthesia, fever, chills
GI: Nausea, vomiting, diarrhea, anorexia, pain, glossitis, bleeding, increased AST, ALT, bilirubin, LDH, alk phosphatase, abdominal pain
GU: Proteinuria, vaginitis, pruritus, candidiasis, increased BUN, ***nephrotoxicity, renal failure***
*HEMA: **Leukopenia, thrombocytopenia, agranulocytosis,** anemia, **neutropenia, lymphocytosis, eosinophilia, pancytopenia, hemolytic anemia***
INTEG: Rash, urticaria, dermatitis, ***anaphylaxis***

Contraindications: Hypersensitivity to cephalosporins, infants <1 mo

Precautions: Hypersensitivity to penicillins, pregnancy (B), lactation, renal disease

Pharmacokinetics:
IV: Onset 5 min
IM: Peak 1 hr
Half-life 4½ hr, excreted in breast milk, 98% protein bound

Interactions/incompatibilities:
• Decreased effects: tetracyclines, erythromycins
• Increased toxicity: aminoglycosides, furosemide, probenecid, sulfinpyrazone, colistin, ethacrynic acid, vancomycin, other cephalosporins

NURSING CONSIDERATIONS
Assess:
• Sensitivity to penicillin and other cephalosporins
• Nephrotoxicity: increased BUN, creatinine
• I&O daily

---

italics = common side effects   ***bold italic*** = life threatening reactions

• Blood studies: AST, ALT, CBC, Hct, bilirubin, LDH, alk phosphatase, Coombs' test monthly if patient is on long-term therapy
• Electrolytes: potassium, sodium, chloride monthly if patient is on long-term therapy
• Bowel pattern qd; if severe diarrhea occurs, drug should be discontinued; may indicate pseudomembranous colitis

Administer:
• IV bolus over 3-5 min
• IV diluted in 50-100 ml compatible IV sol, slight yellowing of sol does not affect potency
• IV, check for irritation, extravasation often
• For 10-14 days to ensure organism death, prevent superimposed infection
• After C&S completed

Evaluate:
• Therapeutic response: decreased fever, fatigue, malaise
• Urine output; if decreasing, notify physician; may indicate nephrotoxicity
• Allergic reactions: rash, urticaria, pruritus, chills, fever, joint pain, angioedema; may occur few days after therapy begins
• Bleeding: ecchymosis, bleeding gums, hematuria, stool guaiac daily
• Overgrowth of infection: perineal itching, fever, malaise, redness, pain, swelling, drainage, rash, diarrhea, change in cough, sputum

Teach patient/family:
• If diabetic, to use Clinistix or Ketodiastix
• Not to use alcohol or meds with alcohol or reaction may occur
• To report sore throat, bruising, bleeding, joint pain; may indicate blood dyscrasias (rare)

Lab test interferences:
Increase (false): Urinary 17-KS

False positive: Urinary protein, direct Coombs', urine glucose
Interference: Cross-matching
Treatment of overdose: Epinephrine, antihistamines, resuscitate if needed (anaphylaxis)

---

cefoperazone sodium
(sef-oh-per'a-zone)
Cefobid

Func. class.: Antibiotic, broad-spectrum
Chem. class.: Cephalosporin (3rd generation)

Action: Inhibits bacterial cell wall synthesis rendering cell wall osmotically unstable
Uses: Gram-negative bacilli: *H. influenzae, E. coli, P. mirabilis, Klebsiella, Enterobacter, Serratia, Citrobacter, Providencia, P. aeruginosa;* lower respiratory tract, urinary tract, skin, bone infections, bacterial septicemia, peritonitis, pelvic inflammatory disease

Dosage and routes:
Mild/moderate infections
• *Adult:* IM/IV 1-2 g q12h
Severe infections
• *Adult:* IM/IV 6-12 g/day divided in 2-4 equal doses
Available forms include: Inj IM, IV, 1, 2 g

Side effects/adverse reactions:
CNS: Headache, dizziness, weakness, paresthesia, fever, chills
GI: Nausea, vomiting, diarrhea, anorexia, pain, glossitis, bleeding, increased AST, ALT, bilirubin, LDH, alk phosphatase, abdominal pain, pseudomembranous colitis
GU: Proteinuria, vaginitis, pruritus, candidiasis, increased BUN, *nephrotoxicity, renal failure*
HEMA: Leukopenia, thrombocytopenia, agranulocytosis, anemia,

---

neutropenia, lymphocytosis, eosinophilia, pancytopenia, hemolytic anemia, bleeding, hypoprothrombinemia
INTEG: Rash, urticaria, dermatitis, *anaphylaxis*
RESP: Dyspnea
Contraindications: Hypersensitivity to cephalosporins, infants <1 mo
Precautions: Hypersensitivity to penicillins, pregnancy (B), lactation, renal disease
Pharmacokinetics:
IV: Onset 5 min, peak 5-20 min, duration 6-8 hr
IM: Peak 1-2 hr, duration 6-8 hr
Half-life 2 hr, 70%-75% is eliminated unchanged in bile, 20%-30% unchanged in urine, excreted in breast milk (small amounts)
Interactions/incompatibilities:
• Do not mix with aminoglycosides in same parenteral fluid
• Decreased effects: tetracyclines, erythromycins
• Increased toxicity: aminoglycosides, furosemide, probenecid, sulfinpyrazone, colistin, ethacrynic acid, vancomycin
• Disulfiram-like reactions if alcohol ingested within 24-72 hr of cefoperazone administration
NURSING CONSIDERATIONS
Assess:
• Sensitivity to penicillin or other cephalosporins
• Nephrotoxicity: increased BUN, creatinine
• I&O daily
• Blood studies: AST, ALT, CBC, Hct, bilirubin, LDH, alk phosphatase, Coombs' test pro-time monthly if patient is on long-term therapy
• Electrolytes: potassium, sodium, chloride monthly if patient is on long-term therapy

• Bowel pattern qd; if severe diarrhea occurs, drug should be discontinued; may indicate pseudomembranous colitis
• IV site for extravasation or phlebitis, change site q72h
Administer:
• IV after diluting 1 g/2.8 ml sterile H_2O for INJ, or 0.9% NaCl; shake; run over 15-30 min; may be further diluted to a concentration of no greater than 25 mg/ml
• IM for concentration of >250 mg/ml, dilute in sterile water, then lidocaine, inject deeply
• For 10-14 days to ensure organism death, prevent superimposed infection
• After C&S completed
Evaluate:
• Therapeutic response: decreased fever, malaise, chills
• Urine output, if decreasing, notify physician; may indicate nephrotoxicity
• Allergic reactions: rash, urticaria, pruritus, chills, fever, joint pain, angioedema; may occur few days after therapy begins
• Bleeding: ecchymosis, bleeding gums, hematuria, stool guaiac daily
• Overgrowth of infection: perineal itching, fever, malaise, redness, pain, swelling, drainage, rash, diarrhea, change in cough, sputum
Teach patient/family:
• Not to drink alcohol for 3 days after use
• To report sore throat, bruising, bleeding, joint pain; may indicate blood dyscrasias (rare)
Lab test interferences:
Increase (false): Urinary 17-KS
False positive: Urinary protein, direct Coombs', urine glucose
Interference: Cross-matching
Treatment of overdose: Epineph-

---

italics = common side effects   ***bold italic*** = life threatening reactions

rine, antihistamines, resuscitate if
needed (anaphylaxis)

ceforanide

(sef-or-aa-nide)
Precef
Func. class.: Antibiotic, broad-
spectrum
Chem. class.: Cephalosporin (2nd
generation)

Action: Inhibits bacterial cell wall
synthesis, rendering cell wall osmotically unstable
Uses: Gram-negative bacilli: *H. influenzae, E. coli, P. mirabilis,
Klebsiella;* gram-positive organisms: *S. pneumoniae, S. aureus;*
lower respiratory tract, urinary
tract, skin, bone infections, septicemia, endocarditis
Dosage and routes:
• *Adult:* IM/IV 0.5-1 g q12h
• *Child:* IM/IV 20-40 mg/kg/day
in 2 equal doses q12h
• Dosage reduction indicated in renal impairment (CrCl < 59 ml/
min)
Available forms include: Powder
for inj IM, IV 500 mg, 1, 10 g
Side effects/adverse reactions:
CNS: Headache, dizziness, weakness, paresthesia, fever, chills
*GI: Nausea, vomiting, diarrhea,
anorexia,* pain, glossitis, bleeding,
increased AST, ALT, bilirubin,
LDH, alk phosphatase, abdominal
pain
GU: Proteinuria, vaginitis, pruritus,
increased BUN, *nephrotoxicity,
renal failure*
*HEMA: Leukopenia, thrombocyto-
penia, agranulocytosis,* anemia,
*neutropenia, lymphocytosis, eo-
sinophilia, pancytopenia, hemolytic anemia*

INTEG: Rash, urticaria, dermatitis,
anaphylaxis
RESP: Dyspnea
Contraindications: Hypersen-
sitivity to cephalosporins, infants <1 mo
Precautions: Hypersensitivity to
penicillins, pregnancy (B), lactation, renal disease
Pharmacokinetics:
IV: Peak 2 hr
IM: Peak 1 hr
Half-life 2½-3 hr, 80% is bound by
plasma proteins, 90% is eliminated
unchanged in urine; crosses pla-
centa, excreted in breast milk
Interactions/incompatibilities:
• Do not mix with aminoglycosides
in same parenteral fluid
• Decreased effects: tetracyclines,
erythromycins
• Increased toxicity: aminoglycosides, furosemide, probenecid,
sulfinpyrazone, colistin, ethacrynic acid, vancomycin
NURSING CONSIDERATIONS
Assess:
• Sensitivity to penicillin or other
cephalosporins
• Nephrotoxicity: increased BUN,
creatinine
• I&O daily
• Blood studies: AST, ALT, CBC,
Hct, bilirubin, LDH alk phosphatase, Coombs' test monthly if patient is on long-term therapy
• Electrolytes: potassium, sodium,
chloride monthly if patient is on
long-term therapy
• Bowel pattern qd; if severe diarrhea occurs, drug should be discontinued; may indicate pseudomembranous colitis
• IV site for extravasation or phlebitis; change site q72h
Administer:
• IV INF diluted 1 g of drug/10 ml
of diluent, shake, give over 3-5 min

---

directly or run over 15-30 min as an infusion

• For 10-14 days to ensure organism death, prevent superimposed infection

• After C&S completed

Evaluate:

• Therapeutic response: decreased fever, malaise, chills

• Urine output, if decreasing, notify physician; may indicate nephrotoxicity

• Allergic reactions: rash, urticaria, pruritus, chills, fever, joint pain, angioedema; may occur few days after therapy begins

• Bleeding: ecchymosis, bleeding gums, hematuria, stool guaiac daily

• Overgrowth of infection: perineal itching, fever, malaise, redness, pain, swelling, drainage, rash, diarrhea, change in cough, sputum

Teach patient/family:

• If diabetic, to use Clinistix, Kefodiastix

• Not to drink alcohol or meds with alcohol as reaction may occur

• To report sore throat, bruising, bleeding, joint pain; may indicate blood dyscrasias (rare)

Lab test interferences:

Increase (false): Urinary 17-KS

False positive: Urinary protein, direct Coombs', urine glucose

Interference: Cross-matching

Treatment of overdose: Epinephrine, antihistamines, resuscitate if needed (anaphylaxis)

---

cefotaxime sodium

(sef-oh-taks'eem)

Claforan

Func. class.: Antibiotic, broad-spectrum

Chem. class.: Cephalosporin (3rd generation)

Action: Inhibits bacterial cell wall synthesis, rendering cell wall osmotically unstable

Uses: Gram-negative organisms: *H. influenzae, E. coli, N. gonorrhea, N. meningitidis, P. mirabilis, Klebsiella, Citrobacter, Serratia, Salmonella, Shigella,* gram-positive organisms: *S. pneumoniae, S. pyogenes, S. aureus,* lower serious respiratory tract, urinary tract, skin, bone, gonococcal infections, bacteremia, septicemia, meningitis

Dosage and routes:

• *Adult:* IM/IV 1 g q8-12h

Severe infections

• *Adult:* IM/IV 2 g q4h, not to exceed 12 g/day

• Uncomplicated gonorrhea, 1 g IM

• Dosage reduction indicated for severe renal impairment (CrCl < 10 ml/min)

Available forms include: Powder for inj IM, IV, 1, 2, 10 g, frozen inj/IV 20, 40 mg/ml

Side effects/adverse reactions:

CNS: Headache, dizziness, weakness, paresthesia, fever, chills

GI: Nausea, vomiting, diarrhea, anorexia, pain, glossitis, bleeding, increased AST, ALT, bilirubin, LDH, alk phosphatase, abdominal pain

GU: Proteinuria, vaginitis, pruritus, candidiasis, increased BUN, *nephrotoxicity, renal failure*

HEMA: Leukopenia, thrombocytopenia, agranulocytosis, anemia, *neutropenia, lymphocytosis, eosinophilia, pancytopenia, hemolytic anemia*

INTEG: Rash, urticaria, dermatitis, *anaphylaxis,* pain, induration (IM), inflammation (IV)

Contraindications: Hypersensitivity to cephalosporins, infants <1 mo

---

italics = common side effects   ***bold italic*** = life threatening reactions

Precautions: Hypersensitivity to penicillins, pregnancy (B), lactation, renal disease

Pharmacokinetics:

IV: Onset 5 min

IM: Onset 30 min

Half-life 1 hr, 35%-65% is bound by plasma proteins, 40%-65% is eliminated unchanged in urine in 24 hr, 25% metabolized to active metabolites, excreted in breast milk (small amounts)

Interactions/incompatibilities:

• Do not mix with aminoglycosides, aminophylline HCO₃ erythromycins in same parenteral fluid

• Decreased effects: tetracyclines, erythromycins

• Increased toxicity: aminoglycosides, furosemide, probenecid, sulfinpyrazone, colistin, ethacrynic acid, vancomycin

NURSING CONSIDERATIONS

Assess:

• Sensitivity to penicillin or other cephalosporins

• Nephrotoxicity: increased BUN, creatinine

• I&O daily

• Blood studies: AST, ALT, CBC, Hct, bilirubin, LDH, alk phosphatase, Coombs' test monthly if patient is on long-term therapy

• Electrolytes: potassium, sodium, chloride monthly if the patient is on long-term therapy

• Bowel pattern qd; if severe diarrhea occurs, drug should be discontinued; may indicate pseudomembranous colitis

• IV site for extravasation or phlebitis, change site q72h

Administer:

• IV after diluting 1g/10 ml and give over 3-5 min; may be diluted further with 50-100 ml of normal saline or D₅W; run over ½-1 hr

• For 10-14 days to ensure organism death, prevent superimposed infection

• After C&S completed

Evaluate:

• Therapeutic response: decreased fever, malaise, chills

• Urine output; if decreasing, notify physician; may indicate nephrotoxicity

• Allergic reactions: rash, urticaria, pruritis, chills, fever, joint pain, angioedema; may occur few days after therapy begins

• Bleeding: ecchymosis, bleeding gums, hematuria, stool guaiac daily

• Overgrowth of infection: perineal itching, fever, malaise, redness, pain, swelling, drainage, rash, diarrhea, change in cough, sputum

Teach patient/family:

• To report sore throat, bruising, bleeding, joint pain; may indicate blood dyscrasias (rare)

• If diabetic, to use Clinistix or Ketodiastix

• Not to use alcohol or meds with alcohol or reaction may occur

Lab test interferences:

Increase (false): Urinary 17-KS

False positive: Urinary protein, direct Coombs', urine glucose

Interference: Cross-matching

Treatment of overdose: Epinephrine, antihistamines, resuscitate if needed (anaphylaxis)

---

cefotetan disodium

(sef'oh-tee-tan)

Cefotan

Func. class.: Antibiotic, broad-spectrum

Chem. class.: Cephalosporin (3rd generation)

Action: Inhibits bacterial cell wall synthesis, which renders cell osmotically unstable

---

Uses: Gram-negative organisms: *H. influenzae, E. coli, E. aerogenes, P. mirabilis, Klebsiella, Citrobacter, Enterobacter, Salmonella, Shigella, Acinetobacter, B. fragilis, Neisseria, Serratia;* gram-positive organisms: *S. pneumoniae, S. pyogenes, S. aureus;* upper, lower, serious respiratory tract, urinary tract, skin, gonococcal, intraabdominal infections, septicemia, meningitis

Dosages and routes:
• *Adult:* IV/IM 1-2g q12h × 5-10 days

Perioperative prophylaxis
• *Adult:* IV 1-2 g ½-1 hr before surgery

Available forms include: Inj (IV, IM)

Side effects/adverse reactions:
CNS: Headache, dizziness, weakness, paresthesia, fever, chills
GI: Nausea, vomiting, diarrhea, anorexia, pain, glossitis, bleeding, increased AST, ALT, bilirubin, LDH, alk phosphatase, *pseudomembranous colitis*
GU: Proteinuria, vaginitis, pruritus, candidiasis, increased BUN, *nephrotoxicity, renal failure*
HEMA: Leukopenia, thrombocytopenia, agranulocytosis, anemia, *neutropenia, lymphocytosis, eosinophilia, pancytopenia, hemolytic anemia*
INTEG: Rash, urticaria, dermatitis
RESP: Dyspnea, *anaphylaxis*
Contraindications: Hypersensitivity to cephalosporins, children
Precautions: Hypersensitivity to penicillins, pregnancy (B), lactation, renal disease
Pharmacokinetics:
IV/IM: Peak 1½-3 hr; half-life 3-5 hr, 70%-90% bound by plasma proteins, 50%-80% eliminated un-

changed in urine, crosses placenta, excreted in milk
Interactions/incompatibilities:
• Do not mix with tetracyclines, erythromycins, aminoglycosides in same parenteral fluid
• Increased toxicity: aminoglycosides
NURSING CONSIDERATIONS
Assess:
• Sensitivity to penicillin or other cephalosporins
• Nephrotoxicity: increased BUN, creatinine
• I&O daily
• Blood studies: AST, ALT, CBC, Hct, bilirubin, LDH, alk phosphatase, Coombs' test monthly if patient is on long-term therapy
• Electrolytes: potassium, sodium, chloride monthly if patient is on long-term therapy
• Bowel pattern qd; if severe diarrhea occurs, drug should be discontinued; may indicate pseudomembranous colitis
• IV site for extravasation, phlebitis, change site q72 h
Administer:
• IV after diluting 1 g/10 ml and give over 3-5 min; may be diluted further with 50-100 ml of normal saline or D₅W; run over ½-1 hr
• For 5-10 days to ensure organism death, prevent superimposed infection
• After C&S is taken
Evaluate:
• Therapeutic response: decreased fever, malaise, chills
• Urine output: if decreasing, notify physician, may indicate nephrotoxicity
• Allergic reactions: rash, urticaria, pruritus, chills, fever; may occur a few days after therapy begins
• Bleeding: ecchymosis, bleeding

gums, hematuria, stool guaiac daily
• Overgrowth of infection: perineal itching, fever, malaise, redness, swelling, drainage, rash, diarrhea, change in cough, sputum

Teach patient/family:
• To report sore throat, bruising, bleeding, joint pain; may indicate blood dyscrasias
• To report severe diarrhea; may indicate pseudomembranous colitis
• To avoid use of alcohol for 3 days after use

Lab test interferences:
Increase (false): Urinary 17-KS
False positive: Urinary protein, direct Coombs' test, urine glucose
Interference: Cross-matching

Treatment of overdose: Epinephrine, antihistamines; resuscitate if needed (anaphylaxis)

---

cefoxitin sodium

(se-fox'i-tin)
Mefoxin
Func. class.: Antibiotic, broad-spectrum
Chem. class.: Cephamycin (2nd generation)

Action: Inhibits bacterial cell wall synthesis rendering cell wall osmotically unstable

Uses: Gram-negative bacilli: *H. influenzae, E. coli, Proteus, Klebsiella, B. fragilis, N. gonorrhoeae;* gram-positive organisms: *S. pneumoniae, S. pyogenes, S. aureus;* anaerobes including *Clostridium,* lower respiratory tract, urinary tract, skin, bone, gonococcal infections, septicemia, peritonitis

Dosage and routes:
• *Adult:* IM/IV 1-2 g q6-8h
• Dosage reduction indicated in renal impairment (CrCl <50 ml/min)
• Uncomplicated gonorrhea 2 g IM

as single dose with 1 g PO probenecid at same time

Severe infections
• *Adult:* IM/IV 2 g q4h

Available forms include: Powder for inj IM, IV 1, 2, 10 g

Side effects/adverse reactions:
CNS: Headache, dizziness, weakness, paresthesia, fever, chills
GI: Nausea, vomiting, diarrhea, anorexia, pain, glossitis, bleeding, increased AST, ALT, bilirubin, LDH, alk phosphatase, abdominal pain
GU: Proteinuria, vaginitis, pruritus, candidiasis, increased BUN, **nephrotoxicity, renal failure**
*HEMA: **Leukopenia, thrombocytopenia, agranulocytosis,** anemia, **neutropenia, lymphocytosis, eosinophilia, pancytopenia, hemolytic anemia***
INTEG: Rash, urticaria, dermatitis, thrombophlebitis
*SYST: **Anaphylaxis***

Contraindications: Hypersensitivity to cephalosporins, infants <1 mo

Precautions: Hypersensitivity to penicillins, pregnancy (B), lactation, renal disease

Pharmacokinetics:
IV: Peak 3 min
IM: Peak 15-60 min
Half-life 1 hr, 55%-75% bound by plasma proteins, 90%-100% eliminated unchanged in urine; crosses placenta, blood-brain barrier, eliminated in milk, not metabolized

Interactions/incompatibilities:
• Do not mix with aminoglycosides in same parenteral fluid
• Decreased effects: tetracyclines, erythromycins
• Increased toxicity: aminoglycosides, furosemide, probenecid,

---

sulfinpyrazone, colistin, etha-crynic acid, vancomycin

NURSING CONSIDERATIONS

Assess:

• Sensitivity to penicillin or other cephalosporins

• Nephrotoxicity: increased BUN, creatinine

• I&O daily

• Blood studies: AST, ALT, CBC, Hct, bilirubin, LDH, alk phosphatase, Coombs' test monthly if patient is on long-term therapy

• Electrolytes: potassium, sodium, chloride monthly if patient is on long-term therapy

• Bowel pattern qd, if severe diarrhea occurs drug should be discontinued (may indicate pseudomembranous colitis)

• IV site for extravasation or phlebitis, change site q72h

Administer:

• IV after diluting 1 g/10 ml and give over 3-5 min; may be diluted further with 50-100 ml of normal saline or D_5W; run over ½-1 hr

• For 10-14 days to ensure organism death, prevent superimposed infection

• After C&S completed

Evaluate:

• Therapeutic response: decreased fever, malaise, chills

• Urine output; if decreasing, notify physician; may indicate nephrotoxicity

• Allergic reactions: rash, urticaria, pruritis, chills, fever, joint pain, angioedema; may occur few days after therapy begins

• Bleeding: ecchymosis, bleeding gums, hematuria, stool guaiac daily

• Overgrowth of infection: perineal itching, fever, malaise, redness, pain, swelling, drainage, rash, diarrhea, change in cough, sputum

Teach patient/family:

• If diabetic, to use Clinistix or Ketodiastix

• Not to use alcohol or meds with alcohol or reaction can occur

• To report severe diarrhea; may indicate pseudomembranous colitis

• To report sore throat, bruising, bleeding, joint pain; may indicate blood dyscrasias (rare)

Lab test interferences:

Increase (false): Creatinine (serum urine), urinary 17-KS

False positive: Urinary protein, direct Coombs', urine glucose

Interference: Cross-matching

Treatment of overdose: Epinephrine, antihistamines, resuscitate if needed (anaphylaxis)

---

ceftazidime

(sef'tay-zi-deem)

Fortaz, Manacef, Tazicef, Tazidime

Func. class.: Antibiotic, broad-spectrum

Chem. class.: Cephalosporin (3rd generation)

Action: Inhibits bacterial cell wall synthesis, which renders cell osmotically unstable

Uses: Gram-negative organisms: *H. influenzae, E. coli, E. aerogenes, P. mirabilis, Klebsiella, Citrobacter, Enterobacter, Salmonella, Shigella, Acinetobacter, B. fragilis, Neisseria, Serratia;* gram-positive organisms: *S. pneumoniae, S. pyogenes, S. aureus;* upper, lower, serious respiratory tract, urinary tract, skin, gonococcal, intraabdominal infections; septicemia, meningitis

Dosage and routes:

• *Adult:* IV/IM 1 g q8-12h × 5-10 days

---

italics = common side effects   ***bold italic*** = life threatening reactions

- *Children:* IV 30-50 mg/kg/day, not to exceed 6 g/day
- *Neonates:* IV 30 mg/kg q12h

Available forms include: Inj (IV, IM)

Side effects/adverse reactions:

CNS: Headache, dizziness, weakness, paresthesia, fever, chills

GI: Nausea, vomiting, diarrhea, anorexia, pain, glossitis, bleeding, increased AST, ALT, bilirubin, LDH, alk phosphatase

GU: Proteinuria, vaginitis, pruritus, candidiasis, increased BUN, *nephrotoxicity, renal failure*

HEMA: Leukopenia, thrombocytopenia, agranulocytosis, anemia, *neutropenia, lymphocytosis, eosinophilia, pancytopenia, hemolytic anemia*

INTEG: Rash, urticaria, dermatitis, *anaphylaxis*

RESP: Dyspnea

Contraindications: Hypersensitivity to cephalosporins, children

Precautions: Hypersensitivity to penicillins, pregnancy (B), lactation, renal disease

Pharmacokinetics:

IV/IM: Peak 1 hr, half-life ½-1 hr, 90% bound by plasma proteins, 80% eliminated unchanged in urine, crosses placenta, excreted in breast milk

Interactions/incompatibilities:

- Do not mix with tetracyclines, erythromycins, aminoglycosides in same parenteral fluid
- Increased toxicity: aminoglycosides

NURSING CONSIDERATIONS

Assess:

- Sensitivity to penicillin or other cephalosporins
- Nephrotoxicity: increased BUN, creatinine
- I&O daily
- Blood studies: AST, ALT, CBC, Hct, bilirubin, LDH, alk phosphatase, Coombs' test monthly if patient is on long-term therapy
- Electrolytes: potassium, sodium chloride monthly if patient is on long-term therapy
- Bowel pattern qd; if severe diarrhea occurs, drug should be discontinued; may indicate pseudomembranous colitis
- IV site for extravasation, phlebitis, change site q72h

Administer:

- IV after diluting 1 g/10 ml and give over 3-5 min; may be diluted further with 50-100 ml of normal saline or D_5W; run over ½-1 hr
- For 5-10 days to ensure organism death, prevent superimposed infection
- After C&S is taken

Evaluate:

- Therapeutic response: decreased fever, malaise, chills
- Urine output: if decreasing, notify physician, may indicate nephrotoxicity
- Allergic reactions: rash, urticaria, pruritus, chills, fever; may occur a few days after therapy begins
- Bleeding: ecchymosis, bleeding gums, hematuria, stool guaiac daily
- Overgrowth of infection: perineal itching, fever, malaise, redness, swelling, drainage, rash, diarrhea, change in cough, sputum

Teach patient/family:

- To report sore throat, bruising, bleeding, joint pain; may indicate blood dyscrasias
- To report severe diarrhea; may indicate pseudomembranous colitis
- If diabetic, to use Clinistix or Ketodiastix
- Not to use alcohol or meds with alcohol or reaction may occur

Lab test interferences:
Increase (false): Urinary 17-KS
False positive: Urinary protein, direct Coombs' test, urine glucose
Interference: Cross-matching
Treatment of overdose: Epinephrine, antihistamines, resuscitate if needed (anaphylaxis)

---

ceftizoxime sodium
(sef-te-zox'eem)
Cefizox
Func. class.: Antibiotic, broad-spectrum
Chem. class.: Cephalosporin (3rd generation)

Action: Inhibits bacterial cell wall synthesis, which renders cell wall osmotically unstable
Uses: Gram-negative organisms: *H. influenzae, E. coli, E. aerogenes, P. mirabilis, Klebsiella, Enterobacter;* gram-positive organisms: *S. pneumoniae, S. pyogenes, S. aureus;* lower serious respiratory tract, urinary tract, skin, intraabdominal infections, septicemia, meningitis, bone, joint infections
Dosage and routes:
• *Adult:* IM/IV 1-2 g q8-12h, may give up to 2g q4h in life-threatening infections.
Available forms include: Inj 1, 2g
Side effects/adverse reactions:
CNS: Headache, dizziness, paresthesia, fever
GI: Nausea, vomiting, diarrhea, anorexia, pain, glossitis, bleeding, increased AST, ALT, bilirubin, LDH, alk phosphatase, abdominal pain, *pseudomembranous colitis*
GU: Proteinuria, vaginitis, pruritus, candidiasis
HEMA: Leukopenia, thrombocytopenia, agranulocytosis, anemia, *neutropenia, eosinophilia, hemolytic anemia*
INTEG: Rash, urticaria, dermatitis
RESP: Dyspnea, *anaphylaxis*
Contraindications: Hypersensitivity to cephalosporins, infants <1 mo
Precautions: Hypersensitivity to penicillins, pregnancy (B), lactation, renal disease
Pharmacokinetics:
IV: Onset 5 min
IM: Peak 1 hr
Half-life 5-8 hr, 90% bound by plasma proteins, 36%-60% is eliminated unchanged in urine, crosses placenta, excreted in milk
Interactions/incompatibilities:
• Do not mix with tetracyclines, erythromycins, aminoglycosides in same parenteral fluid
• Decreased effects: tetracyclines, erythromycins
• Increased toxicity: aminoglycosides, furosemide, probenecid, sulfinpyrazone, colistin, ethacrynic acid

NURSING CONSIDERATIONS
Assess:
• Sensitivity to penicillin or other cephalosporins
• Nephrotoxicity: increased BUN, creatinine
• I&O daily
• Blood studies: AST, ALT, CBC, Hct, bilirubin, LDH, alk phosphatase, Coombs' test monthly if patient is on long-term therapy
• Electrolytes: potassium, sodium, chloride monthly if patient is on long-term therapy
• Bowel pattern qd; if severe diarrhea occurs, drug should be discontinued; may indicate pseudomembranous colitis
• IV site for extravasation, phlebitis; change site q72h

---

italics = common side effects   ***bold italic*** = life threatening reactions

Administer:
• IV after diluting 1 g/10 ml and give over 3-5 min; may be diluted further with 50-100 ml of normal saline or D_5W; run over ½-1 hr
• For 10-14 days to ensure organism death, prevent superimposed infection
• After C&S
Evaluate:
• Therapeutic response: decreased fever, malaise
• Allergic reactions: rash, urticaria, pruritus, chills, fever, joint pain, angioedema; may occur few days after therapy begins
• Bleeding: ecchymosis, bleeding gums, hematuria, stool guaiac daily
• Overgrowth of infection: perineal itching, fever, malaise, redness, pain, swelling, drainage, rash, diarrhea, change in cough, sputum
Teach patient/family:
• If diabetic, to use Clinistix or Ketodiastix
• Not to use alcohol or meds with alcohol or reaction can occur
• To report sore throat, bruising, bleeding, joint pain; may indicate blood dyscrasias (rare)
Lab test interferences:
Increase (false): Urinary 17-KS
False positive: Urinary protein, direct Coombs', urine glucose
Interference: Cross-matching
Treatment of overdose: Epinephrine, antihistamines, resuscitate if needed (anaphylaxis)

---

ceftriaxone sodium
Rocephin

Func. class.: Antibiotic, broad-spectrum
Chem. class.: Cephalosporin (3rd generation)

Action: Inhibits bacterial cell wall synthesis, which renders cell wall osmotically unstable
Uses: Gram-negative organisms: *H. influenzae, E. coli, E. aerogenes, P. mirabilis, Klebsiella, Citrobacter, Enterobacter, Salmonella, Shigella, Acinetobacter, B. Fragilis,* Neisseria, *Serratia;* gram-positive organisms: *S. pneumoniae, S. pyogenes, S. aureus;* lower serious respiratory tract, urinary tract, skin, gonococcal, intraabdominal infections, septicemia, meningitis, bone, joint infections
Dosage and routes:
• *Adult:* IM/IV 1-2 g qd or in two equal doses
• *Child:* IM/IV 50-75 mg/kg/day in equal doses q12h
Uncomplicated Gonorrhea
• 250 mg IM as single dose
• Dosage reduction may be indicated in severe renal impairment (CrCl < 10 ml/min)
Meningitis
• *Adult and child:* IM/IV 100 mg/kg/day in equal doses q12h
Surgical prophylaxis
• Adult: IV 1 g ½-2 hr preop
Available forms include: Inj IM, IV 250, 500 mg, 1, 2, 10 g
Side effects/adverse reactions:
CNS: Headache, dizziness, weakness, paresthesia, fever, chills
GI: Nausea, vomiting, diarrhea, anorexia, pain, glossitis, bleeding, increased AST, ALT, bilirubin, LDH, alk phosphatase, abdominal pain, *pseudomembranous colitis*
GU: Proteinuria, vaginitis, pruritus, candidiasis, increased BUN, ***nephrotoxicity, renal failure***
*HEMA: **Leukopenia, thrombocytopenia, agranulocytosis,** anemia, **neutropenia, lymphocytosis, eosinophilia, pancytopenia, hemolytic anemia***

INTEG: Rash, urticaria, dermatitis
RESP: Dyspnea, ***anaphylaxis***
Contraindications: Hypersensitivity to cephalosporins, infants <1 mo
Precautions: Hypersensitivity to penicillins, pregnancy (B), lactation, renal disease
Pharmacokinetics:
IV: Onset 5 min
IM: Peak 1 hr
Half-life 5-8 hr, 90% bound by plasma proteins, 35%-60% is eliminated unchanged in urine, crosses placenta, excreted in milk
Interactions/incompatibilities:
• Do not mix with tetracyclines, erythromycins, aminoglycosides in same parenteral fluid
• Decreased effects: tetracyclines, erythromycins
• Increased toxicity: aminoglycosides, furosemide, probenecid, sulfinpyrazone, colistin, ethacrynic acid

NURSING CONSIDERATIONS
Assess:
• Sensitivity to penicillin or other cephalosporins
• Nephrotoxicity: increased BUN, creatinine
• I&O daily
• Blood studies: AST, ALT, CBC, Hct, bilirubin, LDH, alk phosphatase, Coombs' test monthly if patient is on long-term therapy
• Electrolytes: potassium, sodium, chloride monthly if patient is on long-term therapy
• Bowel pattern qd; if severe diarrhea occurs, drug should be discontinued; may indicate pseudomembranous colitis
• IV site for extravasation, phlebitis; change site q72h
Administer:
• For 10-14 days to ensure organism death, prevent superimposed infection
• IV after diluting 250 mg/2.4 ml of D_5W, H_2O for inj, 0.9% NaCl; may be further diluted with 50-100 ml of compatible sol; run over ½-1 hr
• After C&S
Evaluate:
• IV after diluting 1 g/10 ml and give over 3-5 min; may be diluted further with 50-100 ml of normal saline or D_5W; run over ½-1 hr
• Therapeutic response: decreased fever, malaise, chills
• Urine output; if decreasing, notify physician; may indicate nephrotoxicity
• Allergic reactions: rash, urticaria, pruritus, chills, fever, joint pain, angioedema; may occur few days after therapy begins
• Bleeding: ecchymosis, bleeding gums, hematuria, stool guaiac daily
• Overgrowth of infection: perineal itching, fever, malaise, redness, pain, swelling, drainage, rash, diarrhea, change in cough, sputum
Teach patient/family:
• If diabetic, to use Clinistix or Ketodiastix
• Not to use alcohol or meds with alcohol or reaction may occur
• To report severe diarrhea; may indicate pseudomembranous colitis
• To report sore throat, bruising, bleeding, joint pain; may indicate blood dyscrasias (rare)
Lab test interferences:
Increase (false): Urinary 17-KS
False positive: Urinary protein, direct Coombs', urine glucose
Interference: Cross-matching
Treatment of overdose: Epinephrine, antihistamines, resuscitate if needed (anaphylaxis)

---

italics = common side effects   ***bold italic*** = life threatening reactions

cefuroxime axetil

(sef-fyoor-ox'eem)

Ceftin

Func. class.: Antibiotic, broad-spectrum

Chem. class.: Cephalosporin (2nd generation)

Action: Inhibits bacterial cell wall synthesis, rendering cell wall osmotically unstable

Uses: Gram-negative bacilli *(H. influenzae, E. coli, Neisseria, P. mirabilis, Klebsiella);* gram-positive organisms *(S. pneumoniae, S. pyogenes, S. aureus);* serious lower respiratory tract, urinary tract, skin, gonococcal infections; septicemia; meningitis

Dosage and routes:

• *Adult and child:* PO 250 mg q12h, may increase to 500 mg q12h in serious infections

Urinary tract infections

• *Adult:* PO 125 mg q12h, may increase to 250 q12h if needed

Otitis media

• Child <2 yr: PO 125 mg bid

• Child >2 yr: PO 250 mg bid

Available forms include: Tabs 125, 250, 500 mg

Side effects / adverse reactions:

CNS: Headache, dizziness, weakness, paresthesia, fever, chills

GI: Nausea, vomiting, diarrhea, anorexia, pain, glossitis, bleeding, increased AST, ALT, bilirubin, LDH, alk phosphatase, abdominal pain, *pseudomembranous colitis*

GU: Proteinuria, vaginitis, pruritus, candidiasis, increased BUN, *nephrotoxicity, renal failure*

HEMA: Leukopenia, thrombocytopenia, agranulocytosis, anemia, *neutropenia, lymphocytosis, eosinophilia, pancytopenia, hemolytic anemia*

INTEG: Rash, urticaria, dermatitis

RESP: Anaphylaxis

Contraindications: Hypersensitivity to cephalosporins, infants <1 mo

Precautions: Hypersensitivity to penicillins, pregnancy (B), lactation, renal disease

Pharmacokinetics:

65% excreted unchanged in urine, half-life 1-2 hr in normal renal function

Interactions / incompatibilities:

• Decreased effects: tetracyclines, erythromycins

• Increased side effects: aminoglycosides, furosemide, probenecid, sulfinpyrazone, colistin, ethacrynic acid

NURSING CONSIDERATIONS

Assess:

• Sensitivity to penicillin or other cephalosporins

• Nephrotoxicity: increased BUN, creatinine

• I&O daily

• Blood studies: AST, ALT, CBC, Hct, bilirubin, LDH, alk phosphatase, Coombs' test monthly if patient is on long-term therapy

• Electrolytes: potassium, sodium, chloride monthly if patient is on long-term therapy

• Bowel pattern qd; if severe diarrhea occurs, drug should be discontinued; may indicate pseudomembranous colitis

• IV site for extravasation, phlebitis; change site q72h

Administer:

• For 10-14 days to ensure organism death, prevent superimpo..d infection

• With food if needed for GI symptoms

• After C&S

Evaluate:

- Therapeutic response: decreased fever, malaise, chills
- Urine output: if decreasing, notify physician; may indicate nephrotoxicity
- Allergic reactions: rash, urticaria, pruritus, chills, fever, joint pain, angioedema; may occur a few days after therapy begins
- Bleeding: ecchymosis, bleeding gums, hematuria, stool guaiac daily
- Overgrowth of infection: perineal itching, fever, malaise, redness, pain, swelling, drainage, rash, diarrhea, change in cough, sputum

Teach patient/family:
- To use yogurt or buttermilk to maintain intestinal flora, decrease diarrhea
- To take all medication prescribed for length of time ordered
- To report sore throat, bruising, bleeding, joint pain; may indicate blood dyscrasias (rare)
- If diabetic, to use Clinistix or Ketodiastix
- Not to use alcohol or meds with alcohol or reaction may occur

Lab test interferences:
Increase (false): Creatinine (serum urine), urinary 17-KS
False positive: Urinary protein, direct Coombs', urine glucose
Interferences: Cross-matching

Treatment of overdose: Epinephrine, antihistamine, resuscitate if needed (anaphylaxis)

---

cefuroxime sodium
(se-fyoor-ox'eem)
Zinacef, Kefurox

Func. class.: Antibiotic, broad-spectrum
Chem. class.: Cephalosporin (2nd generation)

Action: Inhibits bacterial cell wall synthesis, rendering cell wall osmotically unstable

Uses: Gram-negative organisms: *H. influenzae, E. coli, Neisseria, P. mirabilis, Klebsiella;* gram-positive organisms: *S. pneumoniae, S. pyogenes, S. aureus;* serious lower respiratory tract, urinary tract, skin, gonococcal infections, septicemia, meningitis

Dosage and routes:
- *Adult:* IM/IV 750 mg-1.5 g q8h for 5-10 days
Surgical prophylaxis
- *Adult:* IV 1.5 g ½-1 hr preop
Severe infections
- *Adult:* IM/IV 1.5 g q6h; may give up to 3 g q8h for bacterial meningitis
- *Child >3 mo:* IM/IV 50-100 mg/kg/day; may give up to 200-240 mg/kg/day IV in divided doses for bacterial meningitis
- Dosage reduction indicated in severe renal impairment (CrCl < 20 ml/min)
- *Uncomplicated gonorrhea:* 1.5 g IM as single dose with oral probenecid

Available forms include: Inj IM, IV 750 mg, 1.5 g, powder

Side effects/adverse reactions:
CNS: Headache, dizziness, weakness, paresthesia, fever, chills
GI: Nausea, vomiting, diarrhea, anorexia, pain, glossitis, bleeding, increased AST, ALT, bilirubin, LDH, alk phosphatase, abdominal pain, *pseudomembranous colitis*
GU: Proteinuria, vaginitis, pruritus, candidiasis, increased BUN, *nephrotoxicity, renal failure*
HEMA: Leukopenia, thrombocytopenia, agranulocytosis, anemia, *neutropenia, lymphocytosis, eosinophilia, pancytopenia, hemolytic anemia*
INTEG: Rash, urticaria, dermatitis

italics = common side effects   **bold italic** = life threatening reactions

RESP: Dyspnea, ***anaphylaxis***
Contraindications: Hypersensitivity to cephalosporins, infants <1 mo
Precautions: Hypersensitivity to penicillins, pregnancy (B), lactation, renal disease
Pharmacokinetics:
IV: Peak 3 min
IM: Peak 15-60 min
Half-life 1-2 hr, 33%-50% bound by plasma proteins, 70%-100% eliminated unchanged in urine, crosses placenta, blood-brain barrier, excreted in breast milk, not metabolized
Interactions/incompatibilities:
• Do not mix with aminoglycosides in the same parenteral fluid
• Decreased effects: tetracyclines, erythromycins
• Increased toxicity: aminoglycosides, furosemide, probenecid, sulfinpyrazone, colistin, ethacrynic acid, vancomycin

NURSING CONSIDERATIONS
Assess:
• Sensitivity to penicillin or other cephalosporins
• Nephrotoxicity: increased BUN, creatinine
• I&O daily
• Blood studies: AST, ALT, CBC, Hct, bilirubin, LDH, alk phosphatase, Coombs' test monthly if patient is on long-term therapy
• Electrolytes: potassium, sodium, chloride monthly if patient is on long-term therapy
• Bowel pattern qd; if severe diarrhea occurs, drug should be discontinued; may indicate pseudomembranous colitis
• IV site for extravasation, phlebitis; change site q72h
Administer:
• IV after diluting 8 ml/750 mg of sterile H$_2$O for inj and give over 3-

5 min; may be further diluted with 100 ml of compatible sol; run over ½ hr; may also be given by continuous infusion
• For 10-14 days to ensure organism death, prevent superimposed infection
• After C&S
Evaluate:
• Therapeutic response: decreased fever, malaise, chills
• Urine output: if decreasing, notify physician; may indicate nephrotoxicity
• Allergic reactions: rash, urticaria, pruritus, chills, fever, joint pain, angioedema; may occur few days after therapy begins
• Bleeding: ecchymosis, bleeding gums, hematuria, stool guaiac daily
• Overgrowth of infection: perineal itching, fever, malaise, redness, pain, swelling, drainage, rash, diarrhea, change in cough, sputum
Teach patient/family:
• To report severe diarrhea; may indicate pseudomembranous colitis
• If diabetic, to use Clinistix or Ketodiastix
• Not to use alcohol or meds with alcohol or reaction can occur
• To report sore throat, bruising, bleeding, joint pain; may indicate blood dyscrasias (rare)
Lab test interferences:
Increase (false): Urinary 17-KS
False positive: Urinary protein, direct Coombs', urine glucose
Interference: Cross-matching
Treatment of overdose: Epinephrine, antihistamines, resuscitate if needed (anaphylaxis)

---

cellulose sodium phosphate

Calcibind, Calcisorb*

Func. class.: Antihypercalcemia
Chem. class.: Phosphorylated cellulose

Action: Decreases hypercalcium by binding with calcium in bowel, facilitates excretion

Uses: Calcium oxalate or phosphate renal stones associated with absorptive hypercalciuria type I

Dosage and routes:
• *Adult:* PO 15 g/day divided between each meal, then 10 g/day when urine Ca <150 mg/day

Available forms include: Powder 2.5 g packets

Side effects/adverse reactions:
GU: Hypomagnesuria, hyperoxaluria
GI: Nausea, anorexia, diarrhea, dyspepsia
MS: Arthralgia

Contraindications: Hypersensitivity, hyperthyroidism, enteric hyperoxaluria, bone disease, hypocalcemia

Precautions: CHF, ascites, liver disease, pregnancy (C)

Pharmacokinetics:
Not known

Interactions/incompatibilities:
• Decreased action of cellulose: magnesium preparations

NURSING CONSIDERATIONS
Assess:
• Calcium levels (serum, urinary) throughout treatment (therapeutic values: 2.3-2.8 mmol/L, serum; <3.75 mmol/24 hr, urine)

Administer:
• Powder with water, juice; take with meals
• Increase fluids to 3 L/day; urinary output should be >2 L/day

Evaluate:
• Therapeutic response: absence of renal stone formation

Teach patient/family:
• To decrease calcium in diet: dairy products; decrease sodium, citrus fruits in diet; increased excretion of drug will occur; decrease oxalate (chocolate, tea, spinach)
• To increase fluid intake to 3-4 L/day

cephalexin

(sef-a-lex'in)
Ceporex,* Keftab, Keflex, Keflet, Novolexin*

Func. class.: Antibiotic
Chem. class.: Cephalosporin (1st generation)

Action: Inhibits bacterial cell wall synthesis, rendering cell wall osmotically unstable

Uses: Gram-negative bacilli: *H. influenzae, E. coli, P. mirabilis, Klebsiella;* gram-positive organisms: *S. pneumoniae, S. pyogenes, S. aureus;* upper, lower respiratory tract, urinary tract, skin, bone infections, otitis media

Dosage and routes:
• *Adult:* PO 250-500 mg q6h
• *Child:* PO 25-50 mg/kg/day in 4 equal doses

Moderate skin infections
500 mg q12h

Severe infections
• *Adult:* PO 500 mg-1 g q6h
• *Child:* PO 50-100 mg/kg/day in 4 equal doses
• Dosage reduction indicated in renal impairment (CrCl < 50 ml/min)

Available forms include: Caps 250, 500 mg; tabs 250, 500, 1000 mg; pulvules 250 mg; oral susp

---

italics = common side effects   ***bold italic*** = life threatening reactions

125, 250 mg/5ml; pediatric susp 100 mg/5ml

Side effects/adverse reactions:

CNS: Headache, dizziness, weakness, paresthesia, fever, chills

GI: Nausea, vomiting, diarrhea, anorexia, pain, glossitis, bleeding, increased AST, ALT, bilirubin, LDH, alk phosphatase, abdominal pain, *pseudomembranous colitis*

GU: Proteinuria, vaginitis, pruritus, candidiasis, increased BUN, *nephrotoxicity, renal failure*

HEMA: Leukopenia, thrombocytopenia, agranulocytosis, anemia, *neutropenia, lymphocytosis, eosinophilia, pancytopenia, hemolytic anemia*

INTEG: Rash, urticaria, dermatitis

RESP: Dyspnea, *anaphylaxis*

Contraindications: Hypersensitivity to cephalosporins, infants <1 mo.

Precautions: Hypersensitivity to penicillins, pregnancy (B), lactation, renal disease

Pharmacokinetics:

PO: Peak 1 hr, duration 6-8 hr, half-life 30-72 min, 5%-15% bound by plasma proteins, 90%-100% eliminated unchanged in urine, crosses placenta, excreted in breast milk

Interactions/incompatibilities:

• Decreased effects: tetracyclines, erythromycins

• Increased toxicity: aminoglycosides, furosemide, probenecid, sulfinpyrazone, colistin, ethacrynic acid, vancomycin

NURSING CONSIDERATIONS

Assess:

• Sensitivity to penicillin or other cephalosporins

• Nephrotoxicity: increased BUN, creatinine

• I&O daily

• Blood studies: AST, ALT, CBC, Hct, bilirubin, LDH, alk phosphatase, Coombs' test monthly if patient is on long-term therapy

• Electrolytes: potassium, sodium, chloride monthly if patient is on long-term therapy

• Bowel pattern qd; if severe diarrhea occurs, drug should be discontinued; may indicate pseudomembranous colitis

Administer:

• For 10-14 days to ensure organism death, prevent superimposed infection

• With food if needed for GI symptoms

• After C&S

Evaluate:

• Therapeutic response: decreased fever, malaise, chills

• Urine output: if decreasing, notify physician; may indicate nephrotoxicity

• Allergic reactions: rash, urticaria, pruritus, chills, fever, joint pain, angioedema; may occur few days after therapy begins

• Bleeding: ecchymosis, bleeding gums, hematuria, stool guaiac daily

• Overgrowth of infection: perineal itching, fever, malaise, redness, pain, swelling, drainage, rash, diarrhea, change in cough, sputum

Teach patient/family:

• If diabetic, to use Clinistix or Ketodiastix

• Not to use alcohol or meds with alcohol or reaction may occur

• To use yogurt or buttermilk to maintain intestinal flora, decrease diarrhea

• To take all medication prescribed for length of time ordered

• To report sore throat, bruising, bleeding, joint pain; may indicate blood dyscrasias (rare)

• To report severe diarrhea; may indicate pseudomembranous colitis

---

Lab test interferences:
Increase (false): Creatinine (serum urine), urinary 17-KS
False positive: Urinary protein, direct Coombs', urine glucose
Interference: Cross-matching
Treatment of overdose: Epinephrine, antihistamines, resuscitate if needed (anaphylaxis)

---

cephalothin sodium
(sef-a'loe-thin)
Ceporacin,* Keflin, Seffin
Func. class.: Antibiotic, broad-spectrum
Chem. class.: Cephalosporin (1st generation)

Action: Inhibits bacterial cell wall synthesis, rendering cell wall osmotically unstable

Uses: Gram-negative bacilli: *H. influenzae, E. coli, P. mirabilis, Klebsiella, Salmonella, Shigella;* gram-positive organisms: *S. pneumoniae, S. pyogenes, S. aureus;* lower respiratory tract, urinary tract, skin, bone infections, septicemia, endocarditis, bacterial peritonitis

Dosage and routes:
• *Adult:* IM/IV 500 mg-1 g q4-6h
• *Child:* IM/IV 14-27 mg/kg q4h or 20-40 mg/kg, q6h
• Dosage reduction indicated in renal impairment (CrCl < 50 ml/min)
• Uncomplicated gonorrhea 2 g IM as single dose
Severe infections
• *Adult:* IM/IV 1-2 g q4h
Available forms include: Powder for inj IM, IV 1, 2, 4, 10, 20 g; frozen IV 20, 30, 40 mg/ml

Side effects/adverse reactions:
CNS: Headache, dizziness, weakness, paresthesia, fever, chills

GI: Nausea, vomiting, diarrhea, anorexia, pain, glossitis, bleeding, increased AST, ALT, bilirubin, LDH, alk phosphatase, abdominal pain, **pseudomembranous colitis**
GU: Proteinuria, vaginitis, pruritus, candidiasis, increased BUN, **nephrotoxicity, renal failure**
HEMA: **Leukopenia, thrombocytopenia, agranulocytosis,** anemia, **neutropenia, lymphocytosis, eosinophilia, pancytopenia, hemolytic anemia**
INTEG: Rash, urticaria, dermatitis
RESP: Dyspnea, **anaphylaxis**
Contraindications: Hypersensitivity to cephalosporins
Precautions: Hypersensitivity to penicillins, pregnancy (B), lactation, renal disease
Pharmacokinetics:
IV: Peak 15 min
IM: Peak 30 min
Half-life ½-1 hr, 65%-80% bound by plasma proteins, 50%-75% eliminated unchanged in urine in 8 hr, crosses placenta, excreted in breast milk, deacetylated in kidneys, liver
Interactions/incompatibilities:
• Do not mix with tetracyclines, erythromycins, calcium chloride, magnesium salts, aminoglycosides, barbiturates, aminophylline in same parenteral fluid
• Decreased effects: tetracyclines, erythromycins
• Increased toxicity: aminoglycosides, furosemide, probenecid, sulfinpyrazone, colistin, ethacrynic acid, vancomycin
NURSING CONSIDERATIONS
Assess:
• Nephrotoxicity: increased BUN, creatinine
• Sensitivity to penicillin or other cephalosporins
• I&O daily

• Blood studies: AST, ALT, CBC, Hct, bilirubin, LDH, alk phosphatase, Coombs' test monthly if patient is on long-term therapy
• Electrolytes: potassium, sodium, chloride monthly if patient is on long-term therapy
• Bowel pattern qd; if severe diarrhea occurs, drug should be discontinued; may indicate pseudomembranous colitis
• IV site for extravasation, phlebitis; change site q72h

Administer:
• IV after diluting 1 g/10 ml of D_5W normal saline, sterile H_2O for inj; give over 3-5 min; may be further diluted with 50 ml of compatible sol, run over 15-30 min; may also be given by continuous infusion
• For 10-14 days to ensure organism death, prevent superimposed infection
• After C&S

Evaluate:
• Therapeutic response: decreased fever, malaise, chills
• Urine output: if decreasing, notify physician; may indicate nephrotoxicity
• Allergic reactions: rash, urticaria, pruritus, chills, fever, joint pain, angioedema; may occur few days after therapy begins
• Bleeding: ecchymosis, bleeding gums, hematuria, stool guaiac daily
• Overgrowth of infection: perineal itching, fever, malaise, redness, pain, swelling, drainage, rash, diarrhea, change in cough, sputum

Teach patient/family:
• If diabetic, to use Clinistix or Ketodiastix
• Not to use alcohol or meds with alcohol or reaction can occur
• To report sore throat, bruising,

bleeding, joint pain; may indicate blood dyscrasias (rare)
• To report severe diarrhea; may indicate pseudomembranous colitis

Lab test interferences:
Increase (false): Creatinine (serum urine), urinary 17-KS
False positive: Urinary protein, direct Coombs', urine glucose
Interference: Cross-matching

Treatment of overdose: Epinephrine, antihistamines, resuscitate if needed (anaphylaxis)

---

cephapirin sodium
(sef-a-pye′rin)
Cefadyl

Func. class.: Antibiotic, broad-spectrum
Chem. class.: Cephalosporin (1st generation)

Action: Inhibits bacterial cell wall synthesis, rendering cell wall osmotically unstable

Uses: Gram-negative bacilli: *H. influenzae, E. coli, P. mirabilis, Klebsiella;* gram-positive organisms: *S. pneumoniae, S. viridans, S. aureus;* lower respiratory tract, urinary tract, skin infections, septicemia, endocarditis, bacterial peritonitis

Dosage and routes:
• *Adult:* IM/IV 500 mg-1 g q4-6h
• *Child:* IM/IV 20-30 mg/kg, q6h
• Dosage reduction indicated in renal impairment (CrCl < 50 ml/min)

Available forms include: Powder for inj IM, IV 500 mg, 1, 2, 20 g; IV only 1, 2, 4 g

Side effects/adverse reactions:
CNS: Headache, dizziness, weakness, paresthesia, fever, chills
GI: Nausea, vomiting, diarrhea, anorexia, pain, glossitis, bleeding,

increased AST, ALT, bilirubin, LDH, alk phosphatase, abdominal pain, *pseudomembranous colitis*
GU: Proteinuria, vaginitis, pruritus, candidiasis, increased BUN, *nephrotoxicity, renal failure*
HEMA: Leukopenia, thrombocytopenia, agranulocytosis, anemia, *neutropenia, lymphocytosis, eosinophilia, pancytopenia, hemolytic anemia*
INTEG: Rash, urticaria, dermatitis
RESP: Dyspnea, **anaphylaxis**
Contraindications: Hypersensitivity to cephalosporins, infants <1 mo
Precautions: Hypersensitivity to penicillins, pregnancy (B), lactation, renal disease
Pharmacokinetics:
IV: Peak 5 min
IM: Peak 30 min
Half-life 21-47 min, 44%-50% bound by plasma proteins, 40%-70% eliminated unchanged in urine, crosses placenta, excreted in breast milk, metabolized in liver
Interactions/incompatibilities:
• Do not mix with tetracyclines, aminoglycosides in same parenteral fluid
• Decreased effects: tetracyclines, erythromycins
• Increased toxicity: aminoglycosides, furosemide, probenecid, sulfinpyrazone, colistin, ethacrynic acid
NURSING CONSIDERATIONS
Assess:
• Sensitivity to penicillin or other cephalosporins
• Nephrotoxicity: increased BUN, creatinine
• I&O daily
• Blood studies: AST, ALT, CBC, Hct, bilirubin, LDH, alk phosphatase, Coombs' test monthly if patient is on long-term therapy

• Electrolytes: potassium, sodium, chloride monthly if patient is on long-term therapy
• Bowel pattern qd; if severe diarrhea occurs drug should be discontinued; may indicate pseudomembranous colitis
• IV site for extravasation, phlebitis; change site q72h
Administer:
• IV after diluting 1 g/10 ml or more normal saline, D_5W or bacteriostatic H_2O for inj; may be further diluted in 50-100 ml of compatible sol; run over 15 min; may also be given by continous infusion
• For 10-14 days to ensure organism death, prevent superimposed infection
• After C&S
Evaluate:
• Therapeutic response: decreased fever, malaise, chills
• Urine output: if decreasing, notify physician; may indicate nephrotoxicity
• Allergic reactions: rash, urticaria, pruritus, chills, fever, joint pain, angioedema; may occur few days after therapy begins
• Bleeding: ecchymosis, bleeding gums, hematuria, stool guaiac daily
• Overgrowth of infection: perineal itching, fever, malaise, redness, pain, swelling, drainage, rash, diarrhea, change in cough, sputum
Teach patient/family:
• If diabetic, to use Clinistix or Ketodiastix
• Not to use alcohol or meds with alcohol or reaction may occur
• To report severe diarrhea; may indicate pseudomembranous colitis
• To report sore throat, bruising, bleeding, joint pain; may indicate blood dyscrasias (rare)
Lab test interferences:
Increase (false:) Creatinine (serum urine), urinary 17-KS

False positive: Urinary protein, direct Coombs', urine glucose
Interference: Cross-matching
Treatment of overdose: Epinephrine, antihistamines, resuscitate if needed (anaphylaxis)

---

cephradine
(sef'ra-deen)
Anspor, Velosef
Func. class.: Antibiotic
Chem. class.: Cephalosporin (1st generation)

Action: Inhibits bacterial cell wall synthesis, rendering cell wall osmotically unstable
Uses: Gram-negative bacilli: *H. influenzae, E. coli, P. mirabilis, Klebsiella;* gram-positive organisms: *S. pneumoniae, S. pyogenes, S. aureus;* serious respiratory tract, urinary tract, skin infections, otitis media
Dosage and routes:
• *Adult:* IM/IV 500 mg-1 g q4-6h not to exceed 8 g/day; PO 250 mg-1 g q6-12h
• *Child >1 yr.:* IM/IV 12-25 mg/kg q6h; PO 6-12 mg/kg q6h
Available forms include: Powder for inj IM, IV 250, 500 mg, 1 g; caps 250, 500 mg; oral susp 125, 250 mg/5 ml
Side effects/adverse reactions:
CNS: Headache, dizziness, weakness, paresthesia, fever, chills
GI: Nausea, vomiting, diarrhea, anorexia, pain, glossitis, bleeding, increased AST, ALT, bilirubin, LDH, alk phosphatase, abdominal pain, *pseudomembranous colitis*
GU: Proteinuria, vaginitis, pruritus, candidasis, increased BUN, *nephrotoxicity, renal failure*
HEMA: Leukopenia, thrombocytopenia, agranulocytosis, anemia, *neutropenia, lymphocytosis, eosinophilia, pancytopenia, hemolytic anemia*
INTEG: Rash, urticaria, dermatitis
RESP: Dyspnea, *anaphylaxis*
Contraindications: Hypersensitivity to cephalosporins, infants <1 mo
Precautions: Hypersensitivity to penicillins, pregnancy (B), lactation, renal disease
Pharmacokinetics:
PO: Peak 1 hr
IV: Peak 5 min
IM: Peak 1 hr
Half-life 0.75-1.5 h, 20% bound by plasma proteins, 80%-90% eliminated unchanged in urine, crosses placenta, excreted in breast milk
Interactions/incompatibilities:
• Do not mix with tetracyclines, erythromycins, calcium chloride, magnesium salts, aminoglycosides in same parenteral fluid
• Decreased effects: tetracyclines, erythromycins
• Increased toxicity: aminoglycosides, furosemide, probenecid, sulfinpyrazone, colistin, ethacrynic acid, vancomycin

NURSING CONSIDERATIONS
Assess:
• Sensitivity to penicillin or other cephalosporins
• Nephrotoxicity: increased BUN, creatinine
• I&O daily
• Blood studies: AST, ALT, CBC, Hct, bilirubin, LDH, alk phosphatase, Coombs' test monthly if patient is on long-term therapy
• Electrolytes: potassium, sodium, chloride monthly if patient is on long-term therapy
• Bowel pattern qd; if severe diarrhea occurs, drug should be discontinued; may indicate pseudomembranous colitis

---

• IV site for extravasation, phlebitis; change site q72h

Administer:

• IV after diluting 1 g/10 ml of D$_5$W or normal saline; give over 3-5 min; may be further diluted 1 g/10 ml of compatible sol, run over ½-1 hr

• For 10-14 days to ensure organism death, prevent superimposed infection

• With food if needed for GI symptoms

• After C&S

Evaluate:

• Therapeutic response: decreased fever, malaise, chills

• Urine output: if decreasing, notify physician; may indicate nephrotoxicity

• Allergic reactions: rash, urticaria, pruritus, chills, fever, joint pain, angioedema; may occur few days after therapy begins

• Bleeding: ecchymosis, bleeding gums, hematuria, stool guaiac daily

• Overgrowth of infection: perineal itching, fever, malaise, redness, pain, swelling, drainage, rash, diarrhea, change in cough, sputum

Teach patient/family:

• If diabetic, to use Clinistix or Ketodiastix

• Not to use alcohol or meds with alcohol or reaction can occur

• To use yogurt or buttermilk to maintain intestinal flora, decrease diarrhea

• To take all medication prescribed for length of time ordered

• To report sore throat, bruising, bleeding, joint pain; may indicate blood dyscrasias (rare)

Lab test interferences:

Increase (false): Creatinine (serum urine), urinary 17-KS

False positive: Urinary protein, direct Coombs', urine glucose

Interference: Cross-matching

Treatment of overdose: Epinephrine, antihistamines, resuscitate if needed (anaphylaxis)

---

chenodiol

(kee-noe-dye′ole)

Chenix

Func. class.: Antilithic

Chem. class.: Chenodeoxycholic acid

Action: Suppresses synthesis of cholesterol, cholic acid, replacing cholic acid with drug metabolite, which leads to the degradation of gallstones

Uses: Dissolving gallstones instead of surgery

Dosage and routes:

• *Adult:* PO 250 mg bid × 2 wk, then increased by 250 mg/day, not to exceed 16 mg/kg/day × 24 mo

Available forms include: Tabs 250 mg

Side effects/adverse reactions:

*HEMA: **Leukopenia***

GI: Diarrhea, fecal urgency, heartburn, nausea, cramps, increased ALT, AST, LDH, vomiting, dysphagia, absence of taste, ***hepatotoxicity,*** flatulence, dyspepsia

Contraindications: Hypersensitivity, hepatic disease, bile duct obstruction, biliary GI fistula, pregnancy (X)

Precautions: Lactation, children, atherosclerosis

Pharmacokinetics:

Metabolized by liver, excreted in feces (metabolite/unchanged drug), crosses placenta

Interactions/incompatibilities:

• Decreased action of chenodiol. cholestyramine, colestipol, aluminum antacids, estrogens, clofibrate

---

italics = common side effects   ***bold italic*** = life threatening reactions

NURSING CONSIDERATIONS
Assess:
• Vital signs, cardiac status: checking for dysrhythmias increased rate, palpitations
• I&O ratio; check for urinary retention or hesitancy
• Oral cholecystogram or ultrasonogram q6-9 mo
Administer:
• With meals for better absorption
• Antidiarrheals if diarrhea occurs
Perform/provide:
• Storage at room temperature
• Increased fluids, bulk, exercise to patient's lifestyle to decrease constipation
Evaluate:
• Therapeutic response: absence of pain (epigastric), gallstones on diagnostic testing
• GI complaints: nausea, vomiting, anorexia, diarrhea; if diarrhea is severe dosage may need to be decreased
Teach patient/family:
• That stone dissolution may take 6-24 mo, therapy is discontinued in 18 mo if gallstones are still intact
• To notify physician if pregnancy is suspected, birth defects may occur

---

chloral hydrate
(klor-al hye′drate)
Aquachloral Supprettes, Cohidrate, Noctec, Novochlorhydrate*
Func. class.: Sedative-hypnotic
Chem. class.: Chloral derivative

Controlled Substance Schedule IV (USA), Schedule F (Canada)
Action: Reduction product trichloroethanol produces mild cerebral depression, which causes sleep
Uses: Sedation, insomnia

Dosage and routes:
Sedation
• *Adult:* PO/REC 250 mg tid pc
• *Child:* PO 8 mg/kg tid, not to exceed 500 mg tid
Insomnia
• *Adult:* PO/REC 500 mg-1g ½ hr before hs
• *Child:* PO/REC 50 mg/kg in one dose, up to 1 gm
Available forms include: Caps 250, 500 mg; syr 250, 500 mg/5 ml; supp 325, 500, 650 mg
Side effects/adverse reactions:
*HEMA: **Eosinophilia, leukopenia***
CNS: Drowsiness, dizziness, stimulation, nightmares, ataxia, hangover (rare), lightheadedness, headache, paranoia
GI: Nausea, vomiting, flatulence, diarrhea, unpleasant taste, ***gastric necrosis***
INTEG: Rash, urticaria, angioedema, fever, purpura, eczema
CV: Hypotension, dysrhythmias
*RESP: **Depression***
Contraindications: Hypersensitivity to this drug or triclofos, severe renal disease, severe hepatic disease, GI disorders (oral forms), gastritis
Precautions: Severe cardiac disease, depression, suicidal individuals, asthma, intermittent porphyria, pregnancy (C), lactation
Pharmacokinetics:
PO: Onset 30 min-1 hr, duration 4-8 hr
REC: Onset slow, duration 4-6 hr
Metabolized by liver, excreted by kidneys (inactive metabolite) and feces, crosses placenta, excreted in breast milk; metabolite is highly protein bound
Interactions/incompatibilities:
• Increased action of: oral anticoagulants, furosemide

---

*Available in Canada only

• Increased action of both drugs: alcohol, CNS depressants

NURSING CONSIDERATIONS
Assess:
• Blood studies: Hct, Hgb, RBCs serum folate (if on long-term therapy), pro-time in patients receiving anticoagulants
Administer:
• After removal of cigarettes, to prevent fires
• After trying conservative measures for insomnia
• ½-1 hr before hs for sleeplessness
• On empty stomach with full glass of water or juice for best absorption and decrease corrosion (do not chew); after meals to decrease GI symptoms if using for sedation
Perform/provide:
• Assistance with ambulation after receiving dose
• Safety measure: siderails, nightlight, callbell within easy reach
• Checking to see PO medication swallowed
• Storage in dark container, suppositories in refrigerator
Evaluate:
• Therapeutic response: ability to sleep at night, decreased amount of early morning awakening if taking drug for insomnia
• Mental status: mood, sensorium, affect, memory (long, short)
• Physical dependency: more frequent requests for medication, shakes, anxiety
• Respiratory dysfunction: respiratory depression, character, rate, rhythm; hold drug if respirations are <10/min or if pupils are dilated (rare)
• Blood dyscrasias: fever, sore throat, bruising, rash, jaundice, epistaxis (rare)
• Previous history of substance abuse, cardiac disease, or gastritis

Teach patient/family:
• To avoid driving or other activities requiring alertness
• To avoid alcohol ingestion or CNS depressants; serious CNS depression may result
• Not to discontinue medication quickly after long-term use; drug should be tapered over 1-2 wk
• That effects may take 2 nights for benefits to be noticed
• Alternate measures to improve sleep (reading, exercise several hours before hs, warm bath, warm milk, TV, self-hypnosis, deep breathing)

Lab test interferences:
Interferences: Urine catecholamines, urinary 17-OHCS
False Positive: Urine glucose (copper sulfate test)

Treatment of overdose: Lavage, activated charcoal, monitor electrolytes, vital signs

---

chlorambucil

(klor-am′byoo-sil)
Leukeran

Func. class.: Antineoplastic alkylating agent
Chem. class.: Nitrogen mustard

Action: Alkylates DNA, RNA; inhibits enzymes that allow synthesis of amino acids in proteins
Uses: Chronic lymphocytic leukemia, Hodgkin's disease, other lymphomas, macroglobulinemia, nephrotic syndrome, breast carcinoma, choreocarcinoma, ovarian carcinoma
Dosage and routes:
• *Adult:* PO 0.1-0.2 mg/kg/day for 3-6 wk initially, then 2-6 mg/day; maintenance 0.2 mg/kg for 2-4 wk, course may be repeated at 2-4 wk intervals

---

italics = common side effects　　　***bold italic*** = life threatening reactions

• *Child:* PO 0.1-0.2 mg/kg/day in divided doses or 4.5 mg/m²/day as 1 dose or in divided doses

Available forms include: Tabs 2 mg

Side effects/adverse reactions:

*CNS: **Convulsions in children***

*HEMA: **Thrombocytopenia, leukopenia, pancytopenia*** (prolonged use), ***permanent bone marrow depression***

GI: Nausea, vomiting, diarrhea, weight loss

GU: Hyperuremia

INTEG: Alopecia (rare), dermatitis, rash

*RESP: **Fibrosis, pneumonitis***

Contraindications: Radiation therapy within 1 mo, chemotherapy within 1 mo, thrombocytopenia, smallpox vaccination, pregnancy (1st trimester) (D)

Precautions: Pneumococcus vaccination

Pharmacokinetics:

Well absorbed orally, metabolized in liver, excreted in urine; half-life 2 hr

Interactions/incompatibilities:

• Increased toxicity: other antineoplastics, or radiation

NURSING CONSIDERATIONS

Assess:

• CBC, differential, platelet count weekly; withhold drug if WBC is <4000 or platelet count is <75,000; notify physician of results

• Pulmonary functions test, chest x-ray films before, during therapy; chest film should be obtained q2wk during treatment

• Renal function studies: BUN, serum uric acid, urine CrCl before, during therapy

• I&O ratio; report fall in urine output of 30 ml/hr

• Monitor temperature q4h (may indicate beginning infection)

• Liver function tests before, during therapy (bilirubin, AST, ALT, LDH) as needed or monthly

Administer:

• Antacid before oral agent, give drug after evening meal, before bedtime

• Antiemetic 30-60 min before giving drug to prevent vomiting

• Allopurinol or sodium bicarbonate to maintain uric acid levels, alkalinization of urine

• Antibiotics for prophylaxis of infection

Perform/provide:

• Storage in tight container

• Strict medical asepsis, protective isolation if WBC levels are low

• Increase fluid intake to 2-3 L/day to prevent urate deposits, calculi formation

• Diet low in purines: organ meats (kidney, liver), dried beans, peas to maintain alkaline urine

Evaluate:

• Bleeding: hematuria, guaiac, bruising or petechiae, mucosa or orifices q8h

• Food preferences; list likes, dislikes

• Yellowing of skin, sclera, dark urine, clay-colored stools, itchy skin, abdominal pain, fever, diarrhea

• Dyspnea, rales, unproductive cough, chest pain, tachypnea

• Effects of alopecia on body image; discuss feelings about body changes (rare)

Teach patient/family:

• To report signs of infection: increased temperature, sore throat, flu symptoms

• To report signs of anemia: fatigue, headache, faintness, shortness of breath, irritability

• To report bleeding; avoid use of razors or commercial mouthwash

---

*Available in Canada only

- To avoid use of aspirin products or ibuprofen
- Of protective isolation precautions
- To report any changes in breathing or coughing
- That hair may be lost during treatment; a wig or hairpiece may make patient feel better; new hair may be different in color, texture (rare)

---

chloramphenicol/chloramphenicol palmitate/ chloramphenicol sodium succinate

Chloromycetin, Mychel, Novo-chlorocap*

Func. class.: Antibacterial/anti-rickettsial
Chem. class.: Dichoroacetic acid derivative

Action: Binds to 50S ribosomal subunit which interferes with or inhibits protein synthesis
Uses: Infections caused by *H. influenzae, S. typhi, Rickettsia, Neisseria,* mycoplasma
Dosage and routes:
- *Adult and child:* PO/IV 50-100 mg/kg/day in divided doses q6h, not to exceed 100 mg/kg/day
- *Premature infants and neonates:* IV/PO 25 mg/kg/day in divided doses q6h
Available forms include: Inj (IV) 1 g; caps 250, 500 mg; oral susp 150 mg/5 ml
Side effects/adverse reactions:
*HEMA: **Anemia, bone marrow depression, thrombocytopenia, aplastic anemia, granulocytopenia, leukopenia***
EENT: Optic neuritis, blindness
GI: Nausea, vomiting, diarrhea, abdominal pain, xerostomia, glossitis, colitis, pruritus ani

INTEG: Itching, urticaria, contact dermatitis, rash
*CV: **Gray syndrome in newborns: failure to feed, pallid, cyanosis, abdominal distention, irregular respiration, vasomotor collapse***
CNS: Headache, *depression,* confusion
Contraindications: Hypersensitivity, severe renal disease, severe hepatic disease, minor infections
Precautions: Hepatic disease, renal disease, infants, children, bone marrow depression (drug-induced), pregnancy (C), lactation
Pharmacokinetics:
PO/IV: Peak 1-2 hr, duration 8 hr, half-life 1½-4 hr, conjugated in liver, excreted in urine (up to 15% as free drug), breast milk, feces, crosses placenta
Interactions/incompatibilities:
- Increased action of: dicumarol, phenytoin, tolbutamide, chlorpropamide, phenobarbital
- Increased prothrombin time: anticoagulants
- Decreased action of: iron, vitamin B_{12}, folic acid, penicillins
- Do not mix with any drug before consulting package inserts; incompatible with many drugs
- Avoid use with myelosuppressive drugs

NURSING CONSIDERATIONS
Assess:
- Signs of infections, anemia
- Any patient with compromised renal system; drug is excreted slowly in poor renal system function; toxicity may occur rapidly
- Liver studies: AST, ALT
- Blood studies: WBC, RBC, Hct, Hgb, platelets, serum iron, reticulocytes; drug should be discontinued if bone marrow depression occurs

---

italics = common side effects   ***bold italic*** = life threatening reactions

• Renal studies: urinalysis, protein, blood, BUN, creatinine
• C&S before drug therapy; may be taken as soon as culture is taken
• Drug level in impaired hepatic, renal systems

Administer:
• IV after diluting 1 g/10 ml of sterile H_2O for inj or D_5W, give over 1 min; may be further diluted in 50-100 ml of compatible sol; run over ½-1 hr
• Oral form on empty stomach with full glass of water

Perform/provide:
• Storage of capsules in tight container at room temperature, reconstituted solution at room temperature for up to 30 days
• Adrenalin, suction, tracheostomy set, endotracheal intubation equipment on unit
• Adequate intake of fluids (2000 ml) during diarrhea episodes

Evaluate:
• Therapeutic response: decreased temperature, negative C&S
• Bowel pattern before, during treatment
• Skin eruptions, itching, dermatitis after administration
• Respiratory status: rate, character, wheezing, tightness in chest
• Allergies before treatment, reaction of each medication; place allergies on chart, Kardex in bright red letters; notify all people giving drugs
• Neonates for beginning gray syndrome: cyanosis, abdominal distention, irregular respiration, failure to feed; drug should be discontinued immediately

Teach patient/family:
• Aspects of drug therapy: need to complete entire course of medication to ensure organism death (10-14 days); culture may be taken

after complete course of medication
• To report sore throat, fever, fatigue, unusual bleeding, bruising; could indicate bone marrow depression (may occur weeks or months after termination of drug)
• That drug must be taken in equal intervals around clock to maintain blood levels

Treatment of overdose: Withdraw drug, maintain airway, administer epinephrine, aminophylline, O_2, IV corticosteroids

---

chloramphenicol (ophthalmic)

(klor-am-fen'i-kole)
Antibiopto, Chloromycetin Ophthalmic, Chloroptic, Chloroptic SOP, Econochlor Ophthalmic, Fenicol,* Isopto Fenical,* Ophthoclor Ophthalmic, Pentamycin*
Func. class.: Antiinfective

Action: Inhibits bacterial protein synthesis
Uses: Infection of eye
Dosage and routes:
• *Adult and child:* INSTILL 2 gtts in eye qd-qid until desired response; TOP apply oint to conjunctival sac q3-6h as needed or hs if using gtts also
Available forms include: Oint 1%; sol 0.25, 0.5%, 25 mg
Side effects/adverse reactions:
EENT: Poor corneal wound healing, temporary visual haze, overgrowth of nonsusceptible organisms
Contraindications: Hypersensitivity
Precautions: Antibiotic hypersensitivity, pregnancy (C)
NURSING CONSIDERATIONS
Administer:
• After washing hands, cleanse

crusts or discharge from eye before application
• Apply pressure to lacrimal sac for 1 min to prevent systemic absorption

Perform/provide:
• Storage at room temperature, protect from light

Evaluate:
• Therapeutic response: absence of redness, inflammation, tearing
• Allergy: itching, lacrimation, redness, swelling

Teach patient/family:
• To use drug exactly as prescribed
• Not to use eye makeup, towels, washcloths, eye medication of others; reinfection may occur
• That drug container tip should not be touched to eye
• To report itching, increased redness, burning, stinging, swelling; drug should be discontinued
• That drug may cause blurred vision when ointment is applied
• That prolonged or frequent use may lead to serious reactions: hypersensitivity, bone marrow depression

chloramphenicol (otic)
Chloromycetin Otic, Sopamycetin*

Func. class.: Otic, broad-spectrum antibiotic

Action: Inhibits protein synthesis in suspectible microorganisms
Uses: Ear infection (external)
Dosage and routes:
• *Adult and child:* INSTILL 2-3 gtts tid
Available forms include: Sol 0.5%
Side effects/adverse reactions:
EENT: Itching, irritation in ear
INTEG: Rash, urticaria, contact dermatitis, burning, ***angioedema***

*HEMA: **Bone marrow hypoplasia, aplastic anemia***
Contraindications: Hypersensitivity, perforated eardrum

NURSING CONSIDERATIONS
Administer:
• After removing impacted cerumen by irrigation
• After cleaning stopper with alcohol
• After restraining child if necessary
• Warming solution to body temperature; do not warm above body temp; loss of potency will occur

Perform/provide:
• Storage at room temperature, protection from light

Evaluate:
• Therapeutic response: decreased ear pain
• For redness, swelling, pain in ear, which indicates superimposed infection

Teach patient/family:
• Method of instillation, using aseptic technique, including not touching dropper to ear
• That dizziness may occur after instillation

chloramphenicol (topical)
(klor-am-fen'i-kole)
Chloromycetin

Func. class.: Local antiinfective
Chem. class.: Antibacterial

Action: Interferes with bacterial protein synthesis
Uses: Skin infections (bacterial)
Dosage and routes:
• *Adult and child:* TOP apply to affected area bid-qid
Available forms include: Cream 1%

---

italics = common side effects   ***bold italic*** = life threatening reactions

Side effects/adverse reactions:
HEMA: **Blood dyscrasias**
INTEG: Rash, urticaria, stinging, burning, vesicular, maculopapular dermatitis, *angioneurotic edema*
Contraindications: Hypersensitivity
Precautions: Pregnancy (C), lactation
NURSING CONSIDERATIONS
Administer:
• Enough medication to completely cover lesions
• After cleansing with soap, water before each application, dry well
Perform/provide:
• Storage at room temperature in dry place, protect from light
Evaluate:
• Allergic reaction: burning, stinging, swelling, redness
• Therapeutic response: decrease in size, number of lesions
• Signs and symptoms of blood dyscrasias
Teach patient/family:
• To apply with glove to prevent further infection
• To avoid use of OTC creams, ointments, lotions unless directed by physician
• To use medical asepsis (hand washing) before, after each application to prevent further infection
• To notify physician if conditions worsen or if rash or irritation develops
• To watch for superimposed infections

---

chlordiazepoxide HCl
(klor-dye-az-e-pox′ide)
A-poxide, Libritabs, Librium, Medilium,* Novopoxide,* Relaxil, Solium,* Lipoxide, SK-Lygen
Func. class.: Antianxiety
Chem. class.: Benzodiazepine

Controlled Substance Schedule IV

Action: Depresses subcortical levels of CNS, including limbic system, reticular formation
Uses: Short-term management of anxiety, acute alcohol withdrawal, preoperatively for relaxation
Dosage and routes:
Mild anxiety
• *Adult:* PO 5-10 mg tid-qid
• *Child >6 yr:* 5 mg bid-qid, not to exceed 10 mg bid-tid
Severe anxiety
• *Adult:* PO 20-25 mg tid-qid
Preoperatively
• *Adult:* PO 5-10 mg tid-qid on day before surgery; IM 50-100 mg 1 hr before surgery
Alcohol withdrawal
• *Adult:* PO/IM/IV 50-100 mg, not to exceed 300 mg/day
Available forms include: Caps 5, 10, 25 mg; tabs 5, 10, 25 mg; powder for IM inj 100 mg
Side effects/adverse reactions:
CNS: Dizziness, drowsiness, confusion, headache, anxiety, tremors, stimulation, fatigue, depression, insomnia, hallucinations
GI: Constipation, dry mouth, nausea, vomiting, anorexia, diarrhea
INTEG: Rash, dermatitis, itching
CV: Orthostatic hypotension, **ECG changes, tachycardia,** hypotension
EENT: Blurred vision, tinnitus, mydriasis
Contraindications: Hypersensitivity to benzodiazepines, narrow-angle glaucoma, psychosis, pregnancy (D), child <18 yr
Precautions: Elderly, debilitated, hepatic disease, renal disease
Pharmacokinetics:
PO: Onset 30 min, peak ½ hr, duration 4-6 hr, metabolized by liver, excreted by kidneys, crosses placenta, breast milk, half-life 5-30 hr
Interactions/incompatibilities:
• Decreased effects of chlordiaz-

epoxide: oral contraceptives, rifampin, valproic acid
• Increased effects of chlordiazepoxide: CNS depressants, alcohol, cimetidine, disulfiram, oral contraceptives

NURSING CONSIDERATIONS
Assess:
• B/P (lying, standing), pulse; if systolic B/P drops 20 mm Hg, hold drug, notify physician
• Blood studies: CBC during long-term therapy, blood dyscrasias have occurred rarely
• Hepatic studies: AST, ALT, bilirubin, creatinine, LDH, alk phosphatase
• I&O; may indicate renal dysfunction
• For ataxia, oversedation in elderly, debilitated patients

Administer:
• By IV 5 ml saline 100 mg/powder, agitate ampule gently; do not use IM diluent for IV use
• With food or milk for GI symptoms
• Crushed if patient is unable to swallow medication whole
• Sugarless gum, hard candy, frequent sips of water for dry mouth

Perform/provide:
• Assistance with ambulation during beginning therapy, since drowsiness/dizziness occurs
• Safety measure, including siderails
• Check to see PO medication has been swallowed

Evaluate:
• Therapeutic response: decreased anxiety, restlessness, sleeplessness
• Mental status: mood, sensorium, affect, sleeping pattern, drowsiness, dizziness
• Physical dependency, withdrawal symptoms: headache, nausea,

vomiting, muscle pain, weakness after long-term use
• Suicidal tendencies, paradoxical reactions such as excitement, stimulation, and acute rage

Teach patient/family:
• That drug may be taken with food
• Not to be used for everyday stress or used longer than 4 mo, unless directed by physician
• Not to take more than prescribed amount, may be habit-forming
• Avoid OTC preparations unless approved by physician
• To avoid driving, activities that require alertness; drowsiness may occur
• To avoid alcohol ingestion or other psychotropic medications, unless prescribed by physician
• Not to discontinue medication abruptly after long-term use, may precipitate convulsions
• To rise slowly or fainting may occur
• That drowsiness might worsen at beginning of treatment

Lab test interferences:
Increase: AST/ALT, serum bilirubin
False increase: 17-OHCS
Decrease: RAIU

Treatment of overdose: Lavage, VS, supportive care

---

chloroprocaine HCl
(klor'-oh-pro-kane)
Nesacaine, Nesacaine-CE
Func. class.: Local anesthetic
Chem. class.: Ester

Action: Competes with calcium for sites in nerve membrane that control sodium transport across cell membrane; decreases rise of depolarization phase of action potential
Uses: Epidural anesthesia, periph-

eral nerve block, caudal anesthesia, infiltration block

Dosage and routes:
Varies depending on route of anesthesia

Available forms include: Inj 1%, 2%, 3%

Side effects/adverse reactions:
CNS: Anxiety, restlessness, *convulsions, loss of consciousness,* drowsiness, disorientation, tremors, shivering

CV: Myocardial depression, cardiac arrest, dysrhythmias, bradycardia, hypotension, hypertension, fetal bradycardia

GI: Nausea, vomiting

EENT: Blurred vision, tinnitus, pupil constriction

INTEG: Rash, urticaria, allergic reactions, edema, burning, skin discoloration at injection site, tissue necrosis

RESP: Status asthmaticus, respiratory arrest, anaphylaxis

Contraindications: Hypersensitivity, child <12 yr, elderly, severe liver disease

Precautions: Elderly, severe drug allergies, pregnancy (C)

Pharmacokinetics:
Duration ½-1 hr, metabolized by liver, excreted in urine (metabolites)

Interactions/incompatibilities:
• Dysrhythmias: epinephrine, halothane, enflurane
• Hypertension: MAOIs, tricyclic antidepressants, phenothiazines

NURSING CONSIDERATIONS
Assess:
• B/P, pulse, respiration during treatment
• Fetal heart tones if drug is used during labor

Administer:
• Only with crash cart, resuscitative equipment nearby

• Only drugs without preservatives for epidural or caudal anesthesia

Perform/provide:
• Use of new solution, discard unused portions

Evaluate:
• Therapeutic response: anesthesia necessary for procedure
• Allergic reactions: rash, urticaria, itching
• Cardiac status: ECG for dysrhythmias, pulse, B/P during anesthesia

Treatment of overdose: Airway, O₂, vasopressor, IV fluids, anticonvulsants for seizures

---

chloroquine HCl/ chloroquine phosphate
(klor'oh-kwin)

Aralen HCl, Aralen Phosphate, Chlorocon, Novochloroquine*

Func. class.: Antimalarial
Chem. class.: Synthetic 4-aminoquinoline derivative

Action: Inhibits parasite replications, transcription of DNA to RNA by forming complexes with DNA of parasite

Uses: Malaria caused by *Plasmodium vivax, P. malariae, P. ovale, P. falciparum* (some strains), rheumatoid arthritis, amebiasis

Dosage and routes:
Malaria suppression
• *Adult and child:* PO 5 mg/kg/wk on same day of week, not to exceed 300 mg; treatment should begin 2 wk before exposure and for 8 wk after; if treatment begins after exposure, 600 mg for adult and 10 mg/kg for children in 2 divided doses 6 hr apart

Extraintestinal amebiasis
• *Adult:* IM 160-200 mg qd (HCl) up to 12 days, then 1 g (phosphate)

---

* Available in Canada only

qd × 2 days, then 500 mg qd ×
2-3 wk; PO 600 mg qd × 2 days,
then 300 mg qd × 2-3 wk
• *Child:* IM/PO 10 mg/kg qd
(HCl) × 2-3 wk, not to exceed 300
mg/day
Rheumatoid arthritis
• *Adult:* PO 250 mg (phosphate) qd
with evening meal
Available forms include: Tabs 250,
500 mg; inj IM 40 mg/ml
Side effects/adverse reactions:
CV: Hypotension, heart block,
asystole with syncope, ECG
changes
INTEG: Pruritus, pigmentary
changes, skin eruptions, lichen
planus—like eruptions, eczema, *exfoliative dermatitis,* alopecia
CNS: Headache, stimulation, fatigue, irritability, ***convulsion,*** bad
dreams, dizziness, confusion, psychosis, decreased reflexes
*EENT: Blurred vision, corneal
changes, retinal changes, difficulty
focusing,* tinnitus, vertigo, deafness, photophobia, corneal edema
GI: Nausea, vomiting, anorexia,
diarrhea, cramps, weight loss, stomatitis
HEMA: ***Thrombocytopenia, agranulocytosis, hemolytic anemia, leukopenia***
Contraindications: Hypersensitivity, retinal field changes, porphyria, children (long-term)
Precautions: Pregnancy (C), children, blood dyscrasias, severe GI
disease, neurologic disease, alcoholism, hepatic disease, G-6-PD
deficiency, psoriasis, eczema
Pharmacokinetics:
PO: Peak 1-2 hr, half-life 3-5 days,
metabolized in the liver, excreted
in urine, feces, breast milk, crosses
placenta
Interactions/incompatibilities:
• Decreased action of chloroquine:

magnesium or aluminum compounds
NURSING CONSIDERATIONS
Assess:
• Ophthalmic test if long-term
treatment or drug dosage >150
mg/day
• Liver studies q wk: AST, ALT,
bilirubin
• Blood studies: CBC, since blood
dyscrasias occur
• For decreased reflexes: knee, ankle
• ECG during therapy
• Watch for depression of T waves,
widening of QRS complex
Administer:
• Before or after meals at same time
each day to maintain drug level
• IM after aspirating to avoid injection into blood system, which
may cause hypotension, asystole,
heart block; rotate injection sites
Perform/provide:
• Storage in tight, light-resistant
containers at room temperature; injection should be kept in cool environment
Evaluate:
• Allergic reactions: pruritus, rash,
urticaria
• Blood dyscrasias: malaise, fever,
bruising, bleeding (rare)
• For ototoxicity (tinnitus, vertigo,
change in hearing); audiometric
testing should be done before, after
treatment
• For toxicity: blurring vision, difficulty focusing, headache, dizziness, knee, ankle reflexes; drug
should be discontinued immediately
Teach patient/family:
• To use sunglasses in bright sunlight to decrease photophobia
• That urine may turn rust or brown
color
• To report hearing, visual prob-

---

italics = common side effects   ***bold italic*** = life threatening reactions

lems, fever, fatigue, bruising, bleeding, which may indicate blood dyscrasias

Treatment of overdose: Induce vomiting, gastric lavage, administer barbiturate (ultrashort-acting), vasopressin; tracheostomy may be necessary

---

chlorothiazide

(klor-oh-thye′a-zide)
Diachlor, Diurigen, Diuril, Ro-Chlorozide, SK-Chlorothiazide
Func. class.: Diuretic
Chem. class.: Thiazide; sulfonamide derivative

Action: Acts on distal tubule by increasing excretion of water, sodium, chloride, potassium

Uses: Edema, hypertension, diuresis

Dosage and routes:
Edema, hypertension
• *Adult:* PO/IV 500 mg-2 g qd in 2 divided doses
Diuresis
• *Child >6 mo:* PO/IV 20 mg/kg/ day in divided doses
• *Child <6 mo:* PO/IV up to 30 mg/kg/day in 2 divided doses
Available forms include: Tabs 250, 500 mg; oral susp 250 mg/5 ml; inj 500 mg

Side effects/adverse reactions:
GU: Frequency, polyuria, *uremia,* glucosuria
CNS: Drowsiness, paresthesia, anxiety, depression, headache, *dizziness, fatigue, weakness*
GI: Nausea, vomiting, anorexia, constipation, diarrhea, cramps, pancreatitis, GI irritation, *hepatitis*
EENT: Blurred vision
INTEG: Rash, urticaria, purpura, photosensitivity, fever
META: Hyperglycemia, hyperuri-

cemia, hypomagnesemia, increased creatinine, BUN
*HEMA: **Aplastic anemia, hemolytic anemia, leukopenia, agranulocytosis, thrombocytopenia, neutropenia***
CV: Irregular pulse, orthostatic hypotension, palpitations, volume depletion
ELECT: Hypokalemia, hypercalcemia, hyponatremia, hypochloremia

Contraindications: Hypersensitivity to thiazides or sulfonamides, anuria, renal decompensation, pregnancy (D)

Precautions: Hypokalemia, renal disease, hepatic disease, gout, COPD, lupus erythematosus, diabetes mellitus

Pharmacokinetics:
PO: Onset 2 hr, peak 4 hr, duration 6-12 hr; crosses placenta, excreted in breast milk

Interactions/incompatibilities:
• Increased toxicity: lithium, nondepolarizing skeletal muscle relaxants, digitalis
• Decreased effects of: antidiabetics, sulfonylureas
• Decreased absorption of thiazides: cholestyramine, colestipol
• Decreased hypotensive response: indomethacin
• Hyperglycemia, hyperuricemia, hypotension: diazoxide

NURSING CONSIDERATIONS
Assess:
• Weight, I&O daily to determine fluid loss; effect of drug may be decreased if used qd
• Rate, depth, rhythm of respiration, effect of exertion
• B/P lying, standing; postural hypotension may occur
• Electrolytes: potassium, sodium, chloride; include BUN, blood sugar, CBC, serum creatinine,

---

blood pH, ABGs, uric acid, calcium
• Glucose in urine if patient is diabetic

Administer:
• IV after diluting 0.5 g/18 ml of sterile water for inj or more; may be diluted further with compatible IV sol; give over 5 min
• In AM to avoid interference with sleep if using drug as a diuretic
• Potassium replacement if potassium is less than 3.0
• With food if nausea occurs; absorption may be decreased slightly

Evaluate:
• Improvement in edema of feet, legs, sacral area daily if medication is being used in CHF
• Improvement in CVP q8h
• Signs of metabolic alkalosis: drowsiness, restlessness
• Signs of hypokalemia: postural hypotension, malaise, fatigue, tachycardia, leg cramps, weakness
• Rashes, temperature elevation qd
• Confusion, especially in elderly; take safety precautions if needed

Teach patient/family:
• To increase fluid intake 2-3 L/day unless contraindicated, to rise slowly from lying or sitting position
• To notify physician of muscle weakness, cramps, nausea, dizziness
• Drug may be taken with food or milk
• That blood sugar may be increased in diabetics
• Take early in day to avoid nocturia

Lab test interferences:
Increase: BSP retention, calcium, amylase, parathyroid test
Decrease: PBI, PSP

Treatment of overdose: Lavage if taken orally, monitor electrolytes, administer dextrose in saline, monitor hydration, CV, renal status

chlorotrianisene
(klor-oh-trye-an'i-seen)
Tace
Func. class.: Estrogen
Chem. class.: Nonsteroidal synthetic estrogen

Action: Needed for adequate functioning of female reproductive system, it affects release of pituitary gonadotropins, inhibits ovulation, adequate calcium use in bone structures

Uses: Prostatic cancer, menopause, female hypogonadism, atrophic vaginitis, kraurosis vulvae

Dosage and routes:
Prostatic cancer
• *Adult:* PO 12-25 mg qd
Menopause
• *Adult:* PO 12-25 mg qd × 30 days or 3 wk on 1 wk off
Female hypogonadism
• *Adult:* PO 12-25 mg × 21 days, then progesterone 100 mg IM or 5 days of progesterone PO given with last 5 days of medroxyprogesterone 5-10 mg
Vaginitis
• *Adult:* PO 12-25 mg qd × 30-60 days

Available forms include: Caps 12, 25, 72 mg

Side effects/adverse reactions:
CNS: Dizziness, headache, migraines, depression
CV: Hypotension, ***thrombophlebitis,*** edema, ***thromboembolism, stroke, pulmonary embolism, myocardial infarction***
GI: *Nausea,* vomiting, diarrhea, anorexia, pancreatitis, cramps, constipation, increased appetite, in-

creased weight, *cholestatic jaundice*

EENT: Contact lens intolerance, increased myopia, astigmatism

GU: Amenorrhea, cervical erosion, breakthrough bleeding, dysmenorrhea, vaginal candidiasis, breast changes, *gynecomastia, testicular atrophy, impotence*

INTEG: Rash, urticaria, acne, hirsutism, alopecia, oily skin, seborrhea, purpura, melasma

META: Folic acid deficiency, hypercalcemia, hyperglycemia

Contraindications: Breast cancer, thromboembolic disorders, reproductive cancer, genital bleeding (abnormal, undiagnosed), pregnancy (X)

Precautions: Hypertension, asthma, blood dyscrasias, gallbladder disease, CHF, diabetes mellitus, bone disease, depression, migraine headache, convulsive disorders, hepatic disease, renal disease, family history of cancer of the breast or reproductive tract

Pharmacokinetics:

PO: Degraded in liver, excreted in urine, crosses placenta, excreted in breast milk

Interactions/incompatibilities:

• Decreased action of: anticoagulants, oral hypoglycemics

• Toxicity: tricyclic antidepressants

• Decreased action of chlorotrianisene: anticonvulsants, barbiturates, phenylbutazone, rifampin

• Increased action of: corticosteroids

NURSING CONSIDERATIONS
Assess:

• Urine glucose in patient with diabetes, increased urine glucose may occur

• Weight daily, notify physician if weekly weight gain is >5 lb, if increase, diuretic may be ordered

• B/P q4h, watch for increase caused by water and sodium retention

• I&O ratio, be alert for decreasing urinary output and increasing edema

• Liver function studies, including AST, ALT, bilirubin, alk phosphatase

Administer:

• Titrated dose, use lowest effective dose

• In one dose in AM, for prostatic cancer, vaginitis, hypogonadism

• With food or milk to decrease GI symptoms

Evaluate:

• Therapeutic response: reversal of menopause or decrease in tumor size in prostatic cancer

• Edema, hypertension, cardiac symptoms, jaundice

• Mental status: affect, mood, behavioral changes, aggression

• Hypercalcemia

Teach patient/family:

• To weigh weekly, report gain >5 lb

• To report breast lumps, vaginal bleeding, edema, jaundice, dark urine, clay colored stools, dyspnea, headache, blurred vision, abdominal pain, numbness, stiffness, or pain in legs, chest pain; male to report impotence or gynecomastia

• To check with MD before using over-the-counter drugs

Lab test interferences:

Increase: BSP retention test, PBI, T_4, serum sodium, platelet aggressability, thyroxine-binding globulin (TBG), prothrombin, factors VII, VIII, IX, X, triglycerides

Decrease: Serum folate, serum triglyceride, T_3 resin uptake test, glucose tolerance test, antithrombin III, pregnanediol, metyrapone test

---

* Available in Canada only

False positive: LE prep, antinuclear antibodies

---

chlorphenesin carbamate

(klor-fen′e-sin)
Maolate, Mycil*
Func. class.: Skeletal muscle relaxant, central acting
Chem. class.: Carbamate

Action: Unknown; may be related to sedative properties; does not directly relax muscle or depress nerve conduction

Uses: Adjunct for relieving pain in acute, painful musculoskeletal conditions

Dosage and routes:
• *Adult:* PO 800 mg tid, maintenance 400 mg qid, not to exceed 8 wk

Available forms include: Tabs 400 mg

Side effects/adverse reactions:
CNS: Dizziness, weakness, drowsiness, headache, tremor, depression, insomnia, confusion
EENT: Diplopia, temporary loss of vision
HEMA: Blood dyscrasias
CV: Postural hypotension, tachycardia
GI: Nausea, vomiting, hiccups
INTEG: Rash, pruritus, fever, facial flushing
SYST: Anaphylaxis

Contraindications: Hypersensitivity, child <12 yr, intermittent porphyria

Precautions: Renal disease, hepatic disease, addictive personalities, pregnancy (C)

Pharmacokinetics:
PO: Onset ½ hr, peak 1-2 hr, duration 4-6 hr, metabolized by liver, excreted in urine, crosses placenta, excreted in breast milk (large amounts), half-life 4 hr

Interactions/incompatibilities:
• Increased CNS depression: alcohol, tricyclic antidepressants, narcotics, barbiturates, sedatives, hypnotics

NURSING CONSIDERATIONS
Assess:
• Blood studies: CBC, WBC, differential; blood dyscrasias may occur
• Liver function studies: AST, ALT, alk phosphatase; hepatitis may occur
• Kidney function studies
• ECG in epileptic patients; poor seizure control has occurred with patients taking this drug
• B/P lying and standing, postural hypotension may occur

Administer:
• With meals for GI symptoms

Perform/provide:
• Storage in tight container at room temperature
• Assistance with ambulation if dizziness, drowsiness occurs

Evaluate:
• Therapeutic response: decreased pain, spasticity
• Allergic reactions: rash, fever, respiratory distress
• Severe weakness, numbness in extremities
• Psychologic dependency: increased need for medication, more frequent requests for medication, increased pain
• CNS depression: dizziness, drowsiness, psychiatric symptoms

Teach patient/family:
• Not to discontinue medication quickly, insomnia, nausea, headache, spasticity, tachycardia will occur; drug should be tapered off over 1-2 wk

---

italics = common side effects   ***bold italic*** = life threatening reactions

• Not to take with alcohol, other CNS depressants
• To avoid altering activities while taking this drug
• To avoid hazardous activities if drowsiness, dizziness occurs
• To avoid using OTC medication: cough preparations, antihistamines, unless directed by physician
Treatment of overdose: Give physostigmine IV; monitor cardiac function

---

chlorpheniramine maleate

(klor-fen-eer′a-meen)
Alleroid-OD, AL-R, Chlormene, Chlortab, Chlor-Trimeton, Chlor-Tripolon, Novopheniram, Teldrin
Func. class.: Antihistamine
Chem. class.: Alkylamine, H$_1$-receptor antagonist

Action: Acts on blood vessels, GI system, respiratory system, by competing with histamine for H$_1$-receptor site; decreases allergic response by blocking histamine
Uses: Allergy symptoms, rhinitis
Dosage and routes:
• *Adult:* PO 2-4 mg tid-qid, not to exceed 36 mg/day; TIME-REL 8-12 mg bid-tid, not to exceed 36 mg/day; IM/IV/SC 5-40 mg/day
• *Child 6-12 yr:* PO 2 mg q4-6h, not to exceed 12 mg/day; SUS REL 8 mg hs or qd, SUS REL not recommended for child <6 yr
• *Child 2-5 yr:* PO 1 mg q4-6h, not to exceed 4 mg/day
Available forms include: Tabs, chewable 2 mg; tabs 4 mg; tabs, time-rel 8, 12 mg; caps, time-rel 8, 12 mg; syr 2 mg/5 ml; inj IM, SC, IV 10, 100 mg/ml
Side effects/adverse reactions:
CNS: Dizziness, drowsiness, poor coordination, fatigue, anxiety, euphoria, confusion, paresthesia, neuritis
RESP: Increased thick secretions, wheezing, chest tightness
HEMA: Thrombocytopenia, agranulocytosis, hemolytic anemia
GI: Dry mouth, nausea, anorexia, diarrhea
INTEG: Photosensitivity
GU: Retention, dysuria, frequency
EENT: Blurred vision, dilated pupils, tinnitus, nasal stuffiness, dry nose, throat, mouth
Contraindications: Hypersensitivity to H$_1$-receptor antagonists, acute asthma attack, lower respiratory tract disease
Precautions: Increased intraocular pressure, renal disease, cardiac disease, hypertension, bronchial asthma, seizure disorder, stenosed peptic ulcers, hyperthyroidism, prostatic hypertrophy, bladder neck obstruction, pregnancy (B)
Pharmacokinetics:
PO: Onset 20-60 min, duration 8-12 hr; detoxified in liver, excreted by kidneys, (metabolites/free drug), half-life 20-24 hr
Interactions/incompatibilities:
• Increased CNS depression: barbiturates, narcotics, hypnotics, tricyclic antidepressants, alcohol
• Decreased effect of: oral anticoagulants, heparin
• Increased effect of chlorpheniramine: MAOIs
NURSING CONSIDERATIONS
Assess:
• I&O ratio; be alert for urinary retention, frequency, dysuria; drug should be discontinued if these occur
• CBC during long-term therapy
Administer:
• IV undiluted at a rate of 10 mg/1 min or longer

- With meals if GI symptoms occur; absorption may slightly decrease

Perform/provide:
- Hard candy, gum, frequent rinsing of mouth for dryness
- Storage in tight container at room temperature

Evaluate:
- Therapeutic response: absence of running or congested nose or rashes
- Blood dyscrasias: thrombocytopenia, agranulocytosis (rare)
- Respiratory status: rate, rhythm, increase in bronchial secretions, wheezing, chest tightness

Teach patient/family:
- Not to chew or crush sustained release forms
- All aspects of drug use; to notify physician if confusion, sedation, hypotension occurs
- To avoid driving or other hazardous activity if drowsiness occurs
- To avoid concurrent use of alcohol or other CNS depressants

Lab test interferences:
False negative: Skin allergy tests
Treatment of overdose: Administer ipecac syrup or lavage, diazepam, vasopressors, barbiturates (short-acting)

---

chlorpromazine HCl

(klor-proe'ma-zeen)
Chlor-Promanyl, Chlorpromanyl,* Largactil, Promaz, Thorazine
Func. class.: Antipsychotic/neuroleptic
Chem. class.: Phenothiazine-aliphatic

Action: Depresses cerebral cortex, hypothalamus, limbic system, which control activity aggression; blocks neurotransmission produced by dopamine at synapse; exhibits a strong α-adrenergic, anticholinergic blocking action; mechanism for antipsychotic effects is unclear

Uses: Psychotic disorders, mania, schizophrenia, anxiety, intractable hiccups, nausea, vomiting, preoperatively for relaxation, and acute intermittent porphyria, behavioral problems in children

Dosage and routes:
Psychiatry
- *Adult:* PO 10-50 mg q1-4h initially, then increase up to 2000 mg/day if necessary
- *Adult:* IM 10-50 mg q1-4h
- *Child:* PO 0.25 mg/lb q4-6h or 0.5 mg/kg
- *Child:* IM 0.25 mg/lb q6-8h or 0.5 mg/kg
- *Child:* REC 0.5 mg/lb q6-8h or 1 mg/kg

Nausea and vomiting
- *Adult:* PO 10-25 mg q4-6h prn; IM 25-50 mg q3h prn; REC 50-100 mg q6-8h prn, not to exceed 400 mg/day
- *Child:* PO 0.25 mg/lb q4-6h prn, IM 0.25 mg/lb q6-8h prn not to exceed 40 mg/day (<5 yr) or 75 mg/day (5-12 yr); REC 0.5 mg/lb q6-8h prn
- *Adult:* IV 25-50 mg qd-qid
- *Child:* IV 0.55 mg/kg q6-8h

Intractable hiccups
- *Adult:* PO 25-50 mg tid-qid; IM 25-50 mg (used only if PO dose does not work); IV 25-50 mg in 500-1000 ml saline (only for severe hiccups)

Available forms include: Tabs 10, 25, 50, 100, 200 mg; time-release caps 30, 75, 150, 200, 300 mg; syr 10 mg/5ml; conc 30, 100 mg/ml; supp 25, 100 mg; inj IM, IV 25 mg/ml

Side effects/adverse reactions:
*RESP: **Laryngospasm**,* dyspnea, ***respiratory depression***

---

italics = common side effects   ***bold italic*** = life threatening reactions

CNS: Extrapyramidal symptoms: pseudoparkinsonism, akathisia, dystonia, tardive dyskinesia, seizures, *headache*

HEMA: Anemia, **leukopenia, leukocytosis, agranulocytosis**

INTEG: Rash, photosensitivity, dermatitis

EENT: Blurred vision, glaucoma

GI:.Dry mouth, nausea, vomiting, anorexia, constipation, diarrhea, jaundice, weight gain

GU: Urinary retention, urinary frequency, enuresis, impotence, amenorrhea, gynecomastia, breast engorgement

CV: Orthostatic hypotension, hypertension, **cardiac arrest,** ECG changes, **tachycardia**

Contraindications: Hypersensitivity, circulatory collapse, liver damage, cerebral arteriosclerosis, coronary disease, severe hypertension/hypotension, blood dyscrasias, coma, child <2 years, brain damage, bone marrow depression, alcohol and barbiturate withdrawal states

Precautions: Pregnancy (C), lactation, seizure disorders, hypertension, hepatic disease, cardiac disease

Pharmacokinetics:

PO: Onset erratic, peak 2-4 hr, duration may be detected for up to 6 mo after last dose

IM: Onset 15-30 min, peak 15-20 min, duration may be detected for up to 6 mo after last dose

IV: Onset 5 min, peak 10 min, duration may be detected for up to 6 mo after last dose

REC: Onset erratic, peak 3 hr

Metabolized by liver, excreted in urine (metabolites), crosses placenta, enters breast milk; 95% bound to plasma proteins; elimination half-life 10-30 hr

Interactions/incompatibilities:
- Oversedation: other CNS depressants, alcohol, barbiturate anesthetics
- Toxicity: epinephrine
- Decreased absorption: aluminum hydroxide or magnesium hydroxide antacids
- Decreased effects of: levodopa
- Decreased serum chlorpromazine: lithium
- Increased effects of both drugs: β-adrenergic blockers, alcohol
- Increased anticholinergic effects: anticholinergics

NURSING CONSIDERATIONS
Assess:
- Swallowing of PO medication; check for hoarding or giving of medication to other patients
- I&O ratio; palpate bladder if low urinary output occurs
- Bilirubin, CBC, liver function studies monthly
- Urinalysis is recommended before, during prolonged therapy

Administer:
- IV after diluting 1 mg/1 ml with normal saline, give 1 mg/2 min; may be further diluted in 500-1000 ml of compatible sol
- Antiparkinsonian agent, to be used if extrapyramidal symptoms occur
- Drug in liquid form mixed in glass of juice or cola, if hoarding is suspected

Perform/provide:
- Decreased stimuli by dimming lights, avoiding loud noises
- Supervised ambulation until stabilized on medication; do not involve in strenuous exercise program because fainting is possible; patient should not stand still for long periods of time
- Increased fluids to prevent constipation

---

*Available in Canada only

• Sips of water, candy, gum for dry mouth
• Storage in tight, light-resistant container, oral solutions in amber bottles

Evaluate:
• Decrease in: emotional excitement, hallucinations, delusions, paranoia, reorganization of patterns of thought, speech
• Affect, orientation, LOC, reflexes, gait, coordination, sleep pattern disturbances
• B/P standing and lying; take pulse and respirations q4h during initial treatment; establish baseline before starting treatment; report drops of 30 mm Hg
• Dizziness, faintness, palpitations, tachycardia on rising
• For neuroleptic malignant syndrome: hyperpyrexia, muscle rigidity, increased CPK, altered mental status
• Extrapyramidal symptoms including akathisia (inability to sit still, no pattern to movements), tardive dyskinesia (bizarre movements of the jaw, mouth, tongue, extremities), pseudoparkinsonism (rigidity, tremors, pill rolling, shuffling gait)
• Skin turgor daily
• Constipation, urinary retention daily; if these occur, increase bulk, water in diet

Teach patient/family:
• That orthostatic hypotension occurs often, and to rise from sitting or lying position gradually
• To remain lying down after IM injection for at least 30 min
• To avoid hot tubs, hot showers, or tub baths since hypotension may occur
• To avoid abrupt withdrawal of this drug or extrapyramidal symptoms may result; drug should be withdrawn slowly
• To avoid OTC preparations (cough, hayfever, cold) unless approved by physician since serious drug interactions may occur; avoid use with alcohol or CNS depressants; increased drowsiness may occur
• To use a sunscreen and sunglasses during sun exposure to prevent burns
• Regarding compliance with drug regimen
• About extrapyramidal symptoms and necessity for meticulous oral hygiene since oral candidiasis may occur
• To report sore throat, malaise, fever, bleeding, mouth sores; if these occur, CBC should be drawn and drug discontinued
• In hot weather, heat stroke may occur; take extra precautions to stay cool

Lab test interferences:
Increase: Liver function tests, cardiac enzymes, cholesterol, blood glucose, prolactin, bilirubin, PBI, cholinesterase, ^{131}I
Decrease: Hormones (blood and urine)
False positive: Pregnancy tests, PKU
False negative: Urinary steroids, 17-OHCS
Treatment of overdose: Lavage, if orally ingested, provide an airway; *do not induce vomiting or use epinephrine*

---

chlorpropamide
(klor-proe'pa-mide)
Chloronase,* Diabinese, Novopropamide*
Func. class.: Antidiabetic
Chem. class.: Sulfonylurea (1st generation)

Action: Causes functioning β-cells

---

italics = common side effects   ***bold italic*** = life threatening reactions

in pancreas to release insulin, leading to drop in blood glucose levels; may improve insulin binding to insulin receptors or increase the number of insulin receptors; not effective if patient lacks functioning β-cells

Uses: Stable adult-onset diabetes mellitus (type II) NIDDM

Dosage and routes:
• *Adult:* PO 100-250 mg qd, initially, then 100-500 mg maintenance according to response; not to exceed 750 mg/day

Available forms include: Tabs 100, 250 mg

Side effects/adverse reactions:
CNS: Headache, weakness, dizziness, drowsiness, tinnitus, fatigue, vertigo

GI: Hepatotoxicity, cholestatic jaundice, nausea, vomiting, diarrhea, heartburn

HEMA: Leukopenia, thrombocytopenia, agranulocytosis, aplastic anemia, pancytopenia, hemolytic anemia

INTEG: Rash, allergic reactions, pruritus, urticaria, eczema, photosensitivity, erythema

ENDO: Hypoglycemia

Contraindications: Hypersensitivity to sulfonylureas, juvenile or brittle diabetes, pregnancy (D)

Precautions: Elderly, cardiac disease, thyroid disease, renal disease, hepatic disease, severe hypoglycemic reactions

Pharmacokinetics:
PO: Completely absorbed by GI route, onset 1 hr, peak 3-6 hr, duration 60 hr, half-life 36 hr, metabolized in liver, excreted in urine (metabolites and unchanged drug), breast milk, 90%-95% is plasma protein bound

Interactions/incompatibilities:
• Increased hypoglycemic effects:

oral anticoagulants, salicylates, sulfonamides, nonsteroidal antiinflammatories, chloramphenicol, cimetidine, MAOIs, insulin, guanethidine, methyldopa, probenecid, ranitidine

• Increased effects of chlorpropamide: insulin, MAOIs

• Decreased digoxin levels: digoxin

• Decreased effect of both drugs; diazoxide

• Decreased action of chlorpropamide: calcium channel blockers, corticosteroids, oral contraceptives, thiazide diuretics, thyroid preparations, estrogens, phenobarbital, phenytoin, rifampin, sympathomimetics

NURSING CONSIDERATIONS
Administer:
• Drug 30 min before meals

Perform/provide:
• Storage in tight container in cool environment

Evaluate:
• Therapeutic response: decrease in polyuria, polydipsia, polyphagia, clear sensorium, absence of dizziness, stable gait

• Hypoglycemic/hyperglycemic reaction that can occur soon after meals

Teach patient/family:
• To check for symptoms of cholestatic jaundice: dark urine, pruritus, yellow sclera; if these occur, physician should be notified

• To use capillary blood glucose test while on this drug

• To test urine glucose levels with Chemstrip 3 × /day

• Symptoms of hypo/hyperglycemia, what to do about each

• That this drug must be continued on daily basis; explain consequence of discontinuing drug abruptly

• To take drug in morning to pre-

vent hypoglycemic reactions at night
• To avoid OTC medications unless prescribed by physician
• That diabetes is life-long illness, drug will not cure disease
• That all food included in diet plan must be eaten in order to prevent hypoglycemia
• To carry Medic-Alert ID for emergency purposes
• Not to drink alcohol
Treatment of overdose: 10%-50% glucose solution IV

chlortetracycline HCl (topical)
(klor-te-tra-sye'kleen)
Aureomycin
Func. class.: Local antiinfective
Chem. class.: Antibacterial

Action: Interferes with bacterial protein cell synthesis
Uses: Pyogenic skin infections
Dosage and routes:
• *Adult and child:* TOP rub into affected area bid-qid
Available forms include: Oint 3%
Side effects/adverse reactions:
INTEG: Rash, urticaria, stinging, burning, dry skin, photosensitivity, tooth discoloration
Contraindications: Hypersensitivity to this drug or wool
Precautions: Pregnancy (C), lactation
NURSING CONSIDERATIONS
Administer:
• Enough medication to completely cover lesions
• After cleansing with soap, water before each application, dry well
Perform/provide:
• Storage at room temperature in dry place, in light-resistant container

Evaluate:
• Allergic reaction: burning, stinging, swelling, redness
• Therapeutic response: decrease in size, number of lesions
Teach patient/family:
• To watch for superimposed infections
• To apply with glove to prevent further infection
• To avoid use of OTC creams, ointments, lotions unless directed by physician
• To use medical asepsis (hand washing) before, after each application
• To avoid squeezing or poking-lesions or spreading may occur
• To notify physician if condition worsens, or rash, irritation, or swelling occurs
• To avoid sunlight or ultraviolet light
• That skin may be stained
• Long-term use may cause tooth discoloration

chlorthalidone
(klor-thal'i-done)
Hygroton, Hylidone, Novothalidone,* Thalitone
Func. class.: Diuretic
Chem. class.: Thiazide-like; phthalimidine derivative

Action: Acts on distal tubule by increasing excretion of water, sodium, chloride, potassium
Uses: Edema, hypertension, diuresis, CHF
Dosage and routes:
• *Adult:* PO 25-100 mg/day or 100 mg every other day
• *Child:* PO 2 mg/kg 3 ×/wk
Available forms include: Tabs 25, 50, 100 mg

italics = common side effects   ***bold italic*** = life threatening reactions

Side effects/adverse reactions:

GU: Frequency, polyuria, ***uremia,*** glucosuria

CNS: Drowsiness, paresthesia, anxiety, depression, headache, *dizziness, fatigue, weakness*

GI: Nausea, vomiting, anorexia, constipation, diarrhea, cramps, pancreatitis, GI irritation, ***hepatitis***

EENT: Blurred vision

INTEG: Rash, urticaria, purpura, photosensitivity, fever

META: Hyperglycemia, hyperuremia, increased creatinine, BUN

*HEMA: **Aplastic anemia, hemolytic anemia, leukopenia, agranulocytosis, thrombocytopenia, neutropenia***

CV: Irregular pulse, orthostatic hypotension, palpitations, volume depletion

ELECT: Hypokalemia, hypomagnesemia, hypercalcemia, hyponatremia, hypochloremia

Contraindications: Hypersensitivity to thiazides or sulfonamides, anuria, renal decompensation

Precautions: Hypokalemia, renal disease, pregnancy (C), hepatic disease, gout, diabetes mellitus

Pharmacokinetics:

PO: Onset 2 hr, peak 6 hr, duration 24-72 hr; excreted unchanged by kidneys, crosses placenta, enters breast milk, half-life 40 hr

Interactions/incompatibilities:

• Increased toxicity: lithium, nondepolarizing skeletal muscle relaxants

• Decreased effects of: antidiabetics

• Decreased absorption of thiazides: cholestyramine, colestipol

• Decreased hypotensive response: indomethacin

• Hyperglycemia, hyperuricemia, hypotension: diazoxide

NURSING CONSIDERATIONS

Assess:

• Weight, I&O daily to determine fluid loss; effect of drug may be decreased if used qd

• Rate, depth, rhythm of respiration, effect of exertion

• B/P lying, standing; postural hypotension may occur

• Electrolytes: potassium, magnesium, sodium chloride; include BUN, blood sugar, CBC, serum creatinine, blood pH, ABGs, uric acid, calcium

• Glucose in urine if patient is diabetic

Administer:

• In AM to avoid interference with sleep if using drug as a diuretic

• Potassium replacement if potassium is less than 3.0

• With food if nausea occurs; absorption may be decreased slightly

Evaluate:

• Improvement in edema of feet, legs, sacral area daily if medication is being used in CHF

• Improvement in CVP q8h

• Signs of metabolic alkalosis: drowsiness, restlessness

• Signs of hypokalemia: postural hypotension, malaise, fatigue, tachycardia, leg cramps, weakness

• Rashes, temperature elevation qd

• Confusion, especially in elderly; take safety precautions if needed

Teach patient/family:

• To increase fluid intake 2-3 L/day unless contraindicated, to rise slowly from lying or sitting position

• To notify physician of muscle weakness, cramps, nausea, dizziness

• Drug may be taken with food or milk

• That blood sugar may be increased in diabetics

• Take early in day to avoid nocturia

Lab test interferences:

Increase: BSP retention, calcium, cholesterol, triglycerides, amylase

Decrease: PBI, PSP, parathyroid test

Treatment of overdose: Lavage if taken orally, monitor electrolytes, administer dextrose in saline, monitor hydration, CV, renal status

---

chlorzoxazone

(klor-zox'a-zone)

Paraflex, Oxyren, and others

Func. class.: Skeletal muscle relaxant

Chem. class.: Benzoxazole derivative

Action: Inhibits multisynaptic reflex arcs

Uses: Relieving pain, spasm in musculoskeletal conditions

Dosage and routes:

• *Adult:* PO 250-750 mg tid-qid

• *Child:* PO 20 mg/kg/day in divided doses bid-tid

Available forms include: Tabs 250 mg

Side effects/adverse reactions:

GU: Urine discoloration

HEMA: **Granulocytopenia, anemia**

CNS: Dizziness, drowsiness, headache, insomnia, stimulation, malaise

GI: Nausea, vomiting, anorexia, diarrhea, constipation, **hepatotoxicity, jaundice**

INTEG: Rash, pruritus, petechiae, ecchymoses, **angioedema**

SYST: **Anaphylaxis**

Contraindications: Hypersensitivity, impaired hepatic function

Precautions: Pregnancy (C), lactation, hepatic disease

Pharmacokinetics:

PO: Onset 1 hr, peak 3-4 hr, duration 6 hr, half-life 1 hr, metabolized in liver, excreted in urine (metabolites)

Interactions/incompatibilities:

• Increased CNS depression: alcohol, tricylic antidepressants, narcotics, barbiturates, sedatives, hypnotics

NURSING CONSIDERATIONS

Assess:

• Blood studies: CBC, WBC, differential; blood dyscrasias may occur

• Liver function studies: AST, ALT, alk phosphatase; hepatitis may occur; hold dose and notify physician if signs of hepatic function occur

• EEG in epileptic patients; poor seizure control has occurred with patients taking this drug

Administer:

• With meals for GI symptoms

Perform/provide:

• Storage in tight container at room temperature

• Assistance with ambulation if dizziness or drowsiness occurs

Evaluate:

• Therapeutic response: decreased pain, spasticity

• Allergic reactions: rash, fever, respiratory distress

• Severe weakness, numbness in extremities

• Psychologic dependency: increased need for medication, more frequent requests for medication, increased pain

• CNS depression: dizziness, drowsiness, psychiatric symptoms

Teach patient/family:

• Not to discontinue the medication quickly; insomnia, nausea, headache, spasticity, tachycardia will

---

italics = common side effects   ***bold italic*** = life threatening reactions

occur; drug should be tapered off over 1-2 wk
• Not to take with alcohol, other CNS depressants
• To avoid altering activities while taking this drug
• To avoid hazardous activities if drowsiness, dizziness occurs
• To avoid using OTC medication: cough preparations, antihistamines, unless directed by physician
• Urine may be orange or purple
Treatment of overdose: Gastric lavage or induce emesis, then administer activated charcoal; use other supportive treatment as necessary; monitor cardiac function

---

cholestyramine
(koe-less-tir′a-meen)
Questran
Func. class.: Antilipemic
Chem. class.: Bile acid sequestrant

Action: Absorbs, combines with bile acids to form insoluble complex that is excreted through feces; loss of bile acids lowers cholesterol levels
Uses: Primary hypercholesterolemia, pruritus associated with biliary obstruction, diarrhea caused by excess bile acid, digitalis toxicity xanthomas
Dosage and routes:
• *Adult:* PO 4 g ac, and hs, not to exceed 32 g/day
• *Child:* PO 240 mg/kg/day in 3 divided doses; administer with food or drink
Available forms include: Powd 9g/ 4g cholestyramine
Side effects/adverse reactions:
CNS: Headache, dizziness, drowsiness, vertigo, tinnitus
MS: Muscle, joint pain
GI: Constipation, abdominal pain,

nausea, fecal impaction, hemorrhoids, flatulence, vomiting, steatorrhea, peptic ulcer
INTEG: Rash, irritation of perianal area, tongue, skin
HEMA: Decreased vitamin A, D, K, red cell folate content, ***hyperchloremic acidosis, bleeding,*** decreased pro-time
Contraindications: Hypersensitivity, biliary obstruction
Precautions: Pregnancy (C), lactation, children
Pharmacokinetics:
PO: Excreted in feces, maximum effect in 2 wk
Interactions/incompatibilities:
• Decreased absorption of: phenylbutazone, warfarin, thiazides, digitalis, penicillin G, tetracyclines, cephalexin, phenobarbital, folic acid, corticosteroids, iron, thyroid, clindamycin, trimethoprim, chenodiol, fat-soluble vitamins

NURSING CONSIDERATIONS
Assess:
• Cardiac glycoside level, if both drugs are being administered
• For signs of vitamin A, D, K deficiency
• Serum cholesterol, triglyceride levels, electrolytes if on extended therapy
Administer:
• Drug ac, hs; give all other medications 1 hr before cholestyramine or 4 hr after cholestyramine to avoid poor absorption
• Drug mixed/applesauce or stirred into beverage (2-6 oz), do not take dry, let stand for 2 min
• Supplemental doses of vitamins A, D, K, if levels are low
Evaluate:
• Bowel pattern daily; increase bulk, water in diet if constipation develops

---

• Therapeutic response: decreased cholesterol level (hyperlipidemia); diarrhea, pruritus (excess bile area)

Teach patient/family:

• Symptoms of hypothrombinemia: bleeding mucous membranes, dark tarry stools, hematuria, petechiae; report immediately

• Stress patient compliance since toxicity may result if doses are missed

• That risk factors should be decreased: high fat diet, smoking, alcohol consumption, absence of exercise

Lab test interferences:

Increase: Liver function studies, chloride, PO₄

---

choline

(koe'leen)

Func. class.: Miscellaneous GI agent

Action: Acts as a precursor to acetylcholine, a neurotransmitter; a phospholipid

Uses: Hepatic disease, poor fat metabolism

Dosage and routes:

• *Adult and child:* PO 650-750 mg qd

Available forms include: Tabs 250, 500 mg; powder

Side effects/adverse reactions:

CNS: Dizziness, vertigo

GI: GI irritation

META: Ketosis

INTEG: Foul body odor, halitosis

Contraindications: Hypersensitivity

NURSING CONSIDERATIONS

Administer:

• PO, usually in AM

Perform/provide:

• Storage at room temperature

Evaluate:

• Nutritional status: egg yolk, dairy products, beans, peas, beef, liver (high in choline)

Teach patient/family:

• Food high in choline, that diet should contain 500-900 mg/day

---

choline magnesium trisalicylate

(koe'leen)

Trilisate

Func. class.: Nonnarcotic analgesic

Chem. class.: Salicylate

Action: Blocks pain impulses in CNS that occur in response to inhibition of prostaglandin synthesis; antipyretic action results from inhibition of hypothalamic heat-regulating center

Uses: Mild to moderate pain or fever including arthritis, juvenile, rheumatoid arthritis, osteoarthritis

Dosage and routes:

Arthritis

• *Adult:* PO 435-870 mg q4h

• *Child 12-37 kg:* PO 50 mg/kg/day in divided doses

• *Child > 37 kg:* PO 2250 mg in divided doses

Pain/fever

• *Adult:* PO 2-3 g/day in divided doses

• *Child 12-37 kg:* PO 50 mg/kg/day in divided doses

Available forms include: Liq 500, 870 mg/5 ml; tab 500, 750, 1000 mg

Side effects/adverse reactions:

HEMA: ***Thrombocytopenia, agranulocytosis, leukopenia, neutropenia, hemolytic anemia,*** increased pro-time

CNS: Stimulation, drowsiness, dizziness, confusion, convulsion,

---

headache, flushing, hallucinations, *coma*

GI: Nausea, vomiting, GI bleeding, diarrhea, heartburn, anorexia, *hepatitis*

INTEG: Rash, urticaria, bruising

EENT: Tinnitus, hearing loss

CV: Rapid pulse, pulmonary edema

RESP: Wheezing, hyperpnea

ENDO: Hypoglycemia, hyponatremia, hypokalemia

Contraindications: Hypersensitivity to salicylates, GI bleeding, bleeding disorders, children < 3 yr, vitamin K deficiency, children with flu-like symptoms

Precautions: Anemia, hepatic disease, renal disease, Hodgkin's disease, pregnancy (C), lactation

Pharmacokinetics:

PO: Onset 15-30 min, peak 1-2 hr, duration 4-6 hr, metabolized by liver, excreted by kidneys, crosses placenta, excreted in breast milk, half-life 1-3½ hr

Interactions/incompatibilities:

• Decreased effects of choline: antacids, steroids, urinary alkalizers

• Increased blood loss: alcohol, heparin

• Increased effects of: anticoagulants, insulin, methotrexate

• Decreased effects of: probenecid, spironolactone, sulfinpyrazone, sulfonylamides

• Toxic effects: PABA, furosemide, carbonic anhydrase inhibitors

• Decreased blood sugar levels: salicylates

• GI bleeding: steroids, antiinflammatories

NURSING CONSIDERATIONS
Assess:

• Liver function studies: AST, ALT, bilirubin, creatinine if patient is on long-term therapy

• Renal function studies: BUN, urine creatinine if patient is on long-term therapy

• Blood studies: CBC, Hct, Hgb, pro-time if patient is on long-term therapy

• I&O ratio; decreasing output may indicate renal failure (long-term therapy)

Administer:

• To patient crushed or whole; chewable tablets may be chewed

• With food or milk to decrease gastric symptoms; give 30 min before or 2 hr after meals

Evaluate:

• Hepatotoxicity: dark urine, clay-colored stools, yellowing of skin, sclera, itching, abdominal pain, fever, diarrhea if patient is on long-term therapy

• Allergic reactions: rash, urticaria; if these occur, drug may need to be discontinued

• Renal dysfunction: decreased urine output

• Ototoxicity: tinnitus, ringing, roaring in ears; audiometric testing is needed before, after long-term therapy

• Visual changes: blurring, halos, corneal, retinal damage

• Edema in feet, ankles, legs

• Prior drug history; there are many drug interactions

Teach patient/family:

• To report any symptoms of hepatotoxicity, renal toxicity, visual changes, ototoxicity, allergic reactions (long-term therapy)

• Not to exceed recommended dosage; acute poisoning may result

• To read label on other OTC drugs; many contain aspirin

• That therapeutic response takes 2 wk (arthritis)

• To avoid alcohol ingestion; GI bleeding may occur

Lab test interferences:
Increase: Coagulation studies, liver function studies, serum uric acid, amylase, CO_2, urinary protein
Decrease: Serum potassium, PBI, cholesterol
Interfere: Urine catecholamines, pregnancy test
Treatment of overdose: Lavage, activated charcoal, monitor electrolytes, VS

---

choline salicylate
(koe'leen)
Arthropan, Teejel*
Func. class.: Nonnarcotic analgesic
Chem. class.: Salicylate

Action: Blocks pain impulses in CNS that occur in response to inhibition of prostaglandin synthesis; antipyretic action results from inhibition of hypothalamic heat-regulating center to produce vasodilation to allow heat dissipation
Uses: Mild to moderate pain or fever including arthritis, juvenile rheumatoid arthritis
Dosage and routes:
Arthritis
• *Adult:* PO 870-1740 mg qid
Pain/fever
• *Adult:* PO 870 mg q3-4h prn
• *Child 3-6 yr:* PO 105-210 mg q4h prn
Available forms include: Liq 870 mg/5 ml
Side effects/adverse reactions:
*HEMA: **Thrombocytopenia, agranulocytosis, leukopenia, neutropenia, hemolytic anemia,*** increased pro-time
CNS: Stimulation, drowsiness, dizziness, confusion, ***convulsion,*** headache, flushing, hallucinations, ***coma***
*GI: **Nausea, vomiting, GI bleeding, diarrhea, heartburn,** anorexia, **hepatitis***
*INTEG: **Rash,** urticaria, bruising*
EENT: Tinnitus, hearing loss
CV: Rapid pulse, pulmonary edema
RESP: Wheezing, hyperpnea
ENDO: Hypoglycemia, hyponatremia, hypokalemia
Contraindications: Hypersensitivity to salicylates, GI bleeding, bleeding disorders, children < 3 yr, vitamin K deficiency, children with flu-like symptoms
Precautions: Anemia, hepatic disease, renal disease, Hodgkin's disease, pregnancy (C), lactation
Pharmacokinetics:
PO: Onset 15-30 min, metabolized by liver, excreted by kidneys, crosses placenta, excreted in breast milk
Interactions/incompatibilities:
• Decreased effects of choline: antacids, steroids, urinary alkalizers
• Increased blood loss: alcohol, heparin
• Increased effects of: anticoagulants, insulin, methotrexate
• Decreased effects of: probenecid, spironolactone, sulfinpyrazone, sulfonylamides
• Toxic effects: PABA, furosemide, carbonic anhydrase inhibitors
• Decreased blood sugar levels: salicylates
• GI bleeding: steroids, antiinflammatories
NURSING CONSIDERATIONS
Assess:
• Liver function studies: AST, ALT, bilirubin, creatinine if patient is on long-term therapy
• Renal function studies: BUN,

urine creatinine if patient is on long-term therapy
• Blood studies: CBC, Hct, Hgb, pro-time if patient is on long-term therapy
• I&O ratio; decreasing output may indicate renal failure (long-term therapy)

Administer:
• Mixed with fruit juice, carbonated beverage, water

Evaluate:
• Hepatotoxicity: dark urine, clay-colored stools, yellowing of skin, sclera, itching, abdominal pain, fever, diarrhea if patient is on long-term therapy
• Allergic reactions: rash, urticaria; if these occur, drug may need to be discontinued
• Renal dysfunction: decreased urine output
• Ototoxicity: tinnitus, ringing, roaring in ears; audiometric testing needed before, after long-term therapy
• Visual changes: blurring, halos, corneal, retinal damage
• Edema in feet, ankles, legs
• Prior drug history; there are many drug interactions

Teach patient/family:
• To report any symptoms of hepatotoxicity, renal toxicity, visual changes, ototoxicity, allergic reactions (long-term therapy)
• Not to exceed recommended dosage; acute poisoning may result
• To read label on other OTC drugs; many contain aspirin
• That therapeutic response takes 2 wk (arthritis)
• To avoid alcohol ingestion; GI bleeding may occur

Lab test interferences:
Increase: Coagulation studies, liver function studies, serum uric acid, amylase, CO_2, urinary protein

Decrease: Serum potassium, PBI, cholesterol
Interfere: Urine catecholamines, pregnancy test
Treatment of overdose: Lavage, activated charcoal, monitor electrolytes, VS

chorionic gonadotropin, human

(go-nad'oh-troe-pin)
Android HCG, APL, Chorex, Follutein, Glukor, Gonic, Libigen, Pregnyl, Profasi HP, Stemutrolin
Func. class.: Human chorionic gonadotropin
Chem. class.: Polypeptide hormone

Action: Stimulates production of gonadal steroids, androgens; stimulates corpus luteum to produce progesterone
Uses: Infertility, anovulation, hypogonadism, nonobstructive cryptorchidism
Dosage and routes:
Infertility/anovulation
• *Adult:* IM 10,000 U 1 day after last dose of menotropins
Hypogonadism
• *Adult:* IM 500-1000 U 3 × wk × 3 wk, then 2 × wk × 3 wk, or 4000 U 3 × wk × 6-9 mo, then 2000 U 3 × wk × 3 mo
Cryptorchidism
• *Child (boy 4-9 yr):* IM 5000 U qod × 4 doses
Available forms include: Powder for inj 200, 1000, 2000 U/ml
Side effects/adverse reactions:
CNS: Headache, depression, fatigue, anxiety, irritability
GU: Gynecomastia, early puberty, edema, ***ectopic pregnancy***
INTEG: Pain at injection site
Contraindications: Hypersensitiv-

ity, pituitary hypertrophy/tumor, early puberty, prostatic CA

Precautions: Asthma, migraine headache, convulsive disorders, cardiac disease, renal disease

Pharmacokinetics:

IM: Peak 6 hr, half-life 11-24 hr, excreted by kidneys

NURSING CONSIDERATIONS
Assess:

• Weight weekly; notify physician if weekly weight gain is >5 lb

• B/P before, during treatment

• Be alert for decreasing urinary output, increasing edema

Administer:

• Only after clomiphene citrate has been tried on anovulatory client

• After reconstitution with diluent enclosed in package

Perform/provide:

• Refrigeration for up to 2 mo

Evaluate:

• Edema, hypertension

Teach patient/family:

• To report facial, axillary, pubic hair, change in voice, penile enlargement, acne in male, abdominal pain, distention, vaginal bleeding in women

• To report symptoms of ectopic pregnancy: dizziness, pain on one side, shoulder, pallor, weak thready pulse, hemorrhage; shock may proceed rapidly

---

chymopapain

(kye'moe-pa-pane)
Chymodiactin, Discase
Func. class.: Enzyme
Chem. class.: Proteolytic

Action: Hydrolyzes noncollagenous polypeptides that maintain structure of chondromucoprotein; this activity decreases pressure on disk

Uses: Herniated lumbar intervertebral disk

Dosage and routes:

• *Adult:* INJ 2000-4000 U/disk injected intradiskally, not to exceed 10,000 U in a multiple herniation

Available forms include: Powder for inj 4000, 10,000 U/vial

Side effects/adverse reactions:

CNS: ***Paraplegia, cerebral hemorrhage,*** headache, dizziness, paresthesia, numbness of extremities

INTEG: Rash, urticaria, itching

GI: Nausea, paralytic ileus

*MS: Back pain, stiffness, spasm, **acute transverse myelitis,*** weakness, leg pain

SYSTEM: ***Anaphylaxis***

GU: Urinary retention

Contraindications: Hypersensitivity to this drug, papaya, meat tenderizer; severe spondylolisthesis; severe progressing paralysis; spinal cord tumor; cauda equina lesion, previous use

Precautions: Pregnancy, (C) children

Pharmacokinetics:

Onset 30 min, duration 24 hr

Interactions/incompatibilities:

• Dysrhythmias: halothane anesthetics plus epinephrine

NURSING CONSIDERATIONS
Assess:

• RBCs, ESR before treatment

• Respiratory rate, rhythm, depth; notify physician of abnormalities

• Anaphylaxis for several days after injection

• Neuro status after surgery; elimination status, since paralytic ileus can occur

Administer:

• Only with epinephrine available for anaphylaxis

• Only in lumbar spine by physician

• After diluting with sterile water

---

italics = common side effects   ***bold italic*** = life threatening reactions

for injection, use within 60 min
• After completing allergy test
(ChymoFAST)
Evaluate:
• Therapeutic response: absence of
back pain, increased mobility
• For allergies: iodine, papaya,
meat tenderizer; if allergies are
identified, drug should not be used
Teach patient/family
• To report allergic reactions that
have occurred up to 2 wk after in-
jection
• To be aware of possible infection;
redness, swelling, pain

---

chymotrypsin and mixtures

(kye'moe-trip-sen)
Avazyme, Chymoral, Orenzyme
Func. class.: Enzyme
Chem. class.: Proteolytic

Action: Unknown; may increase
tissue permeability in inflamed
areas, restores body fluids, frees
blood flow in inflamed area
Uses: Episiotomy pain
Dosage and routes:
• *Adult:* PO 20,000-40,000 U
(USP) qid
Available forms include: Tabs
20,000, 40,000 USP Units,
50,000, 100,000 Armour Units;
50,000, 100,000 USP Units
Side effects/adverse reactions:
HEMA: Bleeding
CNS: Chills, fever, dizziness
GU: Hematuria, albuminuria
GI: Nausea, diarrhea, vomiting, an-
orexia
INTEG: Rash, itching, urticaria
SYSTEM: Anaphylaxis
Contraindications: Hypersensitiv-
ity to this drug, trypsin; septicemia;
acute infection; hemophilia
Precautions: Severe renal disease,

severe hepatic disease, pregnancy
(C)
Interactions/incompatibilities:
• Increased effect of: anticoagu-
lants
NURSING CONSIDERATIONS
Evaluate:
• Therapeutic response: decreased
episiotomy pain
Teach patient/family
• To notify physician if bleeding
occurs
• That allergic reactions, nausea,
vomiting, diarrhea may occur

---

ciclopirox olamine (topical)

(sye-kloe-peer'ox)
Loprox
Func. class.: Local antiinfective
Chem. class.: Antifungal

Action: Interferes with fungal cell
membrane, which increases per-
meability, leaking of cell nutrients
Uses: Tinea cruris, tinea corporis,
tinea pedis, tinea versicolor, cuta-
neous candidiasis
Dosage and routes:
• *Adult and child >10 yr:* TOP rub
into affected area bid
Available forms include: Cream
1%
Side effects/adverse reactions:
INTEG: Rash, urticaria, stinging,
burning, pruritus, pain
Contraindications: Hypersensi-
tivity
Precautions: Pregnancy (B), lac-
tation, child <10 yr
NURSING CONSIDERATIONS
Administer:
• Enough medication to completely
cover lesions
• After cleansing with soap, water
before each application, dry well

Perform/provide:
• Storage at room temperature in dry place

Evaluate:
• Allergic reaction: burning, stinging, swelling, redness
• Therapeutic response: decrease in size, number of lesions

Teach patient/family:
• To apply with glove to prevent further infection
• To avoid use of OTC creams, ointments, lotions unless directed by physician
• To continue even though condition improves
• To use medical asepsis (hand washing) before, after each application
• Not to cover with occlusive dressing
• To change shoes and socks once a day during treatment of tinea pedis
• To notify physician if area shows signs of increased irritation

---

cimetidine

(sye-met′i-deen)

Tagamet

Func. class.: H₂ Histamine receptor antagonist

Chem. class.: Imidazole derivative

Action: Inhibits histamine at H₂ receptor site in parietal cells, which inhibits gastric acid secretion

Uses: Short-term treatment of duodenal and gastric ulcers and maintenance

Dosage and routes:
• *Adult and child: PO* 300 mg qid with meals, hs × 8 wk or 400 mg bid, 800 mg hs; after 8 wk give hs dose only; IV BOL 300 mg/20 ml 0.9% NaCl over 1-2 min q6h; IV INF 300 mg/50 ml D₅W over 15-20 min; IM 300 mg q6h, not to exceed 2400 mg

Prophylaxis of duodenal ulcer
• *Adult and child >16 yr:* 400 mg hs

Available forms include: Tabs 200, 300, 400, 800 mg; liq 300 mg/15 ml; inj IV 300 mg/2 ml, 300 mg/50 ml 0.9% NaCl

Side effects/adverse reactions:

CNS: Confusion, headache, depression, dizziness, anxiety, weakness, psychosis, tremors, *convulsions*

GI: Diarrhea, abdominal cramps, *paralytic ileus, jaundice*

GU: Gynecomastia, galactorrhea, impotence, increase in BUN, creatinine

CV: Bradycardia, tachycardia

HEMA: Agranulocytosis, thrombocytopenia, neutropenia, aplastic anemia, increase in pro-time

INTEG: Urticaria, rash, alopecia, sweating, flushing, *exfoliative dermatitis*

Contraindications: Hypersensitivity

Precautions: Pregnancy (B), lactation, child <16 yr, organic brain syndrome, hepatic disease, renal disease

Pharmacokinetics:

PO: Peak 1-1½ hr, half-life 1½ hr; metabolized by liver, excreted in urine (unchanged), crosses placenta, enters breast milk

Interactions/incompatibilities:
• Increased toxicity: anticoagulants, benzodiazepines, metoprolol, propranolol, phenytoins, quinidine, theophyllines, tricyclic antidepressants, lidocaine, procainamide
• Decreased absorption of cimetidine: antacids
• Decreased absorption: ketoconazole

---

italics = common side effects   ***bold italic*** = life threatening reactions

NURSING CONSIDERATIONS
Assess:
• Gastric pH (>5 should be maintained)
• I&O ratio, BUN, creatinine
Administer:
• IV after diluting 300 mg/20 ml of normal saline for inj; give over 2 min; may be diluted; 300 mg/50 ml of compatible sol run over 15-20 min
• With meals for prolonged drug effect
• Antacids 1 hr before or 1 hr after cimetidine
• IV slowly, bradycardia may occur, give over 30 min
Perform/provide:
• Storage of diluted solution at room temperature for up to 48 hr
Teach patient/family:
• That gynecomastia, impotence may occur, but is reversible
• Avoid driving or other hazardous activities until patient is stabilized on this medication
• To avoid black pepper, caffeine, alcohol, harsh spices, extremes in temperature of food
• To avoid OTC preparations: aspirin, cough, cold preparations
• That drug must be continued for prescribed time to be effective
• To report bruising, fatigue, malaise; blood dyscrasias may occur
Lab test interferences:
Increase: Alk phosphatase, AST, creatinine
False positive: Gastric bleeding test

---

cinoxacin

(sin-ox′a-sin)
Cinobac
Func. class.: Urinary tract antibacterial

Action: Interferes with conversion of intermediate DNA fragments into high-molecular-weight DNA in bacteria

Uses: Urinary tract infections caused by *E. coli, Klebsiella, Enterobacter, P. mirabilis, P. vulgaris, P. morgani, Serratia, Citrobacter*

Dosage and routes:
• *Adult and child >12 yr:* PO 1 g/day in 2-4 divided doses × 1-2 wk
Available forms include: Caps 250, 500 mg

Side effects/adverse reactions:
INTEG: Pruritus, rash, urticaria, photosensitivity, edema
CNS: Dizziness, headache, agitation, insomnia, confusion
GI: Nausea, vomiting, anorexia, abdominal cramps, diarrhea
EENT: Sensitivity to light, visual disturbances, blurred vision, tinnitus

Contraindications: Hypersensitivity to this drug, anuria, CNS damage

Precautions: Renal disease, hepatic disease, pregnancy (B), nursing mothers

Pharmacokinetics:
PO: Duration 6-8 hr, half-life 1½ hr, excreted in urine (unchanged/inactive metabolites)

Interactions/incompatibilities:
• Increased levels of cinoxacin: probenecid

NURSING CONSIDERATIONS
Assess:
• Kidney, liver function studies: BUN, creatinine, AST, ALT
• I&O ratio,-urine pH; <5.5 is ideal
Administer:
• After clean-catch urine is obtained for C&S
• Two daily doses if urine output is high or if patient has diabetes
Perform/provide:
• Limited intake of alkaline foods,

drugs: milk, dairy products, peanuts, vegetables, alkaline antacids, sodium bicarbonate

Evaluate:

• Therapeutic response: decreased pain, frequency, urgency, C&S absence of infection

• CNS symptoms: insomnia, vertigo, headache, agitation, confusion

• Allergic reactions: fever, flushing, rash, urticaria, pruritus

Teach patient/family:

• That photophobic reactions occur; that patient should avoid sunlight or use sunglasses, sunscreen

• Fluids must be increased to 3 L/day to avoid crystallization in kidneys

• If dizziness occurs, ambulate/activities with assistance

• Complete full course of drug therapy

• Contact physician if adverse reactions occur

• Take with food/milk to decrease GI irritation

Lab test interferences:

Increase: AST/ALT, BUN, creatinine, alk phosphatase

---

ciprofloxacin

(sip-ro-floks′a-sin)

Cipro

Func. class.: Urinary antiinfectives
Chem. class.: Fluoroquinolone antibacterial

Action: Interferes with conversion of intermediate DNA fragments into high-molecular-weight DNA in bacteria

Uses: Adult urinary tract infections (including complicated) caused by *E. coli, E. cloacae, P. mirabilis, K. pneumoniae, P. vulgans, C. freusdil,* group D strep

Dosage and routes:

Uncomplicated urinary tract infections

• *Adult:* PO 250 mg q12h

Complicated/severe urinary tract infections

• *Adult:* PO 500 mg q12h

Respiratory, bone, skin, joint infections

• *Adult:* PO 500 mg q12h

Available forms include: Tabs 250, 500, 750 mg

Side effects/adverse reactions:

CNS: Headache, dizziness, fatigue, insomnia, depression, restlessness
GI: Nausea, constipation, increased ALT, AST, flatulence, insomnia, heartburn, vomiting, diarrhea, oral candidiasis, dysphagia
INTEG: Rash, pruritus, urticaria, photosensitivity, flushing, fever, chills
MS: Blurred vision, tinnitus

Contraindications: Hypersensitivity to quinolones

Precautions: Pregnancy (C), lactation, children, renal disease

Pharmacokinetics:

PO: Peak 1 hr, half-life 3-4 hr; steady state 2 days; excreted in urine as active drug, metabolites

Interactions/incompatibilities:

• Decreased absorption: magnesium antacids, aluminum hydroxide

• Increased serum levels of ciprofloxacin: probenecid

• Increased theophylline levels when used with ciprofloxacin

NURSING CONSIDERATIONS

Assess:

• CNS symptoms: headache, dizziness, fatigue, insomnia, depression

• Kidney, liver function studies: BUN, creatinine, AST, ALT

• I&O ratio, urine pH <5.5 is ideal

Administer:

---

italics = common side effects   ***bold italic*** = life threatening reactions

• After clean-catch urine is obtained for C&S
• Two daily doses if urine output is high or if patient has diabetes
Perform/provide:
• Limited intake of alkaline foods, drugs: milk, dairy products, peanuts, vegetables, alkaline antacids, sodium bicarbonate
Evaluate:
• Therapeutic response: decreased pain, frequency, urgency, C&S—absence of infection
• Allergic reactions: fever, flushing, rash, urticaria, pruritus
Teach patient/family:
• Not to take antacids containing magnesium or aluminum with this drug or within 2 hr of drug
• That photosensitivity occurs; patient should avoid sunlight or use sunscreen to prevent burns
• Fluids must be increased to 3 L/day to avoid crystallization in kidneys
• If dizziness occurs, ambulate, perform activities with assistance
• Complete full course of drug therapy
• Contact physician if adverse reaction occurs
• Take with food, milk to decrease GI irritation
Lab test interferences:
Increase: AST, ALT, BUN, creatinine, alk phosphatase

---

cisplatin

(sis′pla-tin)
Platinol
Func. class.: Antineoplastic alkylating agent
Chem. class.: Inorganic heavy metal

Action: Alkylates DNA, RNA; inhibits enzymes that allow synthesis of amino acids in proteins
Uses: Advanced bladder cancer, adjunctive in metastatic testicular cancer, adjunctive in metastatic ovarian cancer, head, neck cancer, esophagus, prostate, lung and cervical cancer, lymphoma
Dosage and routes:
Testicular cancer
• *Adult:* IV 20 mg/m² qd × 5 days, repeat q3wk for 3 cycles or more, depending on response
Bladder cancer
• *Adult:* IV 50-70 mg/m² q3-4wk
Ovarian cancer
• *Adult:* IV 100 mg/m² q4wk or 50 mg/m² q3wk with doxorubicin therapy; mix with 2 L of NaCl and 37.5 g mannitol over 6 hr
Available forms include: Inj IV 10, 50 mg
Side effects/adverse reactions:
EENT: Tinnitus, hearing loss, vestibular toxicity
*HEMA: **Thrombocytopenia, leukopenia, pancytopenia***
CV: Cardiac abnormalities
GI: Severe nausea, vomiting, diarrhea, weight loss
*GU: **Renal tubular damage,** renal insufficiency, impotence, sterility, amenorrhea, gynecomastia, hyperuremia*
INTEG: Alopecia, dermatitis
*CNS: **Convulsions,** peripheral neuropathy*
*RESP: **Fibrosis***
META: Hypomagnesemia, hypocalcemia, hypokalemia, hypophosphatemia
*SYST: **Hypersensitivity reaction***
Contraindications: Radiation therapy within 1 mo, chemotherapy within 1 mo, thrombocytopenia, smallpox vaccination
Precautions: Pneumococcus vaccination, pregnancy (D)

---

*Available in Canada only

Pharmacokinetics:
Well absorbed orally, metabolized in liver, excreted in urine; half-life 2 hr

Interactions/incompatibilities:
• Increased toxicity: aminoglycosides
• Decreased effects of: phenytoin

NURSING CONSIDERATIONS

Assess:
• CBC, differential, platelet count weekly; withhold drug if WBC is <4000 or platelet count is <75,000; notify physician of results
• Renal function studies: BUN, creatinine, serum uric acid, urine CrCl before, electrolytes during therapy
• I&O ratio; report fall in urine output of 30 ml/hr
• Monitor temperature q4h (may indicate beginning infection)
• Liver function tests before, during therapy (bilirubin, AST, ALT, LDH) as needed or monthly

Administer:
• IV after diluting 10 mg/10 ml sterile H$_2$O for inj; IV INF is given over 5-6 hr; check site for irritation; phlebitis; do not use equipment containing aluminum
• Hydrate patient with 1-2 L of fluids over 8-12 hr before treatment
• Epinephrine for hypersensitivity reaction
• Antiemetic 30-60 min before giving drug to prevent vomiting, and PRN
• Allopurinol or sodium bicarbonate to maintain uric acid levels, alkalinization of urine
• Antibiotics for prophylaxis of infection
• Diuretic (furosemide 40 mg IV) or mannitol after infusion

Perform/provide:
• Strict medical asepsis, protective isolation if WBC levels are low
• Comprehensive oral hygiene
• Storage protected from light in refrigerator (dry powder)
• Deep breathing exercises with patient tid-qid; place in semi-Fowler's position
• Increase fluid intake to 2-3 L/day to prevent urate deposits, calculi formation, elimination of drug
• Diet low in purines: organ meats (kidney, liver), dried beans, peas to maintain alkaline urine

Evaluate:
• Bleeding: hematuria, guaiac, bruising or petechiae, mucosa or orifices q8h, obtain prescription for viscous xylocaine
• Dyspnea, rales, unproductive cough, chest pain, tachypnea
• Food preferences; list likes, dislikes
• Effects of alopecia on body image, discuss feelings about body changes
• Yellowing of skin, sclera, dark urine, clay-colored stools, itchy skin, abdominal pain, fever, diarrhea
• Edema in feet, joint pain, stomach pain, shaking
• Inflammation of mucosa, breaks in skin

Teach patient/family:
• To report signs of infection: increased temperature, sore throat, flu symptoms
• To report signs of anemia: fatigue, headache, faintness, shortness of breath, irritability
• To report bleeding: avoid use of razors or commercial mouthwash
• To avoid use of aspirin or ibuprofen
• Of protective isolation precautions
• To report any complaints or side effects to nurse or physician

---

italics = common side effects   ***bold italic*** = life threatening reactions

• That impotence or amenorrhea can occur, reversible after discontinuing treatment
• To report any changes in breathing or coughing
• That hair may be lost during treatment; a wig or hairpiece may make patient feel better; new hair may be different in color, texture

---

clemastine fumarate

(klem′as-teen)
Tavist, Tavist-1

Func. class.: Antihistamine
Chem. class.: Ethanolamine derivative, H_1-receptor antagonist

---

Action: Acts on blood vessels, GI, respiratory system by competing with histamine for H_1-receptor site; decreases allergic response by blocking histamine
Uses: Allergy symptoms, rhinitis, angioedema, urticaria
Dosage and routes:
• *Adult and child >12 yr:* PO 1.34-2.68 mg bid-tid, not to exceed 8.04 mg/day
Available forms include: Tabs 1.34, 2.68 mg; syr 0.67 mg/ml
Side effects/adverse reactions:
CNS: Dizziness, drowsiness, poor coordination, fatigue, anxiety, euphoria, confusion, paresthesia, neuritis
CV: Hypotension, palpitations, tachycardia
RESP: Increased thick secretions, wheezing, chest tightness
*HEMA: **Thrombocytopenia, agranulocytosis, hemolytic anemia***
GI: Constipation, dry mouth, nausea, vomiting, anorexia, diarrhea
INTEG: Rash, urticaria, photosensitivity
GU: Retention, dysuria, frequency
EENT: Blurred vision, dilated pupils, tinnitus, nasal stuffiness, dry nose, throat, mouth
Contraindications: Hypersensitivity to H_1-receptor antagonists, acute asthma attack, lower respiratory tract disease
Precautions: Increased intraocular pressure, renal disease, cardiac disease, hypertension, bronchial asthma, seizure disorder, stenosed peptic ulcers, hyperthyroidism, prostatic hypertrophy, bladder neck obstruction, pregnancy (B)
Pharmacokinetics:
PO: Peak 5-7 hr, duration 10-12 hr or more; metabolized in liver, excreted by kidneys
Interactions/incompatibilities:
• Increased CNS depression: barbiturates, narcotics, hypnotics, tricyclic antidepressants, alcohol
• Decreased effect of: oral anticoagulants, heparin
• Increased effect of clemastine: MAOIs

NURSING CONSIDERATIONS
Assess:
• I&O ratio; be alert for urinary retention, frequency, dysuria; drug should be discontinued if these occur
• CBC during long-term therapy
Administer:
• With meals if GI symptoms occur; absorption may slightly decrease
Perform/provide:
• Hard candy, gum, frequent rinsing of mouth for dryness
• Storage in tight container at room temperature
Evaluate:
• Therapeutic response: absence of running or congested nose or rashes
• Blood dyscrasias: thrombocytopenia, agranulocytosis (rare)
• Respiratory status: rate, rhythm,

increase in bronchial secretions, wheezing, chest tightness
• Cardiac status: palpitations, increased pulse, hypotension
Teach patient/family:
• All aspects of drug use; to notify physician if confusion, sedation, hypotension occurs
• To avoid driving or other hazardous activity if drowsiness occurs
• To avoid concurrent use of alcohol or other CNS depressants
• To change position slowly, as drug may cause dizziness, hypotension (elderly)
Lab test interferences:
False negative: Skin allergy tests
Treatment of overdose: Administer ipecac syrup or lavage, diazepam, vasopressors, barbiturates (short-acting)

---

clidinium bromide

(kli'di-nee-um)
Quarzan
Func. class.: Gastrointestinal anticholinergic
Chem. class.: Synthetic quaternary ammonium antimuscarinic

Action: Inhibits muscarinic actions of acetylcholine at postganglionic parasympathetic neuroeffector sites
Uses: Treatment of peptic ulcer disease in combination with other drugs
Dosage and routes:
• *Adult:* PO 2.5-5 mg tid-qid ac, hs
• *Elderly:* PO 2.5 mg tid ac
Available forms include: Caps 2.5, 5 mg
Side effects/adverse reactions:
CNS: Confusion, stimulation in elderly, headache, insomnia, dizziness, drowsiness, anxiety, weakness, hallucination
*GI: Dry mouth, constipation, par-**alytic ileus,** heartburn, nausea, vomiting, dysphagia, absence of taste
GU: Hesitancy, retention, impotence
CV: Palpitations, tachycardia
EENT: Blurred vision, photophobia, mydriasis, cycloplegia, increased ocular tension
INTEG: Urticaria, rash, pruritus, anhidrosis, fever, allergic reactions
Contraindications: Hypersensitivity to anticholinergics, narrow-angle glaucoma, GI obstruction, myasthenia gravis, paralytic ileus, GI atony, toxic megacolon
Precautions: Hyperthyroidism, coronary artery disease, dysrhythmias, CHF, ulcerative colitis, hypertension, hiatal hernia, hepatic disease, renal disease, pregnancy (C), urinary retention, prostatic hypertrophy
Pharmacokinetics:
PO: Onset 1 hr, duration 3 hr; ionized, excreted in urine
Interactions/incompatibilities:
• Increased anticholinergic effect: amantadine, tricyclic antidepressants, MAOIs
• Decreased effect of: phenothiazines, levodopa, ketoconazole
NURSING CONSIDERATIONS
Assess:
• VS, cardiac status: checking for dysrhythmias, increased rate, palpitations
• I&O ratio; check for urinary retention or hesitancy
Administer:
• ½-1 hr ac for better absorption
• Decreased dose to elderly patients since their metabolism may be slowed
• Gum, hard candy, frequent rinsing of mouth for dryness of oral cavity

---

italics = common side effects   ***bold italic*** = life threatening reactions

Perform/provide:
• Storage in tight container protected from light
• Increased fluids, bulk, exercise to patient's lifestyle to decrease constipation

Evaluate:
• Therapeutic response: absence of epigastric pain, bleeding, nausea, vomiting
• GI complaints: pain, bleeding (frank or occult), nausea, vomiting, anorexia

Teach patient/family:
• Avoid driving or other hazardous activities until stabilized on medication
• Avoid alcohol or other CNS depressants; will enhance sedating properties of this drug
• To avoid hot environments, stroke may occur, drug suppresses perspiration
• Use sunglasses when outside to prevent photophobia, may cause blurred vision
• Drink plenty of fluids
• To report dysphagia

---

clindamycin HCl/clindamycin palmitate HCl/clindamycin phosphate

(klin-da-mye′sin)
Cleocin, Dalacin C*

Func. class.: Antibacterial macrolide

Chem. class.: Lincomycin derivative

Action: Binds to 50S subunit of bacterial ribosomes, suppresses protein synthesis

Uses: Infections caused by staphylococci, streptococci, pneumococci, *Rickettsia, Fusobacterium, Actinomyces, Peptococcus, Clostridium*

Dosage and routes:
• *Adults:* PO 150-450 mg q6h; IM/IV 300 mg q6-12h, not to exceed 4800 mg/day
• *Child >1 mo:* PO 8-25 mg/kg/day in divided doses q6-8h; IM/IV 15-40 mg/kg/day in divided doses q6-8h

Available forms include: Inj 150 mg/ml; caps 75, 150 mg; oral sol 75 mg/ml

Side effects/adverse reactions:
HEMA: **Leukopenia, eosinophilia, agranulocytosis, thrombocytopenia**
*GI: Nausea, vomiting, abdominal pain, diarrhea, **Pseudomembranous colitis***
GU: Increased AST, ALT, bilirubin, alk phosphatase, jaundice, *vaginitis,* urinary frequency
EENT: Rash, urticaria, pruritus, erythema, pain, abscess at injection site

Contraindications: Hypersensitivity to this drug or lincomycin, ulcerative colitis/enteritis, infants <1 mo

Precautions: Renal disease, liver disease, GI disease, elderly, pregnancy (B), lactation, tartrazine sensitivity

Pharmacokinetics:
PO: Peak 45 min, duration 6 hr
IM: Peak 3 hr, duration 8-12 hr
Half-life 2½ hr, metabolized in liver, excreted in urine, bile, feces as active/inactive metabolites, crosses placenta, excreted in breast milk

Interactions/incompatibilities:
• Increased neuromuscular blockage: nondepolarizing muscle relaxants
• Decreased action of: chloramphenicol, erythromycin

NURSING CONSIDERATIONS
Assess:
• Any patient with compromised

renal system; drug is excreted slowly in poor renal system function; toxicity may occur rapidly

• Liver studies: AST, ALT

• Blood studies: WBC, RBC, Hct, Hgb, platelets, serum iron, reticulocytes; drug should be discontinued if bone marrow depression occurs

• Renal studies: urinalysis, protein, blood, BUN, creatinine

• C&S before drug therapy; drug may be taken as soon as culture is taken

• Drug level in impaired hepatic, renal systems

• B/P, pulse in patient receiving drug parenterally

Administer:

• IV by infusion only; do not administer bolus dose, dilute 300 mg/50 ml of compatible sol; run over >10 min; no more than 1200 mg in a single 1-hr INF

• IM deep injection; rotate sites

• Orally with at least 8 oz water

Perform/provide:

• Storage at room temperature (capsules) and up to 2 wk (reconstituted solution)

• Adrenalin, suction, tracheostomy set, endotracheal intubation equipment on unit

• Adequate intake of fluids (2000 ml) during diarrhea episodes

Evaluate:

• Therapeutic response: decreased temperature, negative C&S

• Bowel pattern before, during treatment

• Skin eruptions, itching, dermatitis after administration

• Respiratory status: rate, character, wheezing, tightness in chest

• Allergies before treatment, reaction of each medication; place allergies on chart, Kardex in bright red letters; notify all people giving drugs

Teach patient/family:

• To take oral drug with full glass of water; may give with food if GI symptoms occur

• Aspects of drug therapy: need to complete entire course of medication to ensure organism death (10-14 days); culture may be taken after completed medication course

• To report sore throat, fever, fatigue; could indicate superimposed infection

• That drug must be taken in equal intervals around clock to maintain blood levels

• To notify nurse of diarrhea

Lab test interferences:

Increase: Alk phosphatase, bilirubin, CPK, AST, ALT

Treatment of hypersensitivity: Withdraw drug, maintain airway, administer epinephrine, aminophylline, O_2, IV corticosteroids

---

clioquinol (iodochlorhydroxyquin)

(klee-oh-kwee′nole)

Quin III, Torofor, Vioform

Func. class.: Local antiinfective

Chem. class.: Halogenated hydroxyquinoline

Action: Increases cell membrane permeability is susceptible organisms by binding sterols; decreases potassium, sodium, and nutrients in cell

Uses: Cutaneous infections: athlete's foot, eczema, and other fungal infections

Dosage and routes:

TOP: apply to affected area bid or tid ×7 days only

Available forms include: cream, oint 3%

---

italics = common side effects   ***bold italic*** = life threatening reactions

Side effects/adverse reactions:
INTEG: Rash, urticaria, stinging, burning, dry skin, pruritus, contact dermatitis, erythema, redness, staining of hair and skin
Contraindications: Hypersensitivity to iodine, chloroxine
Precautions: Pregnancy (C), varicella, viral skin conditions, deep or puncture wounds, serious burns
Pharmacokinetics:
Some absorbed through the skin, excreted in urine (conjugated form), the rest excreted slowly
NURSING CONSIDERATIONS
Administer:
• Enough medication to completely cover lesions
• After cleansing with soap and water before each application, dry well
Perform/provide:
• Storage at room temperature in dry place
Evaluate:
• Allergic reaction: burning, stinging, swelling, redness
• Therapeutic response: decrease in size, number of lesions
Teach patient/family:
• To avoid use of OTC creams, ointments, lotions unless directed by physician
• To use medical asepsis (hand washing) before, after each application to prevent further infection
• Not to cover with occlusive dressing
• To continue even if condition improves
• That drug may stain clothing, skin, hair
Lab test interference:
Interference: Thyroid function tests

clobetasol propionate
(klo-bet′-a-sol)
Temovate
Func. class.: Topical corticosteroid
Chem. class.: Synthetic fluorinated agent, group I potency

Action: Possesses antipruritic, antiinflammatory actions
Uses: Psoriasis, eczema, contact dermatitis, pruritus; usually reserved for severe dermatoses that have not responded to less potent formulation
Dosage and routes:
• *Adult and child:* Apply to affected area bid
Available forms include: Oint 0.05%; cream 0.05%
Side effects/adverse reactions:
INTEG: Burning, dryness, itching, irritation, acne, folliculitis, hypertrichosis, perioral dermatitis, hypopigmentation, atrophy, striae, miliaria, allergic contact dermatitis, secondary infection
Contraindications: Hypersensitivity to corticosteroids, fungal infections
Precautions: Pregnancy (C), lactation, viral infections, bacterial infections
NURSING CONSIDERATIONS
Assess:
• Temperature, if fever develops, drug should be discontinued
Administer:
• Only to affected areas; do not get in eyes
• Leaving uncovered or lightly covered, occlusive dressing is not recommended, systemic absorption may occur
• Only to dermatoses; do not use on weeping, denuded, or infected area
Perform/provide:
• Cleansing before application of drug

---

* Available in Canada only

- Treatment for a few days after area has cleared
- Storage at room temperature

Evaluate:
- Therapeutic response: absence of severe itching, patches on skin, flaking
- For systemic absorption: increased temperature, inflammation, irritation

Teach patient/family:
- To avoid sunlight on affected area; burns may occur
- To limit treatment to 14 days using <50 g/wk

---

clocortolone pivalate

(klo-kort'-oo-lone)
Cloderm
Func. class.: Topical corticosteroid
Chem. class.: Synthetic fluorinated agent, group IV potency

Action: Possesses antipruritic, antiinflammatory actions
Uses: Psoriasis, eczema, contact dermatitis, pruritus
Dosage and routes:
- *Adult and child:* Apply to affected area tid or qid
Available forms include: Cream 0.1%
Side effects/adverse reactions:
INTEG: Burning, dryness, itching, irritation, acne, folliculitis, hypertrichosis, perioral dermatitis, hypopigmentation, atrophy, striae, miliaria, allergic contact dermatitis, secondary infection
Contraindications: Hypersensitivity to corticosteroids, fungal infections
Precautions: Pregnancy (C), lactation, viral infections, bacterial infections

NURSING CONSIDERATIONS
Assess:
- Temperature; if fever develops, drug should be discontinued

Administer:
- Only to affected areas; do not get in eyes
- Medication, then cover with occlusive dressing (only if prescribed), seal to normal skin, change q12h, systemic absorption may occur
- Only to dermatoses; do not use on weeping, denuded, or infected area

Perform/provide:
- Cleansing before application of drug
- Treatment for a few days after area has cleared
- Storage at room temperature

Evaluate:
- Therapeutic response: absence of severe itching, patches on skin, flaking
- For systemic absorption: increased temperature, inflammation, irritation

Teach patient/family:
- To avoid sunlight on affected area; burns may occur

---

clofazimine

(kloe-faaz'-ii-meen)
Lamprene
Func. class.: Leprostatic

Action: Inhibits mycobacterial growth, binds to mycobacterial DNA; exerts antiinflammatory properties in controlling leprosy reactions
Uses: Lepromatous leprosy, dapsone-resistant leprosy, lepromatous leprosy complicated by erythema nodosum leprosum
Dosage and routes:
Erythema nodosum leprosum

---

italics = common side effects   ***bold italic*** = life threatening reactions

• *Adult:* PO: 100-200 mg qd × 3 mo, then taper dosage to 100 mg when disease is controlled, do not exceed 200 mg/day

Dapsone-resistant leprosy

• *Adult:* PO: 100 mg/day in combination with at least one other antileprosy drug × 3 yr, then 100 mg qd clofazimine (only)

Available forms include: Caps 50, 100 mg

Side effects/adverse reactions:

GI: Diarrhea, nausea, vomiting, abdominal pain, intolerance, **GI bleeding, obstruction,** anorexia, constipation, **hepatitis,** jaundice

EENT: Pigmentation of cornea, conjunctive, drying, burning, itching, irritation

INTEG: Pink or brown discoloration, dryness, pruritus, rash, photosensitivity, acne, monilial cheilosis

CNS: Dizziness, headache, fatigue, drowsiness

Precautions: Pregnancy (C), lactation, children, abdominal pain, diarrhea, depression

Pharmacokinetics:

Deposited in fatty tissue, reticuloendothelial system; half-life 70 days, small amount excreted in feces, sputum, sweat

NURSING CONSIDERATIONS

Assess:

• Liver studies q wk: ALT, AST, bilirubin

• Renal studies: BUN, creatinine, I&O, sp gr, urinalysis before; q mo

• Blood level of drug

Administer:

• With meals to decrease GI symptoms

• Antiemetic if vomiting occurs

• After C&S is completed; q mo to detect resistance

Perform/provide:

• Infants to be kept with mother infected with leprosy; breastfeeding during drug therapy is encouraged

Evaluate:

• Mental status often: affect, mood, behavioral changes; psychosis may occur

• Hepatic status: decreased appetite, jaundice, dark urine, fatigue

Teach patient/family:

• That therapeutic effects may occur after 3-6 mo of drug therapy

• That compliance with dosage schedule, length is necessary

• That scheduled appointments must be kept or relapse may occur

• That drug must be taken with meals

• Skin discoloration, although reversible, may take several months or years to disappear

Lab test interferences:

Increase: Albumin, bilirubin, AST, eosinophilia, hypokalemia

---

clofibrate

(kloe-fye'brate)

Atromide-S, Claripen,* Claripex*

Func. class.: Antilipemic

Chem. class.: Aryloxisobutyric acid derivative

Action: Inhibits biosynthesis of VLDL, LDL, which are responsible for triglyceride development, mobilizes triglycerides from tissue, increases excretion of neutral sterols

Uses: Hyperlipidemia, xanthoma tuberosum, type III, IV, V hyperlipidemia

Dosage and routes:

• *Adult:* PO 2 g/day in 4 divided doses

Available forms include: Caps 500 mg

Side effects/adverse reactions:

GI: Nausea, vomiting, dyspepsia, increased liver enzymes, stomatitis, flatulence, hepatomegaly, gastritis, increased cholelithiasis, weight gain

INTEG: Rash, urticaria, pruritus, dry hair and skin, alopecia

*HEMA: **Leukopenia,*** anemia, ***eosinophilia,*** bleeding

CNS: Fatigue, weakness, drowsiness, dizziness

GU: Decreased libido, impotence, dysuria, proteinuria, oliguria, ***hematuria***

MS: Myalgias, arthralgias

CV: Angina, dysrhythmias, thrombophlebitis, ***pulmonary emboli***

MISC: Polyphagia, weight gain

Contraindications: Severe hepatic disease, severe renal disease, primary biliary cirrhosis

Precautions: Peptic ulcer, pregnancy (C), lactation

Pharmacokinetics:

PO: Peak 2-6 hr, plasma protein binding >90%; half-life 6-25 hr, excreted in urine, metabolized in liver

Interactions/incompatibilities:

• Increased effects of: sulfonylureas, insulin

• Increased toxicity of clofibrate: probenecid

• Increased anticoagulant effects of: oral anticoagulants

• Decreased effects of clofibrate: rifampin

NURSING CONSIDERATIONS

Assess:

• Renal and hepatic levels if patient is on long-term therapy

Administer:

• Drug with meals if GI symptoms occur

Evaluate:

• Therapeutic response: decreased triglycerides, diarrhea, pruritus (excess bile area)

• Bowel pattern daily; increase bulk, water in diet if constipation develops

Teach patient/family:

• That patient compliance is needed since toxicity may result if doses are missed

• That risk factors should be decreased: high fat diet, smoking, alcohol consumption, absence of exercise

• Birth control should be practiced while on this drug

• To report GU symptoms: decreased libido, impotence, dysuria, proteinuria, oliguria, hematuria

Lab test interferences:

Increase: Liver function studies, CPK, BSP, thymol turbidity

---

clomiphene citrate

(kloe′mi-feen)

Clomid, Serophene

Func. class.: Ovulation stimulant

Chem. class.: Nonsteroidal antiestrogenic

Action: Increases LH, FSH release from the pituitary, which increase maturation of ovarian follicle, ovulation, development of corpus luteum

Uses: Female infertility

Dosage and routes:

• *Adult:* PO 50-100 mg qd × 5 days or 50-100 mg qd beginning on day 5 of cycle; may be repeated until conception occurs or 3 cycles of therapy have been completed

Available forms include: Tabs 50 mg

Side effects/adverse reactions:

EENT: Blurred vision, diplopia, photophobia

CNS: Headache, depression, rest-

---

italics = common side effects　　　***bold italic*** = life threatening reactions

lessness, anxiety, nervousness, fatigue, insomnia, dizziness, flushing
GI: Nausea, vomiting, constipation, abdominal pain, bloating
INTEG: Rash, dermatitis, urticaria, alopecia
GU: Polyuria, frequency, birth defects, spontaneous abortions, multiple ovulation, breast pain, oliguria, abnormal uterine bleeding
Contraindications: Hypersensitivity, pregnancy (X), hepatic disease, undiagnosed vaginal bleeding
Precautions: Hypertension, depression, convulsions, diabetes mellitus
Pharmacokinetics: Metabolized in liver, excreted in feces
NURSING CONSIDERATIONS
Administer:
• After discontinuing estrogen therapy
• At same time qd to maintain drug level
Teach patient/family:
• Multiple births are common after drug is taken
• To notify physician if low abdominal pain occurs; may indicate ovarian cyst, cyst rupture
• If dose is missed, double at next time; if more than one dose is missed call MD
• Response usually occurs 4-10 days after last day of treatment
• Method for taking, recording basal body temperature to determine whether ovulation has occurred
• If ovulation can be determined (there is a slight decrease in temperature then a sharp increase for ovulation) to attempt coitus 3 days before and qod until after ovulation
• If pregnancy is suspected, physician must be notified immediately
Lab test interferences:
Increase: FSH/LH, BSP, thyroxine, TBG

clomipramine

(klom-ip′ra-meen)
Anafranil
Func. class.: Tricyclic antidepressant
Chem. class.: Tertiary amine

Action: Not known. Potent inhibitor of serotonin uptake, also increases dopamine metabolism
Uses: Depression, dysphoria, phobias, anxiety, agoraphobia, obsessive-compulsive disorder
Dosage and routes:
Obsessive-compulsive disorder
• *Adult:* PO 25 mg hs and increase gradually over 4 wk to a dose of 75-300 mg/day in divided doses
• *Child (10-18 yr):* PO 50 mg/day gradually increased; not to exceed 200 mg/day
Depression
• *Adult:* PO 50-150 mg/day in a single or divided dose
Anxiety/agoraphobia
• *Adult:* PO 25-75 mg/day
Available forms include: Caps 25, 50, 75 mg
Side effects/adverse reactions:
HEMA: Agranulocytosis, neutropenia, pancytopenia
CV: Hypotension, tachycardia, *cardiac arrest*
CNS: Dizziness, tremors, mania, seizures, aggressiveness
ENDO: Galactorrhea, hyperprolactinemia
META: Hyponatremia
GI: Constipation, dry mouth
GU: Delayed ejaculation, anorgasmia, retention
INTEG: Diaphoresis
Contraindications: Pregnancy, hypersensitivity
Precautions: Seizures, suicidal patients

Pharmacokinetics: Extensively bound to tissue and plasma proteins, demethylated in liver (active metabolites), excreted in urine (metabolites); half-life: 21 hr parent compound, 36 hr metabolite

Interactions/incompatibilities:

• Hypotensive antagonism: bethanidine

• Toxicity: phenothiazines, cimetidine

• Ethanol reaction: disulfiram, guanadrel increased or decreased effects

• Increased or decreased effects of clomipramine: estrogens

• Delirium: ethchlorvynol

• Hypertensive crisis, convulsions, hypertensive episode: MAOIs

• Decreased seizure threshold: phenytoin, phenobarbital

NURSING CONSIDERATIONS
Assess:

• B/P (lying, standing), pulse q4h; if systolic B/P drops 20 mm Hg withhold drug, notify physician; take vital signs q4h in patients with cardiovascular disease

• Blood studies: CBC, leukocytes, differential, cardiac enzymes if patient is receiving long-term therapy

• Hepatic studies: AST, ALT, bilirubin, creatinine

Administer:

• Increased fluids, bulk in diet if constipation, urinary retention occur

• With food or milk for GI symptoms

• Gum, hard candy, or frequent sips of water for dry mouth

Perform/provide:

• Storage in tight container at room temperature, do not freeze

• Assistance with ambulation during beginning therapy since drowsiness/dizziness occurs

• Safety measures, including side rails, primarily in elderly

• Checking to see PO medication swallowed

Evaluate:

• Mental status: mood, sensorium, affect, suicidal tendencies; increase in psychiatric symptoms: depression, panic

• Urinary retention, constipation; constipation is more likely to occur in children

• Withdrawal symptoms: headache, nausea, vomiting, muscle pain, weakness; do not usually occur unless drug is discontinued abruptly

• Alcohol consumption; if alcohol is consumed, withhold dose until morning

Teach patient/family:

• That the effects may take 2-3 wk

• Use caution in driving or other activities requiring alertness because of drowsiness, dizziness, blurred vision

• To avoid alcohol ingestion, other CNS depressants

• Not to discontinue medication quickly after long-term use, may cause nausea, headache, malaise

Lab test interferences:

Increase: Prolactin, TBG

Decrease: Serum thryoid hormone

Treatment of overdose: ECG monitoring, induce emesis, lavage, activated charcoal, administer anticonvulsant

---

clonazepam

(kloe-na'zi-pam)
Klonopin, Rivotril

Func. class.: Anticonvulsant
Chem. class.: Benzodiazapine derivative

Controlled Substance Schedule IV

Action: Inhibits spike, wave formation in absence seizures (petit mal), decreases amplitude, frequency, duration, spread of discharge in minor motor seizures

Uses: Absence, atypical absence, akinetic, myoclonic seizures

Dosage and routes:
• *Adult:* PO Not to exceed 1.5 mg/ day in 3 divided doses; may be increased 0.5-1 mg q3 days until desired response, not to exceed 20 mg/day
• *Child <10 yr or 30 kg:* PO 0.01-0.03 mg/kg/day in divided doses q8h, not to exceed 0.05 mg/kg/ day; may be increased 0.25-0.5 mg q3 days until desired response, not to exceed 0.1-0.2 mg/kg/day

Available forms include: Tabs 0.5, 1, 2 mg

Side effects/adverse reactions:
*HEMA: **Thrombocytopenia, leukocytosis, eosinophilia***
CNS: Drowsiness, dizziness, confusion, behavioral changes, tremors, insomnia, headache, suicidal tendencies, slurred speech
GI: Nausea, constipation, polyphagia, anorexia, xerostomia, diarrhea, gastritis, sore gums
INTEG: Rash, alopecia, hirsutism
EENT: Increased salivation, nystagmus, diplopia, abnormal eye movements
*RESP: **Respiratory depression,*** dyspnea, congestion
CV: Palpitations, bradycardia
GU: Dysuria, enuresis, nocturia, retention

Contraindications: Hypersensitivity to benzodiazepines, acute narrow-angle glaucoma

Precautions: Open-angle glaucoma, chronic respiratory disease, pregnancy (C), renal, hepatic disease, elderly

Pharmacokinetics:
PO: Peak 1-2 hr, metabolized by liver, excreted in urine, half-life 18-50 hr

Interactions/incompatibilities:
• Increased CNS depression: alcohol, barbiturates, narcotics, antidepressants, other anticonvulsants
• Decreased effect of: carbamazepine
• Seizures: valproic acid

NURSING CONSIDERATIONS
Assess:
• Renal studies: urinalysis, BUN, urine creatinine
• Blood studies: RBC, Hct, Hgb, reticulocyte counts q wk for 4 wk then q mo
• Hepatic studies: ALT, AST, bilirubin, creatinine
• Drug levels during initial treatment

Administer:
• With food, milk to decrease GI symptoms

Perform/provide:
• Storage at room temperature
• Hard candy, frequent rinsing of mouth, gum for dry mouth
• Assistance with ambulation during early part of treatment; dizziness occurs

Evaluate:
• Therapeutic response: decreased seizure activity, document on patient's chart
• Mental status: mood, sensorium, affect, oversedation, behavioral changes; if mental status changes, notify physician
• Eye problems: need for ophthalmic examinations before, during, after treatment (slit lamp, fundoscopy, tonometry)
• Allergic reaction: red raised rash; if this occurs, drug should be discontinued

---

*Available in Canada only

• Blood dyscrasias: fever, sore throat, bruising, rash, jaundice
• Toxicity: bone marrow depression, nausea, vomiting, ataxia, diplopia, cardiovascular collapse

Teach patient/family:
• To carry ID card to Medic-Alert bracelet stating drugs taken, condition, physician's name, phone number
• To avoid driving, other activities that require alertness
• To avoid alcohol ingestion or CNS depressants, increased sedation may occur
• Not to discontinue medication quickly after long-term use; taper off over several weeks

Lab test interferences:
Increase: AST, alk phosphatase

Treatment of overdose: Lavage, activated charcoal, monitor electrolytes, VS, administer vasopressors

---

clonidine HCl

(kloe′ni-deen)
Catapres, Dixarit*

Func. class.: Antihypertensive
Chem. class.: Central α-adrenergic agonist

Action: Inhibits sympathetic vasomotor center in CNS, which reduces impulses in sympathetic nervous system; blood pressure decreases, pulse rate, cardiac output decreases

Uses: Hypertension

Dosage and routes:
Hypertension
• *Adult:* PO/TRANS 0.1 mg bid, then increase by 0.1 mg/day or 0.2 mg/day until desired response; range 0.2-0.8 mg/day in divided doses

Available forms include: Tabs 0.1, 0.2, 0.3 mg; trans sys 2.5, 5, 7.5

mg delivering 0.1, 0.2, 0.3 mg/24 hr respectively

Side effects/adverse reactions:
CV: Orthostatic hypotension, palpitations, CHF, ECG abnormalities
CNS: Drowsiness, sedation, headache, fatigue, nightmares, insomnia, mental changes, anxiety, depression, hallucinations, delirium
GI: Nausea, vomiting, malaise, constipation, dry mouth
INTEG: Rash, alopecia, facial pallor, pruritus, hives, edema, burning papules, excoriation (transdermal patches)
EENT: Taste change, parotid pain
ENDO: Hyperglycemia
MS: Muscle/joint pain, leg cramps
GU: Impotence, dysuria, *nocturia,* gynecomastia

Contraindications: Hypersensitivity

Precautions: MI (recent), diabetes mellitus, chronic renal failure, Raynaud's disease, thyroid disease, depression, COPD, child <12 (patches), asthma, pregnancy (C), lactation

Pharmacokinetics:
PO: Peak 3-5 hr; half-life 12-16 hr, metabolized by liver (metabolites), excreted in urine (unchanged, inactive metabolites, feces), crosses blood-brain barrier, excreted in breast milk

Interactions/incompatibilities:
• Increased CNS depression: narcotics, sedatives, alcohol, anesthetics
• Decreased hypotensive effects: tricyclic antidepressants, MAOIs, appetite suppressants, other antihypertensives
• Increased hypotensive effects: diuretics

---

italics = common side effects   ***bold italic*** = life threatening reactions

• Increased bradycardia: β-blockers, cardiac glycosides

NURSING CONSIDERATIONS
Assess:

• Blood studies: neutrophils, decreased platelets

• Renal studies: protein, BUN, creatinine; watch for increased levels that may indicate nephrotic syndrome

• Baselines in renal, liver function tests before therapy begins

• K levels, although hyperkalemia rarely occurs

• Dip-stick of urine for protein qd in first morning specimen, if protein is increased, a 24 hr urinary protein should be collected

Administer:

• IV infusion of 0.9% NaCl (as ordered) to expand fluid volume if severe hypotension occurs

• SL if patient is unable to swallow

Perform/provide:

• Storage of patches in cool environment, tablets in tight containers

Evaluate:

• Therapeutic response: decrease in B/P in hypertension

• Edema in feet, legs daily

• Allergic reaction: rash, fever, pruritus, urticaria; drug should be discontinued if antihistamines fail to help

• Allergic reaction from patches: rash, urticaria, angioedema; should not continue to use

• Symptoms of CHF: edema, dyspnea, wet rales, B/P

• Renal symptoms: polyuria, oliguria, frequency

• For retinal degeneration: periodic eye exam

Teach patient/family:

• To avoid hazardous activities, may cause drowsiness

• Administer 1 hr before meals

• Not to discontinue drug abruptly

or withdrawal symptoms may occur: anxiety, increased B/P, headache, insomnia, increased pulse, tremors, nausea, sweating

• Not to use OTC (cough, cold, or allergy) products unless directed by physician

• Tell patient to avoid sunlight or wear sunscreen if in sunlight, photosensitivity may occur

• Stress patient compliance with dosage schedule even if feeling better

• To rise slowly to sitting or standing position to minimize orthostatic hypotension

• Notify physician of: mouth sores, sore throat, fever, swelling of hands or feet, irregular heartbeat, chest pain, signs of angioedema

• Excessive perspiration, dehydration, vomiting; diarrhea may lead to fall in blood pressure—consult physician if these occur

• May cause dizziness, fainting; light-headedness may occur during 1st few days of therapy

• May cause dry mouth, use hard candy, saliva product

• That compliance is necessary, not to skip or stop drug unless directed by physician

• May cause skin rash or impaired perspiration

• That response may take 2-3 days to occur if drug is given transdermally

Lab test interferences:

Increase: Blood glucose

Decrease: VMA, catecholamines, aldosterone

Treatment of overdose: Supportive treatment, administer tolazdine, atropine, dopamine prn

---

* Available in Canada only

clorazepate dipotassium

(klor-az'e-pate)
Tranxene
Func. class.: Antianxiety
Chem. class.: Benzodiazepine

Controlled Substance Schedule IV

Action: Depresses subcortical levels of CNS, including limbic system, reticular formation

Uses: Anxiety, acute alcohol withdrawal, adjunct in seizure disorders

Dosage and routes:

Anxiety
• *Adult:* PO 15-60 mg/day

Alcohol withdrawal
• *Adult:* PO 30 mg then 30-60 mg in divided doses; day 2, 45-90 mg in divided doses; day 3, 22.5-45 mg in divided doses; day 4, 15-30 mg in divided doses; then reduce daily dose to 7.5-15 mg

Seizure disorders
• *Adult and child >12 yr:* PO 7.5 mg tid, may increase by 7.5 mg/wk or less, not to exceed 90 mg/day
• *Child 9-12 yr:* PO 7.5 mg bid, may increase by 7.5 mg/wk or less, not to exceed 60 mg/day

Available forms include: Caps 3.75, 7.5, 15 mg; tabs 3.75, 7.5, 15 mg, single dose tab 11.25, 22.5 mg

Side effects/adverse reactions:

CNS: Dizziness, drowsiness, confusion, headache, anxiety, tremors, stimulation, fatigue, depression, insomnia, hallucinations
GI: Constipation, dry mouth, nausea, vomiting, anorexia, diarrhea
INTEG: Rash, dermatitis, itching
CV: Orthostatic hypotension, ECG changes, tachycardia, hypotension
EENT: Blurred vision, tinnitus, mydriasis

Contraindications: Hypersensitivity to benzodiazepines, narrow-angle glaucoma, psychosis, pregnancy (D), child <18 yr

Precautions: Elderly, debilitated, hepatic disease, renal disease

Pharmacokinetics:

PO: Onset 15 min, peak 1-2 hr, duration 4-6 hr, metabolized by liver, excreted by kidneys, crosses placenta, breast milk, half-life 30-100 hr

Interactions/incompatibilities:

• Decreased effects of clorazepate: valproic acid
• Increased effects of clorazepate: CNS depressants, alcohol, disulfiram, oral contraceptives, antidepressants, MAOIs

NURSING CONSIDERATIONS

Assess:

• B/P (lying, standing), pulse; if systolic B/P drops 20 mm Hg, hold drug, notify physician
• Blood studies: CBC during long-term therapy, blood dyscrasias have occurred rarely
• Hepatic studies: AST, ALT, bilirubin, creatinine, LDH, alk phosphatase
• I&O; may indicate renal dysfunction

Administer:

• With food or milk for GI symptoms
• Crushed if patient is unable to swallow medication whole
• Sugarless gum, hard candy, frequent sips of water for dry mouth

Perform/provide:

• Assistance with ambulation during beginning therapy, since drowsiness/dizziness occurs
• Safety measures, including siderails
• Check to see PO medication has been swallowed

---

italics = common side effects   ***bold italic*** = life threatening reactions

Evaluate:
• Therapeutic response: decreased anxiety, restlessness, insomnia
• Mental status: mood, sensorium, affect, sleeping pattern, drowsiness, dizziness
• Physical dependency, withdrawal symptoms: headache, nausea, vomiting, muscle pain, weakness after long-term use
• Suicidal tendencies

Teach patient/family:
• That drug may be taken with food
• Not to be used for everyday stress or used longer than 4 mo, unless directed by physician; not to take more than prescribed amount, may be habit forming
• Avoid OTC preparations unless approved by physician
• To avoid driving, activities that require alertness; drowsiness may occur
• To avoid alcohol ingestion or other psychotropic medications, unless prescribed by physician
• Not to discontinue medication abruptly after long-term use
• To rise slowly or fainting may occur
• That drowsiness might worsen at beginning of treatment

Lab test interferences:
Increase: AST/ALT, serum bilirubin
Decrease: RAIU
False increase: 17-OHCS

Treatment of overdose: Lavage, VS, supportive care

---

clotrimazole

(kloe-trim′a-zole)
Canesten,* Gyne-Lotrimin, Mycelex, Mycelex-G
Func. class.: Local antiinfective
Chem. class.: Imidazole derivative

Action: Interferes with fungal DNA replication; binds sterols in fungal cell membrane, which increases permeability, leaking of cell nutrients

Uses: Tinea pedis, tinea cruris, tinea corporis, tinea versicolor, *Candida albicans* infection of the vagina, vulva, throat, mouth

Dosage and routes:
• *Adult and child:* TOP rub into affected area bid × 1-8 wk; LOZ dissolve in mouth 5×/day × 2 wk; INTRA VAG 1 applicator/1 tab × 1-2 wk hs, oral troches 10 mg 5×/day × 14 days

Available forms include: Cream, sol, lotion 1%; vag tabs 100, 500 mg; vag cream 1%, troches 10 mg

Side effects/adverse reactions:
INTEG: Rash, urticaria, stinging, burning
OTHER: Abdominal cramps, bloating, urinary frequency, dyspareunia

Contraindications: Hypersensitivity

Precautions: Pregnancy (B), lactation

NURSING CONSIDERATIONS
Administer:
• 1 applicator or 1 tablet intravaginally each night
• Enough medication to completely cover lesions
• After cleansing with soap, water before each application, dry well

Perform/provide:
• Storage at room temperature in dry place

Evaluate:
• Allergic reaction: burning, stinging, swelling, redness
• Therapeutic response: decrease in size, number of lesions, decrease in itching or white patches around vulva

Teach patient/family:
• To apply with glove to prevent further infection

---

* Available in Canada only

C

- To avoid use of OTC creams, ointments, lotions unless directed by physician
- To use medical asepsis (hand washing) before, after each application
- To abstain from sexual intercourse during vaginal/vulvular treatment
- To use continuously even during menstrual period
- To report to physician if infection persists

---

cloxacillin sodium

(klox-a-sill'in)

Apo Cloxi,* Bactopen,* Cloxapen, Novocloxin,* Orbenin,* Tegopen

Func. class.: Broad spectrum antibiotic

Chem. class.: Penicillinase-resistant penicillin

Action: Interferes with cell wall replication of susceptible organisms; the cell wall, rendered osmotically unstable, swells, bursts from osmotic pressure

Uses: Effective for gram-positive cocci *(S. aureus, S. pyogenes, E. pyogenes, S. pneumoniae)*

Dosage and routes:
- *Adult:* PO 1-4 g/day in divided doses q6h
- *Child:* PO 50-100 mg/kg in divided doses q6h

Available forms include: Caps 250, 500 mg; powder for oral susp 125 mg/5 ml

Side effects/adverse reactions:

HEMA: Anemia, increased bleeding time, *bone marrow depression, granulocytopenia*

GI: Nausea, vomiting, diarrhea, increased AST, ALT, abdominal pain, glossitis, colitis

GU: Oliguria, proteinuria, hema-turia, *vaginitis, moniliasis, **glomerulonephritis***

CNS: Lethargy, hallucinations, anxiety, depression, twitching, ***coma, convulsions***

Contraindications: Hypersensitivity to penicillins; neonates

Precautions: Pregnancy (B), hypersensitivity to cephalosporins

Pharmacokinetics:

PO: Peak 1 hr, duration 6 hr; half-life 30-60 min, metabolized in liver, excreted in urine, bile, breast milk, crosses placenta

Interactions/incompatibilities:
- Decreased antimicrobial effectiveness of cloxacillin: tetracyclines, erythromycins
- Increased cloxacillin concentrations: aspirin, probenecid

NURSING CONSIDERATIONS

Assess:
- I&O ratio; report hematuria, oliguria since penicillin in high doses is nephrotoxic
- Any patient with compromised renal system, since drug is excreted slowly in poor renal system function; toxicity may occur rapidly
- Liver studies: AST, ALT
- Blood studies: WBC, RBC, H&H, bleeding time
- Renal studies: urinalysis, protein, blood
- Culture, sensitivity before drug therapy; drug may be taken as soon as culture is taken

Administer:
- After C&S completed

Perform/provide:
- Adrenaline, suction, tracheostomy set, endotracheal intubation equipment on unit
- Adequate intake of fluids (2000 ml) during diarrhea episodes
- Scratch test to assess allergy after securing order from physician; usu-

---

italics = common side effects   – ***bold italic*** = life threatening reactions

ally done when penicillin is only drug of choice
• Storage in tight container; after reconstituting, store in refrigerator for 2 wk, room temperature 1 wk
Evaluate:
• Therapeutic effectiveness: absence of temperature, draining wounds
• Bowel pattern before, during treatment
• Skin eruptions after administration of penicillin to 1 wk after discontinuing drug
• Respiratory status: rate, character, wheezing, tightness in chest
• Allergies before initiation of treatment; reaction of each medication; place allergies on chart, Kardex in bright red
Teach patient/family:
• Aspects of drug therapy including need to complete entire course of medication to ensure organism death (10-14 days); culture may be taken after completed course of medication
• To report sore throat, fever, fatigue (could indicate superimposed infection)
• To wear or carry a Medic Alert ID if allergic to penicillins
• To notify nurse of diarrhea
• To take on an empty stomach with a full glass of water
Lab test interferences:
False positive: Urine glucose, urine protein
Decreased: Uric acid
Treatment of overdose: Withdraw drug, maintain airway, administer epinephrine, aminophylline, O_2, IV corticosteroids for anaphylaxis

clozapine

(kloz-a′pin)
Clozaril
Func. class.: Antipsychotic
Chem. class.: Tricyclic dibenzodiazepine derivative

Action: Interferes with binding of dopamine at D_1 and D_2 receptors with lack of extrapyramidal symptoms, also acts as an adrenergic, cholinergic, histaminergic, serotonergic antagonist
Uses: Management of psychotic symptoms in schizophrenic patients for whom other antipsychotics have failed
Dosage and routes:
• *Adult:* PO 25 mg qd or bid, may increase by 25-50 mg/day, normal range 300-450 mg/day after 2 wk, do not increase dose more than 2 ×/wk, do not exceed 900 mg/day, use lowest dose to control symptoms
Available forms include: Tabs 25, 100 mg
Side effects/adverse reactions:
*CNS: Sedation, salivation, dizziness, headache, tremors, sleep problems, akinesia, fever, **seizures**, sweating, akathisia, confusion, fatigue, insomnia, depression, slurred speech, anxiety*
GI: Dry mouth, constipation, nausea, abdominal discomfort, vomiting, diarrhea, anorexia
MS: Weakness; pain in back, neck, legs; spasm
CV: Tachycardia, hypotension, hypertension, chest pain, ECG changes
GU: Urinary abnormalities, incontinence, ejaculation dysfunction, frequency, urgency, retention
RESP: Dyspnea, nasal congestion, throat discomfort

HEMA: ***Leukopenia, neutropenia, agranulocytosis, eosinophilia***

Contraindications: Hypersensitivity, myeloproliferative disorders, severe granulocytopenia, CNS depression, coma

Precautions: Pregnancy (B), lactation, children <16, hepatic, renal, cardiac disease, seizures

Pharmacokinetics:
Steady state 2.5 hr, 95% protein bound, completely metabolized by the liver, excreted in urine and feces (metabolites), half-life 8-12 hr

Interactions/incompatibilities:
• Increased anticholinergic effects: anticholinergics
• Increased hypotension: antihypertensives
• Increased CNS depression: CNS drugs
• Increased bone marrow suppression: antineoplastics, other drugs suppressing bone marrow
• Increased plasma concentrations: warfarin, digoxin, other highly protein bound drugs

NURSING CONSIDERATIONS
Assess:
• Swallowing of PO medication; check for hoarding or giving of medication to other patients
• I&O ratio; palpate bladder if low urinary output occurs
• Bilirubin, CBC, liver function studies monthly
• Urinalysis is recommended before, during prolonged therapy

Administer:
• Antiparkinsonian agent, to be used if extrapyramidal symptoms occur

Perform/provide:
• Decreased noise input by dimming lights, avoiding loud noises
• Supervised ambulation until stabilized on medication; do not involve in strenuous exercise pro-

gram because fainting is possible; patient should not stand still for long periods of time
• Increased fluids to prevent constipation
• Sips of water, candy, gum for dry mouth
• Storage in tight, light-resistant container

Evaluate:
• Decrease in: emotional excitement, hallucinations, delusions, paranoia, reorganization of patterns of thought, speech
• Affect, orientation, LOC, reflexes, gait, coordination, sleep pattern disturbances
• B/P standing and lying; take pulse and respirations q4h during initial treatment; establish baseline before starting treatment; report drops of 30 mm Hg
• Dizziness, faintness, palpitations, tachycardia on rising
• EPS including akathisia (inability to sit still, no pattern to movements), tardive dyskinesia (bizarre movements of the jaw, mouth, tongue, extremities), pseudoparkinsonism (rigidity, tremors, pill rolling, shuffling gait)
• Skin turgor daily
• Constipation, urinary retention daily, if these occur, increase bulk, water in diet

Teach patient/family:
• That orthostatic hypotension occurs often, and to rise from sitting or lying position gradually
• To avoid hot tubs, hot showers, or tub baths since hypotension may occur
• To avoid abrupt withdrawal of this drug or EPS may result; drug should be withdrawn slowly
• To avoid OTC preparations (cough, hayfever, cold) unless approved by physician since serious

---

italics = common side effects   ***bold italic*** = life threatening reactions

drug interactions may occur; avoid use with alcohol or CNS depressants; increased drowsiness may occur
• Regarding compliance with drug regimen
• About EPS and necessity for meticulous oral hygiene since oral candidiasis may occur
• To report sore throat, malaise, fever, bleeding, mouth sores, if these occur, CBC should be drawn and drug discontinued
• In hot weather, heat stroke may occur; take extra precautions to stay cool
• To avoid driving or other hazardous activities; seizures may occur
Lab test interferences:
Increase: Liver function tests, cardiac enzymes, cholesterol, blood glucose, bilirubin, PBI, cholinesterase, ^{131}I
False positive: Pregnancy tests, PKU
False negative: Urinary steroids, 17-OHCS
Treatment of overdose: Lavage, activated charcoal, provide an airway; do not induce vomiting

---

codeine sulfate/codeine phosphate
(koe'deen)

Func. class.: Narcotic analgesics
Chem. class.: Opiate, phenathrene derivative

Controlled Substance Schedule II
Action: Depresses pain impulse transmission at the spinal cord level by interacting with opioid receptors
Uses: Moderate to severe pain, nonproductive cough
Dosage and routes:
Pain

• *Adult:* PO 15-60 mg q4h prn; IM/SC 15-60 mg q4h prn
• *Child:* PO 3 mg/kg/day in divided doses q4h prn
Cough
• *Adult:* PO 10-20 mg q4-6h, not to exceed 120 mg/day
• *Child:* PO 1-1.5 mg/kg/day in 4 divided doses, not to exceed 60 mg/day
Available forms include: Inj IM, SC 15, 30, 60 mg/ml; tabs 15, 30, 60 mg
Side effects/adverse reactions:
CNS: Drowsiness, sedation, dizziness, agitation, dependency, lethargy, restlessness
GI: Nausea, vomiting, anorexia, constipation
RESP: Respiratory depression, respiratory paralysis
CV: Bradycardia, palpitations, orthostatic hypotension, tachycardia
GU: Urinary retention
INTEG: Flushing, rash, urticaria
Contraindications: Hypersensitivity to opiates, respiratory depression, increased intracranial pressure, seizure disorders, severe respiratory disorders
Precautions: Elderly, cardiac dysrhythmias, pregnancy (C)
Pharmacokinetics: Onset 15-30 min, peak 1-2 hr, duration 4-6 hr; metabolized by liver, excreted by kidneys, crosses placenta, excreted in breast milk, half-life 2½-4 hr
Interactions/incompatibilities:
• Effects may be increased with other CNS depressants: alcohol, narcotics, sedative/hypnotics, antipsychotics, skeletal muscle relaxants
NURSING CONSIDERATIONS
Assess:
• I&O ratio; check for decreasing output; may indicate urinary retention

---

Administer:
• With antiemetic if nausea, vomiting occur
• With milk or food for GI symptoms
• When pain is beginning to return; determine dosage interval by patient response

Perform/provide:
• Storage in light-resistant container at room temperature
• Assistance with ambulation
• Safety measures: siderails, night light, call bell

Evaluate:
• Therapeutic response: decrease in pain, absence of grimacing or decreased cough
• Cough: type, duration, ability to raise secretion
• CNS changes, dizziness, drowsiness, hallucinations, euphoria, LOC, pupil reaction
• Allergic reactions: rash, urticaria
• Respiratory dysfunction: respiratory depression, character, rate rhythm; notify physician if respirations are <10/min
• Need for pain medication, physical dependence

Teach patient/family:
• To report any symptoms of CNS changes, allergic reactions
• That physical dependency may result when used for extended periods of time
• To change position slowly, orthostatic hypotension may occur
• To avoid hazardous activities if drowsiness or dizziness occurs
• To avoid alcohol unless directed by physician

colchicine
(kol'chi-seen)
Colsalide, Novocolchine
Func. class.: Antigout agent
Chem. class.: Colchicum autumnale alkaloid

Action: Inhibits microtubule formation in leukocytes, which decreases phagocytosis and inflammation in joints

Uses: Gout, gouty arthritis (prevention, treatment) to arrest progression of neurologic disability in multiple sclerosis

Dosage and routes:
Prevention
• *Adult:* PO 0.5-1.8 mg qd depending on severity; IV 0.5-1 mg 1-2× day
Treatment
• *Adult:* PO 0.5-1.2 mg, then 0.5-1.2 mg q1h, until pain decreases or side effects occur; IV 2 mg, 0.5 mg q6h, not to exceed 4 mg/24 hr
Available forms include: Tabs 0.5, 0.6 mg; inj IV 1 mg/2 ml

Side effects/adverse reactions:
MISC: Myopathy, alopecia, reversible azoospermia, peripheral neuritis
GU: Hematuria, oliguria, renal damage
HEMA: **Agranulocytosis, thrombocytopenia, aplastic anemia, pancytopenia**
GI: Nausea, vomiting, anorexia, malaise, metallic taste, cramps, peptic ulcer, diarrhea
INTEG: Chills, dermatitis, pruritus, purpura, erythema

Contraindications: Hypersensitivity, serious GI, renal, hepatic, cardiac disorders; blood dyscrasias

Precautions: Severe renal disease, blood dyscrasias, pregnancy (C),

---

italics = common side effects   ***bold italic*** = life threatening reactions

hepatic disease, elderly, lactation, children

Pharmacokinetics:
PO: Peak ½-2 hr, half-life 20 min, deacetylates in liver, excreted in feces (metabolites/active drug)

Interactions/incompatibilities:
• Decreased action of colchicine: acidifying agents
• Decreased action of: vitamin B₁₂
• Increased action of: CNS depressants, sympathomimetics
• Increased action of colchicine: alkalinizers

NURSING CONSIDERATIONS
Assess:
• I&O ratio; observe for decrease in urinary output
• CBC, platelets, reticulocytes before, during therapy (q3 mo)
• Coombs' test to determine Coombs' negative hemolytic anemia

Administer:
• IV undiluted or diluted 1 mg/10-20 ml normal saline or sterile H₂O for inj; give over 2-5 min
• On empty stomach only, to facilitate absorption

Evaluate:
• Therapeutic response: decreased stone formation on x-ray, decreased pain in kidney region, absence of hematuria, decreased pain in joints

Teach patient/family:
• To increase fluids to 3-4 L/day
• To avoid alcohol, OTC preparations that contain alcohol; skin rashes have occurred
• To report any pain, redness, or hard area usually in legs
• Stress patient compliance with medical regimen; bone marrow depression may occur

Lab test interferences:
Increase: Alk phosphatase, AST/ALT
False positive: RBC, Hgb

---

colestipol HCl

(koe-les'ti-pole)
Colestid

Func. class.: Antilipemic
Chem. class.: Bile sequestrant, resin exchange agent

Action: Absorbs, combines with bile acids to form insoluble complex that is excreted through feces; loss of bile acids lowers cholesterol levels

Uses: Primary hypercholesterolemia, xanthomas, digitalis toxicity, pruritus due to biliary obstruction, diarrhea due to bile acids

Dosage and routes:
• *Adult:* PO 15-30 g/day in 2-4 divided doses

Available forms include: Granules

Side effects/adverse reactions:
GI: Constipation, abdominal pain, nausea, fecal impaction, hemorrhoids, flatulence, vomiting, steatorrhea, peptic ulcer
INTEG: Rash, irritation of perianal area, tongue, skin
HEMA: Decreased vitamins A, D, K, red folate content **hyperchloremic acidosis,** bleeding, decreased pro-time

Contraindications: Hypersensitivity, biliary obstruction

Precautions: Pregnancy (B), lactation, children, bleeding disorders

Pharmacokinetics:
PO: Excreted in feces

Interactions/incompatibilities:
• May reduce action of: thiazide, digitalis, warfarin, penicillin G, folic acid, phenylbutazone, tetracycline, corticosteroids, iron, thyroid agents, clindamycin, trimethoprim, chenodiol, fat-soluble vitamins, cephalexin, phenobarbital

---

* Available in Canada only

NURSING CONSIDERATIONS
Assess:
- Cardiac glycoside levels, if both drugs are being administered
- For signs of vitamins A, D, K deficiency
- Serum cholesterol, triglyceride levels, electrolytes if on extended therapy

Administer:
- Drug ac, hs; give all other medications 1 hr before colestipol or 4 hr after colestipol to avoid poor absorption
- Drug mixed in applesauce or stirred into beverage (2-6 oz), do not take dry; let stand for 2 min
- Supplemental doses of vitamins A, D, K if levels are low

Evaluate:
- Therapeutic response: decreased triglycerides, diarrhea, pruritus (excess bile area)
- Bowel pattern daily; increase bulk, water in diet if constipation develops

Teach patient/family:
- Symptoms of hypothrombinemia: bleeding mucous membranes, dark tarry stools, hematuria, petechiae; report immediately
- That patient compliance is needed since toxicity may result if doses are missed
- That risk factors should be decreased: high fat diet, smoking, alcohol consumption, absence of exercise

Lab test interferences:
Increase: Liver function studies, chloride, PO₄

Note: Not all cholesterol lowering agents have been thoroughly tested. Investigate any reaction, however small, immediately.

colfosceril palmitate
Exosurf Neonatal

Func. class.: Synthetic lung surfactant
Chem. class.: dipalmitoylphosphatidylcholine (DPPC)

Action: Surfactant maintains lung inflation and prevents collapse by lowering surface tension

Uses: Treatment of respiratory distress syndrome (RDS) in premature infants

Dosage and routes:
Prophylactic treatment
Endotracheally: 5 ml/kg as soon as possible after birth and repeat doses 12 and 24 hr later to infants remaining on mechanical ventilation

Rescue treatment
Endotracheally: administer in two 5 ml/kg doses; give initial dose after treatment of RDS, then second dose in 12 hr

Available forms include: 10 ml/vial with sterile H₂O for inj and 5 endotracheal tube adapters

Side effects/adverse reactions:
RESP: ***Apnea, pulmonary hemorrhage, pulmonary air leak, congenital pneumonia***
SYST: ***Nonpulmonary fatal infections***

Precautions: Congenital anomalies, prophylactic treatment

Pharmacokinetics: Distributed to all lobes, alveolar spaces, distal airways; alveolar half-life 12 hr; 90% of alveolar phospholipids are recycled

NURSING CONSIDERATIONS
Assess:
- Respiratory rate, rhythm, character, chest expansion, color, transcutaneous saturation, ABGs
- Endotracheal tube placement before dosing

• For apnea after endotracheal administration

• Reflux of drug into the endotracheal tube during administration; stop drug administration if this occurs, and, if needed, increase peak inspiratory pressure on the ventilator by 4-5 cm H_2O until tube is cleared

Administer:

• Infants should be suctioned before administration

• After selecting an adapter size that corresponds to the diameter of the endotracheal tube, insert the adapter into the tube by twisting, connect the breathing circuit to the adapter, remove the cap from the adapter sideport, and attach the syringe to the sideport; after dose is completed, remove the syringe and recap the sideport

• After reconstituting each vial with 8 ml preservative-free sterile water for injection, fill a 10-12 ml syringe with 8 ml preservative-free sterile water for injection, using an 18-19 gauge needle; allow the vacuum in the vial to draw the liquid into the vial; aspirate the 8 ml out of the vial into the syringe while maintaining the vacuum and then release the syringe plunger; repeat the aspiration and release until adequately mixed; draw the dose required into the syringe from below the froth in the vial; do not use if large particles are present

• By endotracheal administration only by persons trained in neonatal intubation and ventilation

Perform/provide:

• Reduction in peak ventilator inspiratory pressures immediately if chest expansion improves substantially after dose

• Reduction in FIO_2 in small, repeated steps when infant becomes pink and transcutaneous oxygen saturation is in excess of 95%; oxygen saturation should remain between 90% and 95%

• Suctioning of all infants before administration to prevent mucus plugging; if endotracheal tube obstruction is suspected, remove the obstruction and replace tube immediately

• Storage at room temperature in dry place

---

colistimethate sodium

(koe-lis-ti-meth′ate)
Coly-Mycin M
Func. class.: Antibacterial
Chem. class.: Polymyxin

Action: Interferes with phospholipids, penetrates cell wall; changes occur immediately in bacterial membrane, causing leakage of essential metabolites; bactericidal

Uses: Serious *P. aeruginosa, E. aerogenes, K. pneumoniae, E. coli, H. influenzae* infections or when other antibiotics cannot be used.

Dosage and routes:

• *Adult/child:* IM/IV 2.5-5 mg/kg/day in 2-4 divided doses, not to exceed 5 mg/kg/day (normal renal function); *Inter IV:* ½ daily dose over 3-5 min q12h; *Cont IV:* ½ daily dose over 3-5 min, add remaining to compatible infusion SOL, run over 1-2 hr

Available forms include: Inj, IV, IM 150 mg/vial

Side effects/adverse reactions:

INTEG: Urticaria, itching

CNS: Dizziness, confusion, weakness, drowsiness, paresthesia, slurred speech, *coma, seizures,* headache, vertigo

RESP: Respiratory arrest

---

*GU: **Proteinuria, hematuria, azotemia, leukocyturia, renal failure, acute tubular necrosis***

MISC: Drug fever, GI upset

Contraindications: Hypersensitivity

Precautions: Pregnancy (B), severe renal disease

Pharmacokinetics:

IM: Peak 1-2 hr, duration 8-12 hr, half-life 2-3 hr, excreted as active metabolites, crosses placenta, excreted in breast milk

Interactions/incompatibilities:

• Increased neuromuscular blockade/muscular paralysis: anesthetics, neuromuscular blockers (tubocurarine, succinylcholine, gallamine)

• Increased nephrotoxicity: cephalothin, aminoglycosides

NURSING CONSIDERATIONS
Assess:

• I&O ratio; report hematuria, oliguria

• Any patient with compromised renal system; drug is excreted slowly in poor renal system function; toxicity may occur rapidly; monitor BUN, creatinine

• Renal studies: urinalysis, protein, blood

• C&S before drug therapy; drug may be taken as soon as culture is taken; C&S may be done after completion of therapy

Administer:

• IV after diluting 150 mg/2 ml sterile water for inj; give dose over 5 min; may be diluted in compatible sol and run at 6 mg/hr

Perform/provide:

• Storage in dark area to room temperature

• Adrenalin, suction, tracheostomy set, endotracheal intubation equipment on unit

Evaluate:

• Therapeutic response: absence of fever, hematuria, burning on urination, urinary frequency, C&S negative

• Skin eruptions, itching; drug should be discontinued

• Respiratory status: rate, character, dyspnea, symptoms of neuromuscular blockade, tightness in chest; discontinue drug if these occur

• Allergies before initiation of treatment, reaction of each medication; note allergies on chart

• For flushing of face, dizziness, disorientation, weakness, paresthesia, blurred vision, slurred speech, restlessness, irritability; indicate neurotoxicity

Teach patient/family:

• To report sore throat, fever, fatigue; could indicate superimposed infection

Treatment of overdose: Withhold drug, maintain airway, administer epinephrine, aminophylline, O_2, IV corticosteroids

---

colistin sulfate (polymyxin E)

(koe-lis'tin)

Coly-Mycin S

Func. class.: Antibacterial
Chem. class.: Polymyxin

Action: Interferes with phospholipids, penetrates cell wall; changes occur immediately in bacterial membrane, causing leakage of essential metabolites; bactericidal

Uses: *E. coli, Shigella,* or when other antibiotics cannot be used

Dosage and routes:

• *Infant/child:* PO 5-15 mg/kg/day divided into 3 doses and given q8h

---

italics = common side effects   ***bold italic*** = life threatening reactions

Available forms include: Powder for oral susp 25 mg/5 ml
Side effects/adverse reaction: Rare with usual dosage
GI: Nausea, vomiting
INTEG: Urticaria
CNS: Dizziness, confusion, weakness, drowsiness, paresthesia, slurred speech, *coma, seizures,* headache
RESP: Paralysis
GU: Proteinuria, hematuria, azotemia, leukocyturia, renal failure, acute tubular necrosis
Contraindications: Hypersensitivity
Precautions: Pregnancy (B), severe renal disease
Pharmacokinetics:
Half-life 2-3 hr, excreted primarily in urine

NURSING CONSIDERATIONS
Assess:
• C&S before drug therapy; drug may be taken as soon as culture is taken; C&S may be done after completion of therapy
Perform/provide:
• Storage in dark area at room temperature
• Adrenalin, suction, tracheostomy set, endotracheal intubation equipment on unit
Evaluate:
• Therapeutic response: absence of fever, purulent drainage, C&S negative
• Skin eruptions, itching; drug should be discontinued
• Allergies before initiation of treatment, reaction of each medication; note allergies on chart and Kardex in bright red letters; notify all people giving drugs
Teach patient/family:
• To report sore throat, fever, fatigue; could indicated superimposed infection

Treatment of overdose: Withhold drug, maintain airway, administer epinephrine, aminophylline, O_2, IV corticosteroids

---

collagenase

(kol′la-je-nase)
Biozyme-C, Santyl
Func. class.: Topical enzyme preparation

Action: Effective in removing debris on skin by digesting collagen deposits
Uses: Debriding dermal ulcers, severely burned areas
Dosage and routes:
• *Adult and child:* TOP apply to lesion qd or qod
Available forms include: Top oint 250 U/g
Side effects/adverse reactions:
INTEG: Pain, burning, redness, irritation, hypersensitivity reactions
Contraindications: Hypersensitivity, elderly
Precautions: Pregnancy (C)
Interactions/incompatibilities:
• Inhibited enzymatic activity of collagenase: benzalkonium chloride, hexachlorophene, nitrofurazone, iodine, heavy metal drugs

NURSING CONSIDERATIONS
Administer:
• After removing debris using hydrogen peroxide solution or modified Dakin solution; use sterile gauze to cover area
• As often as needed if area becomes soiled
• With tongue depressor or wooden spatula to deep wounds, use gauze for superficial wounds
• After covering healthy skin with a protectant such as petrolatum or zinc oxide paste

---

*Available in Canada only

Perform/provide:
• Removal of gauze bandage, cream by applying mineral oil before cleaning area, make sure all cream is removed

Evaluate:
• Therapeutic response: separation of burn eschar; clean, pink ulcer area
• Area of body involved, including time involved, what helps or aggravates condition

Teach patient/family:
• To avoid application on normal skin or getting ointment in eyes
• To discontinue use if rash or irritation occur
• That healing may take 1-2 wk; use only until necrotic tissue is gone, healthy tissue is present

---

corticotropin (ACTH)

(kor-ti-koe-troe′pin)

ACTHAR, Cortigel-40, Cortigel-80, Cortrophin Gel, Cotropic-Gel-40, Cotropic-Gel-80, Cortrophin Zinc, Duracton,* H.P. Acthar Gel

Func. class.: Pituitary hormone
Chem. class.: Adrenocorticotropic hormone

Action: Stimulates adrenal cortex to produce, secrete corticosterone, cortisol

Uses: Testing adrenocortical function, treatment of adrenal insufficiency caused by administration of corticosteroids (long term), multiple sclerosis

Dosage and routes:
Testing of adrenocortical function
• *Adult:* IM/SC up to 80 units in divided doses; IV 10-25 units in 500 ml D_5W given over 8 hr
Inflammation
• *Adult:* SC/IM 40 units in 4 divided doses (aqueous) or 40 units q12-24h (gel/repository form)

Available forms include: Inj IM, IV, SC 25, 40 U/vial, repository inj IM, SC 40, 80/ml

Side effects/adverse reactions:
INTEG: Impaired wound healing, rash, urticaria, hirsutism, petechiae, ecchymoses, sweating, acne, hyperpigmentation
CNS: **Convulsions,** dizziness, euphoria, insomnia, headache, mood swings, behavioral changes, depression, psychosis
GI: Nausea, vomiting, **peptic ulcer perforation,** pancreatitis, distention, ulcerative esophagitis
GU: Water, sodium retention, hypokalemia
EENT: Cataracts, glaucoma
MS: Weakness, osteoporosis, compression fractures, muscle atrophy, steroid myopathy, myalgia, arthralgia
ENDO: Cushingoid symptoms, diabetes mellitus, antibody formation, growth retardation in children, menstrual irregularities

Contraindications: Hypersensitivity, scleroderma, osteoporosis, CHF, peptic ulcer disease, hypertension, systemic fungal infections, smallpox vaccination, recent surgery, ocular herpes simplex, primary adrenocortical insufficiency/hyperfunction

Precautions: Pregnancy (C), lactation, latent TB, hepatic disease, hypothyroiditis, child bearing-age women, psychiatric diagnosis, myasthenia gravis, acute gouty arthritis

Pharmacokinetics:
IV/IM/SC: Onset <6 hr, duration 2-4 hr, repository duration up to 3 days, half life <20 min, excreted in urine

---

italics = common side effects   ***bold italic*** = life threatening reactions

Interactions/incompatibilities:
• Possible ulceration: salicylates, alcohol, corticosteroids
• Hypokalemia: diuretics (K-depleting), amphotericin B
• Hyperglycemia: insulin, or oral hypoglycemic agents

NURSING CONSIDERATIONS
Assess:
• Baseline ECG, B/P, chest x-ray, GTT
• Pulse, B/P
• I&O ratio; weight q wk, report gain over 5 lb/wk
• 2 hr postprandial, chest x-ray, serum potassium, 17 KS, 17-OHCS, cortisol, during long-term treatment

Administer:
• Test for hypersensitivity for individuals allergic to pork products
• Decreased sodium, increase potassium for dependent edema
• Increase protein diet for nitrogen loss
• Gel at room temperature, give deep IM using 21G needle
• May be used to treat edema
• IV; give over 2 min; dilute 25 U/1 ml sterile H₂O or normal saline or 40 U/2 ml; may dilute 10-25 U/500 ml compatible sol; give over 8 hr

Perform/provide:
• Storage in refrigerator of unused portion; use within 24 hr

Evaluate:
• Therapeutic response: absence of inflammation, pain, increased muscle strength in myasthenia gravis
• Dependent edema, moon face, pulmonary edema, cerebral edema
• Infection; drug may mask infections
• Increased stress in patient's life that may require increased corticosteroids
• Mental status: affect, mood, in-creased aggressiveness, irritability; a change in mental status may require decreased steroids
• Growth rate of child
• Hypoadrenalism in neonates if drug was given during pregnancy
• Allergic reaction: rash, urticaria, fever, nausea, vomiting, dyspnea; drug should be discontinued immediately, administer epinephrine 1:1000

Teach patient/family:
• To avoid vaccinations during drug treatment
• To maintain adequate hydration up to 2000 ml/day unless contraindicated
• Avoid OTC products: salicylates, products with alcohol
• Not to discontinue medication abruptly, thyroid crisis may occur; drug should be tapered off over several wk
• To wear Medic Alert ID specifying steroid therapy
• That drug does not cure condition, only decreases symptoms
• To notify physician of infection: increased temperature, sore throat, muscular pain
• To tell patient to notify anyone involved in medical or dental care that this drug is being taken

---

cortisone acetate

(kor'-ti-sone)
Cortone
Func. class.: Corticosteroid, synthetic
Chem. class.: Glucocorticoid, short-acting

Action: Decreases inflammation by suppression of migration of polymorphonuclear leukocytes, fibroblasts, reversal of increased capillary permeability and lysosomal stabilization

Uses: Inflammation, severe allergy, adrenal insufficiency, collagen disorders, respiratory, dermatologic disorders

Dosage and routes:
• *Adult:* PO/IM 25-300 mg qd or q2 days, titrated to patient response
Available forms include: Tabs 5, 10, 25 mg; inj IM 25, 50 mg/ml

Side effects/adverse reactions:
INTEG: Acne, poor wound healing, ecchymosis, bruising, petechiae
CNS: Depression, flushing, sweating, headache, mood changes
*CV: Hypertension, **circulatory collapse, thrombophlebitis, embolism,** tachycardia, **necrotizing angiitis, CHF,** edema*
*HEMA: **Thrombocytopenia***
MS: Fractures, osteoporosis, weakness
*GI: Diarrhea, nausea, abdominal distention, **GI hemorrhage,*** increased appetite, **pancreatitis***
EENT: Fungal infections, increased intraocular pressure, blurred vision

Contraindications: Psychosis, hypersensitivity, idiopathic thrombocytopenia, acute glomerulonephritis, amebiasis, fungal infections, nonasthmatic bronchial disease, child <2 yr, AIDS, TB

Precautions: Pregnancy (C), diabetes mellitus, glaucoma, osteoporosis, seizure disorders, ulcerative colitis, CHF, myasthenia gravis, renal disease, esophagitis, peptic ulcer

Pharmacokinetics:
PO: Peak 2 hr, duration 1½ days
IM: Peak 20-48 hr, duration 1½ days

Interactions/incompatibilities:
• Decreased action of cortisone: cholestyramine, colestipol, barbi-

turates, rifampin, ephedrine, phenytoin, theophylline
• Decreased effects of: anticoagulants, anticonvulsants, antidiabetics, ambenonium, neostigmine, isoniazid, toxoids, vaccines
• Increased side effects: alcohol, salicylates, indomethacin, amphotericin B, digitalis preparations
• Increased action of cortisone: salicylates, estrogens, indomethacin

NURSING CONSIDERATIONS
Assess:
• Potassium, blood sugar, urine glucose while on long-term therapy; hypokalemia and hyperglycemia
• Weight daily, notify physician of weekly gain >5 lb
• B/P q4h, pulse, notify physician if chest pain occurs
• I&O ratio, be alert for decreasing urinary output and increasing edema
• Plasma cortisol levels during long-term therapy (normal level: 138-635 nmol/L SI units if drawn at 8 AM)

Administer:
• After shaking suspension (parenteral)
• Titrated dose, use lowest effective dose
• IM inj deeply in large mass, rotate sites, avoid deltoid, use a 21G needle
• In one dose in AM to prevent adrenal suppression, avoid SC administration, damage may be done to tissue
• With food or milk to decrease GI symptoms

Perform/provide:
• Assistance with ambulation in patient with bone tissue disease to prevent fractures

Evaluate:
• Therapeutic response: ease of res-

pirations, decreased inflammation
• Infection: increased temperature, WBC even after withdrawal of medication; drug masks symptoms of infection
• Potassium depletion: paresthesias, fatigue, nausea, vomiting, depression, polyuria, dysrhythmias, weakness
• Edema, hypertension, cardiac symptoms
• Mental status: affect, mood, behavioral changes, aggression
Teach patient/family:
• That ID as steroid user should be carried at all times
• To notify physician if therapeutic response decreases; dosage adjustment may be needed
• Not to discontinue this medication abruptly or adrenal crisis can result
• To avoid OTC products: salicylates, alcohol in cough products, cold preparations unless directed by physician
• Teach patient all aspects of drug usage, including Cushingoid symptoms
• Symptoms of adrenal insufficiency: nausea, anorexia, fatigue, dizziness, dyspnea, weakness, joint pain
Lab test interferences:
Increase: Cholesterol, sodium, blood glucose, uric acid, calcium, urine glucose
Decrease: Calcium, potassium, T_4, T_3, thyroid ^{131}I uptake test, urine 17-OHCS, 17-KS, PBI
False negative: Skin allergy tests

cosyntropin
(koe-sin-troe'pin)
Cortrosyn, Synacthen Depot*
Func. class.: Pituitary hormone
Chem. class.: Synthetic polypeptide

Action: Stimulates adrenal cortex to produce, secrete corticosterone, cortisol
Uses: Testing adrenocortical function
Dosage and routes:
• *Adult and child >2 yr:* IM/IV 0.25-1 mg between blood sampling
• *Child <2 yr:* IM/IV 0.125 mg
Available forms include: Inj IM, IV 0.25 mg/vial
Side effects/adverse reactions:
INTEG: Rash urticaria, pruritus, flushing
Contraindications: Hypersensitivity
Precautions: Pregnancy (C)
Pharmacokinetics:
IV/IM: Onset 5 min, peak 1 hr, duration 2-4 hr
NURSING CONSIDERATIONS
Assess:
• Plasma cortisol levels at ½-1 hr after drug administered (>5 µg/dl is normal), at end of 1 hr, levels should have doubled
Administer:
• After reconstitution with 1 ml 0.9% NaCl/0.25 mg; may be further diluted in D_5 or normal saline; run 40 mg/hr over 6 hr
Perform/provide:
• Storage at room temperature for 24 hr or refrigerated for 3 wk

---

co-trimoxazole (sulfamethoxazole and trimethoprim)

(koe-trye-mox′a-zole)
Apo-Sulfatrim,* Bactrim, Cotrim, Comoxol, Septra, Sulfatrim, Bethaprim

Func. class.: Antibiotic
Chem. class.: Miscellaneous sulfonamide

Action: Sulfamethoxazole interferes with bacterial biosynthesis of proteins by competitive antagonism of PABA when adequate levels are maintained; trimethoprim blocks synthesis of tetrahydrofolic acid; this combination blocks 2 consecutive steps in bacterial synthesis of essential nucleic acids, protein

Uses: Urinary tract infections, otitis media, acute and chronic prostatitis, shigellosis, *Pneumocystis carinii* pneumonitis, chronic bronchitis, chancroid

Dosage and routes:
Urinary tract infections
• *Adult:* PO 160 mg TMP/800 mg SMZ q12h × 10-14 days
• *Child:* PO 8 mg/kg TMP/40 mg/kg SMZ qd in 2 divided doses q12h
Otitis media
• *Child:* PO 8 mg/kg TMP/40 mg/kg SMZ qd in 2 divided doses q12h × 10 days
Chronic bronchitis
• *Adult:* PO 100 mg TMP/800 mg SMZ q12h × 14 days
Pneumocystis carinii pneumonitis
• *Adult and child:* PO 20 mg/kg TMP/100 mg/kg SMZ qd in 4 divided doses q6h × 14 days; IV 15-20 mg/kg/day (based on TMP) in 3-4 divided doses for up to 14 days
• Dosage reduction necessary in moderate to severe renal impairment (CrCL < 30 ml/min)

Available forms include: Tabs 80 mg trimethoprim/400 mg sulfamethoxazole, 160 mg trimethoprim/800 mg sulfamethoxazole; susp 40 mg/200 mg/5 ml; IV inj 16 mg/80 mg/ml

Side effects/adverse reactions:
*SYST: **Anaphylaxis, SLE***
GI: Nausea, vomiting, abdominal pain, stomatitis, ***hepatitis,*** glossitis, pancreatitis, diarrhea, ***enterocolitis***
CNS: Headache, confusion, insomnia, hallucinations, depression, vertigo, fatigue, anxiety, convulsions, drug fever, chills, aseptic meningitis
*HEMA: **Leukopenia, neutropenia, thrombocytopenia, agranulocytosis, hemolytic anemia, hypoprothrombinemia, Henoch-Schoenler purpura, methenoglobinemia***
INTEG: Rash, dermatitis, urticaria, ***Stevens-Johnson syndrome,*** erythema, photosensitivity, pain, inflammation at injection site
*GU: **Renal failure, toxic nephrosis,*** increased BUN, creatinine, crystalluria
*CV: **Allergic myocarditis***

Contraindications: Hypersensitivity to trimethoprim or sulfonamides, pregnancy at term, megaloblastic anemia, infants <2 mo, CrCl <15 ml/min

Precautions: Pregnancy (C), lactation, renal disease, elderly, G-6-PD deficiency, impaired hepatic function, possible folate deficiency, severe allergy, bronchial asthma

Pharmacokinetics:
PO: Rapidly absorbed, peak 1-4 hr; half-life 8-13 hr, excreted in urine (metabolites and unchanged), breast milk, crosses placenta, highly bound to plasma proteins; TMP achieves high levels in prostatic tissue and fluid

---

italics = common side effects   ***bold italic*** = life threatening reactions

Interactions/incompatibilities:
• Increased hypoglycemic response: sulfonylurea agents
• Increased anticoagulant effects: oral anticoagulants
• Decreased hepatic clearance of: phenytoin
• Increased nephrotoxicity: cyclosporine

NURSING CONSIDERATIONS
Assess:
• I&O ratio; note color, character, pH of urine if drug administered for urinary tract infections; output should be 800 ml less than intake; if urine is highly acidic, alkalization may be needed
• Kidney function studies: BUN, creatinine, urinalysis if on long-term therapy

Administer:
• With full glass of water to maintain adequate hydration; increase fluids to 2000 ml/day to decrease crystallization in kidneys
• Medication after C&S; repeat C&S after full course of medication completed
• After diluting 5 ml of drug/125 ml D_5W, run over 1-1½ hr
• With resuscitative equipment available; severe allergic reactions may occur

Perform/provide:
• Storage in tight, light-resistant containers at room temperature

Evaluate:
• Therapeutic effectiveness: absence of pain, fever, C&S negative
• Blood dyscrasias: skin rash, fever, sore throat, bruising, bleeding, fatigue, joint pain
• Allergic reaction: rash, dermatitis, urticaria, pruritus, dyspnea, bronchospasm

Teach patient/family:
• To take each oral dose with full glass of water to prevent crystalluria

• To complete full course of treatment to prevent superimposed infection
• To avoid sunlight or use sunscreen to prevent burns
• To avoid OTC medications (aspirin, vitamin C) unless directed by physician
• To use alternative contraceptive measures; decreased effectiveness of oral contraceptives may result
• To notify physician if skin rash, sore throat, fever, mouth sores, unusual bruising, bleeding occur

Lab test interferences:
Increase: Alk phosphatase, creatinine, bilirubin
False positive: Urinary glucose test

---

cromolyn sodium
(kroe′moe-lin)
Opticrom 4%
Func. class.: Ophthalmic
Chem. class.: Mast cell stabilizer

Action: Inhibits degranulation of mast cells after contact with antigens, which decreases release of histamine and SRS-A from mast cell

Uses: Vernal keratoconjunctivitis, conjunctivitis, vernal keratitis, allergic keratoconjunctivitis

Dosage and routes:
• *Adult:* INSTILL 1-2 gtts in both eyes q4-6h

Available forms include: Sol 40 mg/ml

Side effects/adverse reactions:
EENT: Stinging, burning, itching, lacrimation, puffiness

Contraindications: Hypersensitivity

Precautions: Pregnancy (B)

NURSING CONSIDERATIONS
Perform/provide:
• Storage at room temperature

Teach patient/family:
• To report stinging, burning, itching, lacrimation, puffiness
• Method of instillation, including pressure on lacrimal sac for 1 min, and not to touch dropper to eye
• Not to wear soft contact lens, use may be reinstituted 4-6 hr after therapy is discontinued

---

cromolyn sodium (disodium cromoglycate)

(kroe'moe-lin)

Intal, Intal p,* Nasalcrom, Rynacrom,* Gastrocrom

Func. class.: Antiasthmatic
Chem. class.: Mast cell stabilizer

Action: Stabilizes the membrane of the sensitized mast cell preventing release of chemical mediators after an antigen-IgE interaction

Uses: Allergic rhinitis, severe perennial bronchial asthma, exercise-induced bronchospasm (prevention), prevention of acute bronchospasm induced by environmental pollutants, mastocytosis

Dosage and routes:

Allergic rhinitis
• *Adult and child >6 yr:* nasal sol 1 spray in each nostril tid-qid, not to exceed 6 doses/day

Bronchospasm
• *Adult and child >5 yr:* INH 20 mg <1 hr before exercise

Bronchial asthma
• *Adult and child >5 yr:* INH 20 mg qid; NEB 20 mg qid by nebulization

Available forms include: Sol 40 mg/ml; inh, caps for inh, 20 mg; oral caps 100 mg, neb sol 20 mg, aerosol 800 µg/actuation

Side effects/adverse reactions:

EENT: Throat irritation, cough, nasal congestion, burning eyes

CNS: Headache, dizziness, neuritis

GU: Frequency, dysuria

GI: Nausea, vomiting, anorexia, dry mouth, bitter taste

INTEG: Rash, urticaria, angioedema

MS: Joint pain/swelling

Contraindications: Hypersensitivity to this drug or lactose, status asthmaticus

Precautions: Pregnancy (B), lactation, renal disease, hepatic disease, child <5 yr

Pharmacokinetics:

INH: Peak 15 min, duration 4-6 hr, excreted unchanged in feces, half-life 80 min

NURSING CONSIDERATIONS

Assess:
• Eosinophil count during treatment

Administer:
• By inhalation/nebulizer only
• Gargle, sip of water to decrease irritation in throat

Evaluate:
• Respiratory status: respiratory rate, rhythm, characteristics, cough, wheezing, dyspnea

Teach patient/family:
• To clear mucous before using
• Proper inhalation technique: exhale, using inhaler, inhale deeply with head tipped back to open airway, remove, hold breath, exhale, repeat until all of drug is inhaled
• That therapeutic effect may take up to 4 wk
• Not to swallow capsule
• That drug is preventative only, not restorative

---

italics = common side effects   ***bold italic*** = life threatening reactions

crotamiton

(kroe-tam'i-tonn)
Eurax

Func. class.: Scabicide
Chem. class.: Synthetic chloroformate salt

Action: Unknown, toxic to *Sarcoptes scabiei*
Uses: Scabies, pruritus
Dosage and routes:
Scabies
• *Adult and child:* CREAM wash area with soap, water; remove visible crusts, apply cream, apply another coat in 24 hr, remove with soap, water in 48 hr; for pruritus, massage into affected area, repeat as necessary
Available forms include: Cream 10%; lotion 10%
Side effects/adverse reactions:
INTEG: Itching, rash, irritation, contact dermatitis
Contraindications: Hypersensitivity, inflammation of skin, abrasions, or breaks in skin, mucous membranes
Precautions: Children, pregnancy (C)
NURSING CONSIDERATIONS
Administer:
• After patient bathes with soap, water; remove all crusts
• To body areas, scalp only, do not apply to face, lips, mouth, eyes, any mucous membrane, anus, or meatus
• Topical corticosteroids as ordered to decrease contact dermatitis
• Lotions of menthol or phenol to control itching
• Topical antibiotics for infection
Perform/provide:
• Storage in tight, light-resistant container
• Isolation until areas on skin,

scalp have cleared; treatment is completed
Evaluate:
• Area of body involved, including crusts, brownish trails on skin, itching papules in skin folds
Teach patient/family:
• To change clothing and bed linen the morning after treatment
• Shake well before using
• To wash all inhabitants' clothing, using hot water, dried in hot dryers for >20 min; preventative treatment may be required of all persons living in same house using lotion or shampoo to decrease spread of infection
• That itching may continue for 4-6 wk
• That drug must be reapplied if accidently washed off or treatment will be ineffective
• To avoid contact with eyes, face, meatus or mucous membranes or irritation may occur
• To discontinue use and notify physician if irritation or sensitization occurs

cyanocobalamin (vitamin B₁₂)/hydroxocobalamin (vitamin B₁₂a)

(sye-an-oh-koe-bal'a-min)
Anacobin,* Bedoce, Bedoz,* Berubigen, Betalin-12, Crystimin, Cyanabin,* Kaybovit, Pernavite, Poyamin, Rubesol, Rubion,* Rubramin, Sigamine/Alpha Rediso, Alpha-Ruvite, Codroxomin, Droxomin, Neo-Betalin 12, Rubesol-LA, Vibedoz

Func. class.: Vitamin B_{12}, water-soluble vitamin

Action: Needed for adequate nerve functioning, protein and carbohydrate metabolism, normal growth, RBC development and cell reproduction

Uses: Vitamin B$_{12}$ deficiency, pernicious anemia, vitamin B$_{12}$ malabsorption syndrome, Schilling test, increased requirements with pregnancy thyrotoxicosis, hemolytic anemia, hemorrhage, renal and hepatic disease

Dosage and routes:
• *Adult:* PO 25 μg qd × 5-10 days, maintenance 100-200 mg IM q mo; IM/SC 30-100 μg qd × 5-10 days, maintenance 100-200 μg IM q mo
• *Child:* PO 1 μg qd × 5-10 days, maintenance 60 μg IM q mo or more; IM/SC 1-30 μg qd × 5-10 days, maintenance 60 μg IM q mo or more

Pernicious anemia/malabsorption syndrome
• *Adult:* IM 100-1000 μg qd × 2 wk, then 100-1000 μg IM q mo
• *Child:* IM 100-500 μg over 2 wk or more given in 100-500 μg doses, then 60 μg IM/SC monthly

Schilling test
• *Adult and child:* IM 1000 μg in one dose

Available forms include: Tabs 25, 50, 100, 250, 500, 1000 μg; inj IM 100, 120, 1000 μg/ml

Side effects/adverse reactions:
CNS: Flushing, optic nerve atrophy
GI: Diarrhea
*CV: **CHF,** peripheral vascular thrombosis, pulmonary edema
INTEG: Itching, rash, pain at site
META: Hypokalemia

Contraindications: Hypersensitivity, optic nerve atrophy
Precautions: Pregnancy (A), lactation, children
Pharmacokinetics: Stored in liver, kidneys, stomach; 50%-90% excreted in urine; crosses placenta, breast milk

Interactions/incompatibilities:
• Decreased absorption: aminoglycosides, anticonvulsants, colchicine, chloramphenicol, aminosalicylic acid, potassium preparation, cimetidine
• Increased absorption: prednisone

NURSING CONSIDERATIONS
Assess:
• GI function: diarrhea, constipation
• Potassium levels during beginning treatment
• CBC for increase in reticulocyte count during 1st week of therapy, then increase in RBC and hemoglobin

Administer:
• With fruit juice to disguise taste
• With meals if possible for better absorption
• By IM injection for pernicious anemia unless contraindicated for life

Perform/provide:
• Protection from light and heat

Evaluate:
• Therapeutic response: decreased anorexia, dyspnea on exertion, palpitations, paresthesias, psychosis, visual disturbances
• Nutritional status: egg yolks, fish, organ meats, dairy products, clams, oysters, which are good sources for vitamin B$_{12}$
• For pulmonary edema, or worsening of CHF in cardiac patients

Teach patient/family
• That treatment must continue for life if diagnosed as having pernicious anemia
• Well balanced diet
• Avoid contact with persons with infection

Lab test interferences:
False positive: Intrinsic factor

---

italics = common side effects   ***bold italic*** = life threatening reactions

Treatment of overdose: Discontinue drug

---

cyclacillin
(sye-kla-sill'in)
Cyclapen-W

Func. class.: Broad-spectrum antibiotic

Chem. class.: Aminopenicillin

Action: Interferes with cell wall replication of susceptible organisms; osmotically unstable cell wall swells, bursts from osmotic pressure

Uses: Otitis media and skin, soft tissue, urinary tract, respiratory tract infections by gram-positive cocci *(S. aureus, S. pneumoniae),* gram-negative cocci, gram-negative bacilli *(E. coli, H. influenzae, P. mirabilis)*

Dosage and routes:
• *Adult:* PO 250-500 mg q6h
• *Child:* PO 50-100 mg/kg/day q6h in equally divided doses

Available forms include: Tabs 250, 500 mg; powder for oral susp 125, 250 mg/5 ml

Side effects/adverse reactions:
HEMA: Anemia, increased bleeding time, *bone marrow depression, granulocytopenia*
GI: Nausea, vomiting, diarrhea, increased AST, ALT, abdominal pain, glossitis, colitis
GU: Oliguria, proteinuria, hematuria, *vaginitis, moniliasis, glomerulonephritis*
CNS: Lethargy, hallucinations, anxiety, depression, twitching, *coma, convulsions*
META: Hyperkalemia, hypokalemia, alkalosis, hypernatremia

Contraindications: Hypersensitivity to penicillins

Precautions: Hypersensitivity to cephalosporins, child <2 mo, pregnancy (B)

Pharmacokinetics:
PO: peak 40-60 min, half-life 30-40 min, metabolized in liver, excreted in urine (unchanged)

Interactions/incompatibilities:
• Decreased antimicrobial effectiveness of cyclacillin: tetracyclines, erythromycins
• Increased cyclacillin concentrations: aspirin, probenecid

NURSING CONSIDERATIONS
Assess:
• I&O ratio; report hematuria, oliguria since penicillin in high doses is nephrotoxic
• Any patient with compromised renal system since drug is excreted slowly in poor renal system function; toxicity may occur rapidly
• Liver studies: AST, ALT
• Blood studies: WBC, RBC, Hct/Hgb, bleeding time
• Renal studies: urinalysis, protein, blood
• C&S before drug therapy; drug may be taken as soon as culture is taken

Administer:
• Drug after C&S has been completed

Perform/provide:
• Adrenalin, suction, tracheostomy set, endotracheal intubation equipment
• Adequate fluid intake (2000 ml) during diarrhea episodes
• Scratch test to assess allergy, after securing order from physician; usually done when penicillin is only drug of choice
• Storage in tight container; after reconstituting, store in refrigerator for up to 2 wk

Evaluate:
• Therapeutic effectiveness: absence of fever, draining wounds

---

*Available in Canada only

- Bowel pattern before, during treatment
- Skin eruptions after administration of penicillin to 1 wk after discontinuing drug
- Respiratory status: rate, character, wheezing, tightness in chest
- Allergies before initiation of treatment, reaction of each medication; highlight allergies on chart, Kardex

Teach patient/family:
- Aspects of drug therapy, including need to complete course of medication to ensure organism death (10-14 days); culture may be taken after completed course
- To report sore throat, fever, fatigue (could indicate superimposed infection)
- To wear or carry Medic Alert ID if allergic to penicillins
- To take on an empty stomach with a full glass of water

Lab test interferences:
False positive: Urine glucose, urine protein

Treatment of overdose: Withdraw drug, maintain airway, administer epinephrine, aminophylline, O_2, IV corticosteroids for anaphylaxis

---

cyclandelate
(sye-klan′da-late)
Cyclospasmol, Cyclan
Func. class.: Peripheral vasodilator
Chem. class.: Nonnitrate

Action: Relaxes vascular smooth muscle, dilates peripheral vascular smooth muscle by direct action
Uses: Intermittent claudication, thrombophlebitis, Raynaud's phenomenon, ischemic cerebrovascular disease, arteriosclerosis obliterans, nocturnal leg cramps

Dosage and routes:
- *Adult:* PO 200 mg qid, not to exceed 400 mg qid; maintenance dose is 400-800 mg/day in 2-4 divided doses
Available forms include: Tabs 200, 400 mg; caps 200, 400 mg
Side effects/adverse reactions:
HEMA: Increased bleeding time (rare)
CV: **Tachycardia**
CNS: Headache, paresthesias, dizziness, weakness
GI: Heartburn, eructation, nausea, pyrosis
INTEG: Sweating, flushing
Contraindications: Hypersensitivity
Precautions: Glaucoma, pregnancy (C), lactation, recent MI, hypertension, severe obliterative coronary artery or cerebrovascular disease
Pharmacokinetics:
PO: Onset 15 min, peak 1½ hr, duration 4 hr
NURSING CONSIDERATIONS
Assess:
- Bleeding time in individuals with bleeding disorders
Administer:
- With meals to reduce GI symptoms
Perform/provide:
- Storage in tight container at room temperature
Evaluate:
- Therapeutic response: ability to walk without pain, increased temperature in extremities, increased pulse volume
- Cardiac status: B/P, pulse, rate, rhythm, character; watch for increasing pulse
Teach patient/family:
- That medication is not cure, may need to be taken continuously
- That it is necessary to quit smok-

italics = common side effects   ***bold italic*** = life threatening reactions

ing to prevent excessive vasoconstriction

• That improvement may be sudden, but usually occurs gradually over several weeks

• To report headache, weakness, increased pulse, as drug may need to be decreased or discontinued

• To avoid hazardous activities until stabilized on medication; dizziness may occur

---

cyclizine HCl/
cyclizine lactate

(sye'kli-zeen)

Marezine, Marzine

Func. class.: Antiemetic, antihistamine, anticholinergic

Chem. class.: H_2-receptor antagonist, piperazine derivative

Action: Acts centrally by blocking chemoreceptor trigger zone, which in turn acts on vomiting center

Uses: Motion sickness, prevention of postoperative vomiting

Dosage and routes:

Vomiting

• *Adult:* IM 50 mg ½ hr before termination of surgery, then q4-6h prn (lactate)

• *Child:* IM 3 mg/kg divided in 3 equal doses

Motion sickness

• *Adult:* PO 50 mg then q4-6h prn, not to exceed 200 mg/day (HCl)

• *Child:* PO 25 mg q4-6h prn

Available forms include: Tabs 50 mg; inj 50 mg/ml

Side effects/adverse reactions:

CNS: Drowsiness, dizziness, vertigo, fatigue, restlessness, headache, insomnia, hallucinations (auditory/visual), hallucinations and *convulsions* in children

GI: Nausea, anorexia

EENT: Dry mouth, blurred vision, tinnitus

Contraindications: Hypersensitivity to cyclizines, shock

Precautions: Children, narrow-angle glaucoma, urinary retention, lactation, prostatic hypertrophy, elderly, pregnancy (B), lactation

Pharmacokinetics:

PO: Duration 4-6 hr, other pharmacokinetics not known

Interactions/incompatibilities:

• May increase effect of: alcohol, tranquilizers, narcotics

NURSING CONSIDERATIONS

Assess:

• VS, B/P

Administer:

• IM injection in large muscle mass, aspirate to avoid IV administration

• Tablets may be swallowed whole, chewed, or allowed to dissolve

Evaluate:

• Signs of toxicity of other drugs or masking of symptoms of disease: brain tumor, intestinal obstruction

• Observe for drowsiness, dizziness

Teach patient/family:

• That a false negative result may occur with skin testing; skin testing procedures should not be scheduled for 4 days after discontinuing use

• To avoid hazardous activities or activities requiring alertness; dizziness may occur; instruct patient to request assistance with ambulation

• Avoid alcohol, other depressants

Lab test interferences:

False negative: Allergy skin testing

---

cyclobenzaprine

(sye-kloe-ben′za-preen)
Flexeril
Func. class.: Skeletal muscle relaxant, central acting
Chem. class.: Tricyclic amine salt

Action: Unknown; may be related to antidepressant effects
Uses: Adjunct for relief of muscle spasm and pain in musculoskeletal conditions
Dosage and routes:
• *Adult:* PO 10 mg tid × 1 wk, not to exceed 60 mg/day × 3 wk
Side effects/adverse reactions:
CNS: Dizziness, weakness, drowsiness, headache, tremor, depression, insomnia, confusion, paresthesia
EENT: Diplopia, temporary loss of vision
CV: Postural hypotension, tachycardia, dysrhythmias
GI: Nausea, vomiting, hiccups, dry mouth
INTEG: Rash, pruritus, fever, facial flushing, sweating
GU: Urinary retention, frequency, change in libido
Contraindications: Acute recovery phase of myocardial infarction, dysrhythmias, heart block, congestive heart failure, hypersensitivity, child <12 yr, intermittent porphyria, thyroid disease
Precautions: Renal disease, hepatic disease, addictive personalities, pregnancy (B), avoid use for more than 2-3 wk
Pharmacokinetics:
PO: Onset 1 hr, peak 3-8 hr, duration 12-24 hr, half-life 1-3 days, metabolized by liver, excreted in urine, crosses placenta, excreted in breast milk

Interactions/incompatibilities:
• Decreased effects of: guanethidine
• Increased CNS depression: alcohol, tricyclic antidepressants, narcotics, barbiturates, sedatives, hypnotics
• Do not use within 14 days of MAOI
NURSING CONSIDERATIONS
Assess:
• Blood studies: CBC, WBC, differential; blood dyscrasias may occur
• Liver function studies: AST, ALT, alk phosphatase; hepatitis may occur
• ECG in epileptic patients; poor seizure control has occurred with patients taking this drug
Administer:
• With meals for GI symptoms
Perform/provide:
• Storage in tight container at room temperature
• Assistance with ambulation if dizziness, drowsiness occurs
Evaluate:
• Therapeutic response: decreased pain, spasticity; muscle spasms of acute, painful musculoskeletal conditions are generally short term, long-term therapy is seldom warranted
• Allergic reactions: rash, fever, respiratory distress
• Severe weakness, numbness in extremities
• Psychologic dependency: increased need for medication, more frequent requests for medication, increased pain
• CNS depression: dizziness, drowsiness, psychiatric symptoms
Teach patient/family:
• Not to discontinue medication quickly; insomnia, nausea, headache, spasticity, tachycardia will

---

italics = common side effects   ***bold italic*** = life threatening reactions

occur; drug should be tapered off over 1-2 wk
• Not to take with alcohol, other CNS depressants
• To avoid altering activities while taking this drug
• To avoid hazardous activities if drowsiness, dizziness occurs
• To avoid using OTC medication: cough preparations, antihistamines, unless directed by physician
• To use gum, frequent sips of water for dry mouth

Treatment of overdose: Empty stomach with emesis, gastric lavage, then administer activated charcoal; use anticonvulsants if indicated; monitor cardiac function

---

cyclopentolate HCl (optic)

(sye-kloe-pen'toe-late)
AK-Pentolate, Cyclogyl
Func. class.: Mydriatic, cycloplegic, anticholinergic

Action: Blocks response of iris sphincter muscle, muscle of accommodation of ciliary body to cholinergic stimulation, resulting in dilation, paralysis of accommodation

Uses: Cycloplegic refraction, mydriasis

Dosage and routes:
• *Adult:* INSTILL SOL 1 gtt of a 1% sol, then 1 gtt in 5 min
• *Child >6 yr:* INSTILL SOL 1 gtt of a 0.5%-2% sol, then 1 gtt in 5 min of a 0.5%-1% sol

Available forms include: Sol 0.5%, 1%, 2%

Side effects/adverse reactions:
SYST: Tachycardia, confusion, fever, flushing, dry skin, dry mouth, abdominal discomfort (infants:

bladder distention, irregular pulse, *respiratory depression)*
EENT: Blurred vision, temporary burning sensation on instillation, eye dryness, photophobia, conjunctivitism, increased intraocular pressure
CNS: Psychotic reaction, behavior disturbances, ataxia, restlessness, hallucinations, somnolence, disorientation, failure to recognize people, *grand mal seizures*
GI: Abdominal distention, vomiting

Contraindications: Hypersensitivity, infants <3 mo, local or systemic glaucoma, conjunctivitis

Precautions: Pregnancy (C)

Pharmacokinetics:
INSTILL: Peak 30-60 min (mydriasis), 25-74 min (cyclopegia), duration ¼-1 day

NURSING CONSIDERATIONS
Administer:
• After shaking vial to mix drug to clear solution, push stopper to mix sterile water with powder
• After cleaning stopper with alcohol (rubbing)
• Immediately after reconstituting, discard unused portion

Teach patient/family:
• To report change in vision, blurring, or loss of sight, trouble breathing, sweating, flushing
• Method of instillation: pressure on lacrimal sac for 1 min, do not touch dropper to eye
• That blurred vision will decrease with repeated use of drug
• That drug will burn when instilled
• Wear dark sunglasses for photophobia
• Not to do hazardous duties until able to see

---

cyclophosphamide

(sye-kloe-foss'fa-mide)

Cytoxan, Neosar, Procytox*

Func. class.: Antineoplastic alkylating agent

Chem. class.: Nitrogen mustard

Action: Alkylates DNA, RNA; inhibits enzymes that allow synthesis of amino acids in proteins; is also responsible for cross linking DNA strands, breast neuroblastoma

Uses: Hodgkin's disease; lymphomas; leukemia; cancer of female reproductive tract, lung, prostate; multiple myeloma; neuroblastoma; retinoblastoma; Ewing's sarcoma

Dosage and routes:

• *Adult:* PO initially 1-5 mg/kg over 2-5 days, maintenance is 1-5 mg/kg; IV initially 40-50 mg/kg in divided doses over 2-5 days, maintenance 10-15 mg/kg q7-10d, or 3-5 mg/kg q3d

• *Child:* PO/IV 2-8 mg/kg or 60-250 mg/m² in divided doses for 6 or more days; maintenance 10-15 mg/kg q7-10d or 30 mg/kg q3-4w; dose should be reduced by half when bone marrow depression occurs

Available forms include: Powder for inj IV 100, 200, 500 mg, 1, 2 g; tabs 25, 50 mg

Side effects/adverse reactions:

CV: **Cardiotoxicity** (high doses)

HEMA: **Thrombocytopenia, leukopenia, pancytopenia; myelosuppression**

GI: *Nausea, vomiting, diarrhea, weight loss,* colitis, **hepatotoxicity**

GU: **Hemorrhagic cystitis,** *hematuria, neoplasms, amenorrhea, azoospermia, impotence, sterility, ovarian fibrosis*

INTEG: *Alopecia,* dermatitis

RESP: **Fibrosis**

ENDO: Syndrome of inappropriate antidiuretic hormone (SIADH)

CNS: Headache, dizziness

Contraindications: Lactation, pregnancy (D)

Precautions: Radiation therapy

Pharmacokinetics:

Metabolized by liver, excreted in urine; half-life 4-6½ hr; 50% bound to plasma proteins

Interactions/incompatibilities:

• Increased toxicity: aminoglycosides

• Increased metabolism of cyclophosphamide: phenobarbital

• Potentiation of cyclophosphamide: succinylcholine

• Increased bone marrow depression: allopurinol, thiazides

• Decreased digoxin levels: digoxin

NURSING CONSIDERATIONS

Assess:

• CBC, differential, platelet count weekly; withhold drug if WBC is <4000 or platelet count is <75,000; notify physician of results

• Pulmonary function tests, chest x-ray films before, during therapy; chest film should be obtained q2wk during treatment

• Renal function studies: BUN, serum uric acid, urine CrCl before, during therapy

• I&O ratio; report fall in urine output of 30 ml/hr

• Monitor temperature q4h (may indicate beginning infection)

• Liver function tests before, during therapy (bilirubin, AST, ALT, LDH) as needed or monthly

Administer:

• Fluids IV or PO before chemotherapy to hydrate patient

• Antacid before oral agent, give

---

italics = common side effects   ***bold italic*** = life threatening reactions

drug after evening meal, before bedtime
• Antiemetic 30-60 min before giving drug to prevent vomiting, and prn
• Allopurinol or sodium bicarbonate to maintain uric acid levels, alkalinization of urine
• Prevent hyperuricemia
• Antibiotics for prophylaxis of infection
• IV after diluting 100 mg/5 ml of sterile H_2O or bacteriostatic H_2O; shake; may be further diluted in up to 250-ml compatible sol
• Slow (over 3 min) IV infusion using 21-, 23-, 25-gauge needle, check site for irritation, phlebitis
• Topical or systemic analgesics for pain
• Local or systemic drugs for infection
• In AM so drug can be eliminated before hs

Perform/provide:
• Storage in tight container at room temperature
• Strict medical asepsis, protective isolation if WBC levels are low
• Special skin care
• Deep breathing exercises with patient tid-qid; place in semi-Fowler's position
• Increase fluid intake to 2-3 L/day to prevent urate deposits, calcuii formation, reduce incidence of hemorrhagic cystitis
• Diet low in purines: organ meats (kidney, liver), dried beans, peas to maintain alkaline urine
• Rinsing of mouth tid-qid with water, club soda; brushing of teeth bid-tid with soft brush or cotton-tipped applicators for stomatitis; use unwaxed dental floss
• Warm compresses at injection site for inflammation

Evaluate:
• Bleeding: hematuria, guaiac, bruising or petechiae, mucosa or orifices q8h
• Dyspnea, rales, unproductive cough, chest pain, tachypnea
• Food preferences; list likes, dislikes
• Effects of alopecia on body image, discuss feelings about body changes
• Yellowing of skin, sclera, dark urine, clay-colored stools, itchy skin, abdominal pain, fever, diarrhea
• Edema in feet, joint pain, stomach pain, shaking
• Inflammation of mucosa, breaks in skin
• Buccal cavity q8h for dryness, sores or ulceration, white patches, oral pain, bleeding, dysphagia, obtain prescription for viscous xylocaine
• Symptoms indicating severe allergic reaction: rash, pruritus, urticaria, purpuric skin lesions, itching, flushing
• Tachypnea, ECG changes, dyspnea, edema, fatigue

Teach patient/family:
• Of protective isolation precautions
• That impotence or amenorrhea can occur, reversible after discontinuing treatment
• To report any changes in breathing or coughing
• That hair may be lost during treatment; a wig or hairpiece may make patient feel better; new hair may be different in color, texture
• To avoid foods with citric acid, hot or rough texture
• To report any bleeding, white spots or ulcerations in mouth to physician; tell patient to examine mouth qd

---

* Available in Canada only

• To report signs of infection: increased temperature, sore throat, flu symptoms
• To report signs of anemia: fatigue, headache, faintness, shortness of breath, irritability
• To report bleeding: avoid use of razors, or commercial mouthwash
• To avoid use of aspirin products or ibuprofen

Lab test interferences:
Increase: Uric acid
False positive: Pap test
False negative: PPD, mumps trichophytin, *Candida*
Decrease: Pseudocholinesterase

---

cycloserine

(sye-kloe-ser'een)
Seromycin Pulvules
Func. class.: Antitubercular
Chem. class.: S. oichidaceus, antibiotic

Action: Inhibits RNA synthesis, decreases tubercle bacilli replication

Uses: Pulmonary tuberculosis, extrapulmonary as adjunctive

Dosage and routes:
• *Adult:* PO 250 mg q12h × 14 days, then 250 mg q8h × 2 wk if there are no signs of toxicity, then 250 mg q6h if there are no signs of toxicity, not to exceed 1 g/day

Available forms include: Caps 250 mg

Side effects/adverse reactions:
INTEG: Dermatitis, photosensitivity
CV: **CHF, dysrhythmias**
CNS: Headache, anxiety, drowsiness, tremors, *convulsions,* lethargy, depression, confusion, psychosis, aggression
EENT: Blurred vision, optic neuritis, photophobia
HEMA: **Megaloblastic anemia,** vitamin B$_{12}$, folic acid deficiency, leukocytosis
GU: Tubular necrosis, hypokalemia, alkalosis

Contraindications: Hypersensitivity, seizure disorders, renal disease, alcoholism (chronic)

Precautions: Pregnancy (C), children

Pharmacokinetics:
PO: Peak 3-4 hr; excreted unchanged in urine, crosses placenta, excreted in breast milk

Interactions/incompatibilities:
• Seizures: alcohol
• May increase toxicity: ethionamide, isoniazid, phenytoin

NURSING CONSIDERATIONS
Assess:
• Liver studies q wk: ALT, AST, bilirubin
• Renal status: before; q mo: BUN, creatinine, output, sp gr, urinalysis
• Blood levels of drug; keep at <30 µg/ml or toxicity may occur

Administer:
• With meals to decrease GI symptoms
• Antiemetic if vomiting occurs
• After C&S is completed, q mo to detect resistance
• Pyridoxine if ordered to prevent neurotoxicity

Perform/provide:
• Storage in tight container at room temperature

Evaluate:
• Mental status often: affect, mood, behavioral changes, psychosis may occur
• Hepatic status: decreased appetite, jaundice, dark urine, fatigue

Teach patient/family:
• Avoid alcohol while taking drug
• That compliance with dosage schedule, length is necessary
• To report neurotoxicity: confusion, headache, drowsiness, trem-

---

italics = common side effects   **bold italic** = life threatening reactions

ors, paresthesias, mental changes
• To avoid hazardous activities if
drowsiness or dizziness occurs
Lab test interferences:
Increase: AST/ALT
Treatment of overdose: Administer vitamin B$_6$, anticonvulsants, lavage, O$_2$, assisted respiration

---

cyclosporine

(sye'kloe-spor-een)
Sandimmune

Func. class.: Immunosuppressant
Chem. class.: Fungus-derived peptide

Action: Produces immunosuppression by inhibiting lymphocytes (T)
Uses: Organ transplants to prevent rejection
Dosage and routes:
• *Adult and child:* PO 15 mg/kg several hours before surgery, daily for 2 wk, reduce dosage by 2.5 mg/kg/wk to 5-10 mg/kg/day; IV 5-6 mg/kg several hours before surgery, daily, switch to PO form as soon as possible
Available forms include: Oral sol 100 mg/ml; inj IV 50 mg/ml
Side effects/adverse reactions:
GI: Nausea, vomiting, diarrhea, *oral Candida, gum hyperplasia, hepatotoxicity,* pancreatitis
INTEG: Rash, acne, *hirsutism*
CNS: Tremors, headache
GU: Albuminuria, hematuria, proteinuria, renal failure
Contraindications: Hypersensitivity
Precautions: Severe renal disease, severe hepatic disease, pregnancy (C)
Pharmacokinetics: Peak 4 hr, highly protein bound, half-life (biphasic) 1.2 hr, 25 hr; metabolized

in liver, excreted in feces, crosses placenta, excreted in breast milk
Interactions/incompatibilities:
• Increased action of cyclosporine: amphotericin B, cimetidine, ketoconazole
• Decreased action of cyclosporine: phenytoin, rifampin
NURSING CONSIDERATIONS
Assess:
• Renal studies: BUN, creatinine at least monthly during treatment, 3 mo after treatment
• Liver function studies: alk phosphatase, AST, ALT, bilirubin
• Drug blood levels during treatment
Administer:
• IV after diluting each 50 mg/20-100 ml of normal saline or D$_5$W; run over 2-6 hr; use an infusion pump
• For several days before transplant surgery
• With corticosteroids
• With meals for GI upset or drug placed in chocolate milk
• With oral antifungal for *Candida* infections
Evaluate:
• Hepatotoxicity: dark urine, jaundice, itching, light-colored stools; drug should be discontinued
Teach patient/family:
• To report fever, chills, sore throat, fatigue since serious infections may occur
• To use contraceptive measures during treatment, for 12 wk after ending therapy

---

cyproheptadine HCl

(si-proe-hep'-ta-deen)
Periactin, Vimicon*

Func. class.: Antihistamine, H$_1$ receptor antagonist
Chem. class.: Piperidine

Action: Acts on blood vessels, GI,

respiratory system by competing with histamine for H_1-receptor site; decreases allergic response by blocking histamine

Uses: Allergy symptoms, rhinitis, pruritus, cold urticaria

Dosage and routes:
• *Adult:* PO 4 mg tid-qid, not to exceed 0.5 mg/kg/day
• *Child 7-14 yr:* PO 4 mg bid-tid, not to exceed 16 mg/day
• *Child 2-6 yr:* PO 2 mg bid-tid, not to exceed 12 mg/day

Available forms include: Tabs 4 mg; syr 2 mg/5 ml

Side effects/adverse reactions:
CNS: Dizziness, drowsiness, poor coordination, fatigue, anxiety, euphoria, confusion, paresthesia, neuritis
CV: Hypotension, palpitations, tachycardia
RESP: Increased thick secretions, wheezing, chest tightness
GI: Constipation, dry mouth, nausea, vomiting, anorexia, diarrhea, weight gain
INTEG: Rash, urticaria, photosensitivity
GU: Retention, dysuria, frequency, increased appetite
EENT: Blurred vision, dilated pupils, tinnitus, nasal stuffiness, dry nose, throat, mouth

Contraindications: Hypersensitivity to H_1-receptor antagonist, acute asthma attack, lower respiratory tract disease

Precautions: Increased intraocular pressure, renal disease, cardiac disease, hypertension, bronchial asthma, seizure disorder, stenosed peptic ulcers, hyperthyroidism, prostatic hypertrophy, bladder neck obstruction, pregnancy (B)

Pharmacokinetics:
PO: Duration 4-6 hr, metabolized in liver, excreted by kidneys, excreted in breast milk

Interactions/incompatibilities:
• Increased CNS depression: barbiturates, narcotics, hypnotics, tricyclic antidepressants, alcohol
• Decreased effect of: oral anticoagulants, heparin
• Increased effect of cyproheptadine: MAOIs

NURSING CONSIDERATIONS
Assess:
• I&O ratio; be alert for urinary retention, frequency, dysuria; drug should be discontinued if these occur
• CBC during long-term therapy

Administer:
• With meals if GI symptoms occur; absorption may slightly decrease

Perform/provide:
• Hard candy, gum, frequent rinsing of mouth for dryness
• Storage in tight container at room temperature

Evaluate:
• Therapeutic response: absence of running or congested nose or rashes
• Respiratory status: rate, rhythm, increase in bronchial secretions, wheezing, chest tightness
• Cardiac status: palpitations, increased pulse, hypotension

Teach patient/family:
• All aspects of drug use; to notify physician if confusion, sedation, hypotension occurs
• To avoid driving or other hazardous activity if drowsiness occurs
• To avoid concurrent use of alcohol or other CNS depressants

Lab test interferences:
False negative: Skin allergy tests

Treatment of overdose: Administer ipecac syrup or lavage, diazepam, vasopressors, barbiturates (short-acting)

---

italics = common side effects   **bold italic** = life threatening reactions

cytarabine (ARA-C, cytosine arabinoside)

(sye-tare′a-been)

Cytosar-U

Func. class.: Antineoplastic, antimetabolite

Chem. class.: Pyrimidine nucleoside

Action: Competes with physiologic substrate that inhibits DNA synthesis; interferes with cell replication at S phase, directly before mitosis

Uses: Acute myelocytic leukemia, acute lymphocytic leukemia, chronic myelocytic leukemia, and in combination for non-Hodgkin's lymphomas in children

Dosage and routes:

Acute myelocytic leukemia

• *Adult:* IV INF 200 mg/m²/day × 5 days; INTRATHECAL 5-50 mg/m²/day × 3 days/wk or 30 mg/m²/day q4 days

In combination

• *Child:* IV INF 100 mg/m²/day × 5-10 days

Available forms include: Inj IV, intrathecal 100, 500 mg, 1, 2 g

Side effects/adverse reactions:

HEMA: Thrombophlebitis, bleeding, thrombocytopenia, leukopenia, myelosuppression, anemia

GI: Nausea, vomiting, anorexia, diarrhea, stomatitis, hepatotoxicity, abdominal pain, hematemesis, *GI hemorrhage*

EENT: Sore throat, conjunctivitis

GU: Urinary retention, *renal failure, hyperuricemia*

INTEG: Rash, fever, freckling, cellulitis

RESP: Pneumonia, dyspnea

CV: Chest pain, *cardiopathy*

CNS: Neuritis, dizziness, headache, personality changes, ataxia, mechanical dysphasia, *coma*

CYTARABINE SYNDROME: Fever, myalgia, bone pain, chest pain, rash, conjunctivitis, malaise (6-12 hr after administration)

Contraindications: Hypersensitivity, infants, pregnancy (1st trimester)

Precautions: Renal disease, hepatic disease, pregnancy (C)

Pharmacokinetics:

INTRATHECAL: Half-life 2 hr, metabolized in liver, excreted in urine (primarily inactive metabolite), crosses blood-brain barrier, placenta

IV: Distribution half-life 10 min, elimination half-life 1-3 hr

Interactions/incompatibilities:

• Increased toxicity: radiation or other antineoplastics

• Decreased effects of: oral digoxin

NURSING CONSIDERATIONS

Assess:

• CBC (RBC, Hct, Hgb), differential, platelet count weekly; withhold drug if WBC is <4000/mm,³ platelet count is <75,000/mm,³ or RBC, Hct, Hgb are low; notify physician of these results

• Renal function studies: BUN, serum uric acid, urine creatinine clearance, electrolytes before and during therapy

• I&O ratio; report fall in urine output to <30 ml/hr

• Monitor temperature q4h; fever may indicate beginning infection; no rectal temperatures

• Liver function tests before and during therapy: bilirubin, ALT, AST, alk phosphatase, as needed or monthly

• Blood uric acid levels during therapy

Administer:

• Antiemetic 30-60 min before giving drug to prevent vomiting, and prn

---

*Available in Canada only

• Allopurinol or sodium bicarbonate to maintain uric acid levels and alkalinization of the urine
• Prevent hyperuricemia
• Antibiotics for prophylaxis of infection
• IV after diluting 100 mg/5 ml of sterile H_2O for inj; may be further diluted in 50-100 ml normal saline or D_5W
• Slow IV infusion using 21-, 23-, 25-gauge needle
• Topical or systemic analgesics for pain
• Transfusion for anemia
• Antispasmodic for GI symptoms

Perform/provide:
• Strict medical asepsis and protective isolation if WBC levels are low
• Increase fluid intake to 2-3 L/day to prevent urate deposits and calculi formation, unless contraindicated
• Diet low in purines: absence of organ meats (kidney, liver), dried beans, peas to prevent increased urate deposits
• Rinsing of mouth tid-qid with water, club soda; brushing of teeth bid-tid with soft brush or cotton-tipped applicators for stomatitis; use unwaxed dental floss
• HOB increased to facilitate breathing if dyspnea or pneumonia occurs

Evaluate:
• Cytarabine syndrome: fever, myalgia, bone pain, chest pain, rash, conjunctivitis, malaise; corticosteroids may be ordered
• Bleeding: hematuria, guaiac, bruising or petechiae, mucosa or orifices q8h
• Dyspnea, rales, unproductive cough, chest pain, tachypnea, fatigue, increased pulse, pallor, lethargy, personality changes, with high doses

• Food preferences; list likes, dislikes
• Edema in feet, joint pain, stomach pain, shaking
• Inflammation of mucosa, breaks in skin
• Yellowing of skin, sclera, dark urine, clay-colored stools, itchy skin, abdominal pain, fever, diarrhea
• Buccal cavity q8h for dryness, sores or ulceration, white patches, oral pain, bleeding, dysphagia
• Local irritation, pain, burning, discoloration at injection site
• GI symptoms: frequency of stools, cramping
• Acidosis, signs of dehydration: rapid respirations, poor skin turgor, decreased urine output, dry skin, restlessness, weakness

Teach patient/family:
• Why protective isolation precautions are necessary
• To report any coughing, chest pain, or changes in breathing, which may indicate beginning pneumonia
• To avoid foods with citric acid, hot or rough texture if stomatitis is present
• To report stomatitis: any bleeding, white spots, ulcerations in mouth; tell patient to examine mouth qd, report any symptoms
• To report signs of infection: increased temperature, sore throat, flu symptoms
• To report signs of anemia: fatigue, headache, faintness, shortness of breath, irritability
• To report bleeding; avoid use of razors or commercial mouthwash
• To avoid use of aspirin products or ibuprofen

---

italics = common side effects   ***bold italic*** = life threatening reactions

dacarbazine (DTIC)

(da-kar'ba-zeen)
DTIC-Dome
Func. class.: Antineoplastic alkylating agent
Chem. class.: Cytotoxic triazine

Action: Alkylates DNA, RNA; inhibits enzymes that allow synthesis of amino acids in proteins; also responsible for cross-linking DNA strands

Uses: Hodgkin's disease, sarcomas, neuroblastoma, malignant melanoma

Dosage and routes:
• *Adult:* IV 2-4.5 mg/kg or 70-160 mg/m² qd × 10 days, repeat q4wk depending on response or 250 mg/m² qd × 5 days, repeat q3wk
Available forms include: Inj IV 100, 200 mg

Side effects/adverse reactions:
*HEMA: **Thrombocytopenia, leukopenia,** anemia*
*GI: Nausea, anorexia, vomiting, **hepatotoxicity***
CNS: Facial paresthesia, flushing, fever, malaise
INTEG: Alopecia, dermatitis, pain at injection site

Contraindications: Lactation
Precautions: Radiation therapy, pregnancy (1st trimester) (C)
Pharmacokinetics:
Metabolized by liver, excreted in urine; half-life 35 min, terminal 5 hr, 5% protein bound
Interactions/incompatibilities:
Decreased effectiveness of dacarbazine: phenytoin, phenobarbital
NURSING CONSIDERATIONS
Assess:
• CBC, differential, platelet count weekly; withhold drug if WBC is <4000 or platelet count is

<75,000; notify physician of results
• Monitor temperature q4h (may indicate beginning infection)
• Liver function tests before, during therapy (bilirubin, AST, ALT, LDH) as needed or monthly
Administer:
• Antiemetic 30-60 min before giving drug to prevent vomiting
• Antibiotics for prophylaxis of infection
• After diluting 100 mg/9.9 ml of sterile H₂O for inj; may be further diluted in 50-250 ml of D₅W or normal saline for inj
• Slow IV infusion using 21-, 23-, 25-gauge needle, watch for extravasation
Perform/provide:
• Storage in light-resistant container, dry area
• Strict medical asepsis, protective isolation if WBC levels are low
• Increase fluid intake to 2-3 L/day to prevent urate deposits, calculi formation
• Warm compresses at injection site for inflammation
Evaluate:
• Bleeding: hematuria, guaiac, bruising or petechiae, mucosa or orifices q8h
• Food preferences; list likes, dislikes
• Effects of alopecia on body image, discuss feelings about body changes
• Yellowing of skin, sclera, dark urine, clay-colored stools, itchy skin, abdominal pain, fever, diarrhea
• Inflammation of mucosa, breaks in skin
Teach patient/family:
• Of protective isolation precautions
• That hair may be lost during treat-

ment; a wig or hairpiece may make the patient feel better; new hair may be different in color, texture
• To report signs of infection: increased temperature, sore throat, flu symptoms
• To report signs of anemia: fatigue, headache, faintness, shortness of breath, irritability
• To report bleeding; avoid use of razors or commercial mouthwash
• To avoid use of aspirin products or ibuprofen

dactinomycin (actinomycin D)

(dak-ti-noe-mye'sin)
Cosmegen

Func. class.: Antineoplastic, antibiotic

Action: Inhibits DNA, RNA, protein synthesis; derived from *Streptomyces parrullus;* replication is decreased by binding to DNA, which causes strand splitting; cell cycle nonspecific; a vesicant

Uses: Sarcomas, melanomas, trophoblastic tumors in women, testicular cancer, Wilms' tumor, rhabdomyosarcoma

Dosage and routes:
• *Adult:* IV 500 μg/m²/day × 5 days; stop drug for 2-4 wk; then repeat cycle
• *Child:* IV 15 μg/kg/day × 5 days, not to exceed 500 μg/day; stop drug until bone marrow recovery, then repeat cycle
Available forms include: Inj IV 500 μg

Side effects/adverse reactions:
*HEMA: **Thrombocytopenia, leukopenia, aplastic anemia***
*GI: Nausea, vomiting, anorexia, stomatitis, **hepatotoxicity,** abdominal pain, diarrhea*

INTEG: Rash, alopecia, pain at injection site, folliculitis, acne, desquamation, ***extravasation***
EENT: Chelitis, dysphagia, esophagitis
CNS: Malaise, fatigue, lethargy, fever
MS: Myalgia
Contraindications: Hypersensitivity, herpes infections, child <6 months
Precautions: Renal disease, hepatic disease, pregnancy (C), lactation, bone marrow depression
Pharmacokinetics: Half-life 36 hr; IV: onset 2-5 min, concentrates in kidneys, liver, spleen; does not cross blood-brain barrier, excreted in feces and urine
Interactions/incompatibilities:
• Increased toxicity: other antineoplastics or radiation

NURSING CONSIDERATIONS
Assess:
• CBC, differential, platelet count weekly; withhold drug if WBC is <4000/mm³ or platelet count is <75,000/mm³; notify physician of these results
• Renal function studies: BUN, serum uric acid, urine CrCl, electrolytes before, during therapy
• I&O ratio; report fall in urine output to <30 ml/hr
• Monitor temperature q4h; fever may indicate beginning infection
• Liver function tests before, during therapy: bilirubin, AST, ALT, alk phosphatase, as needed or monthly
Administer:
• Antiemetic 30-60 min before giving drug to prevent vomiting
• Antibiotics as ordered for prophylaxis of infection
• After diluting 0.5 mg/1.1 ml of sterile H₂O for inj without preservative, may be further diluted in 50

---

italics = common side effects   ***bold italic*** = life threatening reactions

ml D_5W or normal saline for infusion; run over 10-15 min
• Slow IV infusion using 21-, 23-, 25-gauge needle, check for extravasation
• Topical or systemic analgesics for pain
• Local or systemic drugs for infection
• Hydrocortisone, sodium thiosulfate to infiltration area, and ice compress after stopping infusion
• Antispasmodic for GI symptoms
Perform/provide:
• Strict handwashing technique, gloves and protective covering
• Liquid diet: carbonated beverages, gelatin may be added if patient is not nauseated or vomiting
• Rinsing of mouth tid-qid with water, club soda; brushing of teeth bid-qid with soft brush or cotton-tipped applicators for stomatitis; use unwaxed dental floss
• Storage in darkness in cool environment
Evaluate:
• Bleeding: hematuria, guaiac stools, bruising, petechiae, mucosa or orifices q8h
• Food preferences; list likes, dislikes
• Effects of alopecia on body image; discuss feelings about body changes
• Inflammation of mucosa, breaks in skin
• Yellowing of skin, sclera, dark urine, clay-colored stools, itchy skin, abdominal pain, fever, diarrhea
• Buccal cavity q8h for dryness, sores, ulceration, white patches, oral pain, bleeding, dysphagia
• Local irritation, pain, burning at injection site
• Symptoms indicating severe allergic reaction: rash, pruritus, urticaria, purpuric skin lesions, itching, flushing
• GI symptoms: frequency of stools, cramping
• Acidosis, signs of dehydration: rapid respirations, poor skin turgor, decreased urine output, dry skin, restlessness, weakness
Teach patient/family:
• To report any complaints, side effects to nurse or physician
• That hair may be lost during treatment and wig or hairpiece may make patient feel better; tell patient that new hair may be different in color, texture
• To avoid foods with citric acid, hot or rough texture
• To report any bleeding, white spots, ulcerations in mouth to physician; tell patient to examine mouth qd
• To avoid crowds and sources of infection when granulocyte count is low
Lab test interferences:
Increase: Uric acid

---

danazol

(da'na-zole)
Cyclomen,* Danocrine
Func. class.: Androgen
Chem. class.: α-Ethinyl testosterone derivative

Action: Atrophy of endometrial tissue, decreases FSH, LH, which are controlled by pituitary; this leads to amenorrhea/anovulation
Uses: Endometriosis, prevention of hereditary angioedema, fibrocystic breast disease
Dosage and routes:
Endometriosis
• *Adult:* PO initial dose 500 mg bid then decreased to 400 mg bid × 3-9 mo

---

Fibrocystic breast disease
- *Adult:* PO 100-400 mg qd in 2 divided doses × 2-6 mo

Hereditary angioedema
- *Adult:* PO 200 mg bid-tid until desired response, then decrease dose to 100 mg at 1-3 mo intervals

Available forms include: Caps 50, 100, 200 mg

Side effects/adverse reactions:

INTEG: Rash, acneiform lesions, oily hair, skin, flushing, sweating, acne vulgaris, alopecia, hirsutism

CNS: Dizziness, headache, fatigue, tremors, paresthesias, flushing, sweating, anxiety, lability, insomnia

MS: Cramps, spasms

CV: Increased B/P

GU: Hematuria, amenorrhea, atrophic vaginitis, decreased libido, decreased breast size, clitoral hypertrophy, testicular atrophy

GI: Nausea, vomiting, constipation, weight gain, ***cholestatic jaundice***

EENT: Carpal tunnel syndrome, conjunctival edema, nasal congestion

ENDO: Abnormal GTT

Contraindications: Severe renal disease, severe cardiac disease, severe hepatic disease, hypersensitivity, genital bleeding (abnormal)

Precautions: Migraine headaches, seizure disorders, pregnancy (C)

Interactions/incompatibilities:
- Increased effects of: oral antidiabetics, oxyphenbutazone
- Increased prothrombin time: anticoagulants
- Edema: ACTH, adrenal steroids
- Decreased effects of: insulin

NURSING CONSIDERATIONS

Assess:
- Potassium, blood sugar, urine glucose while on long-term therapy

- Weight daily; notify physician if weekly weight gain is >5 lb
- I&O ratio; be alert for decreasing urinary output, increasing edema

Administer:
- With food or milk to decrease GI symptoms

Perform/provide:
- Storage in tight container at room temperature
- ROM exercise for patients who are immobile

Evaluate:
- Therapeutic response: decreased pain in endometriosis, decreased size, pain in fibrocystic breast disease
- Edema, hypertension, cardiac symptoms, jaundice
- Mental status: affect, mood, behavioral changes, aggression, sleep disorders, depression
- Signs of virilization: deepening of voice, decreased libido, facial hair (may not be reversible)
- Hypercalcemia: GI symptoms, polydipsia, polyuria, increased calcium levels, decrease in muscle tone

Teach patient/family:
- To notify physician if therapeutic response decreases
- Not to discontinue medication abruptly but to taper over several weeks
- Women to report menstrual irregularities, that amenorrhea usually occurs but menstruation resumes 2-3 mo after termination of therapy
- Routine breast self-exam, report any increase in nodule size
- Drug should induce anovulation; reversible within 60-90 days after drug is discontinued
- Endometriosis tends to recur after drug is discontinued

Lab test interferences:

Increase: Cholesterol

---

italics = common side effects   ***bold italic*** = life threatening reactions

Decrease: Cholesterol, T$_4$, T$_3$, thyroid ^{131}I uptake test, 17-KS, PBI
Interferes: GTT

---

dantrolene sodium

(dan'troe-leen)
Dantrium, Dantrium IV
Func. class.: Skeletal muscle relaxant, direct acting
Chem. class.: Hydantoin

Action: Interferes with intracellular release of calcium necessary to initiate contraction
Uses: Spasticity in multiple sclerosis, stroke, spinal cord injury, cerebral palsy, malignant hyperthermia
Dosage and routes:
Spasticity
• *Adult:* PO 25 mg/day; may increase by 25-100 mg bid-qid, not to exceed 400 mg/day × 1 wk
• *Child:* PO 1 mg/kg/day given in divided doses bid-tid; may increase gradually, not to exceed 100 mg qid
Malignant hyperthermia
• *Adult and child:* IV 1 mg/kg, may repeat to total dose of 10 mg/kg; PO 4-8 mg/kg/day in 4 divided doses × 3 days to prevent further hyperthermia
Available forms include: Caps 25, 50, 100 mg; powder for inj IV 20 mg/vial
Side effects/adverse reactions:
CNS: Dizziness, weakness, fatigue, drowsiness, headache, disorientation, insomnia, paresthesias, tremors
EENT: Nasal congestion, blurred vision, mydriasis
HEMA: Eosinophilia
CV: Hypotension, chest pain, palpitations
GI: Nausea, constipation, vomiting, increased AST, alk phospha-

tase, abdominal pain, dry mouth, anorexia, hepatitis
GU: Urinary frequency, nocturia, impotence, crystalluria
INTEG: Rash, pruritus, photosensitivity
Contraindications: Hypersensitivity, compromised pulmonary function, active hepatic disease, impaired myocardial function
Precautions: Peptic ulcer disease, renal disease, hepatic disease, stroke, seizure disorder, diabetes mellitus, pregnancy (C); although weakness is a transient side effect, some patients feel excessively weak throughout therapy
Pharmacokinetics:
PO: Peak 5 hr, highly protein bound, half-life 8 hr, metabolized in liver, excreted in urine (metabolites)
Interactions/incompatibilities:
• Increased CNS depression: alcohol, tricylic antidepressants, narcotics, barbiturates, sedatives, hypnotics

NURSING CONSIDERATIONS
Assess:
• For increased seizure activity in epilepsy patient
• I&O ratio; check for urinary retention, frequency, hesitancy
• ECG in epileptic patients; poor seizure control has occurred with patients taking this drug
• Hepatic function by frequent determination of AST, ALT, renal function studies, CBC
Administer:
• With meals for GI symptoms
• Gum, frequent sips of water for dry mouth
• IV after diluting 20 mg/60 ml sterile H$_2$O for inj without bacteriostatic agent; shake; give by rapid IV push through Y-tube or 3-way stopcock

---

* Available in Canada only

Perform/provide:
• Storage in tight container at room temperature
• Assistance with ambulation if dizziness, drowsiness occurs
Evaluate:
• Therapeutic response: decreased pain, spasticity
• Allergic reactions: rash, fever, respiratory distress
• Severe weakness, numbness in extremities
• Psychologic dependency: increased need for medication, more frequent requests for medication, increased pain
• CNS depression: dizziness, drowsiness, psychiatric symptoms
• Signs of hepatitis: jaundice, yellow sclera, pain in abdomen, nausea, fever
Teach patient/family:
• Not to discontinue medication quickly; hallucinations, spasticity, tachycardia will occur; drug should be tapered off over 1-2 wk, notify physician of abdominal pain, jaundiced sclera, clay-colored stools, change in color of urine
• Not to take with alcohol, other CNS depressants
• That if improvement does not occur within 6 wk MD may discontinue
• To avoid altering activities while taking this drug
• To avoid hazardous activities if drowsiness, dizziness occurs
• To avoid using OTC medication: cough preparations, antihistamines, unless directed by physician
Treatment of overdose: Induce emesis of conscious patient, lavage, dialysis

dapsone (DDS)
(dap'sone)
Avlosulfon*
Func. class.: Leprostatic
Chem. class.: Sulfone

Action: Bactericidal and bacteriostatic against *Mycobacterium leprae*
Uses: Hansen's disease
Dosage and routes:
• *Adult:* PO 100 mg qd with rifampin 600 mg qd × 6 mo
Available forms include: Tabs 25, 100 mg
Side effects/adverse reactions:
*INTEG: **Exfoliative dermatitis**,* photosensitivity
CNS: Peripheral neuropathy, headache, anxiety, drowsiness, tremors, ***convulsions,*** lethargy, depression, confusion, psychosis, aggression
GI: Nausea, vomiting, abdominal pain, anorexia
GU: Proteinuria, nephrotic syndrome, renal papillary necrosis
EENT: Blurred vision, optic neuritis, photophobia
*HEMA: **Megaloblastic anemia***
Contraindications: Hypersensitivity to sulfones, severe anemia
Precautions: Renal disease, hepatic disease, G-6-PD deficiency, pregnancy (A), lactation
Pharmacokinetics:
Rapid complete absorption; half-life 25-31 hr; highly bound to plasma protein, metabolized in liver, excreted in urine
Interactions/incompatibilities:
• Increased side effects: hemolytic agents
• Increased action of dapsone: probenecid, folic acid antagonists
• Decreased blood levels of dapsone: rifampin

---

italics = common side effects   ***bold italic*** = life threatening reactions

• Decreased bactericidal action: PABA
• Decreased GI absorption of dapsone: activated charcoal

NURSING CONSIDERATIONS
Assess:
• Temperature, if <101° F, drug should be reduced
• Liver studies q wk: ALT, AST, bilirubin
• Renal status: BUN, creatinine, output, sp gr, urinalysis before; q mo
• Blood levels of drug
• For anemia: Hct, Hgb, fatigue; for peripheral neuritis; or exfoliative dermatitis

Administer:
• With meals to decrease GI symptoms
• Antiemetic if vomiting occurs
• After C&S is completed; q mo to detect resistance

Perform/provide:
• Infants to be kept with mothers infected with leprosy, breastfeeding during drug therapy is encouraged

Evaluate:
• Mental status often: affect, mood, behavioral changes; psychosis may occur
• Hepatic status: decreased appetite, jaundice, dark urine, fatigue

Teach patient/family:
• That therapeutic effects may occur after 3-6 mo of drug therapy
• That compliance with dosage schedule, duration is necessary
• To avoid hazardous machinery if drowsiness occurs

daunorubicin HCl
(daw-noe-roo'bi-sin)
Cerubidine

Func. class.: Antineoplastic, antibiotic
Chem. class.: Anthracycline glycoside

Action: Inhibits DNA synthesis, primarily; derived from *Streptomyces verticillus;* replication is decreased by binding to DNA, which causes strand splitting; cell cycle specific (S phase); a vesicant

Uses: Myelogenous, monocytic leukemia, acute nonlymphocytic leukemia, Ewing's sarcoma, Wilm's tumor, neuroblastoma, rhabdomyosarcoma

Dosage and routes:
Single agent
• *Adult:* IV 60 mg/m^2/day × 3-5 day q4 wk
In combination
• *Adult:* IV 45 mg/m^2/day × 3 days, then 2 days of subsequent courses with cytosine arabinoside

Available forms include: Inj IV 20 mg

Side effects/adverse reactions:
HEMA: Thrombocytopenia, leukopenia, anemia
GI: Nausea, vomiting, anorexia, mucositis, hepatotoxicity
GU: Impotence, sterility, amenorrhea, gynecomastia, hyperuricemia
INTEG: Rash, extravasation, dermatitis, reversible alopecia, cellulitis, thrombophlebitis at injection site
CV: Dysrhythmias, CHF, pericarditis, myocarditis, peripheral edema
CNS: Fever, chills

Contraindications: Hypersensitivity, pregnancy (1st trimester) (D), lactation, systemic infections, cardiac disease

Precautions: Renal, hepatic, gout, bone marrow depression

Pharmacokinetics: Half-life 18½ hr, metabolized by liver, crosses placenta, appears in breast milk, excreted in urine, bile

Interactions/incompatibilities:
• Increased toxicity: other antineoplastics or radiation
• Do not mix with other drugs in solution or syringe

NURSING CONSIDERATIONS
Assess:
• CBC, differential, platelet count weekly; withhold drug if WBC is <4000/mm³ or platelet count is <75,000/mm³; notify physician of these results
• Blood, urine uric acid levels
• Renal function studies: BUN, serum uric acid, urine CrCl, electrolytes before, during therapy
• I&O ratio; report fall in urine output to <30 ml/hr
• Monitor temperature q4h; fever may indicate beginning infection
• Liver function tests before, during therapy: bilirubin, AST, ALT, alk phosphatase as needed or monthly
• ECG; watch for ST-T wave changes, low QRS and T, possible dysrhythmias (sinus tachycardia, heart block, PVCs)

Administer:
• Antiemetic 30-60 min before giving drug and 6-10 hr after treatment to prevent vomiting
• Antibiotics for prophylaxis of infection
• Allopurinol or sodium bicarbonate to reduce uric acid levels, alkalinization of urine
• IV after diluting 20 mg/4 ml sterile H_2O for inj; further dilute in 10-15 ml normal saline; give over 3-5 min; may be further diluted in 50 ml of compatible sol and run over 10-15 min
• Transfusion for anemia
• Antispasmodic for GI symptoms
• Hydrocortisone for extravasation, apply ice compress after stopping infusion

Perform/provide:
• Strict handwashing technique, gloves, protective clothing
• Liquid diet: carbonated beverages, gelatin may be added if patient is not nauseated or vomiting
• Increased fluid intake to 2-3 L/day to prevent urate and calculi formation
• Diet low in purines: absence of organ meats (kidney, liver), dried beans, peas to reduce uric acid level
• Rinsing of mouth tid-qid with water, club soda; brushing of teeth bid-qid with soft brush or cotton-tipped applicators for stomatitis; use unwaxed dental floss
• Storage at room temperature for 24 hr after reconstituting or 48 hr refrigerated

Evaluate:
• Bleeding: hematuria, guaiac stools, bruising or petechiae, mucosa or orifices q8h
• Food preferences; list likes, dislikes
• Effects of alopecia on body image; discuss feelings about body changes
• Inflammation of mucosa, breaks in skin
• Yellowing of skin, sclera, dark urine, clay-colored stools, itchy skin, abdominal pain, fever, diarrhea
• Buccal cavity q8h for dryness, sores or ulceration, white patches, oral pain, bleeding, dysphagia
• Local irritation, pain, burning at injection site

---

italics = common side effects   ***bold italic*** = life threatening reactions

• GI symptoms: frequency of stools, cramping
• Acidosis, signs of dehydration: rapid respirations, poor skin turgor, decreased urine output, dry skin, restlessness, weakness
• Cardiac status: B/P, pulse, character, rhythm, rate

Teach patient/family:
• To report any complaints, side effects to nurse or physician
• That hair may be lost during treatment and wig or hairpiece may make patient feel better; tell patient that new hair may be different in color, texture
• To avoid foods with citric acid, hot or rough texture
• To report any bleeding, white spots, ulcerations in mouth; tell patient to examine mouth qd
• That urine and other body fluids may be red-orange for 48 hr

Lab test interferences:
Increase: Uric acid

---

deferoxamine mesylate
(de-fer-ox'a-meen)
Desferal

Func. class.: Heavy metal antagonist
Chem. class.: Chelating agent

Action: Binds iron ions (ferric ions) to form water-soluble complex that is removed by kidneys
Uses: Acute, chronic iron intoxication, hemochromatosis, hemosiderosis

Dosage and routes:
Acute
• *Adult and child:* IM/IV 1 g, then 500 mg q4h × 2 doses, then 500 mg q4-12h × 2 doses, not to exceed 15 mg/kg/hr or 6 g/24 hr
Chronic
• *Adult and child:* IM 500 mg-1 g/

day plus IV INF 2 g given by separate line with each blood transfusion, not to exceed 15 mg/kg/hr or 6 gm/24 hr; SC 1-2 g over 8-24 hr by SC infusion pump
Available forms include: Powder for inj IV, IM, SC 500 mg/vial

Side effects/adverse reactions:
INTEG: Urticaria, erythema, pruritus, pain at injection site, fever
CV: Hypotension, tachycardia
GI: Diarrhea, abdominal cramps
EENT: Blurred vision, cataracts, decreased healing, *ototoxicity*
MS: Leg cramps
GU: Dysuria, pyelonephritis
SYST: Anaphylaxis

Contraindications: Hypersensitivity, anuria, severe renal disease, child <3 yr
Precautions: Pregnancy (C), lactation

Pharmacokinetics:
Metabolized by plasma enzymes, excreted by kidneys as complex, unchanged drug

NURSING CONSIDERATIONS
Assess:
• Inj site for redness, inflammation, pain
• For blood in stools
• Vision and hearing periodically
• VS
• I&O, kidney function studies: BUN, creatinine, CrCl, serum iron levels

Administer:
• IV (used for shock) after diluting in 500 mg/2 ml H$_2$O for inj; may be further diluted with D$_5$W or LR or NS; run at <15 mg/kg/hr; to be used only for short time; IM is preferred route
• IM after diluting with 2 ml sterile water for injection per 500 mg of drug; rotate injection sites
• Only when epinephrine 1:1000 is on unit for anaphylaxis

Evaluate:
• Allergic reactions: rash, urticaria; if these occur, drug should be discontinued

Teach patient/family:
• Urine may turn red

---

demeclocycline HCl

(dem-e-kloe-sye′kleen)
Declomycin, DMCT, Ledermycin
Func. class.: Broad-spectrum antibiotic/antiinfective
Chem. class.: Tetracycline

Action: Inhibits protein synthesis, phosphorylation in microorganisms by binding to 30S ribosomal subunits, reversibly binding to 50S ribosomal subunits

Uses: Uncommon gram-positive/gram-negative bacteria, protozoa, rickettsia, mycoplasma; diuretic, inappropriate ADH syndrome

Dosage and routes:
• *Adult:* PO 150 mg q6h or 300 mg q12h
• *Child >8 yr:* PO 6-12 mg/kg/day in divided doses q6-12h

Gonorrhea
• *Adult:* PO 600 mg, then 300 mg q12h × 4 days, total 3 g

Inappropriate ADH syndrome
• *Adult:* PO 600-1200 mg/day in divided doses

Available forms include: Tabs 150, 300 mg; caps 150 mg

Side effects/adverse reactions:
CNS: Fever, headache, paresthesia
HEMA: ***Eosinophilia, neutropenia, thrombocytopenia, leukocytosis, hemolytic anemia***
EENT: Dysphagia, glossitis, decreased calcification of deciduous teeth, abdominal pain, oral candidiasis
GI: Nausea, vomiting, diarrhea, anorexia, enterocolitis, ***hepato-toxicity,*** flatulence, abdominal cramps, epigastric burning, stomatitis, ***psuedomembranous colitis***
CV: Pericarditis
GU: Increased BUN, polyuria, polydipsia, ***renal failure, nephrotoxicity***
INTEG: Rash, urticaria, photosensitivity, increased pigmentation, ***exfoliative dermatitis,*** pruritus, angioedema

Contraindications: Hypersensitivity to tetracyclines, children <8 yr, pregnancy (D)

Precautions: Renal disease, hepatic disease, lactation, diabetes insipidus, nephrogenic

Pharmacokinetics:
PO: Peak 3-6 hr, duration 48-72 hr, half-life 10-17 hr, excreted in urine, crosses placenta, excreted in breast milk, 36%-91% bound to serum protein

Interactions/incompatibilities:
• Decreased effect of demeclocycline: antacids, $NaHCO_3$, dairy, alkali products, iron, kaolin, pectin
• Increased effect: anticoagulants
• Decreased effect: penicillins, oral contraceptives
• Nephrotoxicity: methoxyflurane

NURSING CONSIDERATIONS
Assess:
• I&O ratio
• Blood studies: PT, CBC, AST, ALT, BUN, creatinine
• Urine sp gr, sodium
• Signs of infection

Administer:
• On empty stomach 1 hr ac or 2 hr pc with 8 oz of water
• After C&S obtained
• 2 hr before or after laxative or ferrous products; 3 hr after antacid or kaolin-pectin products

Perform/provide:
• Storage in tight, light-resistant container at room temperature

---

italics = common side effects   ***bold italic*** = life threatening reactions

Evaluate:
• Therapeutic response: decreased temperature, absence of lesions, negative C&S
• Allergic reactions: rash, itching, pruritus, angioedema
• Nausea, vomiting, diarrhea; administer antiemetic, antacids as ordered
• Overgrowth of infection: increased temperature, malaise, redness, pain, swelling, drainage, perineal itching, diarrhea, changes in cough, sputum

Teach patient/family:
• To avoid sun exposure since burns may occur; sunscreen does not seem to decrease photosensitivity
• Of diabetic to avoid use of Clinistix, Diastix, or Tes-Tape for urine glucose testing
• That all prescribed medication must be taken to prevent superimposed infection
• To avoid milk products, take with full glass of water

Lab test interferences:
False negative: Urine glucose with Clinistix or Tes-Tape
False increase: Urinary catecholamines, AST, ALT, BUN

---

desipramine HCl
(dess-ip′ra-meen)
Norpramin, Pertofrane
Func. class.: Antidepressant, tricyclic
Chem. class.: Dibenzazepine, secondary amine

Action: Blocks reuptake of norepinephrine, serotonin into nerve endings, increasing action of norepinephrine, serotonin in nerve cells

Uses: Depression

Dosage and routes:
• *Adult:* PO 75-150 mg/day in divided doses, may increase to 300 mg/day or may give daily dose hs
• *Adolescent/geriatric:* PO 25-50 mg/day, may increase to 100 mg/day

Available forms include: Tabs 10, 25, 50, 75, 100, 150 mg; caps 25, 50 mg

Side effects/adverse reactions:
HEMA: **Agranulocytosis, thrombocytopenia, eosinophilia, leukopenia**
CNS: Dizziness, drowsiness, confusion, headache, anxiety, tremors, stimulation, weakness, insomnia, nightmares, EPS (elderly), increased psychiatric symptoms, paresthesia
GI: Diarrhea, dry mouth, nausea, vomiting, **paralytic ileus,** increased appetite, cramps, epigastric distress, jaundice, **hepatitis,** stomatitis
GU: Retention, **acute renal failure**
INTEG: Rash, urticaria, sweating, pruritus, photosensitivity
CV: Orthostatic hypotension, ECG changes, tachycardia, **hypertension,** palpitations
EENT: Blurred vision, tinnitus, mydriasis, ophthalmoplegia

Contraindications: Hypersensitivity to tricyclic antidepressants, recovery phase of myocardial infarction, narrow-angle glaucoma, convulsive disorders, prostatic hypertrophy, child <12 yr

Precautions: Suicidal patients, severe depression, increased intraocular pressure, narrow-angle glaucoma, elderly, pregnancy (C)

Pharmacokinetics:
PO: Steady state 2-11 days; metabolized by liver, excreted by kidneys, crosses placenta, half-life 14-62 hr

---

*Available in Canada only

Interactions/incompatibilities:
• Decreased effects of: guanethidine, clonidine, indirect acting sympathomimetics (ephedrine)
• Increased effects of: direct acting sympathomimetics (epinephrine) alcohol, barbiturates, benzodiazepines, CNS depressants
• Hyperpyretic crisis, convulsions, hypertensive episode: MAOI (pargyline [Eutonyl])

NURSING CONSIDERATIONS
Assess:
• B/P (lying, standing), pulse q4h; if systolic B/P drops 20 mm Hg hold drug, notify physician; take vital signs q4h in patients with cardiovascular disease
• Blood studies: CBC, leukocytes, differential, cardiac enzymes if patient is receiving long-term therapy
• Hepatic studies: AST, ALT, bilirubin, creatinine
• Weight qwk, appetite may increase with drug
• ECG for flattening of T wave, bundle branch block, AV block, dysrhythmias in cardiac patients

Administer:
• Increased fluids, bulk in diet if constipation, urinary retention occur
• With food or milk for GI symptoms
• Crushed if patient is unable to swallow medication whole
• Dosage hs if over-sedation occurs during day; may take entire dose hs; elderly may not tolerate once/day dosing
• Gum, hard candy, or frequent sips of water for dry mouth

Perform/provide:
• Storage at room temperature
• Assistance with ambulation during beginning therapy since drowsiness/dizziness occurs

• Safety measures including side-rails primarily in elderly
• Checking to see PO medication swallowed

Evaluate:
• EPS primarily in elderly: rigidity, dystonia, akathisia
• Mental status: mood, sensorium, affect, suicidal tendencies, an increase in psychiatric symptoms: depression, panic
• Urinary retention, constipation; constipation is more likely to occur in children
• Withdrawal symptoms: headache, nausea, vomiting, muscle pain, weakness; do not usually occur unless drug was discontinued abruptly
• Alcohol consumption; if alcohol is consumed, hold dose until morning

Teach patient/family:
• That therapeutic effects may take 2-3 wk
• Use caution in driving or other activities requiring alertness because of drowsiness, dizziness, blurred vision
• To avoid alcohol ingestion, other CNS depressants
• Not to discontinue medication quickly after long-term use, may cause nausea, headache, malaise
• To wear sunscreen or large hat since photosensitivity occurs

Lab test interferences:
Increase: Serum bilirubin, blood glucose, alk phosphatase
False increase: Urinary catecholamines
Decrease: VMA, 5-HIAA

Treatment of overdose: ECG monitoring, induce emesis, lavage, activated charcoal, administer anticonvulsant

---

italics = common side effects   ***bold italic*** = life threatening reactions

desmopressin acetate

(des-moe-press'in)

DDAVP, Stimate

Func. class.: Pituitary hormone

Chem. class.: Synthetic antidiuretic hormone

Action: Promotes reabsorption of water by action on renal tubular epithelium; causes smooth muscle constriction, resulting in vasopressor effect

Uses: Hemophilia A, von Willebrand's disease Type 1, nonnephrogenic diabetes insipidus, symptoms of polyuria/polydipsia caused by pituitary dysfunction

Dosage and routes:

Diabetes insipidus

• *Adult:* INTRANASAL 0.1-0.4 ml qd in divided doses: IV/SC 0.5-1 ml qd in divided doses

• *Child 3 mo to 12 yr:* INTRANASAL 0.05-0.3 ml qd in divided doses

Hemophilia/von Willebrand's disease

• *Adult and child:* IV 0.3 μg/kg in NaCl over 15-30 min; may repeat if needed

Available forms include: INTRANASAL 0.1 mg/ml; inj IV, SC 4 μg/ml

Side effects/adverse reactions:

EENT: Nasal irritation, congestion, rhinitis

CNS: Drowsiness, headache, lethargy, flushing

GU: Vulval pain

GI: Nausea, heartburn, cramps

CV: Increased B/P

Contraindications: Hypersensitivity, nephrogenic diabetes insipidus

Precautions: Pregnancy (B), CAD, lactation, hypertension, coronary artery disease

Pharmacokinetics:

NASAL: Onset 1 hr, peak 1-2 hr, duration 8-20 hr, half-life 8 min, 76 min (terminal)

Interactions/incompatibilities:

• Increased response: carbamazepine, chlorpropamide, clofibrate

NURSING CONSIDERATIONS

Assess:

• Pulse, B/P when giving drug IV or SC

• I&O ratio; weight daily, check for edema in extremities; if water retention is severe, diuretic may be prescribed

Perform/provide:

• Storage in refrigerator or cool environment

Evaluate:

• Therapeutic response: absence of severe thirst, decreased urine output, osmolality

• Water intoxication: lethargy, behavioral changes, disorientation, neuromuscular excitability

• Intranasal use: nausea, congestion, cramps, headache, usually decreased with decreased dose

Teach patient/family:

• Technique for nasal instillation: to insert tube into nasal cavity to instill drug

• Avoid OTC products: cough, hayfever products since these preparations may contain epinephrine, decrease drug response; do not use with alcohol

• To wear Medic Alert ID specifying therapy

desonide

(dess'oh-nide)

Des Owen, Tridesilon

Func. class.: Topical corticosteroid

Chem. class.: Synthetic nonfluorinated agent, group IV potency

Action: Possesses antipruritic, antiinflammatory actions

---

* Available in Canada only

Uses: Psoriasis, eczema, contact dermatitis, pruritus

Dosage and routes:
• *Adult and child:* Apply to affected area bid-tid

Available forms include: Cream 0.05%; oint 0.05%

Side effects/adverse reactions:
INTEG: Burning, dryness, itching, irritation, acne, folliculitis, hypertrichosis, perioral dermatitis, hypopigmentation, atrophy, striae, miliaria, allergic contact dermatitis, secondary infection

Contraindications: Hypersensitivity to corticosteroids, fungal infections

Precautions: Pregnancy (C), lactation, viral infections, bacterial infections

NURSING CONSIDERATIONS
Assess:
• Temperature; if fever develops, drug should be discontinued

Administer:
• Only to affected areas; do not get in eyes
• Medication, then cover with occlusive dressing (only if prescribed), seal to normal skin, change q12h, systemic absorption may occur
• Only to dermatoses; do not use on weeping, denuded, or infected area

Perform/provide:
• Cleansing before application of drug
• Treatment for a few days after area has cleared
• Storage at room temperature

Evaluate:
• Therapeutic response: absence of severe itching, patches on skin, flaking
• For systemic absorption: increased temperature, inflammation, irritation

Teach patient/family:
• To avoid sunlight on affected area; burns may occur

---

desoximetasone
(des-ox-i-met'a-sone)
Topicort, Topicort LP
Func. class.: Topical corticosteroid
Chem. class.: Synthetic fluorinated agent, group II potency (0.25%), group III potency (0.05%)

Action: Possesses antipruritic, antiinflammatory actions

Uses: Psoriasis, eczema, contact dermatitis, pruritus

Dosage and routes:
• *Adult and child:* Apply to affected area bid-tid

Available forms include: Cream 0.05% (LP), 0.25%; oint 0.25%; gel 0.05%

Side effects/adverse reactions:
INTEG: Burning, dryness, itching, irritation, acne, folliculitis, hypertrichosis, perioral dermatitis, hypopigmentation, atrophy, striae, miliaria, allergic contact dermatitis, secondary infection

Contraindications: Hypersensitivity to corticosteroids, fungal infections

Precautions: Pregnancy (C), lactation, viral infections, bacterial infections

NURSING CONSIDERATIONS
Assess:
• Temperature; if fever develops, drug should be discontinued

Administer:
• Only to affected areas; do not get in eyes
• Medication, then cover with occlusive dressing (only if prescribed), seal to normal skin, change q12h; use occlusive dressing with extreme caution (group II

---

italics = common side effects   ***bold italic*** = life threatening reactions

potency), systemic absorption may occur
- Only to dermatoses; do not use on weeping, denuded, or infected area

Perform/provide:
- Cleansing before application of drug
- Treatment for a few days after area has cleared
- Storage at room temperature

Evaluate:
- Therapeutic response: absence of severe itching, patches on skin, flaking
- For systemic absorption: increased temperature, inflammation, irritation

Teach patient/family:
- To avoid sunlight on affected area; burns may occur

---

desoxycorticosterone acetate/desoxycorticosterone pivalate

(des-ox-i-kor-ti-koe-ster′one)
Doca Acetate, Percorten Acetate/ Percorten Pivalate
Func. class.: Corticosteroid
Chem. class.: Mineralocorticoid

Action: Promotes increased reabsorption of sodium and loss of potassium from the renal tubules

Uses: Adrenal insufficiency, salt-losing adrenogenital syndrome

Dosage and routes:
- *Adult:* IM 2-5 mg qd (acetate); IM 25-100 mg q4wk (pivalate); PELLET 1 pellet/0.5 mg of injected dose

Available forms include: Pellet 125 mg; inj IM 5 mg/ml

Side effects/adverse reactions:
INTEG: Acne, poor wound healing, petechiae, ecchymosis

CNS: Depression, flushing, sweating, headache, mood changes
*CV: Hypertension, **circulatory collapse, thrombophlebitis, embolism,** tachycardia*
*HEMA: **Thrombocytopenia***
MS: Fractures, osteoporosis, weakness
*GI: Diarrhea, nausea, abdominal distention, **GI hemorrhage,** increased appetite, **pancreatitis***
EENT: Fungal infections, increased intraocular pressure, blurred vision

Contraindications: Psychosis, hypersensitivity, idiopathic thrombocytopenia, acute glomerulonephritis, amebiasis, fungal infections, nonasthmatic bronchial disease, child <2 yr

Precautions: Pregnancy (C), diabetes mellitus, glaucoma, osteoporosis, seizure disorders, ulcerative colitis, CHF, myasthenia gravis

Pharmacokinetics:
IM: Duration 24-48 hr
Pellet: Duration 8-12 mo

Interactions/incompatibilities:
- Decreased action of desoxycorticosterone: cholestyramine, colestipol, barbiturates, rifampin, ephedrine, phenytoin, theophylline
- Decreased effects of: anticoagulants, anticonvulsants, antidiabetics, ambenonium, neostigmine, isoniazid, toxoids, vaccines
- Increased side effects: alcohol, salicylates, indomethacin, amphotericin B, digitalis preparations
- Increased action of this drug: salicylates, estrogens, indomethacin

NURSING CONSIDERATIONS
Assess:
- Potassium, blood sugar, urine glucose while on long-term therapy; hypokalemia and hyperglycemia

---

• Weight daily, notify physician of weekly gain >5 lb
• B/P q4h, pulse, notify physician if chest pain occurs
• I&O ratio, be alert for decreasing urinary output and increasing edema
• Plasma cortisol levels during long-term therapy (normal level: 138-635 nmol/L SI units when drawn at 8 AM)

Administer:
• Titrated dose, use lowest effective dose
• IM inj deeply in large mass, rotate sites, avoid deltoid, use 19G needle
• In one dose in AM to prevent adrenal suppression, avoid SC administration, damage may be done to tissue
• With food or milk to decrease GI symptoms

Perform/provide:
• Assistance with ambulation in patient with bone tissue disease to prevent fractures

Evaluate:
• Therapeutic response: ease of respirations, decreased inflammation
• Infection: increased temperature, WBC even after withdrawal of medication; drug masks symptoms of infection
• Potassium depletion: paresthesias, fatigue, nausea, vomiting, depression, polyuria, dysrhythmias, weakness
• Edema, hypertension, cardiac symptoms
• Mental status: affect, mood, behavioral changes, aggression

Teach patient/family:
• That ID as steroid user should be carried
• To notify physician if therapeutic response decreases; dosage adjustment may be needed

• Not to discontinue this medication abruptly or adrenal crisis can result
• To avoid OTC products: salicylates, alcohol in cough products, cold preparations unless directed by physician
• Teach patient all aspects of drug usage, including Cushingoid symptoms
• Symptoms of adrenal insufficiency: nausea, anorexia, fatigue, dizziness, dyspnea, weakness, joint pain

Lab test interferences:
Increase: Cholesterol, sodium, blood glucose, uric acid, calcium, urine glucose
Decrease: Calcium, potassium, T_4, T_3, thyroid ^{131}I uptake test, urine 17-OHCS, 17-KS, PBI
False negative: Skin allergy tests

---

dexamethasone

(dex-a-meth'a-sone)
Aeroseb-Dex, Decaderm, Decaspray

Func. class.: Topical corticosteroid
Chem. class.: Synthetic fluorinated agent

Action: Possesses antipruritic, antiinflammatory actions
Uses: Corticosteroid-responsive dermatoses

Dosage and routes:
• *Adult and child:* TOP apply to affected area bid-qid
Available forms include: Gel 0.1%; aerosol 0.01%, 0.04%

Side effects/adverse reactions:
INTEG: Burning, dryness, itching, irritation, acne, folliculitis, hypertrichosis, perioral dermatitis, hypopigmentation, atrophy, striae, miliaria, allergic contact dermatitis, secondary infection

---

italics = common side effects   ***bold italic*** = life threatening reactions

Contraindications: Hypersensitivity to corticosteroids, fungal infections, viral infections

Precautions: Pregnancy (C), lactation, viral infections, bacterial infections

NURSING CONSIDERATIONS
Assess:
• Temperature, if fever develops drug should be discontinued
Administer:
• Only to affected areas, do not get in eyes
• Then cover with occlusive dressing if ordered, seal to normal skin, change q12h, systemic absorption may occur
• Only to dermatoses, do not use on weeping, denuded or infected area
Perform/provide:
• Cleansing before application of drug
• Treatment for a few days after area has cleared
• Storage at room temperature
Evaluate:
• Systemic absorption: fever, infection, irritation
• Therapeutic response: absence of severe itching, patches on skin, flaking
Teach patient/family:
• To avoid sunlight on affected area, burns may occur

dexamethasone/dexamethasone acetate/dexamethasone sodium phosphate

(dex-a-meth′a-sone)
Decadron, Dexamethasone Intensol, Dexasone,* Dexone, Hexadrol/Dalalone-LA, Decadron-LA, Decaject-LA, Decameth-LA, Dexcen-LA, Dexasone-LA, Dexone-LA/Decadron Phosphate, Decaject, Decameth, Dexacen-4, Dexasone, Dexone, Hexadrol Phosphate

Func. class.: Corticosteroid
Chem. class.: Glucocorticoid, long-acting

Action: Decreases inflammation by suppression of migration of polymorphonuclear leukocytes, fibroblasts, reversal of increase capillary permeability and lysosomal stabilization

Uses: Inflammation, allergies, neoplasms, cerebral edema, shock, collagen disorders

Dosage and routes:
Inflammation
• *Adult:* PO 0.25-4 mg bid-qid IM 4-16 mg q1-3 wk (acetate)
Shock
• *Adult:* IV 1-6 mg/kg or 40 mg q2-6h (phosphate)
Cerebral edema
• *Adult:* IV 10 mg, then 4-6 mg IM q6h × 2-4 days, then taper over 1 wk
• *Child:* PO 0.2 mg/kg/day in divided doses

Available forms include: Tabs 0.25, 0.5, 0.75, 1, 1.5, 3, 4, 6 mg; inj IM acetate 8, 16 mg/ml; inj IV phosphate 4, 10 mg/ml; elix 0.5 mg/5 ml; oral sol 0.5 mg/5 ml, 0.5 mg/1 ml

---

*Available in Canada only

Side effects/adverse reactions:

INTEG: Acne, poor wound healing, ecchymosis, petechiae

CNS: Depression, flushing, sweating, headache, mood changes

*CV: Hypertension, **circulatory collapse, thrombophlebitis, embolism,** tachycardia, edema*

*HEMA: **Thrombocytopenia***

MS: Fractures, osteoporosis, weakness

*GI: Diarrhea, nausea, abdominal distention, **GI hemorrhage,** increased appetite, **pancreatitis***

EENT: Fungal infections, increased intraocular pressure, blurred vision

Contraindications: Psychosis, hypersensitivity, idiopathic thrombocytopenia, acute glomerulonephritis, amebiasis, fungal infections, nonasthmatic bronchial disease, child <2 yr, AIDS, TB

Precautions: Pregnancy (C), diabetes mellitus, glaucoma, osteoporosis, seizure disorders, ulcerative colitis, CHF, myasthenia gravis, renal disease, peptic ulcer, esophagitis

Pharmacokinetics:

PO: Peak 1-2 h, duration 2⅓

IM: Peak 8 h, duration 6 days

Half-life 3-4½ h

Interactions/incompatibilities:

- Decreased action of dexamethasone: cholestyramine, colestipol, barbiturates, rifampin, ephedrine, phenytoin, theophylline, antacids
- Decreased effects of: anticoagulants, anticonvulsants, antidiabetics, ambenonium, neostigmine, isoniazid, toxoids, vaccines
- Increased side effects: alcohol, salicylates, indomethacin, amphotericin B, digitalis preparations
- Increased action of dexamethasone: salicylates, estrogens, indomethacin

NURSING CONSIDERATIONS

Assess:

- Potassium, blood sugar, urine glucose while on long-term therapy; hypokalemia and hyperglycemia
- Weight daily, notify physician of weekly gain >5 lb
- B/P q4h, pulse, notify physician if chest pain occurs
- I&O ratio, be alert for decreasing urinary output and increasing edema
- Plasma cortisol levels during long-term therapy (normal level: 138-635 nmol/L SI units when drawn at 8 AM)

Administer:

- IV after diluting or undiluted; give over 1 min; may be further diluted with normal saline or D₅W
- After shaking suspension (parenteral); do not give suspension IV
- Titrated dose, use lowest effective dose
- IM inj deeply in large mass, rotate sites, avoid deltoid, use 21G needle
- In one dose in AM to prevent adrenal suppression, avoid SC administration, damage may be done to tissue
- With food or milk to decrease GI symptoms

Perform/provide:

- Assistance with ambulation in patient with bone tissue disease to prevent fractures

Evaluate:

- Therapeutic response: ease of respirations, decreased inflammation
- Infection: increased temperature, WBC even after withdrawal of medication; drug masks symptoms of infection
- Potassium depletion: paresthesias, fatigue, nausea, vomiting,

---

italics = common side effects   ***bold italic*** = life threatening reactions

depression, polyuria, dysrhythmias, weakness
• Edema, hypertension, cardiac symptoms
• Mental status: affect, mood, behavioral changes, aggression

Teach patient/family:
• That ID as steroid user should be carried
• To notify physician if therapeutic response decreases; dosage adjustment may be needed
• Not to discontinue this medication abruptly or adrenal crisis can result
• To avoid OTC products: salicylates, alcohol in cough products, cold preparations unless directed by physician
• Teach patient all aspects of drug usage, including Cushingoid symptoms
• Symptoms of adrenal insufficiency: nausea, anorexia, fatigue, dizziness, dyspnea, weakness, joint pain

Lab test interferences:
Increase: Cholesterol, sodium, blood glucose, uric acid, calcium, urine glucose
Decrease: Calcium, potassium, T_4, T_3, thyroid ^{131}I uptake test, urine 17-OHCS, 17-KS, PBI
False negative: Skin allergy tests

---

dexamethasone/dexamethasone sodium phosphate

(dex-a-meth'a-sone)

Ophthalmic Suspension/Decadron Phosphate Ophthalmics, Maxidex Ophthalmic

Func. class.: Ophthalmic antiinflammatory

Action: Results in decreased inflammation, resulting in decreased pain, photophobia, hyperemia, cellular infiltration

Uses: Inflammation of eye, lids, conjunctiva, cornea, uveitis, iridocyclitis, allergic condition, burns, foreign bodies

Dosage and routes:
• *Adult and child:* Instill 1-2 gtts into conjunctival sac q1-4h depending on condition
Available forms include: Oint 0.05%; ophthalmic sol 0.1%

Side effects/adverse reactions:
EENT: Increased intraocular pressure, poor corneal wound healing, increased possibility of corneal infection, glaucoma exacerbation, *optic nerve damage,* decreased acuity, visual field, cataracts

Contraindications: Hypersensitivity, acute superficial herpes simplex, fungal/viral diseases of the eye or conjunctiva, active diabetes mellitus, ocular TB, infections of the eye

Precautions: Corneal abrasions, glaucoma, pregnancy (C)

NURSING CONSIDERATIONS
Perform/provide:
• Storage in light-resistant container

Evaluate:
• Therapeutic response: absence of swelling, redness, exudate

Teach patient/family:
• Instillation method: pressure on lacrimal sac for 1 min
• Not to share eye medications with others
• Not to use if purulent drainage is present
• Shake before using
• Not to discontinue abruptly, taper over 1-2 wk

---

*Available in Canada only

dexamethasone sodium phosphate

(dex-a-meth′a-sone)

Decadron Phosphate

Func. class.: Topical corticosteroid

Chem. class.: Synthetic fluorinated agent, group VI potency

Action: Possesses antipruritic, antiinflammatory actions

Uses: Psoriasis, eczema, contact dermatitis, pruritus

Dosage and routes:

• *Adult and child:* Apply to affected area tid-qid

Available forms include: Cream 0.1%

Side effects/adverse reactions:

INTEG: Burning, dryness, itching, irritation, acne, folliculitis, hypertrichosis, perioral dermatitis, hypopigmentation, atrophy, striae, miliaria, allergic contact dermatitis, secondary infection

Contraindications: Hypersensitivity to corticosteroids, fungal infections

Precautions: Pregnancy (C), lactation, viral infections, bacterial infections

NURSING CONSIDERATIONS

Assess:

• Temperature; if fever develops, drug should be discontinued

Administer:

• Only to affected areas; do not get in eyes

• Medication, then cover with occlusive dressing (only if prescribed), seal to normal skin, change q12h, systemic absorption may occur

• Only to dermatoses; do not use on weeping, denuded, or infected area

Perform/provide:

• Cleansing before application of drug

• Treatment for a few days after area has cleared

• Storage at room temperature

Evaluate:

• Therapeutic response: absence of severe itching, patches on skin, flaking

• For systemic absorption: increased temperature, inflammation, irritation

Teach patient/family:

• To avoid sunlight on affected area; burns may occur

dexamethasone sodium phosphate (nasal)

(dex-a-meth′a-sone)

Decadron Phosphate Turbinaire

Func. class.: Steroid, intranasal

Chem. class.: Glucocorticoid

Action: Long-acting synthetic adrenocorticoid with antiinflammatory activity, minimal mineralocorticoid properties

Uses: Inflammation (not within sinuses), nasal polyps, allergic conditions of nose

Dosage and routes:

• *Adult:* SPRAY 1-2 sprays bid-tid, not to exceed 12/day

• *Child 6-12 yr:* SPRAY 1-2 sprays bid, not to exceed 8/day

Available forms include: 84 µg/metered spray

Side effects/adverse reactions:

EENT: Nasal irritation, dryness, rebound congestion, epistaxis, sneezing, *infarction of nasal mucosa*

INTEG: Urticaria

CNS: Headache, dizziness

SYSTEMIC: **CHF, convulsions,** increased sodium, hypertension

Contraindications: Hypersensitivity, child <12 yr, localized infection of nose, acute status asthmaticus

---

italics = common side effects   ***bold italic*** = life threatening reactions

Precautions: Lactation, nasal trauma, pregnancy (C)

NURSING CONSIDERATIONS

Administer:
• After cleaning daily with warm water, dry thoroughly

Perform/provide:
• Storage in cool environment, do not puncture or incinerate container

Evaluate:
• Adrenal suppression: 17-KS, plasma cortisol for decreased levels
• Nasal passages during long-term treatment for changes in mucus
• For edema, increased B/P, increase in K^+ during treatment, which indicates systemic absorption

Teach patient/family:
• To clear nasal passages if sneezing attack occurs, repeat dose
• To continue using product even if mild nasal bleeding occurs, is usually transient
• Method of instillation after providing written instructions from manufacturer
• To clear nasal passages before administration, use decongestant if needed, shake inhaler, invert, tilt head backward, insert nozzle into nostril, away from septum, hold other nostril closed, depress activator, inhale through nose, exhale through mouth
• To decrease gradually if drug has been used consistently
• That only 1 person should use a single-container drug
• If irritation, dryness, epistaxis occur, drug may need to be discontinued
• Benefit requires regular use, will not occur after several days

dexchlorpheniramine maleate

(dex-klor-fen-eer′a-meen)
Polaramine

Func. class.: Antihistamine
Chem. class.: Alkylamine derivative, H_1-receptor antagonist

Action: Acts on blood vessels, GI, respiratory system by competing with histamine for H_1-receptor site; decreases allergic response by blocking histamine

Uses: Allergy symptoms, rhinitis, pruritus, contact dermatitis

Dosage and routes:
• *Adult:* PO 1-2 mg tid-qid; REPEAT ACTION 4-6 mg bid-tid
• *Child 6-11 yr:* PO 1 mg q4-6h, or TIME REL 4 mg hs
• *Child 2-5 yr:* PO 0.5 mg q4-6h; do not use repeat action form

Available forms include: Tabs 2 mg; repeat-action tab 4, 6 mg; syr 2 mg/5 ml

Side effects/adverse reactions:

CNS: Dizziness, drowsiness, poor coordination, fatigue, anxiety, euphoria, confusion, paresthesia, neuritis

CV: Hypotension, palpitations, tachycardia

RESP: Increased thick secretions, wheezing, chest tightness

GI: Constipation, dry mouth, nausea, vomiting, anorexia, diarrhea

INTEG: Rash, urticaria, photosensitivity

GU: Retention, dysuria, frequency

EENT: Blurred vision, dilated pupils, tinnitus, nasal stuffiness, dry nose, throat, mouth

Contraindications: Hypersensitivity to H_1-receptor antagonist; acute asthma attack, lower respiratory tract disease

Precautions: Increased intraocular pressure, renal disease, cardiac disease, hypertension, bronchial asthma, seizure disorder, stenosed peptic ulcers, hyperthyroidism, prostatic hypertrophy, bladder neck obstruction, pregnancy (B)

Pharmacokinetics:

PO: Onset 15 min, peak 3 hr, duration 3-6 hr, metabolized in liver, excreted by kidneys (inactive metabolites), excreted in breast milk (small amounts)

Interactions/incompatibilities:

• Increased CNS depression: barbiturates, narcotics, hypnotics, tricyclic antidepressants, alcohol

• Decreased effect of: oral anticoagulants, heparin

• Increased effect of dexchlorpheniramine: MAOIs

NURSING CONSIDERATIONS
Assess:

• I&O ratio; be alert for urinary retention, frequency, dysuria; drug should be discontinued if these occur

• CBC during long-term therapy

Administer:

• With meals if GI symptoms occur, absorption may slightly decrease

Perform/provide:

• Hard candy, gum, frequent rinsing of mouth for dryness

• Storage in tight container at room temperature

Evaluate:

• Therapeutic response: absence of running or congested nose or rashes

• Respiratory status: rate, rhythm, increase in bronchial secretions, wheezing, chest tightness

• Cardiac status: palpitations, increased pulse, hypotension

Teach patient/family:

• All aspects of drug use; to notify physician if confusion, sedation, hypotension occurs

• To avoid driving or other hazardous activity if drowsiness occurs

• To avoid concurrent use of alcohol or other CNS depressants

Lab test interferences:

False negative: Skin allergy tests

Treatment of overdose: Administer ipecac syrup or lavage, diazepam, vasopressors, barbiturates (short-acting)

---

dexpanthenol

(dex-pan'the-nole)
Panthoderm

Func. class.: Emollient/protectant
Chem. class.: Pantothenic acid derivative

Action: Prevents irritation of surgical areas by preventing evaporation of moisture

Uses: Diaper rash, decubitus ulcers, itching, eczema, insect bites

Dosage and routes:

• *Adult:* TOP apply qd bid

Available forms include: Cream, lotion 2%

Side effects/adverse reactions: None known

Contraindications: Hemophilia patients, wounds

NURSING CONSIDERATIONS
Administer:

• Only to intact skin, never apply to raw, denuded, blistered, or oozing wounds

Perform/provide:

• Skin cleansing at least qd or more often if needed

Evaluate:

• For infection (increased temperature, redness), often bacteria are trapped underneath

Teach patient/family:

• To report color change on skin, redness, increased temperature

---

italics = common side effects   ***bold italic*** = life threatening reactions

dexpanthenol

(dex-pan'the-nole)
Ilopan, Intrapan, Tonestat
Func. class.: Cholinergic
Chem. class.: Pantothenic acid analog

Action: Action is unknown, but this drug is precursor of pantothenic acid, which is needed for acetylcholine production, which maintains normal intestinal functioning
Uses: Prevention of paralytic ileus, postoperative abdominal distention
Dosage and routes:
Distention
• *Adult and child:* IM 250-500 mg, may repeat in 2 hr, 6 hr; IV INF 500 mg in D_5, or LR slowly
Paralytic ileus
• *Adult and child >16 yr:* IM 500 mg, may repeat in 2 hr, then q4-6h
Available forms include: Inj IM, IV 250 mg/ml
Side effects/adverse reactions:
HEMA: Increased bleeding time
GI: Diarrhea, hyperperistalsis, flatulence
INTEG: Urticaria, rash, pruritus, allergic reactions
Contraindications: Hypersensitivity, hemophilia, GI obstruction
Precautions: Pregnancy (C), children, lactation
Pharmacokinetics: Excreted in urine (pantothenic acid)
NURSING CONSIDERATIONS
Assess:
• Bleeding time, drug should be discontinued if bleeding time is increased
• I&O ratio; check for urinary retention or hesitancy
Administer:
• This drug at least 12 hr after parasympathomimetics

• Increased doses in hypokalemia patient
• IV after dilution, 500 mg or less/500 ml or more D_5W or LR; run over 3-6 hr
Perform/provide:
• Storage at room temperature
• Insertion of rectal tube if ordered
Evaluate:
• Allergic reaction: rash, urticaria; drug should be discontinued
• Therapeutic response: flatulence, bowel sounds present, abdomen soft, absence of pain
Teach patient/family:
• To report flatulence, decreased pain in abdomen

dextran 40

Gentran 40, LMD, Rheomacrodex
Func. class.: Plasma volume expander
Chem. class.: Low molecular weight polysaccharide

Action: Similar to human albumin which expands plasma volume by drawing fluid from interstitial space to intravascular space
Uses: Expand plasma volume, prophylaxis of embolism, thrombosis
Dosage and routes:
Shock
• *Adult:* IV INF 500 ml over 15-30 min, total dose in 24 hr not to exceed 20 ml/kg then subsequent doses given slowly, if given >24 hr, not to exceed 10 ml/kg/day, not to exceed therapy >5 days
Thrombosis/embolism
• *Adult:* IV INF 500-1000 ml, then 500 ml/day × 3 days, then 500 ml q2-3 days × 2 wk if needed
Available forms include: 10% dextran 40/5% dextrose, 10% dextran 40/0.9% sodium chloride

Side effects/adverse reactions:
HEMA: Decreased hematocrit, platelet function, increased bleeding/coagulation times
INTEG: Rash, urticaria, pruritus, angioedema, chills, fever, flushing
RESP: Wheezing, dyspnea, *bronchospasm, pulmonary edema*
CV: Hypotension, *cardiac arrest*
GU: Osmotic nephrosis, renal failure, stasis
GI: Nausea, vomiting, increased AST, ALT
SYST: Anaphylaxis

Contraindications: Hypersensitivity, renal failure, CHF (severe), extreme dehydration

Precautions: Active hemorrhage, pregnancy (C)

Pharmacokinetics:
IV: Expands blood volume 1-2 × amount infused, excreted in urine and feces

NURSING CONSIDERATIONS
Assess:
• VS q5 min × 30 min
• CVP during infusion (5-10 cm H₂O—normal range)
• Urine output q1h; watch for increase in urinary output, which is common; if output does not increase, infusion should be decreased or discontinued
• I&O ratio and specific gravity, urine osmolarity; if specific gravity is very low, renal clearance is low, drug should be discontinued

Administer:
• After crossmatch is drawn, if blood is to be given also
• Dextran 1 (Promit) to prevent anaphylaxis if ordered

Perform/provide:
• Storage at constant temperature 15° C (59° F) to 30° C (86° F); discard unused portions, protect from freezing

Evaluate:
• Allergy: rash, urticaria, pruritus, wheezing, dyspnea, bronchospasm, drug should be discontinued immediately
• Circulatory overload: increased pulse, respirations, SOB, wheezing, chest tightness, chest pain
• Dehydration after infusion: decreased output, decreased sp. gravity of urine, increased temperature, poor skin turgor, increased specific gravity, dry skin

Lab test interferences:
False increase: Blood glucose, urinary protein, bilirubin, total protein
Interference: Rh test, blood typing/crossmatching

---

dextran 70/75

Gentran 75, Macrodex

Func. class.: Plasma volume expander
Chem. class.: High molecular weight polysaccharide

Action: Similar to human albumin, which expands plasma volume by drawing fluid from interstitial spaces to intravascular space
Uses: Expand plasma volume in hypovolemic shock or impending shock

Dosage and routes:
• *Adult:* IV INF 500-1000 ml not to exceed 20-40 ml/min, not to exceed 10 ml/kg/24 hr if therapy >24 hr

Side effects/adverse reactions:
HEMA: Decreased hematocrit, platelet function, increased bleeding/coagulation times
INTEG: Rash, urticaria, pruritus, angioedema, chills, fever, flushing
RESP: Wheezing, dyspnea, *bronchospasm, pulmonary edema*
CV: Hypotension, *cardiac arrest*

italics = common side effects   ***bold italic*** = life threatening reactions

*GU: **Osmotic nephrosis, renal failure, stasis***
GI: Nausea, vomiting, increase AST, ALT
*SYST: **Anaphylaxis***
Contraindications: Hypersensitivity, renal failure, CHF (severe), extreme dehydration
Precautions: Active hemorrhage, pregnancy (C)
Pharmacokinetics:
IV: Expands blood volume 1-2 × amount infused, excreted in urine and feces

NURSING CONSIDERATIONS
Assess:
• VS q5 min × 30 min
• CVP during infusion (5-10 cm H$_2$O—normal range)
• Urine output q1h, watch for increase in urinary output which is common; if output does not increase, infusion should be decreased or discontinued
• I&O ratio and specific gravity, urine osmolarity; if specific gravity is very low, renal clearance is low, drug should be discontinued
Administer:
• After crossmatch is drawn, if blood is to be given also
• Dextran 1 (Promit) to prevent anaphylaxis
Perform/provide:
• Storage at constant temperature <25° C (77° F); discard unused portions, do not use unless clear
Evaluate:
• Allergy: rash, urticaria, pruritus, wheezing, dyspnea, bronchospasm, drug should be discontinued immediately
• Circulatory overload: increased pulse, respirations, SOB, wheezing, chest tightness, chest pain
• Dehydration after infusion: decreased output, increased temperature, poor skin turgor, increased specific gravity, dry skin
Lab test interferences:
False increase: Blood glucose, urinary protein, bilirubin, total protein
Interferes: Rh test, blood typing/crossmatching

---

dextranomer
(dex-tran′oh-mer)
Debrisan
Func. class.: Miscellaneous topical drug
Chem. class.: Hydrophilic dextran polymer

Action: Absorbs exudate, particles from wound surface reducing inflammation, edema
Uses: Cleaning of wet ulcers: decubitus ulcers, surgical wounds, venous stasis ulcers
Dosage and routes:
• *Adult and child:* TOP apply ¼-inch thick on affected area bid, prn, cover with gauze dressing
Available forms include: Topical beads, topical paste
Side effects/adverse reactions:
INTEG: Erythema, pain, irritation, blistering, bleeding when dressings are changed
Contraindications: Hypersensitivity, deep fistulas, sinus tracts
Precautions: Pregnancy
NURSING CONSIDERATIONS
Administer:
• After cleaning wound, do not dry
• Cover with dressing, do not pack wound tightly
• After mixing beads with glycerin, not to be mixed with other substances; do not reuse left-over mixture
Perform/provide:
• Storage in tight, closed container in dry place at room temperature

---

*Available in Canada only

Evaluate:
• Therapeutic response: drying of area, with eventual closure of wound
• Area of body involved, including time involved, what helps or aggravates condition
Teach patient/family:
• That treatment may take 1-2 wk
• To notify physician if condition lasts longer than 2 wk

---

dextroamphetamine sulfate

(dex-troe-am-fet′a-meen)
Dexedrine, Ferndex, Oxydess II, Spancap #1
Func. class.: Cerebral stimulant
Chem. class.: Amphetamine

Controlled Substance Schedule II
Action: Increases release of norepinephrine, dopamine in cerebral cortex to reticular activating system
Uses: Narcolepsy, exogenous obesity, attention deficit disorder with hyperactivity
Dosage and routes:
Narcolepsy
• *Adult:* PO 5-60 mg qd in divided doses
• *Child >12 yr:* PO 10 mg qd increasing by 10 mg/day at weekly intervals
• *Child 6-12 yr:* PO 5 mg qd increasing by 5 mg/wk (max 60 mg/day)
Attention deficit disorder
• *Child >6 yr:* PO 5 mg qd-bid increasing by 5 mg/day at weekly intervals
• *Child 3-6 yr:* PO 2.5 mg qd increasing by 2.5 mg/day at weekly intervals
Obesity
• *Adult:* PO 5-30 mg qd in divided doses 30-60 min before meals

Available forms include: Tabs 5, 10 mg; caps sus rel 5, 10, 15 mg; elix 5 mg/5 ml
Side effects/adverse reactions:
CNS: Hyperactivity, insomnia, restlessness, talkativeness, dizziness, headache, chills, stimulation, dysphoria, irritability, aggressiveness, tremor
GI: Anorexia, dry mouth, diarrhea, constipation, weight loss, metallic taste
GU: Impotence, change in libido
CV: Palpitations, tachycardia, hypertension, decrease in heart rate, dysrhythmias
INTEG: Urticaria
Contraindications: Hypersensitivity to sympathomimetic amines, hyperthyroidism, hypertension, glaucoma hypertrophy, severe arteriosclerosis, drug abuse, cardiovascular disease, anxiety
Precautions: Gilles de la Tourette's disorder, pregnancy (C), lactation, child <3 yr
Pharmacokinetics:
PO: Onset 30 min, peak 1-3 hr, duration 4-20 hr, metabolized by liver, excreted by kidneys, crosses placenta, breast milk, half-life 10-30 hr
Interactions/incompatibilities:
• Hypertensive crisis: MAOIs or within 14 days of MAOIs
• Increased effect of dextroamphetamine: acetazolamide, antacids, sodium bicarbonate, phenothiazines, haloperidol
• Decreased effect of dextroamphetamine: barbiturates, ascorbic acid, ammonium chloride
• Decreased effect of: guanethidine
NURSING CONSIDERATIONS
Assess:
• VS, B/P since this drug may reverse antihypertensives check pa-

---

tients with cardiac disease more often
• CBC, urinalysis; in diabetes: blood sugar, urine sugar; insulin changes may need to be made since eating will decrease
• Height, growth rate in children; growth rate may be decreased

Administer:
• At least 6 hr before hs to avoid sleeplessness
• For obesity only if the patient is on a weight reduction program including dietary changes and exercise; patient will develop tolerance and weight loss won't occur without additional methods, give 30-60 min before meals
• Gum, hard candy, frequent sips of water for dry mouth

Evaluate:
• Therapeutic response: increased CNS stimulation, decreased drowsiness
• Mental status: mood, sensorium, affect, stimulation, insomnia, irritability
• Tolerance or dependency: an increased amount may be used to get same effect; will develop after long-term use
• Overdose: pain, fever, dehydration, insomnia, hyperactivity

Teach patient/family:
• Not to crush or chew sus rel forms
• To decrease caffeine consumption (coffee, tea, cola, chocolate) which may increase irritability, stimulation
• Avoid OTC preparations unless approved by the physician
• To taper off drug over several weeks or depression, increased sleeping, lethargy
• To avoid alcohol ingestion
• To avoid hazardous activities until patient is stabilized on medication

• To get needed rest, patients will feel more tired at end of day
Treatment of overdose: Administer fluids, hemodialysis or peritoneal dialysis; antihypertensive for increased B/P, ammonium Cl for increased excretion

---

dextromethorphan hydrobromide
(dex-troe-meth-or'fan)
Creamcoat, Pertussin 8-hour, Mediquell, Robitussin DM, Sucrets, Hold

Func. class.: Antitussive, nonnarcotic
Chem. class.: Levorphanol derivative

Action: Depresses cough center in medulla
Uses: Nonproductive cough
Dosage and routes:
• *Adult:* PO 10-20 mg q4h, or 30 mg q6-8h, not to exceed 120 mg/day; CON-REL LIQ 60 mg bid, not to exceed 120 mg/day
• *Child 6-12 yr:* PO 5-10 mg q4h; CON-REL LIQ 30 mg bid, not to exceed 60 mg/day
• *Child 2-6 yr:* PO 2.5-5 mg q4h, or 7.5 mg q6-8h, not to exceed 30 mg/day
Available forms include: Loz 5 mg; sol 5, 7.5, 10, 15 mg/5 ml
Side effects/adverse reactions:
CNS: Dizziness
GI: Nausea
Contraindications: Hypersensitivity, asthma/emphysema, productive cough
Precautions: Nausea/vomiting, increased temperature, persistent headache, pregnancy (C)
Pharmacokinetics:
PO: Onset 15-30 min, duration 3-6 hr

---

* Available in Canada only

Interactions/incompatibilities:
• Do not give with MAOIs, penicillins, salicylates, tetracyclines, phenobarbital, iodines (high doses)

NURSING CONSIDERATIONS
Administer:
• Decreased dose to elderly patients; their metabolism may be slowed

Perform/provide:
• Increased fluids to liquefy secretions
• Humidification of patient's room

Evaluate:
• Therapeutic response: absence of cough
• Cough: type, frequency, character including sputum

Teach patient/family:
• Avoid driving or other hazardous activities until patient is stabilized on this medication
• Avoid smoking, smoke-filled rooms, perfumes, dust, environmental pollutants, cleaners that increase cough

---

dextrose (D-glucose)

Func. class.: Caloric

Action: Needed for adequate utilization of amino acids, decreases protein, nitrogen loss, prevents ketosis

Uses: Increases intake of calories, increases fluids in patients unable to take adequate fluids, calories orally

Dosage and routes:
• *Adult and child:* IV depends on individual requirements

Available forms include: Inj IV 2.5%, 5%, 10%, 20%, 40%, 50%

Side effects/adverse reactions:
CNS: Confusion, *loss of consciousness,* dizziness

CV: Hypertension, *CHF, pulmonary edema*
GU: *Glycosuria, osmotic diuresis*
ENDO: Hyperglycemia, rebound hypoglycemia, hyperosmolar syndrome, hyperglycemic nonketotic syndrome
INTEG: Chills, flushing, warm feeling, rash, urticaria, extravasation necrosis

Contraindications: Hyperglycemia, delirium tremens, hemorrhage (cranial/spinal), CHF

Precautions: Renal, liver, cardiac disease, diabetes mellitus

NURSING CONSIDERATIONS
Assess:
• Electrolytes (K, Na, Ca, Cl, Mg), blood glucose, ammonia, phosphate
• Renal, liver function studies: BUN, creatinine, ALT, AST, bilirubin
• Injection site for extravasation: redness along vein, edema at site, necrosis, pain, hard tender area; site should be changed immediately
• Monitor respiratory function q4h: auscultate lung fields bilaterally for rales, respirations, quality, rate, rhythm
• Monitor temperature q4h for increased fever, indicating infection; if infection suspected, infusion is discontinued, tubing, bottle cultured
• Urine glucose q6h using Chemstrips which are not affected by infusion substances

Administer:
• After changing IV catheter, dressing q24h with aseptic technique

Evaluate:
• Therapeutic response: increased weight
• Nutritional status: calorie count by dietitian

---

italics = common side effects   ***bold italic*** = life threatening reactions

Teach patient/family
• Reason for dextrose infusion

---

dextrothyroxine sodium

(dex-troe-thye-rox'een)
Choloxin
Func. class.: Antilipemic
Chem. class.: Hormone isomer

Action: Stimulates hepatic catabolism, excretion of cholesterol; increases bile products into feces
Uses: Hyperlipidemia in euthyroid patients with no evidence of organic heart disease
Dosage and routes:
• *Adult:* PO 1-2 mg/day, may increase 1-2 mg/day q mo, not to exceed 8 mg/day
• *Child:* PO 0.05 mg/kg/day, may increase 0.05 mg/kg/day q mo, not to exceed 4 mg/day
Available forms include: Tabs 1, 2, 4, 6 mg
Side effects/adverse reactions:
GI: Nausea, vomiting, diarrhea, constipation, anorexia, weight loss, jaundice, gallstones
INTEG: Flushing, alopecia, sweating, hyperthermia
CV: Palpitations, dysrhythmias, *myocardial infarction, ischemic myocardial changes,* angina
EENT: Visual disturbances, ptosis, retinopathy, lid lag
GU: Menstrual irregularities, change in libido
CNS: Insomnia, tremors, headache, dizziness, paresthesia, decreased sensorium
Contraindications: Severe hepatic disease, severe renal disease, organic heart disease, Hx of myocardial infarction, cardiac dysrhythmias, rheumatic heart disease, CHF, hypertension, iodism, angina, obesity

Precautions: Hepatic disease, renal disease, pregnancy (C), lactation, surgery
Interactions/incompatibilities:
• Decreased effects of dextrothyroxine: cholestyramine, colestipol
• Increased effects of: digitalis, oral anticoagulants, sympathomimetics
• Increased CNS stimulation: tricyclic antidepressants
• Increased blood sugar levels in patients with diabetes
• Decreased effects of: beta blockers
NURSING CONSIDERATIONS
Assess:
• Renal and hepatic function tests, if patient is on long-term therapy
• CV status: rate, rhythm, character, chest pain
Evaluate:
• Therapeutic response: decreased cholesterol levels, (hyperlipidemia); diarrhea, pruritus (excess bile area)
• Bowel pattern daily; increase bulk, water in diet if constipation develops
Teach patient/family:
• That compliance is needed since toxicity may result if doses are missed
• That risk factors should be decreased: high fat diet, smoking, alcohol consumption, absence of exercise
• Birth control should be practiced while on this drug

---

dezocine

Dalgan
Func. class.: Narcotic agonist-antagonist analgesic
Chem. class.: Opioid, synthetic

Action: Depresses pain impulse

---

*Available in Canada only

transmission at the spinal cord level by interacting with opioid receptors
Uses: Severe pain
Dosage and routes:
Adult: IM 5-20 mg q3-6h, not to exceed 120 mg/day; IV 2.5-10 mg q2-4h
Available forms include: IM, IV inj 5, 10, 15 mg single-dose vials, multiple dose 10 mg/ml
Side effects/adverse reactions:
CV: Hypotension, pulse irregularity, hypertension, chest pain, pallor, edema, thrombophlebitis
CNS: Drowsiness, dizziness, confusion, sedation, anxiety, headache, depression, delirium, sleep disturbances
GI: Nausea, vomiting, anorexia, constipation, cramps, abdominal pain, dry mouth, diarrhea
INTEG: Injection site reactions, pruritus, rash, sweating, chills
*RESP: **Respiratory depression,*** hiccups
GU: Urinary frequency, hesitancy, retention
Contraindications: Hypersensitivity
Precautions: Addictive personality, pregnancy (C), lactation, increased intracranial pressure, respiratory depression, hepatic disease, renal disease, child <18 yr, elderly, biliary surgery, COPD, sulfite sensitivity
Pharmacokinetics: IM: Onset 30 min, peak 50-90 min, duration 2-4 hr; IV: Onset 10 min, peak 30 min, duration 2-4 hr; metabolized by liver, excreted by kidneys, may cross placenta
Interactions/incompatibilities:
• Increased CNS depression: alcohol, narcotics, sedative/hypnotics, antipsychotics, skeletal muscle relaxants, general anesthetics, tranquilizers

NURSING CONSIDERATIONS
Assess:
• I&O ratio; check for decreasing output; may indicate urinary retention
Administer:
• With antiemetic if nausea, vomiting occur
• When pain is beginning to return; determine dosage interval by patient response
Perform/provide:
• Storage in light-resistant area at room temperature
• Assistance with ambulation
• Safety measures: siderails, night light, call bell within easy reach
Evaluate:
• Therapeutic response: decrease in pain
• CNS changes: dizziness, drowsiness, hallucinations, euphoria, LOC, pupil reaction
• Allergic reactions: rash, urticaria
• Respiratory dysfunction: respiratory depression, character, rate, rhythm of respirations; notify physician if respirations are <10/min
• Need for pain medication, physical dependence
Teach patient/family:
• To report any symptoms of CNS changes, allergic reactions
• That physical dependency may result when used for extended periods of time
• Withdrawal symptoms may occur: nausea, vomiting, cramps, fever, faintness, anorexia
Treatment of overdose: Naloxone 0.2-0.8 IV, O₂, IV fluids, vasopressors

---

italics = common side effects   ***bold italic*** = life threatening reactions

diazepam

(dye-az'-e-pam)

D-Tran,* E-Pam,* Meval,* Novo-dipam,* Stress-Pam,* Valium, Valrelease, Vivol*

Func. class.: Antianxiety
Chem. class.: Benzodiazepine

Controlled Substance Schedule IV

Action: Depresses subcortical levels of CNS, including limbic system, reticular formation

Uses: Anxiety, acute alcohol withdrawal, adjunct in seizure disorders, preoperatively

Dosage and routes:
Anxiety/convulsive disorders
• *Adult:* PO 2-10 mg tid-qid; EXT REL 15-30 mg qd
• *Child >6 mo:* PO 1-2.5 mg tid-qid

Tetanic muscle spams
• *Child >5 yr:* IM/IV 5-10 mg q3-4 hr prn
• *Infants >30 days:* IM/IV 1-2 mg q 3-4 hr prn

Status epilepticus
• *Adult:* IV BOLUS 5-20 mg, 2 mg/min, may repeat q5-10 min, not to exceed 60 mg, may repeat in 30 min if seizures reappear
• *Child:* IV BOLUS 0.1-0.3 mg/kg (1 mg/min over 3 min), may repeat q15 min × 2 doses

Available forms include: Tabs 2, 5, 10 mg; caps ext rel 15 mg, IM/IV inj

Side effects/adverse reactions:

CNS: Dizziness, drowsiness, confusion, headache, anxiety, tremors, stimulation, fatigue, depression, insomnia, hallucinations

GI: Constipation, dry mouth, nausea, vomiting, anorexia, diarrhea

INTEG: Rash, dermatitis, itching

*CV: Orthostatic hypotension, **ECG changes, tachycardia,*** hypotension

EENT: Blurred vision, tinnitus, mydriasis

Contraindications: Hypersensitivity to benzodiazepines, narrow-angle glaucoma, psychosis, pregnancy (D), child <18 yr

Precautions: Elderly, debilitated, hepatic disease, renal disease

Pharmacokinetics:

PO: Onset ½, duration 2-3 hr
IM: Onset 15-30 min, duration 1-1½ hr
IV: Onset 1-5 min, duration 15 min

Metabolized by liver, excreted by kidneys, crosses placenta, breast milk, half-life 20-50 hr, more effective by mouth

Interactions/incompatibilities:
• Decreased effects of diazepam: oral contraceptives, rifampin, valproic acid
• Increased effects of diazepam: CNS depressants, alcohol, cimetidine, disulfiram, oral contraceptives
• Incompatible with all drugs in solution or syringe

NURSING CONSIDERATIONS
Assess:
• B/P (lying, standing), pulse; if systolic B/P drops 20 mm Hg, hold drug, notify physician; respirations q5-15 min if given IV
• Blood studies: CBC during long-term therapy, blood dyscrasias have occurred rarely
• Hepatic studies: AST, ALT, bilirubin, creatinine, LDH, alk phosphatase

Administer:
• IV into large vein; do not dilute or mix with any other drug; give IV 5 mg or less/1 min
• With food or milk for GI symptoms

• Crushed if patient is unable to swallow medication whole
• Sugarless gum, hard candy, frequent sips of water for dry mouth
• Reduced narcotic dose by ⅓ if given concomitantly with diazepam
Perform/provide:
• Assistance with ambulation during beginning therapy, since drowsiness/dizziness occurs
• Safety measures, including siderails
• Check to see PO medication has been swallowed
Evaluate:
• Therapeutic response: decreased anxiety, restlessness, insomnia
• Mental status: mood, sensorium, affect, sleeping pattern, drowsiness, dizziness
• Physical dependency, withdrawal symptoms: headache, nausea, vomiting, muscle pain, weakness after long-term use
• Suicidal tendencies
Teach patient/family:
• That drug may be taken with food
• Not to be used for everyday stress or used longer than 4 mo, unless directed by physician; not to take more than prescribed amount, may be habit-forming
• Avoid OTC preparations unless approved by physician
• To avoid driving, activities that require alertness; drowsiness may occur
• To avoid alcohol ingestion or other psychotropic medications, unless prescribed by physician
• Not to discontinue medication abruptly after long-term use
• To rise slowly or fainting may occur
• That drowsiness might worsen at beginning of treatment
Lab test interferences:
Increase: AST/ALT, serum bilirubin

False increase: 17-OHCS
Decrease: RAIU
Treatment of overdose: Lavage, VS, supportive care

---

diazoxide
(dye-az-ox′ide)
Hyperstat
Func. class.: Antihypertensive
Chem. class.: Vasodilator

Action: Vasodilates arteriolar smooth muscle by direct relaxation; a reduction in blood pressure with concomitant increases in heart rate, cardiac output
Uses: Hypertensive crisis when urgent decrease of diastolic pressure required, increase blood glucose levels in hyperinsulinism
Dosage and routes:
• *Adult:* IV BOL 1-3 mg/kg rapidly up to a max of 150 mg in a single injection, dose may be repeated at 5-15 min intervals until desired response is achieved; give IV in 30 sec or less
• *Child:* IV BOL 1-2 mg/kg rapidly; administration same as adult, not to exceed 150 mg
Available forms include: Inj IV 15 mg/ml
Side effects/adverse reactions:
*CV: **Hypotension,*** T wave changes, angina pectoris, palpitations, ***supraventricular tachycardia, edema,*** rebound hypertension
CNS: Headache, sleepiness, euphoria, anxiety, extrapyramidal symptoms, confusion, tinnitus, blurred vision, dizziness, weakness
GI: Nausea, vomiting, dry mouth
INTEG: Rash
HEMA: Decreased hemoglobin, hematocrit, ***thrombocytopenia***
GU: Breast tenderness, increased

italics = common side effects · ***bold italic*** = life threatening reactions

BUN, fluid, electrolyte imbalances, sodium, water retention

ENDO: Hyperglycemia in diabetics, transient hyperglycemia in nondiabetics

Contraindications: Hypersensitivity to thiazides, sulfonamides, hypertension associated with aortic coarctation or AV shunt, pheochromocytoma, dissecting aortic aneurysm

Precautions: Tachycardia, fluid, electrolyte imbalances, pregnancy (B), lactation, impaired cerebral or cardiac circulation, children

Pharmacokinetics:

IV: Onset 1-2 min, peak 5 min, duration 3-12 hr

Half-life 20-36 hr, excreted slowly in urine, crosses blood-brain barrier, placenta

Interactions/incompatibilities:

• Increased effects: thiazide diuretics, antihypertensives, coumadin, guanethidine, sympathomimetics

• Do not mix with any drug in syringe or solution

• Increased effects of: warfarin, other coumarins

• Hyperglycemia/hyperuricemia: thiazides, diuretics

• Decreased pharmacologic effects of both: sulfonylureas

NURSING CONSIDERATIONS

Assess:

• B/P q5 min × 2 hr, then q1h × 2 hr, then q4h

• Pulse, jugular venous distention q4h

• Electrolytes, blood studies: potassium, sodium, chloride, CO_2, CBC, serum glucose

• Weight daily, I&O

Administer:

• Undiluted; give over ½ min or less

• To patient in recumbent position,

keep in that position for 1 hr after administration

Perform/provide:

• Protection from light

Evaluate:

• Therapeutic response: decreased B/P, primarily diastolic pressure

• Edema in feet, legs daily

• Skin turgor, dryness of mucous membranes for hydration status

• Rales, dyspnea, orthopnea

• IV site for extravasation, rate

• Signs of CHF: dyspnea, edema, wet rales

• Postural hypotension, take B/P sitting, standing

Teach patient/family:

• That hirsutism is reversible after drug is discontinued

Treatment of overdose: Administer levarterenol, dopamine, or norepinephrine for hypotension, dialysis

---

diazoxide (oral)

(dye-az-ox'ide)

Proglycem

Func. class.: Hyperglycemic

Chem. class.: Benzothiadiazine

Action: Decreases release of insulin from β-cells in pancreas, resulting in an increase in blood glucose

Uses: Hypoglycemia caused by hyperinsulinism

Dosage and routes:

• *Adult and child:* PO 3-8 mg/kg/day in 3 divided doses q8-12h

• *Infants and neonates:* PO 8-15 mg/kg/day in 2-3 divided doses q8-12h

Available forms include: Caps 50 mg; oral susp 50 mg/ml

Side effects/adverse reactions:

CNS: Headache, weakness, mal-

---

aise, anxiety, dizziness, insomnia, paresthesia

EENT: Diplopia, cataracts, ring scotoma

HEMA: **Thrombocytopenia, leukopenia,** eosinophilia, decreased hemoglobulin, hematocrit

INTEG: Increased hair growth

GI: Nausea, vomiting, anorexia

CV: Dysrhythmias, tachycardia, palpitations, hypotension

META: Hyperuricemia, sodium/fluid retention, ketoacidosis, hyperglycemia

Contraindications: Hypersensitivity to this drug or thiazides, functional hypoglycemia

Precautions: Pregnancy (C), lactation, renal disease, diabetes mellitus, CV disease, gout

Pharmacokinetics:

PO: Onset 1 hr, duration 8 hr, half-life 20-36 min, excreted unchanged by kidneys, crosses blood-brain barrier, placenta

Interactions/incompatibilities:

• Increased effects of diazoxide: phenothiazines

• Decreased effects of: phenytoin

• Increased effects of: antihypertensives, oral anticoagulants

• Decreased effects of diazoxide: α-adrenergic blockers, sulfonylureas

NURSING CONSIDERATIONS
Assess:

• I&O ratio, weight weekly

• Electrolytes (K, Na, Cl), glucose, Hct, Hgb, platelets, differential

• Urine for glucose, ketones qd

Administer:

• Shake before using

Perform/provide:

• Sus storage: protect from light

Evaluate:

• Therapeutic response: adequate blood, urine glucose, absence of ketones in urine

Teach patient/family:

• That if drug is not effective within 2-3 wk, drug may be discontinued

• That if hirsutism occurs, it is reversible after discontinuing treatment

Lab test interferences:

Increase: Bilirubin, uric acid, blood glucose

Decrease: Creatinine, Hgb, Hct, plasma-free fatty acids

---

dibucaine HCl (topical)

(dye′byoo-kane)

D-Caine, Nupercainal

Func. class.: Topical anesthetic

Chem. class.: Amide

Action: Inhibits nerve impulses from sensory nerves, which produces anesthesia

Uses: Pruritus, sunburn, toothache, sore throat, cold sores, oral pain, rectal pain and irritation

Dosage and routes:

• *Adult and child:* TOP apply qid as needed; REC insert tid and after each BM

Available forms include: Cream 0.5%; rec or top oint 1%

Side effects/adverse reactions:

INTEG: Rash, irritation, sensitization

Contraindications: Hypersensitivity, infants <1 yr, application to large areas

Precautions: Child <6 yr, sepsis, pregnancy (C), denuded skin

NURSING CONSIDERATIONS
Administer:

• After cleansing and drying of affected area

Evaluate:

• Allergy: rash, irritation, reddening, swelling

---

italics = common side effects   ***bold italic*** = life threatening reactions

- Therapeutic response: absence of pain, itching of affected area
- Infection: if affected area is infected, do not apply

Teach patient/family:
- To report rash, irritation, redness, swelling
- How to apply cream, ointment

---

diclofenac

(dye-kloe'-fen-ac)
Voltaren

Func. class.: Nonsteroidal antiinflammatory
Chem. class.: Phenylacetic acid

Action: Inhibits prostaglandin synthesis by decreasing enzyme needed for biosynthesis; possesses analgesic, antiinflammatory, antipyretic properties
Uses: Acute, chronic rheumatoid arthritis, osteoarthritis, ankylosing spondylitis
Dosage and routes:
Osteoarthritis
- *Adult:* PO 100-150 mg/day in divided doses

Rheumatoid arthritis
- *Adult:* PO 150-200 mg/day in divided doses

Ankylosing spondylitis
- *Adult:* PO 100-125 mg/day; give 25 mg qid and 25 mg hs if needed

Available forms include: Tabs enteric coated 25, 50, 75 mg
Side effects/adverse reactions:
GI: Nausea, anorexia, vomiting, diarrhea, *jaundice, cholestatic hepatitis,* constipation, flatulence, cramps, dry mouth, peptic ulcer, GI bleeding
CNS: Dizziness, drowsiness, fatigue, tremors, confusion, insomnia, anxiety, depression, nervousness, paresthesia, muscle weakness
CV: CHF, tachycardia, peripheral edema, palpitations, *dysrhythmias,* hypotension, hypertension, fluid retention
INTEG: Purpura, rash, pruritus, sweating, erythema, petechiae, photosensitivity, alopecia
GU: Nephrotoxicity: dysuria, hematuria, oliguria, azotemia, cystitis, UTI
HEMA: Blood dyscrasias, epistaxis, bruising
EENT: Tinnitus, hearing loss, blurred vision
RESP: Dyspnea, hemoptysis, pharyngitis, *bronchospasm, laryngeal edema,* rhinitis, shortness of breath
Contraindications: Hypersensitivity to aspirin, iodides, other nonsteroidal antiinflammatory agents, asthma
Precautions: Pregnancy (B) 1st, 2nd trimester, lactation, children, bleeding disorders, GI disorders, cardiac disorders, hypersensitivity to other antiinflammatory agents
Pharmacokinetics:
PO: Peak 2-3 hr, elimination half-life 1-2 hr, 90% bound to plasma proteins, metabolized in liver to metabolite, excreted in urine
Interactions/incompatibilities:
- Decreased antihypertensive effect: β-blockers, diuretics
- Increased anticoagulant effect: coumarin
- Increased toxicity: phenytoin, sulfonamides, sulfonylurea
- Increased plasma levels of diclofenac: probenecid, potassium-sparing diuretics

NURSING CONSIDERATIONS
Assess:
- Blood counts during therapy, watch for decreasing platelets, if low, therapy may need to be discontinued, restarted after hematologic recovery

Evaluate:
• Blood dyscrasias (thrombocytopenia): bruising, fatigue, bleeding, poor healing

Teach patient/family:
• That drug must be continued for prescribed time to be effective
• To report bleeding, bruising, fatigue, malaise since blood dyscrasias do occur
• To avoid aspirin, alcoholic beverages
• To take with food, milk, or antacids to avoid GI upset, to swallow whole
• Use caution when driving; drowsiness, dizziness may occur
• To take with a full glass of water to enhance absorption

---

dicloxacillin sodium

(dye-klox-a-sill'-in)
Dycill, Dynapen, Pathocil
Func. class.: Broad-spectrum antibiotic
Chem. class.: Penicillinase-resistant penicillin

Action: Interferes with cell wall replication of susceptible organisms; osmotically unstable cell wall swells, bursts from osmotic pressure

Uses: Effective for gram-positive cocci (*S. aureus, S. pyogenes, S. viridans, S. faecalis, S. bovis, S. pneumoniae*), infections caused by penicillinase-producing *Staphylococcus*

Dosage and routes:
• *Adult:* PO 0.5-4 g/day in divided doses q6h
• *Child:* PO 12.5-25 mg/kg in divided doses q6h

Available forms include: Caps 125, 250, 500 mg; powder for oral susp 62.5 mg/5 ml

Side effects/adverse reactions:
HEMA: Anemia, increased bleeding time, **bone marrow depression, granulocytopenia**
GI: Nausea, vomiting, diarrhea, increased AST, ALT, abdominal pain, glossitis, colitis
GU: **Oliguria, proteinuria, hematuria,** vaginitis, moniliasis, **glomerulonephritis**
CNS: Lethargy, hallucinations, anxiety, depression, twitching, **coma, convulsions**

Contraindications: Hypersensitivity to penicillins; neonates

Precautions: Hypersensitivity to cephalosporins, pregnancy (B)

Pharmacokinetics:
PO: Peak 1 hr, duration 4-6 hr, half-life 30-60 min, metabolized in liver, excreted in urine, bile, breast milk, crosses placenta

Interactions/incompatibilities:
• Decreased antimicrobial effectiveness of dicloxacillin: tetracyclines, erythromycins
• Increased dicloxacillin concentrations: aspirin, probenecid

NURSING CONSIDERATIONS
Assess:
• I&O ratio; report hematuria, oliguria since penicillin in high doses is nephrotoxic
• Any patient with compromised renal system since drug is excreted slowly in poor renal system function; toxicity may occur rapidly
• Liver studies: AST, ALT
• Blood studies: WBC, RBC, H&H, bleeding time
• Renal studies: urinalysis, protein, blood
• C&S before drug therapy; drug may be taken as soon as culture is taken

Administer:
• Drug after C&S has been completed

---

italics = common side effects   ***bold italic*** = life threatening reactions

• On an empty stomach with a full glass of water

Perform/provide:

• Adrenalin, suction, tracheostomy set, endotracheal intubation equipment

• Adequate fluid intake (2000 ml) during diarrhea episodes

• Scratch test to assess allergy, after securing order from physician; usually done when penicillin is only drug of choice

• Storage in tight container; after reconstituting, store in refrigerator up to 2 wk

Evaluate:

• Therapeutic effectiveness: absence of fever, draining wounds

• Bowel pattern before, during treatment

• Skin eruptions after administration of penicillin to 1 wk after discontinuing drug

• Respiratory status: rate, character, wheezing, tightness in chest

• Allergies before initiation of treatment, reaction of each medication; highlight allergies on chart, Kardex

Teach patient/family:

• Aspects of drug therapy, including need to complete course of medication to ensure organism death (10-14 days); culture may be taken after completed course

• To report sore throat, fever, fatigue (could indicate superimposed infection)

• To wear or carry Medic Alert ID if allergic to penicillins

• To notify nurse of diarrhea

Lab test interferences:

False positive: Urine glucose, urine protein

Treatment of overdose: Withdraw drug, maintain airway, administer epinephrine, aminophylline, O_2, IV corticosteroids for anaphylaxis

dicyclomine HCl

(dye-sye'kloe-meen)

Antispas, Bentyl, Bentylol,* Dibent, Formulex,* Neoquess, Viserol*

Func. class.: Gastrointestinal anticholinergic

Chem. class.: Synthetic tertiary amine

Action: Inhibits muscarinic actions of acetylcholine at postganglionic parasympathetic neuroeffector sites

Uses: Treatment of peptic ulcer disease in combination with other drugs; infant colic

Dosage and routes:

• *Adult:* PO 10-20 mg tid-qid; IM 20 mg q4-6h

• *Child >2 yr:* PO 10 mg tid-qid

• *Child 6 mo-2 yr:* PO 5 mg tid-qid

Available forms include: Caps 10, 20 mg; tabs 20 mg; syr 10 mg/5 ml; inj IM 10 mg/ml

Side effects/adverse reactions:

CNS: Confusion, stimulation in elderly, headache, insomnia, dizziness, drowsiness, anxiety, weakness, hallucination; *seizures, coma* (child <3 mo)

GI: Dry mouth, constipation, paralytic ileus, heartburn, nausea, vomiting, dysphagia, absence of taste

GU: Hesitancy, rentention, impotence

CV: Palpitations, tachycardia

EENT: Blurred vision, photophobia, mydriasis, cycloplegia, increased ocular tension

INTEG: Urticaria, rash, pruritus, anhidrosis, fever, allergic reactions

Contraindications: Hypersensitivity to anticholinergics, narrow-angle glaucoma, GI obstruction, myasthenia gravis, paralytic ileus, GI atony, toxic megacolon

---

Precautions: Hyperthyroidism, coronary artery disease, dysrhythmias, CHF, ulcerative colitis, hypertension, hiatal hernia, hepatic disease, renal disease, pregnancy (B), urinary retention, prostatic hypertrophy

Pharmacokinetics:

PO: Onset 1-2 hr, duration 3-4 hr; metabolized by liver, excreted in urine

Interactions/incompatibilities:

• Increased anticholinergic effect: amantadine, tricylic antidepressants, MAOIs, H₁ antihistamines
• Decreased effect of: phenothiazines, levodopa, ketoconazole

NURSING CONSIDERATIONS
Assess:

• VS, cardiac status: checking for dysrhythmias, increased rate, palpitations
• I&O ratio; check for urinary retention or hesitancy

Administer:

• ½-1 hr ac for better absorption
• Decreased dose to elderly patients; their metabolism may be slowed
• Gum, hard candy, frequent rinsing of mouth for dryness of oral cavity

Perform/provide:

• Storage in tight container protected from light
• Increased fluids, bulk, exercise to patient's lifestyle to decrease constipation

Evaluate:

• Therapeutic response: absence of epigastric pain, bleeding, nausea, vomiting
• GI complaints: pain, bleeding (frank or occult), nausea, vomiting, anorexia

Teach patient/family:

• Avoid driving or other hazardous activities until stabilized on medication, may cause blurred vision
• Avoid alcohol or other CNS depressants; will enhance sedating properties of this drug
• To avoid hot environments, stroke may occur, drug suppresses perspiration
• Use sunglasses when outside to prevent photophobia
• To drink plenty fluids
• To report dysphagia

---

dienestrol

(dye-en-ess'trole)

DV, Estraguard, Ortho Dienestrol

Func. class.: Estrogen

Chem. class.: Nonsteroidal synthetic estrogen

Action: Needed for adequate functioning of female reproductive system, it affects release of pituitary gonadotropins, inhibits ovulation, adequate calcium use in bone structures

Uses: Atrophic vaginitis, kraurosis vulvae

Dosage and routes:

• *Adult:* VAG CREAM 1-2 applications qd × 2 wk, then ½ dose × 2 wk, then 1 application

Available forms include: Vag cream 0.01%

Side effects/adverse reactions:

CNS: Dizziness, headache, migraines, depression

CV: Hypotension, thrombophlebitis, edema, ***thromboembolism, stroke, pulmonary embolism, myocardial infarction***

GI: Nausea, vomiting, diarrhea, anorexia, pancreatitis, cramps, constipation, increased appetite, increased weight, ***cholestatic jaundice***

EENT: Contact lens intolerance, increased myopia, astigmatism

---

italics = common side effects   ***bold italic*** = life threatening reactions

GU: Amenorrhea, cervical erosion, breakthrough bleeding, dysmenorrhea, vaginal candidiasis, breast changes, gynecomastia, testicular atrophy, impotence

INTEG: Rash, urticaria, acne, hirsutism, alopecia, oily skin, seborrhea, purpura, melasma

META: Folic acid deficiency, hypercalcemia, hyperglycemia

Contraindications: Breast cancer, thromboembolic disorders, reproductive cancer, genital bleeding (abnormal, undiagnosed), pregnancy (X)

Precautions: Hypertension, asthma, blood dyscrasias, gallbladder disease, CHF, diabetes mellitus, bone disease, depression, migraine headache, convulsive disorders, hepatic disease, renal disease, family history of cancer of the breast or reproductive tract

Pharmacokinetics:

TOP: Degraded in liver, excreted in urine, crosses placenta, excreted in breast milk

Interactions/incompatibilities:

• Decreased action of: anticoagulants, oral hypoglycemics

• Toxicity: tricyclic antidepressants

• Decreased action of dienestrol: anticonvulsants, barbiturates, phenylbutazone, rifampin

• Increased action of: corticosteroids

NURSING CONSIDERATIONS
Assess:

• Weight daily; notify physician of weekly weight gain >5 lb

• B/P q4h

• I&O ratio, be alert for decreasing urinary output and increasing edema

• Liver function studies including ALT, AST, bilirubin

Administer:

• At hs for better absorption

• Titrated dose, use lowest effective dose, to prevent adverse reactions

• Dosage reduction should continue at 3-6 month intervals

Perform/provide:

• Storage in tight, light-resistant container in refrigerator

Evaluate:

• Edema, hypertension, cardiac symptoms, jaundice

• Mental status: affect, mood, behavioral changes, aggression

• Hypercalcemia

Teach patient/family:

• How to fill applicator and insert cream

• To check with MD before using any over-the-counter drugs

• To report breast lumps, vaginal bleeding, edema, jaundice, dark urine, clay colored stools, dyspnea, headache, blurred vision, abdominal pain, numbness or stiffness in legs, chest pain

---

diethylpropion HCl
Dospan, Nobesine, Nu-Dispoz, Regibon, Ro-Diet, Tenuate, Tepanil, Ten-Tab, Tepanic

Func. class.: Anorexant

Chem. class.: Amphetamine-like analog

Controlled Substance Schedule IV

Action: Direct stimulation of partial adrenergic pathways to suppress appetite

Uses: Exogenous obesity

Dosage and routes:

• *Adult:* PO 25 mg/hr ac, or 75 mg controlled release qd midmorning

Available forms include: Tabs 25 mg, tabs susp rel 75 mg

Side effects/adverse reactions:

*HEMA: **Bone marrow depression,*** leukopenia, agranulocytosis

CNS: Hyperactivity, restlessness, anxiety, insomnia, dizziness, dysphonia, depression, tremors, headache, blurred vision, incoordination, fatigue, malaise, euphoria, depression, tremor, confusion

GI: Nausea, vomiting, anorexia, dry mouth, diarrhea, constipation

GU: Impotence, change in libido, menstrual irregularities, dysuria, polyuria

CV: Palpitations, tachycardia, hypertension, hypotension, dysrhythmias, pulmonary hypertension, BCG changes

INTEG: Urticaria

Contraindications: Hypersensitivity, hyperthyroidism, hypertension, glaucoma, angina pectoris, drug abuse, cardiovascular disease, children <12 yr, severe arteriosclerosis, agitated states

Precautions: Convulsive disorders, pregnancy (B), lactation

Pharmacokinetics:

PO: Duration 4 hr

CONT REL: Duration 10-14 hr; metabolized by liver, excreted by kidneys, crosses placenta, breast milk, half-life 1-3½ hr

Interactions/incompatibilities:

• Hypertensive crisis: MAOIs or within 14 days of MAOIs

• Increased effect of diethylpropion: acetazolamide, antacids, sodium bicarbonate, ascorbic acid, ammonium chloride

• Decreased effects of diethylpropion: barbiturates, tricyclics

• Decreased effects of: guanethidine, other antihypertensives

NURSING CONSIDERATIONS
Assess:

• VS, B/P since this drug may reverse antihypertensives; check patients with cardiac disease more often

• CBC, urinalysis, in diabetes: blood sugar, urine sugar; insulin changes may need to be made since eating will decrease

• Height, growth rate in children; growth rate may be decreased

Administer:

• At least 6 hr before hs to avoid sleeplessness

• For obesity only if patient is on weight reduction program, including dietary changes, exercise; patient will develop tolerance, and weight loss won't occur without additional methods, give 1 hour before meals

• Gum, hard candy, frequent sips of water for dry mouth

Evaluate:

• Mental status: mood, sensorium, affect, stimulation, insomnia, aggressiveness

• Physical dependency: should not be used for extended time; dose should be discontinued gradually, drug tolerance occurs after long-term use

• Withdrawal symptoms: headache, nausea, vomiting, muscle pain, weakness

Teach patient/family:

• To not crush or chew sus rel preps; not to take more frequently than prescribed

• To decrease caffeine consumption (coffee, tea, cola, chocolate); may increase irritability, stimulation

• Avoid OTC preparations unless approved by physician

• To taper off drug over several weeks, or depression, increased sleeping, lethargy will occur

• To avoid alcohol ingestion

• To avoid hazardous activities un-

---

italics = common side effects   ***bold italic*** = life threatening reactions

til patient is stabilized on medication
• To get needed rest, patients will feel more tired at end of day
Treatment of overdose: Administer fluids, hemodialysis for peritoneal dialysis; antihypertensive for increased B/P; ammonium Cl for increased excretion

---

diethylstilbestrol/diethylstilbestrol diphosphate

(dye-eth-il-stil-bess′trole)
DES, Stilboestrol*/Honvol,* Stilphostrol
Func. class.: Estrogen
Chem. class.: Nonsteroidal synthetic estrogen

Action: Needed for adequate functioning of female reproductive system, it affects release of pituitary gonadotropins, inhibits ovulation, adequate calcium use in bone structures

Uses: Atrophic vaginitis, kraurosis vulvae, menopause, postcoital contraception, hypogonadism, castration, primary ovarian failure, breast engorgement, breast cancer, prostatic cancer

Dosage and routes:
Atrophic vaginitis/kraurosis vulvae
• *Adult:* VAG SUPP 0.1-1 mg qd × 10-14 days with oral therapy or up to 5 mg q wk
Menopause
• *Adult:* PO 0.1-2 mg qd 3 wk on, 1 wk off
Contraception
• *Adult:* PO 25 mg bid × 5 days, within 72 hr of intercourse
Hypogonadism/castration/ovarian failure
• *Adult:* PO 0.2-0.5 mg qd
Breast engorgement

• *Adult:* PO 5 mg qd-tid, not to exceed 30 mg
Prostatic cancer
• *Adult:* PO 1-3 mg qd, then 1 mg qd; PO 50-200 mg tid (diphosphate); IM 5 mg 2×/wk, then 4 mg 2×/wk; IV 0.25-1 g qd × 5 days, then 1-2×/wk
Breast cancer
• *Adult:* PO 15 mg qd
Available forms include: Tabs 1, 5 mg; tabs enteric coated 0.1, 0.25, 0.5, 1, 5 mg; vag supp 0.1, 0.5 mg
Side effects/adverse reactions:
CNS: Dizziness, headache, migraines, depression
CV: Hypotension, thrombophlebitis, edema, *thromboembolism, stroke, pulmonary embolism, myocardial infarction*
GI: Nausea, vomiting, diarrhea, anorexia, pancreatitis, cramps, constipation, increased appetite, increased weight, *cholestatic jaundice*
EENT: Contact lens intolerance, increased myopia, astigmatism
GU: Amenorrhea, cervical erosion, breakthrough bleeding, dysmenorrhea, vaginal candidiasis, breast changes, *gynecomastia, testicular atrophy, impotence*
INTEG: Rash, urticaria, acne, hirsutism, alopecia, oily skin, seborrhea, purpura, melasma
META: Folic acid deficiency, hypercalcemia, hyperglycemia
Contraindications: Breast cancer, thromboembolic disorders, reproductive cancer, genital bleeding (abnormal, undiagnosed), pregnancy (X)
Precautions: Hypertension, asthma, blood dyscrasias, gallbladder disease, CHF, diabetes mellitus, bone disease blocking agents
Interactions/incompatibilities:
• Decreased action of: anticoagulants, oral hypoglycemics

• Toxicity: tricyclic antidepressants

• Decreased action of diethylstilbestrol: anticonvulsants, barbiturates, phenylbutazone, rifampin

• Increased action of: corticosteroids

NURSING CONSIDERATIONS

Assess:

• Urine glucose in patient with diabetes; increased urine glucose may occur

• Weight daily, notify physician of weekly weight gain >5 lb; if increase, diuretic may be ordered

• B/P q4h, watch for increase caused by water and sodium retention

• I&O ratio, be alert for decreasing urinary output and increasing edema

• Liver function studies, including AST, ALT, bilirubin, alk phosphatase

Administer:

• IV after diluting in 300 ml of dextrose or saline sol; give at a rate of 20 g hs/min × 15 min; may increase rate to complete infusion 1 hr after starting

• Titrated dose, use lowest effective dose

• IM injection deeply in large muscular mass

• In one dose in AM for prostatic cancer, vaginitis, hypogonadism

• With food or milk to decrease GI symptoms

Evaluate:

• Therapeutic response: absence of breast engorgement, reversal of menopause or decrease in tumor size in prostatic cancer

• Edema, hypertension, cardiac symptoms, jaundice

• Mental status: affect, mood, behavioral changes, aggression

• Hypercalcemia

Teach patient/family:

• To weigh weekly, report gain >5 lb

• To report breast lumps, vaginal bleeding, edema, jaundice, dark urine, clay colored stools, dyspnea, headache, blurred vision, abdominal pain, numbness or stiffness in legs, chest pain; male to report impotence or gynecomastia

• To check with MD before taking any over-the-counter drugs

Lab test interferences:

Increase: BSP retention test, PBI, T_4, serum sodium, platelet aggressability, thyroxine-binding globulin (TBG), prothrombin, factors VII, VIII, IX, X, triglycerides

Decrease: Serum folate, serum triglyceride, T_3 resin uptake test, glucose tolerance test, antithrombin III, pregnanediol, metyraponetest

False positive: LE prep, antinuclear antibodies

---

difenoxin HCl with atropine sulfate

(dye-fen-ox' -in)

Motofen

Func. class.: Antidiarrheal

Chem. class.: Phenylpiperidine de-

Controlled Substance Schedule IV

Action: Slows intestinal motility by local action on GI wall

Uses: Acute nonspecific and acute exacerbations of chronic functional diarrhea

Dosage and routes:

• *Adult:* PO 2 mg, then 1 mg after each loose stool or 1 mg q3-4h as needed, not to exceed 8 mg/24 hr

Available forms include: Tab 1 mg difenoxin HCl, 0.025 mg atropine sulfate

---

italics = common side effects   ***bold italic*** = life threatening reactions

Side effects/adverse reactions:
CNS: Dizzines, drowsiness, headache, fatigue, nervousness, insomnia, confusion
GI: Nausea, vomiting, dry mouth, epigastric distress, constipation
EENT: Burning eyes, blurred vision
Contraindications: Hypersensitivity, pseudomembranous enterocolitis, glaucoma, child <2 yr, severe electrolyte imbalances, diarrhea associated with organisms that penetrate intestinal mucosa
Precautions: Hepatic disease, renal disease, ulcerative colitis, pregnancy (C), lactation, severe liver disease
Pharmacokinetics:
PO: Peak 40-60 min, duration 3-4 hr, metabolized in liver to inactive metabolite; excreted in urine, feces
Interactions/incompatibilities:
• Do not use with MAOIs; hypertensive crisis may occur
• Increased action of: alcohol, narcotics, barbituates, other CNS depressants, anticholinergics
NURSING CONSIDERATIONS
Assess:
• Electrolytes (K, Na, Cl) if on long-term therapy
Administer:
• For 48 hr only
Evaluate:
• Therapeutic response: decreased diarrhea
• Bowel pattern before; for rebound constipation after termination of medication
• Response after 48 hr; if no response, drug should be discontinued
• Abdominal distention, toxic megacolon, which may occur in ulcerative colitis
Teach patient/family:
• To avoid OTC products unless directed by physician; may contain alcohol
• Not to exceed recommended dose
• May be habit forming

---

diflorasone diacetate

(die-floor'-a-sone)
Florone, Futone, Maxifloor, Psorcon
Func. class.: Topical corticosteroid
Chem. class.: Synthetic fluorinated agent, group II potency

Action: Possesses antipruritic, antiinflammatory actions
Uses: Psoriasis, eczema, contact dermatitis, pruritus
Dosage and routes:
• *Adult and child:* Apply to affected area qd-tid
Available forms include: Cream 0.05%; oint 0.05%
Side effects/adverse reactions:
INTEG: Burning, dryness, itching, irritation, acne, folliculitis, hypertrichosis, perioral dermatitis, hypopigmentation, atrophy, striae, miliaria, allergic contact dermatitis, secondary infection
Contraindications: Hypersensitivity to corticosteroids, fungal infections
Precautions: Pregnancy (C), lactation, viral infections, bacterial infections
NURSING CONSIDERATIONS
Assess:
• Temperature; if fever develops, drug should be discontinued
Administer:
• Only to affected areas; do not get in eyes
• Medication, then cover with occlusive dressing (only if prescribed), seal to normal skin, change q12h; use occlusive dress-

ing with extreme caution, systemic absorption may occur
• Only to dermatoses; do not use on weeping, denuded, or infected area

Perform/provide:
• Cleansing before application of drug
• Treatment for a few days after area has cleared
• Storage at room temperature

Evaluate:
• Therapeutic response: absence of severe itching, patches on skin, flaking
• For systemic absorption: increased temperature, inflammation, irritation

Teach patient/family:
• To avoid sunlight on affected area; burns may occur

---

diflunisal

(dye-floo'ni-sal)
Dolobid
Func. class.: Nonsteroidal anti-inflammatory
Chem. class.: Salicylate derivative

Action: May block pain impulses in CNS that occur in response to inhibition of prostaglandin synthesis; antipyretic action results from inhibition of hypothalamic heat-regulating center to produce vasodilation to allow heat dissipation
Uses: Mild to moderate pain or fever including arthritis, juvenile rheumatoid arthritis, 3-4 times more potent than aspirin
Dosage and routes:
Pain/fever
• *Adult:* PO loading dose 1 g then 500-1000 mg/day in 2 divided doses, q12h, not to exceed 1500 mg/day

Available forms include: Tabs 250, 500 mg
Side effects/adverse reactions:
*HEMA: **Thrombocytopenia, agranulocytosis, leukopenia, neutropenia, hemolytic anemia,*** increased pro-time
CNS: Stimulation, drowsiness, dizziness, confusion, convulsion, headache, flushing, hallucinations, coma
GI: Nausea, vomiting, GI bleeding, diarrhea, heartburn, anorexia, ***hepatitis***
INTEG: Rash, urticaria, bruising
EENT: Blurred vision, decreased acuity, corneal deposits
CV: Rapid pulse, pulmonary edema
RESP: Wheezing, hyperpnea
ENDO: Hypoglycemia, hyponatremia, hypokalemia
Contraindications: Hypersensitivity to salicylates, GI bleeding, bleeding disorders, children <3 yr, vitamin K deficiency
Precautions: Anemia, hepatic disease, renal disease, Hodgkin's disease, pregnancy (C), lactation
Pharmacokinetics:
PO: Onset 15-30 min, peak 2-3 hr, half-life 10-12 hr, metabolized by liver, excreted by kidneys, crosses placenta, 99% protein bound, excreted in breast milk
Interactions/incompatibilities:
• Decreased effects of diflunisal: antacids, steroids, urinary alkalizers
• Increased blood loss: alcohol, heparin
• Increased effects of: anticoagulants, insulin, methotrexate, hydrochlorothiazide, acetaminophen
• Decreased effects of: probenecid, spironolactone, sulfinpyrazone, sulfonylmides
• Toxic effects: PABA

---

italics = common side effects   ***bold italic*** = life threatening reactions

• Decreased blood sugar levels: salicylates

NURSING CONSIDERATIONS
Assess:

• Liver function studies: AST, ALT, bilirubin, creatinine if patient is on long-term therapy

• Renal function studies: BUN, urine creatinine if patient is on long-term therapy

• Blood studies: CBC, Hct, Hgb, pro-time if patient is on long-term therapy

• I&O ratio; decreasing output may indicate renal failure (long-term therapy)

Administer:

• To patient whole

• With food or milk to decrease gastric symptoms

Evaluate:

• Hepatotoxicity: dark urine, clay-colored stools, yellowing of skin, sclera, itching, abdominal pain, fever, diarrhea if patient is on long-term therapy

• Allergic reactions: rash, urticaria; if these occur, drug may need to be discontinued

• Renal dysfunction: decreased urine output

• Ototoxicity: tinnitus, ringing, roaring in ears; audiometric testing is needed before, after long-term therapy

• Visual changes: blurring, halos, corneal, retinal damage

• Edema in feet, ankles, legs

• Prior drug history; there are many drug interactions

Teach patient/family:

• To report any symptoms of hepatotoxicity, renal toxicity, visual changes, ototoxicity, allergic reactions (long-term therapy)

• Not to exceed recommended dosage; acute poisoning may result

• To read label on other OTC drugs; many contain aspirin

• That therapeutic response takes 2 wk (arthritis)

• To avoid alcohol ingestion; GI bleeding may occur

Lab test interferences:

Increase: Coagulation studies, liver function studies, serum uric acid, amylase, CO_2, urinary protein

Decrease: Serum potassium, PBI, cholesterol

Interfere: Urine catecholamines, pregnancy test

Treatment of overdose: Lavage, activated charcoal, monitor electrolytes, VS

---

digitoxin

(di-ji-tox′in)
Crystodigin, Digitaline,* Purodigin*
Func. class.: Antidysrhythmic, cardiac glycoside cardiotonic
Chem. class.: Digitalis preparation

Action: Acts by increased influx of calcium ions from extracellular to intracellular cytoplasm, increasing force of contraction and cardiac output

Uses: Congestive heart failure, atrial fibrillation, atrial flutter, atrial tachycardia, rapid digitalization in these disorders

Dosage and routes:

• *Adult and child >12 yr:* 1.2-1.6 initially; give in divided doses over 24 hr; 150 μg qd

Available forms include: Powder, tabs 50, 100, 150, 200 μg

Side effects/adverse reactions:

CNS: Headache, drowsiness, apathy, confusion, disorientation, fatigue, depression, hallucinations

CV: Dysrhythmias, hypotension, bradycardia, AV block

GI: *Nausea, vomiting, anorexia,* abdominal pain, diarrhea
EENT: *Blurred vision, yellow-green halos,* photophobia, diplopia
MS: Muscular weakness
Contraindications: Hypersensitivity to digitalis, ventricular fibrillation, ventricular tachycardia, carotid sinus syndrome
Precautions: Hepatic disease, acute MI, AV block, hypokalemia, hypomagnesemia, sinus node disease, lactation, severe respiratory disease, hypothyroidism, elderly, pregnancy (C)
Pharmacokinetics:
PO: Onset ½-2 hr, peak 4-12 hr; duration 2-3 wk, half-life 5-7 days metabolized in liver, excreted in urine
Interactions/incompatibilities:
• Hypokalemia: diuretics
• Increased blood levels: spironolactone
• Decreased effects: hydantoins, aminoglutethimide, rifampin, phenylbutazone, barbiturates, cholestyramine, colestipol
• Toxicity: adrenergics, diuretics, succinylcholine, quinidine, thioamines
• Decreased level of digitoxin: thyroid agents
NURSING CONSIDERATIONS
Assess:
• Apical pulse for 1 min before giving drug; if pulse <60, take again in 1 hr; if <60, call physician
• Electrolytes: potassium, sodium, chloride, calcium; renal function studies: BUN, creatinine; blood studies: ALT, AST, bilirubin
• Monitor drug levels (therapeutic level 25-35 ng/ml)
Administer:
• Potassium supplements if ordered for potassium levels <3.0

Evaluate:
• Cardiac status: apical pulse, character, rate, rhythm
• Therapeutic response: decreased weight, edema, pulse, respiration and increased urine output
Teach patient/family:
• Not to stop drug abruptly; teach all aspects of drug
• To avoid OTC medications, since many adverse drug interactions may occur
Lab test interferences:
Increase: CPK
Treatment of overdose: Discontinue drug, administer potassium, monitor EKG

---

digoxin
(di-jox'in)
Lanoxicaps, Lanoxin
Func. class.: Antidysrhythmic, cardiac glycoside
Chem. class.: Digitalis preparation

Action: Acts by inhibiting the sodium-potassium ATPase, which makes more calcium available for contractile proteins, resulting in increased cardiac contractility and cardiac output
Uses: Congestive heart failure, atrial fibrillation, atrial flutter, atrial tachycardia, rapid digitalization in these disorders
Dosage and routes:
• *Adult:* IV 0.5 mg given over >5 mins then PO 0.125-0.5 mg qd in divided doses q4-6h as needed
• *Elderly:* PO 0.125 qd maintenance
• *Child >2 yr:* PO 0.02-0.04 mg/kg divided q8h over 24 hr, maintenance 0.006-0.012 mg/kg qd in divided doses q12hr; IV loading dose 0.015-0.035 mg/kg over >5 min

italics = common side effects   ***bold italic*** = life threatening reactions

• *Child 1 mo-2 yr:* IV 0.03-0.05 mg/kg in divided doses over >5 min q4-8h, change to PO as soon as possible; PO 0.035-0.060 mg/kg divided in 3 doses over 24 hr, maintenance 0.01-0.02 mg/kg in divided doses q12h

• *Neonates:* IV loading dose 0.02-0.03 mg/kg over >5 min in divided doses q4-8h; change to PO as soon as possible; PO loading dose 0.035 mg/kg divided q8h, over 24h, maintenance 0.01 mg/kg in divided doses q12h

• *Premature infants:* IV 0.015-0.025 mg/kg divided in 3 doses over 24 hr, given over >5 min maintenance 0.003-0.009 mg/kg in divided doses q12h

Available forms include: Caps 50, 100, 200 μg; elix 50 μg/ml; tabs 125, 250, 500 μg; inj 100, 250 μg/ml

Side effects/adverse reactions:

CNS: Headache, drowsiness, apathy, confusion, disorientation, fatigue, depression, hallucinations

CV: Dysrhythmias, hypotension, bradycardia, *AV block*

GI: Nausea, vomiting, anorexia, abdominal pain, diarrhea

EENT: Blurred vision, yellow-green halos, photophobia, diplopia

MS: Muscular weakness

Contraindications: Hypersensitivity to digitalis, ventricular fibrillation, ventricular tachycardia, carotid sinus syndrome

Precautions: Renal disease, acute MI, AV block, severe respiratory disease, hypothyroidism, elderly, pregnancy (C), sinus nodal disease, lactation

Pharmacokinetics:

IV: Onset 5-30 min, peak 1-5 hr, duration variable, half-life 1.5 days excreted in urine

Interactions/incompatibilities:

• Hypokalemia: diuretics, amphotericin B, carbenicillin, ticarcillin, corticosteroids

• Decreased digoxin level: thyroid agents

• Increased blood levels: propantheline bromide, spironolactone quinidine, verapamil, aminoglycosides PO, amiodarone, anticholinergics, quinine

• Toxicity: adrenergics, amphotericin, corticosteroids, diuretics, glucose, insulin, reserpine, succinylcholine, quinidine, thioamines

• Incompatible with all medications in syringe or solution

NURSING CONSIDERATIONS

Assess:

• Apical pulse for 1 min before giving drug; if pulse <60, take again in 1 hr; if <60, call physician

• Electrolytes: potassium, sodium chloride, magnesium, calcium; renal function studies: BUN, creatinine; blood studies: ALT, AST, bilirubin

• I&O ratio, daily weights

• Monitor drug levels (therapeutic level 0.5-2 ng/ml)

Administer:

• Potassium supplements if ordered for potassium levels <3.0

• IV undiluted or 1 ml of drug/4 ml sterile H_2O, D_5, or normal saline; give over >5 min through Y-tube or 3-way stopcock

Evaluate:

• Cardiac status: apical pulse, character, rate, rhythm

• Therapeutic response: decreased weight, edema, pulse, respiration and increased urine output

Teach patient/family:

• Not to stop drug abruptly; teach all aspects of drug

• To avoid OTC medications, since many adverse drug interactions

---

*Available in Canada only

may occur; do not take antacid at same time

• To notify physician if loss of appetite, lower stomach pain, diarrhea, weakness, drowsiness, headache, blurred or yellow vision, rash, depression; toxicity is occurring

Lab test interferences:
Increase: CPK

Treatment of overdose: Discontinue drug, administer potassium, monitor EKG, administer an adrenergic blocking agent

---

digoxin immune FAB (ovine)
Digibind

Func. class.: Antidote—digoxin specific

Action: Fragments bind to free digoxin to reverse digoxin toxicity by not allowing digoxin to bind to sites of action

Uses: Life-threatening digoxin or digitoxin toxicity

Dosage and routes:
Digoxin
• *Adult:* IV dose (mg) = Dose ingested (mg) × 0.8; if ingested amount is unknown, give 800 mg IV

Available forms include: Inj 40 mg/vial (binds 0.6 mg digoxin or digitoxin)

Side effects/adverse reactions:
CV: CHF, ventricular rate increase, *atrial fibrillation,* low cardiac output
RESP: Impaired respiratory function, rapid respiratory rate
META: Hypokalemia
INTEG: Hypersensitivity, allergic reactions

Contraindications: Mild digoxin toxicity

Precautions: Children, lactation, cardiac disease, renal disease, pregnancy (C)

Pharmacokinetics:
IV: Peaks after completion of infusion, onset 30 min (variable); not known if crosses placenta, breast milk; half-life biphasis—14-20 hr; prolonged in renal disease; excreted by kidneys

NURSING CONSIDERATIONS
Assess:
• Potassium levels, may decrease rapidly

Administer:
• After diluting 40 mg/4 ml of sterile H₂O for inj; mix; may be further diluted with normal saline
• By bolus if cardiac arrest is eminent, or IV over 30 min using a 0.22 μm filter

Perform/provide:
• Storage of reconstituted solution for up to 4 hr, in refrigerator

Evaluate:
• Therapeutic response: correction of digoxin toxicity, check digoxin levels

Lab test interferences:
Interfere: Immunoassay digoxin

---

dihydroergotamine mesylate
(dye-hye-droe-er-got'a-meen)
D.H.E. 45

Func. class.: α-Adrenergic blocker
Chem. class.: Ergot alkaloid (dihydrogenated)

Action: Constricts smooth muscle in periphery, cranial blood vessels; inhibits norepinephrine uptake

Uses: Vascular headache (migraine or histamine)

Dosage and routes:
• *Adult:* IM/IV 1 mg, may repeat

q1-2 hr if needed, not to exceed 3 mg/day or 6 mg/wk

Available forms include: Inj 1 mg/ml

Side effects/adverse reactions:

CNS: Numbness in fingers, toes, weakness

CV: Transient tachycardia, chest pain, bradycardia, increase or decrease in B/P, *gangrene*

GI: Nausea, vomiting

MS: Muscle pain

Contraindications: Hypersensitivity to ergot preparations, occlusion (peripheral, vascular), CAD, hepatic disease, pregnancy (X), renal disease, peptic ulcer, hypertension, lactation, children, uremia

Pharmacokinetics:

IM: Onset 15-30 min, peak 2 hr, duration 3-4 hr

IV: Onset 5 min, peak 45 min, duration 3-4 hr

Half-life 1.3-4 hr

Interactions/incompatibilities:

• Increased effects: troleandomycin

• Increased vasoconstriction: beta blockers

NURSING CONSIDERATIONS
Assess:

• Weight daily, check for peripheral edema in feet, legs

Administer:

• IV undiluted; give 1 mg or less/min

• IM dose, which takes 20 min for effect, or use IV for immediate effect

• At beginning of headache, dose must be titrated to patient response

• Only to women who are not pregnant, harm to fetus may occur

Perform/provide:

• Storage in dark area, do not use discolored solutions

• Quiet, calm environment with decreased stimulation for noise, or bright light or excessive talking

Evaluate:

• Therapeutic response: decrease in frequency, severity of headache

• For stress level, activity, recreation, coping mechanisms of patient

• Neurological status: LOC, blurring vision, nausea, vomiting, tingling in extremities that occur preceding the headache

• Ingestion of tyramine foods (pickled products, beer, wine, aged cheese), food additives, preservatives, colorings, artificial sweeteners, chocolate, caffeine, which may precipitate these types of headaches

Teach patient/family:

• Not to use OTC medications; serious drug interactions may occur

• To report side effects: increased vasoconstriction starting with cold extremities, then paresthesia, weakness

• That an increase in headaches may occur when this drug is discontinued after long-term use

• Keep drug out of reach of children; death may occur

---

dihydrotachysterol

(dye-hye-droe-tak-iss'ter-ole)

DHT Intensol, DHT Oral Solution, Hytakerol

Func. class.: Parathyroid agent (calcium regulator)

Chem. class.: Vitamin D analog

Action: Increases intestinal absorption of calcium for bones, increases renal tubular absorption of phosphate

Uses: Renal osteodystrophy, hypoparathyroidism, pseudo hypo-

---

parathyroidism, familial hypophosphatemia, postoperative tetany

Dosage and routes:

Hypophosphatemia

• *Adult and child:* PO 0.5-2 mg qd, maintenance 0.3-1.5 mg qd

Hypoparathyroidism/pseudohypoparathyroidism

• *Adult:* PO 0.8-2.4 mg qd × 1 wk, maintenance 0.2-2 mg qd regulated by serum Ca levels

• *Child:* PO 1-5 mg qd × 1 wk, maintenance 0.2-1 mg qd regulated by serum Ca levels

Renal osteodystrophy

• *Adult:* PO 0.1-0.6 mg qd

Available forms include: Tabs 0.125, 0.2, 0.4 mg; caps 0.125 mg; oral sol 0.2, 0.25 mg/5 ml

Side effects/adverse reactions:

EENT: Tinnitus

CNS: Drowsiness, headache, vertigo, fever, lethargy

GI: Nausea, diarrhea, vomiting, jaundice, anorexia, dry mouth, constipation, cramps, metallic taste

MS: Myalgia, arthralgia, decreased bone development

GU: Polyuria, hypercalciuria, hyperphosphatemia, *hematuria*

Contraindications: Hypersensitivity, renal disease, hyperphosphatemia, hypercalcemia

Precautions: Pregnancy (C), renal calculi, lactation, CV disease

Pharmacokinetics:

PO: Onset 2 wk; metabolized by liver, excreted in feces (active/inactive)

Interactions/incompatibilities:

• Decreased absorption of dihydrotachysterol: cholestyramine, colestipol, HCl, mineral oil

• Hypercalcemia: thiazide diuretics, calcium supplements

• Cardiac dysrhythmias: cardiac glycosides, verapamil

• Decreased effect of dihydrota-chysterol: corticosteroids, phenytoin, barbiturates

NURSING CONSIDERATIONS

Assess:

• BUN, urinary calcium, AST, ALT, cholesterol, creatinine, uric acid, chloride, magnesium, electrolytes, urine pH, phosphate; may increase calcium, should be kept at 9-10 mg/dl, vitamin D 50-135 IU/dl, phosphate 70 mg/dl

• Alk phosphatase; may be decreased

• For increased blood level since toxic reactions may occur rapidly

Administer:

• PO, may be increased q4wk depending on blood level

Perform/provide:

• Storage in tight, light-resistant containers at room temperature

• Restriction of sodium, potassium if required

• Restriction of fluids if required for chronic renal failure

Evaluate:

• For dry mouth, metallic taste, polyuria, bone pain, muscle weakness, headache, fatigue, tinnitus, change in LOC, irregular pulse, dysrhythmias, increased respirations, anorexia, nausea, vomiting, cramps, diarrhea, constipation; may indicate hypercalcemia

• Renal status: decreased urinary output (oliguria, anuria), edema in extremities, weight gain 5 lb, periorbital edema

• Nutritional status, diet for sources of vitamin D (milk, some seafood), calcium (dairy products, dark green vegetables), phosphates (dairy products) must be avoided

Teach patient/family:

• The symptoms of hypercalcemia

• Foods rich in calcium

Lab test interferences:

False increase: Cholesterol

---

italics = common side effects   ***bold italic*** = life threatening reactions

dihydroxyaluminum sodium carbonate
(dye-hye-drox'-ee-a-loom-aa-nim)
Rolaids
Func. class.: Antacid
Chem. class.: Aluminum product

Action: Neutralizes gastric acidity, reduces pepsin
Uses: Antacid
Dosage and routes:
• *Adult:* PO 1-2 as needed; may give up to 2-4 tabs
Available forms include: Chewable tab 334 mg
Side effects/adverse reactions:
GI: Constipation, obstruction
Contraindications: Hypersensitivity to aluminum products
Precautions: Elderly, sodium/fluid restriction, decreased GI motility, GI obstruction, dehydration, severe renal disease, CHF, pregnancy (C)
Pharmacokinetics:
PO: Onset 20-40 min, excreted in feces
Interactions/incompatibilities:
• Decreased effectiveness of: tetracyclines, ketoconazole, isoniazid, phenothiazines, iron salts, digitalis
NURSING CONSIDERATIONS
Administer:
• Laxatives or stool softeners if constipation occurs
Evaluate:
• Therapeutic response: absence of pain, decreased acidity
• Constipation; increase bulk in the diet if needed
Teach patient/family:
• Increase fluids to 2000 ml/day unless contraindicated
• To avoid long-term usage

diltiazem HCl
(dil-tye'a-zem)
Cardizem, Cardizem SR
Func. class.: Calcium channel blocker
Chem. class.: Benzothiazepine

Action: Inhibits calcium ion influx across cell membrane during cardiac depolarization; produces relaxation of coronary vascular smooth muscle, dilates coronary arteries, decreases SA/AV node conduction times, dilates peripheral arteries
Uses: Chronic stable angina pectoris, vasospastic angina, coronary artery spasm, hypertension
Dosage and routes:
• *Adult:* PO 30 mg qid, increasing dose gradually to 180-360 mg/day in divided doses or 60-120 mg bid; may increase to 240-360 mg/day
Available forms include: Tabs 30, 60, 90, 120 mg, sus rel 60, 90, 120, 150 mg
Side effects/adverse reactions:
CV: Dysrhythmia, edema, CHF, bradycardia, hypotension, palpitations, heart block, peripheral edema, angina
GI: Nausea, vomiting, diarrhea, gastric upset, constipation, increased liver function studies
GU: Nocturia, polyuria, acute renal failure
INTEG: Rash, pruritus, flushing, photosensitivity
CNS: Headache, fatigue, drowsiness, dizziness, depression, weakness, insomnia, tremor, paresthesia
Contraindications: Sick sinus syndrome, 2nd or 3rd degree heart block, hypotension less than 90 mm Hg systolic, acute MI, pulmonary congestion

---

Precautions: CHF, hypotension, hepatic injury, pregnancy (C), lactation, children, renal disease

Pharmacokinetics: Onset 30-60 min, peak 2-3 hr, immediate rel, 6-11 sus rel, half-life 3½-9 hr; metabolized by liver, excreted in urine (96% as metabolites)

Interactions/incompatibilities:
• Increased effects of: β-blockers, digitalis, lithium, carbamazepine, cyclosporine
• Increased effects of diltiazem: cimetidine

NURSING CONSIDERATIONS
Assess:
• Blood levels (therapeutic levels: 0.025-0.1 μg/ml)
Administer:
• Before meals, hs
Perform/provide:
• Storage in tight container at room temperature
Evaluate:
• Therapeutic response: decreased anginal pain, decreased B/P
• Cardiac status: B/P, pulse, respiration, ECG and intervals PR, QRS, QT
Teach patient/family:
• To carry nitrites at all times
• How to take pulse before taking drug; record or graph should be kept
• To avoid hazardous activities until stabilized on drug; dizziness is no longer a problem
• To limit caffeine consumption
• To avoid OTC drugs unless directed by a physician
• Stress patient compliance to all areas of medical regimen: diet, exercise, stress reduction, drug therapy
Treatment of overdose: Defibrillation, atropine for AV block, vasopressor for hypotension

dimenhydrinate

(dye-men-hye′dri-nate)

Calm-X, Dimen, Dimentabs, Dipendrate, Dramamine, Dramamine Junior, Dymenate, Gravol,* Hydrate, Nauseal,* Nauseatol,* Novodimenate,* Marmine, Reidamine, Travamine,* Vertiban

Func. class.: Antiemetic, antihistamine, anticholinergic

Chem. class.: H₁-receptor antagonist, ethanolamine derivative

Action: Acts centrally by blocking chemoreceptor trigger zone, which in turn acts on vomiting center

Uses: Motion sickness, nausea, vomiting

Dosage and routes:
• *Adult:* PO 50-100 mg q4h; REC 100 mg qd or bid; IM/IV 50 mg as needed
• *Child:* IM/PO 5 mg/kg divided in 4 equal doses

Available forms include: Tabs 50 mg; inj 500 mg/ml; liq 12.5/4 ml; supp 50, 100 mg

Side effects/adverse reactions:

CNS: Drowsiness, restlessness, headache, dizziness, insomnia, confusion, nervousness, tingling, vertigo, hallucinations and *convulsions* in young children

GI: Nausea, anorexia, diarrhea, vomiting, constipation

CV: Hypertension, hypotension, palpitation

INTEG: Rash, urticaria, fever, chills, flushing

EENT: Dry mouth, blurred vision, diplopia, nasal congestion, photosensitivity

Contraindications: Hypersensitivity to narcotics, shock

Precautions: Children, cardiac dysrhythmias, elderly, asthma,

---

pregnancy (B), prostatic hypertrophy, bladder-neck obstruction, narrow-angle glaucoma, stenosing peptic ulcer, pyloroduodenal obstruction

Pharmacokinetics:

IM/PO: Duration 4-6 hr

Interactions/incompatibilities:

• Increased effect: alcohol, other CNS depressants

• May mask ototoxic symptoms associated with aminoglycosides

NURSING CONSIDERATIONS
Assess:

• VS, B/P; check patients with cardiac disease more often

Administer:

• IV after diluting 50 mg/10 ml of NaCl inj; give 50 mg or less over 2 min

• IM injection in large muscle mass; aspirate to avoid IV administration

• Tablets may be swallowed whole, chewed, or allowed to dissolve

Evaluate:

• Signs of toxicity of other drugs or masking of symptoms of disease: brain tumor, intestinal obstruction

• Observe for drowsiness, dizziness

Teach patient/family:

• That a false negative result may occur with skin testing; these procedures should not be scheduled for 4 days after discontinuing use

• Avoid hazardous activities, activities requiring alertness; dizziness may occur; instruct patient to request assistance with ambulation

• Avoid alcohol, other depressants

Lab test interferences:

False negative: Allergy skin testing

dimercaprol

(dye-mer-kap′role)
BAL in Oil, British Anti-Lewisite*

Func. class.: Heavy metal antagonist

Chem. class.: Chelating agent (dithiol compound)

Action: Binds ions from arsenic, gold, mercury, lead, copper to form water-soluble complex removed by kidneys

Uses: Arsenic, gold, mercury, lead poisoning

Dosage and routes:

Severe gold/arsenic poisoning

• *Adult:* IM 3 mg/kg q4h × 2 days, then qid × 1 day, then bid × 10 days

Mild gold/arsenic poisoning

• *Adult:* IM 2.5 mg/kg qid × 2 days, then bid × 1 day, then qd × 10 days

Acute lead poisoning

• *Adult:* IM 4 mg/kg, then q4h with edetate calcium disodium 12.5 mg/kg IM, not to exceed 5 mg/kg/dose

Mercury poisoning

• *Adult:* IM 5 mg/kg, then 2.5 mg/kg/day or bid × 10 days

Available forms include: Inj IM 100 mg/ml

Side effects/adverse reactions:

CNS: Headache, paresthesia, anxiety, tremors, **convulsions, shock**

INTEG: Urticaria, erythema, pruritus, pain at injection site, fever

CV: Hypertension, tachycardia

GI: Nausea, vomiting, salivation

EENT: Rhinorrhea, throat pain or constriction, lacrimation

GU: Burning sensation in penis, **nephrotoxicity**

*SYST: **Anaphylaxis,*** metabolic acidosis

---

*Available in Canada only

Contraindications: Hypersensitivity, anuria, hepatic insufficiency, poisoning of other metals, severe renal disease, child <3 yr
Precautions: Hypertension, pregnancy (D), lactation
Pharmacokinetics:
Metabolized by plasma enzymes, excreted by kidneys as complex, unchanged drug
Interactions/incompatibilities:
• Increased toxicity: iron, selenium, uranium, cadmium
NURSING CONSIDERATIONS
Assess:
• B/P, increasing B/P or tachycardia, respirations, pulse
• Monitor I&O, kidney function studies: BUN, creatinine, CrCl; report decreases in output
• Urine: pH, albumin, casts, blood
• Metal levels daily, temperature
Administer:
• IM in deep muscle mass; rotate injection sites if giving EDTA also, give in separate site; observe for sterile abscesses
• Only when epinephrine 1:1000 is on unit for anaphylaxis
• Being careful not to allow drug to touch skin; contact dermatitis can occur
• Acetazolamide or sodium citrate to decrease pH of urine, which decreases renal damage
Evaluate:
• Therapeutic response: decreasing level of metal exposed to in the blood
• Allergic reactions (rash, urticaria); if these occur, drug should be discontinued
Teach patient/family:
• That breath may be odorous
Lab test interferences:
Decrease: RAIU test

dinoprostone

(dye-noe-prost′one)
PGE₂, Prepidil Gel*, Prostin E₂
Func. class.: Oxytocic
Chem. class.: Prostaglandin E₂

D

Action: Stimulates uterine contractions causing abortion; acts within 30 hr for complete abortion
Uses: Abortion during 2nd trimester, benign hydatidiform mole, expulsion of uterine contents in fetal deaths to 28 wk, missed abortion
Dosage and routes:
• *Adult:* VAG SUPP 20 mg, repeat q3-5h until abortion occurs
Available forms include: Vag supp 20 mg
Side effects/adverse reactions:
CNS: Headache, dizziness, chills, fever
CV: Hypotension
GI: Nausea, vomiting, diarrhea
GU: Vaginitis, vaginal pain, vulvitis, vaginismus
INTEG: Rash, skin color changes
MS: Leg cramps, joint swelling, weakness
EENT: Blurred vision
Contraindications: Hypersensitivity, uterine fibrosis, cervical stenosis, pelvic surgery, pelvic inflammatory disease (PID), respiratory disease
Precautions: Hepatic disease, renal disease, cardiac disease, asthma, anemia, jaundice, diabetes mellitus, convulsive disorders, hypertension, hypotension
Pharmacokinetics:
SUPP: Onset 10 min, duration 2-3 hr; metabolized in spleen, kidney, lungs, excreted in urine
NURSING CONSIDERATIONS
Assess:
• Respiratory rate, rhythm, depth;

notify physician of abnormalities, pulse, B/P, temperature
• Vaginal discharge: check for itching, irritation; indicates vaginal infection

Administer:
• Antiemetic/antidiarrheal before administration of this drug
• High in vagina
• After warming suppository by running warm water over package

Evaluate:
• For length, duration of contraction; notify physician of contractions lasting over 1 min or absence of contractions
• For fever, chills: increase fluids, or give tepid sponge bath or blanket

Teach patient/family:
• To remain supine for 10-15 min after insertion
• To report excessive cramping, bleeding, chills, fever
• Methods of pain, comfort control

---

diphenhydramine HCl

(dye-fen-hye′dra-meen)
Allerdryl, Baramine, Bax, Benachlor, Benadryl, Benahist, Bendylate, Benylin, Bentract, Compoz, Diphenacen, Fenylhist, Nordryl, Rohydra, Span-Lanin, Valdrene, Wehdryl
Func. class.: Antihistamine
Chem. class.: Ethanolamine derivative, H_1-receptor antagonist

Action: Acts on blood vessels, GI, respiratory system by competing with histamine for H_1-receptor site; decreases allergic response by blocking histamine

Uses: Allergy symptoms, rhinitis, motion sickness, antiparkinsonism, nighttime sedation, infant colic, nonproductive cough

Dosage and routes:
• *Adult:* PO 25-50 mg q4-6h, not to exceed 400 mg/day; IM/IV 10-50 mg, not to exceed 400 mg/day
• *Child >12 kg:* PO/IM/IV 5 mg/kg/day in 4 divided doses, not to exceed 300 mg/day

Available forms include: Caps 25, 50 mg; tabs 50 mg; elix 12.5 mg/5 ml; syr 12.5 mg/5ml; inj IM, IV 10, 50 mg/ml

Side effects/adverse reactions:
CNS: Dizziness, drowsiness, poor coordination, fatigue, anxiety, euphoria, confusion, paresthesia, neuritis
RESP: Increased thick secretions, wheezing, chest tightness
HEMA: Thrombocytopenia, agranulocytosis, hemolytic anemia
GI: Dry mouth, nausea, anorexia, diarrhea
INTEG: Photosensitivity
GU: Retention, dysuria, frequency
EENT: Blurred vision, dilated pupils, tinnitus, nasal stuffiness, dry nose, throat, mouth

Contraindications: Hypersensitivity to H_1-receptor antagonist, acute asthma attack, lower respiratory tract disease

Precautions: Increased intraocular pressure, renal disease, cardiac disease, hypertension, bronchial asthma, seizure disorder, stenosed peptic ulcers, hyperthyroidism, prostatic hypertrophy, bladder neck obstruction, pregnancy (C)

Pharmacokinetics:
PO: Peak 1-3 hr, duration 4-7 hr; *IM:* onset ½ hr, peak 1-4 hr, duration 4-7 hr; *IV:* onset immediate, duration 4-7 hr, metabolized in liver, excreted by kidneys, crosses placenta, excreted in breast milk, half-life 2-7 hr

Interactions/incompatibilities:
• Increased CNS depression: bar-

biturates, narcotics, hypnotics, tricyclic antidepressants, alcohol
• Decreased effect of: oral anticoagulants, heparin
• Increased effect of diphenhydramine: MAOIs

NURSING CONSIDERATIONS
Assess:
• I&O ratio; be alert for urinary retention, frequency, dysuria; drug should be discontinued if these occur
• CBC during long-term therapy
Administer:
• With meals if GI symptoms occur, absorption may slightly decrease
• IV undiluted; give 25 mg/1 min
• Deep IM in large muscle; rotate site
• hs only if using for sleep aid
Perform/provide:
• Hard candy, gum, frequent rinsing of mouth for dryness
• Storage in tight container at room temperature
Evaluate:
• Therapeutic response: absence of running or congested nose or rashes, improved sleep
• Respiratory status: rate, rhythm, increase in bronchial secretions, wheezing, chest tightness
Teach patient/family:
• All aspects of drug use; to notify physician if confusion, sedation, hypotension occurs
• To avoid driving or other hazardous activity if drowsiness occurs
• To avoid concurrent use of alcohol or other CNS depressants
Lab test interferences:
False negative: Skin allergy tests
Treatment of overdose: Administer ipecac syrup or lavage, diazepam, vasopressors, barbiturates (short-acting)

diphenidol
(dye-fen′-i-dole)
Vontrol
Func. class.: Antiemetic
Chem. class.: Trihexyphenidyl derivative

Action: May act as dopamine antagonist at chemoreceptor trigger zone to inhibit vomiting
Uses: Nausea, vomiting, peripheral dizziness
Dosage and routes:
• *Adult:* PO 25-50 mg q4h
• *Children >23 kg:* PO 25 mg q4h prn; do not exceed 5.5 mg/kg/24 hr
Available forms include: Tabs 25 mg
Side effects/adverse reactions:
CNS: Drowsiness, fatigue, restlessness, tremor, headache, stimulation, dizziness, insomnia, twitching, disorientation, confusion, sleep disturbance, auditory, visual hallucination, depression
GI: Nausea, indigestion
CV: Hypotension
INTEG: Rash
EENT: Dry mouth, blurred vision
Contraindications: Hypersensitivity, psychosis, anuria
Precautions: Children, prostatic hypertrophy, glaucoma, pyloric and duodenal stenosis, elderly
Pharmacokinetics:
PO: Onset 30-45 min, duration 3-6 hr, metabolized by liver, excreted by kidneys
NURSING CONSIDERATIONS
Assess:
• VS, B/P; check patients with cardiac disease more often
• Observe for CNS adverse effects: confusion, hallucination
• Monitor I&O (90% excreted in urine)

---

italics = common side effects   ***bold italic*** = life threatening reactions

Administer:
• Tabs may be swallowed whole, chewed, or allowed to dissolve
Evaluate:
• Signs of toxicity of other drugs or masking of symptoms of disease: brain tumor, intestinal obstruction
• Drowsiness, dizziness
Teach patient/family:
• To avoid alcohol, other depressants
• That drug should be used only under close supervision

---

diphenoxylate HCl with atropine sulfate

(dye-fen-ox′i-late)
Diphenatol, Lofene, Lomotil, Lo-Trol

Func. class.: Antidiarrheal
Chem. class.: Phenylipeperidine derivative, opiate agonist

Controlled Substance Schedule V
Action: Inhibits gastric motility by acting on mucosal receptors responsible for peristalsis
Uses: Diarrhea (cause undetermined)
Dosage and routes:
• *Adult:* PO 2.5-5 mg qid, titrated to patient response
• *Child 2-12 yr:* PO 0.3-0.4 mg/kg/day in divided doses
Available forms include: Tabs 2.5 mg
Side effects/adverse reactions:
CNS: Drowsiness, headache, sedation, depression, weakness, lethargy, flushing, hyperthermia
GI: Nausea, vomiting, abdominal pain, glossitis, colitis, *paralytic ileus, toxic megacolon,* dry mucous membranes
EENT: Blurred vision, nystagmus, mydriasis

INTEG: Rash, urticaria, pruritus, *angioneurotic edema*
CV: Tachycardia
GU: Urine retention
Contraindications: Hypersensitivity, severe liver disease, pseudomembranous enterocolitis, glaucoma, child <2 yr, electrolyte imbalances
Precautions: Hepatic disease, renal disease, ulcerative colitis, pregnancy (C), lactation, elderly
Pharmacokinetics:
PO: Onset 45-60 min, peak 2 hr, duration 3-4 hr, half-life 2½ hr; metabolized in liver to active, inactive metabolites; excreted in urine, feces, breast milk
Interactions/incompatibilities:
• Do not use with MAOIs; hypertensive crisis may occur
• Increased action of: alcohol, narcotics, barbiturates, other CNS depressants, anticholinergics
NURSING CONSIDERATIONS
Assess:
• Electrolytes (K, Na, Cl) if on long-term therapy
Administer:
• For 48 hr only
Evaluate:
• Therapeutic response: decreased diarrhea
• Bowel pattern before; for rebound constipation after termination of medication
• Response after 48 hr; if no response, drug should be discontinued
• Dehydration in children
• Abdominal distention, toxic megacolon, which may occur in ulcerative colitis
Teach patient/family:
• To avoid OTC products unless directed by physician; may contain alcohol

---

- Not to exceed recommended dose
- May be habit forming

---

diphtheria and tetanus toxoids and pertussis vaccine (DPT)

Tri-Immunol

Func. class.: Vaccine/toxoid

Action: Provide immunity to diphtheria, tetanus, pertussis by stimulating antibody/antitoxin production

Uses: Prevention of diphtheria, tetanus, pertussis

Dosage and routes:
- *Child >6 wk-6 yr:* IM 0.5 ml at 2, 4, 6 mos, 1½ yr; booster needed 0.5 ml at age 6

Available forms include: Inj IM diphtheria 12.5 LfU, tetanus 5 LfU, pertussis 4 U/0.5 ml

Side effects/adverse reactions:
GI: Nausea, vomiting, anorexia
INTEG: Skin abscess, urticaria, itching, swelling, erythema, edema at site
CV: Tachycardia, hypotension
SYST: Lymphadenitis, ***anaphylaxis,*** fever, chills, malaise
CNS: Crying, fretfulness, fever, drowsiness, ***seizures***
MS: Osteomyelitis

Contraindications: Hypersensitivity, active infection, poliomyelitis outbreak, immunosuppression, febrile illness

Precautions: Pregnancy

Interactions/incompatibilities:
- Decreased response to toxoid: immunosuppressive agents: antineoplastics, corticosteroids, radiation therapy; alkylating agents

NURSING CONSIDERATIONS
Assess:
- For skin reactions: swelling, rash, urticaria

Administer:
- At least 4 wk apart × 3 doses
- Only with epinephrine 1:1000 on unit to treat laryngospasm
- IM only; not to be given SC (vastus lateralis in infants, deltoid in adults)

Perform/provide:
- Storage in refrigerator, do not freeze

Evaluate:
- For history of allergies, skin conditions (eczema, psoriasis, dermatitis), reactions to vaccinations
- For anaphylaxis: inability to breathe, bronchospasm

Teach patient/family:
- That doses are given at least 4 wk apart × 3 doses, booster needed at 10 yr intervals, diphtheria/tetanus

---

dipivefrin HCl

(dye-pi've-frin)

Propine

Func. class.: Adrenergic agonist
Chem. class.: Diesterified epinephrine

Action: Converted to epinephrine, which decreases aqueous production and increases outflow

Uses: Open-angle glaucoma

Dosage and routes:
- *Adult:* INSTILL 1 gtt q12h

Available forms include: Sol 0.1%

Side effects/adverse reactions:
CV: Hypertension, tachycardia, dysrhythmias
EENT: Burning, stinging, mydriasis, photophobia

Contraindications: Hypersensitivity, narrow-angle glaucoma

Precautions: Pregnancy (B), lactation, children, aphakia

Pharmacokinetics:
INSTILL: Onset 30 min, duration 1 hr

NURSING CONSIDERATIONS
Perform/provide:
• Storage at room temperature
Teach patient/family:
• To report stinging, burning, itching, lacrimation, puffiness
• Method of instillation, including pressure on lacrimal sac for 1 min and not to touch dropper to eye

---

dipyridamole

(dye-peer-id'a-mole)
Persantine, Pyridamole
Func. class.: Coronary vasodilator, antiplatelet
Chem. class.: Nonnitrate

Action: Increases oxygen saturation in coronary tissues, coronary blood flow; acts on small resistance vessels with little effect on vascular resistance; may increase development of collateral circulation
Uses: Prevention of transient ischemic attacks, inhibition of platelet adhesion to prevent myocardial reinfarction, thromboembolism, with warfarin in prosthetic heart valves, prevention of coronary bypass graft occlusion with aspirin; possibly effective for long-term therapy of chronic angina pectoris
Dosage and routes:
TIA
• *Adult:* PO 50 mg tid, 1 hr ac, not to exceed 400 mg qd
Inhibition of platelet adhesion
• *Adult:* PO 50-75 mg qid in combination with aspirin or warfarin
Available forms include: Tabs 25, 50, 75 mg
Side effects/adverse reactions:
CV: Postural hypotension
CNS: Headache, dizziness, weakness, fainting, syncope
GI: Nausea, vomiting, anorexia, diarrhea

INTEG: Rash, flushing
Contraindications: Hypersensitivity, hypotension
Precautions: Pregnancy (C)
Pharmacokinetics:
PO: Peak 2-2½ hr, duration 6 hr
Therapeutic response may take several months, metabolized in liver, excreted in bile, undergoes enterohepatic recirculation
Interactions/incompatibilities:
• Additive antiplatelet effects: ASA, NSAID
• Increased bleeding: Coumadin
NURSING CONSIDERATIONS
Assess:
• B/P, pulse during treatment until stable; take B/P lying, standing; orthostatic hypotension is common
Administer:
• On an empty stomach: 1 hr before meals or 2 hr after
Perform/provide:
• Storage at room temperature
Evaluate:
• Therapeutic response: decreased chest pain (angina), decreased platelet adhesion
• Cardiac status: chest pain, what aggravates or ameliorates condition
Teach patient/family:
• That medication is not cure, may need to be taken continuously
• That it is necessary to quit smoking to prevent excessive vasoconstriction
• To avoid hazardous activities until stabilized on medication; dizziness may occur
Treatment of overdose: Administer IV phenylephrine

---

disopyramide

(dye-soe-peer'a-mide)
Rythmodan, Norpace, DSP, Napamide, Norpace CR, Norpaceor
Func. class.: Antidysrhythmic (Class IA)
Chem. class.: Nonnitrate

Action: Increases action potential duration and effective refractory period; reduces disparity in refractory between normal and infarcted myocardium

Uses: PVCs, ventricular tachycardia

Dosage and routes:
• *Adult:* PO 100-200 mg q6h, in renal dysfunction 100 mg q6h; SUS REL CAPS 200 mg q12h
• *Child 12-18 yr:* PO 6-15 mg/kg/day, in divided doses q6h
• *Child 4-12 yr:* PO 10-15 mg/kg/day, in divided doses q6h
• *Child 1-4 yr:* PO 10-20 mg/kg/day, in divided doses q6h
• *Child <1 yr:* PO 10-30 mg/kg/day, in divided doses q6h
Available forms include: Caps 100, 150 mg (as phosphate), caps, sus rel 100, 150 mg

Side effects/adverse reactions:
GU: Retention, hesitancy, impotence, urinary frequency, urgency
CNS: Headache, dizziness, psychosis, fatigue, depression, paresthesias, anxiety, insomnia
GI: Dry mouth, constipation, nausea, anorexia, flatulence, diarrhea, vomiting
CV: Hypotension, bradycardia, angina, PVCs, tachycardia, increases QRS, QT segments, ***cardiac arrest,*** edema, weight gain, AV block, ***CHF,*** syncope, chest pain
META: Hypoglycemia
INTEG: Rash, pruritus, urticaria

MS: Weakness, pain in extremities
EENT: Blurred vision, dry nose, throat, eyes, narrow-angle glaucoma
*HEMA: **Thrombocytopenia, agranulocytosis,*** anemia (rare), decreased hemoglobin, hematocrit
Contraindications: Hypersensitivity, 2nd/3rd degree block, cardiogenic shock, CHF (uncompensated), sick sinus syndrome, QT prolongation
Precautions: Pregnancy (C), lactation, diabetes mellitus, renal disease, children, hepatic disease, myasthenia gravis, narrow-angle glaucoma, cardiomyopathy, conduction abnormalities

Pharmacokinetics:
PO: Peak 30 min-3 hr, duration 6-12 hr
Half-life 4-10 hr, metabolized in liver, excreted in feces, urine, breast milk, crosses placenta
Interactions/incompatibilities:
• Increased effects of disopyramide: quinidine, procainamide, propranolol, lidocaine, atenolol, other antidysrhythmics
• Do not administer within 48 hr of verapamil
• Increased side effects of disopyramide: anticholinergics
• Decreased effects of disopyramide: phenytoin, rifampin

NURSING CONSIDERATIONS
Assess:
• Apical pulse for 1 min, if less than 60 check again in 1 hr; if still less than 60, notify physician
• ECG, check for increased QT, widening QRS; drug should be discontinued
• Blood level during treatment (therapeutic level 2-8 µg/ml)
• Weight daily, a rapid weight gain should be reported
• For dehydration or hypovolemia,

---

italics = common side effects   ***bold italic*** = life threatening reactions

I&O ratio, electrolytes (Na, K, Cl)
• Liver, kidney function studies (AST, ALT, bilirubin, BUN, creatinine) during treatment
• Diabetics for signs of hypoglycemia
• B/P continuously for hypotension, hypertension

Administer:
• Sugar-free gum, frequent sips of water for dry mouth
• Reduced dosage slowly with ECG monitoring

Evaluate:
• Increase in QRS, QT; drug should be discontinued
• For rebound hypertension after 1-2 hr
• Constipation, increase bulk in diet, water, stool softeners or laxatives needed
• Cardiac rate, respiration: rate, rhythm, character
• Urinary hesitancy, frequency or a change in I&O ratio; check for edema daily; check for toxicity

Teach patient/family:
• To take drug exactly as prescribed
• To avoid alcohol or severe hypotension may occur; to avoid OTC drugs or serious drug interactions may occur
• To make position change slowly during early therapy to prevent fainting
• To avoid hazardous activities if dizziness or blurred vision occurs
• Stress patient compliance with drug regimen; tell patient that this drug does not cure condition

Treatment of overdose: O₂, artificial ventilation, ECG, administer dopamine for circulatory depression, administer diazepam or thiopental for convulsions

Lab test interferences:

Increase: Liver enzymes, lipids, BUN, creatinine
Decrease: Hgb/Hct, blood glucose

---

disulfiram

(dye-sul'fi-ram)
Antabuse, Cronetal, Ro-Sulfiram
Func. class.: Alcohol deterrent
Chem. class.: Aldehyde dehydrogenase inhibitor

Action: Blocks oxidation of alcohol at acetaldehyde stage; accumulation of acetaldehyde produces the disulfiram-alcohol reaction
Uses: Chronic alcoholism (as adjunct)
Dosage and routes:
• *Adult:* PO 250-500 mg qd × 1-2 wk, then 125-500 mg qd until fully socially recovered
Available forms include: Tabs 250, 500 mg
Side effects/adverse reactions:
CNS: Headache, drowsiness, restlessness, dizziness, fatigue, tremors, psychosis, neuritis, sweating, *convulsions, death,* peripheral neuropathy
GI: Nausea, vomiting, anorexia, severe thirst, *hepatotoxicity,* metallic, garliclike after taste
INTEG: Rash, dermatitis, urticaria
RESP: Respiratory depression, hyperventilation
CV: Tachycardia, chest pain, hypotension, *dysrhythmias*
Disulfiram: Alcohol reaction: flushing, throbbing, headache, respiratory difficulty, nausea, vomiting, sweating, thirst, chest pain, palpitations, dyspnea, hyperventilation, tachycardia, confusion, CV collapse, MI, CHF, convulsions, death
Contraindications: Hypersensitivity, alcohol intoxication, psycho-

ses, CV disease, pregnancy (X)
Precautions: Hypothyroidism, hepatic disease, diabetes mellitus, seizure disorders, nephritis
Pharmacokinetics:
PO: Onset 12 hr, oxidized by liver, excreted unchanged in feces
Interactions/incompatibilities:
• Increased effects of: tricyclic antidepressants, diazepam, oral anticoagulants, paraldehyde, phenytoin, chloriazepoxide, isoniazid, caffeine
• Disulfiram reaction: alcohol
• Psychosis: metronidazole
NURSING CONSIDERATIONS
Assess:
• Liver function studies q2 wk during therapy: AST, ALT
• CBC, SMA q3-6 mo to detect any abnormality including increased cholesterol
Administer:
• Only with patient's knowledge; do not give to intoxicated individuals
• Vitamin B₆ to decrease cholesterol levels, which often increase with this drug
• Once per day in the AM or hs if drowsiness occurs
• Only after patient has not been drinking for >12 hr
Evaluate:
• Mental status: affect, mood, drug history, ability to follow treatment, abstain from alcohol
• For signs of hepatotoxicity: jaundice, dark urine, clay-colored stools, abdominal pain
Teach patient/family:
• Effect of this drug if alcohol is taken; written consent for disulfiram therapy should be obtained
• That shaving lotions, creams, lotin, cough preparations, skin products must be checked for alcohol

content; even in small amount, alcohol can produce a reaction
• That tolerance will not develop if treatment is prolonged
• That reaction may occur for 2 wk after last dose
• That tablets can be crushed, mixed with beverage
• To carry ID listing disulfiram therapy
• To avoid driving or hazardous tasks if drowsiness occurs
• That disulfiram reaction can be fatal, occurs 15 min after drinking
Lab test interferences:
Increase: Cholesterol
Decrease: ¹³¹I uptake, PBI, VMA
Treatment of overdose: IV vitamin C, ephedrine sulfate, antihistamines, O₂

---

dobutamine HCl
(doe-byoo′ta-meen)
Dubutrex
Func. class.: Adrenergic direct-acting β₁-agonist
Chem. class.: Catecholamine

Action: Causes increased contractility, increased coronary blood flow and heart rate by acting on β-1 receptors in heart
Uses: Cardiac surgery, refractory heart failure
Dosage and routes:
• *Adult:* IV INF 2.5-10 μg/kg/min, may increase to 40 μg/kg/min if needed
Available forms include: Inj 250 mg vial IV
Side effects/adverse reactions:
CNS: Anxiety, headache, dizziness
CV: Palpitations, tachycardia, hypertension, PVCs, angina
GI: Heartburn, nausea, vomiting
MS: Muscle cramps (leg)
Contraindications: Hypersensitiv-

ity, idiopathic hypertropic subaortic stenosis

Precautions: Pregnancy (C), lactation, children, hypertension

Pharmacokinetics:

IV: Onset 1-5 min, peak 10 min, half-life 2 min, metabolized in liver (inactive metabolites), excreted in urine

Interactions/incompatibilities:
• Dysrhythmias: general anesthetics
• Decreased action of dobutamine: other β-blockers
• Increased B/P: oxytocics
• Increased pressor effect and dysrhythmias: tricyclic antidepressant, MAOIs
• Incompatible with alkaline solutions: Na HCO₃

NURSING CONSIDERATIONS

Assess:
• I&O ratio
• ECG during administration continuously; if B/P increases, drug is decreased
• B/P and pulse q5min after parenteral route
• CVP or PWP during infusion if possible

Administer:
• IV diluting each 250 mg/10 ml of sterile H₂O or D₅ for inj; may be further diluted to 50 ml or more
• Plasma expanders for hypovolemia
• Parenteral (IV) dose slowly, after reconstituting, then diluting with at least 50 ml of D₅W, 0.9% NS, or Na lactate

Perform/provide:
• Storage of reconstituted solution if refrigerated for no longer than 24 hr

Evaluate:
• Therapeutic response: increased B/P with stabilization

Teach patient/family:
• Reason for drug administration

Treatment of overdose: Administer a β-1 adrenergic blocker

---

docusate calcium/docusate potassium/docusate sodium

(dok′yoo-sate)

Surfak/Kasof/Bu-lax, Colace, Dialose, Diocto, DioSul, Doxinate, D.S.S., Laxinate, Regulex*, Regutol, Roctate, Sulfolax

Func. class.: Laxative, emollient

Chem. class.: Anionic surface

Action: Increases water, fat penetration in intestine; allows for easier passage of stool

Uses: To soften stools

Dosage and routes:
• *Adult:* PO 50-300 mg qd (sodium) or 240 mg (calcium or potassium) prn; ENEMA 5 ml (potassium)
• *Child >12 yr:* ENEMA 2 ml (potassium)
• *Child 6-12 yr:* PO 40-120 mg qd (sodium)
• *Child 3-6 yr:* PO 20-60 mg qd (sodium)
• *Child <3 yr:* PO 10-40 mg qd (sodium)

Available forms include: Caps 50, 100, 240, 250, 300 mg; tabs 50, 100 mg; oral sol 10, 50 mg/ml, 16.7, 20 mg/5 ml

Side effects/adverse reactions:

GI: Nausea, anorexia, cramps, diarrhea

INTEG: Rash

EENT: Bitter taste, throat irritation

Contraindications: Hypersensitivity, obstruction, fecal impaction, nausea/vomiting

Precautions: Pregnancy (C)

---

*Available in Canada only

NURSING CONSIDERATIONS
Assess:
• Blood, urine electrolytes if drug is used often by patient
• I&O ratio to identify fluid loss
Administer:
• Alone with 8 oz water only for better absorption; do not take within 1 hr of other drugs or within 1 hr of antacids, milk, or H_2 blockers
• In morning or evening (oral dose)
Perform/provide:
• Storage in cool environment, do not freeze
Evaluate:
• Therapeutic response: decrease in constipation
• Cause of constipation; identify whether fluids, bulk, or exercise is missing from lifestyle
• Cramping, rectal bleeding, nausea, vomiting; if these symptoms occur, drug should be discontinued
Teach patient/family:
• Swallow tabs whole; do not chew
• That normal bowel movements do not always occur daily
• Do not use in presence of abdominal pain, nausea, vomiting
• Notify physician if constipation unrelieved or if symptoms of electrolyte imbalance occur: muscle cramps, pain, weakness, dizziness, excessive thirst
• Keep out of children's reach

---

dopamine HCl

(doe′pa-meen)
Dopastat, Intropin, Revimine*
Func. class.: Agonist
Chem. class.: Catecholamine

Action: Causes increased cardiac output; acts on α-receptors, causing vasoconstriction in blood vessels; when low doses are administered, causes renal and mesenteric vasodilation
Uses: Shock, increase perfusion, hypotension
Dosage and routes:
• *Adult:* IV INF 2-5 μg/kg/min, not to exceed 50 μg/kg/min, titrate to patient's response
Available forms include: Inj 0.8, 1.6, 40, 80, 160 mg/ml
Side effects/adverse reactions:
CNS: Headache
CV: Palpitations, tachycardia, hypertension, ectopic beats, angina, wide QRS complex, peripheral vasoconstriction
GI: Nausea, vomiting, diarrhea
INTEG: Necrosis, tissue sloughing with extravasation, ***gangrene***
RESP: Dyspnea
Contraindications: Hypersensitivity, ventricular fibrillation, tachydysrhythmias, pheochromocytoma
Precautions: Pregnancy (C), lactation, arterial embolism, peripheral vascular disease
Pharmacokinetics:
IV: Onset 5 min, duration <10 min, metabolized in liver, excreted in urine (metabolites)
Interactions/incompatibilities:
• Do not use within 2 wk of MAOIs, phenytoin, barbiturates, or hypertensive crisis may result
• Dysrhythmias: general anesthetics
• Decreased action of dopamine: other β-blockers
• Increased B/P: oxytocics
• Increased pressor effect: tricyclic antidepressant, MAOIs
• Incompatible with alkaline solutions: Na HCO_3
• Additive effect: diuretics
NURSING CONSIDERATIONS
Assess:
• I&O ratio
• ECG during administration con-

---

italics = common side effects   ***bold italic*** = life threatening reactions

tinuously; if B/P increases, drug is decreased
• B/P and pulse q5min after parenteral route
• CVP or PWP during infusion if possible

Administer:
• Plasma expanders for hypovolemia
• IV after diluting 200 mg/250-500 ml of compatible sol
• Parenteral IV dose slowly, after reconstituting, use infusion pump, flush line before infusing, infuse as secondary IV line

Perform/provide:
• Storage of reconstituted solution if refrigerated for no longer than 24 hr
• Do not use discolored solutions

Evaluate:
• Paresthesias and coldness of extremities, perpiperal blood flow may decrease
• Injection site: tissue sloughing; if this occurs, administer phentolamine mixed with NS
• Therapeutic response: increased B/P with stabilization

Teach patient/family:
• Reason for drug administration

Treatment of overdose: Administer a β-1 adrenergic blocker

---

doxapram HCl

(dox'a-pram)
Dopram
Func. class.: Analeptic

Action: Respiratory stimulation through activation of peripheral carotid chemoreceptor; with higher doses medullary respiratory centers are stimulated

Uses: Chronic obstructive pulmonary disease (COPD), postanesthesia respiratory stimulation,

acute hypercapnia, drug-induced CNS depression

Dosage and routes:
Post anesthesia
• *Adult:* IV INJ 0.5-1 mg/kg, not to exceed 1.5 mg/kg total as a single injection; IV INF 250 mg in 250 ml sol, not to exceed 4 mg/kg, run at 1-3 mg/min

Drug-induced CNS depression
Priming IV dose of 2mg/kg, repeated in 5 min. Repeat q1-2 h till pt awakes; IV INF priming dose 2mg/kg at 1-3 mg/min, not to exceed 3 g/day

COPD
• *Adult:* IV INF 1-2 mg/min, not to exceed 3 mg/min for no longer than 2 hr

Available forms include: Inj IV 20 mg/ml

Side effects/adverse reactions:
CNS: Convulsions, (clonus/generalized), *headache,* restlessness, dizziness, confusion, paresthesias, flushing, sweating, bilateral Babinski's sign, rigidity, depression
GI: Nausea, vomiting, diarrhea, hiccups
GU: Retention, incontinence
CV: Chest pain, hypertension, change in heart rate, lowered T waves, tachycardia
INTEG: Pruritus, irritation at injection site
EENT: Pupil dilation, sneezing
RESP: Laryngospasm, bronchospasm, rebound hypoventilation, dyspnea, cough

Contraindications: Hypersensitivity, seizure disorders, severe hypertension, severe bronchial asthma, severe dyspnea, severe cardiac disorders, pneumothorax, pulmonary embolism, severe respiratory disease

Precautions: Bronchial asthma,

---

*Available in Canada only

hyperthyroidism, pheochromocytoma, severe tachycardia, dysrhythmias, pregnancy (C), hypertension, lactation, children

Pharmacokinetics:
IV: Onset 20-40 sec, peak 1-2 min, duration 5-10 min; metabolized by liver, excreted by kidneys (metabolites), half-life 2.5-4 hr

Interactions/incompatibilities:
• Synergistic pressor effect: MAOIs, sympathomimetics
• Cardiac dysrhythmias: halothane, cyclopropane, enflurane
• Do not mix in alkaline solution including thiopental sodium, bicarbonate, aminophylline

NURSING CONSIDERATIONS
Assess:
• BP, HR, deep tendon reflexes, ABGs before administration, q30min
• PO_2, Pco_2, O_2 saturation during treatment

Administer:
• IV undiluted or diluted with equal parts of sterile H_2O for inj; may be diluted 250 mg/250 ml of D_5W, $D_{10}W$ and run as infusion
• IV at 1-3 mg/min, adjust for desired respiratory response, using infusion pump IV
• Only after adequate airway is established
• After O_2, IV barbiturates, resuscitative equipment is available

Perform/provide:
• Placing patient in Sims' position to prevent aspiration of vomitus
• Discontinue infusion if side effects occur; narrow margin of safety

Evaluate:
• Hypertension, dysrhythmias, tachycardia, dyspnea, skeletal muscle hyperactivity; may indicate overdosage; discontinue if these occur

• Respiratory stimulation: increased respiratory rate, abnormal rhythm
• Extravasation, change IV site q48h

Treatment of overdose: Lavage, activated charcoal, monitor electrolytes, vital signs

---

doxazosin mesylate
Cardura
Func. class.: Peripheral α-adrenergic blocker
Chem. class.: Quinozoline

Action: Peripheral blood vessels are dilated, peripheral resistance lowered; reduction in blood pressure results from α-adrenergic receptors being blocked

Uses: Hypertension

Dosage and routes:
Adult: PO 1 mg q d, increasing up to 16 mg q d if required; usual range 4-16 mg/day

Available forms include: Tabs 1, 2, 4, 8 mg

Side effects/adverse reactions:
CV: Palpitations, orthostatic hypotension, tachycardia, edema, dysrhythmias, chest pain
CNS: Dizziness, headache, drowsiness, anxiety, depression, vertigo, weakness, fatigue, asthenia
GI: Nausea, vomiting, diarrhea, constipation, abdominal pain
GU: Incontinence, polyuria
EENT: Epistaxis, tinnitus, dry mouth, red sclera, pharyngitis, rhinitis

Contraindications: Hypersensitivity to quinazolines

Precautions: Pregnancy (C), children, lactation, hepatic disease

Pharmacokinetics:
PO: Onset 2 hr, peak 2-6 hr, duration 6-12 hr; half-life 22 hr, metabolized in liver, excreted via bile/

---

feces (<63%) and in urine (9%); extensively protein bound (98%)
Interaction/incompatibilities:
• Increased hypotensive effects: Beta-blockers, indomethacin, verapamil

NURSING CONSIDERATIONS
Assess:
• B/P 2-6 hr after each dose and with each increase; postural effects may occur
• Pulse, jugular venous distention q4h
• BUN, uric acid if on long-term therapy
• Weight daily, I&O
Administer:
• Whole; do not chew or crush tablets
Perform/provide:
• Storage in tight containers in cool environment
Evaluate:
• Edema in feet, legs daily
• Skin turgor, dryness of mucous membranes for hydration status
• Rales, dyspnea, orthopnea q30 min
Teach patient/family:
• That fainting occasionally occurs after 1st dose; do not drive or operate machinery for 4 hr after 1st dose or take 1st dose hs
Treatment of overdose: Administer volume expanders or vasopressors; discontinue drug; place in supine position

---

doxepin HCl
(dox'e-pin)
Adapin, Sinequan, Triadapin*

Func. class.: Antidepressant, tricyclic
Chem. class.: Dibenzoxepin, tertiary amine

Action: Blocks reuptake of nor-epinephrine, serotonin into nerve endings, increasing action of norepinephrine, serotonin in nerve cells
Uses: Major depression, anxiety
Dosage and routes:
• *Adult:* PO 50-75 mg/day in divided doses, may increase to 300 mg/day or may give daily dose hs
Available forms include: Caps 10, 25, 50, 75, 100, 150 mg; oral conc 10 mg/ml
Side effects/adverse reactions:
*HEMA: **Agranulocytosis, thrombocytopenia, eosinophilia, leukopenia***
CNS: Dizziness, drowsiness, confusion, headache, anxiety, tremors, stimulation, weakness, insomnia, nightmares, EPS (elderly), increased psychiatric symptoms, paresthesia
GI: Diarrhea, dry mouth, nausea, vomiting, ***paralytic ileus,*** increased appetite, cramps, epigastric distress, jaundice, ***hepatitis,*** stomatitis
*GU: Retention, **acute renal failure***
INTEG: Rash, urticaria, sweating, pruritus, photosensitivity
*CV: Orthostatic hypotension, ECG changes, tachycardia, **hypertension,*** palpitations
EENT: Blurred vision, tinnitus, mydriasis, ophthalmoplegia, glossitis
Contraindications: Hypersensitivity to tricyclic antidepressants, urinary retention, narrow-angle glaucoma, prostatic hypertrophy
Precautions: Suicidal patients, elderly, pregnancy (C)
Pharmacokinetics:
PO: Steady state 2-8 days; metabolized by liver, excreted by kidneys, crosses placenta, excreted in breast milk, half-life 8-24 hr
Interactions/incompatibilities:
• Decreased effects of: guanethi-

dine, clonidine, indirect acting sympathomimetics (ephedrine)
• Increased effects of: direct acting sympathomimetics (epinephrine), alcohol, barbiturates, benzodiazepines, CNS depressants
• Hyperpyretic crisis, convulsions, hypertensive episode: MAOI (pargyline [Eutonyl])

NURSING CONSIDERATIONS

Assess:
• B/P (lying, standing), pulse q4h; if systolic B/P drops 20 mm Hg hold drug, notify physician; take vital signs q4h in patients with cardiovascular disease
• Blood studies: CBC, leukocytes, differential, cardiac enzymes if patient is receiving long-term therapy
• Hepatic studies: AST, ALT, bilirubin, creatinine
• Weight qwk, appetite may increase with drug
• ECG for flattening of T wave, bundle branch block, AV block, dysrhythmias in cardiac patients

Administer:
• Increased fluids, bulk in diet if constipation, urinary retention occur
• With food or milk for GI symptoms
• Dosage hs if over-sedation occurs during day; may take entire dose hs; elderly may not tolerate once/day dosing
• Gum, hard candy, or frequent sips of water for dry mouth
• Concentrate with fruit juice, water, or milk to disguise taste

Perform/provide:
• Storage protected from direct sunlight, in tight container
• Assistance with ambulation during beginning therapy since drowsiness/dizziness occurs
• Safety measures including siderails primarily in elderly

• Checking to see PO medication swallowed

Evaluate:
• EPS primarily in elderly: rigidity, dystonia, akathisia
• Mental status: mood, sensorium, affect, suicidal tendencies, an increase in psychiatric symptoms: depression, panic
• Urinary retention, constipation; constipation is more likely to occur in children
• Withdrawal symptoms: headache, nausea, vomiting, muscle pain, weakness; do not usually occur unless drug was discontinued abruptly
• Alcohol consumption; if alcohol is consumed, hold dose until morning

Teach patient/family:
• That therapeutic effects may take 2-3 wk
• Use caution in driving or other activities requiring alertness because of drowsiness, dizziness, blurred vision
• To avoid alcohol ingestion, other CNS depressants
• Not to discontinue medication quickly after long-term use, may cause nausea, headache, malaise
• To wear sunscreen or large hat since photosensitivity occurs

Lab test interferences:
Increase: Serum bilirubin, blood glucose, alk phosphatase
False increase: Urinary catecholamines
Decrease: VMA, 5-HIAA

Treatment of overdose: ECG monitoring, induce emesis, lavage, activated charcoal, administer anticonvulsant

doxorubicin HCl

(dox-oh-roo'bi-sin)
Adriamycin
Func. class.: Antineoplastic, antibiotic
Chem. class.: Anthracycline glycoside

Action: Inhibits DNA synthesis, primarily; derived from *Streptomyces peucetius;* replication is decreased by binding to DNA, which causes strand splitting; active throughout entire cell cycle, a vesicant

Uses: Wilms' tumor, bladder, breast, cervical, head, neck, liver, lung, ovarian, prostatic, stomach, testicular, thyroid cancer, Hodgkin's disease, acute lymphoblastic leukemia, myeloblastic leukemia, neuroblastomas, lymphomas, sarcomas

Dosage and routes:
• *Adult:* 60-75 mg/m² q3 wk, or 30 mg/m² on days 1-3 of 4-wk cycle, not to exceed 550 mg/m² cumulative dose

Available forms include: Inj IV 10, 20, 50 mg

Side effects/adverse reactions:
HEMA: Thrombocytopenia, leukopenia, anemia
GI: Nausea, vomiting, anorexia, mucositis, *hepatotoxicity*
GU: Impotence, sterility, amenorrhea, gynecomastia, hyperuricemia
INTEG: Rash, necrosis at injection site, dermatitis, reversible alopecia, cellulitis, thrombophlebitis at injection site
CV: Increased B/P, *sinus tachycardia, PVCs,* chest pain, *bradycardia, extra systoles*
Contraindications: Hypersensitivity, pregnancy (1st trimester) (D), lactation, systemic infections

Precautions: Renal, hepatic, cardiac disease, gout, bone marrow depression (severe)

Pharmacokinetics: Triphasic pattern of elimination; half-life 12 min, 3⅓ hr, 29⅔ hr, metabolized by liver, crosses placenta, appears in breast milk, excreted in urine, bile

Interactions/incompatibilities:
• Increased toxicity: other antineoplastics or radiation
• Do not mix with other drugs in solution or syringe or use same IV tubing
• Decreased serum digoxin levels: digoxin

NURSING CONSIDERATIONS
Assess:
• CBC, differential, platelet count weekly; withhold drug if WBC is <4000/mm³ or platelet count is <75,000/mm³; notify physician of these results
• Blood, urine uric acid levels
• Renal function studies: BUN, serum uric acid, urine CrCl, electrolytes before, during therapy
• I&O ratio; report fall in urine output to <30 ml/hr
• Monitor temperature q4h; fever may indicate beginning infection
• Liver function tests before, during therapy: bilirubin, AST, ALT, alk phosphatase as needed or monthly
• ECG; watch for ST-T wave changes, low QRS and T, possible dysrhythmias (sinus tachycardia, heart block, PVCs)

Administer:
• Hydrocortisone, dexamethasone or sodium bicarbonate (1 mEq/1 ml) for extravasation, apply ice compresses
• Antiemetic 30-60 min before giving drug to prevent vomiting
• Allopurinol or sodium bicarbon-

---

* Available in Canada only

ate to maintain uric acid levels, alkalinization of urine
• IV after diluting 10 mg/5 ml of NaCl for inj; shake; give over 3-5 min; give through Y-tube or 3-way stopcock
• Slow IV infusion using 20-, 21-gauge needle
• Topical or systemic analgesics for pain
• Transfusion for anemia
• Antispasmodic for GI symptoms
Perform/provide:
• Strict handwashing technique, gloves, protective clothing
• Liquid diet: carbonated beverages, Jello may be added if patient is not nauseated or vomiting
• Increased fluid intake to 2-3 L/day to prevent urate, calculi formation
• Diet low in purines: absence of organ meats (kidney, liver), dried beans, peas to maintain alkaline urine
• Rinsing of mouth tid-qid with water, club soda; brushing of teeth bid-tid with soft brush or cotton-tipped applicators for stomatitis; use unwaxed dental floss
• Storage at room temperature for 24 hr after reconstituting or 48 hr refrigerated
Evaluate:
• Bleeding: hematuria, guaiac, bruising or petechiae, mucosa or orifices q8h
• Food preferences; list likes, dislikes
• Effects of alopecia on body image; discuss feelings about body changes
• Inflammation of mucosa, breaks in skin
• Yellowing of skin, sclera, dark urine, clay-colored stools, itchy skin, abdominal pain, fever, diarrhea

• Buccal cavity q8h for dryness, sores, ulceration, white patches, oral pain, bleeding, dysphagia
• Alkalosis if severe vomiting is present
• Local irritation, pain, burning at injection site
• GI symptoms: frequency of stools, cramping
• Acidosis, signs of dehydration: rapid respirations, poor skin turgor, decreased urine output, dry skin, restlessness, weakness
• Cardiac status: B/P, pulse, character, rhythm, rate, ABGs, ECG
Teach patient/family:
• To report any complaints, side effects to nurse or physician
• That hair may be lost during treatment and wig or hairpiece may make the patient feel better; tell patient that new hair may be different in color, texture
• To avoid foods with citric acid, hot or rough texture
• To report any bleeding, white spots, ulcerations in mouth to physician; tell patient to examine mouth qd
• That urine and other body fluids may be red-orange for 48 hr
• To avoid crowds and persons with infections when granulocyte count is low
Lab test interferences:
Increase: Uric acid

---

doxycycline hyclate
(dox-i-sye'kleen)
Doryx, Doxy-Caps, Doxychel, Doxycin,* Doxy-Tabs, Vibramycin, Vibra-Tabs, Vivox
Func. class.: Broad spectrum antibiotic/antiinfective
Chem. class.: Tetracycline

Action: Inhibits protein synthesis,

prosphorylation in microorganisms by binding to 30S ribosomal subunits, reversibly binding to 50S ribosomal subunits

Uses: Syphilis, chlamydia trachomatis, gonorrhea, lymphogranuloma venereum, uncommon gram negative/positive organisms

Dosage and routes:
• *Adult:* PO 100 mg q12h on day 1, then 100 mg/day; IV 200 mg in 1-2 inf on day 1, then 100-200 mg/day
• *Child >8 yr:* PO/IV 4.4 mg/kg/day in divided doses q12h on day 1, then 2.2-4.4 mg/kg/day

Gonorrhea (uncomplicated)
• *Adult:* PO 200 mg, then 100 mg hs and 100 mg bid × 3 days or 300 mg, then 300 mg in 1 hr
• Disseminated; 100 mg PO bid × at least 7 days

Chlamydia trachomatis
• *Adult:* PO 100 mg bid × 7 days

Syphilis
• *Adult:* PO 300 mg/day in divided doses × 10 days

Available forms include: Tabs 100 mg; caps 50, 100 mg; syr 50 mg/ml; powder for inj IV 100, 200 mg

Side effects/adverse reactions:
CNS: Fever, headache, paresthesia
HEMA: Eosinophilia, neutropenia, thrombocytopenia, leukocytosis, hemolytic anemia
EENT: Dysphagia, glossitis, decreased calcification of deciduous teeth, abdominal pain, oral candidiasis
GI: Nausea, vomiting, diarrhea, anorexia, enterocolitis, *hepatotoxicity,* flatulence, abdominal cramps, gastric burning, stomatitis, *pseudomembranous colitis*
CV: Pericarditis
GU: Increased BUN, polyuria, polydipsia, *renal failure, nephrotoxicity*

INTEG: Rash, urticaria, photosensitivity, increased pigmentation, exfoliative dermatitis, pruritus, *angioedema*

Contraindications: Hypersensitivity to tetracyclines, children <8 yr, pregnancy (D)

Precautions: Hepatic disease, lactation

Pharmacokinetics:
PO: Peak 1½-4 hr, half-life 15-22 hr; excreted in bile, 25%-93% protein bound

Interactions/incompatibilities:
• Do not mix with other drugs
• Decreased effects of doxycycline: antacids, $NaHCO_3$, dairy products, alkali products, iron, kaolin/pectin, barbiturates, carbemazine, phenytoin
• Increased effect: anticoagulants
• Decreased effects: penicillins, oral contraceptives

NURSING CONSIDERATIONS
Assess:
• I&O ratio
• Blood studies: PT, CBC, AST, ALT, BUN, creatinine
• Signs of infection

Administer:
• IV after diluting 100 mg or less/10 ml of sterile H_2O or normal saline for inj; further dilute with 100-1000 ml of compatible sol; run 100 mg or less over 1-4 hr
• On empty stomach 1 hr ac or 2 hr pc with 8 oz of water
• After C&S obtained
• 2 hr before or after laxative or ferrous products; 3 hr after antacid or kaolin-pectin products

Perform/provide:
• Storage in tight, light-resistant container at room temperature

Evaluate:
• Therapeutic response: decreased temperature, absence of lesions, negative C&S

---

*Available in Canada only

- Allergic reactions: rash, itching, pruritus, angioedema
- Nausea, vomiting, diarrhea; administer antiemetic, antacids as ordered
- Overgrowth of infection: increased temperature, malaise, redness, pain, swelling, drainage, perineal itching, diarrhea, changes in cough or sputum
- IV site for phlebitis/thrombosis; drug is highly irritating

Teach patient/family:
- To avoid sun exposure since burns may occur; sunscreen does not seem to decrease photosensitivity
- If diabetic to avoid use of Clinistix, Diastix, or Tes-Tape for urine glucose testing
- That all prescribed medication must be taken to prevent superimposed infection
- Take with a full glass of water

Lab test interferences:
False negative: Urine glucose with Clinistix or Tes-Tape
False increase: Urinary catecholamines; ALT, AST

D-penicillamine

(pen-i-sill'a-meen)
Cuprimine, Depen

Func. class.: Heavy metal antagonist
Chem. class.: Chelating agent (thiol compound)

Action: Binds with ions of lead, mercury, copper, iron, zinc to form a water-soluble complex excreted by kidneys
Uses: Wilson's disease, rheumatoid arthritis, cystinuria, lead poisoning

Dosage and routes:
Cystinuria

- *Adult:* PO 250 mg qid ac, not to exceed 5 g/day
- *Child:* PO 30 mg/kg/day in divided doses qid ac

Wilson's disease
- *Adult:* PO 250 mg qid ac
- *Child:* PO 20 mg/kg/day in divided doses ac

Rheumatoid arthritis
- *Adult:* PO 125-250 mg/day, then increased 250 mg q2-3 mo if needed, not to exceed 1 g/day

Available forms include: Caps 125, 250 mg; tabs 250 mg

Side effects/adverse reactions:
HEMA: **Thrombocytopenia, granulocytopenia, leukopenia, eosinophilia,** Lupus-syndrome, increased sedimentation rate
INTEG: Urticaria, erythema, pruritus, fever, ecchymosis
CV: Hypotension, tachycardia
GI: Diarrhea, abdominal cramping, nausea, vomiting, **hepatotoxicity**
EENT: Tinnitus, optic neuritis
MS: Arthralgia
GU: **Proteinuria, nephrotic syndrome, glomerulonephritis**
SYST: **Anaphylaxis**
RESP: Pneumonitis

Contraindications: Hypersensitivity to penicillins, anuria, agranulocytosis, severe renal disease, pregnancy (D)

Pharmacokinetics:
PO: Peak 1 hr, metabolized in liver, excreted in urine

Interactions/incompatibilities:
- Increased side effects: oxyphenbutazone, phenylbutazone, gold salts, antimalarials, cytotoxics
- Decreased absorption of D-penicillamine: oral iron

NURSING CONSIDERATIONS
Assess:
- Monitor hepatic, renal studies:

---

italics = common side effects   **bold italic** = life threatening reactions

AST/ALT, alk phosphatase, BUN, creatinine
• Monitor I&O, temperature
• Monitor platelet, neutropenia, WBC, H&H; if WBC <3500/mm³ or if platelets <100,000/mm³, drug should be discontinued

Administer:
• On an empty stomach, ½-1 hr before meals or at least 2 hr after meals
• Vitamin B₆ daily, depleted when this drug is used
• Only when epinephrine 1:1000 is on unit for anaphylaxis
• Fluids to 3 L/day to prevent renal failure

Evaluate:
• Therapeutic response: absence of pain, rigidity in joints (rheumatoid arthritis)
• Allergic reactions (rash, urticaria); if these occur, drug should be discontinued

Teach patient/family:
• That urine may be red in color
• That therapeutic effect may take 1-3 mo
• To report sore throat, easy bruising, bleeding from mucous membranes; may indicate bone marrow depression

---

droperidol

(droe-per'i-dole)
Inapsine

Func. class.: General anesthetic
Chem. class.: Butyrophenone derivative

Action: Acts on CNS at subcortical levels, produces tranquilization, sleep

Uses: Premedication for surgery, induction, maintenance in general anesthesia

Dosage and routes:
Induction
• *Adult:* IV 2.5 mg/20-25 lb given with analgesic or general anesthetic
• *Child 2-12 yr:* IV 1-1.5 mg/20-25 lb, titrated to response needed
Premedication
• *Adult:* IM 2.5-10 mg ½-1 hr before surgery
• *Child 2-12 yr:* IM 1-1.5 mg/20-25 lb
Maintaining general anesthesia
• *Adult:* IV 1.25-2.5 mg
Available forms include: Inj IM, IV 2.5 mg/ml

Side effects/adverse reactions:
RESP: **Laryngospasm, bronchospasm**
CNS: Dystonia, akathisia, flexion of arms, fine tremors, dizziness, anxiety, drowsiness, restlessness, hallucination, depression
CV: Tachycardia, hypotension
EENT: Upward rotation of eyes, oculogyric crisis
INTEG: Chills, facial sweating, shivering

Contraindications: Hypersensitivity, child <2 yr, pregnancy (C)
Precautions: Elderly, cardiovascular disease (hypotension, bradydysrhythmias), renal disease, liver disease, Parkinson's disease

Pharmacokinetics:
IM/IV: Onset 3-10 min, peak ½ hr, duration 3-6 hr; metabolized in liver, excreted in urine as metabolites, crosses placenta

Interactions/incompatibilities:
• Increased CNS depression: alcohol, narcotics, barbiturates, antipsychotics or other CNS depressants
• Decreased effects of: amphetamines, anticonvulsants, anticoagulants, when given with this drug
• Increased intraocular pressure:

---

* Available in Canada only

anticholinergics, antiparkinson drugs

• Increased side effects of: lithium

• Do not mix with barbiturates in solution

NURSING CONSIDERATIONS
Assess:

• VS q10 min during IV administration, q30 min after IM dose

Administer:

• IV undiluted; give through Y-tube or 3-way stopcock; may be given as an infusion 20 mg/1000 ml LR, D₅W, 0.9% NaCl

• Anticholinergics (benztropine, diphenhydramine) for extrapyramidal reaction

• Only with crash cart, resuscitative equipment nearby

• IV slowly only

Perform/provide:

• Slow movement of patient to avoid orthostatic hypotension

Evaluate:

• Therapeutic response: decreased anxiety, absence of vomiting during surgery

• Extrapyramidal reactions: dystonia, akathisia

• For increasing heart rate or decreasing B/P, notify physician at once; do not place patient in Trendelenburg position or sympathetic blockade may occur causing respiratory arrest

---

dyclonine HCl (topical)

(dye-kloe-neen)

Dyclone

Func. class.: Topical anesthetic
Chem. class.: Organic ketone

Action: Inhibits nerve impulses from sensory nerves, which produces anesthesia

Uses: Topical anesthesia prior to diagnostic examination, suppress

gag reflex, itching of pruritus ani or vulvae

Dosage and routes:

• *Adult and child:* TOP apply tid-qid; INSTILL 10 ml sol into urethra after cysturethroscopy

Available forms include: Sol 0.5%, 1%

Side effects/adverse reactions:

INTEG: Rash, irritation, sensitization, edema, urticaria, burning

Contraindications: Hypersensitivity, infants, application to large areas

Precautions: Children, sepsis, pregnancy (C), denuded skin

NURSING CONSIDERATIONS
Administer:

• After cleansing and drying of affected area

• With diphenhydramine elixir for stomatitis

Evaluate:

• Allergy: rash, irritation, reddening, swelling

• Therapeutic response: anesthesia of area, absence of gag reflex

Teach patient/family:

• To report rash, irritation, redness, swelling

---

dyphylline

(dye′fi-lin)

Asminyl, Dilin, Dilor, Dyflex, Dylline, Lufyllin, Neothylline, Oxystat, Protophylline*

Func. class.: Spasmolytic
Chem. class.: Xanthine, ethylenediamide

Action: Relaxes smooth muscle of respiratory system by blocking phosphodiesterase, which increases cyclic AMP

Uses: Bronchial asthma, bronchospasm in chronic bronchitis, COPD

Dosage and routes:
• *Adult:* PO 200-800 mg q6h; IM 250-500 mg q6h injected slowly
• *Child >6 yr:* PO 4-7 mg/kg/day in 4 divided doses
Available forms include: Tabs 200, 400 mg; elix 100, 160 mg/15 ml; inj IM 250 mg/ml

Side effects/adverse reactions:
CNS: Anxiety, restlessness, insomnia, dizziness, convulsions, headache, light-headedness, muscle twitching
CV: Palpitations, sinus tachycardia, hypotension, flushing, dysrhythmias
GI: Nausea, vomiting, anorexia, dyspepsia, epigastric pain
INTEG: Flushing, urticaria
RESP: Tachypnea
Other: Fever, dehydration, *albuminuria,* hyperglycemia

Contraindications: Hypersensitivity to xanthines, tachydysrhythmias
Precautions: Elderly, CHF, cor pulmonale, hepatic disease, active peptic ulcer disease, diabetes mellitus, hyperthyroidism, hypertension, children, renal disease, pregnancy (C), glaucoma

Pharmacokinetics:
Peak 1 hr, half-life 2 hr, excreted in urine unchanged

Interactions/incompatibilities:
• Do not mix in syringe with other drugs
• Increased action of dyphylline: cimetidine, propranolol, erythromycin, troleandomycin
• May increase effects of: anticoagulants
• Cardiotoxicity: β-blockers
• Increased metabolism: barbiturates, phenytoin
• Decreased elimination of dyphylline: uricosurics

NURSING CONSIDERATIONS
Assess:
• Dyphylline blood levels; toxicity may occur with small increase above 20 μg/ml
• Monitor I&O; diuresis occurs, dehydration may result in elderly or children
• Whether theophylline was given recently

Administer:
• PO after meals to decrease GI symptoms; absorption may be affected
• Avoid IM injection; pain occurs

Perform/provide
• Storage protected from light, at room temperature

Evaluate:
• Therapeutic response: decreased dyspnea, respiratory rate, rhythm
• Auscultate lung fields bilaterally; notify physician of abnormalities
• Allergic reactions: rash, urticaria; if these occur, drug should be discontinued

Teach patient/family
• To check OTC medications, current prescription medications for ephedrine; will increase stimulation; not to drink alcohol or caffeine
• To avoid hazardous activities; dizziness, drowsiness, blurred vision may occur
• If GI upset occurs, to take drug with 8 oz of water; avoid food, since absorption may be decreased

---

echothiophate iodide
(ek-oh-thye'oh-fate)
Phospholine Iodide, Echodide
Func. class.: Miotic
Chem. class.: Cholinesterase inhibitor, irreversible

Action: Prevents breakdown of neurotransmitter acetylcholine, which then accumulates, causing enhancement, prolongation of its physiologic effects

Uses: Glaucoma (open-angle), accommodative esotropia, treatment of obstructed aqueous outflow; extremely effective in control of chronic wide-angle glaucoma, aphakic glaucoma, congenital glaucoma

Dosage and routes:
• *Adult and child:* INSTILL 1 gtt of 0.03%, or 0.125% sol qd in conjunctival sac, not to exceed 1 gtt bid
Available forms include: Powder for reconstitution, 1.5 mg (0.03%), 3 mg (0.06%), 6.25 mg (0.125%), 12.5 mg (0.25%) with 5 ml diluent

Side effects/adverse reactions:
GU: Frequency
CV: Hypotension, bradycardia, *cardiac arrest*
INTEG: Sweating, pallor, cyanosis
RESP: *Bronchospasm*
GI: Nausea, vomiting, abdominal cramps, diarrhea
EENT: Blurred vision, stinging, burning, lacrimation, lid muscle twitching, conjunctival, ciliary redness, browache, headache, induced myopia, iris cysts, hyperemia, hyphema

Contraindications: Hypersensitivity, ureitis

Precautions: Asthma, bradycardia, parkinsonism, peptic ulcer, pregnancy (C)

Interactions/incompatibilities:
• Decreased effect of echothiophate: pilocarpine
• Increased effect of both drugs: ambenonium, edrophonium, neostigmine, physostigmine, pyridostigmine
• Increased effects of: general anesthetics

NURSING CONSIDERATIONS
Administer:
• After checking vial for concentration

• Immediately after reconstituting; discard unused portion

Evaluate:
• Specific condition being treated
• History of patient's previous/current conditions (e.g., asthma, cardiac), possible sensitivity, contraindications, drug interactions

Teach patient/family:
• Instruct as to why patient is receiving medication; patient, family should have a clear regimen as well as name of medication
• To report change in vision, blurring or loss of sight, trouble breathing, sweating, flushing
• Method of instillation, including pressure on lacrimal sac for 1 min, not to touch dropper to eye
• That long-term therapy may be required
• That blurred vision will decrease with repeated use of drug
• That they may experience stinging sensation, dull ache or tearing which should subside in a few minutes; if it persists, contact physician
• Patient may experience decreased visual ability at night; instruct not to drive
• To use drops at night to eliminate hazardous, transient blurring

---

econazole nitrate (topical)

(e-kone′a-zole)
Ecostatin, Spectazole

Func. class.: Local antiinfective
Chem. class.: Imidazole derivative, antifungal

Action: Interferes with fungal cell membrane, which increases permeability, leaking of cell nutrients
Uses: Tinea pedis, tinea cruris, tinea corporis, tinea versicolor, cutaneous candidiasis

---

italics = common side effects   ***bold italic*** = life threatening reactions

Dosage and routes:
• *Adult and child:* TOP apply to affected area bid-qid depending on condition
Available forms include: Cream 1%
Side effects/adverse reactions:
INTEG: Rash, urticaria, stinging, burning, pruritus
Contraindications: Hypersensitivity
Precautions: Pregnancy (C), lactation
NURSING CONSIDERATIONS
Administer:
• Enough medication to completely cover lesions
• After cleansing with soap, water before each application, dry well
Perform/provide:
• Storage at room temperature in dry place
Evaluate:
• Allergic reaction: burning, stinging, swelling, redness
• Therapeutic response: decrease in size, number of lesions
Teach patient/family:
• To apply with glove to prevent further infection
• To avoid use of OTC creams, ointments, lotions unless directed by physician
• To use medical asepsis (hand washing) before, after each application
• Not to cover with occlusive dressing
• To continue even though condition improves
• To notify physician if condition worsens

edetate calcium disodium

(ed′e-tate)
Calcium Disodium Versenate, Calcium EDTA
Func. class.: Heavy metal antagonist
Chem. class.: Chelating agent

Action: Binds ions of lead to form a water-soluble complex that is removed by kidneys
Uses: Lead poisoning, acute lead encephalopathy
Dosage and routes:
Acute lead encephalopathy
• *Adult and child:* 1.5 g/m²/day × 3-5 days, with dimercaprol, may be given again after 4 days off drug
Lead poisoning
• *Adult:* IV 1 g/250-500 ml D_5W or 0.9% NaCl over 1-2 hr or q12h × 3-5 days, may repeat after 2 days, not to exceed 50 mg/kg/day, may be given as a continuous infusion over 8-24 hr
• *Child:* IM 35 mg/kg/day in divided doses q8-12 hr, not to exceed 50 mg/kg/day
Available forms include: Inj IM, IV 200 mg/ml
Side effects/adverse reactions:
CNS: Headache, paresthesia, numbness
INTEG: Urticaria, erythema, pruritus, pain at injection site, fever, cheilosis
CV: Hypotension, dysrhythmias, thrombophlebitis
GI: Vomiting, *diarrhea, abdominal cramps, anorexia,* cheilosis, histamine-like reaction with GI distress
EENT: Nasal congestion, sneezing
MS: Leg cramps, myalgia, arthralgia, weakness

*GU: **Hematuria, renal tubular necrosis, proteinuria***

Contraindications: Hypersensitivity, anuria, hepatic insufficiency, poisoning of other metals, severe renal disease, child <3 yr

Precautions: Hypertension, pregnancy (C), lactation, gout, active TB

Pharmacokinetics:
Not metabolized, excreted in urine, half-life: 20-60 min (IV), 90 min (IM)

NURSING CONSIDERATIONS
Assess:
• VS, B/P, pulse, respirations, weigh daily
• Monitor I&O, kidney function studies: BUN, creatinine, CrCl; watch for decreasing urine output
• Neuro status: Watch for paresthesias, beginning convulsions
• Urine: pH, albumin, casts, blood, coproporphyrins, calcium
• For febrile reactions that may occur 4-8 hr following drug therapy

Administer:
• EDTA, BAL separately
• IV slowly, IM is preferred route
• IM in large muscle mass; rotate injection sites, procaine Hcl should be added to IM injection (1 ml of procaine 1% to each ml of concentrated drug) to minimize pain at injection site
• Only when epinephrine 1 : 1000 is on unit for anaphylaxis
• IV fluids to ensure adequate hydration before administration of drug

Evaluate:
• Cardiac abnormalities: dysrhythmias, hypotension, tachycardia
• Allergic reactions (rash, urticaria); if these occur drug should be discontinued

Teach patient/family:
• That compliance to dosage schedule must be followed

Lab test interferences:
Decrease: Cholesterol/triglycerides, potassium

---

edetate disodium
(ed′e-tate)
Disodium EDTA, Disotate, Endrate
Func. class.: Metal antagonist
Chem. class.: Chelating agent

Action: Binds with ions of calcium, zinc, magnesium to form a water-soluble complex excreted from kidneys

Uses: Hypercalcemic crisis

Dosage and routes:
• *Adult and child:* IV INF 15-50 mg/kg/500 ml of D₅W or 0.9% NaCl, given over 3-4 hr, not to exceed 3 g/day (adult) or 70 mg/kg/day (child)

Available forms include: Inj conc 150 mg/ml

Side effects/adverse reactions:
*CNS: Headache, paresthesia, **convulsions***

INTEG: Urticaria, erythema, pain at injection site, hypertension

CV: Hypotension, ***exfoliative dermatitis,*** thrombophlebitis

GI: Nausea, vomiting, anorexia, diarrhea, abdominal cramps

GU: Dysuria, pyelonephritis, ***nephrotoxicity,*** hyperuricemia, hypomagnesemia, polyuria, ***proteinuria, renal tubular necrosis, hypocalcemia***

Contraindications: Hypersensitivity, anuria, hepatic insufficiency, poisoning of other metals, severe renal disease, child <3 yr, seizure disorders, active/inactive TB

Precautions: Hypertension, pregnancy (C), lactation

Pharmacokinetics:
Excreted in urine as calcium chelate

---

italics = common side effects   ***bold italic*** = life threatening reactions

NURSING CONSIDERATIONS
Assess:
• VS, B/P, pulse; if hypotension occurs, drug should be discontinued
• Monitor I&O, kidney function studies: BUN, creatinine, CrCl, calcium (must be done following each administration)
Administer:
• Only when IV calcium preparation is on unit for emergency use
• EDTA, BAL separately
• IV slowly, use infusion pump, rotate infusion sites, observe site for redness, inflammation
• IV fluids to ensure adequate hydration before administration of drug
Perform/provide:
• Assistance with ambulation
Evaluate:
• Therapeutic response: calcium levels between 9-10 mg/dl; absence of hypercalemic symptoms
• Hypocalcemia: numbness of feet, hands, tongue, lips; positive Chvostek's, Trousseau's signs; convulsions; stupor
• Cardiac abnormalities: dysrhythmias, hypotension, tachycardia
• Allergic reactions (rash, urticaria); if these occur, drug should be discontinued
Teach patient/family:
• To remain recumbent for ½ hr to prevent postural hypotension
• To make position changes slowly to prevent fainting
• That compliance to dosage schedule must be followed
• That breath may be odorous
Lab test interferences:
False decrease: Calcium
Decrease: Magnesium, alk phosphatase

edrophonium chloride
(ed-roe-foe'nee-um)
Enlon, Tensilon
Func. class.: Cholinergics, anticholinesterase
Chem. class.: Quaternary ammonium compound

Action: Inhibits destruction of acetylcholine, which increases concentration at sites where acetylcholine is released; this facilitates transmission of impulses across myoneural junction
Uses: To diagnose myasthenia gravis, curare antagonist, differentiation of myasthenic crisis from cholinergic crisis
Dosage and routes:
Tensilon test
• *Adult:* IV 1-2 mg over 15-30 sec, then 8 mg if no response, IM: 10 mg; if cholinergic reaction occurs, retest after ½ hr with 2 mg IM
• *Child >34 kg:* IV 2 mg, if no response in 45 sec then 1 mg q45 sec, not to exceed 10 mg
• *Child <34 kg:* IV 1 mg, if no response in 45 sec, then 1 mg q45 sec, not to exceed 5 mg
• *Infant:* IV 0.5 mg
Curare antagonist
• *Adult:* IV 10 mg over 30-45 sec, may repeat, not to exceed 40 mg
Differentiation of myasthenic crisis from cholinergic crisis
• *Adult:* IV 1 mg, if no response in 1 min, may repeat
Available forms include: Inj IV 10 mg/ml
Side effects/adverse reactions:
INTEG: Rash, urticaria
CNS: Dizziness, headache, sweating, confusion, weakness, *convulsions,* incoordination, *paralysis*
GI: Nausea, diarrhea, vomiting, cramps

---

*Available in Canada only

CV: Tachycardia, dysrythmias, bradycardia, hypotension AV block, ECG changes, ***cardiac arrest***

GU: Frequency, incontinence

RESP: ***Respiratory depression, bronchospasm, constriction, laryngospasm, respiratory arrest***

EENT: Miosis, blurred vision, lacrimation

Contraindications: Obstruction of intestine, renal system, hypersensitivity

Precautions: Seizure disorders, bronchial asthma, coronary occlusion, hyperthyroidism, dysrhythmias, peptic ulcer, megacolon, poor GI motility, pregnancy (C), bradycardia, hypotension

Pharmacokinetics:

IV: Onset 30-60 sec, duration 6-24 min

IM: Onset 2-10 min, duration 12-45 min

Interactions/incompatibilities:

• Decreased action of edrophonium: procainamide, quinidine, aminoglycosides, anesthetics, mecamylamine, polymyxin, magnesium, corticosteroids, antidysrythmics

• Bradycardia: digitalis

NURSING CONSIDERATIONS

Assess:

• VS, respiration during test

• Diabetic patient carefully since this drug lowers blood glucose

Administer:

• IV undiluted or given as continuous infusion

• Only with atropine sulfate available for cholinergic crisis

• Only after all other cholinergics have been discontinued

Perform/provide:

• Storage at room temperature

Evaluate:

• Therapeutic response: increased muscle strength, hand grasp, improved gait, absence of labored breathing (if severe)

Teach patient/family:

• To wear Medic Alert ID specifying myasthenia gravis, drugs taken

Treatment of overdose:

Respiratory support, atropine 1-4 mg (IV)

emetine HCl

(em'e-teen)

Func. class.: Amebicide

Chem. class.: Ipecac alkaloid

Action: Inhibits protein synthesis in developing trophozoites

Uses: Amebic dysentery (acute fulminating), amebic hepatitis, amebic abscess

Dosage and routes:

Amebic dysentery

• *Adult:* SC/IM 1 mg/kg/day, not to exceed 60 mg/day × 3-5 days simultaneously with another amebicide

• *Child:* IM 1 mg/kg/day in 2 divided doses × 5 days, not to exceed 60 mg/day

Amebic hepatitis/abscess

• *Adult:* SC/IM 60 mg/day × 10 days

• *Child:* IM 1 mg/kg in 2 doses × 5 days, not to exceed 60 mg/day (use only if other amebicides have failed)

Available forms include: Inj SC/IM 65 mg/ml

Side effects/adverse reactions:

CV: Hypotension, tachycardia, dysrhythmia, pericarditis, ECG abnormalities, ***CHF,*** chest pain, gallop rhythm, palpitations, hypotension, myocarditis, ***cardiac arrest,*** T wave inversion, increased QT, widening QRS

---

italics = common side effects   ***bold italic*** = life threatening reactions

HEMA: ***Thrombocytopenia***
INTEG: Rash, pruritus, necrosis, abscesses
GI: *Nausea, vomiting,* diarrhea, epigastric distress, anorexia
CNS: Weakness, tremors, aching, fatigue, depression, paresthesia, ***paralysis,*** encephalitis
Contraindications: Hypersensitivity, renal disease, hepatic disease, pregnancy (X)
Precautions: Elderly, lactation, surgery patients, hypotension, children
Pharmacokinetics:
SC/IM: Metabolized in liver, excreted in urine slowly over 40-60 days

NURSING CONSIDERATIONS
Assess:
• Stools during entire treatment; should be clear at end of therapy; stools must be clear for 1 yr before patient is considered cured
• ECG q2-3 days before, after 5th dose, after last therapy dose, 1 wk after; be aware that inversion of T waves occurs
• Vision by ophthalmalogic exam during, after therapy; vision problems occur often
• Injection site for irritation, absence of necrosis q8h
• I&O, stools for number, frequency, character
• B/P, pulse q4h; watch for decrease in B/P; discontinue
Administer:
• Being careful not to get drug in eyes; causes mucous membrane irritation
• Cleansing enema if ordered before beginning treatment
• SC or IM, never IV; rotate injection sites
• PO after meals to avoid GI symptoms

Perform/provide:
• Storage in tight, light-resistant container
Evaluate:
• Allergic reaction: fever, rash, itching, chills; drug should be discontinued if these occur
• Superimposed infection, fever, monilial growth, fatigue, malaise
• Tachycardia, decreasing B/P, GI symptoms, weakness, neuromuscular symptoms
• Diarrhea for 2-3 days
Teach patient/family:
• Proper hygiene after BM: handwashing technique
• Avoid contact of drug with eyes, mouth, nose, other mucous membranes
• Need for compliance with dosage schedule, duration of treatment

---

enalapril maleate
(en-al-a′prel)
Vasotec, Vasotec IV
Func. class.: Antihypertensive
Chem. class.: Renin-angiotensin antagonist

Action: Selectively suppresses renin-angiotensin-aldosterone system; inhibits ACE, prevents conversion of angiotensin I to angiotensin II, dilation of arterial, venous vessels
Uses: Hypertension
Dosage and routes:
• *Adult:* PO 5 mg/day, may increase or decrease to desired response range 10-40 mg/day
Hypertension
• *Adult:* IV 1.25 mg q6h over 5 min
Patients on diuretics
• *Adult:* IV 0.625 over 5 min, may give additional doses of 1.25 mg q6h

---

E

Renal impairment
• *Adult:* 1.25 mg q6hr with CrCl <3 mg/dl or 0.625 mg if CrCl >3 mg/dl

Available forms include: Tabs 5, 10, 20 mg, inj 1.25 mg/ml

Side effects/adverse reactions:
CV: Hypotension, chest pain, tachycardia, dysrhythmias

CNS: Insomnia, dizziness, paresthesias, headache, fatigue, anxiety

GI: Nausea, vomiting, colitis, cramps, diarrhea, constipation flatulence, dry mouth, loss of taste

INTEG: Rash, purpura, alopecia, hyperhidrosis

*HEMA: **Agranulocytosis, neutropenia***

EENT: Tinnitus, visual changes, sore throat, double vision, dry burning eyes

*GU: **Proteinuria, renal failure,*** increased frequency of polyurea or oliguria

RESP: Dyspnea, cough, rales, angioedema

META: Hyperkalemia

Contraindications: Pregnancy (C), lactation

Precautions: Renal disease, hyperkalemia

Pharmacokinetics:
PO: Peak 4-6 hr; half-life 1½ hr; metabolized by liver to active metabolite, excreted in urine

IV: Onset 5-15 min, peak up to 4 hr

Interactions/incompatibilities:
• Hypersensitivity: allopurinol
• Severe hypotension: diuretics, other antihypertensives
• Decreased effects of enalapril: aspirin, antacids
• Increased potassium levels: salt substitutes, potassium-sparing diuretics, potassium supplements
• May increase effects of: ergots, neuromuscular blocking agents, antihypertensives, hypoglycemics, barbiturates, reserpine, levodopa
• Effects may be increased by phenothiazines, diuretics, phenytoin, quinidine, nifedipine

NURSING CONSIDERATIONS
Assess:
• B/P, pulse q4h; note rate, rhythm, quality
• Electrolytes: K, Na, Cl
• Baselines in renal, liver function tests before therapy begins

Administer:
• By slow IV, over 5 min, use diluent provided or 50 ml of D_5W, 0.9% NaCl, 0.9% NaCl in D_5W or LR, Isolyte E

Evaluate:
• Edema in feet, legs daily
• Skin turgor, dryness of mucous membranes for hydration status
• Symptoms of CHF: edema, dyspnea, wet rales

Teach patient/family:
• Administer 1 hr before meals
• Not to use OTC (cough, cold, or allergy) products unless directed by physician
• Tell patient to avoid sunlight or wear sunscreen if in sunlight, photosensitivity may occur
• Stress patient compliance with dosage schedule, even if feeling better
• Notify physician of: mouth sores, sore throat, fever, swelling of hands or feet, irregular heartbeat, chest pain, signs of angioedema
• Excessive perspiration, dehydration, vomiting, diarrhea may lead to fall in blood pressure—consult physician if these occur
• May cause dizziness, fainting; light-headedness may occur during 1st few days of therapy
• May cause skin rash or impaired perspiration
• Not to discontinue drug abruptly

---

italics = common side effects   ***bold italic*** = life threatening reactions

• Not to use OTC products unless directed by physician
• To rise slowly to sitting or standing position to minimize orthostatic hypotension

Lab test interferences:
Interference: Glucose/insulin tolerance tests

Treatment of overdose: Lavage, IV atropine for bradycardia, IV theophylline for bronchospasm, digitalis, O_2, diuretic for cardiac failure, hemodialysis

---

encainide HCl

(en-kay'nide)
Enkaid

Func. class.: Antidysrhythmics—Class IC

Action: Unknown; able to slow conduction, reduce membrane responsiveness, inhibit automaticity, increase ratio of effective refractory period to action potential duration

Uses: Life-threatening dysrhythmias, frequent PVCs, sustained ventricular tachycardia

Dosage and routes:
• *Adult:* PO 25 mg q8h, then increase to 35 mg tid after 3-5 days, if needed, then increase to 50 mg tid after 3-5 more days if needed, not to exceed 75 mg qid

Available forms include: Caps 25, 35, 50 mg

Side effects/adverse reactions:
CV: Dysrhythmias, palpitations, CHF, chest pain, peripheral edema
CNS: Headache, dizziness, insomnia, anxiety, tremors, syncope
GI: Pain, constipation, diarrhea, *nausea, vomiting,* dyspepsia
RESP: Dyspnea, cough
EENT: Blurred vision, altered taste, tinnitus

MISC: Asthenia, paresthesia, skin rash, pain in extremities

Contraindications: 2-3 degree AV block, right bundle branch block, cardiogenic shock, hypersensitivity, symptomatic nonsustained ventricular dysrhythmias, frequent PVCs

Precautions: CHF, hypokalemia, hyperkalemia, sick-sinus syndrome, pregnancy (B), lactation, children, impaired hepatic, renal disease

Pharmacokinetics:
Peak ½-1½ hr, elimination via kidneys, active metabolites; half-life 1-2 hr

Interactions/incompatibilities:
• Increased effect of encainide: cimetidine, diuretics, other CV agents

NURSING CONSIDERATIONS
Assess:
• GI status: bowel pattern, number of stools
• Cardiac status: rate, rhythm, quality
• Chest x-ray, pulmonary function test during treatment
• I&O ratio; check for decreasing output
• B/P for fluctuations
• Lung fields; bilateral rales may occur in CHF patient
• Increased respiration, increased pulse; drug should be discontinued

Evaluate:
• Therapeutic response: absence of dysrhythmias
• Toxicity: fine tremors, dizziness
• Cardiac rate: respiration, rate, rhythm, character continuously

Lab test interferences:
Increase: CPK

Treatment of overdose: O_2, artificial ventilation, ECG, administer dopamine for circulatory depression, administer diazepam or thiopental for convulsions

---

ephedrine sulfate

(e-fed′rin)

Vatronol Nose Drops, Efedron Nasal

Func. class.: Nasal decongestant
Chem. class.: Indirect/direct sympathomimetic amine

Action: Relaxes bronchial smooth muscle, increases diameter of nasal passage by action on β-2 adrenergic receptors
Uses: Nasal congestion associated with colds, hayfever, sinusitis, other allergic conditions, adjunct in middle ear infections
Dosage and routes:
• *Adult and child:* INSTILL 3-4 gtts, q4h or small amount of gel in each nostril q4h
Available forms include: Sol 0.5% sulfate, gel 0.6% HCl
Side effects/adverse reactions:
GI: Nausea, vomiting, anorexia
EENT: Irritation, burning, sneezing, stinging, dryness, rebound congestion
INTEG: Contact dermatitis
CNS: Anxiety, restlessness, tremors, weakness, insomnia, dizziness, fever, headache
Contraindications: Hypersensitivity to sympathomimetic amines
Precautions: Child <6 yr, elderly, diabetes, cardiovascular disease, hypertension, hyperthyroidism, increase ICP, prostatic hypertrophy, pregnancy (C)
Interactions/incompatibilities:
• Hypertension: MAOIs, β-adrenergic blockers
• Hypotension: methyldopa, mecamylamine, reserpine

NURSING CONSIDERATIONS
Administer:
• No more than q4h
• For <4 consecutive days
Perform/provide:
• Environmental humidification to decrease nasal congestion, dryness
• Storage in light-resistant containers; do not expose to high temperatures
Evaluate:
• Redness, swelling, pain in nasal passages
Teach patient/family:
• Stinging may occur for a few applications; drying of mucosa may be decreased by environmental humidification
• To notify physician if irregular pulse, insomnia, dizziness, or tremors occur
• Proper administration to avoid systemic absorption

---

ephedrine sulfate

(e-fed′rin)

Efedrin, Vatronol

Func. class.: Adrenergic, mixed direct and indirect effects
Chem. class.: Phenylisopropylamine

Action: Causes increased contractility and heart rate by acting on β-receptors in the heart; also, acts on α-receptors, causing vasoconstriction in blood vessels
Uses: Shock, increase perfusion, hypotension, bronchodilation
Dosage and routes:
• *Adult:* IM/SC 25-50 mg, not to exceed 150 mg/24 hr
IV 10-25 mg, not to exceed 150 mg/24 hr
• *Child:* SC/IV 3 mg/kg/day in divided doses q4-6h

---

italics = common side effects   ***bold italic*** = life threatening reactions

Bronchodilator
- *Adult:* PO 12.5-50 mg bid-qid, not to exceed 400 mg/day
- *Child:* PO 2-3 mg/kg/day in 4-6 divided doses

Available forms include: Inj 25, 50 mg/ml, IM, SC, IV; caps 25, 50 mg; syr 11, 20 mg/5 ml

Side effects/adverse reactions:

CNS: Tremors, anxiety, insomnia, headache, dizziness, confusion, hallucinations, ***convulsions, CNS depression***

GU: Dysuria, urinary retention

CV: Palpitations, tachycardia, hypertension, chest pain, ***dysrhythmias***

GI: Anorexia, nausea, vomiting

RESP: ***Dyspnea***

Contraindications: Hypersensitivity to sympathomimetics, narrow-angle glaucoma

Precautions: Pregnancy (C), cardiac disorders, hyperthyroidism, diabetes mellitus, prostatic hypertrophy

Pharmacokinetics:

PO: Onset 15-60 min, duration 2-4 hr

IV: Onset 5 min, duration 2 hr

Metabolized in liver, excreted in urine (unchanged), crosses blood-brain barrier, placenta, breast milk

Interactions/incompatibilities:
- Do not use with MAOIs or tricyclic antidepressants; hypertensive crisis may occur
- Decreased effect of ephedrine: methyldopa, urinary acidifiers, rauwolfia alkaloids
- Increased effect of this drug: urinary alkalizers
- Dysrhythmia: halothane, anesthetics, digitalis
- Decreased effect of: guanethidine

NURSING CONSIDERATIONS

Assess:
- I&O ratio

- ECG during administration continuously, if B/P increases, drug is decreased
- B/P and pulse q5 min after parenteral route
- CVP or PWP during infusion if possible

Administer:
- IV undiluted given through Y-tube or 3-way stopcock; give 10 mg or less over 1 min
- Plasma expanders for hypovolemia

Perform/provide:
- Storage of reconstituted solution if refrigerated for no longer than 24 hr
- Do not use discolored solutions

Evaluate:
- For paresthesias and coldness of extremities, peripheral blood flow may decrease
- Injection site: tissue sloughing if this occurs administer phentolamine mixed with NS
- Therapeutic response: increased B/P with stabilization

Teach patient/family:
- Reason for drug administration

Treatment of overdose: Administer phentolamine for hypertension, diazepam for convulsions

---

epinephrine/ epinephrine bitartrate/ epinephrine HCl

(ep-i-nef′rin)

Bronkaid Mist, Primatene Mist/ AsthmaHaler, Medihaler-Epi/ Adrenalin, Sus-Phrine, Vaponefrin*

Func. class.: Adrenergic
Chem. class.: Catecholamine

Action: β₁ and β₂ agonist causing increased levels of cyclic AMP producing bronchodilation, cardiac, and CNS stimulation; large doses cause vaso-constriction; small doses can cause vasodilation via β₂-vascular receptors

Uses: Acute asthmatic attacks, hemostasis, bronchospasm, anaphylaxis, allergic reactions, cardiac arrest

Dosage and routes:
• *Adult:* IM/SC 0.1-0.5 ml of 1:1000 sol, may repeat q10-15 min IV 0.1-0.25 ml of 1:1000 sol
• *Child:* SC 0.01 ml of 1:1000/kg, may repeat q20 min to 4 hr; INH 0.005 ml/kg of 1:200 solution, may repeat q8-12h

Asthma
• *Adult and child:* INH 1-2 puffs of 1:100 or 2.25% racemic q1-5 min

Hemostasis
• *Adult:* TOP 1:50,000-1:1000 applied as needed to stop bleeding

Cardiac arrest
• *Adult:* IC 0.5-1 mg followed by IV INF at 1-4 μg/min
• *Child:* IC 10 μg/kg or 5-10 μg/kg

Available forms include: Aerosol 0.16 mg/spray, 0.2 mg/spray, 0.25 mg/spray, inj 1:1000 (1 mg/ml), 1:200 (5 mg/ml) IM, IV, SC; sol for nebulization 1:100, 1.25% 2.25% (base)

Side effects/adverse reactions:
GU: Urinary retention
CNS: Tremors, anxiety, insomnia, headache, dizziness, confusion, hallucinations, ***cerebral hemorrhage***
CV: Palpitations, tachycardia, hypertension, *dysrhythmias,* increase T-wave
GI: Anorexia, nausea, vomiting
RESP: Dyspnea

Contraindications: Hypersensitivity to sympathomimetics, narrow-angle glaucoma

Precautions: Pregnancy (C), cardiac disorders, hyperthyroidism, diabetes mellitus, prostatic hypertrophy

Pharmacokinetics:
SC: Onset 3-5 min, duration 20 min
PO, INH: Onset 1 min

Interactions/incompatibilities:
• Do not use with MAOIs or tricyclic antidepressants; hypertensive crisis may occur
• Decreased effect of epinephrine: methyldopa, urinary acidifiers, rauwolfia alkaloids
• Increased effect of epinephrine: urinary alkalizers

NURSING CONSIDERATIONS
Assess:
• ECG during administration continuously; if B/P increases, drug is decreased
• B/P and pulse q5 min after parenteral route
• CVP or PWP during infusion if possible

Administer:
• Parenteral IV dose slowly, after reconstituting 1 mg (1:1000 sol)/10 ml or more normal saline; for maintenance may be further diluted in 500 ml D₅W; give 1 mg or less over 1 min or more through Y-tube or 3-way stopcock

Perform/provide:
• Storage of reconstituted sol if refrigerated for no longer than 24 hr
• Do not use discolored solutions

Evaluate:
• Injection site: tissue sloughing; if this occurs administer phentolamine mixed with NS
• Therapeutic response: increased B/P with stabilization or ease of breathing

Teach patient/family:
• Reason for drug administration

---

italics = common side effects   ***bold italic*** = life threatening reactions

- To rinse mouth after use to prevent dryness
- Not to take OTC preparations

Treatment of overdose: Administer an α-blocker, and a β blocker

---

epinephrine bitartrate/ epinephrine HCl/ epinephryl borate (optic)

(ep-i-nef'rin)

Epitrate, Mytrate/Epifrin, Glaucon/Epinal, Eppy*

Func. class.: Mydriatic
Chem. class.: Sympathomimetic amine

Action: Blocks response of iris sphincter muscle, muscle of accommodation of ciliary body to cholinergic stimulation, resulting in dilation, paralysis of accommodation

Uses: During ocular surgery, open-angle glaucoma

Dosage and routes:
- *Adult and child:* INTRAOCULAR INJ 0.1-0.2 ml of a 0.01 or 0.1% sol (HCl); INSTILL SOL 1-2 gtts of a 1%-2% sol, determined by tonometric reading (Bitartrate); 1 gtt of a 0.5%-2% sol (HCl) or 0.5%-1% (Borate)

During surgery
- *Adult and child:* INSTILL SOL 1 or more gtts of a 0.1% sol (HCl) up to 3 × /day

Available forms include: Sol 0.1% (HCl)

Side effects/adverse reactions:
CV: Palpitations, tachycardia
EENT: Blurred vision, eye pain, ocular irritation, and tearing

Contraindications: Hypersensitivity to sympathomimetic amines, narrow-angle glaucoma, dysrhyth-

mias, cardiogenic shock, cerebral arteriosclerosis

Precautions: Elderly, prostatic hypertrophy, diabetes mellitus, hyperthymus, TB, Parkinson's disease, pregnancy (C)

Pharmacokinetics:
INSTILL: Onset 1 hr, peak 4-8 hr, duration 12-24 hr

Interactions/incompatibilities:
- Dysrhythmias: cyclopropane, halogenated hydrocarbons
- Increased pressor effects: tricyclic antidepressants, antihistamines, beta-blockers, MAOIs

NURSING CONSIDERATIONS
Assess:
- Tonometer readings during long-term treatment
- B/P, pulse, respirations

Evaluate:
- Allergic reaction: itching, edema of eyelids, eye discharge; drug should be discontinued

Teach patient/family:
- To report change in vision, blurring or loss of sight, trouble breathing, sweating, pallor
- Method of instillation: pressure on lacrimal sac for 1 min, do not touch dropper to eye
- That long-term therapy may be required if using for glaucoma
- Check OTC drugs for other sympathetic nervous system stimulants (e.g., phenylephrine)

---

epinephrine HCl (nasal)

(ep-i-nef'rin)

Adrenalin Chloride

Func. class.: Nasal decongestant
Chem. class.: Sympathomimetic amine

Action: Relaxes bronchial smooth muscle, increases diameter of nasal passage by action on β-adrenergics

---

Uses: Nasal congestion, superficial bleeding

Dosage and routes:

• *Adult and child >6 yr old:* TOP apply to affected area with sterile swab

Available forms include: Sol 0.1%

Side effects/adverse reactions:

GI: Nausea, vomiting, anorexia

EENT: Irritation, burning, sneezing, stinging, dryness, rebound congestion

INTEG: Contact dermatitis

CNS: Anxiety, restlessness, tremors, weakness, insomnia, dizziness, fever, headache

Contraindications: Hypersensitivity to sympathomimetic amines

Precautions: Child <6 yr, elderly, diabetes, cardiovascular disease, hypertension, hyperthyroidism, increased ICP, prostatic hypertrophy, pregnancy (C)

Interactions/incompatibilities:

• Hypertension: MAOIs, β-adrenergic blockers

• Hypotension: methyldopa, mecamylamine, reserpine

NURSING CONSIDERATIONS

Administer:

• No more than q4h

• For <4 consecutive days

Perform/provide:

• Environmental humidification to decrease nasal congestion, dryness

• Storage in light-resistant containers; do not expose to high temperatures

Evaluate:

• For redness, swelling, pain in nasal passages

Teach patient/family:

• Stinging may occur for a few applications; drying of mucosa may be decreased by environmental humidification

• To notify physician if irregular pulse, insomnia, dizziness, or tremors occur

• Proper administration to avoid systemic absorption

---

ergoloid mesylate

(er′goe-loid mess′i-late)

Deapril-ST, Gerimal, Hydergine, Hydroloid-G, Niloric

Func. class.: Migraine agent

Chem. class.: Ergot alkaloid–amino acid

Action: May increase cerebral metabolism and blood flow

Uses: Senile dementia, Alzheimer's dementia, multiinfarct dementia, primary progressive dementia

Dosage and routes:

• *Adult:* PO/SL 1 mg tid, may increase to 4.5-12 mg/day

Available forms include: Tabs SL 0.5, 1 mg, tabs 1 mg, cap 1 mg, liquid 1 mg/ml

Side effects/adverse reactions:

GI: Nausea, vomiting, sublingual irritation

Contraindications: Hypersensitivity to ergot preparations; psychosis

Precautions: Acute intermittent porphyria, pregnancy (C)

Pharmacokinetics:

PO: Peak 1 hr; metabolized in liver, excreted as metabolites in feces, crosses blood-brain barrier; half-life 3½ hr

NURSING CONSIDERATIONS

Assess:

• Weigh daily, check for peripheral edema in feet, legs

• B/P and pulse, check regularly

Administer:

• With meals or after meals to avoid GI symptoms; do not crush or chew SL tab

---

italics = common side effects   ***bold italic*** = life threatening reactions

Perform/provide:
• Storage in well-closed container at room temperature
Evaluate:
• Therapeutic response: decreased forgetfulness, increased mental alertness and ability for self-care
• Neurological status: LOC, blurring vision, nausea, vomiting, tingling in extremities that occur preceding the headache
• Toxicity: dyspnea; hypotension or hypertension; rapid, weak pulse; delirium; nausea; vomiting; bradycardia
Teach family/patient:
• To change positions slowly, and to move extremities before walking
• To maintain dosage at approved level, not to increase drug
• To report side effects, including increased vasoconstriction starting with cold extremities, then paresthesia, weakness
• That 6 months of treatment may be required, some improvement occurs in one month
• Keep drug out of reach of children, death may occur
Treatment of overdose: Induce emesis if orally ingested, or gastric lavage, administer saline cathartic, keep warm

---

ergonovine maleate

(er-goe-noe′veen)
Ergotrate Maleate
Func. class.: Oxytocic
Chem. class.: Ergot alkaloid

Action: Stimulates uterine contractions, decreases bleeding
Uses: Treatment of hemorrhage associated with postpartum or postabortion
Dosage and routes:
• *Adult:* IM 0.2 mg q2-4h, not to

exceed 5 doses; IV 0.2 mg given over 1 min; PO 0.2-0.4 mg q6-12h × 2-7 days after initial IM or IV dose
Available forms include: Inj IM, IV 0.2 mg/ml; tabs 0.2 mg
Side effects/adverse reactions:
CNS: Headache, dizziness, fainting
CV: Hypertension, chest pain
GI: Nausea, vomiting
INTEG: Sweating
RESP: Dyspnea
EENT: Tinnitus
GU: Cramping
Contraindications: Hypersensitivity to ergot medication, augmentation of labor, before delivery of placenta, spontaneous abortion (threatened), pelvic inflammatory disease (PID)
Precautions: Hepatic disease, renal disease, cardiac disease, asthma, anemia, convulsive disorders, hypertension, glaucoma, obliterative vascular disease
Pharmacokinetics:
PO: Onset 5-25 min, duration 3 hr
IM: Onset 2-5 min, duration 3 hr
IV: Onset immediate, duration 45 min
Metabolized in liver, excreted in urine
Interactions/incompatibilities:
• Hypertension: sympathomimetics, ergots
NURSING CONSIDERATIONS
Assess:
• B/P, pulse; watch for change that may indicate hemorrhage
• Respiratory rate, rhythm, depth; notify physician of abnormalities
• Fundal tone, nonphasic contractions, check for relaxation
Administer:
• IV undiluted through Y-tube or 3-way stopcock
• IM in deep muscle mass, rotate

---

injection sites if additional doses are given

• After having crash cart available on unit

Evaluate:

• Therapeutic response: decreased blood loss, severe cramping

Teach patient/family:

• To report increased blood loss, increased temperature or foul-smelling lochia, that cramping is normal

---

ergotamine tartrate

(er-got′a-meen)

Ergomar, Ergostat, Gynergen, Medihaler-Ergotamine, Wigrettes

Func. class.: α-Adrenergic blocker

Chem. class.: Ergot alkaloid-amino acid

Action: Constricts smooth muscle in peripheral, cranial blood vessels, relaxes uterine muscle

Uses: Vascular headache (migraine or histamine)

Dosage and routes:

• *Adult:* 2 mg, then 1-2 mg qh or q½ hr for SL, not to exceed 6 mg/day or 10 mg/wk; INH 1 puff, may repeat in 5 min, not to exceed 6/24 hr

Available forms include: SL tabs 2 mg; tabs 1 mg; oral inh 360 μg/dose

Side effects/adverse reactions:

CNS: Numbness in fingers, toes, headache, weakness

CV: Transient tachycardia, chest pain, bradycardia, edema, claudication, increase or decrease in B/P

GI: Nausea, vomiting

MS: Muscle pain

Contraindications: Hypersensitivity to ergot preparations, occlusion (peripheral, vascular), CAD, hepatic disease, renal disease, peptic ulcer, hypertension, pregnancy (X)

Precautions: Lactation, children, anemia

Pharmacokinetics:

PO: Peak 30 min-3 hr; metabolized in liver, excreted as metabolites in feces, crosses blood-brain barrier, excreted in breast milk

Interactions/incompatibilities:

• Increased effects: troleandomycin

• Increased vasoconstriction: β-blockers

NURSING CONSIDERATIONS

Assess:

• Weight daily, check for peripheral edema in feet, legs

• Check for coldness of extremities and tingling of fingers, drug should be discontinued

Administer:

• At beginning of headache, dose must be titrated to patient response

• By SL route if possible for better, faster absorption

• With meals or after meals to avoid GI symptoms

• Only to women who are not pregnant, harm to fetus may occur

Perform/provide:

• Quiet, calm environment with decreased stimulation for noise, or bright light or excessive talking

Evaluate:

• Therapeutic response: decrease in frequency, severity of headache

• For stress level, activity, recreation, coping mechanisms of patient

• Neurological status: LOC, blurring vision, nausea, vomiting, tingling in extremities that occur preceding the headache

• Ingestion of tyramine foods (pickled products, beer, wine, aged cheese), food additives, preservatives, colorings, artificial sweeteners, chocolate, caffeine, which

---

italics = common side effects   ***bold italic*** = life threatening reactions

may precipitate these types of headaches
• Toxicity: dyspnea, hypotension or hypertension, rapid, weak pulse, delirium, nausea, vomiting
Teach patient/family:
• Not to use OTC medications, serious drug interactions may occur
• To maintain dose at approved level, not to increase even if drug does not relieve headache
• To report side effects including increased vasoconstriction starting with cold extremities, then paresthesia, weakness
• That an increase in headaches may occur when this drug is discontinued after long-term use
• Keep drug out of reach of children, death may occur
Treatment of overdose: Induce emesis if orally ingested, orgastric lavage, administer saline cathartic, keep warm

---

erythrityl tetranitrate
(e-ri′thri-till)
Cardilate
Func. class.: Vasodilator, coronary
Chem. class.: Nitrate

Action: Decreases preload, afterload, which is responsible for decreasing left ventricular end diastolic pressure, systemic vascular resistance, improve exercise tolerance
Uses: Chronic stable angina pectoris, prophylaxis of angina pain
Dosage and routes:
• *Adult:* PO 10-30 mg tid; SL 5-15 mg before stress
Available forms include: Chew tabs 10 mg; tabs PO, SL 5, 10 mg
Side effects/adverse reactions:
CV: Postural hypotension, tachycardia, ***collapse,*** syncope

GI: Nausea, vomiting
INTEG: Pallor, sweating, rash
*CNS: Headache, flushing, dizziness **weakness, fainting***
MISC: Twitching, hemolytic anemia, ***methemoglobinemia***
Contraindications: Hypersensitivity to this drug or nitrites, severe anemia, increased intracranial pressure, cerebral hemorrhage, acute MI
Precautions: Postural hypotension, pregnancy (C), lactation, children
Pharmacokinetics:
PO: Onset 30 min, peak 1-1½ hr, duration 6 hr
SL: Onset 5-10 min, peak 30-45 min, duration 3 hr
Metabolized by liver, excreted in urine
Interactions/incompatibilities:
• Increased effects: β-blockers, diuretics, antihypertensives, alcohol
NURSING CONSIDERATIONS
Assess:
• B/P, supine and sitting, pulse, respirations during beginning therapy
Administer:
• With 8 oz of water on empty stomach (oral tablet)
Evaluate:
• Pain: duration, time started, activity being performed, character
• Tolerance if taken over long period of time
• Headache, lightheadedness, decreased B/P; may indicate a need for decreased dosage
Teach patient/family:
• Keep tabs in original container
• If 3 SL tabs do not relieve pain, get to ER
• Avoid alcohol
• May cause headache; tolerance occurs over time
• That drug may be taken before

---

stressful activity: exercise, sexual activity
• That SL may sting when drug comes in contact with mucous membranes
• To avoid hazardous activities if dizziness occurs
• Stress patient compliance with complete medical regimen
• To make position changes slowly to prevent fainting

---

erythromycin (ophthalmic)

(er-ith-roe-mye′sin)
Ilotycin Ophthalmic
Func. class.: Antiinfective

Action: Inhibits bacterial protein synthesis
Uses: Infection of eye
Dosage and routes:
• *Adult and child:* Apply oint qd-qid as needed
Ophthalmia neonatorum
• *Neonates:* Apply oint to conjunctival sacs immediately after delivery
Available forms include: Oint 0.5%
Side effects/adverse reactions:
EENT: Poor corneal wound healing, temporary visual haze, overgrowth of nonsusceptible organisms
Contraindications: Hypersensitivity
Precautions: Antibiotic hypersensitivity
NURSING CONSIDERATIONS
Administer:
• After washing hands, cleanse crusts or discharge from eye before application
Perform/provide:
• Storage at room temperature, in tight container

Evaluate:
• Therapeutic response: absence of redness, inflammation, tearing
• Allergy: itching, lacrimation, redness, swelling
Teach patient/family:
• To use drug exactly as prescribed
• Not to use eye makeup, towels, washcloths, eye medication of others; reinfection may occur
• That drug container tip should not be touched to eye
• To report itching, increased redness, burning, stinging, swelling; drug should be discontinued
• That drug may cause blurred vision when ointment is applied

---

erythromycin (topical)

(er-ith-roe-mye′sin)
Akne-mycin, A/T/S, Eryderm, Staticin
Func. class.: Local antiinfective
Chem. class.: Macrolide antibacterial

Action: Interferes with bacterial protein synthesis
Uses: Pyoderma, acne vulgaris
Dosage and routes:
• Adult and child: TOP apply to affected area tid-qid
Available forms include: Top sol, ointment 1.5%, 2%
Side effects/adverse reactions:
INTEG: Rash, urticaria, stinging, burning, pruritus, dry or oily skin
EENT: Eye irritation, tenderness
Contraindications: Hypersensitivity
Precautions: Pregnancy (C), lactation
Interactions/incompatibilities:
Avoid use with clindamycin, abrasive agents, acids, alkaline media

---

NURSING CONSIDERATIONS
Administer:
- Enough medication to completely cover lesions
- After cleansing with soap, water before each application, dry well

Perform/provide:
- Storage at room temperature in dry place

Evaluate:
- Allergic reaction: burning, stinging, swelling, redness
- Therapeutic response: decrease in size, number of lesions

Teach patient/family:
- To apply with glove to prevent further infection
- To avoid use of OTC creams, ointments, lotions unless directed by physician
- To use medical asepsis (hand washing) before, after each application
- To avoid use near eyes, nose, mouth
- To monitor for superimposed infection

---

erythromycin base, erythromycin estolate, erythromycin ethylsuccinate, erythromycin glucceptate, erythromycin lactobionate, erythromycin stearate

(er-ith-roe-mye'sin)

E-Mycin, ERYC, Ery-Tab, Erythromid,* Ethril, Ilotycin, Novorythro,* Robimycin, Staticin, Ilosone, E.E.S., Erythrocin, Pediamycin, Wyamycin Liquid, E-Biotic, Erypar, Wintrocin, Wyamycin

Func. class.: Antibacterial
Chem. class.: Macrolide antibiotic

Action: Binds to 50S ribosomal subunits of susceptible bacteria and suppresses protein synthesis

Uses: Infections caused by *N. gonorrhoeae,* mild to moderate respiratory tract, skin, soft tissue infections caused by *D. pneumoniae, M. pneumoniae, C. diphtheriae, B. pertussis, L. monocytogenes,* syphilis, Legionnaire's disease, *C. trachomatis, H. influenzae*

Dosage and routes:
Soft tissue infections
- *Adult:* PO 250-500 mg q6h (base, estolate, stearate); PO 400-800 mg q6h (ethylsuccinate); IV INF 15-20 mg/kg/day (lactobionate)
- *Child:* PO 30-50 mg/kg/day in divided doses q6h (salts); IV 15-20 mg/kg/day in divided doses q4-6h (lactobionate)

N. gonorrhoeae/PID
- *Adult:* IV 500 mg q6h × 3 days (glucceptate, lactobionate), then PO 250 mg (base, estolate, stearate) or 400 mg (ethylsuccinate) q6h × 1 wk

Syphilis
Adult: PO 20 g in divided doses over 15 days (base, estolate, stearate)

Chlamydia
- *Adult:* PO 500 mg q6h × 1 wk or 250 mg qid × 2 wk
- *Infant:* PO 50 mg/kg/day in 4 divided doses × 3 wk or more
- *Newborn:* PO 50 mg/kg/day in 4 divided doses × 2 wk or more

Intestinal amebiasis
- *Adult:* PO 250 mg q6h × 10-14 days (base, estolate, stearate)
- *Child:* PO 30-50 mg/kg/day in divided doses q6h × 10-14 days (base, estolate, stearate)

Available forms include: Base: tabs, enteric-coated 250, 333, 500 mg; tabs film-coated 250, 500 mg; caps, enteric-coated 125, 250 mg; estolate: tabs chewable 125, 250

mg; tabs 500 mg; caps 125, 250 mg; drops 100 mg/ml; susp 125, 250 mg/5ml; stearate: tabs, film-coated 250, 500 mg; ethylsuccinate: tabs, chewable 200 mg; tabs, film-coated 400 mg/2.5 ml, 200, 400 mg/5 ml; susp 200, 400 mg powder for suspension 100 mg/2.5 ml, 200 and 400 mg/5 ml powder for inj 500 mg and 1 g (lactobionate), 250 mg, 500 mg, 1 g (as gluceptate)

Side effects/adverse reactions:

INTEG: Rash, urticaria, pruritus

GI: Nausea, vomiting, diarrhea, ***hepatotoxicity,*** abdominal pain, stomatitis, heartburn, anorexia, pruritus ani

GU: Vaginitis, moniliasis

EENT: Hearing loss, tinnitus

Contraindications: Hypersensitivity

Precautions: Pregnancy (C), hepatic disease, lactation

Pharmacokinetics: Peak 4 hr, duration 6 hr, half-life 1-3 hr, metabolized in liver, excreted in bile, feces

Interactions/incompatabilities:

• Increased action of: oral anticoagulants, digitalis, theophylline, methylprednisolone, cyclosporine

• Decreased action of: clindamycin, penicillins

• Toxicity: carbamazepine

NURSING CONSIDERATIONS

Assess:

• I&O ratio; report hematuria, oliguria in renal disease

• Liver studies: AST, ALT

• Renal studies: urinalysis, protein, blood

• C&S before drug therapy; drug may be taken as soon as culture is taken; C&S may be repeated after treatment

Administer:

• IV after diluting 500 mg or less/

10 ml sterile H$_2$O without preservatives; dilute further in 80-250 ml of compatible sol; may be further diluted to 1 mg/ml and given as continuous infusion; run 1 g or less/100 ml over ½-1 hr; continuous infusion over 6 hr

• Enteric-coated tablets may be given with food

Perform/provide:

• Storage at room temperature

• Adequate intake of fluids (2000 ml) during diarrhea episodes

Evaluate:

• Bowel pattern before, during treatment

• Skin eruptions, itching

• Respiratory status: rate, character, wheezing, tightness in chest; discontinue drug if these occur

• Allergies before treatment, reaction of each medication; place allergies on chart, Kardex in bright red letters; notify all people giving drugs

Teach patient/family:

• To take oral drug with full glass of water; may give with food if GI symptoms occur

• Do not take with fruit juice

• To report sore throat, fever, fatigue; could indicate superimposed infection

• To notify nurse of diarrhea stools, dark urine, pale stools, yellow discoloration of eyes or skin, and severe abdominal pain

• To take at evenly spaced intervals; complete dosage regimen

Lab test interferences:

False increase: 17-OHCS/17-KS, AST/ALT

Decrease: Folate assay

Treatment of overdose: Withdraw drug, maintain airway, administer epinephrine, aminophylline, O$_2$, IV corticosteroids

---

italics = common side effects   ***bold italic*** = life threatening reactions

erythropoietin recombinant

(er-ith-row-poe'-ee-tin)
rHU-EPO, eprex*
Func. class.: Hormone
Chem. class.: Amino acid polypeptide

Action: Erythropoietin is one factor controlling rate of red cell production; drug is developed by recombinant DNA technology

Uses: Anemia caused by reduced endogenous erythropoietin production, primarily end-stage renal disease; to correct hemostatic defect in uremia

Dosage and routes:
• *Adult:* IV 5-500 U/kg 3 × /wk

Side effects/adverse reactions:
CV: Hypertension, **hypertension encephalopathy**
CNS: **Seizures,** coldness, sweating
MS: Bone pain

Contraindications: Hypersensitivity

Pharmacokinetics:
IV: Metabolized in body, extent of metabolism unknown, onset of increased reticulocyte count 1-2 wk

NURSING CONSIDERATIONS

Assess:
• Renal studies: urinalysis, protein, blood, BUN, creatinine
• Blood studies: reticulocyte count weekly
• I&O, report drop in output to <50 ml/hr
• CNS symptoms: coldness, sweating
• CV status: B/P; hypertension may occur rapidly leading to hypertension encephalopathy

Evaluate:
• Therapeutic response: increase in reticulocyte count in 1-2 wk, increased appetite, enhanced sense of well-being

esmolol HCl

(ess'moe-lol)
Brevibloc
Func. class.: β-Adrenergic blocker

Action: Competitively blocks stimulation of β_1-adrenergic receptors in the myocardium; produces negative chronotropic, inotropic activity (decreases rate of SA node discharge, increases recovery time), slows conduction of AV node, decreases heart rate, decreases O_2 consumption in myocardium; also, decreases renin-aldosterone-angiotensin system at high doses, inhibits β-2 receptors in bronchial system slightly

Uses: Supraventricular tachycardia, noncompensatory tachycardia

Dosage and routes:
• *Adult:* IV loading dose—500 µg/kg/min for 1 min; maintenance—50 µg/kg/min for 4 min; may repeat q5min

Available forms include: Inj IV 10 mg, 250 mg/ml

Side effects/adverse reactions:
INTEG: Induration, inflammation at site, discoloration, edema, erythema, burning pallor, flushing, rash, pruritus, dry skin, alopecia
CNS: Confusion, lightheadedness, paresthesia, somnolence, fever, dizziness, fatigue, headache, depression, anxiety
GI: Nausea, vomiting, anorexia, gastric pain, flatulence, constipation, heartburn, bloating
CV: Hypotension, bradycardia, chest pain, peripheral ischemia, shortness of breath, CHF, conduction disturbances

---

* Available in Canada only

GU: Urinary retention, impotence, dysuria

*RESP: **Bronchospasm,*** dyspnea, cough, wheeziness, nasal stuffiness

Contraindications: Second- or third-degree heart block, cardiogenic shock, CHF, cardiac failure, hypersensitivity

Precautions: Hypotension, pregnancy (C), peripheral vascular disease, diabetes, hypoglycemia, thyrotoxicosis, renal disease, lactation

Pharmacokinetics:
Metabolized in liver, excreted via kidneys

Interactions/incompatibilities:
• Increased digoxin levels: digoxin
• Increased esmolol levels: morphine
• Do not mix with other drugs in syringe or solution
• Reversal of esmolol effects: isoproterenol, norepinephrine, dopamine, dobutamine
• Increased effects of both drugs: disopyramide
• Increased effects of lidocaine

NURSING CONSIDERATIONS
Assess:
• I&O ratio, weight daily
• B/P, pulse q4h; note rate, rhythm, quality; rapid changes can cause shock; if systolic >100 or diastolic <60, notify physician before giving drug
• Apical/radial pulse before administration; notify physician if less than 60 bpm
• Baselines in renal, liver function tests before therapy begins
• Breath sounds and respiratory pattern

Administer:
• Reduced dosage in cool environment
• IV diluted 5 g/20 ml of compatible sol; further dilute in the remaining 480 ml and give as infusion

Perform/provide:
• Storage protected from light, moisture; place in cool environment

Evaluate:
• Therapeutic response: decreased B/P immediately
• Respiratory pattern: wheezing from bronchospasm
• Edema in feet, legs daily
• Skin turgor, dryness of mucous membranes for hydration status

Lab test interferences:
Interference: Glucose/insulin tolerance test

Treatment of overdose: Discontinue drug

---

essential crystalline amino acid solution

Aminosyn-RF, Nephramine, Ren-Amine 6.5

Func. class.: Nitrogen product

Action: Needed for anabolism to maintain structure, decrease catabolism, promote healing

Uses: Renal decompensation

Dosage and routes:
• *Adult:* CENT IV 0.3-0.5 g/kg, 250 ml of amino acid/500 ml D70, given at rate of 20-30 ml/hr, increased by 10 ml/hr q24h, not to exceed 100 ml/hr
• *Child:* CENT IV 1 g/kg/day or less, depending on patient's needs

Available forms include: Inj central line only, many types

Side effects/adverse reactions:
CNS: Dizziness, *headache,* confusion, ***loss of consciousness***
CV: Hypertension, ***CHF, pulmonary edema***
GI: Nausea, vomiting, liver fat deposits, abdominal pain

---

italics = common side effects   ***bold italic*** = life threatening reactions

GU: Glycosuria, osmotic diuresis
ENDO: Hyperglycemia, rebound hypoglycemia, electrolyte imbalances, hyperosmolar syndrome, hyperosmolar hyperglycemic non-ketotic syndrome, alkalosis, acidosis, hypophosphatemia, hyperammonemia, dehydration, hypocalcemia
INTEG: Chills, flushing, warm feeling, rash, urticaria, extravasation necrosis, phlebitis at injection site
Contraindications: Hypersensitivity, severe electrolyte imbalances, anuria, severe liver damage, maple syrup urine disease, PKU
Precautions: Renal disease, pregnancy (C), children, diabetes mellitus, CHF

NURSING CONSIDERATIONS
Assess:
• Electrolytes (K, Na, Ca, Cl, Mg), blood glucose, ammonia, phosphate
• Renal, liver function studies: BUN, creatinine, ALT, AST, bilirubin
• Injection site for extravasation: redness along vein, edema at site, necrosis, pain, hard tender area, site should be changed immediately
• Monitor respiratory function q4h: auscultate lung fields bilaterally for rales, respirations, quality, rate, rhythm
• Monitor temperature q4h for increased fever, indicating infection; if infection suspected, infusion is discontinued, tubing, bottle cultured
• Urine glucose q6h using Tes-Tape, Clinistix, Keto-Diastix, which are not affected by infusion substances
Administer:
• TPN must be used only mixed with dextrose to promote protein synthesis

• Immediately after mixing in pharmacy under strict aseptic technique using laminar flowhood; use infusion pump, in-line filter
• Using careful monitoring technique; do not speed up infusion; pulmonary edema, glucose overload will result
Perform/provide:
• Storage depends on type of solution, consult manufacturer
• Changing dressing, IV tubing to prevent infection q24-48h
Evaluate:
• Hyperammonemia: nausea, vomiting, malaise, tremors, anorexia, convulsions
• Therapeutic response: weight gain, decreased jaundice in liver disorders, increased serum albumin
Teach patient/family:
• Reason for use of TPN
• If chills, sweating are experienced, they should be reported at once

---

estazolam
ProSom

Func. class.: Sedative-hypnotic
Chem. class.: Benzodiazepine derivative

Controlled Substance Schedule IV (US)
Action: Produces CNS depression at the limbic, thalamic, hypothalamic levels of the CNS; may be mediated by neurotransmitter γ-aminobutyric acid (GABA); results are sedation, hypnosis, skeletal muscle relaxation, anticonvulsant activity, anxiolytic action
Uses: Insomnia
Dosage and routes:
Adult: PO 1-2 mg hs
Available forms include: Tabs 1 mg

Side effects/adverse reactions:
INTEG: Dermatitis, allergy, sweating, flushing, pruritus
*HEMA: **Leukopenia, granulocytopenia** (rare)*
CNS: Lethargy, drowsiness, daytime sedation, dizziness, confusion, lightheadedness, headache, anxiety, irritability, weakness, tremors, depression, lack of coordination
GI: Nausea, vomiting, diarrhea, heartburn, abdominal pain, constipation, anorexia, taste alteration
CV: Chest pain, pulse changes, palpitations, tachycardia
MISC: Joint pain, congestion
Contraindications: Hypersensitivity to benzodiazepines, pregnancy (X), sleep apnea
Precautions: Hepatic disease, renal disease, suicidal individuals, drug abuse, elderly, psychosis, child <18, lactation, depression, pulmonary insufficiency
Pharmacokinetics: Onset 15-45 min, peaks 1½-2 hr, duration 7-8 hr; metabolized by liver, excreted by kidneys (inactive/active metabolites), crosses placenta, excreted in breast milk
Interactions/incompatibilities:
• Increased effects of estazolam: cimetidine, disulfiram, isonizid, probenecid
• Increased CNS depression: alcohol, CNS depressants
• Decreased effect of estazolam: theophylline, rifampin
NURSING CONSIDERATIONS
Assess:
• Blood studies: Hct, Hgb, RBCs (if on long-term therapy)
• Hepatic studies: AST, ALT, bilirubin
Administer:
• After removal of cigarettes, to prevent fire

• After trying conservative measures for insomnia
• ½-1 hr before hs for sleeplessness
• On empty stomach for fast onset, but may be taken with food if GI symptoms occur
Perform/provide:
• Assistance with ambulation after receiving dose
• Safety measures: siderails, night light, call bell within easy reach
• Checking to see PO medication has been swallowed
• Storage in tight container in cool environment
Evaluate:
• Therapeutic response: ability to sleep at night, decreased amount of early morning awakenings
• Mental status: mood, sensorium, affect, memory (long, short)
• Blood dyscrasias: fever, sore throat, bruising, rash, jaundice, epistaxis (rare)
• Type of sleep problem: falling asleep, staying asleep
Teach patient/family:
• To avoid driving or other activities requiring alertness until drug is stabilized

---

esterified estrogens

Climestrone,* Estabs, Estratab, Menest, Ms-Med, Neo-Estrone*
Func. class.: Estrogen
Chem. class.: Nonsteroidal synthetic estrogen

Action: Needed for adequate functioning of female reproductive system; affects release of pituitary gonadotropins, inhibits ovulation, adequate calcium use in bone structures
Uses: Menopause, breast cancer, prostatic cancer hypogonadism, castration, primary ovarian failure

italics = common side effects   ***bold italic*** = life threatening reactions

Dosage and routes:
Menopause
- *Adult:* PO 0.3-3.75 mg qd 3 wk on, 1 wk off

Hypogonadism/castration/ovarian failure
- *Adult:* PO 2.5 mg qd-tid 3 wk on, 1 wk off

Prostatic cancer
- *Adult:* PO 1.25-2.5 mg tid

Breast cancer
- *Adult:* PO 10 mg tid × 3 months or longer

Available forms include: Tabs 0.3, 0.625, 1.25, 2.5 mg

Side effects/adverse reactions:
CNS: Dizziness, headache, migraines, depression
CV: Hypotension, thrombophlebitis, edema, *thromboembolism, stroke, pulmonary embolism, myocardial infarction*
GI: Nausea, vomiting, diarrhea, anorexia, pancreatitis, cramps, constipation, increased appetite, increased weight, *cholestatic jaundice*
EENT: Contact lens intolerance, increased myopia, astigmatism
GU: Amenorrhea, cervical erosion, breakthrough bleeding, dysmenorrhea, vaginal candidiasis, breast changes, *gynecomastia, testicular atrophy, impotence*
INTEG: Rash, urticaria, acne, hirsutism, alopecia, oily skin, seborrhea, purpura, melasma
META: Folic acid deficiency, hypercalcemia, hyperglycemia

Contraindications: Breast cancer, thromboembolic disorders, reproductive cancer, genital bleeding (abnormal, undiagnosed), pregnancy (X)

Precautions: Hypertension, asthma, blood dyscrasias, gallbladder disease, CHF, diabetes mellitus, bone disease, depression, migraine headache, convulsive disorders, hepatic disease, renal disease, family history of cancer of breast or reproductive tract

Pharmacokinetics:
PO: Degraded in liver, excreted in urine, crosses placenta, excreted in breast milk

Interactions/incompatibilities:
- Decreased action of: anticoagulants, oral hypoglycemics
- Toxicity: tricyclic antidepressants
- Decreased action of estrogens: anticonvulsants barbiturates, phenylbutazone, rifampin
- Increased action of: corticosteroids

NURSING CONSIDERATIONS
Assess:
- Urine glucose in patient with diabetes, increased urine glucose may occur
- Weight daily, notify physician of weekly weight gain >5 lb; if increase, diuretic may be ordered
- B/P q4h, watch for increase caused by water and sodium retention
- I&O ratio, be alert for decreasing urinary output and increasing edema
- Liver function studies, including AST, ALT, bilirubin, alk phosphatase

Administer:
- Titrated dose, use lowest effective dose
- With food or milk to decrease GI symptoms

Evaluate:
- Therapeutic response: reversal of menopause or decrease in tumor size in prostatic cancer
- Edema, hypertension, cardiac symptoms, jaundice
- Mental status: affect, mood, behavioral changes, aggression
- Hypercalcemia

Teach patient/family:
• To weigh weekly, report gain >5 lb
• To check with MD before using over-the-counter drugs
• To report breast lumps, vaginal bleeding, edema, jaundice, dark urine, clay colored stools, dyspnea, headache, blurred vision, abdominal pain, numbness or stiffness in legs, chest pain, male to report impotence or gynecomastia

estradiol/estradiol cypionate/estradiol valerate

(ess-tra-dye′ole)

Estrace/Depo-Estradiol Cypionate, Depogen, Dura Estrin, E-lonate PA, Estro-Cyp, Estroject-LA/ Delestrogen,* Dioval Duragen, Estradiol LA, Estraval, Retestrin, Valergen, Hormogen Depot, Deladiol

Func. class.: Estrogen
Chem. class.: Nonsteroidal synthetic estrogen

Action: Needed for adequate functioning of female reproductive system; affects release of pituitary gonadotropins, inhibits ovulation, adequate calcium use in bone structures

Uses: Menopause, breast cancer, prostatic cancer, atrophic vaginitis, kraurosis vulvae, hypogonadism, castration, primary ovarian failure

Dosage and routes:
Menopause/hypogonadism/castration/ovarian failure
• *Adult:* PO 1-2 mg qd 3 wk on, 1 wk off or 5 days on, 2 days off; IM 0.2-1 mg q wk

Prostatic cancer
• *Adult:* IM 30 mg q 1-2 wk (valerate); PO 1-2 mg tid (oral estradiol)
Breast cancer
• *Adult:* PO 10 mg tid × 3 mo or longer
Atropic vaginitis
• *Adult:* VAG CREAM 2-4 g qd × 1-2 wk, then 1 g 1-3 ×/wk
Kraurosis valvae
• *Adult:* IM 1-1.5 mg 1-2 ×/wk
Available forms include: Estradiol-tabs 1, 2 mg; cypionate-injection IM 1, 5 mg/ml; valerate-injection IM 10, 20, 40 mg/ml
Side effects/adverse reactions:
CNS: Dizziness, headache, migraines, depression
CV: Hypotension, thrombophlebitis, edema, *thromboembolism, stroke, pulmonary embolism, myocardial infarction*
GI: Nausea, vomiting, diarrhea, anorexia, pancreatitis, cramps, constipation, increased appetite, increased weight, *cholestatic jaundice*
EENT: Contact lens intolerance, increased myopia, astigmatism
GU: Amenorrhea, cervical erosion, breakthrough bleeding, dysmenorrhea, vaginal candidiasis, breast changes, *gynecomastia, testicular atrophy, impotence*
INTEG: Rash, urticaria, acne, hirsutism, alopecia, oily skin, seborrhea, purpura, melasma
META: Folic acid deficiency, hypercalcemia, hyperglycemia
Contraindications: Breast cancer, thromboembolic disorders, reproductive cancer, genital bleeding (abnormal, undiagnosed), pregnancy (X)
Precautions: Hypertension, asthma, blood dyscrasias, gallbladder disease, CHF, diabetes

E

mellitus, bone disease, depression, migraine headache, convulsive disorders, hepatic disease, renal disease, family history of cancer of breast or reproductive tract

Pharmacokinetics:

PO/IH/TOP: Degraded in liver, excreted in urine, crosses placenta, excreted in breast milk

Interactions/incompatibilities:

• Decreased action of: anticoagulants, oral hypoglycemics
• Toxicity: tricyclic antidepressants
• Decreased action of estramustine: anticonvulsants, barbiturates, phenylbutazone, rifampin, milk products, calcium
• Increased action of: corticosteroids

NURSING CONSIDERATIONS
Assess:

• Urine glucose in patient with diabetes, increased urine glucose may occur
• Weight daily, notify physician of weekly weight gain >5 lb; if increase, diuretic may be ordered
• B/P q4h, watch for increase caused by water and sodium retention
• I&O ratio, be alert for decreasing urinary output and increasing edema
• Liver function studies, including AST, ALT, bilirubin, alk phosphatase

Administer:

• Titrated dose, use lowest effective dose
• IM injection deeply in large muscle mass
• With food or milk to decrease GI symptoms (oral)

Evaluate:

• Therapeutic response: reversal of menopause or decrease in tumor size in prostatic cancer
• Edema, hypertension, cardiac symptoms, jaundice, hypercalcemia
• Mental status: affect, mood, behavioral changes, aggression

Teach patient/family:

• To weigh weekly, report gain >5 lb
• To report breast lumps, vaginal bleeding, edema, jaundice, dark urine, clay-colored stools, dyspnea, headache, blurred vision, abdominal pain, numbness or stiffness in legs, chest pain; male to report impotence or gynecomastia

Lab test interferences:

Increase: BSP retention test, PBI, T_4, serum sodium, platelet aggregation, thyroxine-binding globulin (TBG), prothrombin, factors VII, VIII, IX, X, triglycerides

Decrease: Serum folate, serum triglyceride, T_3 resin uptake test, glucose tolerance test, antithrombin III, pregnanediol, metyrapone test

False positive: LE prep, antinuclear antibodies

---

estramustine phosphate sodium

(ess-tra-muss'teen)
Emcyt

Func. class.: Antineoplastic
Chem. class.: Hormone: estrogen

Action: Precise actions unknown
Uses: Metastatic prostate cancer
Dosage and routes:

• *Adult:* PO 10-16 mg/kg in 3-4 divided doses; treatment may continue for 3 mo or more

Available forms include: Caps 140 mg (12.5 mg sodium/cap)

Side effects/adverse reactions:
GI: Nausea, vomiting, anorexia,
hepatotoxicity
GU: **Renal failure,** impotence, gynecomastia
INTEG: Rash, urticaria, pruritus,
flushing, alopecia
RESP: Dyspnea, **emboli,** hoarseness
CV: **Myocardial infarction,** hypertension, **CHF, CVA**
CNS: Headache, anxiety, seizures,
insomnia, mood swings
Contraindications: Hypersensitivity to estradiol, thromboembolic
disorders, pregnancy (D)
Precautions: Edema, hepatic dis-
ease, CVA, MI, seizures, hyperten-
sion, diabetes mellitus
Pharmacokinetics:
PO: Peak 1-2 hr, metabolized in
liver, excreted in bile, half-life 20
hr (terminal)
NURSING CONSIDERATIONS
Assess:
• Renal function studies: BUN, se-
rum uric acid, urine CrCl, electrolytes before, during therapy
• I&O ratio; report fall in urine output of 30 ml/hr
• Liver function tests before, during therapy (bilirubin, AST, ALT,
LDH) as needed or monthly
• Monitor ECG before, during
treatment
Administer:
• Antacid before oral agent; give
drug after evening meal before
bedtime
Evaluate:
• Dyspnea, chest pain, tachy-
pnea, fatigue, increased pulse,
pallor, lethargy
• Food preferences; list likes,
dislikes
• Edema in feet, joint, stomach
pain, shaking
• Inflammation of mucosa, breaks
in skin

• Yellowing of skin and sclera,
dark urine, clay-colored stools,
itchy skin, abdominal pain, fever,
diarrhea
• Symptoms indicating severe allergic reaction: rash, pruritus, urticaria, purpuric skin lesions, itching, flushing
• Tachycardia, ECG changes, dyspnea, edema, fatigue, leg cramps;
may indicate cardiac toxicity
Teach patient/family:
• To report any complaints, side effects to nurse or physician
• That gynecomastia, impotence
can occur and are reversible after
discontinuing treatment
• To report any changes in breathing, coughing
• Importance of immediately re-
porting GI bleeding
• To use contraception during use,
positive mutagenic effects

---

estrogenic substances, conjugated
C.E.S.,* Estrocon, Premarin, Pro-
gens
Func. class.: Estrogen
Chem. class.: Nonsteroidal syn-
thetic estrogen

Action: Needed for adequate functioning of female reproductive system; it affects release of pituitary
gonadotropins, inhibits ovulation,
adequate calcium use in bone structures
Uses: Menopause, breast cancer,
prostatic cancer, abnormal uterine
bleeding, hypogonadism, castration, primary ovarian failure, osteoporosis
Dosage and routes:
Menopause
• *Adult:* PO 0.3-1.25 mg qd 3 wk
on, 1 wk off

Prostatic cancer
- *Adult:* PO 1.25-2.5 mg tid

Breast cancer
- *Adult:* PO 10 mg tid × 3 mo or longer

Abnormal uterine bleeding
- *Adult:* IV/IM 25 mg, repeat in 6-12 hr

Castration/primary ovarian failure/osteoporosis
- *Adult:* PO 1.25 mg qd 3 wk on, 1 wk off

Hypogonadism
- *Adult:* PO 2.5 mg bid-tid × 20 days/mo

Available forms include: Tabs 0.3, 0.625, 0.9, 1.25, 2.5 mg

Side effects/adverse reactions:
CNS: Dizziness, headache, migraine, depression
CV: Hypotension, thrombophlebitis, edema, *thromboembolism, stroke, pulmonary embolism, myocardial infarction*
GI: *Nausea,* vomiting, diarrhea, anorexia, pancreatitis, cramps, constipation, increased appetite, increased weight, *cholestatic jaundice*
EENT: Contact lens intolerance, increased myopia, astigmatism
GU: Amenorrhea, cervical erosion, breakthrough bleeding, dysmenorrhea, vaginal candidiasis, breast changes, *gynecomastia, testicular atrophy, impotence*
INTEG: Rash, urticaria, acne, hirsutism, alopecia, oily skin, seborrhea, purpura, melasma
META: Folic acid deficiency, hypercalcemia, hyperglycemia

Contraindications: Breast cancer, thromboembolic disorders, reproductive cancer, genital bleeding (abnormal, undiagnosed), pregnancy (X), lactation

Precautions: Hypertension, asthma, blood dyscrasias, gallbladder disease, CHF, diabetes mellitus, bone disease, depression, migraine headache, convulsive disorders, hepatic disease, renal disease, family history of cancer of breast or reproductive tract

Pharmacokinetics:
PO/IV/IM: Degraded in liver, excreted in urine, crosses placenta, excreted in breast milk

Interactions/incompatibilities:
- Decreased action of: anticoagulants, oral hypoglycemics
- Toxicity: tricyclic antidepressants
- Decreased action of estrogens: anticonvulsants, barbiturates, phenylbutazone, rifampin
- Increased action of: corticosteroids

NURSING CONSIDERATIONS
Assess:
- Urine glucose in patient with diabetes; increased urine glucose may occur
- Weight daily, notify physician of weekly weight gain >5 lb; if increase, diuretic may be ordered
- B/P q4h; watch for increase caused by water and sodium retention
- I&O ratio, be alert for decreasing urinary output and increasing edema
- Liver function studies, including AST, ALT, bilirubin, alk phosphatase

Administer:
- Titrated dose, use lowest effective dose
- IM injection deeply in large muscle mass
- With food or milk to decrease GI symptoms PO

Evaluate:
- Therapeutic response: absence of breast engorgement, reversal of

menopause, or decrease in tumor size in prostatic cancer
• Edema, hypertension, cardiac symptoms, jaundice, hypercalcemia
• Mental status: affect, mood, behavioral changes, aggression

Teach patient/family:
• To avoid breastfeeding, since drug is secreted in breast milk
• To weigh weekly, report gain >5 lb
• To report breast lumps, vaginal bleeding, edema, jaundice, dark urine, clay-colored stools, dyspnea, headache, blurred vision, abdominal pain, numbness or stiffness in legs, chest pain; male to report impotence or gynecomastia
• To avoid sunlight or wear sunscreen; burns may occur

---

estrone
(ess'trone)
Bestrone, Femogen Forte,* Kestrone-5, Theelin Aqeous, Esmone A
Func. class.: Estrogen
Chem. class.: Nonsteroidal synthetic estrogen

Action: Needed for adequate functioning of female reproductive system; affects release of pituitary gonadotropins, inhibits ovulation, promotes adequate calcium use in bone structures

Uses: Menopause, prostatic cancer, atrophic vaginitis, hypogonadism, primary ovarian failure

Dosage and routes:
Menopause/atrophic vaginitis
• *Adult:* IM 0.1-0.5 mg 2-3 × /wk
Prostatic cancer
• *Adult:* IM 2-4 mg 2-3 × /wk
Female hypogonadism/primary ovarian failure

• *Adult:* IM 0.1-1 mg q wk in one dose or divided doses
Available forms include: Inj IM 2, 5 mg/ml

Side effects/adverse reactions:
CNS: Dizziness, headache, migraine, depression
CV: Hypotension, thrombophlebitis, edema, *thromboembolism, stroke, pulmonary embolism, myocardial infarction*
GI: Nausea, vomiting, diarrhea, anorexia, pancreatitis, cramps, constipation, increased appetite, increased weight, *cholestatic jaundice*
EENT: Contact lens intolerance, increased myopia, astigmatism
GU: Amenorrhea, cervical erosion, breakthrough bleeding, dysmenorrhea, vaginal candidiasis, breast changes, *gynecomastia, testicular atrophy, impotence*
INTEG: Rash, urticaria, acne, hirsutism, alopecia, oily skin, seborrhea, purpura, melasma
META: Folic acid deficiency, hypercalcemia, hyperglycemia

Contraindications: Breast cancer, thromboembolic disorders, reproductive cancer, genital bleeding (abnormal, undiagnosed), pregnancy (X)

Precautions: Hypertension, asthma, blood dyscrasias, gallbladder disease, CHF, diabetes mellitus, bone disease, depression, migraine headache, convulsive disorders, hepatic disease, renal disease, family history of cancer of the breast or reproductive tract

Pharmacokinetics:
IM: Degraded in liver, excreted in urine, crosses placenta, excreted in breast milk

Interactions/incompatibilities:
• Decreased action of: anticoagulants, oral hypoglycemics

---

italics = common side effects   **bold italic** = life threatening reactions

• Toxicity: tricyclic antidepressants
• Decreased action of estrone: anticonvulsants, barbiturates, phenylbutazone, rifampin
• Increased action of: corticosteroids

NURSING CONSIDERATIONS
Assess:
• Urine glucose in patient with diabetes; increased urine glucose may occur
• Weight daily, notify physician of weekly weight gain >5 lb; if increase, diuretic may be ordered
• B/P q4h, watch for increase caused by water and sodium retention
• I&O ratio, be alert for decreasing urinary output and increasing edema
• Liver function studies, including AST, ALT, bilirubin, alk phosphatase

Administer:
• Titrated dose, use lowest effective dose
• IM injection deeply in large muscle mass

Evaluate:
• Therapeutic response: absence of breast engorgement, reversal of menopause, or decrease in tumor size in prostatic cancer
• Edema, hypertension, cardiac symptoms, jaundice, hypercalcemia
• Mental status: affect, mood, behavioral changes, aggression

Teach patient/family:
• To weigh weekly, report gain >5 lb
• To report breast lumps, vaginal bleeding, edema, jaundice, dark urine, clay-colored stools, dyspnea, headache, blurred vision, abdominal pain, numbness or stiffness in legs, chest pain; male to report impotence or gynecomastia
• To avoid sunlight or wear sunscreen, burns may occur

---

ethacrynate sodium/ ethacrynic acid
(eth-a-kri'nate)
Sodium Edecrin
Func. class.: Loop diuretic
Chem. class.: Ketone derivative

Action: Acts on loop of Henle by increasing excretion of chloride, sodium
Uses: Pulmonary edema, edema in CHF, liver disease, nephrotic syndrome, ascites
Dosage and routes:
• *Adult:* PO 50-200 mg/day may give up to 200 mg bid
• *Child:* PO 25 mg, increased by 25 mg/day until desired effect occurs
Pulmonary edema
• *Adult:* IV 50 mg given over several minutes or 0.5-1 mg/kg
Available forms include: Tabs 25, 50 mg; powder for inj 50 mg
Side effects/adverse reactions:
GU: Polyuria, **renal failure,** glycosuria
ELECT: Hypokalemia, hypochloremic alkalosis, hypomagnesemia, hyperuricemia, hypocalcemia, hyponatremia
CNS: Headache, fatigue, weakness, vertigo
GI: Nausea, severe diarrhea, dry mouth, vomiting, anorexia, cramps, upset stomach, abdominal pain, **acute pancreatitis,** jaundice, **GI bleeding**
EENT: **Loss of hearing,** ear pain, tinnitus, blurred vision
INTEG: Rash, pruritus, purpura, **Stevens-Johnson syndrome,** sweating, photosensitivity

MS: Cramps, arthritis, stiffness
ENDO: Hyperglycemia
HEMA: ***Thrombocytopenia, agranulocytosis, leukopenia, neutropenia***
CV: Chest pain, hypotension, ***circulatory collapse,*** ECG changes
Contraindications: Hypersensitivity to sulfonamides, anuria, hypovolemia, lactation, electrolyte depletion, infants
Precautions: Dehydration, ascites, severe renal disease, pregnancy (D), hypoproteinemia
Pharmacokinetics:
PO: Onset ½ hr, peak 2 hr, duration 6-8 hr
IV: Onset 5 min, peak 15-30 min, duration 2 hr
Excreted by kidneys, crosses placenta, half-life 30-70 min
Interactions/incompatibilities:
• Increased hypotension: antihypertensives
• Decreased diuretic effect: indomethacin
• Increased ototoxicity: cisplatin, aminoglycosides
• Increased toxicity: lithium, nondepolarizing skeletal muscle relaxants
• Increased anticoagulant activity: warfarin

NURSING CONSIDERATIONS
Assess:
• Weight, I&O daily to determine fluid loss; effect of drug may be decreased if used qd
• Rate, depth, rhythm of respiration, effect of exertion
• B/P lying, standing; postural hypotension may occur
• Electrolytes: potassium, sodium, chloride; include BUN, blood sugar, CBC, serum creatinine, blood pH, ABGs, uric acid, calcium, magnesium

• Glucose in urine if patient is diabetic
• Hearing when giving high doses
Administer:
• IV after diluting with 50 ml NaCl inj; give through Y-tube or 3-way stopcock, give 10 mg or less over 1 min or run infusion over ½ hr
• In AM to avoid interference with sleep if using drug as a diuretic
• Potassium replacement if potassium is less than 3.0
• With food, if nausea occurs, absorption may be decreased slightly
• PO, IV only, do not give IM/SC
Evaluate:
• Improvement in edema of feet, legs, sacral area daily if medication is being used in CHF
• Improvement in CVP q8h
• Signs of metabolic alkalosis: drowsiness, restlessness
• Signs of hypokalemia: postural hypotension, malaise, fatigue, tachycardia, leg cramps, weakness
• Rashes, temperature elevation qd
• Confusion, especially in elderly, take safety precautions if needed
Teach patient/family:
• To increase fluid intake 2-3 L/day unless contraindicated; to rise slowly from lying or sitting position
• Adverse reactions: muscle cramps, weakness, nausea, dizziness
• Take with food or milk for GI symptoms
• Take early in day to prevent nocturia
Treatment of overdose: Lavage if taken orally, monitor electrolytes, administer dextrose in saline, monitor hydration, CV, renal status

E

---

italics = common side effects   ***bold italic*** = life threatening reactions

ethambutol HCl

(e-tham'byoo-tole)

Etibi,* Myambutol

Func. class.: Antitubercular

Chem. class.: Diisopropylethylene diamide derivative

Action: Inhibits RNA synthesis, decreases tubercle bacilli replication

Uses: Pulmonary tuberculosis, as an adjunct

Dosage and routes:

• *Adult and child >13 yr:* PO 15 mg/kg/day as a single dose

Retreatment

• *Adult and child >13 yr:* PO 25 mg/kg/day as single dose × 2 mo with at least 1 other drug, then decrease to 15 mg/kg/day as single dose

Available forms include: Tabs 100, 400 mg

Side effects/adverse reactions:

GI: Abdominal distress

INTEG: Dermatitis, photosensitivity

CV: **CHF, dysrhythmias**

CNS: Headache, anxiety, drowsiness, tremors, **convulsions,** lethargy, depression, confusion, psychosis, aggression

EENT: Blurred vision, optic neuritis, photophobia, decreased visual acuity

HEMA: **Megaloblastic anemia,** vitamin B$_{12}$, folic acid deficiency

Contraindications: Hypersensitivity, optic neuritis, child <13 yr

Precautions: Pregnancy (D), renal disease, diabetic retinopathy, cataracts, ocular defects

Pharmacokinetics:

PO: Peak 2-4 hr, half-life 3 hr; metabolized in liver, excreted in urine (unchanged drug/inactive metabolites, feces)

Interactions/incompatibilities:

• Increased toxicity: aminoglycosides, cisplatin, aluminum salts

NURSING CONSIDERATIONS

Assess:

• Liver studies q wk: ALT, AST, bilirubin

• Renal status: before, q mo: BUN, creatinine, output, sp gr, urinalysis

• Blood level of drug

• Signs of anemia: Hct, Hgb, fatigue

Administer:

• With meals to decrease GI symptoms

• Antiemetic if vomiting occurs

• After C&S is completed; q mo to detect resistance

Evaluate:

• Ototoxicity: tinnitus, vertigo, change in hearing

• Mental status often: affect, mood, behavioral changes; psychosis may occur

• Hepatic status: decreased appetite, jaundice, dark urine, fatigue

Teach patient/family:

• That compliance with dosage schedule, duration is necessary

• That scheduled appointments must be kept or relapse may occur

ethchlorvynol

(eth-klor-vi'nole)

Placidyl

Func. class.: Sedative-hypnotic

Chem. class.: Tertiary acetylenic alcohol

Controlled Substance Schedule IV (USA), Schedule F (Canada)

Action: Produces cerebral depression, exact action is unknown

Uses: Sedation, insomnia

Dosage and routes:

Sedation

• *Adult:* PO 100-200 mg bid or tid

Insomnia
• *Adult:* PO 500 mg-1g ½ hr before hs, may repeat 100-200 mg if needed

Medication for EEG
• *Child:* PO 25 mg/kg in one dose not to exceed 1 g

Available forms include: Caps 100, 200, 500, 750 mg

Side effects/adverse reactions:
HEMA: **Thrombocytopenia**
CNS: Fatigue, drowsiness, dizziness, sedation, ataxia, nightmares, hangover, giddiness, weakness, hysteria
GI: Nausea, vomiting
INTEG: Rash, urticaria
EENT: Blurred vision, bitter aftertaste
CV: Hypotension

Contraindications: Hypersensitivity to this drug, severe pain, porphyria, pregnancy (C)

Precautions: Depression, hepatic disease, renal disease, suicidal individual, pregnancy (3rd trimester) (C), elderly

Pharmacokinetics:
PO: Onset 15-30 min, peak 1-1½ hr, duration 5 hr; metabolized by liver, excreted by kidneys; half-life 10-20 hr, 21-100 hr terminal

Interactions/incompatibilities:
• Decreased hypoprothrombinemic effect: dicumarol, warfarin
• Increased CNS effects of ETOH, barbiturates, other CNS depressants, MAOIs

NURSING CONSIDERATIONS
Assess:
• Blood studies: Hct, Hgb, RBCs before and after treatment if blood dyscrasias are suspected
• Hepatic studies: AST, ALT, bilirubin if hepatic disease is present

Administer:
• After removal of cigarettes, to prevent fires

• After trying conservative measures for insomnia
• ½-1 hr before hs for sleeplessness
• With food or meals to decrease dizziness, giddiness
• For only 1 wk, not intended for long-term treatment

Perform/provide:
• Assistance with ambulation after receiving dose
• Safety measures: siderails, nightlight, callbell within easy reach
• Checking to see PO medication swallowed
• Storage in tight, light-resistant container in cool environment

Evaluate:
• Therapeutic response: ability to sleep at night, decreased amount of early morning awakenings if taking drug for insomnia
• Mental status: mood, sensorium, affect, memory (long, short)
• Physical dependency: more frequent requests for medication, shakes, anxiety
• Toxicity: hypotension, hypothermia, weakness, poor muscle coordination, visual problems; drug should be discontinued
• Respiratory dysfunction: respiratory depression, character, rate, rhythm; hold drug if respirations are <10/min or if pupils are dilated (rare)
• Blood dyscrasias: fever, sore throat, bruising, rash, jaundice, epistaxis (rare)
• Allergy to tartrazine: this drug contains tartrazine and should not be used in patients allergic to this dye

Teach patient/family:
• To avoid driving or other activities requiring alertness
• To avoid alcohol ingestion or CNS depressants; serious CNS depression may result

---

italics = common side effects   ***bold italic*** = life threatening reactions

• That effects may take 2 nights for benefits to be noticed
• Alternate measures to improve sleep: reading, exercise several hours before hs, warm bath, warm milk, TV, self-hypnosis, deep breathing
Treatment of overdose: Lavage, activated charcoal, monitor electrolytes, vital signs
Lab test interferences:
Interferes: Clinitest

---

ethinyl estradiol

(eth'in-il ess-tra-dye'ole)
Estinyl, Feminone
Func. class.: Estrogen
Chem. class.: Nonsteroidal synthetic estrogen

Action: Needed for adequate functioning of female reproductive system; affects release of pituitary gonadotropins, inhibits ovulation, promotes adequate calcium use in bone structures
Uses: Menopause, prostatic cancer, breast cancer, breast engorgement, hypogonadism
Dosage and routes:
Menopause
• *Adult:* PO 0.02-0.5 mg qd 3 wk on, 1 wk off
Prostatic cancer
• *Adult:* PO 0.15-2 mg qd
Hypogonadism
• *Adult:* PO 0.05 mg qd-tid × 2 wk/mo, then 2 wk progesterone, then 3-6 mo cycles, then 2 mo off
Breast cancer
• *Adult:* PO 1 mg tid
Breast engorgement
• *Adult:* PO 0.5-1 mg qd × 3 days, then tapered off over 7 days
Available forms include: Tabs 0.02, 0.05, 0.5 mg

Side effects/adverse reactions:
CNS: Dizziness, headache, migraine, depression
CV: Hypotension, thrombophlebitis, edema, *thromboembolism, stroke, pulmonary embolism, myocardial infarction*
GI:Nausea, vomiting, diarrhea, anorexia, pancreatitis, cramps, constipation, increased appetite, increased weight, *cholestatic jaundice*
EENT: Contact lens intolerance, increased myopia, astigmatism
GU: Amenorrhea, cervical erosion, breakthrough bleeding, dysmenorrhea, vaginal candidiasis, breast changes, *gynecomastia, testicular atrophy, impotence*
INTEG: Rash, urticaria, acne, hirsutism, alopecia, oily skin, seborrhea, purpura, melasma
META: Folic acid deficiency, hypercalcemia, hyperglycemia
Contraindications: Breast cancer, thromboembolic disorders, reproductive cancer, genital bleeding (abnormal, undiagnosed), pregnancy (X)
Precautions: Hypertension, asthma, blood dyscrasias, gallbladder disease, CHF, diabetes mellitus, bone disease, depression, migraine headache, convulsive disorders, hepatic disease, renal disease, family history of cancer of breast or reproductive tract
Pharmacokinetics:
PO: Degraded in liver, excreted in urine, crosses placenta, excreted in breast milk
Interactions/incompatibilities:
• Decreased action of: anticoagulants, oral hypoglycemics
• Toxicity: tricyclic antidepressants
• Decreased action of estradiol: an-

---

ticonvulsants, barbiturates, phenylbutazone, rifampin
• Increased action of: corticosteroids

NURSING CONSIDERATIONS
Assess:
• Urine glucose in patient with diabetes; increased urine glucose may occur
• Weight daily, notify physician of weekly weight gain >5 lb; if increase, diurectic may be ordered
• B/P q4h, watch for increase caused by water and sodium retention
• I&O ratio, be alert for decreasing urinary output and increasing edema
• Liver function studies: AST, ALT, bilirubin, alk phosphatase
Administer:
• Titrated dose, use lowest effective dose
• IM injection deeply in large muscle mass
• With food or milk to decrease GI symptoms
Evaluate:
• Therapeutic response: absence of breast engorgement, reversal of menopause, or decrease in tumor size in prostatic cancer
• Edema, hypertension, cardiac symptoms, jaundice, hypercalcemia
• Mental status: affect, mood, behavioral changes, aggression
Teach patient/family:
• To weigh weekly, report gain >5 lb
• To report breast lumps, vaginal bleeding, edema, jaundice, dark urine, clay-colored stools, dyspnea, headache, blurred vision, abdominal pain, numbness or stiffness in legs, chest pain; male to report impotence or gynecomastia

ethionamide
(e-thye-on-am-ide)
Trecator SC
Func. class.: Antitubercular
Chem. class.: Thiomine derivative

Action: Inhibits RNA synthesis, decreases tubercle bacilli replication
Uses: Pulmonary, extrapulmonary tuberculosis when other antitubercular drugs are not feasible
Dosage and routes:
• *Adult:* PO 500 mg-1 g qd in divided doses, with another antitubercular drug and pyridoxine
• *Child:* PO 12-15 mg/kg/day in 3-4 doses, not to exceed 750 mg
Available forms include: Tabs 250 mg
Side effects/adverse reactions:
INTEG: Dermatitis, photosensitivity
CV: **CHF, dysrhythmias**
CNS: Headache, anxiety, drowsiness, tremors, **convulsions,** lethargy, depression, confusion, psychosis, aggression
GI: **Anorexia, nausea, vomiting, diarrhea,** metallic taste
EENT: Blurred vision, optic neuritis, photophobia
HEMA: **Megaloblastic anemia,** vitamin B_{12}, folid acid deficiency
Contraindications: Hypersensitivity, optic neuritis
Precautions: Pregnancy (D), renal disease, diabetic retinopathy, cataracts, ocular defects, child <13 yr
Pharmacokinetics:
PO: Peak 3 hr, duration 9 hr, half-life 3 hr; metabolized in liver, excreted in urine (unchanged drug/inactive), crosses placenta
Interactions/incompatibilities:
• Increased neurotoxicity: cycloserine, ethyl alcohol

---

italics = common side effects   **bold italic** = life threatening reactions

• Increased adverse reactions: TB test agents, anti-TB drugs

Assess:
• Signs of anemia: Hgb, Hct, fatigue
• Liver studies q wk: ALT, AST, bilirubin
• Renal status: before, q mo: BUN, creatinine, output, sp gr, urinalysis
Administer:
• With meals to decrease GI symptoms
• Antiemetic if vomiting occurs
• After C&S is completed, q mo to detect resistance
• Pyridoxine to prevent neuritis
Evaluate:
• Ototoxicity: tinnitus, vertigo, change in hearing
• Mental status often: affect, mood, behavioral changes; psychosis may occur
• Hepatic status: decreased appetite, jaundice, dark urine, fatigue
Teach patient/family:
• That compliance with dosage schedule, duration is necessary
• Avoid alcohol while taking this drug
• To notify physician of depression, mood changes, which are symptoms of toxicity

---

ethosuximide
(eth-oh-sux'i-mide)
Zarontin
Func. class.: Anticonvulsant
Chem. class.: Succinimide

Action: Inhibits spike, wave formation in absence seizures (petit mal), decreases amplitude, frequency, duration, spread of discharge in minor motor seizures
Uses: Absence seizures, partial seizures, tonic-clonic seizures.

Dosage and routes:
• *Adult and child >6 yr:* PO 250 mg bid initially; may increase by 250 mg q4-7 days, not to exceed 1.5 g/day
• *Child 3-6 yr:* PO 250 mg/day or 125 mg bid; may increase by 250 mg q4-7 days, not to exceed 1.5 g/day
Available forms include: Caps 250 mg, syr 250 mg/5 ml
Side effects/adverse reactions:
HEMA: **Agranulocytosis, aplastic anemia, thrombocytopenia, leukocytosis, eosinophilia, pancytopenia**
CNS: Drowsiness, dizziness, fatigue, euphoria, lethargy, anxiety, aggressiveness, irritability, depression, insomnia, headache
GI: Nausea, vomiting, heartburn, anorexia, diarrhea, abdominal pain, cramps, constipation, hiccups, weight loss, gum hypertrophy, tongue swelling
GU: Vaginal bleeding, ***hematuria, renal damage***
INTEG: Urticaria, pruritic erythema, hirsutism, ***Stevens-Johnson syndrome***
EENT: Myopia, blurred vision
Contraindications: Hypersensitivity to succinimide derivatives
Precautions: Lactation, pregnancy (C), hepatic disease, renal disease
Pharmacokinetics:
PO: Peak 1-7 hr, steady state 4-7 days, metabolized by liver, excreted in urine, bile, feces, half-life 24-60 hr
Interactions/incompatibilities:
• Antagonist effect: tricyclic antidepressants (imipramine, doxepin)
• Decreased effects of: estrogens, oral contraceptives

---

*Available in Canada only

NURSING CONSIDERATIONS
Assess:
- Renal studies: urinalysis, BUN, urine creatinine
- Blood studies: CBC, Hct, Hgb, reticulocyte counts q wk for 4 wk, then q mo
- Hepatic studies: AST, ALT, bilirubin, creatinine
- Drug levels during initial treatment, therapeutic range (40-80 µg/ml

Administer:
- With food, milk to decrease GI symptoms

Perform/provide:
- Hard candy, frequent rinsing of mouth, gum for dry mouth
- Assistance with ambulation during early part of treatment; dizziness occurs

Evaluate:
- Therapeutic response: decreased seizure activity, document on patient's chart
- Mental status: mood, sensorium, affect, behavioral changes; if mental status changes, notify physician
- Eye problems: need for ophthalmic examinations before, during, after treatment (slit lamp, fundoscopy, tonometry)
- Allergic reaction: red raised rash, exfoliative dermatitis; if these occur, drug should be discontinued
- Blood dyscrasias: fever, sore throat, bruising, rash, jaundice
- Toxicity: bone marrow depression, nausea, vomiting, ataxia, diplopia, cardiovascular collapse, Stevens-Johnson syndrome

Teach patient/family:
- To carry ID card or Medic-Alert bracelet stating drugs taken, condition, physician's name, phone number
- To avoid driving, other activities that require alertness
- To avoid alcohol ingestion, CNS depressants; increased sedation may occur
- Not to discontinue medication quickly after long-term use

Lab test interferences:
False positive: Direct Coombs' test

Treatment of overdose: Lavage, activated charcoal, monitor electrolytes, VS

---

ethotoin
(eth'oh-toyin)
Peganone
Func. class.: Anticonvulsant
Chem. class.: Hydantoin derivative

Action: Inhibits nerve in impulses in the motor cortex by decreasing sodium ion influx, limiting tetanic stimulation

Uses: Generalized tonic-clonic or complex-partial seizures

Dosage and routes:
- *Adult:* PO 250 mg qid initially; may increase over several days to 3 g/day in divided doses
- *Child:* PO 250 mg bid; may increase by 250 mg qid

Available forms include: Tabs 250, 500 mg

Side effects/adverse reactions:
HEMA: ***Agranulocytosis, thrombocytopenia, leukopenia, pancytopenia, megaloblastic anemia,*** lymphadenopathy
CNS: *Fatigue, insomnia, numbness, fever, headache, dizziness*
GI: *Nausea, vomiting, diarrhea,* gingival hypertrophy
INTEG: *Rash*
EENT: *Nystagmus, diplopia*
CV: *Chest pain*

Contraindications: Hypersensitivity to hydantoins, blood dyscrasias, hematologic disease, hepatic disease, pregnancy (D)

---

italics = common side effects   ***bold italic*** = life threatening reactions

Pharmacokinetics: Metabolized by liver, excreted in urine, half-life 3-9 hr

Interactions/incompatibilities:
• Decreased effects of: rifampin, chronic alcohol, barbiturates, antihistamines, antacids, other anticonvulsants antineoplastics, calcium products, folic acid, oxacillin
• Increased effects of: benzodiazepines, cimetidine, salicylates, sulfonamide, pyrazolones, phenothiazines, estrogens, disulfiram, chloramphenicol, anticoagulants
• Seizures: valproic acid
• Myocardial depressions: lidocaine, propranolol, sympathomimetics

NURSING CONSIDERATIONS
Assess:
• Renal studies: urinalysis, BUN, urine creatinine
• Blood studies: RBC, Hct, Hgb, reticulocyte counts q wk for 4 wk then q mo
• Hepatic studies: AST, ALT, bilirubin, creatinine periodically
• Drug levels during initial treatment, therapeutic level (15-50 μg/ml)

Administer:
• With food, milk to decrease GI symptoms
• After meals

Perform/provide:
• Hard candy, frequent rinsing of mouth, gum for dry mouth
• Assistance with ambulation during early part of treatment; dizziness occurs

Evaluate:
• Therapeutic response: decreased seizure activity, document on patient's chart
• Mental status: mood, sensorium, affect, behavioral changes; if mental status changes, notify physician
• Eye problems: need for ophthalmic examinations before, during, after treatment (slit lamp, fundoscopy, tonometry)
• Allergic reaction: red raised rash; if this occurs, drug should be discontinued
• Blood dyscrasias: fever, sore throat, bruising, rash, jaundice
• Toxicity: bone marrow depression, nausea, vomiting, ataxia, diplopia, cardiovascular collapse, Stevens-Johnson syndrome, lupuslike syndrome

Teach patient/family:
• To carry ID card or Medic-Alert bracelet stating drugs taken, condition, physician's name, phone number
• To avoid driving, other activities that require alertness
• To avoid alcohol ingestion, CNS depressants; increased sedation may occur
• Not to discontinue medication quickly after long-term use, taper off over several weeks

Lab test interferences:
Increase: Serum glucose, BSP, alk phosphatase
Decrease: Urinary steroids, PBI, dexamethasone/metyrapone tests

Treatment of overdose: Lavage, activated charcoal, monitor electrolytes, VS

---

ethylestrenol
(eth-il-ess′tre-nole)
Maxibolin
Func. class.: Androgenic anabolic steroid
Chem. class.: Hydantoin derivative

Action: Increases weight by building body tissue, increases potassium, phosphorus, chloride, and nitrogen levels, increases bone development
Uses: To increase weight, combat

tissue depletion, osteoporosis, immobility, refractory anemias, catabolic effects of corticosteroid therapy

Dosage and routes:
• *Adult:* PO 4-8 mg qd, decreased at beginning clinical response
• *Child:* PO 1-3 mg qd, not to exceed treatment of 6 wk, lupuslike syndrome

Available forms include: Tabs 2 mg; elix 2 mg/5 ml

Side effects/adverse reactions:
INTEG: Rash, acneiform lesions, oily hair, skin, flushing, sweating, acne vulgaris, alopecia, hirsutism
CNS: Dizziness, headache, fatigue, tremors, paresthesias, flushing, sweating, anxiety, lability, insomnia
MS: Cramps, spasms
CV: Increased B/P
GU: **Hematuria,** amenorrhea, vaginitis, decreased libido, decreased breast size, clitoral hypertrophy, testicular atrophy
GI: Nausea, vomiting, constipation, weight gain, ***cholestatic jaundice***
EENT: Carpal tunnel syndrome, conjunctional edema, nasal congestion
ENDO: Abnormal GTT

Contraindications: Severe renal disease, severe cardiac disease, severe hepatic disease, hypersensitivity, pregnancy (C), lactation, genital bleeding (abnormal)

Precautions: Migraine headaches, seizure disorders

Pharmacokinetics:
PO: Metabolized in liver, excreted in urine, crosses placenta, excreted in breast milk

Interactions/incompatibilities:
• May increase effects of: oral anticoagulants, antidiabetics, oxyphenbutazone, phenylbutazone

• May decrease effect of ethylestrenol: barbiturates

NURSING CONSIDERATIONS
Assess:
• Weight daily, notify physician if weekly weight gain is >5 lb
• B/P q4h
• I&O ratio; be alert for decreasing urinary output, increasing edema
• Growth rate in children since growth rate may be uneven (linear/bone growth) used for extended periods of time; periodic x-rays are done to assure changes in bone growth
• Electrolytes: K, Na, Cl; cholesterol
• Liver function studies; ALT, AST, bilirubin
• Blood sugar in diabetes (may become hypoglycemic)

Administer:
• Increased calcium, Vitamin D in diet for osteoporosis, decrease in high phosphorus foods (bread, soft drinks, phosphate-based preservatives)
• Titrated dose, use lowest effective dose
• With food or milk to decrease GI symptoms

Perform/provide:
• Diet with increased calories, protein; decrease sodium if edema occurs

Evaluate:
• Therapeutic response: increased appetite, increased stamina
• Edema, hypertension, cardiac symptoms, jaundice
• Mental status: affect, mood, behavioral changes, aggression
• Signs of masculinization in female: increased libido, deepening of voice, breast tissue, enlarged clitoris, menstrual irregularities; male: gynecomastia, impotence, testicular atrophy

---

italics = common side effects   ***bold italic*** = life threatening reactions

• Hypercalcemia: lethargy, poly-uria, polydipsia, nausea, vomiting, constipation, drug may need to be decreased

• Hypoglycemia in diabetics, since oral anticoagulant action is de-creased

Teach patient/family:

• Drug needs to be combined with complete health plan: diet, rest, ex-ercise

• To notify physician if therapeutic response decreases

• Not to discontinue medication abruptly

• Teach patient about change in sex characteristics

Lab test interferences:

Increase: Cholesterol

Decrease: Cholesterol, T_4, T_3, thy-roid ^{131}I uptake test, 17-KS, PBI

Interferes: GTT

---

ethylnorepinephrine HCl

(eth-il-nor-ep-i-nef'rin)
Bronkephrine

Func. class.: Adrenergic
Chem. class.: Catecholamine

Action: α-Stimulation with vaso-constriction, pressor response, na-sal decongestion and β_2-stimulation with vasodilation and bronchial di-lation

Uses: Bronchospasm

Dosage and routes:

• *Adult:* IM/SC 0.5-1 ml

• *Child:* IM/SC 0.1-0.5 ml

Available forms include: Inj 2 mg/ml IM, SC

Side effects/adverse reactions:

CNS: Tremors, anxiety, insomnia, headache, dizziness, confusion, *CV:* Palpitations, tachycardia, hy-pertension, chest pain, ***dysrhyth-mias***

GI: Anorexia, nausea, vomiting

Contraindications: Hypersensitiv-ity to sympathomimetics, narrow-angle glaucoma

Precautions: Pregnancy (C), car-diac disorders, hyperthyroidism, diabetes mellitus, prostatic hyper-trophy

Pharmacokinetics:

IM/SC: Onset 6-12 min, duration 1-2 hr

Interactions/incompatibilities:

• Do not use with MAOIs or tri-cyclic antidepressants; hyperten-sive crisis may occur

• Decreased effect of ethylnorepi-nephrine when used with methyl-dopa, urinary acidifiers, rauwolfia alkaloids

• Increased effect of ethylnorepi-nephrine when used with urinary alkalizers

NURSING CONSIDERATIONS

Assess:

• B/P and pulse q5 min after par-enteral route

Perform/provide:

• Storage of reconstituted solution if refrigerated for no longer than 24 hr

• Do not use discolored solutions

Evaluate:

• Therapeutic response: Ease of breathing after several mins

Teach patient/family:

• The reason for drug administra-tion

---

etidocaine HCl

(et-ee'-doe-kane)
Duranest

Func. class.: Local anesthetic
Chem. class.: Amide

Action: Competes with calcium for sites in nerve membrane that con-trol sodium transport across cell

---

membrane; decreases rise of depolarization phase of action potential

Uses: Peripheral nerve block, caudal anesthesia, central neural block, vaginal block

Dosage and routes:

Varies depending on route of anesthesia

Available forms include: Inj 1%, 1.5%

Side effects/adverse reactions:

CNS: Anxiety, restlessness, *convulsions, loss of consciousness,* drowsiness, disorientation, tremors, shivering

CV: Myocardial depression, cardiac arrest, dysrhythmias, bradycardia, hypotension, hypertension, fetal bradycardia

GI: Nausea, vomiting

EENT: Blurred vision, tinnitus, pupil constriction

INTEG: Rash, urticaria, allergic reactions, edema, burning, skin discoloration at injection site, tissue necrosis

RESP: Status asthmaticus, respiratory arrest, anaphylaxis

Contraindications: Hypersensitivity, child <12 yr, elderly, severe liver disease

Precautions: Elderly, severe drug allergies, pregnancy (B)

Pharmacokinetics:

Onset 2-8 min, duration 3-6 hr; metabolized by liver, excreted in urine (metabolites)

Interactions/incompatibilities:

• Dysrhythmias: epinephrine, halothane, enflurane

• Hypertension: MAOIs, tricyclic antidepressants, phenothiazines

• Decreased action of etidocaine: chloroprocaine

NURSING CONSIDERATIONS

Assess:

• B/P, pulse, respiration during treatment

• Fetal heart tones if drug is used during labor

Administer:

• Only with crash cart, resuscitative equipment nearby

• Only drugs without preservatives for epidural or caudal anesthesia

Perform/provide:

• Use of new solution, discard unused portions

Evaluate:

• Therapeutic response: anesthesia necessary for procedure

• Allergic reactions: rash, urticaria, itching

• Cardiac status: ECG for dysrhythmias, pulse, B/P during anesthesia

Treatment of overdose: Airway, O_2, vasopressor, IV fluids, anticonvulsants for seizures

---

etidronate disodium

(e-ti-droe'nate)
Didronel, Didronel IV

Func. class.: Parathyroid agents (calcium regulator)

Chem. class.: Diphosphate

Action: Decreases bone resorption and new bone development (accretion)

Uses: Paget's disease, heterotopic ossification, hypercalcemia of malignancy

Dosage and routes:

Paget's disease

• *Adult:* PO 5-10 mg/kg/day 2 hr ac with water, not to exceed 20 mg/kg/day, max 6 mo

Heterotropic ossification

• *Adult:* PO 20 mg/kg qd × 2 wk, then 10 mg/kg/day for 10 wk, total 12 wk

Available forms include: Tabs 200, 400 mg

---

italics = common side effects   ***bold italic*** = life threatening reactions

Side effects/adverse reactions:
GI: Nausea, diarrhea
MS: Bone pain, hypocalcemia, decreased mineralization of noneffected bones
Contraindications: Pathologic fractures, children, colitis, severe renal disease with creatinine >5 mg/dl
Precautions: Pregnancy (B), renal disease, lactation, restricted vitamin D/calcium
Pharmacokinetics: Not metabolized, excreted in urine/feces, therapeutic response: 1-3 mo
NURSING CONSIDERATIONS
Assess:
• I&O ratio, check for decreased output in renal patients
• BUN, creatinine, uric acid, phosphate chloride, electrolytes, pH, urine calcium, magnesium, alk phosphatase, urinalysis, calcium should be kept at 9-10 mg/dl, vitamin D 50-135 IU/dl
Administer:
• On empty stomach with water 2 hr ac
• Drug therapy should not last longer than 6 mo
• IV after diluting in 250 ml or more of normal saline; give over 2 hr or longer
• Food, especially high in calcium and vitamins with mineral supplements or antacids high in metals should not be given within 2 hr of dose
Evaluate:
• Muscle spasm, laryngospasm, paresthesias, facial twitching, colic; may indicate hypocalcemia
• Nutritional status, diet for sources of vitamin D (milk, some seafood), calcium (dairy products, dark green vegetables), phosphates—adequate intake is necessary
• Persistent nausea or diarrhea

Teach patient/family:
• Avoid OTC products
• Therapeutic response may take 1-3 mo, effects persist for months after drug is discontinued
• Adequate intake of Ca^+, vitamin D is necessary

---

etomidate
(e-tom'i-date)
Amidate, Hypnomidate
Func. class.: General anesthetic
Chem. class.: Nonbarbiturate hypnotic

Action: Acts at level of reticular-activating system to produce anesthesia
Uses: Induction of general anesthesia
Dosage and routes:
• *Adult and child >10 yr:* IV 0.2-0.6 mg/kg over ½-1 min
Available forms include: Inj IV 2 mg/ml
Side effects/adverse reactions:
GI: Nausea, vomiting (postoperatively)
CNS: Tonic movements, myoclonic movements, averting movements
CV: Tachycardia, hypotension, hypertension, bradycardia
ENDO: Decreases steroid production
RESP: Laryngospasm
INTEG: Pain on administration
Contraindications: Hypersensitivity, labor/delivery
Precautions: Pregnancy (C), child <10 yr, lactation
Pharmacokinetics:
IV: Onset 20 sec, peak 1 min, duration 3-5 min; half-life 75 min, metabolized in liver, excreted in urine

NURSING CONSIDERATIONS
Assess:
• I&O ratio for increasing urine output
• VS q10 min during IV administration, q30 min after IM dose
• Plasma cortisol levels if administered over several hours (5-20 μg/100 ml normal level of cortisol)
Administer:
• Corticosteroids for severe hypotension
• Only with crash cart, resuscitative equipment nearby
• IV slowly only, muscular twitching is reduced with fentanyl before anesthesia induction
Evaluate:
• Increasing or decreasing heart rate or dysrhythmias shown on ECG

---

etoposide (VP-16)
(e-toe-poe′side)
VePesid

Func. class.: Antineoplastic
Chem. class.: Semisynthetic podophyllotoxin

Action: Inhibits mitotic activity through metaphase to mitosis; also inhibits cells from entering mitosis, depresses DNA, RNA synthesis
Uses: Leukemias, lung, testicular cancer, lymphomas, neuroblastoma, melanoma, ovarian cancer
Dosage and routes:
• *Adult:* IV 45-75 mg/m²/day × 3-5 days given q3-5 wk or 200-250 mg/m²/wk, or 125-140 mg/m²/day 3 × wk, q5 wk
Available forms include: Inj IV 20 mg/ml, caps 50 mg
Side effects/adverse reactions:
*HEMA: **Thrombocytopenia, leukopenia, myelosuppression, anemia***

*GI: Nausea, vomiting, anorexia, **hepatotoxicity***
INTEG: Rash, alopecia, phlebitis
*RESP: **Bronchospasm***
CV: Hypotension
CNS: Headache, *fever*
*GU: **Nephrotoxicity***
Contraindications: Hypersensitivity, bone marrow depression, severe hepatic disease, severe renal disease, bacterial infection, pregnancy (D)
Precautions: Renal disease, hepatic disease, lactation, children, gout
Pharmacokinetics: Half-life 3 hr, terminal 15 hr, metabolized in liver, excreted in urine, crosses placental barrier
Interactions/incompatibilities:
• Do not use with radiation
• Do not use with dextrose solution
• Increased protime: warfarin
NURSING CONSIDERATIONS
Assess:
• CBC, differential, platelet count weekly; withhold drug if WBC is <4000 or platelet count is <75,000; notify physician of results
• Renal function studies: BUN, serum uric acid, urine CrCl, electrolytes before, during therapy
• I&O ratio, report fall in urine output of 30 ml/hr
• Monitor temperature q4h; may indicate beginning infection
• Liver function tests before, during therapy (bilirubin, AST, ALT, LDH) as needed or monthly
• RBC, Hct, Hgb since these may be decreased
Administer:
• After diluting 100 mg/250 ml or more D₅W or NaCl to a concentration of 0.2-0.4 mg/ml, infuse over 30-60 min
• Antiemetic 30-60 min before giv-

---

italics = common side effects   ***bold italic*** = life threatening reactions

ing drug and prn to prevent vomiting

• Allopurinol or sodium bicarbonate to maintain uric acid levels, alkalinization of urine

• Hyaluronidase 150 U/ml to 1 ml NaCl to infiltration area, ice compress

• Transfusion for anemia

• Antispasmodic

Perform/provide:

• Liquid diet: cola, Jell-O; dry toast or crackers may be added if patient is not nauseated or vomiting

• Increase fluid intake to 2-3 L/day to prevent urate deposits, calculi formation

• Diet low in purines: organ meats (kidney, liver), dried beans, peas to maintain alkaline urine

• Nutritious diet with iron, vitamin supplements

• HOB increased to facilitate breathing

Evaluate:

• Bleeding: hematuria, guaiac stools, bruising or petechiae, mucosa or orifices q8h

• Food preferences; list likes, dislikes

• Effects of alopecia on body image; discuss feelings about body changes

• Yellowing of skin and sclera, dark urine, clay-colored stools, itchy skin, abdominal pain, fever, diarrhea

• Buccal cavity q8h for dryness, sores or ulceration, white patches, oral pain, bleeding, dysphagia

• Local irritation, pain, burning, discoloration at injection site

• Symptoms indicating severe allergic reaction: rash, pruritus, urticaria, purpuric skin lesions, itching, flushing

• Symptoms of anaphylaxis: flushing, restlessness, coughing, difficulty breathing

• Frequency of stools, characteristics: cramping, acidosis; signs of dehydration: rapid respirations, poor skin turgor, decreased urine output, dry skin, restlessness, weakness

Teach patient/family:

• To report any complaints or side effects to nurse or physician

• To report any changes in breathing or coughing

• That hair may be lost during treatment, a wig or hairpiece may make patient feel better; tell patient that new hair may be different in color, texture

• To make position changes slowly to prevent fainting

---

etretinate

(e-tret′-in-ate)

Tegison

Func. class.: Systemic antipsoriatic

Chem. class.: Retinol derivative

Action: Unknown; drug is related to retinol

Uses: Severe recalcitrant psoriasis, including erythrodermic and generalized pustular types

Dosage and routes:

• *Adult:* PO 0.75-1 mg/kg/day in divided doses, not to exceed 1.5 mg/kg/day; maintenance dose 0.5-0.75 mg/kg/day

Available forms include: Caps 10, 25 mg

Side effects/adverse reactions:

INTEG: Alopecia; peeling of palms, soles, fingertips; itching; rash; dryness; red scaling face; bruising; sunburn; pyogenic granuloma; paronychia; onycholysis; perspiration change

---

CNS: Fatigue, headache, dizziness, fever, pain, anxiety, amnesia, depression
EENT: Eye irritation, pain, double vision, change in lacrimation, earache, otitis externa
*GI: Anorexia, abdominal pain, nausea, **hepatitis,** constipation, diarrhea, flatulence*
*CV: Edema, **CV obstruction, atrial fibrillation,** chest pain, coagulation disorders*
RESP: Dyspnea, cough
*GU: WBC in urine, **proteinuria,** glycosuria, increased BUN, creatinine, **hematuria,** casts, **acetonuria, hemoglobinuria***
MET: Increase or decrease potassium, calcium, phosphate, sodium, chloride
MS: Hyperostosis, bone pain, cramps, myalgia, gout, hypertonia
Contraindications: Pregnancy (X)
Precautions: Lactation, children, hepatic disease
Pharmacokinetics:
99% plasma protein binding; excreted in bile, urine; terminal half-life 120 days; stored in fatty tissue
Interactions/incompatibilities:
• Increased absorption of etretinate: milk or high lipid diet
NURSING CONSIDERATIONS
Assess:
• For pseudotumor cerebri: headache, nausea, vomiting, visual problems, papilledema
• Hepatic studies: AST, ALT, LDH, since hepatotoxicity may occur
• Visual problems: blurring, decreased night vision, poor visual acuity; drug should be discontinued and opthalmologist consulted
• Lipids before, q1-2 wk during treatment; after discontinuing treatment, lipids will return to normal

Evaluate:
• Therapeutic response: decrease in scaling, itching, amount of psoriasis
Teach patient/family:
• To take with food
• Not to use during pregnancy; contraception must be used for 1 mo before or after therapy
• Not to take vitamin A supplements
• That contact lens-intolerance is common

---

factor IX complex (human)
Konyne HT, Profilnine Heat-Treated, Proplex T, Proplex SX-T
Func. class.: Hemostatic
Chem. class.: Factors II, VII, IX, X

Action: Causes an increase in blood levels of clotting factors II, VII, IX, X
Uses: Hemophilia B (Christmas disease), factor IX deficiency, anticoagulant reversal, control bleeding in factor VIII inhibitors
Dosage and routes:
• *Adult and child:* IV 1 U/kg × desired % increase
Available forms include: Inj IV (number of units noted on label)
Side effects/adverse reactions:
GI: Nausea, vomiting, abdominal cramps, jaundice, ***viral hepatitis***
INTEG: Rash, flushing, *urticaria*
CNS: Headache, dizziness, malaise, paresthesia, *lethargy, chills, fever, flushing*
HEMA: ***Thrombosis, hemolysis, AIDS***
CV: Hypotension, tachycardia, *MI,* ***venous thrombosis, pulmonary embolism***
RESP: ***Bronchospasm***

---

italics = common side effects   ***bold italic*** = life threatening reactions

Contraindications: Hypersensitivity, hepatic disease, DIC, elective surgery, mild factor IX deficiency
Precautions: Neonates/infants, pregnancy (C)
Pharmacokinetics:
IV: Half-life factor VII—3-6 hr, factor IX—24-36 hr
NURSING CONSIDERATIONS
Assess:
• Blood studies (coagulation factors assays by % normal: 5% prevents spontaneous hemorrhage, 30%-50% for surgery, 80%-100% for severe hemorrhage)
• Increased B/P, pulse
Administer:
• IV slowly, with plastic syringe only
• After dilution with provided diluent, 50 U/ml or 25 U/ml; give not to exceed 10 ml/min
• After crossmatch is completed if patient has blood type A, B, AB, to determine incompatibility with factor
Perform/provide:
• Storage of reconstituted solution for 3 hr at room temp or up to 2 yr refrigeration (powder); check expiration date
Evaluate:
• Allergic or pyrogenic reaction: fever, chills, rash, itching, slow infusion rate if not severe
• DIC: bleeding, ecchymosis, hypersensitivity, changes in coagulation tests
Teach patient/family:
• To report any signs of bleeding: gums, under skin, urine, stools, emesis
• Risk of viral hepatitis, AIDS
• That immunization for hepatitis B may be given first
• To be tested q 2-3 mo for HIV

famotidine

(fam-oo'-te-dine)
Pepcid, Pepcid IV
Func. class.: H₂ histamine receptor antagonist

Action: Competitively inhibits histamine at histamine H₂ receptor site, decreasing gastric secretion while pepsin remains at stable level
Uses: Short-term treatment of active duodenal ulcer, maintenance therapy for duodenal ulcer, Zollinger-Ellison syndrome, multiple endocrine adenomas, gastric ulcers
Dosage and routes:
Duodenal ulcer
• *Adult:* PO 40 mg qd hs × 4-8 wk, then 20 mg qd hs if needed (maintenance); IV 20 mg q12h if unable to take PO
Hypersecretory conditions
• *Adult:* PO 20 mg q6h, may give 160 mg q6h if needed; IV 20 mg q12h if unable to take PO
Available forms include: Tabs 20, 40 mg; powder for oral susp 40 mg/5 ml; inj IV 10 mg/ml
Side effects/adverse reactions:
*HEMA: **Thrombocytopenia***
CNS: Headache, dizziness, paresthesia, seizure, depression, anxiety, somnolence, insomnia, fever
GI: Constipation, nausea, vomiting, anorexia, cramps, abnormal liver enzymes
*RESP: **Bronchospasm***
EENT: Taste change, tinnitus, orbital edema
INTEG: Rash
MS: Myalgia, arthralgia
Contraindications: Hypersensitivity
Precautions: Pregnancy (B), lactation, children, severe renal disease, severe hepatic function, elderly

Pharmacokinetics:
PO: Peak 1-3 hr, plasma protein-binding 15%-20%; metabolized in liver (active metabolites), excreted by kidneys, half-life 2.5-3.5 hr
Interactions/incompatibilities:
• Decreased absorption: ketoconazole
• Decreased absorption of famotidine: antacids
NURSING CONSIDERATIONS
Assess:
• Blood counts during therapy, watch for decreasing platelets, if low, therapy may need to be discontinued and restarted after hematologic recovery
Administer:
• Antacids 1 hr before or 2 hr after famotidine
• IV after diluting with water for injection
• IV after diluting 2 ml of drug in IV solution to total volume of 5-10 ml, inject over >2 min
• IV infusion after diluting 2 ml of drug in 100 ml of IV solution and run over 15-30 min
Perform/provide:
• Storage in cool environment (oral), IV solution is stable for 48 hr at room temperature
Evaluate:
• Blood dyscrasias (thrombocytopenia): bruising, fatigue, bleeding, poor healing
Teach patient/family:
• That drug must be continued for prescribed time to be effective
• To report bleeding, bruising, fatigue, malaise since blood dyscrasias do occur
• Discuss possibility of decreased libido, reversible after discontinuing therapy
• To avoid irritating foods and extreme temperatures of foods

fat emulsions

Intralipid 10%, 20%; Liposyn 10%, 20%; Soyacal 10%, 20%; Travamulsion 10%, 20%

Func. class.: Caloric
Chem. class.: Fatty acid, long chain

Action: Needed for energy, heat production; consist of neutral triglycerides, primarily unsaturated fatty acids
Uses: Increase calorie intake, fatty acid deficiency, prevention
Dosage and routes:
Deficiency
• *Adult and child:* IV 8%-10% of required calorie intake (intralipid)
Adjunct to TPN
• *Adult:* IV 1 ml/min over 15-30 min (10%) or 0.5 ml/min over 15-30 min (20%); may increase to 500 ml over 4-8 hr if no adverse reactions occur, not to exceed 2.5 gm/kg
• *Child:* IV 0.1 ml/min over 10-15 min (10%) or 0.05 ml/min over 10-15 min (20%); may increase to 1 g/kg over 4 hr if no adverse reactions occur, not to exceed 4 gm/kg
Prevention of deficiency
• *Adult:* IV 500 ml twice a wk (10%), given 1 ml/min for 30 min, not to exceed 500 ml over 6 hr
• *Child:* IV 5-10 ml/kg/day (10%), given 0.1 ml/min for 30 min, not to exceed 100 ml/hr
Available forms include: Inj IV many types
Side effects/adverse reactions:
CNS: Dizziness, headache, drowsiness, focal seizures
*CV: **Shock***
GI: Nausea, vomiting, ***hepatomegaly***
RESP: Dyspnea, ***fat in lung tissue***
HEMA: ***Hyperlipemia, hyperco-***

---

italics = common side effects   ***bold italic*** = life threatening reactions

agulation, thrombocytopenia, leukopenia, leukocytosis

Contraindications: Hypersensitivity, hyperlipemia, lipid necrosis, acute pancreatitis accompanied by hyperlipemia, hyperbilirubinemia of the newborn

Precautions: Severe liver disease, diabetes mellitus, thrombocytopenia, gastric ulcers, premature, term newborns, pregnancy (C), sepsis

Interactions/incompatibilities:

• Do not mix with any drug, electrolytes, solutions, vitamin, unless added to TPN

NURSING CONSIDERATIONS
Assess:

• Triglycerides, free fatty acid levels, platelet counts daily to prevent fat overload, thrombocytopenia

• Liver function studies: AST, ALT

Administer:

• After changing IV tubing at each infusion: infection may occur with old tubing

• With infusion pump: do not use in-line filter; clogging will occur

Perform/provide:

• Use of mixed solutions that are not separated or oily looking

Evaluate:

• Therapeutic response: increased weight

• Nutritional status: calorie count by dietician

Teach patient/family

• Reason for use of lipids

---

fenfluramine HCl

(fen-fluer′a-meen)
Pondimin

Func. class.: Anorexant
Chem. class.: Amphetamine derivative

Controlled Substance Schedule IV

Action: Influences serotonin pathways in central nervous system

Uses: Exogenous obesity

Dosage and routes:

• *Adult:* PO 20 mg ac, not to exceed 40 mg tid

Available forms include: Tabs 20 mg

Side effects/adverse reactions:

HEMA: Bone marrow depression, leukopenia, agranulocytosis

MISC: Hair loss, flushing, fever

EENT: Mydriasis, blurred vision

CNS: Insomnia, talkativeness, dizziness, drowsiness, headache, irritability, confusion, mood changes, anxiety, weakness, vivid dreams, uncoordination, depression, fatigue, malaise, euphoria, tremor, confusion

GI: Nausea, vomiting, anorexia, *dry mouth, diarrhea,* constipation, abdominal pain

GU: Impotence, change in libido, dysuria, urinary frequency

CV: Palpitations, tachycardia, hypertension, hypotension, dysrythmias, pulmonary hypertension

INTEG: Urticaria, rash, burning, sweating, chills, fever, erythma

Contraindications: Hypersensitivity to sympathomimetic amine, glaucoma, drug abuse, cardiovascular disease, alcoholism, children <12 yr, hypertension, hyperthyroidism, severe arteriosclerosis

Precautions: Diabetes mellitus, hypertension, depression, pregnancy (C), lactation

Pharmacokinetics:

PO: Onset 1-2 min, duration 4-6 hr, metabolized by liver, excreted by kidneys, half-life 20 hr

Interactions/incompatibilities:

• Hypertensive crisis: MAOIs or within 14 days of MAOIs

• Increased effect of fenfluramine: acetazolamide, antacids, sodium

---

bicarbonate, ascorbic acid, ammonium chloride
• Decreased effects of fenfluramine: tricyclics
• Decrease effects of: guanethidine, other antihypertensives

NURSING CONSIDERATIONS
Assess:
• VS, B/P since this drug may reverse antihypertensives; check patients with cardiac disease more often
• CBC, urinalysis, in diabetes: blood sugar, urine sugar; insulin changes may need to be made since eating will decrease
• Height, growth rate in children; growth rate may be decreased

Administer:
• At least 6 hr before hs to avoid sleeplessness
• For obesity only if patient is on weight reduction program, including dietary changes, exercise; patient will develop tolerance and weight loss won't occur without additional methods, give 1 hr before meals
• Gum, hard candy, frequent sips of water for dry mouth

Perform/provide:
• Check to see PO medication has been swallowed

Evaluate:
• Mental status: mood, sensorium, affect, stimulation, insomnia, aggressiveness may occur
• Physical dependency: should not be used for extended time; dose should be discontinued gradually, drug tolerance will occur after long-term use
• Withdrawal symptoms: headache, nausea, vomiting, muscle pain, weakness

Teach patient/family:
• Not to take more frequently than prescribed

• To decrease caffeine consumption (coffee, tea, cola, chocolate); may increase irritability, stimulation
• Avoid OTC preparations unless approved by physician
• To taper off drug over several weeks, or depression, increased sleeping, lethargy may ensue
• To avoid alcohol ingestion
• To avoid hazardous activities until patient is stabilized on medication
• To get needed rest; patients will feel more tired at end of day

Treatment of overdose: Administer fluids, gastric lavage, hemodialysis or peritoneal dialysis; antihypertensive for increased B/P; ammonium Cl for increased excretion

---

fenoprofen calcium
(fen-oh-proe'fen)
Nalfon
Func. class.: Nonsteroidal antiinflammatory
Chem. class.: Propionic acid derivative

Action: May inhibit prostaglandin synthesis by decreasing enzyme needed for biosynthesis; possesses analgesic, antiinflammatory, antipyretic properties

Uses: Mild to moderate pain, osteoarthritis, rheumatoid arthritis, acute gout, arthritis, ankylosing spondylitis, inflammation, dysmenorrhea

Dosage and routes:
Pain
• *Adult:* PO 200 mg q4-6h as needed
Arthritis
• *Adult:* PO 300-600 mg qid, not to exceed 3.2 g/day

---

italics = common side effects   **bold italic** = life threatening reactions

Available forms include: Caps 200, 300 mg; tabs 600 mg

Side effects/adverse reactions:

GI: Nausea, anorexia, vomiting, diarrhea, jaundice, *cholestatic hepatitis,* constipation, flatulence, cramps, dry mouth, peptic ulcer

CNS: Dizziness, headache, drowsiness, fatigue, tremors, confusion, insomnia, anxiety, depression

CV: Tachycardia, peripheral edema, palpitations, dysrhythmias

INTEG: Purpura, rash, pruritus, sweating

GU: Nephrotoxicity: dysuria, hematuria, oliguria, azotemia

HEMA: Blood dyscrasias

EENT: Tinnitus, hearing loss, blurred vision

Contraindications: Hypersensitivity, asthma, severe renal disease, severe hepatic disease

Precautions: Pregnancy, (B) 1st and 2nd trimester, lactation, children, bleeding disorders, GI disorders, cardiac disorders, hypersensitivity to other antiinflammatory agents

Pharmacokinetics:

PO: Peak 2 hr, half-life 3-3½ hr, metabolized in liver, excreted in urine (metabolites), breast milk, 99% plasma protein binding

Interactions/incompatibilities:

• May increase the action of: coumarin, sulfonamides, salicyates

• May decrease effects of fenoprofen: phenobarbital, probenecid

NURSING CONSIDERATIONS

Assess:

• Renal, liver, blood studies: BUN, creatinine, AST, ALT, Hgb, before treatment, periodically thereafter

• Audiometric, ophthalmic exam before, during, after treatment

Administer:

• With food to decrease GI symptoms; however, best to take on empty stomach to facilitate absorption

Perform/provide:

• Storage at room temperature

Evaluate:

• Therapeutic response: decreased pain, stiffness in joints, decreased swelling in joints, ability to move more easily

• For eye, ear problems: blurred vision, tinnitus; may indicate toxicity

Teach patient/family:

• To report blurred vision, ringing, roaring in ears; may indicate toxicity

• To avoid driving, other hazardous activities if dizziness, drowsiness occurs

• To report change in urine pattern, increased weight, edema, increased pain in joints, fever, blood in urine; indicates nephrotoxicity

• That therapeutic effects may take up to 1 mo

• To take with a full glass of water to enhance absorption

---

fentanyl citrate

(fen'ta-nill)

Sublimaze

Func. class.: Narcotic analgesics

Chem. class.: Opiate, synthetic phenylpiperidine derivative

Controlled Substance Schedule II

Action: Inhibits ascending pain pathways in CNS, increases pain threshold, alters pain perception

Uses: Preoperatively, postoperatively; adjunct to general anesthetic, when combined with droperidol

Dosage and routes:

Anesthetic

• *Adult:* IV 0.05-0.1 mg q2-3min prn

Preoperatively

- *Adult:* IM 0.05-0.1 mg q30-60 min before surgery

Postoperatively
- *Adult:* IM 0.05-0.1 mg ql-2h prn
- *Child:* IM 0.02-0.03 mg/9 kg

Available forms include: Inj IM, IV 0.05 mg/ml

Side effects/adverse reactions:

CNS: Dizziness, delirium, euphoria
GI: Nausea, vomiting
MS: Muscle rigidity
EENT: Blurred vision, miosis
CV: **Bradycardia, arrest,** hypotension or hypertension
RESP: **Respiratory depression, arrest, laryngospasm**

Contraindications: Hypersensitivity to opiates, myasthenia gravis
Precautions: Elderly, respiratory depression, increased intracranial pressure, seizure disorders, severe respiratory disorders, cardiac dysrhythmias, pregnancy (C)

Pharmacokinetics:
IM: Onset 7-15 min, peak 30 min, duration 1-2 hr
IV: Onset immediate, peak 3-5 min, duration ½-1 hr
Metabolized by liver, excreted by kidneys, crosses placenta, excreted in breast milk, half-life 2½-4 hr, 80% bound to plasma proteins

Interactions/incompatibilities:
- Effects may be increased with other CNS depressants: alcohol, narcotics, sedative/hypnotics, antipsychotics, skeletal muscle relaxants

NURSING CONSIDERATIONS
Assess:
- VS after parenteral route, note muscle rigidity
Administer:
- By injection (IM, IV), give slowly to prevent rigidity
- Only with resuscitative equipment available

- IV; may be diluted with compatible sol and given as an infusion
Perform/provide:
- Storage in light-resistant area at room temperature
- Coughing, turning, deep breathing for postoperative patients
- Safety measures: siderails, night light, call bell within reach
Evaluate:
- CNS changes: dizziness, drowsiness, hallucinations, euphoria, LOC, pupil reaction
- Allergic reactions: rash, urticaria
- Respiratory dysfunction: respiratory depression, character, rate, rhythm; notify physician if respirations are <10/min

fentanyl citrate/droperidol combination

(fen'ta-nil) (droe-per'i-dole)
Innovar

Func. class.: General anesthetic/narcotic analgesic
Chem. class.: Phenylpiperone derivative

Controlled Substance Schedule II
Action: Action at subcortical levels to reduce motor activity, produces analgesia
Uses: Premedication, adjunct to general anesthesia, maintenance of anesthesia
Dosage and routes:
Induction
- *Adult:* IV 1 ml/20-25 lb
- *Child:* IV 0.5 ml/20 lb
Premedication
- *Adult:* IM 0.5-2 ml 45-60 min before surgery or procedure
- *Child:* IM 0.25 ml/20 lb 45-60 min before surgery or procedure

Available forms include: Inj IM, IV 0.05 mg fentanyl, 2.5 mg droperidol/ml

Side effects/adverse reactions:
*RESP: **Laryngospasm, broncho-spasm, respiratory arrest***
CNS: Dystonia, akathisia, flexion of arms, fine tremors, dizziness, anxiety, drowsiness, restlessness, hallucination, depression
CV: Tachycardia, hypotension, circulatory depression
EENT: Upward rotation of eyes, oculogyric crisis, blurred vision
INTEG: Chills, facial sweating, shivering, diaphoresis
GI: Nausea, vomiting

Contraindications: Hypersensitivity, child < 2 yr, myasthenia gravis

Precautions: Elderly, increased intracranial pressure, cardiovascular disease (bradydysrhythmias), renal disease, liver disease, Parkinson's disease, COPD, pregnancy (C)

Pharmacokinetics:
IV: Onset 20 sec, peak 2-5 min, duration ½-2 hr
IM: Onset 7 min, duration 1-2 hr, metabolized in liver, excreted in urine metabolites (90%)

Interactions/incompatibilities:
• Increased CNS depression: alcohol, narcotics, barbiturates, antipsychotics or other CNS depressants
• Decreased effects of: amphetamines, anticonvulsants, anticoagulants
• Increased intraocular pressure: anticholinergics, antiparkinson drugs
• Increased side effects of: lithium
• Do not mix with barbiturates in solution

NURSING CONSIDERATIONS
Assess:
• VS q10 min during IV administration, q30 min after IM dose
Administer:
• Anticholinergics (benztropine,

diphenhydramine) for extrapyramidal reaction
• Only with crash cart, resuscitative equipment nearby
• IV slowly only
Perform/provide:
• Slow movement of patient to avoid orthostatic hypotension
Evaluate:
• Therapeutic response: decreased anxiety, absence of vomiting, maintenance of anesthesia
• Rigidity of skeletal muscles
• Extrapyramidal reactions: dystonia, akathisia
• Increasing heart rate or decreasing B/P, notify physician at once; do not place patient in Trendelenburg position or sympathetic blockade may occur causing respiratory arrest
Teach patient/family:
• To use deep breathing, turning, coughing after surgery to prevent increased secretions in lungs

---

fentanyl transdermal
Duragesic

Func. class.: Narcotic analgesic
Chem. class.: Opiate, synthetic phenylpiperidine

Controlled Substance Schedule II

Action: Inhibits ascending pain pathways in CNS, increases pain threshold, alters pain perception
Uses: Management of chronic pains for those requiring opioid analgesia

Dosage and routes:
Adult: 25 μg/hr; may increase until pain relief occurs; apply patch to flat surface on upper torso and wear for 72 hr; apply new patch on different site for continued relief

Available forms include: Patch 2.5, 5, 7.5, 10 mg

Side effects/adverse reactions:

CNS: Dizziness, delirium, euphoria, lightheadedness, sedation, dysphoria, agitation, anxiety

GI: Nausea, vomiting, diarrhea, cramps

EENT: Blurred vision, miosis

CV: Bradycardia, **cardiac arrest,** hypotension or hypertension, facial flushing, chills

RESP: **Respiratory depression, laryngospasm, bronchospasm**

Contraindications: Hypersensitivity to opiates, myasthenia gravis

Precautions: Elderly, respiratory depression, increased intracranial pressure, seizure disorders, severe respiratory disorders, cardiac dysrhythmias, pregnancy (C)

Interactions/incompatibilities:

• Effects may be increased with other CNS depressants: alcohol, narcotics, sedative/hypnotics, antipsychotics, skeletal muscle relaxants

NURSING CONSIDERATIONS

Assess:

• Pain contol; check for duration, site, character of pain

Administer:

• q72h for continuous pain relief

Perform/provide:

• Safety measures: siderails, night light, call bell within reach

Evaluate:

• CNS changes: dizziness, drowsiness, hallucinations, euphoria, LOC, pupil reaction

• Allergic reactions: rash, urticaria

• Respiratory dysfunction: respiratory depression, character, rate, rhythm; notify physician if respirations are <10/min

ferrous fumarate/ferrous gluconate/ferrous sulfate

Eldofe, Farbegen, Fecot, Femiron, Feostat, Ferranol,* Fersamal, Fumasorb, Fumerin, Hemocyte, Ircon, Laud-Iron, Maniron, Neofer, Novofumar,* Palafer,* Palmiron/Fergon, Ferralet, Fertinic,* Novoferrogluc*, Simiron/Fer-in-Sol, Feosol, Fero-Grad,* Fero-Gradumet, Ferolix, Ferospace, Fesofor,* Irospan, Mol-Iron, Novoferrosulfa,* Slow-Fe, Telefon

Func. class.: Hematinic

Chem. class.: Iron preparation

Action: Replaces iron stores needed for red blood cell development, energy and O_2 transport, utilization; fumarate contains 33% elemental iron; gluconate, 12%; sulfate, 20%; iron, 30%; ferrous sulfate exsicated

Uses:

Iron deficiency anemia, prophylaxis for iron deficiency in pregnancy

Dosage and routes:

Fumarate

• *Adult:* PO 200 mg tid-qid

• *Child:* 2-12 yr: PO 3 mg/kg/day (elemental iron) tid-qid

• *Child 6 mo-2 yr:* PO up to 6 mg/kg/day (elemental iron) tid-qid

• *Infants:* PO 10-25 mg/day (elemental iron) tid-qid

Gluconate

• *Adult:* PO 200-600 mg tid

• *Child 6-12 yr:* 300-900 mg qd

• *Child <6 yr:* 100-300 mg qd

Sulfate

• *Adult:* PO 0.750-1.5 g/day in divided doses tid

• *Child 6-12 yr:* 600 mg/day in divided doses

---

italics = common side effects   **bold italic** = life threatening reactions

Pregnancy
• *Adult:* PO 300-600 mg/day in divided doses
Available forms include:
Fumarate
Tabs 63, 195, 200, 324, 325 mg; tabs chewable 100 mg; tabs controlled-release 300 mg; oral susp 100 ml/5 ml, 45 mg/0.6 ml
Gluconate
Tabs 300, 320, 325 mg; caps 86, 325, 435 mg; tabs film-coated 300 mg; elix 300 mg/5 ml
Sulfate
Tabs, 195, 300, 325 mg; tabs enteric-coated 325 mg; tabs extended-release, time-release caps, 525 mg
Side effects/adverse reactions:
GI: Nausea, constipation, epigastric pain, black and red tarry stools, vomiting, diarrhea
INTEG: Temporarily discolored tooth enamel and eyes
Contraindications: Hypersensitivity, ulcerative colitis/regional enteritis, hemosiderosis/hemochromatosis, peptic ulcer disease, hemolytic anemia, cirrhosis
Precautions: Anemia (long-term), pregnancy (A)
Pharmacokinetics:
PO: Excreted in feces, urine, skin, breast milk, enters bloodstream, bound to transferrin, crosses placenta
Interactions/incompatibilities:
• Decreased absorption of: tetracycline, penicillamine, antacids
• Decreased absorption of iron preparations: chloramphenicol, antacids
• Increased absorption of iron preparation: ascorbic acid
NURSING CONSIDERATIONS
Assess:
• Blood studies: Hct, Hgb, reticulocytes, bilirubin before treatment, at least monthly

Administer:
• Only with vitamin E supplements to infants or hemolytic anemia may occur
• Between meals for best absorption, may give with juice; do not give with antacids or milk, delay at least 1 hr; if GI symptoms occur, give PC even if absorption is decreased
• Through plastic straw to avoid discoloration of tooth enamel; dilute thoroughly
• At least 1 hr before hs since corrosion may occur in stomach
• For <6 months for anemia
Perform/provide:
• Storage in tight, light-resistant container
Evaluate:
• Toxicity: nausea, vomiting, diarrhea (green then tarry stools), hematemesis, pallor, cyanosis, shock, coma
• Elimination; if constipation occurs, increase water, bulk, activity
• Nutrition: amount of iron in diet (meat, dark green leafy vegetables, dried beans, dried fruits, eggs)
• Cause of iron loss or anemia, including salicylates, sulfonamides, antimalarials, quinidine
• Therapeutic response: improvement in Hct, Hgb, reticulocytes, decreased fatigue, weakness
Teach patient/family:
• That iron will change stools black or dark green
• That iron poisoning may occur if increased beyond recommended level
• Not to crush; swallow tablet whole
• Keep out of reach of children
• Do not substitute one iron salt for another; elemental iron content differs (e.g., 300 mg ferrous fumarate contains about 100 mg elemental

iron, whereas 300 mg ferrous gluconate contains only about 30 mg elemental iron)

• Avoid reclining position for 15-30 min after taking drug to avoid esophageal corrosion

Lab test interferences:
False-positive: Occult blood

Treatment of overdose: Induce vomiting; give eggs, milk until lavage can be done

---

fibrinolysin/desoxyribonuclease

(fye-bri-noe-lye'sin)
Elase
Func. class.: Enzyme
Chem. class.: Proteolytic-bovine

Action: Dissolves fibrin in clots, attacks DNA in areas of disintegrating cells

Uses: Debridement of wounds, intravaginally; irrigating wounds, topically

Dosage and routes:
Debridement/intravaginally
• *Adult:* OINT 5 g
Irrigating
• *Adult:* IRIG dilution depends on type of wound

Available forms include: Fibrinolysin with desoxyribonuclease 666.6 U/g; top sol fibrinolysin 25 U/desoxyribonuclease 15,000 U

Side effects/adverse reactions:
INTEG: Hyperemia

Contraindications: Hypersensitivity to bovine or mercury products, hematoma

Precautions: Pregnancy (C)

NURSING CONSIDERATIONS
Assess:
• For signs of irritation and inflammation; drug should be discontinued

Administer:
• After reconstituting with 10 ml sterile Nacl solution, use only fresh solution
• After removing necrotic debris, dry eschar
• Wet dressing by mixing 1 vial elase/10-50 ml saline solution, saturate gauze with solution, pack area, remove in 6-8 hr, repeat tid-qid

Perform/provide:
• Cleaning of wound using aseptic technique, cover with drug, cover, change at least qid

Evaluate:
• Therapeutic response: decrease in wound scarring, tissue necrosis
• Wound: drainage, color, odor

---

flavoxate HCl

(fla-vox'ate)
Urispas
Func. class.: Spasmolytic
Chem. class.: Flavone derivative

Action: Relaxes smooth muscles in urinary tract

Uses: Relief of nocturia, incontinence, suprapubic pain, dysuria, frequency associated with urologic conditions (symptomatic only)

Dosage and routes:
• *Adult and child >12 yr:* PO 100-200 mg tid-qid

Available forms include: Tabs 100 mg

Side effects/adverse reactions:
HEMA: **Leukopenia, eosinophilia**
CNS: Anxiety, restlessness, dizziness, **convulsions,** headache, drowsiness, confusion, decreased concentration
CV: Palpitations, sinus tachycardia, hypotension
GI: Nausea, vomiting, anorexia, abdominal pain, constipation

---

italics = common side effects   ***bold italic*** = life threatening reactions

GU: Dysuria
INTEG: Urticaria, dermatitis
EENT: Blurred vision, increased intraocular tension, dry mouth, throat
Contraindications: Hypersensitivity, GI obstruction, GI hemorrhage, GU obstruction
Precautions: Pregnancy (B), lactation, suspected glaucoma, children <12 yr
Pharmacokinetics: Excreted in urine

NURSING CONSIDERATIONS
Evaluate:
• Urinary status: dysuria, frequency, nocturia, incontinence
• Allergic reactions: rash, urticaria; if these occur, drug should be discontinued
Teach patient/family
• To avoid hazardous activities; dizziness may occur

---

flecainide acetate

(fle-kay'nide)
Tambocor

Func. class.: Antidysrhythmic (Class IC)

Action: Decreases conduction in all parts of the heart, with greatest effect on His-Purkinje system, which stabilizes cardiac membrane
Uses: Life-threatening ventricular dysrhythmias
Dosage and routes:
• *Adult:* PO 100 mg q12h, may increase q4 days by 50 mg bid to desired response, not to exceed 400 mg/day
Available forms include: Tabs 100 mg
Side effects/adverse reactions:
CNS: Headache, dizziness, involuntary movement, confusion, psychosis, restlessness, irritability, paresthesias, ataxia, flushing, som-

nolence, depression, anxiety, malaise
EENT: Tinnitus, *blurred vision,* hearing loss
GI: Nausea, vomiting, anorexia, constipation, abdominal pain, flatulence, change in taste
CV: Hypotension, bradycardia, angina, PVCs, *heart block, cardiovascular collapse, arrest, dysrhythmias, CHF*
RESP: Dyspnea, *respiratory depression*
INTEG: Rash, urticaria, edema, swelling
HEMA: Leukopenia, thrombocytopenia
GU: Impotence, decreased libido, polyuria, urinary retention
Contraindications: Hypersensitivity, severe heart block, cardiogenic shock, nonsustained ventricular dysrhythmias, frequent PVCs
Precautions: Pregnancy (C), lactation, children, renal disease, liver disease, CHF, respiratory depression, myasthenia gravis
Pharmacokinetics:
PO: Peak 3 hr; half-life 12-27 hr; metabolized by liver, excreted unchanged by kidneys (10%), excreted in breast milk
Interactions/incompatibilities:
• Increased levels of both drugs: propranolol
• Increased negative inotropic effects: disopyramide, verapamil
• Increased digoxin level: digoxin
NURSING CONSIDERATIONS
Assess:
• For hypokalemia, hyperkalemia before administration; correct electrolytes
• Blood levels: trough (0.2-1 µg/ml)
• B/P continuously for fluctuations
Administer:
• Reduced dosage as soon as dysrhythmia is controlled

Evaluate:
• Malignant hyperthermia: tachypnea, tachycardia, changes in B/P, increased temperature
• Cardiac rate, respiration: rate, rhythm, character, continuously
• Respiratory status: rate, rhythm, lung fields for rales
• CNS effects: dizziness, confusion, psychosis, paresthesias, convulsions; drug should be discontinued
• Increased respiration, increased pulse; drug should be discontinued
Lab test interferences:
Increase: CPK
Treatment of overdose: O$_2$, artificial ventilation, ECG, administer dopamine for circulatory depression, administer diazepam or thiopental for convulsions

---

floxuridine

(flox-yoor'i-deen)
FUDR
Func. class.: Antineoplastic, antimetabolite
Chem. class.: Pyrimidine antagonist

Action: Inhibits DNA synthesis; interferes with cell replication by competitively inhibiting thymidylate synthesis
Uses: GI adenocarcinoma metastatic to liver, cancer of breast, head, neck, liver, brain, gallbladder, bile duct
Dosage and routes:
• *Adult:* INTRAARTERIAL 0.1-0.6 mg/kg/day × 1-6 wk; HEPATIC ARTERY INJ 0.4-0.6 mg/kg/day × 1-6 wk
Available forms include: Powder for inj (intraarterial, hepatic artery) 500 mg/5 ml vial

Side effects/adverse reactions:
*HEMA: **Thrombocytopenia, leukopenia, myelosuppression, anemia***
GI: Anorexia, diarrhea, nausea, vomiting, ***hemorrhage***
*GU: **Renal failure***
EENT: Epistaxis
INTEG: Rash, fever
CNS: Lethargy, malaise, weakness
Contraindications: Hypersensitivity, myelosuppression, pregnancy (D), poor nutritional states, serious infections
Precautions: Renal disease, hepatic disease, bone marrow depression
Pharmacokinetics: Half-life 10-20 min, 20 hr terminal, metabolized in liver, excreted in urine (active metabolite), crosses blood-brain barrier
Interactions/incompatibilities:
• Increased toxicity: radiation or other antineoplastics

NURSING CONSIDERATIONS
Assess:
• CBC, differential, platelet count weekly; withhold drug if WBC is <3500/mm^3 or platelet count is <100,000/mm^3; notify physician of these results; drug should be discontinued
• Renal function studies: BUN, serum uric acid, urine CrCl, electrolytes before, during therapy
• I&O ratio: report fall in urine output to <30 ml/hr
• Monitor temperature q4h; fever may indicate beginning infection
• Liver function tests before, during therapy: bilirubin, alk phosphatase, AST, ALT, LDH; as needed or monthly
Administer:
• By intraarterial infusion pump after diluting 5 ml drug/5 ml sterile H$_2$O for inj, dilute further with

italics = common side effects   ***bold italic*** = life threatening reactions

D$_5$W or normal saline to required dilution
• Antiemetic 30-60 min before giving drug to prevent vomiting and prn
• Antibiotics for prophylaxis of infection
• Topical or systemic analgesics for pain
• Transfusion for anemia
• Antispasmodic for diarrhea
Perform/provide:
• Wrapping solution, do not expose to light
• Strict medical asepsis and protective isolation if WBC levels are low
• Increased fluid intake to 2-3 L/day to prevent dehydration unless contraindicated
• Rinsing of mouth tid-qid with water, club soda, brushing of teeth bid-tid with soft brush or cotton-tipped applicators for stomatitis; use unwaxed dental floss
• Nutritious diet with iron, vitamin supplements, low fiber, and no dairy products as ordered
Evaluate:
• Bleeding: hematuria, guaiac, bruising or petechiae, mucosa or orifices q8h
• Food preferences; list likes, dislikes
• Inflammation of mucosa, breaks in skin
• Buccal cavity q8h for dryness, sores or ulceration, white patches, oral pain, bleeding, dysphagia
• Symptoms indicating severe allergic reaction: rash, urticaria, itching, flushing
• GI symptoms: frequency of stools, cramping; low residue diet with elimination of milk products when used in conjunction with 5FUDR/radiation therapy
• Acidosis, signs of dehydration: rapid respirations, poor skin turgor, decreased urine output, dry skin, restlessness, weakness
Teach patient/family:
• Why protective isolation precautions are necessary
• To report signs of infection: increased temperature, sore throat, flu symptoms
• To report signs of anemia: fatigue, headache, faintness, shortness of breath, irritability
• To report bleeding: avoid use of razors, or commercial mouthwash
• To avoid use of aspirin products or ibuprofen
• To report stomatitis: any bleeding, white spots, ulcerations in mouth; tell patient to examine mouth qd, report symptoms
Lab test interferences:
Increase: Liver function studies

---

fluconazole

(floo-con'-a-zole)
Diflucan
Func. class.: Anti-fungal

Action: Inhibits ergosterol biosynthesis, causes direct damage to membrane phospholipids
Uses: Oropharyngeal candidiasis in AIDS patients, chronic mucocutaneous candidiasis, urinary candidiasis, cryptococcal meningitis
Dosage and routes:
Vaginal candidiasis
• *Adult:* PO 150 mg as a single dose
Serious fungal infections
• *Adult:* PO/IV 50-400 mg qd
Oropharyngeal candidiasis in AIDS patients:
• *Adult:* PO 50 mg qd
Available forms include: Tabs 50, 100, 200 mg, IV inj 200, 400 mg
Side effects/adverse reactions:
GI: Nausea, vomiting, diarrhea,

cramping, flatus, increased AST, ALT

Contraindications: Hypersensitivity

Precautions: Renal disease, pregnancy (B)

Interactions/incompatibilities:
• Potentiation of anticoagulation: warfarin
• Increased renal dysfunction: cyclosporines

NURSING CONSIDERATIONS
Assess:
• VS q15-30min during first infusion, note changes in pulse, B/P
• I&O ratio, watch for decreasing urinary output, change in sp gr; discontinue drug to prevent renal damage
• Weigh weekly; if weight gain >2 lb/wk and edema is present, renal damage should be considered

Administer:
• After diluting according to package directions
• IV using an in-line filter, using distal veins; check for extravasation and necrosis q2h
• Drug only after C&S confirms organism, drug needed to treat condition

Perform/provide:
• Storage, protected from moisture and light, diluted solution is stable for 24 hr

Evaluate:
• Therapeutic response: decreasing oral candidiasis, fever, malaise, rash, negative C&S for infection organism
• Renal toxicity: increasing BUN, serum creatinine; if BUN is >40 mg/dl or if serum creatinine is >3 mg/dl, drug may be discontinued or dosage reduced
• For hepatotoxicity: increasing AST, ALT, alk phosphatase, bilirubin

Teach patient/family:
• That long-term therapy may be needed to clear infection

---

flucytosine

(floo-sye'toe-seen)
Ancobon, Ancotil*

Func. class.: Antifungal
Chem. class.: Pyrimidine (fluorinated)

Action: Converted to fluorouracil after entering fungi, which inhibits DNA synthesis

Uses: *Candida* infections (septicemia, endocarditis, pulmonary, urinary tract infections), *Cryptococcus* (meningitis, pulmonary, urinary tract infections)

Dosage and routes:
• *Adult and child >50 kg:* PO 50-150 mg/kg/day q6h
• *Adult and child <50 kg:* PO 1.5-4.5 g/m²/day in 4 divided doses

Available forms include: Caps 250, 500 mg

Side effects/adverse reactions:
INTEG: Rash

CNS: Headache, confusion, dizziness, sedation

GI: Nausea, vomiting, anorexia, diarrhea, cramps, enterocolitis, increased AST, ALT, alk phosphatase, *bowel perforation* (rare)

*HEMA: **Thrombocytopenia, agranulocytosis, anemia, leukopenia, pancytopenia***

GU: Increased BUN, creatinine

Contraindications: Hypersensitivity

Precautions: Renal disease, bone marrow depression, blood dyscrasias, radiation/chemotherapy, pregnancy (C)

Pharmacokinetics:
PO: Peak 2½-6 hr, half-life 3-6 hr, excreted in urine (unchanged),

---

italics = common side effects   ***bold italic*** = life threatening reactions

well-distributed to CSF, aqueous humor, joints
Interactions/incompatibilities:
• Synergisim: Amphotericin B
NURSING CONSIDERATIONS
Assess:
• VS q15-30 min during first infusion, note changes in pulse and B/P
• Blood studies: CBC, including platelets
• Drug level during treatment (therapeutic level 25-100 µg/ml); if renal impairment is present level usually kept <100 µg/ml
Administer:
• Drug only after C&S confirms organism, drug needed to treat condition
• Few caps at a time to decrease nausea, vomiting over 15 min
Perform/provide:
• Symptomatic treatment as ordered for adverse reactions: aspirin, antihistamines, antiemetics, antispasmodics
• Storage in tight, light-resistant containers at room temperature
Evaluate:
• Therapeutic response: decreased fever, malaise, rash, negative C&S for infecting organism
• For renal toxicity: increasing BUN, serum creatinine; if serum creatinine >1.7 mg/100 dl, dosage may be reduced
• For hepatotoxicity: increasing AST, ALT, alk phosphatase
• For allergic reaction: dermatitis, rash; drug should be discontinued, antihistamines (mild reaction) or epinephrine (severe reaction) administered
• For blood dyscrasias, fatigue, bruising, malaise, dark urine
Teach patient/family:
• That long-term therapy may be needed to clear infection (1-2 mo depending on type of infection)
• To report symptoms of blood dyscrasias: fatigue, bruising, malaise, dark urine
Lab test interferences:
False-increase: Creatinine

---

fludrocortisone acetate

(floo-droe-kor′ti-sone)
Florinef Acetate
Func. class.: Corticosteroid
Chem. class.: Mineralocorticoid

Action: Promotes increased reabsorption of sodium and loss of potassium from the renal tubules
Uses: Adrenal insufficiency, salt-losing adrenogenital syndrome
Dosage and routes:
• *Adult:* PO 0.1-0.2 mg qd
Available forms include: Tabs 0.1 mg
Side effects/adverse reactions:
CNS: Flushing, sweating, headache
CV: Hypertension, **circulatory collapse, thrombophlebitis, embolism,** tachycardia
MS: Fractures, osteoporosis, weakness
Contraindications: Hypersensitivity, acute glomerulonephritis, amebiasis
Precautions: Pregnancy (C), osteoporosis, CHF
Pharmacokinetics:
PO: Half-life 3.5 hr, metabolized by liver, excreted in urine
Interactions/incompatibilities:
• Decreased action of fludrocortisone: cholestyramine, colestipol, barbiturates, rifampin, ephedrine, phenytoin, theophylline
• Decreased effects of: diuretics, K-sparing diuretics, potassium supplements
• Increased side effects: sodium-

containing food or medication, digitalis preparations

NURSING CONSIDERATIONS
Assess:
• Potassium, while on long-term therapy; hypokalemia
• Weight daily, notify physician of weekly gain >5 lb
• B/P q4h, pulse, notify physician if chest pain occurs
• I&O ratio, be alert for decreasing urinary output and increasing edema

Administer:
• Titrated dose, use lowest effective dose
• With food or milk to decrease GI symptoms

Perform/provide:
• Assistance with ambulation in patient with bone tissue disease to prevent fractures

Evaluate:
• Potassium depletion: paresthesias, fatigue, nausea, vomiting, depression, polyuria, dysrhythmias, weakness
• Edema, hypertension, cardiac symptoms

Teach patient/family:
• That ID as steroid user should be carried
• Not to discontinue this medication abruptly

Lab test interferences:
Increase: Potassium, sodium
Decrease: Hematocrit

---

flunisolide
(floo-niss'oh-lide)
AeroBid,* Nasalide Nasal Solution, Rhinalar*

Func. class.: Steroid, intranasal
Chem. class.: Glucocorticoid

Action: Long-acting synthetic adrenocorticoid with antiinflammatory activity, minimal mineralocorticoid properties

Uses: Rhinitis (seasonal or perennial)

Dosage and routes:
• *Adult:* INSTILL 2 sprays in each nostril bid, then increase to tid if needed, not to exceed 8 sprays in each nostril/day
• *Child 6-14 yr:* INSTILL 1 spray in each nostril tid or 2 sprays bid, not to exceed 4 sprays in each nostril/day

Available forms include: Aerosol 25µg/spray

Side effects/adverse reactions:
EENT: Nasal irritation, dryness, rebound congestion, epistaxis, sneezing
INTEG: Urticaria
CNS: Headache, dizziness
SYST: ***Congestive heart failure, convulsions,*** increased sodium, hypertension

Contraindications: Hypersensitivity, child <12 yr, fungal, bacterial infection of nose

Precautions: Lactation, pregnancy (C)

Pharmacokinetics:
AERO: Half-life 6 min, terminal half-life 1.8 hr, metabolized in liver, excreted in urine

NURSING CONSIDERATIONS
Administer:
• No more than q4h

Perform/provide:
• Storage in light-resistant container; discard open container after 3 mo

Evaluate:
• Redness, swelling, pain in nasal passages

Teach patient/family:
• Stinging may occur for several applications; drying of mucosa may be decreased by environmental humidification

---

italics = common side effects   ***bold italic*** = life threatening reactions

• To notify physician if irregular pulse, insomnia, dizziness, or tremors occur
• Proper administration to avoid systemic absorption
• To check with physician before using any other nasal medications

---

flunisolide

(floo-niss'oh-lide)
AeroBid, Nasalide

Func. class.: Corticosteroid
Chem. class.: Glucocorticoid

Action: Decreases inflammation by suppression of migration of polymorphonuclear leukocytes, fibroblasts, reversal of increased capillary permeability and lysosomal stabilization; does not depress hypothalamus

Uses: Rhinitis, allergies, nasal polyps

Dosage and routes:
• *Adult and child >6 yr:* SPRAY 2 puffs bid, not to exceed 4 puffs bid
Available forms include: Nasal sol 25 μg/metered dose (Nasalide), 250 μg/metered dose (AeroBid)

Side effects/adverse reactions:
CNS: Headache, nervousness, restlessness
EENT: Hoarseness, candida infection of oral cavity, sore throat
GI: Nausea, vomiting, dry mouth
Contraindications: Hypersensitivity, child <6 yr
Precautions: Nonasthmatic bronchial disease, bacterial, fungal, viral infections of mouth, throat, lungs, respiratory TB, untreated fungal, bacterial, or viral infections, pregnancy (C), glaucoma
Pharmacokinetics:
INH: Duration 1 hr

NURSING CONSIDERATIONS
Administer:
• Titrated dose, use lowest effective dose
Evaluate:
• Therapeutic response: ease of respirations, decreased inflammation
• Infection: increased temperature, WBC, even after withdrawal of medication; drug masks symptoms of infection
Teach patient/family:
• To use gum; rinse mouth after each dose
• That ID as steroid user should be carried
• To notify physician if therapeutic response decreases; dosage adjustment may be needed
• Proper administration technique, shake well before use
• Compliance to therapy
• Teach patient about cushingoid symptoms
• Symptoms of adrenal insufficiency: nausea, anorexia, fatigue, dizziness, dyspnea, weakness, joint pain

---

fluocinonide

(floo-oh-sin'oh-nide)
Lidex, Lidex-E, Lidemol*/Topsyn

Func. class.: Topical corticosteroid
Chem. class.: Synthetic fluorinated agent, group II potency

Action: Possesses antipruritic, antiinflammatory actions
Uses: Psoriasis, eczema, contact dermatitis, pruritus
Dosage and routes:
• *Adult and child:* Apply to affected area tid-qid
Available forms include: Oint 0.05%; cream 0.05%; sol 0.05%; gel 0.05%

Side effects/adverse reactions:

INTEG: Burning, dryness, itching, irritation, acne, folliculitis, hypertrichosis, perioral dermatitis, hypopigmentation, atrophy, striae, miliaria, allergic contact dermatitis, secondary infection

Contraindications: Hypersensitivity to corticosteroids, fungal infections

Precautions: Pregnancy (C), lactation, viral infections, bacterial infections

NURSING CONSIDERATIONS
Assess:

• Temperature; if fever develops, drug should be discontinued

Administer:

• Only to affected areas; do not get in eyes

• Medication, then cover with occlusive dressing (only if prescribed), seal to normal skin, change q12h; use occlusive dressings with extreme caution

• Only to dermatoses; do not use on weeping, denuded, or infected area

Perform/provide:

• Cleansing before application of drug

• Treatment for a few days after area has cleared

• Storage at room temperature

Evaluate:

• Therapeutic response: absence of severe itching, patches on skin, flaking

Teach patient/family:

• To avoid sunlight on affected area; burns may occur

fluorescein sodium

(flure'e-seen)

Fluorescite, Fluor-I-Strip, Ful-Glo, Funduscein Injections

Func. class.: Diagnostic agent, optic

Chem. class.: Fluorescent dye

Action: Allows breaks in the corneal tissue to absorb dye and show up as bright green under cobalt blue light

Uses: Diagnostic aid in identifying foreign bodies, fitting hard contact lenses, fundus photography, tonometry, identifying corneal abrasions, retinal angiography

Dosage and routes:

• *Adult:* INSTILL 1 gtt of 2% sol, irrigate or wet strip with sterile water and touch conjunctiva or fornix, flush eye with irrigating sol

Retinal angiography

• *Adult:* IV 5 ml 10% sol or 3 ml 25% sol injected in antecubital vein

• *Child:* IV 0.077 ml 10% sol or 0.044 ml 25% sol injected in antecubital vein

Available forms include: Inj IV 10%, 25%; sol 2%; strips 0.6, 9 mg

Side effects/adverse reactions:

CNS: Headache, dizziness, paresthesia, ***convulsions***

CV: Bradycardia, ***shock, cardiac arrest,*** hypertension

RESP: ***Dyspnea, acute pulmonary edema***

GI: Nausea, vomiting

EENT: Stinging, burning, conjunctival redness

Contraindications: Hypersensitivity

Precautions: Bronchial asthma, pregnancy (C), lactation

---

italics = common side effects   ***bold italic*** = life threatening reactions

NURSING CONSIDERATIONS
Administer:
• Only after soft contact lens are removed
• Solution, have patient close eyelids for 1 min
• Only with resuscitative equipment nearby
• Test dose (IV) before angiography
• Epinephrine 1:1000 for IV, IM route; an antihistamine and O₂ should always be available

Perform/provide:
• Storage at room temperature

Evaluate:
• IV site for redness, inflammation, swelling
• Eye color after application: epithelial defects are green while normal precorneal tear film appears bright yellow
• For allergic reaction: rash, urticaria, pruritus, angioedema

Teach patient/family:
• To report stinging, burning, itching, lacrimation, puffiness
• Urine will be yellow after IV dose

---

fluorometholone

(flure-oh-meth'oh-lone)
FML Liquifilm Ophthalmic
Func. class.: Ophthalmic antiinflammatory

Action: Decreases inflammation, resulting in decreased pain, photophobia, hyperemia, cellular infiltration
Uses: Inflammation of eye, lids, conjunctiva, cornea, uveitis, iridocyclitis, allergic condition, burns, foreign bodies, postoperatively in cataract
Dosage and routes:
• *Adult and child:* Instill 1-2 gtts

into conjunctival sac 1hr × 2 days, if needed, then bid-qid
Available forms include: Oint 0.1%; ophthalmic susp 0.1%, 0.25%
Side effects/adverse reactions:
*EENT: **Increased intraocular pressure,*** poor corneal wound healing, increased possibility of corneal infections, glaucoma exacerbation, ***optic nerve damage,*** decreased acuity, visual field
Contraindications: Hypersensitivity, acute superficial herpes simplex, fungal/viral diseases of the eye or conjunctiva, active diabetes mellitus, ocular TB, infections of the eye
Precautions: Corneal abrasions, glaucoma, pregnancy (C)
NURSING CONSIDERATIONS
Evaluate:
• Therapeutic response: absence of swelling, redness, exudate
Administer:
• After shaking
Perform/provide:
• Storage in tight, light-resistant container
Teach patient/family:
• Instillation method: pressure on lacrimal sac for 1 min
• Not to share eye medications with others
• Not to use if purulent drainage is present
• Not to discontinue steroids abruptly, they should be tapered over 1-2 wks

---

fluorouracil

(flure-oh-yoor'a-sil)
Efudex, Fluoroplex
Func. class.: Topical antineoplastic
Chem. class.: Antimetabolite

Action: Inhibits synthesis of DNA, RNA in susceptible cells

Uses: Keratosis (multiple/actinic), basal cell carcinoma

Dosage and routes:
• *Adult and child:* TOP apply to affected area bid

Available forms include: Sol 1%, 2%, 5%; cream 1%, 5%

Side effects/adverse reactions:
INTEG: Rash, irritation, pain, burning, contact dermatitis, scaling, swelling, soreness, hyperpigmentation, pruritus

Contraindications: Hypersensitivity, pregnancy (D)

NURSING CONSIDERATIONS
Assess:
• WBC, platelets at least monthly
Administer:
• Only 5% sol/cream for basal cell carcinoma
• Using gloves or applicator
• A low residue diet with no dairy product where radiation is also used
Perform/provide:
• Covering of lesion with porous gauze dressing only
• Washing of hands after application if gloves or applicator are not used
• Storage at room temperature
Evaluate:
• Therapeutic response: decreased size of lesion
• Area of body involved for redness, swelling
• Check oral cavity qd for stomatitis; if present discontinue drug
Teach patient/family:
• To avoid application on normal skin or getting cream in eyes
• To discontinue use if rash or irritation occurs
• To avoid sunlight or use sunscreen, photosensitivity may occur
• To wash hands after application
• Not to change application and use exactly as prescribed
• Lesion will disappear in 1-2 mo

fluorouracil (5-fluoro-uracil)

(flure-oh-yoor′a-sil)
Adrucil, 5-FU

Func. class.: Antineoplastic, antimetabolite
Chem. class.: Pyrimidine antagonist

Action: Inhibits DNA synthesis; interferes with cell replication by competitively inhibiting thymidylate synthesis, a vesicant

Uses: Cancer of breast, colon, rectum, stomach, pancreas, liver, ovary, cervix

Dosage and routes:
• *Adult:* IV 12 mg/kg/day × 4 days, not to exceed 800 mg/day; may repeat with 6 mg/kg on day 6, 8, 10, 12; maintenance is 10-15 mg/kg/wk as a single dose, not to exceed 1 g/wk

Available forms include: Inj IV 50 mg/ml

Side effects/adverse reactions:
*HEMA: **Thrombocytopenia, leukopenia, myelosuppression, anemia***
GI: Anorexia, stomatitis, diarrhea, nausea, vomiting, ***hemorrhage***
*GU: **Renal failure***
EENT: Epistaxsis
INTEG: Rash, fever
CNS: Lethargy, malaise, weakness

Contraindications: Hypersensitivity, myelosuppression, pregnancy (D), poor nutritional states, serious infections

Precautions: Renal disease, hepatic disease, bone marrow depression

Pharmacokinetics: Half-life 10-20 min, 20 hr terminal, metabolized in the liver, excreted in the urine, crosses blood-brain barrier

Interactions/incompatibilities:
• Increased toxicity: radiation or other antineoplastics

NURSING CONSIDERATIONS
Assess:
• CBC, differential, platelet count weekly; withhold drug if WBC is <3500/mm³ or platelet count is <100,000/mm³; notify physician of these results; drug should be discontinued
• Renal function studies: BUN, serum uric acid, urine CrCl, electrolytes before, during therapy
• I&O ratio: report fall in urine output to <30 ml/hr
• Temperature q4h; fever may indicate beginning infection
• Liver function tests before, during therapy: bilirubin, alk phosphatase, AST, ALT, LDH; as needed or monthly

Administer:
• IV undiluted, may inject through Y-tube or 3-way stopcock; give over 1-3 min
• Antiemetic 30-60 min before giving drug to prevent vomiting
• Antibiotics for prophylaxis of infection
• Topical or systemic analgesics for pain
• Transfusion for anemia
• Antispasmodic for diarrhea

Perform/provide:
• Protection from light
• Strict medical asepsis, protective isolation if WBC levels are low
• Increase fluid intake to 2-3 L/day to prevent dehydration, unless contraindicated
• Changing of IV site q48hrs.
• Rinsing of mouth tid-qid with water, club soda; brushing of teeth bid-tid with soft brush or cotton-tipped applicators for stomatitis; use unwaxed dental floss
• Nutritious diet with iron, vitamin supplements, low fiber, few dairy products especially when combined with radiotherapy as ordered

Evaluate:
• Bleeding: hematuria, guaiac, bruising or petechiae, mucosa or orifices q8h
• Food preferences; list likes, dislikes
• Inflammation of mucosa, breaks in skin
• Buccal cavity q8h for dryness, sores or ulceration, white patches, oral pain, bleeding, dysphagia
• Symptoms indicating severe allergic reaction: rash, urticaria, itching, flushing
• GI symptoms: frequency of stools, cramping
• Acidosis, signs of dehydration: rapid respirations, poor skin turgor, decreased urine output, dry skin, restlessness, weakness

Teach patient/family:
• Why protective isolation precautions are necessary
• To avoid foods with citric acid, hot or rough texture if stomatitis is present
• To report stomatitis: any bleeding, white spots, ulcerations in mouth; tell patient to examine mouth qd, report symptoms
• To report signs of infection: increased temperature, sore throat, flu symptoms
• To report signs of anemia: fatigue, headache, faintness, shortness of breath, irritability
• To report bleeding: avoid use of razors, or commercial mouthwash
• To avoid use of aspirin products or ibuprofen

Lab test interferences:
Increase: Liver function studies, 6-HIAA
Decrease: Albumin

---

fluoxetine

(floo-ox'e-teen)
Prozac
Func. class.: Bicyclic antidepressant

Action: Inhibits CNS neuron uptake of serotonin, but not of norepinephrine
Uses: Major depressive disorder
Dosage and routes:
• *Adult:* PO 20 mg qd in AM; after 4 wk if no clinical improvement is noted, dose may be increased to 20 mg bid in AM, afternoon, not to exceed 80 mg/day
Available forms include: Pulvules 20 mg
Side effects/adverse reactions:
*CNS: Headache, nervousness, insomnia, drowsiness, anxiety, tremor, dizziness, fatigue, sedation, poor concentration, abnormal dreams, agitation, **convulsions**,* apathy, euphoria, hallucinations, delusions, psychosis
GI: Nausea, diarrhea, dry mouth, anorexia, dyspepsia, constipation, cramps, vomiting, taste changes, flatulence, decreased appetite
INTEG: Sweating, rash, pruritus, acne, alopecia, urticaria
RESP: Infection, pharyngitis, nasal congestion, sinus headache, sinusitus, cough, dyspnea, bronchitis, asthma, hyperventilation, pneumonia
CV: Hot flashes, palpitations, angina pectoris, ***hemorrhage,*** hypertension, tachycardia, first-degree AV block, bradycardia, *MI,* thrombophlebitis
MS: Pain, arthritis, twitching
GU: Dysmenorrhea, decreased libido, urinary frequency, urinary tract infection, amenorrhea, cystitis, impotence

EENT: Visual changes, ear/eye pain, photophobia, tinnitus
SYST: Asthenia, viral infection, fever, allergy, chills
Contraindications: Hypersensitivity
Precautions: Pregnancy (B), lactation, children, elderly
Pharmacokinetics:
PO: Peak 6-8 hr; metabolized in liver, excreted in urine; half-life 2-7 days
Interactions/incompatibilities:
• Do not use with MAOIs
• Increased agitation: L-Tryptophan
• Increased side effects: highly protein bound drugs (i.e. fluoxetine)
• Increased half-life of: diazepam
NURSING CONSIDERATIONS
Assess:
• Mental status: mood, sensorium, affect, suicidal tendencies, increase in psychiatric symptoms, depression, panic
• B/P (lying/standing), pulse q4h; if systolic B/P drops 20 mm Hg, hold drug, notify physician; take vital signs q4h in patients with cardiovascular disease
• Blood studies: CBC, leukocytes, differential, cardiac enzymes if patient is receiving long-term therapy
• Hepatic studies: AST, ALT, bilirubin, creatinine
• Weight qwk, appetite may decrease with drug
• ECG for flattening of T wave, bundle branch, AV block, dysrhythmias in cardiac patients
Administer:
• Increased fluids, bulk in diet if constipation, urinary retention occur
• With food or milk for GI symptoms
• Crushed if patient is unable to swallow medication whole

---

italics = common side effects   ***bold italic*** = life threatening reactions

• Dosage hs if over-sedation occurs during the day; may take entire dose hs; elderly may not tolerate once/day dosing
• Gum, hard candy, frequent sips of water for dry mouth
Perform/provide:
• Storage at room temperature, do not freeze
• Assistance with ambulation during therapy since drowsiness, dizziness occur
• Safety measures including side rails, primarily in elderly
• Checking to see PO medication swallowed
Evaluate:
• EPS primarily in elderly, rigidity, dystonia, akathisia
• Urinary retention, constipation
• Withdrawal symptoms: headache, nausea, vomiting, muscle pain, weakness; do not usually occur unless drug was discontinued abruptly
• Alcohol consumption; if alcohol is consumed, hold dose until morning
Teach patient/family:
• That therapeutic effect may take 2-3 wk
• Use caution in driving or other activities requiring alertness because of drowsiness, dizziness, or blurred vision
• Not to discontinue medication quickly after long-term use, may cause nausea, headache, malaise
• To avoid alcohol ingestion or other CNS depressants
• To notify physician if pregnant or plan to become pregnant or breastfeed
Lab test interferences:
Increase: Serum bilirubin, blood glucose, alk phosphatase
Decrease: VMA, 5-HIAA

False increase: Urinary catecholamines

---

fluoxymesterone
(floo-ox-ee-mess'te-rone)
Android-F, Halotestin, Ora-Testryl
Func. class.: Androgenic anabolic steroid
Chem. class.: Halogenated testosterone derivative

Action: Increases weight by building body tissue, increases potassium, phosphorus, chloride, nitrogen levels, increases bone development
Uses: Impotence from testicular deficiency, hypogonadism, breast engorgement, palliative treatment of female breast cancer
Dosage and routes:
Hypogonadism/impotence
• *Adult:* PO 2-10 mg qd
Breast engorgement
• *Adult:* PO 2.5 mg qd, then 5-10 mg qd × 5 days
Breast cancer
• *Adult:* PO 15-30 mg qd in divided doses until therapeutic effect occurs, then dosage should be reduced
Available forms include: Tabs 2, 5, 10 mg
Side effects/adverse reactions:
INTEG: Rash, acneiform lesions, oily hair, skin, flushing, sweating, acne vulgaris, alopecia, hirsutism
CNS: Dizziness, headache, fatigue, tremors, paresthesias, flushing, sweating, anxiety, lability, insomnia
MS: Cramps, spasms
CV: Increased B/P
GU: **Hematuria,** amenorrhea, vaginitis, decreased libido, decreased breast size, clitoral hypertrophy, testicular atrophy

---

GI: Nausea, vomiting, constipation, weight gain, ***cholestatic jaundice***

EENT: Carpal tunnel syndrome, conjunctival edema, nasal congestion

ENDO: Abnormal GTT

Contraindications: Severe renal disease, severe cardiac disease, severe hepatic disease, hypersensitivity, pregnancy (X), lactation, genital bleeding (abnormal)

Precautions: Diabetes mellitus, CV disease, MI

Pharmacokinetics:

PO: Metabolized in liver, excreted in urine, crosses placenta, excreted in breast milk

Interactions/incompatibilities:

- Increased effects of: oral antidiabetics, oxyphenbutazone
- Increased PT: anticoagulants
- Edema: ACTH, adrenal steroids
- Decreased effects of: insulin

NURSING CONSIDERATIONS

Assess:

- Weight daily, notify physician if weekly weight gain is >5 lb
- B/P q4h
- I&O ratio; be alert for decreasing urinary output, increasing edema
- Growth rate in children since growth rate may be uneven (linear/bone growth) if used for extended periods of time
- Electrolytes: K, Na, Cl, cholesterol
- Liver function studies: ALT, AST, bilirubin

Administer:

- Titrated dose, use lowest effective dose
- With food or milk to decrease GI symptoms

Perform/provide:

- Diet with increased calories, protein; decrease sodium, if edema occurs

Evaluate:

- Therapeutic response: increased appetite, stamina
- Edema, hypertension, cardiac symptoms, jaundice
- Mental status: affect, mood, behavioral changes, aggression
- Signs of masculinization in female: increased libido, deepening of voice, breast tissue, enlarged clitoris, menstrual irregularities; male: gynecomastia, impotence, testicular atrophy
- Hypercalcemia: lethargy, polyuria, polydipsia, nausea, vomiting, constipation, drug may need to be decreased
- Hypoglycemia in diabetics, since oral anticoagulant action is decreased

Teach patient/family:

- Drug needs to be combined with complete health plan: diet, rest, exercise
- To notify physician if therapeutic response decreases
- Not to discontinue medication abruptly
- Teach patient about change in sex characteristics
- Females to report menstrual irregularities
- 1-3 mo course is necessary for response in breast cancer
- That steroids should not be used for body building

Lab test interferences:

Increase: Serum cholesterol, blood glucose, urine glucose

Decrease: Serum calcium, serum potassium, T_4, T_3, thyroid ^{131}I uptake test, urine 17-OHCS, 17-KS, PBI, BSP

---

fluphenazine decanoate/fluphenazine enanthate/fluphenazine HCl

(floo-fen-'a-zeen)

Modecate Decanoate,* Prolixin Decanoate/Moditen Enanthate,* Prolixin Enanthate/Moditen HCl,* Permitil HCl, Prolixin HCl

Func. class.: Antipsychotic/neuroleptic

Chem. class.: Phenothiazine, piperazine

Action: Depresses cerebral cortex, hypothalamus, limbic system, which control activity and aggression; blocks neurotransmission produced by dopamine at synapse; exhibits strong α-adrenergic and anticholinergic blocking action; mechanism for antipsychotic effects is unclear

Uses: Psychotic disorders, schizophrenia

Dosage and routes:

Enanthate, decanoate

• *Adult and child >12 yr:* SC 12.5-25 mg ql-3wk

HCl

• *Adult:* PO 2.5-10 mg, in divided doses q6-8h, not to exceed 20 mg qd; IM initially 1.25 mg then 2.5-10 mg in divided doses q6-8h

Available forms include: HCl Tabs 1, 2.5, 5, 10 mg; elix 2.5 mg/5 ml; conc 5 mg/ml; inj IM 10 mg/ml, enanthate, decanoate, inj SC, IM 25 mg/ml

Side effects/adverse reactions:

RESP: Laryngospasm, dyspnea, *respiratory depression*

CNS: Extrapyramidal symptoms: pseudoparkinsonism, akathisia, dystonia, tardive dyskinesia, drowsiness, headache, sei-zures, *neuroleptic malignant syndrome*

HEMA: Anemia, *leukopenia, leukocytosis, agranulocytosis*

INTEG: Rash, photosensitivity, dermatitis

EENT: Blurred vision, glaucoma

GI: Dry mouth, nausea, vomiting, anorexia, constipation, diarrhea, jaundice, weight gain

GU: Urinary retention, urinary frequency, enuresis, impotence, amenorrhea, gynecomastia

CV: Orthostatic hypotension, hypertension, *cardiac arrest,* ECG changes, *tachycardia*

Contraindications: Hypersensitivity, circulatory collapse, liver damage, cerebral arteriosclerosis, coronary disease, severe hypertension/hypotension, blood dyscrasias, coma, child <12 yr, brain damage, bone marrow depression, alcohol and barbiturate withdrawal states

Precautions: Pregnancy (C), lactation, seizure disorders, hypertension, hepatic disease, cardiac disease

Pharmacokinetics:

PO/IM (HCl): Onset 1 hr, peak 2-4 hr, duration 6-8 hr

SC (enanthate): Onset 1-2 days, peak 2-3 days, duration 1-3 wk, half-life 3.5-4 days; decanoate: onset 1-3 days, peak 1-2 days, duration over 4 wk, half-life (single dose) 6.8-9.6 days, (multiple dose) 14.3 days Metabolized by liver, excreted in urine (metabolites), crosses placenta, enters breast milk

Interactions/incompatibilities:

• Oversedation: other CNS depressants, alcohol, barbiturate anesthetics

• Toxicity: epinephrine

• Decreased effects of: levodopa, lithium

---

* Available in Canada only

• Increased effects of both drugs: β-adrenergic blockers, alcohol
• Increased anticholinergic effects: anticholinergics

NURSING CONSIDERATIONS
Assess:
• Swallowing of PO medication; check for hoarding or giving of medication to other patients
• I&O ratio; palpate bladder if low urinary output occurs
• Bilirubin, CBC, liver function studies monthly
• Urinalysis is recommended before and during prolonged therapy

Administer:
• Concentrate with juice, milk or uncaffeinated drinks
• Antiparkinsonian agent, to be used if extrapyramidal symptoms occur
• IM injection into large muscle mass, to minimize postural hypotension give injection with patient seated or recumbent
• Use dry needle or solution will become cloudy; use No. 21 G or larger due to viscosity

Perform/provide:
• Decreased noise input by dimming lights, avoiding loud noises
• Supervised ambulation until stabilized on medication; do not involve in strenuous exercise program because fainting is possible; patient should not stand still for long periods of time
• Increased fluids to prevent constipation
• Sips of water, candy, gum for dry mouth
• Storage in tight, light-resistant container in cool environment

Evaluate:
• Therapeutic response: decrease in emotional excitement, hallucinations, delusions, paranoia, reorganization of patterns of thought, speech
• Affect, orientation, LOC, reflexes, gait, coordination, sleep pattern disturbances
• B/P standing and lying; take pulse and respirations q4h during initial treatment; establish baseline before starting treatment; report drops of 30 mm Hg
• Dizziness, faintness, palpitations, tachycardia on rising
• Extrapyramidal symptoms including akathisia (inability to sit still, no pattern to movements), tardive dyskinesia (bizarre movements of jaw, mouth, tongue, extremities), pseudoparkinsonism (rigidity, tremors, pill rolling, shuffling gait)
• Skin turgor daily
• Constipation, urinary retention daily; if these occur, increase bulk, water in diet

Teach patient/family:
• That orthostatic hypotension occurs often, to rise from sitting or lying position gradually
• To avoid hot tubs, hot showers, or tub baths since hypotension may occur
• To avoid abrupt withdrawal of this drug or extrapyramidal symptoms may result; drug should be withdrawn slowly
• To avoid OTC preparations (cough, hayfever, cold) unless approved by physician since serious drug interactions may occur; avoid use with alcohol or CNS depressants; increased drowsiness may occur
• To use a sunscreen during sun exposure to prevent burns
• Regarding compliance with drug regimen
• About extrapyramidal symptoms and necessity for meticulous oral

---

italics = common side effects   ***bold italic*** = life threatening reactions

hygiene since oral candidiasis may occur
• To report sore throat, malaise, fever, bleeding, mouth sores; if these occur, CBC should be drawn and drug discontinued
• In hot weather heat stroke may occur; take extra precautions to stay cool

Lab test interferences:

Increase: Liver function tests, cardiac enzymes, cholesterol, blood glucose, prolactin, bilirubin, PBI, cholinesterase, ^{131}I

Decrease: Hormones (blood and urine)

False positive: Pregnancy tests, PKU

False negative: Urinary steroids, 17-OHCS

Treatment of overdose: Lavage, if orally injested, provide an airway; *do not induce vomiting*

---

flurandrenolide

(flure-an-dren'oh-lide)

Cordran, Drenison 1/4,* Drenison Tape*

Func. class.: Topical corticosteroid
Chem. class.: Synthetic fluorinated agent

Action: Possesses antipruritic, antiinflammatory actions

Uses: Corticosteroid-responsive dermatoses, pruritus

Dosage and routes:
• *Adult and child:* TOP apply to affected area tid-qid; apply tape q12-24h

Available forms include: Oint 0.025%, 0.05%; cream 0.025%, 0.05%; lotion 0.05%; tape 4 μg/cm²

Side effects/adverse reactions:

INTEG: Burning, dryness, itching, irritation, acne, folliculitis, hypertrichosis, perioral dermatitis, hypopigmentation, atrophy, striae, miliaria, allergic contact dermatitis, secondary infection

Contraindications: Hypersensitivity to corticosteroids, fungal infections, viral infections

Precautions: Pregnancy (C), lactation, viral infections, bacterial infections

NURSING CONSIDERATIONS

Assess:
• Temperature, if fever develops drug should be discontinued

Administer:
• Only to affected areas, do not get in eyes
• Then cover with occlusive dressing if ordered, seal to normal skin, change q12h, systemic absorption may occur
• Only to dermatoses, do not use on weeping, denuded or infected area
• Tape after cutting with scissors, apply only to clean dry wounds

Perform/provide:
• Cleansing before application of drug
• Treatment for a few days after area has cleared
• Storage at room temperature

Evaluate:
• Systemic absorption: fever, infection, irritation
• Therapeutic response: absence of severe itching, patches on skin, flaking

Teach patient/family:
• To avoid sunlight on affected area, burns may occur

---

* Available in Canada only

flurandrenolide

(flure-an-dren'oh-lide)
Cordan, Cordran SP, Cordran Tape
Func. class.: Topical corticosteroid
Chem. class.: Synthetic fluorinated
agent, group III potency (0.05%),
group IV potency (0.025%)

Action: Possesses antipruritic, antiinflammatory actions
Uses: Psoriasis, eczema, contact
dermatitis, pruritus
Dosage and routes:
• *Adult and child:* Apply to affected area tid-qid; apply tape q12h
Available forms include: Oint
0.025%, 0.05%; cream 0.025%,
0.05%; lotion 0.05%, tape 4 μg/
cm²
Side effects/adverse reactions:
INTEG: Burning, dryness, itching,
irritation, acne, folliculitis, hypertrichosis, perioral dermatitis, hypopigmentation, atrophy, striae,
miliaria, allergic contact dermatitis, secondary infection
Contraindications: Hypersensitivity to corticosteroids, fungal infections
Precautions: Pregnancy (C), lactation, viral infections, bacterial infections
NURSING CONSIDERATIONS
Assess:
• Temperature; if fever develops,
drug should be discontinued
Administer:
• Only to affected areas; do not get
in eyes
• Medication, then cover with occlusive dressing (only if prescribed), seal to normal skin,
change q12h, systemic absorption
may occur
• Only to dermatoses; do not use
on weeping, denuded, or infected
area

Perform/provide:
• Cleansing before application of
drug
• Treatment for a few days after
area has cleared
• Storage at room temperature
Evaluate:
• Therapeutic response: absence of
severe itching, patches on skin,
flaking
• For systemic absorption: in-
creased temperature, inflamma-
tion, irritation
Teach patient/family:
• To avoid sunlight on affected
area; burns may occur

flurazepam HCl

(flure-az'e-pam)
Dalmane, Durapam, Somnol*
Func. class.: Sedative-hypnotic
Chem. class.: Benzodiazepine de-
rivative

**Controlled Substance Schedule
IV (USA), Schedule F (Canada)**
Action: Produces CNS depression
at the limbic, thalamic, hypothalamic levels of CNS; may be mediated by neurotransmitter gamma
aminobutyric acid (GABA); results
are sedation, hypnosis, skeletal
muscle relaxation, anticonvulsant
activity, anxiolytic action
Uses: Insomnia
Dosage and routes:
• *Adult:* PO 15-30 mg hs, may repeat dose once if needed
• *Geriatric:* PO 15 mg hs, may increase if needed
Available forms include: Caps 15,
30 mg
Side effects/adverse reactions:
HEMA: **Leukopenia, granulocytopenia** (rare)
CNS: Lethargy, drowsiness, daytime sedation, dizziness, confu-

italics = common side effects   ***bold italic*** = life threatening reactions

sion, lightheadedness, headache, anxiety, irritability

GI: Nausea, vomiting, diarrhea, heartburn, abdominal pain, constipation

CV: Chest pain, pulse changes

Contraindications: Hypersensitivity to benzodiazepines, pregnancy, lactation, intermittent porphyria, uncontrolled pain

Precautions: Anemia, hepatic disease, renal disease, suicidal individuals, drug abuse, elderly, psychosis, child <15 yr

Pharmacokinetics:

PO: Onset 15-45 min, duration 7-8 hr; metabolized by liver, excreted by kidneys (inactive/active metabolites), crosses placenta, excreted in breast milk; half-life 47-100 hr, additional 100 hr for active metabolites

Interactions/incompatibilities:

• Increased effects of flurazepam: cimetidine, disulfiram

• Increased action of both drugs: alcohol, CNS depressants

• Decreased effect of flurazepam: antacids

NURSING CONSIDERATIONS
Assess:

• Blood studies: Hct, Hgb, RBCs (if on long-term therapy)

• Hepatic studies: AST, ALT, bilirubin

Administer:

• After removal of cigarettes, to prevent fires

• After trying conservative measures for insomnia

• ½-1 hr before hs for sleeplessness

• On empty stomach for fast onset, but may be taken with food if GI symptoms occur

Perform/provide:

• Assistance with ambulation after receiving dose

• Safety measure: siderails, night-

light, callbell within easy reach

• Checking to see PO medication has been swallowed

• Storage in tight container in cool environment

Evaluate:

• Therapeutic response: ability to sleep at night, decreased amount of early morning awakening if taking drug for insomnia

• Mental status: mood, sensorium, affect, memory (long, short)

• Blood dyscrasias: fever, sore throat, bruising, rash, jaundice, epistaxis (rare)

• Type of sleep problem: falling asleep, staying asleep

Teach patient/family:

• To avoid driving or other activities requiring alertness until drug is stabilized

• To avoid alcohol ingestion or CNS depressants; serious CNS depression may result

• That effects may take 2 nights for benefits to be noticed

• Alternate measures to improve sleep: reading, exercise several hours before hs, warm bath, warm milk, TV, self-hypnosis, deep breathing

• That hangover is common in elderly, but less common than with barbiturates

Lab test interferences:

Increase: AST/ALT, serum bilirubin

False increase: Urinary 17-OHCS
Decrease: RAI uptake

Treatment of overdose: Lavage, activated charcoal, monitor electrolytes, vital signs

flurbiprofen sodium

(flure-bi'proe-fen)
Ocufen

Func. class.: Nonsteroidal antiinflammatory ophthalmic
Chem. class.: Phenylalkanoic acid

Action: Inhibits enzyme system necessary for biosynthesis of prostaglandins; inhibits miosis
Uses: Inhibition of intraoperative miosis, corneal edema
Dosage and routes:
• *Adult:* 1 gtt q½h 2 hr before surgery (4 gtts total)
Available forms include: Sol 0.03%
Side effects/adverse reactions:
EENT: Burning, stinging in the eye, irritation, bleeding or redness
Contraindications: Hypersensitivity, epithelial herpes simplex keratitis
Precautions: Pregnancy (C), lactation, child, aspirin or nonsteroidal antiinflammatory drug hypersensitivity, allergy, bleeding disorder
NURSING CONSIDERATIONS
Administer:
• Excess solution must be wiped away promptly to prevent its flow into lacrimal system, producing systemic symptoms
Perform/provide:
• Protect solution from sun
Teach patient/family:
• To report change in vision, blurring, or loss of sight during miosis
• Not to use for any other condition than prescribed

flutamide

(floo'-ta-mide)
Eulexin

Func. class.: Antineoplastic-hormone
Chem. class.: Antiandrogen

Action: Interferes with testosterone at the cellular level. Inhibits androgen uptake by inhibiting nuclear binding or by interfering with androgen in target tissues. Prostatic carcinoma is androgen-sensitive, which results in arrested tumor growth
Uses: Metastatic prostatic carcinoma, stage D2 in combination with LHRH agonistic analogs
Dosage and routes:
• *Adult:* PO 250 mg q8h tid, for a daily dosage of 750 mg
Available forms: cap 125 mg
Side effects/adverse reactions:
CNS: Hot flashes, drowsiness, confusion, depression, anxiety
GU: Decreased libido, impotence, gynecomastia
GI: Diarrhea, nausea, vomiting, increased liver function studies, ***hepatitis,*** anorexia
INTEG: Irritation at site, rash, photosensitivity
MISC: Edema, hematopoietic symptoms, neuromuscular and pulmonary symptoms, hypertension
Contraindications: Hypersensitivity, pregnancy (D)
Pharmacokinetics: Rapidly and completely absorbed. Excreted in urine and feces as metabolites. Half-life 6 hr, geriatric half-life 8 hrs, 94% bound to plasma proteins
NURSING CONSIDERATIONS
Assess:
• Liver function studies: AST, ALT, alk phosphatase, which may be elevated

---

italics = common side effects   ***bold italic*** = life threatening reactions

• For CNS symptoms: drowsiness, confusion, depression, anxiety
Evaluate:
• Therapeutic response: decrease in prostatic tumor size
Treatment of overdose: Induce vomiting, provide supportive care

---

fluticasone propionate
Cutivate

Func. class.: Topical corticosteroid
Chem. class.: Synthetic fluorinated agent, group VI potency

Action: Possesses antipruritic, antiinflammatory actions
Uses: Psoriasis, eczema, contact dermatitis, pruritus
Dosage and routes:
• Adult and child: Apply to affected area tid-qid
Available forms include: Cream 0.05%; oint 0.005%
Side effects/adverse reactions:
INTEG: Burning, dryness, itching, irritation, acne, folliculitis, hypertrichosis, perioral dermatitis, hypopigmentation, atrophy, striae, miliaria, allergic contact dermatitis, secondary infection
Contraindications: Hypersensitivity to corticosteroids, fungal infections
Precautions: Pregnancy (C), lactation, viral infections, bacterial infections

NURSING CONSIDERATIONS
Assess:
• Temperature: if fever develops, drug should be discontinued
Administer:
• Only to affected areas; do not get in eyes
• Medication, then cover with occlusive dressing (only if prescribed); seal to normal skin; change q12h; systemic absorption may occur
• Only to dermatoses; do not use on weeping, denuded, or infected area
Perform/provide:
• Cleansing before application of drug
• Treatment for a few days after area has cleared
• Storage at room temperature
Evaluate:
• Therapeutic response: absence of severe itching, patches on skin, flaking
• For systemic absorption: increased temperature, inflammation, irritation
Teach patient/family:
• To avoid sunlight on affected area; burns may occur

---

folic acid (vitamin B₉)
Apo-Folic, Folvite, Novofolacid*

Func. class.: Vitamin B complex group

Action: Needed for erythropoiesis; increases RBC, WBC, and platelet formation in megaloblastic anemias
Uses: Megaloblastic or macrocytic anemia caused by folic acid deficiency; liver disease, alcoholism, hemolysis, intestinal obstruction, pregnancy
Dosage and routes:
Supplement
• *Adult:* PO/IM/SC 0.1 mg qd
• *Child:* PO 0.05 mg qd
Megaloblastic/macrocytic anemia
• *Adult and child >4 yr:* PO/SC/IM 1 mg qd × 4-5 days
• *Child <4 yr:* PO/SC/IM 0.3 mg or less qd
• *Pregnancy/lactation:* PO/SC/IM 0.8 mg qd
Prevention of megaloblastic/macrocytic anemia

• *Pregnancy:* PO/SC/IM 1 mg qd
Available forms include: Tabs 0.1,
0.4, 0.8, 1 mg; inj SC, IM 5, 10
mg/ml
Side effects/adverse reactions:
RESP: **Bronchospasm**
Contraindications: Hypersensitivity, anemias other than megaloblastic/macrocytic anemia, vitamin B$_{12}$ deficiency anemia
Precautions: Pregnancy (A)
Pharmacokinetics:
PO: Peak ½-1 hr, bound to plasma proteins, excreted in breast milk, methylated in liver, excreted in urine (small amounts)
Interactions/incompatibilities:
• Decreased folate levels: chloramphenicol
• Increased metabolism of: phenobarbital, hydantoins
• Do not use with methotrexate unless leucovorin rescue is available
NURSING CONSIDERATIONS
Assess:
• Folate levels: 6-15 μg/ml
Perform/provide:
• Storage in light-resistant container
Evaluate:
• Therapeutic response: increased weight, oriented well-being, absence of fatigue
• Nutritional status: bran, yeast, dried beans, nuts, fruits, fresh vegetables, asparagus
• Drugs currently taken: alcohol, oral contraceptives, hydantoins, trimethoprim, these drugs may cause increased folic acid use by body and contribute to a deficiency
Teach patient/family:
• To take drug exactly as prescribed
• To notify physician of side effects

furazolidone

(fur-a-zoe'li-done)
Furoxone
Func. class.: Antibacterial
Chem. class.: Nitrofuran

Action: Interferes with enzyme systems in bacteria
Uses: Gastroenteritis, cholera (as an adjunctive)
Dosage and routes:
• *Adult:* PO 100 mg qid
• *Child 5-12 yr:* PO 25-50 mg qid
• *Child 1-4 yr:* PO 17-25 mg qid
• *Child 1 mo-1 yr:* PO 8-17 mg qid,
• Not to exceed 8.8 mg/kg/day
Available forms include: Tabs 100 mg; liq 50 mg/15 ml
Side effects/adverse reactions:
INTEG: Urticaria, angioedema, rash
CNS: Headache, malaise, fever
GI: Nausea, vomiting, anorexia, diarrhea, abdominal pain
Allergic: Hypotension, urticaria, arthralgia, rash
Contraindications: Hypersensitivity, infant <1 mo
Precautions: Pregnancy, lactation, G-6-PD deficiency
Pharmacokinetics: Metabolized, inactivated in intestine, only 5% in urine
Interactions/incompatibilities:
• Avoid use with alcohol, MAOIs, narcotics, indirect-acting sympathomimetic amines, ephedrine, phenylephrine, sedatives, antihistamines, guanethidine, tyramine, other CNS depressants, levodopa, antidepressants
• Increased hypoglycemic effect: insulin, sulfonylureas
• Disulfiram-like reaction: alcohol
NURSING CONSIDERATIONS
Assess:
• C&S before drug therapy; drug

---

italics = common side effects   ***bold italic*** = life threatening reactions

may be taken as soon as culture is taken

• Electrolytes: K, Na, Cl

Administer:

• With full glass of water

Perform/provide:

• Storage protected from light in tight container

• Adequate intake of fluids (2000 ml) during diarrhea episodes

Evaluate:

• Bowel pattern before, during treatment

• Skin eruptions, itching

• Allergies before treatment, reaction of each medication; place allergies on chart, Kardex in bright red letters, notify all people giving drugs

• Nausea, vomiting; if severe may require decrease in dosage

Teach patient/family:

• To avoid alcohol during, for 4 days after completion of therapy, including cough, cold remedies, anorexiants

• Urine may turn brown

• To avoid high tyramine foods: pickled products, aged cheese, figs, bananas, chocolate, yeast products

Treatment of overdose: Withdraw drug, maintain airway, administer epinephrine, aminophylline, O_2, IV corticosteroids

---

furosemide

(fur-oh'se-mide)

Lasix, Novosemide,* Uritol*

Func. class.: Loop diuretic

Chem. class.: Sulfonamide derivative

Action: Acts on loop of Henle by increasing excretion of chloride, sodium

Uses: Pulmonary edema, edema in CHF, liver disease, nephrotic syndrome, ascites, hypertension

Dosage and routes:

• *Adult:* PO 20-80 mg/day in AM, may give another dose in 6 hr, up to 600 mg/day; IM/IV 20-40 mg, increased by 20 mg q2h until desired response

• *Child:* PO/IM/IV 2 mg/kg, may increase by 1-2 mg/kg/q6-8h up to 6 mg/kg

Pulmonary edema

• *Adult:* IV 40 mg given over several minutes, repeated in 1 hr; increase to 80 mg if needed

Available forms include: Tabs 20, 40, 80 mg; oral sol 10 mg/ml; inj IM, IV 10 mg/ml

Side effects/adverse reactions:

*GU: Polyuria, **renal failure,** glycosuria*

ELECT: Hypokalemia, hypochloremic alkalosis, hypomagnesemia, hyperuricemia, hypocalcemia, hyponatremia

CNS: Headache, fatigue, weakness, vertigo, paresthesias

GI: Nausea, diarrhea, dry mouth, vomiting, anorexia, cramps, oral, gastric irritations

*EENT: **Loss of hearing,** ear pain, tinnitus, blurred vision*

*INTEG: Rash, pruritus, purpura, **Stevens-Johnson syndrome,** sweating, photosensitivity, urticaria*

MS: Cramps, arthritis, stiffness

ENDO: Hyperglycemia

*HEMA: **Thrombocytopenia, agranulocytosis, leukopenia, neutropenia, anemia***

CV: Orthostatic hypotension, chest pain, ECG changes, **circulatory collapse**

Contraindications: Hypersensitivity to sulfonamides, anuria, hypovolemia, infants, lactation, electrolyte depletion

---

Precautions: Diabetes mellitus, dehydration, ascites, severe renal disease, pregnancy (C)
Pharmacokinetics:
PO: Onset 1 hr, peak 1-2 hr, duration 6-8 hr
IV: Onset 5 min, peak ½ hr, duration 2 hr
Excreted in urine, feces, crosses placenta, excreted in breast milk
Interactions/incompatibilities:
• Increased toxicity: lithium, nondepolarizing skeletal muscle relaxants
• Increased action of: antihypertensives
• Increased ototoxicity: aminoglycosides, cisplatin
• Decreased antihypertensive effect of furosemide: indomethacin
NURSING CONSIDERATIONS
Assess:
• Hearing when giving high doses
• Weight, I&O daily to determine fluid loss; effect of drug may be decreased if used qd
• Rate, depth, rhythm of respiration, effect of exertion
• B/P lying, standing; postural hypotension may occur
• Electrolytes: potassium, sodium, chloride; include BUN, blood sugar, CBC, serum creatinine, blood pH, ABGs, uric acid, calcium, magnesium
• Glucose in urine if patient is diabetic
• Hearing when giving high doses
Administer:
• IV undiluted may be given through Y-tube or 3-way stopcock; give 20 mg or less/min
• In AM to avoid interference with sleep if using drug as a diuretic
• Potassium replacement if potassium is less than 3.0
• With food, if nausea occurs, absorption may be decreased slightly

Evaluate:
• Improvement in edema of feet, legs, sacral area daily if medication is being used in CHF
• Improvement in CVP q8h
• Signs of metabolic alkalosis: drowsiness, restlessness
• Signs of hypokalemia: postural hypotension, malaise, fatigue, tachycardia, leg cramps, weakness
• Rashes, temperature elevation qd
• Confusion, especially in elderly, take safety precautions if needed
Teach patient/family:
• To increase fluid intake 2-3 L/day unless contraindicated, to rise slowly from lying or sitting position
• Adverse reactions: muscle cramps, weakness, nausea, dizziness
• Take with food or milk for GI symptoms
• Take early in day to prevent nocturia
Lab test interferences:
Interfere: GTT
Treatment of overdose: Lavage if taken orally, monitor electrolytes, administer dextrose in saline, monitor hydration, CV, renal status

gallamine triethiodide
(gal'a-meen)
Flaxedil
Func. class.: Neuromuscular blocker (nondepolarizing)

Action: Inhibits transmission of nerve impulses by binding with cholinergic receptor sites, antagonizing action of acetylcholine
Uses: Facilitation of endotracheal intubation, skeletal muscle relaxation during mechanical ventilation, surgery, or general anesthesia
Dosage and routes:
• *Adult and child >1 mo:* IV 1 mg/

kg, not to exceed 100 mg, then 0.5-1 mg/kg q30-40 min

• *Child <1 mo, >5 kg:* IV 0.25-0.75 mg/kg, then 0.01-0.05 mg/kg q30-40 min

Available forms include: Inj IV 20 mg/ml

Side effects/adverse reactions:

CV: Bradycardia, tachycardia, increased, decreased B/P

*RESP: **Prolonged apnea, bronchospasm, cyanosis, respiratory depression***

EENT: Increased secretions

INTEG: Rash, flushing, pruritus, urticaria

*CNS: **Malignant hyperthermia***

GI: Decreased motility

Contraindications: Hypersensitivity to iodides

Precautions: Pregnancy (C), thyroid disease, collagen disease, cardiac disease, lactation, children <2 yr, electrolyte imbalances, dehydration, neuromuscular disease (myasthenia gravis), respiratory disease

Pharmacokinetics:

IV: Onset 2 min, duration 20-60 min; half-life 2 min, 29 min (terminal), excreted in urine, feces (metabolites), crosses placenta

Interactions/incompatibilities:

• Increased neuromuscular blockade: aminoglycosides, clindamycin, lincomycin, quinidine, local anesthetics, polymyxin antibiotics, lithium, narcotic analgesics, thiazides, enflurane, isoflurane; used with cyclopropane, may provoke ventricular dysrhythmias

• Dysrhythmias: theophylline

• Do not mix with barbiturates in solution or syringe

• May be added to Pentothal, but not vice versa; do not use syringe previously used for Pentothal

• Do not use yellow colored solutions of the drug

NURSING CONSIDERATIONS
Assess:

• For electrolyte imbalances (K, Mg); may lead to increased action of this drug

• Vital signs (B/P, pulse, respirations, airway) q15 min until fully recovered; rate, depth, pattern of respirations, strength of hand grip

• I&O ratio; check for urinary retention, frequency, hesitancy

Administer:

• Using nerve stimulator by anesthesiologist to determine neuromuscular blockade

• Anticholinesterase to reverse neuromuscular blockade

• IV undiluted over 1-2 min (only by qualified person, usually an anesthesiologist)

• Only slight discolored solution

Perform/provide:

• Storage in light-resistant, cool area

• Reassurance if communication is difficult during recovery from neuromuscular blockade

Evaluate:

• Therapeutic response: paralysis of jaw, eyelid, head, neck, rest of body

• Recovery: decreased paralysis of face, diaphragm, leg, arm, rest of body

• Allergic reactions: rash, fever, respiratory distress, pruritus; drug should be discontinued

Treatment of overdose: Edrophonium or neostigmine, atropine, monitor VS; may require mechanical ventilation

gancyclovir (DHPG)

(gan-sy-clo-ver)

Cytovene

Func. class.: Antiviral

Chem. class.: Synthetic nucleoside analog

Action: Inhibits replication of herpes viruses in vitro; in vivo by selective inhibition of the human CMV DNA polymerase and by direct incorporation into viral DNA

Uses: Cytomegalovirus (CMV) retinitis in immunocompromised persons, including those with AIDS, after indirect ophthalmoscopy confirms diagnosis

Dosage and routes:

Induction treatment

• *Adult:* IV 5 mg/kg given over 1 hr, q12h × 2-3 wks

Maintenance treatment

• *Adult:* IV INF 5 mg/kg given over 1 hr, qd × 7 days each wk; or 6 mg/kg qd × 5 days each wk

• Dosage must be reduced in renal impairment

Available forms: powder 500 mg/vial gancyclovir

Side effects/adverse reactions:

*HEMA: **Granulocytopenia, thrombocytopenia, irreversible neutropenia,** anemia, eosinophilia*

*GI: Abnormal LFTs, nausea, vomiting, anorexia, diarrhea, abdominal pain, **hemorrhage***

INTEG: Rash, alopecia, pruritis, urticaria, pain at site, phlebitis

*CNS: Fever, chills, **coma,** confusion, abnormal thoughts, dizziness, bizarre dreams, headache, psychosis, tremors, somnolence, paresthesia*

CV: Dysrhythmia, hypertension/hypotension

RESP: Dyspnea

EENT: Retinal detachment in CMV retinitis

*GU: **Hematuria,** increased creatinine, BUN*

Contraindications: Hypersensitivity to acyclovir or gancyclovir

Precautions: Preexisting cytopenias, renal function impairment, pregnancy (C), lactation, children <6 mo, elderly, platelet count <25,000/mm

Pharmacokinetics: Half-life 3-4½ hr, excreted by the kidneys (unchanged drug), crosses blood-brain barrier

Interactions/incompatibilities:

• Decreased renal clearance of gancyclovir: probenecid

• Increased toxicity: dapsone, pentamidine, flucytosine, vincristine, vinblastine, adriamycin, doxorubicin, amphotericin B, trimethoprim/sulfa combinations, or other nucleoside analogs

• Severe granulocytopenia: zidovudine; do not give together

• Increased seizures: imipenem-cilastatin

NURSING CONSIDERATIONS

Assess:

• For leukopenia/neutropenia/thrombocytopenia: WBCs, platelets q2d during twice a day dosing and q1wk thereafter

• For leukopenia with gd WBC count in patients with prior leukopenia with other nucleoside analogs or for whom leukopenia counts are <1,000 cells/mm³ at start of treatment

• Serum creatinine or creatine clearance at least q2wk

Administer:

• IV after diluting 500 mg/10 ml sterile H₂O for injection, shake, further dilute in 100 ml compatible sol and run over 1 hr

---

italics = common side effects   ***bold italic*** = life threatening reactions

• Slowly; do not give by bolus IV, IM, SC injection
• Using diluted solution within 24 hr

Teach patient/family:
• That drug does not cure condition, that regular ophthalmologic examinations are necessary
• That major toxicities may necessitate discontinuing drug
• To use contraception during treatment and that infertility may occur; men should use barrier contraception for 90 days after treatment

Treatment of overdose: Discontinue drug, use hemodialysis, and increase hydration

---

gemfibrozil

(gem-fi'broe-zil)
Lopid

Func. class.: Antilipemic
Chem. class.: Aryloxisobutyric acid derivative

Action: Inhibits biosynthesis of VLDL, LDL, which are responsible for cholesterol development

Uses: Type III/IV, V hyperlipidemia

Dosage and routes:
• *Adult:* PO 1200 mg in divided doses bid 30 min before meals

Available forms include: Caps 300 mg

Side effects/adverse reactions:
GI: Nausea, vomiting, dyspepsia, diarrhea, abdominal pain
INTEG: Rash, urticaria, pruritus
HEMA: Leukopenia, anemia, eosinophilia
CNS: Dizziness, blurred vision

Contraindications: Severe hepatic disease, pre-existing gall bladder disease, severe renal disease, primary biliary cirrhosis, hypersensitivity

Precautions: Monitor hematologic

and hepatic function, pregnancy (B), lactation

Pharmacokinetics:
PO: Peak 1-2 hr, plasma protein binding >90%, half-life 1.5 hr, excreted in urine, metabolized in liver

Interactions/incompatibilities:
• May increase anticoagulant properties: oral anticoagulants
• Increased risk of myositis, myalgia: lovastatin

NURSING CONSIDERATIONS

Assess:
• Renal, hepatic levels if patient is on long-term therapy

Administer:
• 30 min before morning and evening meals

Evaluate:
• Bowel pattern daily; increase bulk, water in diet if constipation develops

Teach patient/family:
• That compliance is needed since toxicity may result if doses are missed
• That risk factors should be decreased: high fat diet, smoking, alcohol consumption, absence of exercise
• Birth control should be practiced while on this drug

Lab test interferences:
Increase: Liver function studies, CPK, BSP, thymol turbidity, glucose
Decrease: Hgb, Hct, WBC

Note: Not all cholesterol lowering agents have been thoroughly tested. Investigate any reaction, however small, immediately.

---

gentamicin sulfate

(jen-ta-mye'sin)
Alcomicin,* Apogen, Cidomycin,* Garamycin, Jenamicin, U-Gencin

Func. class.: Antibiotic
Chem. class.: Aminoglycoside

Action: Interferes with protein synthesis in bacterial cell by binding to ribosomal subunit, causing misreading of genetic code; inaccurate peptide sequence forms in protein chain, causing bacterial death

Uses: Severe systemic infections of CNS, respiratory, GI, urinary tract, bone, skin, soft tissues caused by susceptible strains of *P. aeruginosa, Proteus, Klebsiella, Serratia, E. coli, Enterobacter, Acinetobacter, Citrobacter, Staphylococcus*

Dosage and routes:
Severe systemic infections
• *Adult:* IV INF 3-5 mg/kg/day in 3 divided doses q8h; dilute in 50-200 ml NS or D₅W given over 30 min-2 hr; IM 3 mg/kg/day in divided doses q8h
• *Adult:* INTRATHECAL 4-8 mg qd
• *Child:* IV/IM 2-2.5 mg/kg q8h
• *Neonates and infants:* IV/IM 2.5 mg/kg q8h
• *Neonates <1 wk:* 2.5 mg/kg q12h
• *Infants and child >3 months:* INTRATHECAL 1-2 mg qd
Dental/respiratory procedures/ GI/GU surgery (prophylaxis endocarditis)
• *Adult:* IM 1.5 mg/kg ½-1 hr before procedure with ampicillin
• *Child:* IM 2.5 mg/kg ½-1 hr before procedure with ampicillin
Available forms include: Inj IM, IV 10, 40 mg; intrathecal 2 mg/ml
Side effects/adverse reactions:
GU: Oliguria, hematuria, renal damage, azotemia, renal failure, nephrotoxicity
CNS: Confusion, depression, numbness, tremors, *convulsions,* muscle twitching, *neurotoxicity*
EENT: Ototoxicity, deafness, visual disturbances
HEMA: Agranulocytosis, throm-

bocytopenia, leukopenia, eosinophilia, anemia
GI: Nausea, vomiting, anorexia, increased ALT, AST, bilirubin, hepatomegaly, *hepatic necrosis,* splenomegaly
CV: Hypotension, hypertension, palpitations
INTEG: Rash, burning, urticaria, photosensitivity, dermatitis
Contraindications: Severe renal disease, hypersensitivity
Precautions: Neonates, mild renal disease, pregnancy (C), hearing deficits, myasthenia gravis, lactation, elderly
Pharmacokinetics:
IM: Onset rapid, peak 1-2 hr
IV: Onset immediate, peak 1-2 hr
Plasma half-life 1-2 hr; duration 6-8 hr, not metabolized, excreted unchanged in urine; crosses placental barrier
Interactions/incompatibilities:
• Increased ototoxicity, neurotoxicity, nephrotoxicity: other aminoglycosides, amphotericin B, polymyxin, vancomycin, ethacrynic acid, furosemide, mannitol, methoxyflurane, cisplatin, cephalosporins
• Decreased effects of: parenteral penicillins, digoxin, vitamin B₁₂
• Do not mix in solution or syringe: carbenicillin, ticarcillin, amphotericin B, cephalothin, erythromycin, heparin
• Increased effects: nondepolarizing muscle relaxants
NURSING CONSIDERATIONS
Assess:
• Weight before treatment; calculation of dosage is usually done based on ideal body weight, but may be calculated on actual body weight
• I&O ratio, urinalysis daily for proteinuria, cells, casts; report sud-

---

italics = common side effects   ***bold italic*** = life threatening reactions

den change in urine output, toxicity is increased in patients with decreased renal function if high doses are given

• VS during infusion, watch for hypotension, change in pulse

• IV site for thrombophlebitis including pain, redness, swelling q30 min, change site if needed; apply warm compresses to discontinued site

• Serum peak, drawn at 30-60 min after IV infusion or 60 min after IM injection, and trough level drawn just before next dose; blood level should be 2-4 times bacteriostatic level

• Urine pH if drug is used for UTI; urine should be kept alkaline

Administer:

• IV after diluting in 50-200 ml of normal saline or D_5W, sol concentration should be 1 mg/ml or less, run over ½-1 hr (adults) or 2 hr (children)

• IM injection in large muscle mass, rotate injection sites

• Drug in evenly spaced doses to maintain blood level

• Bicarbonate to alkalinize urine if ordered for UTI, as drug is most active in alkaline environment

Perform/provide:

• Adequate fluids of 2-3 L/day unless contraindicated to prevent irritation of tubules

• Flush of IV line with NS or D_5W after infusion

• Supervised ambulation, other safety measures with vestibular dysfunction

Evaluate:

• Therapeutic effect: absence of fever, draining wounds, negative C&S after treatment

• Renal impairment by securing urine for CrCl testing, BUN, serum creatinine; lower dosage should be given in renal impairment (CrCl <80 ml/min)

• Deafness by audiometric testing, ringing, roaring in ears, vertigo; assess hearing before, during, after treatment

• Dehydration: high sp gr, decrease in skin turgor, dry mucous membranes, dark urine

• Overgrowth of infection including increased temperature, malaise, redness, pain, swelling, perineal itching, diarrhea, stomatitis, change in cough or sputum

• C&S before starting treatment to identify infecting organism

• Vestibular dysfunction: nausea, vomiting, dizziness, headache; drug should be discontinued if severe

• Injection sites for redness, swelling, abscesses; use warm compresses at site

Teach patient/family:

• To report headache, dizziness, symptoms of overgrowth of infection, renal impairment

• To report loss of hearing, ringing, roaring in ears or feeling of fullness in head

Treatment of overdose: Hemodialysis, monitor serum levels of drug

---

gentamicin sulfate (ophthalmic)

(jen-ta-mye'sin)

Garamycin Ophthalmic, Genoptic

Func. class.: Antiinfective ophthalmic

Action: Inhibits bacterial protein synthesis

Uses: Infection of external eye

Dosage and routes:

• *Adult and child:* INSTILL 1 or 2 gtts q2-4h; TOP apply oint to conjunctival sac bid-qid

Available forms include: Oint, sol 3%

Side effects/adverse reactions:
EENT: Poor corneal wound healing, temporary visual haze, overgrowth of nonsusceptible organisms

Contraindications: Hypersensitivity

Precautions: Antibiotic hypersensitivity, pregnancy (C)

NURSING CONSIDERATIONS
Administer:
• After washing hands, cleanse crusts or discharge from eye before application

Perform/provide:
• Storage at room temperature

Evaluate:
• Therapeutic response: absence of redness, inflammation, tearing
• Allergy: itching, lacrimation, redness, swelling, photosensitivity

Teach patient/family:
• To use drug exactly as prescribed
• Not to use eye makeup, towels, washcloths, eye medication of others; reinfection may occur
• That drug container tip should not be touched to eye
• To report itching, increased redness, burning, stinging, swelling; drug should be discontinued
• That drug may cause blurred vision when ointment is applied

---

gentamicin sulfate (topical)

(jen-ta-mye′sin)
Garamycin

Func. class.: Local antiinfective
Chem. class.: Aminoglycoside

Action: Interferes with bacterial protein synthesis
Uses: Skin infections
Dosage and routes:
• *Adult and child:* TOP rub into affected area tid-qid

Available forms include: Cream, oint 0.1%

Side effects/adverse reactions:
INTEG: Rash, urticaria, stinging, burning, photosensitivity, pruritus

Contraindications: Hypersensitivity

Precautions: Pregnancy (C), lactation

NURSING CONSIDERATIONS
Administer:
• Enough medication to completely cover lesions
• After cleansing with soap, water before each application, dry well

Perform/provide:
• Storage at room temperature in dry place

Evaluate:
• Allergic reaction: burning, stinging, swelling, redness, photosensitivity
• Therapeutic response: decrease in size, number of lesions

Teach patient/family:
• To apply with glove to prevent further infection
• To avoid use of OTC creams, ointments, lotions unless directed by physician
• To use medical asepsis (hand washing) before, after each application
• To avoid sunlight or wear sunscreen to prevent burns
• Not to use in eyes or external ear if eardrum is perforated
• To notify physician if condition worsens

---

glipizide

(glip-i′zide)
Glucotrol

Func. class.: Antidiabetic
Chem. class.: Sulfonylurea (2nd generation)

Action: Causes functioning β-cells

---

italics = common side effects   ***bold italic*** = life threatening reactions

in pancreas to release insulin, leading to drop in blood glucose levels; may improve insulin binding to insulin receptors or increase the number of insulin receptors; not effective if patient lacks functioning β-cells

Uses: Stable adult-onset diabetes mellitus (type II) NIDDM

Dosage and routes:
• *Adult:* PO 5 mg initially, then increased to desired response, do not exceed 15 mg once a day dose, 40 mg/day in divided doses
• *Elderly:* PO 2.5 mg initially, then increased to desired response, max 40 mg/day in divided doses or 15 mg once a day dose

Available forms include: Tabs 5, 10 mg

Side effects/adverse reactions:
CNS: Headache, weakness, dizziness, drowsiness, tinnitus, fatigue, vertigo
GI: Hepatotoxicity, cholestatic jaundice, nausea, vomiting, diarrhea, heartburn
HEMA: Leukopenia, thrombocytopenia, agranulocytosis, aplastic anemia, increased AST, ALT, alk phosphatase, *pancytopenia, hemolytic anemia*
INTEG: Rash, allergic reactions, pruritus, urticaria, eczema, photosensitivity, erythema
ENDO: Hypoglycemia

Contraindications: Hypersensitivity to sulfonylureas, juvenile or brittle diabetes

Precautions: Pregnancy (C), elderly, cardiac disease, severe renal disease, severe hepatic disease, thyroid disease

Pharmacokinetics:
PO: Completely absorbed by GI route, onset 1-1½ hr, duration 10-24 hr, half-life 2-4 hr, metabolized in liver, excreted in urine, 90%-95% is plasma protein bound

Interactions/incompatibilities:
• Increased hypoglycemic effects: insulin, MAOIs, cimetidine, chloramphenicol, guanethidine, methyldopa, non-steroidal antiinflammatories, salicylates, probenecid
• Decreased action of glipizide: calcium channel blockers, corticosteroids, oral contraceptives, thiazide diuretics, thyroid preparations, estrogens, phenothiazines, phenytoin, rifampin, isoniazide, phenobarbital, sympathomimetics
• Disulfiram-like reaction: alcohol
• Decreased effects of both drugs: diazoxide

NURSING CONSIDERATIONS
Assess:
• Blood, urine glucose levels during treatment to determine diabetes control
Administer:
• Drug 30 min before meals
Perform/provide:
• Storage in tight light-resistant containers at room temperature
Evaluate:
• Therapeutic response: decrease in polyuria, polydipsia, polyphagia, clear sensorium, absence of dizziness, stable gait
• Hypoglycemic/hyperglycemic reaction that can occur soon after meals
Teach patient/family:
• Not to drink alcohol
• To check for symptoms of cholestatic jaundice: dark urine, pruritus, yellow sclera; if these occur physician should be notified
• To use a capillary blood glucose test while on this drug
• To test urine glucose levels with Chemstrip 3 × /day
• The symptoms of hypo/hyperglycemia, what to do about each

---

* Available in Canada only

• That drug must be continued on daily basis; explain consequence of discontinuing drug abruptly
• To take drug in morning to prevent hypoglycemic reactions at night
• To avoid OTC medications unless prescribed by a physician
• That diabetes is a life-long illness; drug will not cure disease
• That all food included in diet plan must be eaten in order to prevent hypoglycemia
• To carry Medic-Alert ID for emergency purposes
• To test urine for glucose/ketones tid if this drug is replacing insulin
• To continue weight control, dietary restrictions, exercise, hygiene
Treatment of overdose: 10%-50% glucose solution or 1 mg glucagon

glutamic acid HCl
(gloo-tam'ik)
Acidulin
Func. class.: Digestant
Chem. class.: Amino acid

Action: Increases gastric acidity when needed for replacement
Uses: Hypoacidity
Dosage and routes:
• *Adult:* PO 1-3 caps tid ac
Available forms include: Pulvules 340 mg
Side effects/adverse reactions:
MET: Metabolic acidosis
Contraindications: Peptic ulcer disease
Precautions: Pregnancy (C)
NURSING CONSIDERATIONS
Assess:
• Acid-base, gastric pH during treatment
Administer:
• Before or during meals with 8 oz of water

Perform/provide:
• Storage in tight container at room temperature
Evaluate:
• For achlorhydria: belching, nausea, vomiting, diarrhea, epigastric distress

glutethimide
(gloo-teth'i-mide)
Doriden, Rolathimide
Func. class.: Sedative-hypnotic
Chem. class.: Piperidine derivative

Controlled Substance Schedule III (USA), Schedule F (Canada)
Action: Depresses activity in brain cells primarily in reticular activating system in brainstem, also selectively depresses neurons in posterior hypothalamus, limbic structures
Uses: Insomnia, labor (stage 1), preoperatively for relaxation
Dosage and routes:
Insomnia
• *Adult:* PO 250-500 mg hs, may repeat dose >4 hr before usual awakening, not to exceed 1 g
Preoperatively
• *Adult:* PO 500 mg hs the night before surgery, then 500 mg-1 g 1 hr before surgery
Labor
• *Adult:* PO 500 mg given at the onset of labor, may repeat
Available forms include: Tabs 250, 500 mg; caps 500 mg
Side effects/adverse reactions:
*HEMA: **Thrombocytopenia, aplastic anemia, leukopenia, megaloblastic anemia***
CNS: Residual sedation, dizziness, ataxia, stimulation, headache, hangover
GI: Nausea, vomiting, hiccups, diarrhea, jaundice

italics = common side effects   ***bold italic*** = life threatening reactions

GU: Porphyria

INTEG: Rash, urticaria, purpura, ***exfoliative dermatitis (rare)***

EENT: Dry mouth, blurred vision

Contraindications: Hypersensitivity to this drug or piperidine derivatives, severe pain, severe renal disease, porphyria

Precautions: Depression, suicidal individuals, drug abuse, cardiac dysrhythmias, narrow-angle glaucoma, prostatic hypertrophy, stenosed peptic ulcer, pyloroduodenal/bladder neck obstruction, pregnancy (C)

Pharmacokinetics:

PO: Onset 30 min, peak 1-2 hr, duration 4-8 hr; metabolized by liver, excreted by kidneys (metabolites), crosses placenta, excreted in breast milk; half-life 4 hr, 10-20 hr terminal

Interactions/incompatibilities:

• Decreased hypoprothrombinemic effect: oral anticoagulants

• Increased CNS depression: alcohol and other CNS depressants

• Increased anticholinergic effect: tricyclic antidepressants

NURSING CONSIDERATIONS
Assess:

• Blood studies: Hct, Hgb, RBCs (if on long-term therapy)

• Hepatic studies: AST, ALT, bilirubin

Administer:

• After removal of cigarettes, to prevent fires

• After trying conservative measures for insomnia

• ½-1 hr before hs for sleeplessness

• Several hours before patient is to arise (to avoid hangover)

Perform/provide:

• Assistance with ambulation after receiving dose

• Safety measures: siderails, nightlight, callbell within easy reach

• Checking to see PO medication has been swallowed

• Storage in tight container in cool environment

Evaluate:

• Therapeutic response: ability to sleep at night, decreased amount of early morning awakening if taking drug for insomnia

• Mental status: mood, sensorium, affect, memory (long, short)

• Blood dyscrasias: fever, sore throat, bruising, rash, jaundice, epistaxis (rare)

• Type of sleep problem: falling asleep, staying asleep

Teach patient/family:

• To avoid driving or other activities requiring alertness until drug is stabilized

• To avoid alcohol ingestion or CNS depressants; serious CNS depression may result

• Not to discontinue medication quickly after long-term use, drug should be tapered over 1-2 wk

• That effects may take 2 nights for benefits to be noticed

• Alternate measures to improve sleep: reading, exercise several hours before hs, warm bath, warm milk, TV, self-hypnosis, deep breathing

• That hangover is common in elderly, but less common than with barbiturates

• Withdrawal: nausea, vomiting, anxiety, hallucinations, insomnia, tachycardia, fever, cramps, tremors, seizures

• Blood dyscrasias: fever, sore throat, bruising, rash, jaundice (rare)

• Allergic reaction: rash, discontinue drug if rash occurs

Lab test interferences:

*Interferes: 17-*OHCS

Treatment of overdose: Lavage,

---

activated charcoal, monitor electrolytes, vital signs

---

glyburide

(glye′byoor-ide)
DiaBeta,* Micronase
Func. class.: Antidiabetic
Chem. class.: Sulfonylurea (2nd generation)

Action: Causes functioning β-cells in pancreas to release insulin, leading to drop in blood glucose levels; may improve insulin binding to insulin receptors and increase number of insulin receptors; not effective if patient lacks functioning β-cells
Uses: Stable adult-onset diabetes mellitus (type II) NIDDM
Dosage and routes:
• *Adult:* PO 2.5-5 mg initially, then increased to desired response
• *Elderly:* PO 1.25 mg initially, then increased to desired response; max 20 mg/day, maintenance 1.25-20 mg/qd
Available forms include: Tabs 1.25, 2.5, 5 mg
Side effects/adverse reactions:
CNS: Headache, weakness, paresthesia, tinnitus, fatigue, vertigo
GI: Nausea, fullness, heartburn, **hepatotoxicity, cholestatic jaundice,** vomiting, diarrhea
HEMA: Leukopenia, thrombocytopenia, agranulocytosis, aplastic anemia, increased AST, ALT, alk phosphatase
INTEG: Rash, allergic reactions, pruritus, urticaria, eczema, photosensitivity, erythema
ENDO: Hypoglycemia
MS: Joint pains
Contraindications: Hypersensitivity to sulfonylureas, juvenile or brittle diabetes
Precautions: Pregnancy (B), el-

derly, cardiac disease, severe renal disease, severe hepatic disease, thyroid disease, severe hypoglycemic reactions
Pharmacokinetics:
PO: Completely absorbed by GI route, onset 2-4 hr, peak 2-8 hr, duration 24 hr; half-life 10 hr, metabolized in liver, excreted in urine, feces (metabolites), crosses placenta, 90%-95% is plasma protein bound
Interactions/incompatibilities:
• Both drugs effects may be decreased: diazoxide
• Decreased digoxin level: digoxin
• Increased hypoglycemic effects: insulin, MAOIs, cimetidine, oral anticoagulants, chloramphenicol, guanethidine, methyldopa, nonsteroidal anti-inflammatories, salicylates, probenecid
• Decreased action of glyburide: calcium channel blockers, corticosteroids, oral contraceptives, thiazide diuretics, thyroid preparations, estrogens, phenothiazines, phenytoin, rifampin, isoniazide, phenobarbital, sympathomimetics
• Disulfiram-like reaction: alcohol
NURSING CONSIDERATIONS
Administer:
• With breakfast
Perform/provide:
• Storage in tight container in cool environment
Evaluate:
• Therapeutic response: decrease in polyuria, polydipsia, polyphagia, clear sensorium, absence of dizziness, stable gait
• Hypoglycemic/hyperglycemic reaction that can occur soon after meals
Teach patient/family:
• Not to drink alcohol
• To check for symptoms of cholestatic jaundice: dark urine, pru-

---

italics = common side effects   **bold italic** = life threatening reactions

ritus, yellow sclera; if these occur a physician should be notified
• To use a capillary blood glucose test while on this drug
• To test urine glucose levels with Chemstrip 3 × /day
• The symptoms of hypo/hyperglycemia, what to do about each
• That drug must be continued on daily basis; explain consequence of discontinuing drug abruptly
• To take drug in morning to prevent hypoglycemic reactions at night
• To avoid OTC medications unless prescribed by a physician
• That diabetes is a life-long illness, drug will not cure disease
• That all food included in diet plan must be eaten in order to prevent hypoglycemia
• To carry a Medic-Alert ID for emergency purposes
Treatment of overdose: 10%-50% glucose solution or 1 mg glucagon

---

glycerin
(gli'ser-in)
Glycerol, Glyrol, Osmoglyn
Func. class.: Laxative, hyperosmotic
Chem. class.: Trihydric alcohol

Action: Increases osmotic pressure, draws fluid into colon
Uses: Constipation
Dosage and routes:
• *Adult and child >6 yr:* REC SUPP 3 g; ENEMA 5-15 ml
• *Child <6 yr:* REC SUPP 1-1.5 g; ENEMA 2-5 ml
Available forms include: Rec sol 4 ml/applicator; supp
Side effects/adverse reactions: None known

Contraindications: Hypersensitivity
Precautions: Pregnancy (C)

NURSING CONSIDERATIONS
Administer:
• In morning or evening (oral dose)
Perform/provide:
• Storage in cool environment, do not freeze
Evaluate:
• Therapeutic response: decrease in constipation
• Cause of constipation; identify whether fluids, bulk, or exercise is missing from lifestyle
• Cramping, rectal bleeding, nausea, vomiting; if these symptoms occur, drug should be discontinued
Teach patient/family:
• Not to use laxatives for long-term therapy; bowel tone will be lost
• That normal bowel movements do not always occur daily
• Do not use in presence of abdominal pain, nausea, vomiting
• Notify physician if constipation unrelieved or if symptoms of electrolyte imbalance occur: muscle cramps, pain, weakness, dizziness, excessive thirst

---

glycerin, anhydrous
(gli'ser-in)
Ophthalgan
Func. class.: Opthalmic
Chem. class.: Trihydric alcohol

Action: Reduces corneal edema by osmosis of water through corneal epithelium which is semipermeable
Uses: Reduce corneal edema
Dosage and routes:
• *Adult:* INSTILL 1-2 gtts after local anesthetic
Available forms include: Sol
Side effects/adverse reactions:
EENT: Eye pain
Contraindications: Hypersensitivity
Precautions: Pregnancy (C)

Pharmacokinetics: Onset 10 min, peak 20 min, duration 6-8 hr
NURSING CONSIDERATIONS
Administer:
• Anesthetic (tetracaine or proparacaine) before instillation to decrease pain
Perform/provide:
• Storage in tight container
Teach patient/family:
• Method of instillation, including pressure on lacrimal sac for 1 min, and not to touch dropper to eye

---

glycopyrrolate

(glye-koe-pye'roe-late)
Robinul, Robinul Forte
Func. class.: Cholinergic blocker
Chem. class.: Quaternary ammonium compound

Action: Inhibits acetylcholine at receptor sites in autonomic nervous system, which controls secretions, free acids in stomach
Uses: Decreased secretions before surgery, reversal of neuromuscular blockade, peptic ulcer disease, irritable bowel syndrome
Dosage and routes:
Preoperatively
• *Adult:* IM 0.002 mg/lb ½-1 hr before surgery
• *Child 2-12 yr:* IM 0.002-0.004 mg/lb
• *Child <2 yr:* IM 0.004 mg/lb
Reversal of neuromuscular blockage
• *Adult:* IV 0.2 mg for each 1 mg of neostigmine or 5 mg IV of pyridostigmine simultaneously
GI disorders
• *Adult:* PO 1-2 mg bid-tid; IM/IV 0.1-0.2 mg tid-qid, titrated to patient response
Available forms include: Tabs 1, 2 mg; inj 0.2 mg/ml

Side effects/adverse reactions:
INTEG: Urticaria, allergic reactions
MISC: Suppression of lactation, nasal congestion, decreased sweating
CNS: Confusion, anxiety, restlessness, irritability, delusions, hallucinations, headache, sedation, depression, incoherence, dizziness, lethargy, flushing, weakness
EENT: Blurred vision, photophobia, dilated pupils, difficulty swallowing, increased intraocular pressure, mydriasis, cycloplegia
CV: Palpitations, tachycardia, postural hypotension, paradoxical bradycardia
GI: Dryness of mouth, constipation, nausea, vomiting, abdominal distress, paralytic ileus, altered taste perception
GU: Hesitancy, retention, impotence
Contraindications: Hypersensitivity, narrow-angle glaucoma, myasthenia gravis, GI/GU obstruction, child <3 yr, tachycardia, myocardial ischemia, hepatic disease, ulcerative colitis, toxic megacolon
Precautions: Pregnancy (C), elderly, lactation, prostatic hypertrophy, renal disease, CHF, pulmonary disease, hyperthyroidism
Pharmacokinetics:
PO: Peak 1 hr, duration 6 hr
IM: Peak 30-45 min, duration 7 hr
IV: Peak 10-15 min, duration 4 hr
Excreted in urine, bile, feces (unchanged)
Interactions/incompatibilities:
• Increased anticholinergic effect: alcohol, antihistamines, phenothiazines, amantadine, tricyclics
• Do not mix with diazepam, chloramphenicol, pentobarbital, sodium bicarbonate, sodium chloride in syringe or solution

---

italics = common side effects   ***bold italic*** = life threatening reactions

NURSING CONSIDERATIONS
Assess:
• I&O ratio; retention commonly causes decreased urinary output
Administer:
• IV undiluted, give through a Y-tube or 3-way stopcock; give 0.2 mg or less over 1-2 min
• Parenteral dose with patient recumbent to prevent postural hypotension
• With or after meals to prevent GI upset; may give with fluids other than water
• Parenteral dose slowly; keep in bed for at least 1 hr after dose, monitor vital signs
• After checking dose carefully, even slight overdose could lead to toxicity
Perform/provide:
• Storage at room temperature
• Hard candy, frequent drinks, sugarless gum to relieve dry mouth
Evaluate:
• Urinary hesitancy, retention: palpate bladder if retention occurs
• Constipation; increase fluids, bulk, exercise if this occurs
• For tolerance over long-term therapy; dose may need to be increased or changed
• Mental status: affect, mood, CNS depression, worsening of mental symptoms during early therapy
Teach patient/family:
• Not to discontinue this drug abruptly; to taper off over 1 wk
• To avoid driving or other hazardous activities; drowsiness may occur
• To avoid OTC medication: cough, cold preparations with alcohol, antihistamines unless directed by physician

gonadorelin acetate
Lutrepulse

Func. class.: Gonadotropin
Chem. class.: Synthetic endogenous gonadotropin-releasing hormone (GnRH)

Action: Induces ovulation in women by release of LH in the anterior pituitary gland
Uses: Primary hypothalamic amenorrhea
Dosage and routes:
• IV Pump: 5 μg/min, × 21 days; after three treatment intervals, it may be necessary to raise the dose in a stepwise program
Available forms include: Powder for inj, IV 0.8, 3.2 mg
Side effects/adverse reactions:
INTEG: Inflammation at injection site, phlebitis, hematoma at catheter site
SYST: Anaphylaxis (bronchospasm, tachycardia, flushing, urticaria, induration of injection site)
REPRO: Ovarian hyperstimulation, multiple pregnancy
Contraindications: Hypersensitivity; patients with ovarian cysts or hormonally dependent tumors; causes of anovulation other than those of hypothalamic origin
Precautions: Pregnancy (B)
Pharmacokinetics: Excreted by kidneys, half-life (initial) 2-10 min, (terminal 10-40 min)
Interaction/incompatibilities:
• Ovulation stimulators should not be used with this drug
NURSING CONSIDERATIONS
Assess:
• Effects by ovarian ultrasound—baseline, after 1 wk, after 2 wk, midluteal phase serum progesterone

---

Administer:

• Using Lutrepulse pump only; detailed instructions are given with pump

• After reconstituting 8 ml of diluent provided and transferring to plastic reservoir, withdraw 8 ml of diluent and inject into lyophile drug cake; shake, fill reservoir bag with reconstituted solution, and administer IV using pump provider

Perform/provide:

• Storage at room temperature; use prepared solution within 24 hr

Evaluate:

• Therapeutic effect: absence of amenorrhea with drug use

---

gonadorelin HCl

(goe-nad-oh-rell′in)

Factrel

Func. class.: Gonadotropin

Chem. class.: Synthetic luteinizing hormone–releasing hormone

---

Action: Combination luteinizing hormone (releasing hormone) that acts on anterior pituitary

Uses: Evaluation of response of gonadotropic hormone

Dosage and routes:

• *Adult:* SC/IV 100 μg usually given between day 1-7 of menstrual cycle

• *Child:* SC/IV 2 μg/kg

Available forms include: Powder for inj SC, IV 100, 500 μg/vial

Side effects/adverse reactions:

CNS: Dizziness, headache, flushing

GI: Nausea

INTEG: Inflammation at injection site

Contraindications: Hypersensitivity

Precautions: Pregnancy (B)

Pharmacokinetics: Excreted by kidneys

Interactions/incompatibilities:

• Increased level of gonadorelin: levodopa, spironolactone

• Decreased level of gonadorelin: digoxin, oral contraceptives

• May produce false test results when used with androgens, glucocorticoids, estrogens, progestins

NURSING CONSIDERATIONS

Assess:

• Test result: pituitary/hypothalamus dysfunction (decreased LH); postmenopausal (increased LH)

Administer:

• After reconstituting with sterile diluent (1 ml)/100 μg enclosed in package; give over 30 sec

• Repeated doses may be necessary to elevate pituitary gonadotropin reserve

Perform/provide:

• Storage at room temperature; use prepared solution within 24 hr

---

goserelin acetate

Zoladex

Func. class.: Gonadotropin-releasing hormone

Chem. class.: Synthetic decapeptide analog of LHRH

Action: Inhibitor of pituitary gonadotropin secretion. Initially increases LH and FSH with increases in testosterone, and reduction in sex steroid levels

Uses: Advanced prostate cancer, premenopausal breast cancer

Dosage and routes:

• *Adult:* SC 3.6 mg q28 days

Available forms include: Depot inj 3.6 mg

Side effects/adverse reactions:

CNS: Headaches, ***spinal cord compression,*** anxiety, depression

CV: Dysrhythmia, ***cerebrovascular***

---

italics = common side effects   ***bold italic*** = life threatening reactions

accident, hypertension, *MI*, chest pain

ENDO: Gynecomastia, breast tenderness, hot flashes

GI: Nausea, vomiting, constipation, diarrhea, ulcer

GU: Spotting, breakthrough bleeding, decreased libido, renal insufficiency, urinary obstruction, urinary tract infection

INTEG: Rash, pain on injection

MS: Osteoneuralgia

Contraindications: Hypersensitivity, pregnancy

Pharmacokinetics: Peak serum concentrations in 12-15 days

NURSING CONSIDERATIONS

Assess:

• For relief of bone pain

Evaluate:

• Therapeutic response: more normal levels of prostate-specific antigen, acid phosphatase, alk phosphatase, testosterone level of <25 ng/dl

Teach patient/family:

• That gynecomastia and postmenopausal symptoms may occur, but will decrease after treatment is discontinued

Lab test interferences:

Increased: Alk phosphatase, estradiol, FSH, LH, testosterone levels

Decreased: Testosterone levels, progesterone

---

griseofulvin microsize/ griseofulvin ultramicrosize

(gri-see-oh-ful'vin)

Fulvicin-U/F, Grifulvin-V, Grasactin, Grisovin-FP, Fulvicin P/G, Grisactin-Ultra, Gris-PEG

Func. class.: Antifungal

Chem. class.: Penicillium griseofulvum derivative

Action: Arrests fungal cell division

at metaphase, binds to human keratin making it resistant to disease

Uses: Mycotic infections: Tinea corporis, pedis, cruris, barbae, capitis, unguium if caused by *Epidermophyton, Microsporum, Trichophyton*

Dosage and routes:

• *Adult:* PO 500-1000 mg qd in single or divided doses (microsize), 125-165 mg bid (ultramicrosize) or 250-330 mg qd; may need 500-660 mg in divided doses for severe infections

• *Child:* PO 10 mg/kg/day or 30 mg/m^2/day (microsize) or 5 mg/kg/day (ultramicrosize)

Available forms include: Microcaps 125, 250 mg; tabs 250, 500 mg; oral susp 125 mg/ml; ultratabs 125, 165, 250, 330 mg

Side effects/adverse reactions:

INTEG: Rash, urticaria, photosensitivity, lichen planus, angioedema

CNS: Headache, peripheral neuritis, paresthesias, confusion, dizziness, fatigue, insomnia, psychosis

EENT: Blurred vision, oral candidiasis, furry tongue, transient hearing loss

GU: Proteinuria, cylinduria, precipitate porphyria, increased thirst

GI: Nausea, vomiting, anorexia, diarrhea, cramps, dry mouth, flatulence

HEMA: Leukopenia, granulocytopenia, neutropenia, monocytosis

Contraindications: Hypersensitivity, porphyria, hepatic disease, lupus erythematosus

Precautions: Penicillin sensitivity, pregnancy (C)

Pharmacokinetics:

PO: Peak 4 hr, half-life 9-24 hr, metabolized in liver, excreted in urine (inactive metabolites), feces, perspiration

Interactions/incompatibilities:
• Tachycardia: alcohol
• Decreased action of griseofulvin: barbiturates
• Decreased action of: warfarin, anticoagulants (oral)

NURSING CONSIDERATIONS
Assess:
• I&O ratio
• Liver studies q wk (ALT, AST, bilirubin, alk phosphatase)
• Renal studies: BUN, serum creatinine
• Blood studies: CBC, platelets, q2 wk
• Drug level during treatment

Administer:
• Drug carefully, making sure there is no confusion with dosage form (microsize vs ultrasize)
• With meals to decrease GI symptoms
• Until 3 separate cultures are negative for infective organism

Perform/provide:
• Storage in tight, light-resistant containers at room temperature

Evaluate:
• Therapeutic response: decreased fever, malaise, rash, negative C&S for infecting organism
• For history of penicillin allergy; may be cross-sensitive to this drug
• For renal toxicity: increasing BUN, serum creatinine, proteinuria, cylinduria
• For hepatotoxicity: increasing ALT, AST, bilirubin, alk phosphatase
• For blood dyscrasias: fatigue, malaise, dark urine, bruising

Teach patient/family:
• That long-term therapy may be needed to clear infection (2 wk-6 mo depending on organism)
• Proper hygiene: handwashing technique, nail care, use of con-

comitant topical agents if prescribed
• Stress compliance even after feeling better
• To avoid alcohol since nausea, vomiting, hypertension may occur
• To use sunscreen or avoid direct sunlight to prevent photosensitivity
• To notify physician of sore throat, fever, skin rash, which may indicate overgrowth of organisms

G

guaifenesin
(gwye-fen′e-sin)
Anti-Tuss, Balminil,* Bowtussin, Breonesin, Colrex, Cosin-GG, Dilyn, Glycotuss, Gly-O-Tussin, Glytuss, G-Tussin, Hytuss, Malotuss, Nortussin Proco, Recsei-Tuss, Resyl,* Robitussin, Tursen, Wal-Tussin DM

Func. class.: Expectorant

Action: Acts as an expectorant by stimulating a gastric mucosal reflex to increase the production of lung mucus
Uses: Dry, nonproductive cough
Dosage and routes:
• *Adult:* PO 100-400 mg q4-6h, not to exceed 1.2 g/day
• *Child:* PO 12 mg/kg/day in 6 divided doses
Available forms include: Tabs 100, 200 mg; caps 200 mg; syr 100 mg/5 ml
Side effects/adverse reactions:
CNS: Drowsiness
GI: Nausea, anorexia, vomiting
Contraindications: Hypersensitivity, persistent cough
Precautions: Pregnancy (C)
NURSING CONSIDERATIONS
Perform/provide:
° Storage at room temperature
• Increased fluids, room humidification to liquefy secretions

---

italics = common side effects   ***bold italic*** = life threatening reactions

Evaluate:
- Therapeutic response: absence of cough
- Cough: type, frequency, character including sputum

Teach patient/family:
- Avoid driving, other hazardous activities if drowsiness occurs (rare)
- Avoid smoking, smoke-filled room, perfumes, dust, environmental pollutants, cleansers

---

guanabenz acetate

(gwan'a-benz)
Wytensin

Func. class.: Antihypertensive
Chem. class.: Central α_2-adrenergic agonist

Action: Stimulates central α_2-adrenergic receptors resulting in decreased sympathetic outflow from brain

Uses: Hypertension

Dosage and routes:
- *Adult:* PO 4 mg bid, increasing in increments of 4-8 mg/day q1-2 wk, not to exceed 32 mg bid

Available forms include: Tabs 4, 8, 16 mg

Side effects/adverse reactions:
CV: Severe rebound hypertension, chest pain, dysrhythmias, palpitations

CNS: Drowsiness, dizziness, sedation, headache, depression, weakness

EENT: Dry mouth, nasal congestion, blurred vision

GI: Nausea, diarrhea, constipation

GU: Impotence

Contraindications: Hypersensitivity to guanabenz

Precautions: Pregnancy (C), lactation, children <12 yr, severe coronary insufficiency, recent myocardial infarction, cerebrovascular disease, severe hepatic or renal failure

Pharmacokinetics:
PO: Peak 2-4 hr; half-life 6 hr, excreted in urine

Interactions/incompatibilities:
- Increased sedation: CNS depressants

NURSING CONSIDERATIONS
Assess:
- Renal studies: protein, BUN, creatinine, watch for increased levels; may indicate nephrotic syndrome
- Baselines in renal, liver function tests before therapy begins
- K levels, although hyperkalemia rarely occurs
- Dip-stick of urine for protein qd in first morning specimen, if protein is increased a 24 hr urinary protein should be collected
- B/P during beginning treatment, periodically thereafter

Evaluate:
- Therapeutic response: decrease in B/P
- Edema in feet and legs daily
- Allergic reaction: rash, fever, pruritus, urticaria; drug should be discontinued if antihistamines fail to help
- Renal symptoms: polyuria, oliguria, frequency

Teach patient/family:
- To avoid hazardous activities, sedation may occur
- Not to discontinue drug abruptly or withdrawal symptoms may occur: anxiety, increased B/P, headache, insomnia, increased pulse, tremors, nausea, sweating
- Not to use OTC (cough, cold, or allergy) products unless directed by physician
- Stress patient compliance with dosage schedule even if feeling better

---

• Notify physician of: swelling of hands or feet, irregular heartbeat, chest pain
• Excessive perspiration, dehydration, vomiting, diarrhea; may lead to fall in blood pressure—consult physician if these occur
• May cause dizziness, fainting; light-headedness may occur during 1st few days of therapy
• That compliance is necessary, not to skip or stop drug unless directed by physician
• May cause skin rash or impaired perspiration

Treatment of overdose: Administer vasopressor, discontinue drug, supine position

---

guanadrel sulfate

(gwahn′a-drel)
Hylorel

Func. class.: Antihypertensive
Chem. class.: Adrenergic blocker, peripheral guinidine derivative

---

Action: Inhibits sympathetic vasoconstriction by inhibiting release of norepinephrine, depletes norepinephrine stores in adrenergic nerve endings

Uses: Hypertension

Dosage and routes:
• *Adult:* PO 5 mg bid, adjusted to desired response, may need 20-75 mg/day in divided doses

Available forms include: Tabs 10, 25 mg

Side effects/adverse reactions:

*CV: Orthostatic hypotension, bradycardia, **CHF,** palpitations,* chest pain, tachycardia, dysrhythmias

CNS: Drowsiness, fatigue, weakness, feeling of faintness, insomnia, dizziness, mental changes, memory loss, hallucinations, *depression,* anxiety, *confusion, paresthesias, headache*

GI: Nausea, cramps, diarrhea, constipation, dry mouth, anorexia, indigestion

INTEG: Rash, purpura, alopecia

EENT: Nasal stuffiness, tinnitus, visual changes, sore throat, double vision, dry burning eyes

GU: Ejaculation failure, impotence, dysuria, nocturia, frequency

*RESP: **Bronchospasm,** dyspnea,* cough, rales, SOB

MS: Leg cramps, aching, pain, inflammation

Contraindications: Hypersensitivity, pregnancy (B), pheochromocytoma, lactation, CHF, child <18 yr

Precautions: Elderly, bronchial asthma, peptic ulcer, electrolyte imbalances, vascular disease

Pharmacokinetics:
PO: Onset 0.5-2 hr, peak 1½-2 hr, duration 4-14 hr; half-life 10-12 hr, excreted in urine (50% unchanged)

Interactions/incompatibilities:
• Increased hypotension: diuretics, other antihypertensives
• Do not use with MAOIs
• Increased orthostatic hypotension: alcohol, opioids
• Decreased hypotensive effect: tricyclic antidepressants, phenothiazines, ephedrine, phenylpropanolamine

NURSING CONSIDERATIONS

Assess:
• Renal function studies in renal impairment (BUN, creatinine)
• Bleeding time, check for ecchymosis, thrombocytopenia, purpura
• I&O in renal disease patient

Evaluate:
• Cardiac status: B/P lying and standing, pulse, watch for hypotension

---

• Edema in feet, legs daily; take weight daily
• Skin turgor, dryness of mucous membranes for hydration status
• Symptoms of CHF: edema, dyspnea, wet rales

Teach patient/family:
• To avoid driving, hazardous activities if drowsiness occurs
• Not to discontinue drug abruptly
• Not to use OTC products unless directed by physician: cough, cold preparations
• To report bradycardia, dizziness, confusion, depression, fever or sore throat
• That impotence, gynecomastia may occur but are reversible
• To rise slowly to sitting or standing position to minimize orthostatic hypotension
• That therapeutic effect may take 2-4 wk

---

guanethidine sulfate

(gwahn-eth'i-deen)
Ismelin

Func. class.: Antihypertensive
Chem. class.: Antiadrenergic agent, peripheral

Action: Inhibits norepinephrine release, depleting norepinephrine stores in adrenergic nerve endings
Uses: Moderate to severe hypertension

Dosage and routes:
• *Adult:* PO 10 mg qd, increase by 10 mg qwk at monthly intervals; may require 25-50 mg qd
• *Adult:* (Hospitalized) 25-50 mg; may increase by 25-50 mg/day or every other day
• *Child:* PO 200 μg/kg/day; increase q7-10 days, not to exceed 3000 μg/kg/24 hr

Available forms include: Tabs 10, 25 mg

Side effects/adverse reactions:
CV: Orthostatic hypotension, dizziness, weakness, lassitude, bradycardia, **CHF,** fatigue, angina, heart block, chest paresthesia
CNS: Depression
GI: Nausea, vomiting, *diarrhea,* constipation, dry mouth, weight gain, anorexia
INTEG: Dermatitis, loss of scalp hair
HEMA: **Thrombocytopenia, leukopenia**
EENT: Nasal congestion, ptosis, blurred vision
GU: Ejaculation failure, impotence, nocturia, edema, retention, increased BUN
RESP: Dyspnea

Contraindications: Hypersensitivity, pheochromocytoma, recent MI, CHF, cardiac failure, sinus bradycardia
Precautions: Pregnancy (B), lactation, peptic ulcer, asthma

Pharmacokinetics:
PO: Therapeutic level: 1-3 wk; half-life 5 days, metabolized by liver, excreted in urine (metabolites), breast milk

Interactions/incompatibilities:
• Increased hypotension: diuretics, other antihypertensives
• Do not use with MAOIs
• Increased orthostatic hypotension: alcohol
• Decreased hypotensive effect: tricyclic antidepressants, phenothiazines, ephedrine, phenylpropanolamine, oral contraceptives, thiothixine, doxepin, haloperidol, amphetamines

NURSING CONSIDERATIONS
Assess:
• Renal function studies in renal impairment (BUN, creatinine)

---

* Available in Canada only

- Bleeding time, check for ecchymosis, thrombocytopenia, purpura
- I&O in renal disease patient

Evaluate:
- Cardiac status: B/P, pulse, watch for hypotension
- Edema in feet, legs daily; take weight daily
- Skin turgor, dryness of mucous membranes for hydration status
- Symptoms of CHF: edema, dyspnea, wet rales

Teach patient/family:
- To avoid driving, hazardous activities if drowsiness occurs
- Not to discontinue drug abruptly
- Not to use OTC products unless directed by physician: cough, cold preparations
- To report bradycardia, dizziness, confusion, depression, fever, sore throat
- That impotence, gynecomastia may occur, but are reversible
- To rise slowly to sitting or standing position to minimize orthostatic hypotension, more common in AM, hot weather, exercise or when using alcohol
- That therapeutic effect may take 2-4 wk
- Notify MD of severe diarrhea

Lab test interferences:
Increase: BUN
Decrease: Blood glucose, VMA excretion, urinary norepinephrine

Treatment of overdose: Lavage, vasopressors given cautiously

---

guanfacine HCl
(gwahn'fa-seen)
Tenex

Func. class.: Antihypertensive
Chem. class.: α-2 Adrenergic receptor agonist

Action: Stimulates central α-adrenergic receptors resulting in decreased sympathetic outflow from brain

Uses: Hypertension in individual using a thiazide diuretic

Dosage and routes:
- *Adult:* PO 1 mg/day hs, may increase dose in 2-3 wk to 2-3 mg/day

Available forms include: Tabs 1 mg

Side effects/adverse reactions:
GI: Dry mouth, constipation, cramps, nausea, diarrhea
CNS: Somnolence, dizziness, headache, fatigue
GU: Impotence, urinary incontinence
EENT: Taste change, tinnitus, vision change, rhinitis
MS: Leg cramps
RESP: Dyspnea
INTEG: Dermatitis, pruritus, purpura
CV: Bradycardia, chest pain

Contraindications: Hypersensitivity

Precautions: Pregnancy (B), lactation, children <12 yr, severe coronary insufficiency, recent MI, renal or hepatic disease, CVA

Pharmacokinetics:
Peak 1-4 hr, 70% bound to plasma proteins, half-life 17 hr, eliminated via kidney unchanged and as metabolites

Interactions/incompatibilities:
- Increased sedation: CNS depressants, other antihypertensives

NURSING CONSIDERATIONS
Assess:
- Blood studies: neutrophils, decrease in platelets
- Renal studies: protein, BUN, creatinine; watch for increased levels that may indicate nephrotic syndrome

---

italics = common side effects   ***bold italic*** = life threatening reactions

• Baselines in renal, liver function tests before therapy begins
• Potassium levels, although hyperkalemia rarely occurs
• Dip-stick of urine for protein in first morning specimen, if protein is increased, a 24 hr urinary protein should be collected
• B/P before, during, after treatment; notify physician of significant changes

Perform/provide:
• Storage of tablets in tight containers

Evaluate:
• Therapeutic response: decreased B/P in hypertension
• Edema in feet, legs daily
• Allergic reaction: rash, fever, pruritus, urticaria; drug should be discontinued if antihistamines fail to help
• Symptoms of CHF: edema, dyspnea, wet rales, B/P
• Renal symptoms: polyuria, oliguria, frequency

Teach patient/family:
• To avoid hazardous activities
• Not to discontinue drug abruptly or withdrawal symptoms may occur: anxiety, increased B/P, headache, insomnia, increased pulse, tremors, nausea, sweating
• Not to use OTC (cough, cold, or allergy) products unless directed by physician
• Tell patient to avoid sunlight or to wear sunscreen; photosensitivity may occur
• Stress patient compliance with dosage schedule even if feeling better

haemophilus b vaccines (polysaccharide, conjugate)
(hee-moef'ii-lus)
Hib-Imune, HibVAX (polysaccharide), b-Capsa 1, ProHIBIT (conjugate)
Func. class.: Vaccine
Chem. class.: Haemophilus influenzae capsular polysaccharide

Action: Stimulates antibody production to *Haemophilus influenzae b*

Uses: Polysaccharide immunization of children 2-6 yr against *H. influenzae b,* conjugate immunization of child 1½-5 yr against invasive disease of *H. influenzae b*

Dosage and routes:
• *Child:* SC 0.5 ml (polysaccharide), IM 0.5 mg (conjugate)
Available forms include: Polysaccharide powder for injection 25 μg/0.5 ml after reconstituting; conjugate powder for injection 25 μg polysaccharide and 18 μg conjugated diphtheria toxoid/0.5 ml

Side effects/adverse reactions:
INTEG: Redness, soreness at injection site, rash
SYST: Low-grade fever

Contraindications: Hypersensitivity

Precautions: Pregnancy (C)

NURSING CONSIDERATIONS
Assess:
• For skin reactions: swelling, rash, urticaria

Administer:
• After diluting with 0.6 ml diluent, which will yield 10 doses of 0.5 ml
• Only with epinephrine 1:1000 on unit to treat laryngospasm
• Only by SC or IM route

Perform/provide:
• Storage in refrigerator
Evaluate:
• For history of allergies, skin conditions (eczema, psoriasis, dermatitis), reactions to vaccinations
• For anaphylaxis: inability to breathe, bronchospasm
Teach patient/family:
• That usually one dose is required
Lab test interferences:
Interference: Latex agglutination, countercurrent immunoelectrophoresis

---

halazepam
(hal-az′e-pam)
Paxipam
Func. class.: Antianxiety
Chem. class.: Benzodiazepine

Controlled Substance Schedule IV
Action: Depresses subcortical levels of CNS, including limbic system, reticular formation
Uses: Anxiety
Dosage and routes:
• *Adult:* PO 20-40 mg tid-qid
• *Geriatric:* PO 20 mg qd-bid
Available forms include: Tabs 20, 40 mg
Side effects/adverse reactions:
CNS: Dizziness, drowsiness, confusion, headache, anxiety, tremors, stimulation, fatigue, depression, insomnia, hallucinations
GI: Constipation, dry mouth, nausea, vomiting, anorexia, diarrhea
INTEG: Rash, dermatitis, itching
*CV: Orthostatic hypotension, **ECG changes, tachycardia,*** hypotension
EENT: Blurred vision, tinnitus, mydriasis
Contraindications: Hypersensitivity to benzodiazepines, narrow-angle glaucoma, psychosis, pregnancy (D), child <18 yr
Precautions: Elderly, debilitated, hepatic disease, renal disease
Pharmacokinetics:
PO: Peak 1-3 hr, duration 3-6 hr, metabolized by liver, excreted by kidneys, crosses placenta, breast milk, half-life 14 hr
Interactions/incompatibilities:
• Decreased effects of halazepam: oral contraceptives, valproic acid
• Increased effects of halazepam: CNS depressants, alcohol, disulfiram, oral contraceptives

NURSING CONSIDERATIONS
Assess:
• B/P (lying, standing), pulse; if systolic B/P drops 20 mm Hg, hold drug, notify physician, respirations q5-15 min if given IV
• Blood studies: CBC during long-term therapy, blood dyscrasias have occurred rarely
• Hepatic studies: AST, ALT, bilirubin, creatinine, LDH, alk phosphatase
Administer:
• With food or milk for GI symptoms
• Crushed if patient is unable to swallow medication whole
• Sugarless gum, hard candy, frequent sips of water for dry mouth
Perform/provide:
• Assistance with ambulation during beginning therapy, since drowsiness/dizziness occurs
• Safety measures, including side-rails
• Check to see PO medication has been swallowed
Evaluate:
• Therapeutic response: decreased anxiety, restlessness, sleeplessness
• Mental status: mood, sensorium, affect, sleeping pattern, drowsiness, dizziness

H

---

italics = common side effects **bold italic** = life threatening reactions

- Physical dependency, withdrawal symptoms: headache, nausea, vomiting, muscle pain, weakness after long-term use
- Suicidal tendencies

Teach patient/family:
- That drug may be taken with food
- Not to be used for everyday stress or used longer than 4 mo, unless directed by physician, not to take more than prescribed amount, may be habit forming
- Avoid OTC preparations (hay fever, cough, cold) unless approved by physician
- To avoid driving or other activities that require alertness; drowsiness may occur
- To avoid alcohol ingestion or other psychotropic medications, unless prescribed by physician
- Not to discontinue medication abruptly after long-term use
- To rise slowly or fainting may occur
- That drowsiness might worsen at beginning of treatment

Lab test interferences:
Increase: AST/ALT, serum bilirubin
False increase: 17-OHCS
Decrease: RAIU

Treatment of overdose: Lavage, VS, supportive care

---

halcinonide

(hal-sin'oo-nide)
Halciderm, Halog
Func. class.: Corticosteroid, synthetic
Chem. class.: Fluorinated corticosteroid

Action: Antiinflammatory, antipruritic, vasoconstrictor actions
Uses: Inflammation of corticosteroid-responsive dermatoses

Dosage and routes:
- *Adult:* TOP apply to affected area bid-tid
Available forms include: Cream 0.025%, 0.1%; oint 0.1%; sol 0.1%

Side effects/adverse reactions:
INTEG: Acne, atrophy, epidermal thinning, purpura, striae
Contraindications: Hypersensitivity, viral infections, fungal infections
Precautions: Pregnancy (C)

NURSING CONSIDERATIONS
Administer:
- Using an occlusive dressing, systemic absorption may occur
- For 3-5 days after lesions are gone

Perform/provide:
- Washing of skin before application
- Dressing change qd, check area for redness, rash, inflammation, discoloration; do not leave dressing in place over 16 hr

Evaluate:
- Therapeutic response: decreased inflammation
- Infection: increased temperature, WBC, even after withdrawal of medication; keep in mind these may be systemically absorbed

Teach patient/family:
- Not to get drug in eyes or mucous membranes

---

halobetasol propionate

Untravate
Func. class.: Topical corticosteroid
Chem. class.: Synthetic fluorinated agent, group VI potency

Action: Possesses antipruritic, antiinflammatory actions
Uses: Psoriasis, eczema, contact dermatitis, pruritus

Dosage and routes:
• *Adult and child:* Apply to affected area tid-qid
Available forms include: Cream 0.05%; oint 0.005%
Side effects/adverse reactions:
INTEG: Burning, dryness, itching, irritation, acne, folliculitis, hypertrichosis, perioral dermatitis, hypopigmentation, atrophy, striae, miliaria, allergic contact dermatitis, secondary infection
Contraindications: Hypersensitivity to corticosteroids, fungal infections
Precautions: Pregnancy (C), lactation, viral infections, bacterial infections
NURSING CONSIDERATIONS
Assess:
• Temperature: if fever develops, drug should be discontinued
Administer:
• Only to affected areas; do not get in eyes
• Medication, then cover with occlusive dressing (only if prescribed); seal to normal skin; change q12h; systemic absorption may occur
• Only to dermatoses: do not use on weeping, denuded, or infected area
Perform/provide:
• Cleansing before application of drug
• Treatment for a few days after area has cleared
• Storage at room temperature
Evaluate:
• Therapeutic response: absence of severe itching, patches on skin, flaking
• For systemic absorption: increased temperature, inflammation, irritation
Teach patient/family:
• To avoid sunlight on affected area: burns may occur

haloperidol/haloperidol decanoate

(ha-loe-per'idole)
Haldol, Peridol/Haloperidol Decanoate
Func. class.: Antipsychotic/neuroleptic
Chem. class.: Butyrophenone

Action: Depresses cerebral cortex, hypothalamus, limbic system, which control activity and aggression; blocks neurotransmission produced by dopamine at synapse; exhibits strong α-adrenergic, anticholinergic blocking action; mechanism for antipsychotic effects is unclear.
Uses: Psychotic disorders, control of tics, vocal utterances in Tourette syndrome, short-term treatment of hyperactive children showing excessive motor activity, prolonged parenteral therapy in chronic schizophrenia
Dosage and routes:
Psychosis
• *Adult:* PO 0.5-5 mg bid or tid initially depending on severity of condition; dose is increased to desired dose, max 100 mg/day; IM 2-5 mg q1-8h
• *Child 3-12 yr:* PO/IM 0.05-0.15 mg/kg/day
• *Decanoate:* Initial dose IM is 10-15 x daily oral dose at 4 wk interval; do not administer IV, not to exceed 100 mg
Chronic schizophrenia
• *Adult:* IM 10-15 times the PO dose q4 wk (decanoate)
• *Child 3-12 yr:* PO/IM 0.05-0.15 mg/kg/day
Tics/vocal utterances
• *Adult:* PO 0.5-5 mg bid or tid increased until desired response occurs

---

italics = common side effects   ***bold italic*** = life threatening reactions

- *Child 3-12 yr:* PO 0.05-0.075 mg/kg/day
Hyperactive children
- *Child 3-12 yr:* PO 0.05-0.075 mg/kg/day
Available forms include: Tabs 0.5, 1, 2, 5, 10, 20 mg; conc 2 mg/ml; inj IM 5 mg/ml
Side effects/adverse reactions:
*RESP: **Laryngospasm,** dyspnea, **respiratory depression***
*CNS: Extrapyramidal symptoms: pseudoparkinsonism, akathisia, dystonia, tardive dyskinesia, drowsiness, headache, **seizures neuroleptic malignant syndrome***
INTEG: Rash, photosensitivity, dermatitis
EENT: Blurred vision, glaucoma
GI: Dry mouth, nausea, vomiting, anorexia, constipation, diarrhea, jaundice, weight gain
GU: Urinary retention, urinary frequency, enuresis, impotence, amenorrhea, gynecomastia
CV: Orthostatic hypotension, hypertension, **cardiac arrest,** ECG changes, **tachycardia**
Contraindications: Hypersensitivity, blood dyscrasias, coma, child <3 yr, brain damage, bone marrow depression, alcohol and barbiturate withdrawal states, Parkinson's disease, angina, epilepsy, urinary retention
Precautions: Pregnancy (C), lactation, seizure disorders, hypertension, hepatic disease, cardiac disease
Pharmacokinetics:
PO: Onset erratic, peak 2-6 hr, half-life 24 hr
IM: Onset 15-30 min, peak 15-20 min, half-life 21 hr
IM (Decanoate): Peak 4-11 days, half-life 3 wk
Metabolized by liver, excreted in urine, bile, crosses placenta, enters breast milk
Interactions/incompatibilities:
- Oversedation: other CNS depressants, alcohol, barbiturate anesthetics
- Toxicity: epinephrine
- Toxicity: with lithium, neurotoxicity and brain damage possible
- Decreased effects of: lithium, levodopa
- Increased effects of both drugs: β-adrenergic blockers, alcohol
- Increased anticholinergic effects: anticholinergics

NURSING CONSIDERATIONS
Assess:
- Swallowing of PO medication; check for hoarding or giving of medication to other patients
- I&O ratio; palpate bladder if low urinary output occurs
- Bilirubin, CBC, liver function studies monthly
- Urinalysis is recommended before and during prolonged therapy
Administer:
- Antiparkinsonian agent, to be used if extrapyramidal symptoms occur
- IM injection into large muscle mass, use No. 21G needle; give no more than 3 ml/injection site
- Oral liquid use calibrated dropper, do not mix in coffee or tea
- PO with food or milk
Perform/provide:
- Decreased noise input by dimming lights, avoiding loud noises
- Supervised ambulation until stabilized on medication; do not involve in strenuous exercise program because fainting is possible; patient should not stand still for long periods of time
- Increased fluids to prevent constipation

• Sips of water, candy, gum for dry mouth
• Storage in tight, light-resistant container

Evaluate:
• Therapeutic response: decrease in emotional excitement, hallucinations, delusions, paranoia, reorganization of patterns of thought, speech
• For depression in bipolar patients; rapid mood swings may occur with this drug
• Affect, orientation, LOC, reflexes, gait, coordination, sleep pattern disturbances
• B/P standing and lying; take pulse and respirations q4h during initial treatment; establish baseline before starting treatment; report drops of 30 mm Hg
• Dizziness, faintness, palpitations, tachycardia on rising
• Extrapyramidal symptoms including akathisia (inability to sit still, no pattern to movements), tardive dyskinesia (bizarre movements of jaw, mouth, tongue, extremities), pseudoparkinsonism (rigidity, tremors, pill rolling, shuffling gait)
• Skin turgor daily
• For neuroleptic malignant syndrome: hyperthermia, muscle rigidity, altered mental status, increased CPK
• Constipation, urinary retention daily; if these occur, increase bulk, water in diet

Teach patient/family:
• That orthostatic hypotension occurs often, and to rise from sitting or lying position gradually
• To remain lying down after IM injection for at least 30 min
• To avoid hot tubs, hot showers, or tub baths since hypotension may occur

• To avoid abrupt withdrawal of this drug or extrapyramidal symptoms may result; drug should be withdrawn slowly
• To avoid OTC preparations (cough, hayfever, cold) unless approved by physician since serious drug interactions may occur; avoid use with alcohol or CNS depressants, increased drowsiness may occur
• To use a sunscreen during sun exposure to prevent burns
• Regarding compliance with drug regimen
• About EPS and necessity for meticulous oral hygiene since oral candidiasis may occur
• To report impaired vision, jaundice, tremors, muscle twitching
• In hot weather, heat stroke may occur; take extra precautions to stay cool

Lab test interferences:
Increase: Liver function tests, cardiac enzymes, cholesterol, blood glucose, prolactin, bilirubin, PBI, cholinesterase, ^{131}I
Decrease: Hormones (blood, urine)
False positive: Pregnancy tests, PKU
False negative: Urinary steroids
Treatment of overdose: Induce emesis, activated charcoal lavage, if orally injested, provide an airway; *do not induce vomiting*

haloprogin (topical)
(ha-loe-proe'jin)
Halotex
Func. class.: Local antiinfective, antifungal
Chem. class.: Iodinated phenolic ester

Action: Interferes with fungal cell membrane permeability

italics = common side effects   ***bold italic*** = life threatening reactions

Uses: Tinea pedis, tinea cruris, tinea corporis, tinea manus, tinea versicolor

Dosage and routes:
• *Adult and child:* TOP apply to affected area bid × 14-21 days

Available forms include: Cream, sol 1%

Side effects/adverse reactions:
INTEG: Rash, urticaria, stinging, burning, vesiculation, maceration, pruritus, erythema, scaling, folliculitis sensitization

Contraindications: Hypersensitivity

Precautions: Pregnancy (B), lactation, children

NURSING CONSIDERATIONS
Administer:
• Enough medication to completely cover lesions
• After cleansing with soap, water before each application, dry well

Perform/provide:
• Storage at room temperature in dry place

Evaluate:
• Allergic reaction: burning, stinging, swelling, redness, vesiculation, scaling
• Therapeutic response: decrease in size, number of lesions

Teach patient/family:
• To apply with glove to prevent further infection
• To avoid use of OTC creams, ointments, lotions unless directed by physician
• To use medical asepsis (hand washing) before, after each application
• To avoid contact with eyes
• To continue even though condition improves
• Discontinue use and notify physician if condition worsens

---

heparin calcium/heparin sodium
(hep'a-rin)
Calciparine,* Calcilean,* Liquaemin/Hepalean,* Hep Lock
Func. class.: Anticoagulant

Action: Prevents conversion of fibrinogen to fibrin, and prothrombin to thrombin by enhancing inhibitory effects of antithrombin III

Uses: Deep vein thrombosis, pulmonary emboli, myocardial infarction, open heart surgery, disseminated intravascular clotting syndrome, atrial fibrillation with embolization, as an anticoagulant in transfusion and dialysis procedures

Dosage and routes:
Deep vein thrombosis/MI
• *Adult:* IV PUSH 5000-7000 U q4h then titrated to PTT or ACT level, IV BOL 5000-7500 U, then IV INF; IV INF After bolus dose, then 1000 U/hr titrated to PTT or ACT level
• *Child:* IV INF 50 U/kg, maintenance 100 U/kg q4h or 20,000 U/m² qd

Pulmonary embolism
• *Adult:* IV PUSH 7500-10,000 q4h then titrated to PTT or ACT level; IV BOL 7500-10,000, then IV INF; IV INF After bolus dose, then 1000 U/hr titrated to PTT or ACT level
• *Child:* IV INF 50 U/kg, maintenance 100 U/kg q4h or 20,000 U/m² qd

Open heart surgery
• *Adult:* IV INF 150-300 U/kg

Available forms include: (Heparin sodium) inj 1000, 2500, 5000, 7500, 10,000, 15,000, 20,000, 40,000 U/ml; (Heparin calcium) inj 5000, 12,500, 20,000 U/dose

---

*Available in Canada only

Side effects/adverse reactions:
GI: Diarrhea, nausea, vomiting, anorexia, stomatitis, abdominal cramps, ***hepatitis***
*GU: **Hematuria***
INTEG: Rash, dermatitis, urticaria, alopecia, pruritus
CNS: Fever, chills
*HEMA: **Hemorrhage, thrombocytopenia***
Contraindications: Hypersensitivity, hemophilia, leukemia with bleeding, peptic ulcer disease, thrombocytopenic purpura, hepatic disease (severe), renal disease (severe), blood dyscrasias, pregnancy, severe hypertension, subacute bacterial endocarditis, acute nephritis
Precautions: Alcoholism, elderly, pregnancy (C)
Pharmacokinetics:
IV: Peak 5 min, duration 2-6 hr
SC: Onset 20-60 min, duration 8-12 hr
Half-life 1½ hr, excreted in urine, 95% bound to plasma proteins
Interactions/incompatibilities:
• Decreased action of: corticosteroids
• Increased action of: diazepam
• Decreased action of heparin: digitalis, tetracyclines, antihistamines
• Increased action of heparin: oral anticoagulants, salicylates, dextran, steroids, non-steroidal antiinflammatories

NURSING CONSIDERATIONS
Assess:
• Blood studies (Hct, platelets, occult blood in stools) q3 mo
• Partial prothrombin time, which should be 1½-2 × control, PTT; often done qd, APTT, ACT
• B/P, watch for increasing signs of hypertension
Administer:
• IV undiluted or diluted in compatible sol and given by direct, in-

termittent, or continuous infusion; give 1000 U or less over 1 min; then 5000 U or less over 1 min; infusion may run from 4-24 hr
• At same time each day to maintain steady blood levels
• Do not massage area or aspirate when giving SC injection, give in abdomen between pelvic bone, rotate sites; do not pull back on plunger, leave in for 10 sec
• Changing needles is not recommended
• Avoiding all IM injections that may cause bleeding
Perform/provide:
• Storage in tight container
Evaluate:
• Therapeutic response: decrease of deep vein thrombosis
• Bleeding gums, petecchiae, ecchymosis, black tarry stools, hematuria
• Fever, skin rash, urticaria
• Needed dosage change q 1-2 wk
Teach patient/family:
• To avoid OTC preparations that may cause serious drug interactions unless directed by physician
• Drug may be held during active bleeding (menstruation), depending on condition
• To use soft-bristle toothbrush to avoid bleeding gums
• To carry a Medic-Alert ID identifying drug taken
• To report any signs of bleeding: gums, under skin, urine, stools
Lab test interferences:
Increase: T_3 uptake
Decrease: Uric acid
Treatment of overdose:
Protamine SO_4 1:1 solution

---

hepatitis B vaccine
Heptavax-B
Func. class.: Vaccine

Action: Provides active immunity to hepatitis B

---

italics = common side effects   ***bold italic*** = life threatening reactions

Uses: Prevention of hepatitis B virus

Dosage and routes:
• *Adult and child >10 yr:* IM 1 ml, then 1 ml after 1 mo, then 1 ml 6 mo after initial dose
• *Child 3 mo-10 yr:* IM 0.5 ml, then 0.5 ml after 1 mo, then 0.5 ml 6 mo after initial dose
• *Patients with decreased immunity:* IM 2 ml, then 2 ml after 1 mo, then 2 ml 6 mo after initial dose
Available forms include: Inj IM 10 mg/0.5 ml, 20 μg/ml

Side effects/adverse reactions:
INTEG: Soreness at injection site, urticaria, erythema, swelling
SYST: Induration
CNS: Headache, dizziness, fever
GI: Nausea, vomiting

Contraindications: Hypersensitivity

Precautions: Pregnancy, elderly, lactation, children; active infection, compromised cardiac or pulmonary status

NURSING CONSIDERATIONS
Assess:
• For skin reactions: rash, induration, urticaria

Administer:
• After rotating vial, do not shake
• Only with epinephrine 1:1000 on unit to treat laryngospasm
• In deltoid for better protection

Evaluate:
• For history of allergies, skin conditions (eczema, psoriasis, dermatitis), reactions to vaccinations
• For anaphylaxis: inability to breathe, bronchospasm

---

hetastarch

(het'a-starch)
Hespan, HES, Volex
Func. class.: Plasma expander
Chem. class.: Synthetic polymer

Action: Similar to human albumin, which expands plasma volume by colloidal osmotic pressure

Uses: Plasma volume expander, leukapheresis

Dosage and routes:
• *Adult:* IV INF 500-1000 ml, total dose not to exceed 1500 ml/day, not to exceed 20 ml/kg/hr (hemorrhagic shock)

Leukapheresis
• *Adult:* IV INF 250-700 ml infused in 1:8 ratio with whole blood, may be repeated 2/wk up to 10 treatments
Available forms include: 6% hetastarch/0.9% NaCl

Side effects/adverse reactions:
HEMA: Decreased hematocrit, platelet function, increased bleeding/coagulation times, increased sed rate
INTEG: Rash, urticaria, pruritus, angioedema, chills, fever, flushing
RESP: Wheezing, dyspnea, *bronchospasm, pulmonary edema*
GI: Nausea, vomiting
SYST: **Anaphylaxis**
CNS: Headache

Contraindications: Hypersensitivity, severe bleeding disorders, renal failure, CHF (severe)

Precautions: Pregnancy (C), liver disease

Pharmacokinetics:
IV: Expands blood volume 1-2 × amount infused, excreted in urine

NURSING CONSIDERATIONS
Assess:
• VS q5 min × 30 min
• CVP during infusion (5-10 cm H_2O normal range)
• Urine output q1h, watch for increase in urinary output, which is common; if output does not increase, infusion should be decreased or discontinued
• I&O ratio and specific gravity,

urine osmolarity; if specific gravity is very low, renal clearance is low, drug should be discontinued
Administer:
• IV, run at 20 ml/kg/hr; reduced rate in septic shock, burns
Perform/provide:
• Storage at room temperature; discard unused portions, do not freeze, do not use if turbid, deep brown, or precipitate forms
Evaluate:
• Allergy: rash, urticaria, pruritus, wheezing, dyspnea, bronchospasm, drug should be discontinued immediately
• For circulatory overload: increased pulse, respirations, SOB, wheezing, chest tightness, chest pain
• For dehydration after infusion: decreased output, increased temperature, poor skin turgor, increased specific gravity, dry skin
Lab test interferences:
False increase: Blood glucose, bilirubin

---

hexamethylmelamine
Hexalen
Func. class.: Antineoplastic, alkylating agent

Action: Responsible for inhibition of cell DNA and RNA synthesis, cell death; rapidly degraded; cell-cycle nonspecific
Uses: Resistant or recurrent ovarian cancer; may be used alone or in combination
Dosage and routes:
Adult: PO 260 mg/m²; average dose 400 q d × 14 days, then rest for 14 days; cycle should continue until patient no longer responds
Available forms include: Caps 50 mg

Side effects/adverse reactions:
EENT: Tinnitus, hearing loss
HEMA: **Thrombocytopenia, leukopenia**
GI: Nausea, vomiting, diarrhea, stomatitis, weight loss, colitis, hepatotoxicity, anorexia
CNS: Headache, dizziness, drowsiness, paresthesia, peripheral neuropathy, coma, hyporeflexia, muscle weakness
INTEG: Alopecia, pruritus, herpes zoster
Contraindications: Lactation, pregnancy (first trimester) (D), myelosuppression, acute herpes zoster, hypersensitivity
Precautions: Radiation therapy, leukopenia, thrombocytopenia
Pharmacokinetics: Metabolized in liver, excreted in urine
Interactions/incompatibilities:
• Increased toxicity: antineoplastics, radiation
• Reduced efficiency: influenza vaccine, pneumococcal vaccine
NURSING CONSIDERATIONS
Assess:
• CBC, differential, platelet count weekly; withhold drug if WBC is <4000 or platelet count is 75,000; notify physician of these results
• Renal function studies: BUN, serum uric acid, urine CrCl before, during therapy
• I&O ratio: report fall in urine output to <30 ml/hr
• Monitor temperature q4h; fever may indicate beginning infection, no rectal temperatures
• Liver function tests before, during therapy: (bilirubin, AST, ALT, LDH) as needed or monthly
Administer:
• As divided daily doses 1-2 hr pc and hs
• Antiemetic 30-60 min before giv-

ing drug to prevent vomiting and prn
• Topical or systemic analgesics for pain
• Local or systemic drugs for infection

Perform/provide:
• Storage at room temperature in dry form
• Strict medical asepsis, protective isolation if WBC levels are low
• Special skin care
• Increase fluid intake to 2-3 L/day to prevent urate deposits, calculi information
• Diet low in purines: organ meats (kidney, liver), dried beans, peas to maintain alkaline urine
• Rinsing of mouth tid-qid with water, club soda; brushing of teeth bid-tid with soft brush or cotton-tipped applicators for stomatitis; use unwaxed dental floss

Evaluate:
• Bleeding: hematuria, guaiac, bruising, or petechiae, mucosa or orifices q8h
• Food preferences: list likes, dislikes
• Yellowing of skin, sclera, dark urine, clay-colored stools, itchy skin, abdominal pain, fever, diarrhea
• Effects of alopecia on body image; discuss feelings about body changes
• Inflammation of mucosa, breaks in skin
• Buccal cavity q8h for dryness, sores, or ulceration, white patches, oral pain, bleeding, dysphagia
• Symptoms indicating severe allergic reaction: rash, pruritus, urticaria, purpuric skin lesions, itching, flushing

Teach patient/family:
• Of protective isolation precautions

• That sterility, amenorrhea can occur; reversible after discontinuing treatment
• That hair may be lost during treatment; a wig or hairpiece may make patient feel better; new hair may be different in color, texture
• To avoid foods with citric acid, hot or rough texture
• To report any bleeding, white spots, or ulcerations in mouth to physician: tell patient to examine mouth qd
• To report signs of infection: increased temperature, sore throat, flu symptoms
• To report signs of anemia: fatigue, headache, faintness, shortness of breath, irritability

hexocyclium methylsulfate

(hex-oh-sye'klee-um)
Tral

Func. class.: Gastrointestinal anticholinergic
Chem. class.: Synthetic quaternary ammonium compound

Action: Inhibits muscarinic actions of acetylcholine at postganglionic parasympathetic neuroeffector sites
Uses: Treatment of peptic ulcer disease in combination with other drugs; other GI disorders

Dosage and routes:
• *Adult:* PO 25 mg qid ac, hs
Available forms include: Tabs 25 mg

Side effects/adverse reactions:
CNS: Confusion, stimulation in elderly, headache, insomnia, dizziness, drowsiness, anxiety, weakness, hallucination
*GI: Dry mouth, constipation, **paralytic ileus,** heartburn, nausea,*

vomiting, dysphagia, absence of taste

GU: Hesitancy, retention, impotence

CV: Palpitations, tachycardia

EENT: Blurred vision, photophobia, mydriasis, cycloplegia, increased ocular tension

INTEG: Urticaria, rash, pruritus, anhidrosis, fever, allergic reactions

Contraindications: Hypersensitivity to anticholinergics, narrow-angle glaucoma, GI obstruction, myasthenia gravis, paralytic ileus, GI atony, toxic megacolon

Precautions: Hyperthyroidism, coronary artery disease, dysrhythmias, CHF, ulcerative colitis, hypertension, hiatal hernia, hepatic disease, renal disease, pregnancy (C), urinary retention, prostatic hypertrophy, elderly

Pharmacokinetics:

PO: Onset 1 hr, duration 3-4 hr; metabolized by liver, excreted in urine

Interactions/incompatibilities:

• Increased anticholinergic effect: amantadine, tricyclic antidepressants, MAOIs

• Decreased effect of: phenothiazines, levodopa, ketoconazole

NURSING CONSIDERATIONS

Assess:

• VS, cardiac status: checking for dysrhythmias, increased rate, palpitations

• I&O ratio; check for urinary retention or hesitancy

Administer:

• ½-1 hr ac for better absorption

• Decreased dose to elderly patients; their metabolism may be slowed

• Gum, hard candy, frequent rinsing of mouth for dryness of oral cavity

Perform/provide:

• Storage in tight container protected from light

• Increased fluids, bulk, exercise to patient's lifestyle to decrease constipation

Evaluate:

• Therapeutic response: absence of epigastric pain, bleeding, nausea, vomiting

• GI complaints: pain, bleeding (frank or occult), nausea, vomiting, anorexia

Teach patient/family:

• Avoid driving or other hazardous activities until stabilized on medication

• Avoid alcohol or other CNS depressants; will enhance sedating properties of drug

• To avoid hot environments, stroke may occur, drug suppresses perspiration

• Use sunglasses when outside to prevent photophobia, may cause blurred vision

• To drink plenty of fluids

• To report dysphagia

---

homatropine hydrobromide (optic)

(hoe'ma-troe-peen)

Homatrocel, Isopto Homatropine, Murrocoll Homatropine

Func. class.: Mydriatic

Chem. class.: Synthetic alkaloid

Action: Blocks response of iris sphincter muscle, muscle of accommodation of ciliary body to cholinergic simulation, resulting in dilation, paralysis of accommodation

Uses: Uveitis, iritis

Dosage and routes:

• *Adult and child:* INSTILL 1-2

gtts repeat in 5-10 min for refraction or q3-4h for uveitis

Available forms include: Sol 2%, 5%

Side effects/adverse reactions:

CV: Tachycardia

CNS: Confusion, somnolence, flushing, fever

EENT: Blurred vision, photophobia, increased intraocular pressure, irritation, edema

Contraindications: Hypersensitivity, children <6 yr, narrow-angle glaucoma, increased intraocular pressure, infants

Precautions: Children, elderly, hypertension, hyperthyroidism, diabetes, pregnancy (C)

Pharmacokinetics:

INSTILL: Peak ½-1 hr, duration 1-3 days

NURSING CONSIDERATIONS
Evaluate:

• Therapeutic response: decrease in inflammation or cycloplegic refraction

• Eye pain, discontinue use

Teach patient/family:

• To report change in vision, blurring or loss of sight, trouble breathing, sweating, flushing

• Method of instillation: pressure on lacrimal sac for 1 min, do not touch dropper to eye

• That blurred vision will decrease with repeated use of drug

• Not to engage in hazardous activities until able to see

• Wait 5 min to use other drops

• Do not blink more than usual

---

hyaluronidase

(hye-l-yoor-on'i-dase)

Wydase

Func. class.: Enzyme

Action: Hydrolyzes hyaluronic

within areas filled with exudates

Uses: Hypodermoclysis, subcutaneous urography, adjunct to dispersion of other drugs

Dosage and routes:

Adjunct

• *Adult and child:* INJ 150 U with other drug

Urography

• *Adult and child:* SC 75 U over scapula, then contrast medium is injected at same site

Hypodermoclysis

• *Adult and child >3 yr:* SC 150 U/L of clysis sol for 1000 ml of clysis sol

Available forms include: Inj powder 150, 1500 U; inj sol 150 U/ml

Side effects/adverse reactions:

INTEG: Rash, urticaria, itching

OTHER: Overhydration (hyperdermoclysis)

Contraindications: Hypersensitivity to bovine products, CHF, hypoproteinemia

Precautions: Pregnancy (C)

NURSING CONSIDERATIONS
Assess:

• Site before administration (hypodermoclysis)

Administer:

• After test dose: 0.02 ml of 150 u/ml solution is injected if wheal develops, itching test is positive

• Right after mixing since solution is unstable

• To child <3 yr, not exceeding 200 ml, in neonates not exceeding 2 ml/min

Evaluate:

• Therapeutic response: absence of swelling, pain after hypodermoclysis

• For overhydration in child <3 yr

---

hydralazine HCl

(hye'dral'a-zeen)
Apresoline, Hydralyn, Rolazine
Func. class.: Antihypertensive, direct-acting peripheral vasodilator
Chem. class.: Phthalazine

Action: Vasodilates arteriolar smooth muscle by direct relaxation; reduction in blood pressure with reflex increases in cardiac function
Uses: Essential hypertension; *parenteral:* severe essential hypertension

Dosage and routes:
• *Adult:* PO 10 mg qid 2-4 days, then 25 mg for rest of 1st wk, then 50 mg qid individualized to desired response, not to exceed 300 mg; IV/IM BOL 20-40 mg q4-6h, administer PO as soon as possible; IM 20-40 mg q4-6h
• *Child:* PO 0.75 mg/kg qd 0.75-3 mg/kg/day in 4 divided doses; max 7.5 mg/kg/24 hr; IV BOL 0.1-0.2 mg/kg q4-6h; IM 0.1-0.2 mg/kg q4-6h
Available forms include: Inj IV, IM 20 mg/ml; tabs 10, 25, 50, 100 mg
Side effects/adverse reactions:
MISC: Nasal congestion, muscle cramps, *lupus-like symptoms*
CV: Palpitations, *reflex tachycardia, angina,* **shock,** edema, rebound hypertension
CNS: Headache, tremors, dizziness, anxiety, peripheral neuritis, depression
GI: Nausea, vomiting, anorexia, diarrhea, constipation
INTEG: Rash, pruritus
HEMA: **Leukopenia, agranulocytosis,** anemia
GU: Impotence, urinary retention, sodium, water retention
Contraindications: Hypersensitiv-

ity to hydralazines, coronary artery disease, mitral valvular rheumatic heart disease, rheumatic heart disease
Precautions: Pregnancy (C), CVA, advanced renal disease
Pharmacokinetics:
PO: Onset 20-30 min, peak 1 hr, duration 2-4 hr
IM: Onset 5-10 min, peak 1 hr, duration 2-4 hr
IV: Onset 5-20 min, peak 10-80 min, duration 2-6 hr
Half-life 2-8 hr, metabolized by liver, less than 10% present in urine
Interactions/incompatibilities:
• Increased tachycardia, angina: sympathomimetics (epinephrine, norepinephrine)
• Increased effects of: β-blockers
• Use MAOIs with caution in patients receiving hydralazine
• Do not mix with any drug in syringe or solution
NURSING CONSIDERATIONS
Assess:
• B/P q5 min × 2 hr, then q1h × 2 hr, then q4h
• Pulse, jugular venous distention q4h
• Electrolytes, blood studies: potassium, sodium, chloride, CO_2, CBC, serum glucose
• Weight daily, I&O
• LE prep, ANA titer before starting therapy
Administer:
• IV undiluted; give through Y-tube or 3-way stopcock each 10 mg or less/min
• To patient in recumbent position, keep in that position for 1 hr after administration
Evaluate:
• Edema in feet, legs daily
• Skin turgor, dryness of mucous membranes for hydration status
• Rales, dyspnea, orthopnea

---

italics = common side effects   ***bold italic*** = life threatening reactions

- IV site for extravasation, rate
- Fever, joint pain, tachycardia, palpitations, headache, nausea
- Mental status: affect, mood, behavior, anxiety; check for personality changes

Teach patient/family:
- To take with food to increase bioavailability
- To avoid OTC preparations unless directed by physician
- To notify physician if chest pain, severe fatigue, fever, muscle or joint pain occurs

Treatment of overdose: Administer vasopressors, volume expanders for shock; if PO lavage or give activated charcoal, digitalization

---

hydrochlorothiazide

(hye-droe-klor-oh-thye′a-zide)
Chlorzide, Diaqua, Diu-Scrip, Diuchlor H,* Esidrix, Hydrodiuril, Hydromal, Hydroz-50, Hydrozide,* Hyperetic, Neo-Codema,* Novohydrazide,* Oretic, Urozide*
Func. class.: Thiazide diuretic
Chem. class.: Sulfonamide derivative

Action: Acts on distal tubule by increasing excretion of water, sodium, chloride, potassium
Uses: Edema, hypertension, diuresis, CHF

Dosage and routes:
- *Adult:* PO 25-100 mg/day
- *Child >6 mo:* PO 2.2 mg/kg/day in divided doses
- *Child <6 mo:* PO up to 3.3 mg/kg/day in divided doses
Available forms include: Tabs 25, 50, 100 mg; sol 50 mg/5 ml, 100 mg/ml

Side effects/adverse reactions:
GU: Frequency, polyuria, ***uremia, glucosuria***

CNS: Drowsiness, paresthesia, anxiety, depression, headache, *dizziness, fatigue, weakness*
GI: Nausea, vomiting, anorexia, constipation, diarrhea, cramps, pancreatitis, GI irritation, ***hepatitis***
EENT: Blurred vision
INTEG: Rash, urticaria, purpura, photosensitivity, fever
META: Hyperglycemia, hyperuricemia, increased creatinine, BUN
*HEMA: **Aplastic anemia, hemolytic anemia, leukopenia, agranulocytosis, thrombocytopenia, neutropenia***
CV: Irregular pulse, orthostatic hypotension, palpitations, volume depletion
ELECT: Hypokalemia, hypercalcemia, hyponatremia, hypochloremia, hypomagnesemia

Contraindications: Hypersensitivity to thiazides or sulfonamides, anuria, renal decompensation, hypomagnesium
Precautions: Hypokalemia, renal disease, pregnancy (D), hepatic disease, gout, COPD, lupus erythematosus, diabetes mellitus
Pharmacokinetics:
PO: Onset 2 hr, peak 4 hr, duration 6-12 hr; excreted unchanged by kidneys, crosses placenta, enters breast milk
Interactions/incompatibilities:
- Increased toxicity of: lithium, nondepolarizing skeletal muscle relaxants, digitalis
- Decreased effects of: antidiabetics
- Decreased absorption of thiazides: cholestyramine, colestipol
- Decreased hypotensive response: indomethacin
- Hyperglycemia, hyperuricemia, hypotension: diazoxide

NURSING CONSIDERATIONS
Assess:
- Weight, I&O daily to determine

---

fluid loss; effect of drug may be decreased if used qd
• Rate, depth, rhythm of respiration, effect of exertion
• B/P lying, standing; postural hypotension may occur
• Electrolytes: potassium, magnesium, sodium chloride; include BUN, blood sugar, CBC, serum creatinine, blood pH, ABGs, uric acid, calcium
• Glucose in urine if patient is diabetic

Administer:
• In AM to avoid interference with sleep if using drug as a diuretic
• Potassium replacement if potassium is less than 3.0
• With food, if nausea occurs, absorption may be decreased slightly

Evaluate:
• Improvement in edema of feet, legs, sacral area daily if medication is being used in CHF
• Improvement in CVP q8h
• Signs of metabolic alkalosis: drowsiness, restlessness
• Signs of hypokalemia: postural hypotension, malaise, fatigue, tachycardia, leg cramps, weakness, dehydration
• Rashes, temperature elevation qd
• Confusion, especially in elderly; take safety precautions if needed

Teach patient/family:
• To increase fluid intake 2-3 L/day unless contraindicated; to rise slowly from lying or sitting position
• To notify physician of muscle weakness, cramps, nausea, dizziness
• Drug may be taken with food or milk
• That blood sugar may be increased in diabetics
• Take early in day to avoid nocturia

Lab test interferences:
Increase: BSP retention, amylase, parathyroid test
Decrease: PBI, PSP
Treatment of overdose: Lavage if taken orally, monitor electrolytes, administer dextrose in saline, monitor hydration, CV, renal status

---

hydrocodone bitartrate

(hye-droe-koe′done)
Dihydrocodeinone bitartrate, Hycodan,* Robidone*

Func. class.: Narcotic analgesic
Chem. class.: Opiate

Controlled Substance III
Action: Acts directly on cough center in medulla to suppress cough
Uses: Hyperactive and nonproductive cough, mild pain

Dosages and routes:
• *Adults:* PO 5 mg q4h prn
• *Child:* 2-12 mg PO, 1.25-5 mg q4h prn
Available forms include: Caps 5 mg, susp 5 mg/ml, tabs 5 mg

Side effects/adverse reactions:
CNS: Drowsiness, dizziness, lightheadedness, confusion, headache, sedation, euphoria, dysphoria, weakness, hallucinations, disorientation, *convulsions*
GI: Nausea, vomiting, anorexia, constipation, cramps, dry mouth
GU: Increased urinary output, dysuria, urinary retention
INTEG: Rash, urticaria, flushing, pruritus
EENT: Tinnitus, blurred vision, miosis, diplopia
CV: Palpitations, tachycardia, bradycardia, change in B/P, *circulatory depression,* syncope
RESP: Respiratory depression
Contraindications: Hypersensitivity, addiction (narcotic)

---

italics = common side effects   ***bold italic*** = life threatening reactions

Precautions: Addictive personality, pregnancy (C), lactation, increased intracranial pressure, MI (acute), severe heart disease, respiratory depression, hepatic disease, renal disease, child <18 yr
Pharmacokinetics: Onset 10-20 min, duration 3-6 hr; half-life 3-4 hr, metabolized in the liver, excreted in urine, crosses placenta
Interactions/incompatibilities:
• Increased CNS depression: alcohol, narcotics, sedative/hypnotics, phenothiazines, skeletal muscle relaxants, general anesthetics, tricyclic antidepressants
NURSING CONSIDERATIONS
Assess:
• I&O ratio; check for decreasing output; may indicate urinary retention
Administer:
• With antiemetic after meals if nausea or vomiting occur
Perform/provide:
• Storage in light-resistant area at room temperature
• Assistance with ambulation
• Safety measures: siderails, night light, call bell within easy reach
Evaluate:
• Therapeutic response: decrease in pain or cough
• CNS changes: dizziness, drowsiness, hallucinations, euphoria, LOC, pupil reaction
• Allergic reactions: rash, urticaria
• Respiratory dysfunction: respiratory depression, character, rate, rhythm; notify physician if respirations are <10/min
• Need for pain medication, physical dependence
Teach patient/family:
• To report any symptoms of CNS changes, allergic reactions
• That physical dependency may

result when used for extended periods of time
• Withdrawal symptoms may occur: nausea, vomiting, cramps, fever, faintness, anorexia
Lab test interferences:
Increase: Amylase
Treatment of overdose: Narcan 0.2-0.8 IV, O_2, IV fluids, vasopressors

---

hydrocortisone/hydrocortisone acetate

(hye-droe-kor'ti-sone)
Cortamed,* Otall
Func. class.: Otic
Chem. class.: Synthetic steroid

Action: Antiinflammatory, antipruritic
Uses: Ear canal inflammation
Dosage and routes:
• *Adult and child:* INSTILL 3-4 gtts bid-qid
Available forms include: Otic sol 0.25%, 0.5%, 1%
Side effects/adverse reactions:
EENT: Itching, irritation in ear
INTEG: Rash, urticaria
Contraindications: Hypersensitivity, perforated eardrum
Precautions: Pregnancy (C)
NURSING CONSIDERATIONS
Administer:
• After removing impacted cerumen by irrigation
• After cleaning stopper with alcohol
• After restraining child if necessary
• Warming solution to body temperature
Evaluate:
• Therapeutic response: decreased ear pain, inflammation
• For redness, swelling, fever, pain in ear, which indicates infection

Teach patient/family:
• Method of instillation using aseptic technique, including not touching dropper to ear
• That dizziness may occur after instillation

---

hydrocortisone/hydrocortisone acetate/hydrocortisone valerate

(hye-droe-kor'ti-sone)

Acticort, Aeroseb-HC, Carmol HC, Cetacort, Cort-Dome, Delacort, Dermicort, Dermolate, Proctocort, Cortaid, Cortef, Cortifoam, Epifoam, My-Cort, Proctofoam-HC, Westcort Cream

Func. class.: Topical corticosteroid
Chem. class.: Natural nonfluorinated, group IV potency (Valerate), group VI potency (acetate and plain)

Action: Possesses antipruritic, antiinflammatory actions
Uses: Psoriasis, eczema, contact dermatitis, pruritus
Dosage and routes:
• *Adult and child >2 yr:* Apply to affected area qd-qid
Available forms include: Hydrocortisone—oint 0.5%, 1%, 2.5%; cream 0.25%, 0.5%, 1%, 2.5%; lotion 0.25%, 0.5%, 1%, 2%, 2.5%; gel 1%; sol 1%; aerosol/pump spray 0.5%; *acetate*—oint 0.5%, 1%, 2.5%; cream 0.5%; lotion 0.05%; aerosol 1%; *valerate*—oint 0.2%; cream 0.2% (many others)
Side effects/adverse reactions:
INTEG: Burning, dryness, itching, irritation, acne, folliculitis, hypertrichosis, perioral dermatitis, hypopigmentation, atrophy, striae, miliaria, allergic contact dermatitis, secondary infection

Contraindications: Hypersensitivity to corticosteroids, fungal infections
Precautions: Pregnancy (C), lactation, viral infections, bacterial infections
NURSING CONSIDERATIONS
Assess:
• Temperature; if fever develops, drug should be discontinued
Administer:
• Only to affected areas; do not get in eyes
• Medication, then cover with occlusive dressing (only if prescribed), seal to intact skin, change q12h, systemic absorption may occur, use gloves
• Only to dermatoses; do not use on weeping, denuded, or infected area
• Apply aerosol at distance 15 cm for 1-2 sec
Perform/provide:
• Cleansing before application of drug
• Treatment for a few days after area has cleared
• Storage at room temperature
Evaluate:
• Therapeutic response: absence of severe itching, patches on skin, flaking
• For systemic absorption: increased temperature, inflammation, irritation
Teach patient/family:
• To avoid sunlight on affected area; burns may occur
• Not to use other OTC products unless approved by physician

H

---

italics = common side effects   **bold italic** = life threatening reactions

hydrocortisone/hydrocortisone acetate/hydrocortisone sodium phosphate/hydrocortisone sodium succinate

(hye-dro-kor′ti-sone)

Cortef, Hydrocortone/ Cortef Acetate, Hydrocortone Acetate/Hydrocortone Phosphate/A-Hydrocort, Solu-Cortef, Cortenema

Func. class.: Corticosteroid
Chem. class.: Glucocorticoid, short-acting

Action: Decreases inflammation by suppression of migration of polymorphonuclear leukocytes, fibroblasts, reversal of increased capillary permeability and lysosomal stabilization

Uses: Severe inflammation, shock, adrenal insufficiency, ulcerative colitis, collagen disorders

Dosage and routes:
Adrenal insufficiency/inflammation
• *Adult:* PO 5-30 mg bid-qid; IM/IV 100-250 mg (succinate), then 50-100 mg IM as needed; IM/IV 15-240 mg q12h (phosphate)
Shock
• *Adult:* 500 mg-2 g q2-6h, (succinate)
• *Child:* IM/IV 0.16-1 mg/kg bid-tid (succinate)
Colitis
• *Adult:* ENEMA 100 mg nightly for 21 days
Available forms include: Retention enema 100 mg/60 ml; tabs 5, 10, 20 mg; inj 25, 50 mg/ml; inj 50 mg/ml; phosphate inj 100, 250, 500, 1000 mg/vial; succinate inj 25, 50 mg/ml

Side effects/adverse reactions:
INTEG: Acne, poor wound healing, ecchymosis, petechiae

CNS: Depression, flushing, sweating, headache, mood changes
*CV: Hypertension, **circulatory collapse, thrombophlebitis, embolism,*** tachycardia, edema
*HEMA: **Thrombocytopenia***
MS: Fractures, osteoporosis, weakness
GI: Diarrhea, nausea, abdominal distention, *GI hemorrhage,* increased appetite, *pancreatitis*
EENT: Fungal infections, increased intraocular pressure, blurred vision
Contraindications: Psychosis, hypersensitivity, idiopathic thrombocytopenia, acute glomerulonephritis, amebiasis, fungal infections, nonasthmatic bronchial disease, child <2 yr, AIDS, TB
Precautions: Pregnancy (C), diabetes mellitus, glaucoma, osteoporosis, seizure disorders, ulcerative colitis, CHF, myasthenia gravis, renal disease, esophagitis, peptic ulcer
Pharmacokinetics:
PO: Onset 1-2 hr, peak 1 hr, duration 1-1½ days
IM/IV: Onset 20 min, peak 4-8 hr, duration 1-1½ days
REC: Onset 3-5 days
Metabolized by liver, excreted in urine (17-OHCS, 17-KS), crosses placenta
Interactions/incompatibilities:
• Decreased action of hydrocortisone: cholestyramine, colestipol, barbiturates, rifampin, ephedrine, phenytoin, theophylline
• Decreased effects of: anticoagulants, anticonvulsants, antidiabetics, ambenonium, neostigmine, isoniazid, toxoids, vaccines
• Increased side effects: alcohol, salicylates, indomethacin, amphotericin B, digitalis preparations
• Increased action of hydrocorti-

sone: salicylates, estrogens, indomethacin

NURSING CONSIDERATIONS
Assess:
• Potassium, blood sugar, urine glucose while on long-term therapy; hypokalemia and hyperglycemia
• Weight daily, notify physician of weekly gain >5 lb
• B/P q4h, pulse, notify physician if chest pain occurs
• I&O ratio, be alert for decreasing urinary output and increasing edema
• Plasma cortisol levels during long-term therapy (normal level: 138-635 nmol/L SI units when drawn at 8 AM)

Administer:
• IV undiluted or added to dextrose or saline inj and given by infusion; give 25 mg or less/min
• After shaking suspension (parenteral)
• Titrated dose, use lowest effective dose
• IM inj deeply in large mass, rotate sites, avoid deltoid, use 21G needle
• In one dose in AM to prevent adrenal suppression, avoid SC administration, damage may be done to tissue
• With food or milk to decrease GI symptoms

Perform/provide:
• Assistance with ambulation in patient with bone tissue disease to prevent fractures

Evaluate:
• Therapeutic response: ease of respirations, decreased inflammation
• Infection: increased temperature, WBC, even after withdrawal of medication; drug masks symptoms of infection
• Potassium depletion: paresthesias, fatigue, nausea, vomiting, depression, polyuria, dysrhythmias, weakness
• Edema, hypertension, cardiac symptoms
• Mental status: affect, mood, behavioral changes, aggression

Teach patient/family:
• That ID as steroid user should be carried
• To notify physician if therapeutic response decreases; dosage adjustment may be needed
• Not to discontinue this medication abruptly or adrenal crisis can result
• To avoid OTC products: salicylates, alcohol in cough products, cold preparations unless directed by physician
• Teach patient about cushingoid symptoms
• Symptoms of adrenal insufficiency: nausea, anorexia, fatigue, dizziness, dyspnea, weakness, joint pain

Lab test interferences:
Increase: Cholesterol, sodium, blood glucose, uric acid, calcium, urine glucose
Decrease: Calcium, potassium, T_4, T_3, thyroid ^{131}I uptake test, urine 17-OHCS, 17-KS, PBI
False negative: Skin allergy tests

---

hydrogen peroxide
(per-ox'ide)

Func. class.: Disinfectant
Chem. class.: Oxidizing drug

Action: Destroys bacteria (primarily anaerobic) by mechanical action
Uses: Douche, cleansing wounds, mouthwash for Vincent's stomatitis, removal of ear wax

Dosage and routes:
• *Adult and child:* SOL Use as needed

Available forms include: Top sol 1.5%, 3%

Side effects/adverse reactions:

CV: Oxygen emboli

INTEG: Irritation

EENT: Black hairy tongue, decalcification of tooth enamel

Contraindications: Hypersensitivity to this drug, closed wounds

Precautions: 3rd-degree burns, deep wounds

Pharmacokinetics:

TOP: Duration to end of bubbling

NURSING CONSIDERATIONS
Administer:

• To ear canal to facilate removal of cerumen

• As mouthwash for Vincent's stomatitis; do not use everyday as mouthwash

• After dilution with water or salt water solution

• Only when oxygen can flow in and out of wound; emboli may result

Evaluate:

• Area of body involved: irritation, rash, breaks, dryness, scales

---

hydromorphone HCl

(hye-droe-mor′fone)
Dilaudid

Func. class.: Narcotic analgesics
Chem. class.: Opiate, semisynthetic phenanthrene

Controlled Substance Schedule II

Action: Inhibits ascending pain pathways in CNS, increases pain threshold, alters pain perception

Uses: Moderate to severe pain

Dosage and routes:

• *Adult:* PO 1-6 mg q4-6h prn; IM/SC/IV 2-4 mg q4-6h; REC 3 mg hs prn

Available forms include: Inj IM, IV 1, 2, 3, 4 mg/ml; tabs 1, 2, 3, 4 mg; rec supp 3 mg

Side effects/adverse reactions:

CNS: Drowsiness, dizziness, confusion, headache, sedation, euphoria

GI: Nausea, vomiting, anorexia, constipation, cramps

GU: Increased urinary output, dysuria, urinary retention

INTEG: Rash, urticaria, bruising, flushing, diaphoresis, pruritus

EENT: Tinnitus, blurred vision, miosis, diplopia

CV: Palpitations, bradycardia, change in B/P

RESP: Respiratory depression

Contraindications: Hypersensitivity, addiction (narcotic)

Precautions: Addictive personality, pregnancy (C), lactation, increased intracranial pressure, MI (acute), severe heart disease, respiratory depression, hepatic disease, renal disease, child <18 yr

Pharmacokinetics:

Onset 15-30 min, peak ½-1½ hr, duration 4-5 hr; metabolized by liver, excreted by kidneys, crosses placenta, excreted in breast milk

Interactions/incompatibilities:

• Effects may be increased with other CNS depressants: alcohol, narcotics, sedative/hypnotics, antipsychotics, skeletal muscle relaxants

NURSING CONSIDERATIONS
Assess:

• I&O ratio; check for decreasing output; may indicate urinary retention

• Need for drug

Administer:

• IV diluted with 5 ml of sterile H₂O or normal saline; give through Y-tube, or 3-way stopcock; give 2 mg or less/5 min

---

• With antiemetic if nausea, vomiting occur
• When pain is beginning to return; determine dosage interval by patient response

Perform/provide:
• Storage in light-resistant area at room temperature
• Assistance with ambulation
• Safety measures: siderails, night light, call bell within easy reach

Evaluate:
• Therapeutic response: decrease in pain
• CNS changes: dizziness, drowsiness, hallucinations, euphoria, LOC, pupil reaction
• Allergic reactions: rash, urticaria
• Respiratory dysfunction: respiratory depression, character, rate, rhythm; notify physician if respirations are <10/min
• Need for pain medication, physical dependence

Teach patient/family:
• To report any symptoms of CNS changes, allergic reactions
• That physical dependency may result when used for extended periods of time
• Withdrawal symptoms may occur: nausea, vomiting, cramps, fever, faintness, anorexia

Lab test interferences:
Increase: Amylase

Treatment of overdose: Narcan 0.2-0.8 IV, O$_2$, IV fluids, vasopressors

---

hydromorphone HCl
(hye-droe-mor′fone)
Dilaudid Cough Syrup
Func. class.: Antitussive, narcotic
Chem. class.: Phenanthrene derivative, guaifenesin

Controlled Substance Schedule II

Action: Increases respiratory tract fluid by decreasing surface tension, adhesiveness, which increases removal of mucus; possesses analgesic, antitussive properties

Uses: Cough

Dosage and routes:
• *Adult:* PO 1 mg q3-4h prn
• *Child 6-12 yr:* PO 0.5 mg q3-4h prn

Available forms include: Syr 1 mg/5 ml

Side effects/adverse reactions:
CNS: Dizziness, drowsiness
GI: Nausea, constipation, vomiting, anorexia
CV: Hypotension
INTEG: Urticaria, rash
RESP: **Respiratory depression**

Contraindications: Hypersensitivity, increased intracranial pressure, status asthmaticus

Precautions: Hypothyroidism, Addison's disease, CNS depression, brain tumor, asthma, hepatic disease, renal disease, COPD, psychosis, alcoholism, convulsive disorders, pregnancy (C)

Pharmacokinetics: Metabolized by liver, half-life 2-4 hr

Interactions/incompatibilities:
• Enhanced CNS depression: barbiturates, narcotics, antipsychotics, antidepressants

NURSING CONSIDERATIONS
Assess:
• VS, cardiac status including hypotension
• Respiratory rate, depth

Administer:
• Decreased dose to elderly patients; their metabolism may be slowed

Perform/provide:
• Storage at room temperature
• Increased fluids, bulk, exercise to patient's lifestyle to decrease constipation

---

Evaluate:
- Therapeutic response: absence of cough
- Cough: type, frequency, character including sputum

Teach patient/family:
- Avoid driving, other hazardous activities until patient is stabilized on this medication if drowsiness occurs
- Avoid alcohol, other CNS depressants; will enhance sedating properties of this drug

---

hydroquinone
(hye′droe-kwin-one)
Derma-Blanch, Eldopaque, Eldoquin, Esoterica Medicated Cream, Melanex, Quinnone, Porcelana, Solaquin

Func. class.: Depigmentating agent
Chem. class.: Enzyme inhibitor

Action: Inhibits production of tyrosine, which is needed in formation of melanin
Uses: Bleaching skin, including old-age spots, freckles, lentigo, chloasma
Dosage and routes:
- *Adult and child:* TOP apply to affected area qd-bid
Available forms include: Top cream 2%, 4%; top lotion 2%; gel 4%; sol 3%
Side effects/adverse reactions:
INTEG: Rash, dryness, fissures, stinging, contact dermatitis, erythema, irritation
Contraindications: Hypersensitivity, inflamed skin, prickly heat, sunburn
Precautions: Pregnancy (C), lactation, child <1 yr

NURSING CONSIDERATIONS
Administer:
- Topical corticosteroid for irritation
- Test dose to be applied to area 25 mm in diameter, check site after 24 hr; if itching or excessive inflammation occurs, drug should not be used

Perform/provide:
- Storage at room temperature in tight container

Evaluate:
- Therapeutic response: fading of spots over time
- Area of body involved, including time involved, what helps or aggravates condition

Teach patient/family:
- To avoid application on normal skin or getting cream in eyes
- To use opaque sunscreen during day on exposed areas or bleaching effect may be reversed
- That minor redness is not a contraindication
- To continue to use sunscreen after bleaching is complete

---

hydroxocobalamin (vitamin B$_{12}$)
Acti-B$_{12}$,* Alpha Redisol, Alpha-Ruvite, Codrozomin, Droxomin, Neo-Betalin 12, Rubesol-LA

Func. class.: Vitamin
Chem. class.: B$_{12}$—water-soluble vitamin

Action: Needed for adequate nerve functioning, protein and carbohydrate metabolism, normal growth, RBC development
Uses: Vitamin B$_{12}$ deficiency, pernicious anemia, vitamin B$_{12}$ malabsorption syndrome, Schilling test
Dosage and routes:
- *Adult:* IM 30-100 µg qd × 5-10

---

*Available in Canada only

days, maintenance 100-200 mg IM q mo
• *Child:* IM 1-30 μg qd × 5-10 days, maintenance 60 μg IM q mo or more
Pernicious anemia/malabsorption syndrome
• *Adult:* IM 100-1000 μg qd × 2 wk, then 100-1000 μg IM q mo
• *Child:* IM 1000-5000 μg × 2 wk or more given in 100-500 μg doses, then 60 μg IM/SC mo
Schilling test
• *Adult and child:* IM 1000μg in one dose
Available forms include: Inj IM 100, 120, 1000 μg/ml
Side effects/adverse reactions:
CNS: Flushing, optic nerve atrophy
GI: Diarrhea
CV: **CHF,** peripheral vascular thrombosis, pulmonary edema
INTEG: Itching, rash
Contraindications: Hypersensitivity, optic nerve atrophy
Precautions: Pregnancy (A), lactation, children
Pharmacokinetics: Stored in liver, kidneys, stomach; 50%-90% excreted in urine, crosses placenta, breast milk
Interactions/incompatibilities:
• Decreased absorption of hydroxocobalamin: aminoglycosides, anticonvulsants, colchicine, chloramphenicol, aminosalicylic acid, potassium preparations
• Increased absorption of this drug: prednisone
NURSING CONSIDERATIONS
Assess:
• Potassium levels during beginning treatment
• CBC for increased reticulocyte count during 1st week of therapy, then increase RBC and hemoglobin after that

Administer:
• With fruit juice to disguise taste
• With meals if possible for better absorption
• By IM inj for pernicious anemia unless contraindicated
Evaluate:
• Therapeutic response: decreased anorexia, dyspnea on excretion, palpitations, paresthesias, psychosis, visual disturbances
• Nutritional status: egg yolks, fish, organ meats, dairy products, clams, oysters, which are good sources for Vitamin B_{12}
• For pulmonary edema, or worsening of CHF in cardiac patients
Teach patient/family
• That treatment must continue for life if diagnosed as having pernicious anemia
• Well-balanced diet
• Avoid persons with infections
Lab test interferences:
False positive: Intrinsic factor

---

hydroxychloroquine sulfate
(hye-drox-ee-klor′oh-kwin)
Plaquenil Sulfate
Func. class.: Antimalarial
Chem. class.: 4-aminoquinoline derivative

Action: Inhibits parasite replications, transcription of DNA to RNA by forming complexes with DNA of parasite
Uses: Malaria caused by *Plasmodium vivax, P. malariae, P. ovale, P. falciparum* (some strains): lupus erythematosus, rheumatoid arthritis
Dosage and routes:
Malaria
• *Adult and child:* PO 5 mg/kg/wk on same day of week, not to exceed

300 mg; treatment should begin 2 wk before entering endemic area, continue 8 wk after leaving; if treatment begins after exposure, 600 mg for adult, 10 mg/kg for children in 2 divided doses 6 hr apart

Lupus erythematosus
• *Adult:* PO 400 mg qd-bid, length depends on patient response; maintenance 200-400 mg qd

Rheumatoid arthritis
• *Adult:* PO 400-600 mg qd, then 200-300 mg qd after good response
Available forms include: Tabs 200 mg

Side effects/adverse reactions:
CV: Hypotension, heart block, *asystole with syncope*
INTEG: Pruritus, pigmentation changes, skin eruptions, lichen planus–like eruptions, eczema, *exfoliative dermatitis,* alopecia
CNS: Headache, stimulation, fatigue, irritability, *convulsion,* bad dreams, dizziness, confusion, psychosis, decreased reflexes
EENT: Blurred vision, corneal changes, retinal changes, difficulty focusing, tinnitus, vertigo, deafness, photophobia, corneal edema
GI: Nausea, vomiting, anorexia, diarrhea, cramps
HEMA: Thrombocytopenia, agranulocytosis, hemolytic anemia, leukopenia

Contraindications: Hypersensitivity, retinal field changes, prophyria, children (long-term)
Precautions: Blood dyscrasias, severe GI disease, neurologic disease, alcoholism, hepatic disease, G-6-PD deficiency, psoriasis, eczema, pregnancy (C)
Pharmacokinetics:
PO: Peak 1-2 hr, half-life 3-5 days, metabolized in liver, excreted in urine, feces, breast milk, crosses placenta

Interactions/incompatibilities:
• Decreased action of hydroxychloroquine: magnesium or aluminum compounds

NURSING CONSIDERATIONS
Assess:
• Ophthalmic test if long-term treatment or drug dosage >150 mg/day
• Liver studies q wk: AST, ALT, bilirubin
• Blood studies: CBC, since blood dyscrasias occur
• For decreased reflexes: knee, ankle
• ECG during therapy
• Watch for depression of T waves, widening of QRS complex

Administer:
• Before or after meals at same time each day to maintain drug level
• IM after aspirating to avoid injection into blood system, which may cause hypotension, asystole, heart block; rotate injection sites

Perform/provide:
• Storage in tight, light-resistant containers at room temperature; injection should be kept in cool environment

Evaluate:
• Allergic reactions: pruritus, rash, urticaria
• Blood dyscrasias: malaise, fever, bruising, bleeding (rare)
• For ototoxicity (tinnitus, vertigo, change in hearing); audiometric testing should be done before, after treatment
• For toxicity: blurring vision, difficulty focusing, headache, dizziness, knee, ankle reflexes; drug should be discontinued immediately

---

* Available in Canada only

Teach patient/family:
• To use sunglasses in bright sunlight to decrease photophobia
• That urine may turn rust or brown color
• To report hearing, visual problems, fever, fatigue, bruising, bleeding, which may indicate blood dyscrasias
Treatment of overdose: Induce vomiting, gastric lavage, administer barbiturate (ultrashort-acting), vasopressin; tracheostomy may be necessary

---

hydroxyprogesterone caproate

(hye-drox-ee-proe-jess'te-rone)
Delalutin, Dura-lutin
Func. class.: Progestogen, hormone

Action: Inhibits secretion of pituitary gonadotropins, which prevents follicular maturation, ovulation, stimulates growth of mammary tissue, antineoplastic action against endometrial cancer
Uses: Uterine cancer, menstrual disorders
Dosage and routes:
• *Adult:* IM 125-375 mg q4 wk, discontinue after 4 cycles
Uterine cancer
• *Adult:* IM 1-5 g/wk
Available forms include: Inj IM 125, 250 mg/ml
Side effects/adverse reactions:
CNS: Dizziness, headache, migraines, depression, fatigue
CV: Hypotension, thrombophlebitis, edema, *thromboembolism, stroke, pulmonary embolism, myocardial infarction*
GI: Nausea, vomiting, anorexia, cramps, increased weight, *cholestatic jaundice*
EENT: Diplopia
GU: Amenorrhea, cervical erosion, breakthrough bleeding, dysmenorrhea, vaginal candidiasis, breast changes, *gynecomastia, testicular atrophy, impotence,* endometriosis, *spontaneous abortion*
INTEG: Rash, urticaria, acne, hirsutism, alopecia, oily skin, seborrhea, purpura, melasma, photosensitivity
META: Hyperglycemia
Contraindications: Breast cancer, hypersensitivity, thromboembolic disorders, reproductive cancer, genital bleeding (abnormal, undiagnosed), pregnancy (X)
Precautions: Lactation, hypertension, asthma, blood dyscrasias, gallbladder disease, HF, diabetes mellitus, bone disease, depression, migraine headache, convulsive disorders, hepatic disease, renal disease, family history of breast or reproductive tract cancer
Pharmacokinetics:
IM: Half-life 5 min, duration 24 hr, excreted in urine, feces, metabolized in liver
NURSING CONSIDERATIONS
Assess:
• Weight daily, notify physician of weekly weight gain >5 lb
• B/P at beginning of treatment and periodically
• I&O ratio; be alert for decreasing urinary output, increasing edema
• Liver function studies: ALT, AST, bilirubin, periodically during long-term therapy
Administer:
• Titrated dose, use lowest effective dose
• Oil solution deeply in large muscle mass (IM), rotate sites
• In one dose in AM
• With food or milk to decrease GI symptoms

---

italics = common side effects   ***bold italic*** = life threatening reactions

• After warming to dissolve crystals

Perform/provide:
• Storage in dark area

Evaluate:
• Therapeutic response: decreased abnormal uterine bleeding, absence of amenorrhea
• Edema, hypertension, cardiac symptoms, jaundice
• Mental status: affect, mood, behavioral changes, depression
• Hypercalcemia

Teach patient/family:
• To avoid sunlight or use sunscreen; photosensitivity can occur
• About cushingoid symptoms
• To report breast lumps, vaginal bleeding, edema, jaundice, dark urine, clay-colored stools, dyspnea, headache, blurred vision, abdominal pain, numbness or stiffness in legs, chest pain; male to report impotence or gynecomastia
• To report suspected pregnancy

Lab test interferences:
Increase: Alk phosphatase, nitrogen (urine), pregnanediol, amino acids
Decrease: GTT, HDL

---

hydroxyurea

(hye-drox′ee-yoo-ree-ah)
Hydrea

Func. class.: Antineoplastic-antimetabolite
Chem. class.: Synthetic urea analog

Action: Acts by inhibiting DNA synthesis without interfering with RNA or protein synthesis; incorporates thymidine into DNA, causing direct damage to DNA strands
Uses: Melanoma, chronic myelocytic leukemia, recurrent or metastatic ovarian cancer, squamous cell carcinoma of the head and neck

Dosage and routes:
Solid tumors
• *Adult:* PO 80 mg/kg as a single dose q3 days or 20-30 mg/kg as a single dose qd
In combination with radiation
• *Adult:* PO 80 mg/kg as a single dose q3 days
Resistant chronic myelocytic leukemia
• *Adult:* PO 20-30 mg/kg/day as a single daily dose
Available forms include: Caps 500 mg

Side effects/adverse reactions:
HEMA: **Leukopenia, anemia, thrombocytopenia**
GI: Nausea, vomiting, anorexia, diarrhea, stomatitis, constipation
GU: Increased BUN, uric acid, creatinine, temporary renal function impairment
INTEG: Rash, urticaria, pruritus, dry skin
CV: Angina, ischemia
CNS: Headache, confusion, hallucinations, dizziness, ***convulsions***
Contraindications: Hypersensitivity, leukopenia (<2500/mm³), thrombocytopenia (<100,000/mm³), anemia (severe), pregnancy (D)
Precautions: Renal disease (severe)
Pharmacokinetics: Readily absorbed when taken orally, peak level in 2 hr, degraded in liver, excreted in urine, almost totally eliminated in 24 hr; readily crosses blood-brain barrier
Interactions/incompatibilities:
• Increased toxicity: radiation or other antineoplastics

NURSING CONSIDERATIONS
Assess:
• CBC, differential, platelet count

---

weekly; withhold drug if WBC is <3500/mm³ or platelet count is <100,000/mm³; notify physician of these results; drug should be discontinued
• Renal function studies: BUN, serum uric acid, urine CrCl, electrolytes before, during therapy
• I&O ratio, report fall in urine output to <30 ml/hr
• Monitor temperature q4h; fever may indicate beginning infection
• Liver function tests before, during therapy: bilirubin, alk phosphatase, AST, ALT, LDH; as needed or monthly
• B/P q3-4h; check for chest pain; angina, ischemia may occur

Administer:
• Allopurinol or NaHCO₃ concurrently to prevent high uric acid levels; extra fluids
• Antiemetic 30-60 min before giving drug to prevent vomiting and prn
• Antibiotics for prophylaxis of infection
• Transfusion for anemia

Perform/provide:
• Rinsing of mouth tid-qid with water, club soda; brushing of teeth bid-tid with soft brush or cotton-tipped applicators for stomatitis; use unwaxed dental floss
• Nutritious diet with iron, vitamin supplements as ordered

Evaluate:
• Bleeding: hematuria, guaiac, bruising or petechiae, mucosa or orifices q8h
• Food preferences; list likes, dislikes
• Inflammation of mucosa, breaks in skin
• Buccal cavity q8h for dryness, sores or ulceration, white patches, oral pain, bleeding, dysphagia
• Symptoms indicating severe al-

lergic reaction: rash, urticaria, itching, flushing
• Neurotoxicity: headaches, hallucinations, convulsions, dizziness

Teach patient/family:
• To report signs of infection: increased temperature, sore throat, flu symptoms
• To report signs of anemia: fatigue, headache, faintness, shortness of breath, irritability
• To report bleeding: avoid use of razors, or commercial mouthwash
• To avoid use of aspirin products or ibuprofen
• To avoid foods with citric acid, hot or rough texture if stomatitis is present
• To report stomatitis: any bleeding, white spots, ulcerations in the mouth; tell patient to examine mouth qd, report symptoms
• Contraceptive measures are recommended during therapy
• To drink 10-12 glasses of fluid/day
• Notify physician of fever, chills, sore throat, nausea, vomiting, anorexia, diarrhea, bleeding, bruising; may indicate blood dyscrasias

Lab test interferences:
Increase: Renal function studies

---

hydroxyzine HCl/ hydroxyzine pamoate
(hye-drox′i-zeen)
Atarax, Durrax, Orgatrax, Quiess, Vistaril/Vistaril IM

Func. class.: Antianxiety
Chem. class.: Piperazine derivative

Action: Depresses subcortical levels of CNS, including limbic system, reticular formation
Uses: Anxiety, preoperatively, postoperatively to prevent nausea,

---

vomiting, to potentiate narcotic analgesics, sedation, pruritus

Dosage and routes:
- *Adult:* PO 25-100 mg tid-qid
- *Child >6 yr:* 50-100 mg/day in divided doses
- *Child <6 yr:* 50 mg/day in divided doses

Preoperatively/postoperatively
- *Adult:* IM 25-100 mg q4-6h
- *Child:* IM 1.1 mg/kg q4-6h

Available forms include: Tabs 10, 25, 50, 100 mg; caps 25, 50, 100 mg; syrup 10 mg/5 ml; oral susp 25 mg/5 ml; IM inj

Side effects/adverse reactions:
CNS: Dizziness, drowsiness, confusion, headache, tremors, fatigue, depression, convulsions
GI: Dry mouth

Contraindications: Hypersensitivity, pregnancy (C)

Precautions: Elderly, debilitated, hepatic disease, renal disease

Pharmacokinetics:
PO: Onset 15-30 min, duration 4-6 hr, half-life 3 hr

Interactions/incompatibilities:
- Increased CNS depressant effect: barbiturates, narcotics, analgesics, alcohol

NURSING CONSIDERATIONS
Assess:
- B/P (lying, standing), pulse; if systolic B/P drops 20 mm Hg, hold drug, notify physician
- Blood studies: CBC
- Hepatic studies: AST, ALT, bilirubin, creatinine

Administer:
- By Z-track injection in large muscle for IM to decrease pain, chance of necrosis
- With food or milk for GI symptoms
- Crushed if patient is unable to swallow medication whole

- Gum, hard candy, frequent sips of water for dry mouth

Perform/provide:
- Assistance with ambulation during beginning therapy, since drowsiness/dizziness occurs
- Safety measures, including side-rails
- Checking to see PO medication has been swallowed

Evaluate:
- Mental status: mood, sensorium, affect
- Increased sedation

Teach patient/family:
- Not to be used for everyday stress or used longer than 4 mo
- Avoid OTC preparations (cold, cough, hay fever) unless approved by physician
- To avoid driving, activities that require alertness
- To avoid alcohol ingestion, or other psychotropic medications
- Not to discontinue medication quickly after long-term use
- To rise slowly or fainting may occur

Lab test interferences:
False increase: 17-OHCS

Treatment of overdose: Lavage if orally ingested; VS, supportive care; IV norepinephrine for hypotension

---

hyoscyamine sulfate
(hye-oh-sye′a-meen)
Anaspaz, Levsin, Levsinex
Func. class.: Gastrointestinal anticholinergic
Chem. class.: Belladonna alkaloid

Action: Inhibits muscarinic actions of acetylcholine at postganglionic parasympathetic neuroeffector sites
Uses: Treatment of peptic ulcer disease in combination with other

drugs; other GI disorders, other spastic disorders

Dosage and routes:
• *Adult:* PO/SL 0.125-0.25 mg tid-qid ac, hs; TIME REL 0.375 q12h; IM/SC/IV 0.25-0.5 mg q6h
• *Child 2-10 yr:* ½ adult dose
• *Child <2 yr:* ¼ adult dose
Available forms include: Tabs 0.125, 0.13, 0.15 mg; caps time rel 0.375 mg; sol 0.125 mg/ml; elix 0.125 mg/5 ml; inj IM, IV, SC 0.5 mg/ml

Side effects/adverse reactions:
CNS: Confusion, stimulation in elderly, headache, insomnia, dizziness, drowsiness, anxiety, weakness, hallucination
GI: Dry mouth, constipation, paralytic ileus, heartburn, nausea, vomiting, dysphagia, absence of taste
GU: Hesitancy, retention, impotence
CV: Palpitations, tachycardia
EENT: Blurred vision, photophobia, mydriasis, cycloplegia, increased ocular tension
INTEG: Urticaria, rash, pruritus, anhidrosis, fever, allergic reactions
Contraindications: Hypersensitivity to anticholinergics, narrow-angle glaucoma, GI obstruction, myasthenia gravis, paralytic ileus, GI atony, toxic megacolon, prostatic hypertrophy
Precautions: Hyperthyroidism, coronary artery disease, dysrhythmias, CHF, ulcerative colitis, hypertension, hiatal hernia, hepatic disease, renal disease, pregnancy (C), urinary retention
Pharmacokinetics:
PO: Duration 4-6 hr; metabolized by liver, excreted in urine, half-life 3.5 hr
Interactions/incompatibilities:
• Decreased effect of hyoscyamine: antacids
• Increased anticholinergic effect: amantadine, tricyclic antidepressants, MAOIs, H_1 antihistamines
• Decreased effect of: phenothiazines, levodopa, ketoconazole

NURSING CONSIDERATIONS
Assess:
• VS, cardiac status: checking for dysrhythmias, increased rate, palpitations
• I&O ratio; check for urinary retention or hesitancy
Administer:
• ½ hr ac for better absorption
• Decreased dose to elderly patients; their metabolism may be slowed
• Gum, hard candy, frequent rinsing of mouth for dryness of oral cavity
Perform/provide:
• Storage is tight container protected from light
• Increased fluids, bulk, exercise to patient's lifestyle to decrease constipation
Evaluate:
• Therapeutic response: absence of epigastric pain, bleeding, nausea, vomiting
• GI complaints: pain, bleeding (frank or occult), nausea, vomiting, anorexia
Teach patient/family:
• Avoid driving or other hazardous activities until stabilized on medication
• Avoid alcohol or other CNS depressants; will enhance sedating properties of this drug
• To avoid hot environments, stroke may occur, drug suppresses perspiration
• Use sunglasses when outside to prevent photophobia, may cause blurred vision

H

---

italics = common side effects   ***bold italic*** = life threatening reactions

ibuprofen

(eye-byoo'proe-fen)

Amersol, Motrin, Rufen

Func. class.: Nonsteroidal antiinflammatory

Chem. class.: Propionic acid derivative

Action: Inhibits prostaglandin synthesis by decreasing enzyme needed for biosynthesis; possesses analgesic, antiinflammatory, antipyretic properties

Uses: Rheumatoid arthritis, osteoarthritis, primary dysmenorrhea, gout, dental pain, musculoskeletal disorders

Dosage and routes:

• *Adult:* PO 200-800 mg qid, not to exceed 3.2 g/day

Available forms include: Tabs 200, 300, 400, 600, 800 mg

Side effects/adverse reactions:

GI: Nausea, anorexia, vomiting, diarrhea, jaundice, *cholestatic hepatitis,* constipation, flatulence, cramps, dry mouth, peptic ulcer

CNS: Dizziness, drowsiness, fatigue, tremors, confusion, insomnia, anxiety, depression

CV: Tachycardia, peripheral edema, palpitations, dysrhythmias

INTEG: Purpura, rash, pruritus, sweating

GU: Nephrotoxicity: dysuria, hematuria, oliguria, azotemia

HEMA: Blood dyscrasias

EENT: Tinnitus, hearing loss, blurred vision

Contraindications: Hypersensitivity, asthma, severe renal disease, severe hepatic disease

Precautions: Pregnancy (B) 1st and 2nd trimester, lactation, children, bleeding disorders, GI disorders, cardiac disorders, hypersensitivity to other antiinflammatory agents

Pharmacokinetics:

PO: Peak 1-2 hr, half-life 2-4 hr, metabolized in liver (inactive metabolites), excreted in urine (inactive metabolites), 90%-99% plasma protein binding

Interactions/incompatibilities:

• May increase action of: coumarin, phenytoin, sulfonamides

• Decreased action of ibuprofen: salicylates

NURSING CONSIDERATIONS

Assess:

• Renal, liver, blood studies: BUN, creatinine, AST, ALT, Hgb, before treatment, periodically thereafter

• Audiometric, ophthalmic exam before, during, after treatment

• Cardiac status: edema (peripheral), tachycardia, palpitations; monitor B/P, pulse for character, quality, rhythm

• For past history of peptic ulcer disorder

Administer:

• With food to decrease GI symptoms; however, best to take on empty stomach to facilitate absorption

Perform/provide:

• Storage at room temperature

Evaluate:

• Therapeutic response: decreased pain, stiffness in joints, decreased swelling in joints, ability to move more easily

• For eye, ear problems: blurred vision, tinnitus; may indicate toxicity

Teach patient/family:

• To report blurred vision, ringing, roaring in ears; may indicate toxicity

• To avoid driving, other hazardous activities if dizziness, drowsiness occurs

• To report change in urine pattern,

increased weight, edema, increased pain in joints, fever, blood in urine; indicate nephrotoxicity

• That therapeutic effects may take up to 1 mo

• To avoid alcohol, salicylates; bleeding may occur

• To avoid sun or sun lamp exposure

---

idarubicin HCl

Idamycin

Func. class.: Antineoplastic, antibiotic

Chem. class.: Anthracycline glycoside

Action: Inhibits DNS synthesis derived from daunorubicin by binding to DNA, which causes strand splitting; cell cycle specific (S phase); a vesicant

Uses: Used in combination with other antineoplastics for acute myelocytic leukemia in adults

Dosage and routes:

Adult: IV 12 mg/m²/day × 3 days in combination with cytosine arabinoside, or 25 mg/m² IV bolus followed by 200 mg/m²/day × 5 days by continuous INF

Available forms include: inj IV 5, 10 mg

Side effects/adverse reactions:

*HEMA: **Thrombocytopenia, leukopenia, anemia***

GI: Nausea, vomiting, abdominal pain, mucositis, diarrhea, hepatoxicity

INTEG: Rash, extravasation, dermatitis, reversible alopecia, urticaria, thrombophlebitis at injection site

CV: Dysrhythmias, CHF, pericarditis, myocarditis, peripheral edema

CNS: Fever, chills, headache

Contraindications: Hypersensitivity

Precautions: Renal and hepatic disease, gout, bone marrow depression, children

Pharmacokinetics: Half-life 22 hr, metabolized by liver, crosses placenta, excreted in bile, urine (primarily as metabolites)

Interactions/incompatibilities:

• Increased toxicity: other antineoplastics or radiation

• Do not mix with other drugs in solution or syringe

NURSING CONSIDERATIONS

Assess:

• CBC, differential, platelet count weekly; withhold drug if WBC is 4000/mm³ or platelet count is 75,000/mm³; notify physician of these results

• Blood, urine, uric acid levels

• Renal function studies: BUN, serum uric acid, urine CrCl, electrolytes before, during therapy

• I&O ratio: report fall in urine output to <30 ml/hr

• Monitor temperature q4h; fever may indicate beginning infection

• Liver function tests before, during therapy: bilirubin, AST, ALT, alk phosphatase as needed or monthly

• ECG: watch for ST-T wave changes, low QRS and T, possible dysrhythmias (sinus tachycardia, heart block, PVCs)

Administer:

• Antiemetic 30-60 min before giving drug and 6-10 hr after treatment to prevent vomiting

• After reconstituting 5 mg vial with 5 ml 0.9% NaCl (1 mg/1 ml), give over 10-15 min

• Antibiotics for prophylaxis of infection

• Allopurinol or sodium bicarbon-

---

italics = common side effects   ***bold italic*** = life threatening reactions

ate to reduce uric acid levels, alkalinization, or urine
• Transfusion for anemia
• Hydrocortisone for extravasation; apply ice compress after stopping infusion

Perform/provide:
• Strict handwashing technique, gloves, protective clothing
• Liquid diet: carbonated beverages, gelatin may be added if patient is not nauseated or vomiting
• Increase fluid intake to 2-3 L/day to prevent urate and calculi formation
• Diet low in purines: absence of organ meats (kidney, liver), dried beans, peas to reduce uric acid level
• Rinsing of mouth tid-qid with water, club soda; brushing of teeth tid-qid with soft brush or cotton-tipped applicators for stomatitis; use unwaxed dental floss
• Storage at room temperature for 3 days after reconstituting or 7 days refrigerated

Evaluate:
• Bleeding: hematuria, guaiac stools, bruising or petechiae, mucosa or orifices q8h
• Food preferences: list likes, dislikes
• Effects of alopecia on body image; discuss feelings about body changes
• Inflammation of mucosa, breaks in skin
• Yellowing of skin, sclera, dark urine, clay-colored stools, itchy skin, abdominal pain, fever, diarrhea
• Buccal cavity q8h for dryness, sores, or ulceration, white patches, oral pain, bleeding, dysphagia
• Local irritation, pain, burning at injection site
• GI symptoms: frequency of stools, cramping

• Acidosis, signs of dehydration: rapid respirations, poor skin turgor, decreased urine output, dry skin, restlessness, weakness
• Cardiac status: B/P, pulse, character, rhythm, rate

Teach patient/family:
• To report any complaints, side effects to nurse or physician
• That hair may be lost during treatment and wig or hairpiece may make patient feel better; tell patient that new hair may be different in color, texture
• To avoid foods with citric acid, hot or rough texture
• To report any bleeding, white spots, ulcerations in mouth; tell patient to examine mouth q d
• That urine may be red-orange for 48 hr

Lab test interferences:
Increase: Uric acid

---

idoxuridine-IDU (ophthalmic)

Dendrid Herplex, IDU Stoxil

Func. class.: Antiviral
Chem. class.: Pyrimidine nucleoside

Action: Inhibits viral replication by interfering with viral DNA synthesis
Uses: Herpes simplex keratitis, cytomegalovirus, varicella-zoster alone or with corticosteroids

Dosage and routes:
• *Adult and child:* INSTILL 1 gtt q1h during day and 2 hr during night; TOP apply oint q4h × 1 wk, if no response, discontinue

Available forms include: Oint 0.5%, sol 0.1%

Side effects/adverse reactions:
EENT: Poor corneal wound healing,

temporary visual haze, overgrowth of nonsusceptible organisms

Contraindications: Hypersensitivity

Precautions: Antibiotic hypersensitivity, pregnancy (C)

Interactions/incompatibilities:
• Do not use boric acid with this drug

NURSING CONSIDERATIONS
Administer:
• After washing hands, cleanse crusts or discharge from eye before application

Perform/provide:
• Storage in refrigerator, in light-resistant container until used

Evaluate:
• Therapeutic response: absence of redness, inflammation, tearing, photophobia
• Allergy: itching, lacrimation, redness, swelling

Teach patient/family:
• To use drug exactly as prescribed
• Not to use eye makeup, towels, washcloths, eye medication of others; reinfection may occur
• That drug container tip should not be touched to eye
• To report itching, increased redness, burning, stinging, swelling; drug should be discontinued
• That drug may cause blurred vision when ointment is applied

---

imipramine HCl
(im-ip′ra-meen)
Impril,* Janimine, Novopramine,* Presamine, Ropramine, Tipramine, Tofranil

Func. class.: Antidepressant—tricyclic
Chem. class.: Dibenzazepine—tertiary amine

Action: Blocks reuptake of nor-epinephrine, serotonin into nerve endings, increasing action of nor-epinephrine, serotonin in nerve cells

Uses: Depression, enuresis in children

Dosage and routes:
• *Adult:* PO/IM 75-100 mg/day in divided doses, may increase by 25-50 mg to 200 mg, not to exceed 300 mg/day; may give daily dose hs
• *Child:* PO 25-75 mg/day

Available forms include: Tabs 10, 25, 50 mg; inj IM 25 mg/2 ml

Side effects/adverse reactions:
*HEMA: **Agranulocytosis, thrombocytopenia, eosinophilia, leukopenia***
CNS: Dizziness, drowsiness, confusion, headache, anxiety, tremors, stimulation, weakness, insomnia, nightmares, EPS (elderly), increased psychiatric symptoms, paresthesia
GI: Diarrhea, dry mouth, nausea, vomiting, **paralytic ileus,** increased appetite, cramps, epigastric distress, jaundice, **hepatitis,** stomatitis
*GU: Retention, **acute renal failure***
INTEG: Rash, urticaria, sweating, pruritus, photosensitivity
*CV: Orthostatic hypotension, ECG changes, tachycardia, **hypertension,** palpitations*
EENT: Blurred vision, tinnitus, mydriasis

Contraindications: Hypersensitivity to tricyclic antidepressants, recovery phase of myocardial infarction, convulsive disorders, prostatic hypertrophy

Precautions: Suicidal patients, severe depression, increased intraocular pressure, narrow-angle glaucoma, urinary retention, cardiac disease, hepatic disease, hyperthy-

---

italics = common side effects   ***bold italic*** = life threatening reactions

roidism, electroshock therapy, elective surgery, elderly, pregnancy (C)

Pharmacokinetics:
PO: Steady state 2-5 days; metabolized by liver, excreted by kidneys, feces, crosses placenta, excreted in breast milk, half-life 6-20 hr

Interactions/incompatibilities:
• Decreased effects of: guanethidine, clonidine, indirect acting sympathomimetics (ephedrine)
• Increased effects of: direct acting sympathomimetics (epinephrine), alcohol, barbiturates, benzodiazepines, CNS depressants
• Hyperpyretic crisis, convulsions, hypertensive episode: MAOI (pargyline [Eutonyl])

NURSING CONSIDERATIONS
Assess:
• B/P (lying, standing), pulse q4h; if systolic B/P drops 20 mm Hg hold drug, notify physician; take vital signs q4h in patients with cardiovascular disease
• Blood studies: CBC, leukocytes, differential, cardiac enzymes if patient is receiving long-term therapy
• Hepatic studies: AST, ALT, bilirubin, creatinine
• Weight qwk, appetite may increase with drug
• ECG for flattening of T wave, bundle branch block, AV block, dysrhythmias in cardiac patients

Administer:
• Increased fluids, bulk in diet if constipation, urinary retention occur
• With food or milk for GI symptoms
• Dosage hs if over-sedation occurs during day; may take entire dose hs; elderly may not tolerate once/day dosing
• Gum, hard candy, or frequent sips of water for dry mouth

Perform/provide:
• Storage in tight container at room temperature, do not freeze
• Assistance with ambulation during beginning therapy since drowsiness/dizziness occurs
• Safety measures including side rails primarily in elderly
• Checking to see PO medication swallowed

Evaluate:
• EPS primarily in elderly: rigidity, dystonia, akathisia
• Mental status: mood, sensorium, affect, suicidal tendencies, increase in psychiatric symptoms: depression, panic
• Urinary retention, constipation; constipation is more likely to occur in children
• Withdrawal symptoms: headache, nausea, vomiting, muscle pain, weakness; do not usually occur unless drug was discontinued abruptly
• Alcohol consumption; if alcohol is consumed, hold dose until morning

Teach patient/family:
• That therapeutic effects may take 2-3 wk
• Use caution in driving or other activities requiring alertness because of drowsiness, dizziness, blurred vision
• To avoid alcohol ingestion, other CNS depressants
• Not to discontinue medication quickly after long-term use, may cause nausea, headache, malaise
• To wear sunscreen or large hat since photosensitivity occurs

Lab test interferences:
Increase: Serum bilirubin, alk phosphatase, blood glucose

---

*Available in Canada only

Decrease: 5-HIAA, VMA, urinary catecholamines

Treatment of overdose: ECG monitoring, induce emesis, lavage, activated charcoal, administer anticonvulsant

---

immune globulin

Gamastan, Gamimune, Gammar, Immuglobin, Sandoglobulin

Func. class.: Immune serum
Chem. class.: IgG

Action: Provides passive immunity to hepatitis A, measles, varicella, rubella, immune globulin deficiency

Uses: Agammaglobulinemia, hepatitis A exposure, measles exposure, measles vaccine complications, purpura, rubella exposure, chicken pox exposure

Dosage and routes:
• *Adult:* IM 30-50 ml q mo; IV 100 mg/kg q mo, 0.01-0.02 ml/kg/ min × ½ hr (Gamimune); IV 200 mg/kg q, 0.05-1 ml/min × 15-30 min, then increase to 1.5-2.5 ml/ min (Sandoglobulin)
• *Child:* IM 20-40 ml qmo

Hepatitis A exposure
• *Child and adult:* IM 0.02-0.04 ml/kg or 0.1 mg/kg if treatment is delayed

Hepatitis B exposure
• *Adult and child:* IM 0.06 ml/kg within 1 wk, q month

Measles
• *Child:* IM 0.25 ml/kg within 6 days

Immunoglobulin deficiency
• *Child:* IM 1.3 ml/kg, then 0.66 ml/kg after 2-4 wk and q2-4 wk thereafter

Idiopathic thrombocytopenia purpura
• *Adult:* IV 0.4 g/kg × 5 days

Available forms include: IV, IM inj 2, 10 ml/vial

Side effects/adverse reactions:
INTEG: Pain at injection site, rash, pruritus, chills, chest pain
MS: Arthralgia
SYST: Lymphadenopathy, ***anaphylaxis***
CNS: Headache, fatigue, malaise
GI: Abdominal pain

Contraindications: Hypersensitivity

Precautions: Pregnancy (C)

Interactions/incompatibilities:
• Do not administer live virus vaccines within 3 mo of this drug

NURSING CONSIDERATIONS
Administer:
• Gamimune: IV undiluted or dilute with D₅; give 0.01 ml/kg/ min; may increase to 0.02-0.04 ml/kg/ min
• Sandoglobulin: IV diluted with provided diluent; give 0.5-1 ml/ min × 15-30 min; may increase to 1.5-2.5 ml/min
• IM 3 ml or < in one site, use large muscle mass
• Only after epinephrine 1:1000, resuscitation equipment are available
• Only within 2 wk of exposure to hepatitis A

Perform/provide:
• Storage at 2°-8° C

Teach patient/family:
• Passive immunity is temporary

---

indapamide

(in-dap′a-mide)
Lozol, Lozide*

Func. class.: Diuretic—Thiazide-like
Chem. class.: Indoline

Action: Acts on proximal section of distal renal tubule by inhibiting

---

italics = common side effects   ***bold italic*** = life threatening reactions

reabsorption of sodium; may act by direct vasodilation caused by blocking of calcium channel

Uses: Edema, hypertension, diuresis

Dosage and routes:
• *Adult:* PO 2.5 mg qd in AM, may be increased to 5 mg qd if needed
Available forms include: Tabs 2.5 mg

Side effects/adverse reactions:
GU: Polyuria, dysuria, frequency
ELECT: Hypochloremic alkalosis, hypomagnesemia, hyperuricemia, hypercalcemia, hyponatremia, hypokalemia, hyperglycemia
CNS: Headache, dizziness, fatigue, weakness, paresthesias, depression
GI: Nausea, diarrhea, dry mouth, vomiting, anorexia, cramps, constipation, pancreatitis, abdominal pain, jaundice, hepatitis
EENT: Loss of hearing, tinnitus, blurred vision, nasal congestion, increased intraocular pressure
INTEG: Rash, pruritus, photosensitivity, alopecia, urticaria
MS: Cramps
*HEMA: **Thrombocytopenia, agranulocytosis, leukopenia, neutropenia, anemia***
CV: Orthostatic hypotension, volume depletion, palpitations

Contraindications: Hypersensitivity, anuria

Precautions: Hypokalemia, dehydration, ascites, hepatic disease, severe renal disease, pregnancy (B)

Pharmacokinetics:
PO: Onset 1-2 hr, peak 2 hr, duration up to 36 hr; excreted in urine, feces, half-life 14-18 hr

Interactions/incompatibilities:
• Hyperglycemia, hyperuricemia, hypotension: diazoxide
• Muscle relaxants, steroids, lithium, digitalis
• Decreased potassium: steroids

NURSING CONSIDERATIONS
Assess:
• Weight daily, I&O daily to determine fluid loss; effect of drug may be decreased if used qd
• Rate, depth, rhythm of respiration, effect of exertion
• B/P lying, standing; postural hypotension may occur
• Electrolytes: potassium, magnesium, sodium chloride; include BUN, CBC, serum creatinine, blood pH, ABGs, uric acid, calcium, glucose

Administer:
• In AM to avoid interference with sleep
• With food, if nausea occurs, absorption may be decreased slightly

Evaluate:
• Improvement in edema of feet, legs, sacral area daily if medication is being used in CHF
• Improvement in CVP q8h
• Signs of metabolic alkalosis
• Signs of hypokalemia
• Rashes, temperature elevation qd
• Confusion, especially in elderly; take safety precautions if needed
• Hydration: skin turgor, thirst, dry mucous membranes

Teach patient/family:
• To increase fluid intake 2-3 L/day unless contraindicated; to rise slowly from lying or sitting position
• Adverse reactions: muscle cramps, weakness, nausea, dizziness
• Take with food or milk for GI symptoms
• Take early in day to prevent nocturia

Lab test interferences:
Increase: Calcium, parathyroid test
Treatment of overdose: Lavage if taken orally, monitor electrolytes, administer IV fluids, monitor hydration, CV, renal status

---

* Available in Canada only

indecainide HCl

(in-de-kane'ide)
Decabid
Func. class.: Antidysrhythmic,
(Class I)

Action: Unknown; able to slow
conduction, reduce membrane responsiveness, inhibits automatic-
ity, increases ratio of effective refractory period to action potential
duration
Uses: Life-threatening dysrhythmias, sustained ventricular tachycardia
Dosage and routes:
• *Adult:* PO 100-200 mg/day in divided dose bid
Available forms include: Caps 25,
35, 50 mg
Side effects/adverse reactions:
CV: **Dysrhythmias, CHF**
CNS: Headache, dizziness, lightheadedness
GI: Constipation, nausea
GU: Impotence
EENT: Blurred vision, diplopia
Contraindications: 2nd-3rd degree AV block, right bundle branch
block, cardiogenic shock, hypersensitivity
Precautions: Severe CHF, hypokalemia, hyperkalemia, sick-sinus
syndrome, pregnancy (B), lacta-
tion, children, impaired hepatic or
renal disease
Pharmacokinetics:
Half-life 9-10 hr metabolized by
the liver; 63% of drug recovered in
urine
Interactions/incompatibilities:
• Increased effect of indecainide:
cimetidine
• Increased serum concentrations
of: digoxin

NURSING CONSIDERATIONS
Assess:
• GI status: bowel pattern, number
of stools
• Cardiac status: rate, rhythm,
quality
• Chest x-ray, pulmonary function
test during treatment
• I&O ratio; check for decreasing
output
• B/P for fluctuations
• Lung fields; bilateral rales may
occur in CHF patient
• Increased respiration, increased
pulse; drug should be discontinued
Evaluate:
• Therapeutic response: absence of
dysrhythmias
• Cardiac rate: respiration, rate,
rhythm, character continuously
Lab test interferences:
Increase: CPK
Treatment of overdose: O_2, arti-
ficial ventilation, ECG, administer
dopamine for circulatory depression, administer diazepam or thiopental for convulsions

indomethacin/
indomethacin sodium
trihydrate

(in-doe-meth'a-sin)
Indocid, Indocin, Indocin SR, In-
domed/Indocin IV
Func. class.: Nonsteroidal
Chem. class.: Propionic acid deriv-
ative

Action: Inhibits prostaglandin synthesis by decreasing enzyme
needed for biosynthesis; possesses
analgesic, antiinflammatory, antipyretic properties
Uses: Rheumatoid arthritis, ankylosing rheumatoid spondylitis,
acute gouty arthritis, closure of pa-

italics = common side effects   ***bold italic*** = life threatening reactions

tent ductus arteriosus in premature infants

Dosage and routes:

Arthritis

• *Adult:* PO/REC 25 mg bid-tid, may increase by 25 mg/day q1 wk, not to exceed 200 mg/day; SUS REL 75 mg qd, may increase to 75 mg bid

Acute arthritis

• *Adult:* PO/REC 50 mg tid; use only for acute attack, then reduce dose

Patent ductus arteriosus

• *Infant <2 days:* IV 0.2 mg/kg, then 0.1 mg/kg q12-24 hr

• *Infant 2-7 days:* IV 0.2 mg/kg, then 0.2 mg × 2 doses after 12, 24 hr

• *Infant >7 days:* IV 0.2 mg/kg, then 0.25 mg/kg × 2 doses after 12, 24 hr

Available forms include: Caps 25, 50 mg; caps ext rel 75 mg; susp 25 mg/5 ml; rec supp 50 mg

Side effects/adverse reactions:

GI: Nausea, anorexia, vomiting, diarrhea, jaundice, ***cholestatic hepatitis,*** constipation, flatulence, cramps, dry mouth, peptic ulcer

CNS: Dizziness, drowsiness, fatigue, tremors, confusion, insomnia, anxiety, depression

CV: Tachycardia, peripheral edema, palpitations, dysrhythmias

INTEG: Purpura, rash, pruritus, sweating

*GU: **Nephrotoxicity: dysuria, hematuria, oliguria, azotemia***

*HEMA: **Blood dyscrasias***

EENT: Tinnitus, hearing loss, blurred vision

Contraindications: Hypersensitivity, asthma, severe renal disease, severe hepatic disease

Precautions: Pregnancy, lactation, children, bleeding disorders, GI disorders, cardiac disorders, hypersensitivity to other antiinflammatory agents, pregnancy (B) 1st and 2nd trimesters, depression

Pharmacokinetics:

PO: Onset 1-2 hr, peak 3 hr, duration 4-6 hr; metabolized in liver, kidneys, excreted in urine, bile, feces, crosses placenta, excreted in breast milk, 99% plasma protein binding

Interactions/incompatibilities:

• Increased action of: coumarin, phenytoin, sulfonamides

• Toxicity: lithium, methotrexate

• Decreased action of: triamterene

• Do not give with antacids

NURSING CONSIDERATIONS

Assess:

• Renal, liver, blood studies: BUN, creatinine, AST, ALT, Hgb, before treatment, periodically thereafter

• Audiometric, ophthalmic exam before, during, after treatment

Administer:

• IV after diluting 1 mg/ml or more normal saline or sterile H_2O for inj without preservative; give over 5-10 sec

• With food to decrease GI symptoms; however, best to take on empty stomach to facilitate absorption

Perform/provide:

• Storage at room temperature

Evaluate:

• Therapeutic response: decreased pain, stiffness in joints, decreased swelling in joints, ability to move more easily

• For eye, ear problems: blurred vision, tinnitus; may indicate toxicity

• For confusion, mood changes, hallucinations

Teach patient/family:

• To report blurred vision, ringing, roaring in ears; may indicate toxicity

• To avoid driving, other hazardous

activities if dizziness, drowsiness occurs

• To report change in urine pattern, increased weight, edema, increased pain in joints, fever, blood in urine; indicate nephrotoxicity

• That therapeutic effects may take up to 1 mo

• To avoid alcohol, salicylates; bleeding may occur

---

influenza virus vaccine, trivalent A & B (whole virus/split virus)

Fluzone, Fluogen, Fluviral*
Func. class.: Vaccine

Action: Produces antibodies to influenza virus by production of antibodies; split virus vaccine causes less adverse reactions

Uses: Prevention of Russian, Chile, Philippine influenza

Dosage and routes:

• *Adult and child >12 yr:* IM 0.5 ml in 1 dose

• *Child 3-12 yr:* IM 0.5 ml, repeat in 1 mo (split) unless 1978-1985 vaccine was given

• *Child 6 mo to 3 yr:* IM 0.25 ml, repeat in 1 mo (split) unless 1978-1985 vaccine was given

Available forms include: Inj IM 100 µg/ml

Side effects/adverse reactions:

CNS: Fever, Guillian-Barré syndrome

INTEG: Urticaria, induration, erythema

SYST: Anaphylaxis, malaise

MS: Myalgia

Contraindications: Hypersensitivity, active infection, chicken, egg allergy, Guillain-Barré syndrome

Precautions: Elderly, immunosuppression, pregnancy

NURSING CONSIDERATIONS

Assess:

• For skin reactions: rash, induration, erythema

Administer:

• Only with epinephrine 1:1000 on unit to treat laryngospasm

• Only IM

Evaluate:

• For history of allergies, skin conditions (eczema, psoriasis, dermatitis), reactions to vaccinations

• For anaphylaxis: inability to breathe, bronchospasm

---

insulin, isophane suspension (NPH)

Beef NPH Iletin II, Humulin N, Iletin NPH,* Insulatard NPH, NPH Iletin I, Pork NPH Iletin II, Protaphane NPH, Novolin N,* NPH Insulin, NPH Purified Pork

Func. class.: Antidiabetic
Chem. class.: Exogenous unmodified insulin

Action: Decreases blood sugar, and indirectly increases blood pyruvate, lactate, decreases phosphate, potassium

Uses: Ketoacidosis, Type I (IDDM), Type II (NIDDM) diabetes mellitus, hyperkalemia

Dosage and routes:

• *Adult:* SC dosage individualized by blood, urine glucose, usual dose 7-26 U, may increase by 2-10 U/day if needed

Available forms include: SC 40, 100 U/ml

Side effects/adverse reactions:

CNS: Headache, lethargy, tremors, weakness, fatigue, delirium, sweating

CV: Tachycardia, palpitations

EENT: Blurred vision, dry mouth

GI: Hunger, nausea

---

italics = common side effects   ***bold italic*** = life threatening reactions

META: Hypoglycemia
INTEG: Flushing, rash, urticaria, warmth, lipodystrophy, lipohypertrophy
SYST: **Anaphylaxis**

Contraindications: Hypersensitivity

Precautions: Pregnancy (B)

Interactions/incompatibilities:
• Increased hypoglycemia: salicylate, alcohol, β-blockers, anabolic steroids, fenfluramine, phenylbutazone, sulfinpyrazone, guanethidine, oral hypoglycemics, MAOIs, tetracycline
• Decreased hypoglycemia: thiazides, thyroid hormones, oral contraceptives, corticosteroids, estrogens, dobutamine, epinephrine

Pharmacokinetics:
SC: Onset 1-2 hr, peak 4-12 hr, duration 18-24 hr
Metabolized by liver, muscle, kidneys; excreted in urine

NURSING CONSIDERATIONS
Assess:
• Fasting blood glucose, 2 hr PP (60-100 mg/dl normal fasting level) (70-130 mg/dl-normal 2 hr level)
• Urine ketones during times of illness; insulin requirements may increase during times of stress, illness

Administer:
• After warming to room temperature by rotating in palms to prevent lipodystrophy from injecting cold insulin
• Increased doses if tolerance occurs
• Human insulin to those allergic to beef or pork

Perform/provide:
• Storage at room temperature for <1 mo, keep away from heat and sunlight, refrigerate all other supply, do not use if discolored; do not freeze
• Rotation of injection sites: abdomen, upper back, thighs, upper arm, buttocks; keep record of sites

Evaluate:
• Therapeutic response: decrease in polyuria, polydipsia, polyphagia, clear sensorium, absence of dizziness, stable gait
• Hypoglycemic reaction that can occur during peak time

Teach patient/family:
• That blurred vision occurs, not to change corrective lens until vision is stabilized 1-2 mo
• To keep insulin, equipment available at all times
• That drug does not cure diabetes, but controls symptoms
• To carry Medic Alert ID as diabetic
• Hypoglycemia reaction: headache, tremors, fatigue, weakness
• Dosage, route, mixing instructions, if any diet restrictions, disease process
• To carry candy or lump sugar to treat hypoglycemia
• Symptoms of ketoacidosis: nausea, thirst, polyuria, dry mouth, decreased B/P, dry, flushed skin, acetone breath, drowsiness, Kussmaul respirations
• That a plan is necessary for diet, exercise; all food on diet should be eaten, exercise routine should not vary
• Urine glucose testing, make sure patient is able to determine glucose, acetone levels
• The pregnant patient to use glucose oxidase reagents
• To avoid OTC drugs unless directed by physician

Lab test interferences:
Increase: VMA
Decrease: Potassium, calcium

Interference: Liver function studies, thyroid function studies
Treatment of overdose: 10%-50% glucose PO if conscious or IV if comatose or 1 mg glucagon

---

insulin, isophane suspension and regular insulin

Humulin 70/30, Mixtard, Novolin 70/30

Func. class.: Antidiabetic
Chem. class.: Exogenous unmodified insulin

Action: Decreases blood sugar, indirectly increases blood pyruvate, lactate, decreases phosphate, potassium
Uses: Ketoacidosis, Type I (IDDM), Type II (NIDDM) diabetes mellitus, hyperkalemia
Dosage and routes:
• *Adult:* SC individualized dose
Available forms include: 70 units/ml isophane insulin with 30 units/ml regular insulin = 100 units/ml
Side effects/adverse reactions:
CNS: Headache, lethargy, tremors, weakness, fatigue, delirium, sweating
CV: Tachycardia, palpitations
EENT: Blurred vision, dry mouth
GI: Hunger, nausea
META: Hypoglycemia
INTEG: Flushing, rash, urticaria, warmth, lipodystrophy, lipohypertrophy
SYST: **Anaphylaxis**
Contraindications: Hypersensitivity
Precautions: Pregnancy (B)
Interactions/incompatibilities:
• Increased hypoglycemia: salicylate, alcohol, β-blockers, anabolic steroids, fenfluramine, guanethi-

dine, sulfinpyrazone, oral hypoglycemics, MAOIs, tetracycline
• Decreased hypoglycemia: thiazides, thyroid hormones, oral contraceptives, corticosteroids, estrogens, dobutamine, epinephrine, smoking, dextrothyroxine
Pharmacokinetics:
SC: Onset 30 min, peak 4-8 hr, duration 12-24 hr
Metabolized by liver, muscle, kidneys; excreted in urine
NURSING CONSIDERATIONS
Assess:
• Fasting blood glucose, 2 hr PP (60-100 mg/dl normal fasting level) (70-130 mg/dl-normal 2 hr level)
• Urine ketones during times of illness; insulin requirement increases during times of stress; illness
Administer:
• After warming to room temperature by rotating in palms to prevent lipodystrophy from injecting cold insulin
• Increased doses if tolerance occurs
• Human insulin to those allergic to beef or pork
Perform/provide:
• Storage at room temperature for <1 mo, keep cool and away from heat, refrigerate all other supply, do not use if discolored
• Rotation of injection sites: abdomen, upper back, thighs, upper arm, buttocks, keep record of sites
Evaluate:
• Therapeutic response: decrease in polyuria, polydipsia, polyphagia, clear sensorium, absence of dizziness, stable gait
• Hypoglycemic reaction that can occur during peak time
Teach patient/family:
• That blurred vision occurs, not to

---

change corrective lens until vision is stabilized 1-2 mo
• To keep insulin, equipment available at all times
• That drug does not cure diabetes, but controls symptoms
• To carry Medic Alert ID as diabetic
• Hypoglycemia reaction: headache, tremors, fatigue, weakness
• Dosage, route, mixing instructions, if any diet restrictions, disease process
• To carry candy or lump sugar to treat hypoglycemia
• Symptoms of ketoacidosis: nausea, thirst, polyuria, dry mouth, decreased B/P, dry, flushed skin, acetone breath, drowsiness, Kussmaul respirations
• That a plan is necessary for diet, exercise; all food on diet should be eaten, exercise routine should not vary
• Urine glucose testing, make sure patient is able to determine glucose, acetone levels
• The pregnant patient to use glucose oxidase reagents
• To avoid OTC drugs unless directed by physician

Lab test interferences:
Increase: VMA
Decrease: Potassium, calcium
Interference: Liver function studies, thyroid function studies

Treatment of overdose: 10%-50% glucose PO if conscious or IV if comatose or glucogon 1 mg

---

insulin, protamine zinc suspension (PZI)

Beef Protamine Zinc Iletin II, Iletin PZI,* Pork Protamine Zinc Iletin II, Protamine Zinc Iletin I

Func. class.: Antidiabetic
Chem. class.: Exogenous unmodified insulin

Action: Decreases blood sugar, in-

directly increases blood pyruvate, lactate, decreases phosphate, potassium

Uses: Ketoacidosis, Type I (IDDM), Type II (NIDDM) diabetes mellitus, hyperkalemia

Dosage and routes:
• *Adult:* SC 7-26 U q30-60 min before breakfast, individualized
Available forms include: SC 40, 100 U/ml

Side effects/adverse reactions:
CNS: Headache, lethargy, tremors, weakness, fatigue, delirium, sweating
CV: Tachycardia, palpitations
EENT: Blurred vision, dry mouth
GI: Hunger, nausea
META: Hypoglycemia
INTEG: Flushing, rash, urticaria, warmth, lipodystrophy, lipohypertrophy
SYST: Anaphylaxis

Contraindications: Hypersensitivity

Precautions: Pregnancy (B)

Pharmacokinetics:
SC: Onset 4-8 hr, peak 14-24 hr, duration 24-36 hr
Metabolized by liver, muscle, kidneys; excreted in urine

Interactions/incompatibilities:
• Increased hypoglycemia: salicylate, alcohol, β-blockers, anabolic steroids, fenfluramine, guanethidine, oral hypoglycemics, MAOIs, tetracycline
• Decreased hypoglycemia: thiazides, thyroid hormones, oral contraceptives, corticosteroids, estrogens, dobutamine, epinephrine, smoking, dextrothyroxine

NURSING CONSIDERATIONS
Assess:
• Fasting blood glucose, 2 hr PP (60-100 mg/dl normal fasting level) (70-130 mg/dl-normal 2 hr level)   •

---

* Available in Canada only

• Urine ketones during times of illness; insulin requirements increase during times of illness, stress

Administer:

• After warming to room temperature by rotating in palms to prevent lipodystrophy from injecting cold insulin

• Increased doses if tolerance occurs

Perform/provide:

• Storage at room temperature for current vial <1mo, in cool area, refrigerate all other supply, do not use if discolored; do not freeze

• Rotation of injection sites: abdomen, upper back, thighs, upper arm, buttocks; keep record of sites

Evaluate:

• Therapeutic response: decrease in polyuria, polydipsia, polyphagia, clear sensorium, absence of dizziness, stable gait

• Hypoglycemic reaction that can occur during peak time

Teach patient/family:

• That blurred vision occurs, not to change corrective lens until vision is stabilized 1-2 mo

• To keep insulin, equipment available at all times

• That drug does not cure diabetes, but controls symptoms

• To carry Medic Alert ID as diabetic

• Hypoglycemia reaction: headache, tremors, fatigue, weakness

• Dosage, route, mixing instructions, if any diet restrictions, disease process

• To carry candy or lump sugar to treat hypoglycemia

• Symptoms of ketoacidosis: nausea, thirst, polyuria, dry mouth, decreased B/P, dry, flushed skin, acetone breath, drowsiness, Kussmaul respirations

• That a plan is necessary for diet, exercise; all food on diet should be eaten, exercise routine should not vary

• Urine glucose testing; make sure patient is able to determine glucose, acetone levels

• The pregnant patient to use glucose oxidase reagents

• To avoid OTC drugs unless directed by physician

Lab test interferences:

Increase: VMA

Decrease: Potassium, calcium

Interference: Liver function studies, thyroid function studies

Treatment of overdose: 10%-50% glucose PO if conscious or IV if comatose or 1 mg glucagon

---

insulin, zinc suspension (Lente)

Beef Lente Iletin II, Lente Iletin I, Lente Insulin, Pork Lente Iletin II, Lentard Monotard,* Novolin L, Humulin L, Lente Purified Pork Insulin

Func. class.: Antidiabetic

Chem. class.: Exogenous unmodified insulin

Action: Decreases blood sugar, indirectly increases blood pyruvate, lactate, decreases phosphate, potassium

Uses: Ketoacidosis, Type I (IDDM), Type II (NIDDM) diabetes mellitus, hyperkalemia

Dosage and routes:

• *Adult:* SC individualized

Available forms include: SC 40, 100 U/ml

Side effects/adverse reactions:

CNS: Headache, lethargy, tremors, weakness, fatigue, delirium, sweating

CV: Tachycardia, palpitations

EENT: Blurred vision, dry mouth

GI: Hunger, nausea
META: Hypoglycemia
INTEG: Flushing, rash, urticaria, warmth, lipodystrophy, lipohypertrophy
SYST: **Anaphylaxis**
Contraindications: Hypersensitivity
Precautions: Pregnancy (B)
Pharmacokinetics:
SC: Onset 1-2½ hr, peak 7-15 hr, duration 12-24 hr
Metabolized by liver, muscle, kidneys; excreted in urine
Interactions/incompatibilities:
• Increased hypoglycemia: salicylate, alcohol, β-blockers, anabolic steroids, fenfluramine, guanethidine, oral hypoglycemics, MAOIs, tetracycline, sulfinpyrazone
• Hyperglycemia: thiazides, thyroid hormones, oral contraceptives, corticosteroids, estrogens, dobutamine, epinephrine, smoking, dextrothyroxine

NURSING CONSIDERATIONS
Assess:
• Fasting blood glucose, 2 hr PP (60-100 mg/dl normal fasting level) (70-130 mg/dl-normal 2 hr level)
• Urine ketones during times of illness; insulin requirements increase during times of illness, stress
Administer:
• After warming to room temperature by rotating in palms to prevent lipodystrophy from injecting cold insulin
• Increased doses if tolerance occurs
• Human insulin to those allergic to beef or pork
Perform/provide:
• Storage at room temperature for <1 mo, keep in cool area, refrigerate all other supply, do not use if discolored

• Rotation of injection sites: abdomen, upper back, thighs, upper arm, buttocks; keep record of sites
Evaluate:
• Therapeutic response: decrease in polyuria, polydipsia, polyphagia, clear sensorium, absence of dizziness, stable gait
• Hypoglycemic reaction that can occur during peak time
Teach patient/family:
• That blurred vision occurs, not to change corrective lens until vision is stabilized 1-2 mo
• To keep insulin, equipment available at all times
• That drug does not cure diabetes, but controls symptoms
• To carry Medic Alert ID as diabetic
• Hypoglycemia reaction: headache, tremors, fatigue, weakness
• Dosage, route, mixing instructions, if any diet restrictions, disease process
• To carry candy or lump sugar to treat hypoglycemia
• Symptoms of ketoacidosis: nausea, thirst, polyuria, dry mouth, decreased B/P, dry, flushed skin, acetone breath, drowsiness, Kussmaul respirations
• That a plan is necessary for diet, exercise; all food on diet should be eaten, exercise routine should not vary
• Urine glucose testing, make sure patient is able to determine glucose, acetone levels
• The pregnant patient to use glucose oxidase reagents
• To avoid OTC drugs unless directed by physician
Lab test interferences:
Increase: VMA
Decrease: Potassium, calcium

Interference: Liver function studies, thyroid function studies
Treatment of overdose: 10%-50% glucose PO if conscious or IV if comatose or 1 mg glucagon

---

insulin, zinc suspension extended (Ultralente)

Iletin Ultralente,* Ultralente,* Ultralente Iletin I, Ultralente Insulin, Ultralente Purified Beef

Func. class.: Antidiabetic
Chem. class.: Exogenous unmodified insulin

Action: Decreases blood sugar, indirectly increases blood pyruvate, lactate, decreases phosphate, potassium
Uses: Ketoacidosis, Type I (IDDM), Type II (NIDDM) diabetes mellitus, hyperkalemia
Dosage and routes:
• *Adult:* SC individualized
Available forms include: SC 40, 100 U/ml
Side effects/adverse reactions:
CNS: Headache, lethargy, tremors, weakness, fatigue, delirium, sweating
CV: Tachycardia, palpitations
EENT: Blurred vision, dry mouth
GI: Hunger, nausea
META: Hypoglycemia
INTEG: Flushing, rash, urticaria, warmth, lipodystrophy, lipohypertrophy
*SYST: **Anaphylaxis***
Contraindications: Hypersensitivity
Precautions: Pregnancy (C)
Pharmacokinetics:
SC: Onset 4-8 hr, peak 10-30 hr, duration 7-36 hr
Metabolized by liver, muscle, kidneys, excreted in urine

Interactions/incompatibilities:
• Increased hypoglycemia: salicylate, alcohol, β-blockers, anabolic steroids, fenfluramine, guanethidine, oral hypoglycemics, MAOIs, tetracycline, sulfinpyrazone
• Decreased hypoglycemia: thiazides, thyroid hormones, oral contraceptives, corticosteroids, estrogens, dobutamine, epinephrine, smoking, dextrothyroxine
NURSING CONSIDERATIONS
Assess:
• Fasting blood glucose, 2 hr PP (60-100 mg/dl normal fasting level) (70-130 mg/dl-normal 2 hr level)
• Urine ketones during illness; insulin requirements increase during times of stress, illness
Administer:
• After warming to room temperature by rotating in palms to prevent lipodystrophy from injecting cold insulin
• Increased doses if tolerance occurs
Perform/provide:
• Storage at room temperature for <1 mo, refrigerate all other supply, do not use if discolored
• Rotation of injection sites: abdomen, upper back, thighs, upper arm, buttocks, keep record of sites
Evaluate:
• Therapeutic response: decrease in polyuria, polydipsia, polyphagia, clear sensorium, absence of dizziness, stable gait
• Hypoglycemic reaction that can occur during peak time
Teach patient/family:
• That blurred vision occurs, not to change corrective lens until vision is stabilized 1-2 mo
• To keep insulin, equipment available at all times

---

italics = common side effects   ***bold italic*** = life threatening reactions

• That drug does not cure diabetes, but controls symptoms
• To carry Medic Alert ID as diabetic
• Hypoglycemia reaction: headache, tremors, fatigue, weakness
• Dosage, route, mixing instructions, if any diet restrictions, disease process
• To carry candy or lump sugar to treat hypoglycemia
• Symptoms of ketoacidosis: nausea, thirst, polyuria, dry mouth, decreased B/P, dry, flushed skin, acetone breath, drowsiness, Kussmaul respirations
• That a plan is necessary for diet, exercise; all food on diet should be eaten, exercise routine should not vary
• Urine glucose testing, make sure patient is able to determine glucose, acetone levels
• The pregnant patient to use glucose oxidase reagents
• To avoid OTC drugs unless directed by physician

Lab test interferences:
Increase: VMA
Decrease: Potassium, calcium
Interference: Liver function studies, thyroid function studies
Treatment of overdose: 10%-50% glucose PO if conscious or IV if comatose or 1 mg glucagon

---

insulin, zinc suspension, prompt (semilente)

Semilente Iletin I, Semilente Insulin, Semilente Purified Pork

Func. class.: Antidiabetic
Chem. class.: Exogenous unmodified insulin

Action: Decreases blood sugar, indirectly increases blood pyruvate, lactate, decreases phosphate, potassium

Uses: Ketoacidosis, Type I (IDDM), Type II (NIDDM) diabetes mellitus, hyperkalemia

Dosage and routes:
• *Adult:* SC dosage individualized by blood, urine glucose qd-tid
Available forms include: SC 40, 100 U/ml

Side effects/adverse reactions:
CNS: Headache, lethargy, tremors, weakness, fatigue, delirium, sweating
CV: Tachycardia, palpitations
EENT: Blurred vision, dry mouth
GI: Hunger, nausea
META: Hypoglycemia
INTEG: Flushing, rash, urticaria, warmth, lipodystrophy, lipohypertrophy
*SYST: **Anaphylaxis***

Contraindications: Hypersensitivity
Precautions: Pregnancy (B)
Pharmacokinetics:
SC: Onset 1-1½ min, peak 5-10 hr, duration 12-16 hr
Metabolized by liver, muscle, kidneys; excreted in urine

Interactions/incompatibilities:
• Increased hypoglycemia: salicylate, alcohol, β-blockers, anabolic steroids, fenfluramine, guanethidine, oral hypoglycemics, MAOIs, tetracycline, sulfinpyrazone
• Hyperglycemia: thiazides, thyroid hormones, oral contraceptives, corticosteroids, estrogens, dobutamine, epinephrine, smoking, dextrothyroxine

NURSING CONSIDERATIONS
Assess:
• Fasting blood glucose, 2 hr PP (60-100 mg/dl normal fasting level) (70-130 mg/dl-normal 2 hr level)

---

* Available in Canada only

• Urine ketones during illness; insulin requirements increase during times of stress, illness

Administer:

• After warming to room temperature by rotating in palms, to prevent lipodystrophy from injecting cold insulin

• Increased doses if tolerance occurs

Perform/provide:

• Storage at room temperature for <1 mo in cool area, refrigerate all other supply, do not use if discolored

• Rotation of injection sites: abdomen, upper back, thighs, upper arm, buttocks; keep record of sites

Evaluate:

• Therapeutic response: decrease in polyuria, polydipsia, polyphagia, clear sensorium, absence of dizziness, stable gait

• Hypoglycemic reaction that can occur during peak time

Teach patient/family:

• That blurred vision occurs, not to change corrective lens until vision is stabilized 1-2 mo

• To keep insulin, equipment available at all times

• That drug does not cure diabetes, but controls symptoms

• To carry Medic Alert ID as diabetic

• Hypoglycemia reaction: headache, tremors, fatigue, weakness

• Dosage, route, mixing instructions, if any diet restrictions, disease process

• To carry candy or lump sugar to treat hypoglycemia

• Symptoms of ketoacidosis: nausea, thirst, polyuria, dry mouth, decreased B/P, dry, flushed skin, acetone breath, drowsiness, Kussmaul respirations

• That a plan is necessary for diet, exercise; all food on diet should be eaten, exercise routine should not vary

• Urine glucose testing, make sure patient is able to determine glucose, acetone levels

• The pregnant patient to use glucose oxidase reagents

• To avoid OTC drugs unless directed by physician

Lab test interferences:

Increase: VMA

Decrease: Potassium, calcium

Interference: Liver function studies, thyroid function studies

Treatment of overdose: 10%-50% glucose PO if conscious or IV if comatose or 1 mg glucagon

---

interferon alfa-2a/interferon alfa-2b

(in-ter-ferón)

Roferon-a/Intron-a

Func. class.: Miscellaneous antineoplastic

Chem. class.: Protein product

Action: Antiviral action inhibits viral replication by reprogramming virus; antitumor action suppresses cell proliferation; immunomodulating action phagocytizes target cells

Uses: Hairy cell leukemia in persons >18 yr, condylomata acuminata, metastatic melanoma, AIDS

Dosage and routes:

• *Adult:* SC/IM (interferon alfa-2a) 3,000,000 IU × 16-24 wk, then 3,000,000 IU 3 × wk maintenance; SC/IM (interferon alfa-2b) 2,000,000 IU/m² 3 × wk; if severe adverse reactions occur, dose should be skipped or reduced by ½

Available forms include: alfa-2a inj 3, 18 million IU/vial; alfa-2b inj 3, 5, 10, 25 million IU/vial

Side effects/adverse reactions:

CNS: Dizziness, confusion, numbness, parethesias, hallucinations, ***convulsions, coma,*** amnesia, anxiety, mood changes

CV: Edema, hypotension, hypertension, chest pain, palpitations, dysrhythmias, ***CHF, MI, CVA***

INTEG: Rash, dry skin, itching, alopecia, flushing

GI: Weight loss, taste changes

GU: Impotence

MISC: Flu-like syndrome; fever, fatigue, myalgias, headache, chills

Contraindications: Hypersensitivity

Precautions: Severe hypotension, dysrhythmia, tachycardia, pregnancy (C), lactation, children, severe renal or hepatic disease, convulsion disorder

Pharmacokinetics:

Half-life (interferon alfa-2a) 3.7-8.5 hr, peak 3-4 hr; half-life (interferon alfa-2b) 2-7 hr, peak 6-8 hr

NURSING CONSIDERATIONS

Assess:

• For symptoms of infection, may be masked by drug fever

• CNS reaction: LOC, mental status, dizziness, confusion

Administer:

• At hs for minimizing side effects

• Acetaminophen as ordered to alleviate fever and headache

Perform/provide:

• Storage of reconstituted solution for 1 mo in refrigerator

• Increased fluid intake to 2-3 L/day

Evaluate:

• Therapeutic response: decrease in tumor size, increase in ease of breathing

Teach patient/family:

• To avoid hazardous tasks, since confusion, dizziness may occur

• That brands of this drug should not be changed; each form is different with different doses

• That fatigue is common, activity may need to be altered

• Not to become pregnant while taking drug

• To report signs of infection: sore throat, fever, diarrhea, vomiting

Lab test interferences:

Interference: AST, ALT, LDH, alk phosphatase, WBC, platelets, granulocytes, creatinine

---

Interferon alfa-n 3

(in-ter-feer'on)

Alferon N

Func. class.: Antineoplastic

Chem. class.: Human interferon alfa protein

Action: Binds interferon to membrane receptors on cell surface with high specificity; this produces protein synthesis, inhibition of virus replication, suppression of cell proliferide, and increased phagocytosis

Uses: Condylomata acuminata (veneral/genital warts)

Dosages and routes:

• *Adult:* 0.05 ml (250,000 IU) per wart, given 2 ×/wk × 8 wk; not to exceed 0.5 ml (2.5 million IU); inject into base of wart

Available forms include: Inj 5 m IU/1 ml vial with 3.3 mg/ml phenol and 1 mg/ml human albumin

Side effects/adverse reactions:

CNS: Fever, headache, sweating, vasovagal reaction, chills, fatigue, dizziness, insomnia, sleepiness, depression

GI: Nausea, vomiting, heartburn, diarrhea, constipation, anorexia, stomatitis, dry mouth

MS: Myalgias, arthralgia, back pain
INTEG: Pain at injection site, pruritis
CV: Chest pain, hypotension
Contraindications: Hypersensitivity to this product, egg protein, IgG, neomycin
Precautions: Pregnancy (C), lactation, children, CHF, angina (unstable), COPD, diabetes mellitus with ketoacidosis, hemophilia, pulmonary embolism, thrombophlebitis, bone marrow depression, convulsive disorder
Pharmacokinetics: Unable to detect
NURSING CONSIDERATIONS
Assess:
• For symptoms of infection, may be masked by drug fever
• CNS reaction: LOC, mental status, dizziness, confusion
Administer:
• Acetaminophen to alleviate fever and headache
Perform/provide:
• Storage of reconstituted solution for 1 mo in refrigerator
• Increased fluid intake to 2-3 L/day
Evaluate:
• Therapeutic response: decrease in wart size
Teach patient/family:
• To avoid hazardous tasks, since confusion, dizziness may occur
• That brands of this drug should not be changed; each form is different with different doses
• That fatigue is common, activity may need to be altered
• Not to become pregnant while taking drug
• To report signs of infection: sore throat, fever, diarrhea, vomiting
• Signs of hypersensitivity: liver, urticaria, wheezing, dyspnea; notify physician immediately
Lab test interferences:
Interferences: AST, ALT, LDH, alk phosphatase, WBC, platelets, granulocytes, creatinine

---

iodinated glycerol
Organidin, Isophen Elixir
Func. class.: Expectorant
Chem. class.: Iodopropylidene glycerol isom

Action: Increases respiratory tract fluid by decreasing surface tension, adhesiveness, which increases removal of mucus
Uses: Bronchial asthma, emphysema, bronchitis
Dosage and routes:
• *Adult:* PO 60 mg qid; SOL 20 gtts qid; ELIX 5 ml qid
• *Child:* PO up to half adult dose, depending on weight
Available forms include: Tabs 30 mg; sol 50 mg/ml, 60 mg/5 ml
Side effects/adverse reactions:
EENT: Burning mouth, throat, eye irritation, swelling of eyelids
GI: Gastric irritation
ENDO: Iodism, goiter, myxedema
RESP: Pulmonary edema
INTEG: **Angioedema,** rash
CNS: Frontal headache, ***CNS depression,*** fever, parkinsonism
Contraindications: Hypersensitivity to iodides, pulmonary TB, pregnancy (X), hyperthyroidism, hyperkalemia, newborns, lactation, acute bronchitis
Precautions: Hypothyroidism, cystic fibrosis, lactation
Pharmacokinetics: Excreted in urine
Interactions/incompatibilities:
• Increased hypothyroid effects: lithium, antithyroid drugs

---

italics = common side effects   ***bold italic*** = life threatening reactions

• Dysrhythmias, hyperkalemia: potassium-sparing diuretics, potassium-containing medication
NURSING CONSIDERATIONS
Administer:
• Orally in solution or tablet form
Perform/provide:
• Increased fluids to liquefy secretions
Evaluate:
• Therapeutic response: absence of cough
• Cough: type, frequency, character including sputum
Teach patient/family:
• Not to use if pregnant or if any potential for pregnancy
• Symptoms of iodism: eruptions, burning of oral cavity, eye irritation
• Symptoms of hyperthyroidism: CNS depression, fever, glomerulonephritis

---

iodoquinol

(eye-oh-do-kwin'ole)
Diodoquin,* Yodoxin, Amebaquine

Func. class.: Amebicide
Chem. class.: Dihalogenated derivative of 8-hydroxyquinoline

Action: Direct-acting amebicide; action occurs in intestinal lumen
Uses: Intestinal amebiasis
Dosage and routes:
• *Adult:* PO 630-650 mg tid × 20 days, not to exceed 2 g/day
• *Child:* PO 30-40 mg/kg/day in 2-3 divided doses × 20 days; do not repeat treatment before 2-3 wk
Available forms include: Tabs 210, 650 mg; powder
Side effects/adverse reactions:
HEMA: Agranulocytosis (rare)
INTEG: Rash, pruritus, discolored skin, alopecia
CNS: Headache, dizziness, ataxia

EENT: Blurred vision, sore throat, retinal edema, subacute myelooptic neuropathy
GI: Nausea, vomiting, diarrhea, epigastric distress, anorexia, gastritis, constipation, abdominal cramps, rectal irritation, itching
Contraindications: Hypersensitivity to this drug or iodine, renal disease, hepatic disease, severe thyroid disease, preexisting optic neuropathy
Precautions: Pregnancy (C)
NURSING CONSIDERATIONS
Assess:
• Stools during entire treatment; should be clear at end of therapy, stools should be free of parasites for 1 yr before patient is considered cured
• I&O, stools for number, frequency, character
Administer:
• PO after meals to avoid GI symptoms
Perform/provide:
• Storage in tight container
Evaluate:
• Iodism: skin eruption, urticaria, discoloring of hair, nails
• Allergic reaction: fever, rash, itching, chills; drug should be discontinued if these occur
• Blurred vision
• Superimposed infection, fever, monilial growth, fatigue, malaise
• Diarrhea for 2-3 days
Teach patient/family:
• Proper hygiene after BM: handwashing technique
• Avoid contact of drug with eyes, mouth, nose, other mucous membranes
• Need for compliance with dosage schedule, duration of treatment
Lab test interferences:
False positive: PKU

Increase: PBI
Decrease: ^{131}I uptake test

ipecac syrup
(ip′e-kak)

Func. class.: Emetic
Chem. class.: Cephaelis ipecacuanha derivative

Action: Acts on chemoreceptor trigger zone to induce vomiting, irritates gastric mucosa
Uses: In poisoning to induce vomiting
Dosage and routes:
• *Adult:* PO 15 ml, then 200-300 ml water
• *Child >1 yr:* PO 15 ml, then 200-300 ml water
• *Child <1 yr:* PO 5-10 ml, then 100-200 ml water; may repeat dose if needed
Available forms include: Liq
Side effects/adverse reactions:
CNS: Depression, convulsions, coma
GI: Nausea, vomiting, bloody diarrhea
CV: Circulatory failure, atrial fibrillation, fatal myocarditis, dysrhythmias
Contraindications: Hypersensitivity, unconscious/semiconscious, depressed gag reflex, poisoning with petroleum products or caustic substances, convulsions
Precautions: Lactation, pregnancy (C)
Pharmacokinetics:
PO: Onset 15-30 min
Interactions/incompatibilities:
• Do not administer with activated charcoal; effect will be decreased
NURSING CONSIDERATIONS
Assess:
• VS, B/P; check patients with cardiac disease more often

Administer:
• Ipecac *syrup* **not ipecac,** which is 14 times stronger; death may occur
• Then bounce child to increase emetic effect
• Activated charcoal if this drug doesn't work; may begin lavage after 10-15 min
Evaluate:
• Type of poisoning; do not administer if petroleum products or caustic substances have been ingested: kerosene, gasoline, lye, Drano
• Respiratory status before, during, after administration of emetic; check rate, rhythm, character; respiratory depression can occur rapidly with elderly or debilitated patients

ipratropium bromide
(eye-pra-troep′ee-um)
Atrovent

Func. class.: Anticholinergic
Chem. class.: Synthetic quaternary ammonium compound

Action: Inhibits interaction of acetylcholine at receptor sites on the bronchial smooth muscle, resulting in bronchodilation
Uses: Bronchodilation during bronchospasm in those with COPD
Dosage and routes:
• *Adult:* 2 INH 4 × day, not to exceed 12 INH/24 hr
Available forms include: Aerosol 18 μg/actuation
Side effects/adverse reactions:
GI: Nausea, vomiting, cramps
EENT: Dry mouth, blurred vision
CNS: Anxiety, dizziness, headache
RESP: Cough, worsening of symptoms
INTEG: Rash
CV: Palpitation

---

italics = common side effects   ***bold italic*** = life threatening reactions

Contraindications: Hypersensitivity to this drug or atropine

Precautions: Pregnancy (B), lactation, children <12 yr, narrow-angle glaucoma, prostatic hypertrophy, bladder neck obstruction

Pharmacokinetics:
Half-life 2 hr, does not cross blood-brain barrier

NURSING CONSIDERATIONS
Assess:
• For palpitations; if severe, drug may need to be changed

Perform/provide:
• Storage at room temperature
• Hard candy, frequent drinks, sugarless gum to relieve dry mouth

Evaluate:
• Therapeutic response: ability to breathe adequately
• For tolerance over long-term therapy; dose may need to be increased or changed

Teach patient/family:
• Compliance is necessary with number of inhalations/24 hr, or overdose may occur
• To shake before using
• Correct method of inhalation

---

iron dextran
Dextraron, Feostat, Hematran, Hydextran, Imferon, Irodex, K-Feron, Proferdex, Rocyte, Nor-Feran

Func. class.: Hematinic
Chem. class.: Ferric hydroxide complexed with dextran

Action: Iron is carried by transferrin to the bone marrow where it is incorporated into hemoglobin

Uses: Iron deficiency anemia

Dosage and routes:
• *Adult and child:* IM 0.5 ml as a test dose by Z-track, then no more than the following per day
• *Adult <50 kg:* IM 100 mg

• *Adult >50 kg:* IM 250 mg
• *Infant <5 kg:* IM 25 mg
• *Child <9 kg:* IM 50 mg
• *Adult:* IV 0.5 ml test dose then 100 mg qd after 2-3 days; IV 250/1000 ml of NaCl, give 25 mg test dose, wait 5 min, then infuse over 6-12 hr or follow equation

$$\frac{0.3 \times \text{wt (lb)} \times \frac{100\text{-Hgb (g/dl)} \times 100}{14.8}}{} = \text{mg iron}$$

<30 lb should be given 80% of above formula dose

Available forms include: Inj IM/IV 50 mg/ml, inj IM only 50 mg/ml

Side effects/adverse reactions:
CNS: Headache, paresthesia, dizziness, shivering, weakness, ***seizures***
GI: Nausea, vomiting, metallic taste, abdominal pain
INTEG: Rash, pruritus, urticaria, fever, sweating, chills, brown skin discoloration at injection site, necrosis, sterile abscesses, phlebitis
CV: Chest pain, ***shock,*** hypotension, tachycardia
RESP: Dyspnea
*HEMA: **Leukocytosis***
*Other: **Anaphylaxis***

Contraindications: Hypersensitivity, all anemias excluding iron deficiency anemia, hepatic disease

Precautions: Acute renal disease, children, asthma, lactation, rheumatoid arthritis (IV), infants <4 mo, pregnancy (C)

Pharmacokinetics:
IM: Excreted in feces, urine, bile, breast milk, crosses placenta, most absorbed through lymphatics, can be gradually absorbed over weeks/months from fixed locations

Interactions/incompatibilities:
• Not to mix with other drugs in syringe or D_5W

• Decreased reticulocyte response: chloramphenicol
• Increased toxicity: oral iron—do not use

NURSING CONSIDERATIONS
Assess:
• Blood studies: Hct, Hgb, reticulocytes, bilirubin before treatment, at least monthly
Administer:
• Only after test dose of 25 mg by preferred route; wait at least 1 hr before giving remaining portion
• IM deeply in large muscle mass, use Z-track method and a 19-20 G 2-3 inch needle; ensure needle is long enough to place drug deep in muscle
• IV, after flushing with 10 ml of NS; give undiluted; may be diluted in 50-250 normal saline for infusion
• IV injection requires single dose vial without preservative; verify on label IV use is approved
• Only with epinephrine available in case of anaphylactic reaction during dose

Perform/provide:
• Storage at room temperature in cool environment
• Recumbent position 30 min after injection

Evaluate:
• Allergy: *anaphylaxis*, rash, pruritus, fever, chills
• Cardiac status: anginal pain, hypotension, tachycardia
• Nutrition: amount of iron in diet (meat, dark green leafy vegetables, dried beans, dried fruits, eggs)
• Cause of iron loss or anemia including salicylates, sulfonamides

Teach patient/family:
• That iron poisoning may occur if increased beyond recommended level

Lab test interferences:
False increase: Serum bilirubin
False decrease: Serum calcium
False positive: ^{99m}Tc diphosphate bone scan, iron test (large doses >2 ml)

---

isocarboxazid
(eye-soe-kar-box'a-zid)
Marplan
Func. class.: Antidepressant—MAOI
Chem. class.: Hydrazine

Action: Increases concentrations of endogenous epinephrine, norepinephrine, serotonin, dopamine in storage sites in CNS by inhibition of MAO; increased concentration reduces depression
Uses: Depression, when uncontrolled by other means
Dosage and routes:
• *Adult:* PO 30 mg/day in divided doses, reduce dose to lowest effective dose when condition improves
Available forms include: Tabs 10 mg
Side effects/adverse reactions:
HEMA: Anemia
CNS: Dizziness, drowsiness, confusion, headache, anxiety, tremors, stimulation, weakness, hyperreflexia, mania, insomnia, fatigue, weight gain
GI: Constipation, dry mouth, nausea, vomiting, *anorexia,* diarrhea, weight gain
GU: Change in libido, frequency
INTEG: Rash, flushing, increased perspiration, jaundice
CV: Orthostatic hypotension, hypertension, dysrhythmias, hypertensive crisis
EENT: Blurred vision
ENDO: SIADH-like syndrome
Contraindications: Hypersensitiv-

---

italics = common side effects   ***bold italic*** = life threatening reactions

ity to MAOIs, elderly, hypertension, CHF, severe hepatic disease, pheochromocytoma, severe renal disease, severe cardiac disease

Precautions: Suicidal patients, convulsive disorders, severe depression, schizophrenia, hyperactivity, diabetes mellitus, pregnancy (C)

Pharmacokinetics:

PO: Duration up to 2 wk; metabolized by liver, excreted by kidneys

Interactions/incompatibilities:

• Increased pressor effects: guanethidine, clonidine, indirect acting sympathomimetics (ephedrine)

• Increased effects of: direct acting sympathomimetics (epinephrine), alcohol, barbiturates, benzodiazepines, CNS depressants, levodopa

• Hyperpyretic crisis, convulsions, hypertensive episode: tricyclic antidepressants, meperidine

• Hypoglycemic effect: increased insulin

NURSING CONSIDERATIONS

Assess:

• B/P (lying, standing), pulse; if systolic B/P drops 20 mm Hg hold drug, notify physician

• Blood studies: CBC, leukocytes, cardiac enzymes if patient is receiving long-term therapy

• Hepatic studies: ALT, AST, bilirubin, creatinine, hepatotoxicity may occur

Administer:

• Increased fluids, bulk in diet if constipation, urinary retention occur

• With food or milk for GI symptoms

• Crushed if patient is unable to swallow medication whole

• Dosage hs if over-sedation occurs during day

• Gum, hard candy, or frequent sips of water for dry mouth

• Phentolamine for severe hypertension

Perform/provide:

• Storage in tight container in cool environment

• Assistance with ambulation during beginning therapy since drowsiness/dizziness occurs

• Safety measures including siderails

• Checking to see PO medication swallowed

Evaluate:

• Toxicity: increased headache, palpitation; discontinue drug immediately; prodromal signs of hypertensive crisis

• Mental status: mood, sensorium, affect, memory (long, short), increase in psychiatric symptoms

• Urinary retention, constipation, edema, take weight weekly

• Withdrawal symptoms: headache, nausea, vomiting, muscle pain, weakness

Teach patient/family:

• That therapeutic effects may take 1-4 wk

• To avoid driving or other activities requiring alertness

• To avoid alcohol ingestion, CNS depressants or OTC medications: cold, weight, hay fever, cough syrup

• Not to discontinue medication quickly after long-term use

• To avoid high tyramine foods: cheese (aged), sour cream, beer, wine, pickled products, liver, raisins, bananas, figs, avocados, meat tenderizers, chocolate, yogurt; increase caffeine

• Report headache, palpitation, neck stiffness

Treatment of overdose: Lavage, activated charcoal, monitor electrolytes, vital signs, diazepam IV, $NaHCO_3$

isoetharine HCl/ isoetharine mesylate

(eye-soe-eth'a-reen)

Beta-Z solution, Bronkosol/Bronkometer

Func. class.: Adrenergic β_2 agonist

Action: Causes bronchodilation by β_2 stimulation, resulting in increased levels of cAMP, causing relaxation of bronchial smooth muscle with very little effect on heart rate

Uses: Bronchospasm, asthma

Dosage and routes:

• *Adult:* INH 3-7 puffs undiluted, IPPB 0.5 ml diluted 1:3 with NS

Available forms include: Sol for nebulization 0.06%, 0.08%, 0.1%, 0.125%, 0.17%, 0.2%, 0.25%, 0.5%, 10%

Side effects/adverse reactions:

CNS: Tremors, anxiety, insomnia, headache, dizziness, stimulation

CV: Palpitations, tachycardia, hypertension, *cardiac arrest,* dysrhythmias

GI: Nausea

• *META:* Hyperglycemia

Contraindications: Hypersensitivity to sympathomimetics, narrow-angle glaucoma

Precautions: Pregnancy (C), cardiac disorders, hyperthyroidism, diabetes mellitus, prostatic hypertrophy

Pharmacokinetics:

INH: Onset immediate, peak 5-15 min, duration 1-4 hr, metabolized in liver, GI tract, lungs, excreted in urine

Interactions/incompatibilities:

• Increased effects of both drugs: other sympathomimetics

• Decreased action when used with other β-blockers

• Hypertensive crisis: MAOIs

NURSING CONSIDERATIONS

Assess:

• Respiratory function: vital capacity, forced expiratory volume, ABGs, pulse, B/P

Administer:

• 2 hr before hs to avoid sleeplessness

Perform/provide:

• Storage at room temperature. Do not use solution if brown or contains a precipitate

Evaluate:

• Paresthesias and coldness of extremities, peripheral blood flow may decrease

• Therapeutic response: ease of breathing

Teach patient/family:

• Not to use OTC medications, extra stimulation may occur

• Use of inhaler, review package insert with patient

• To avoid getting aerosol in eyes

• To wash inhaler in warm water and dry qd

• On all aspects of drug; avoid smoking, smoke-filled rooms, persons with respiratory infections

isoflurophate

(eye-soe-flure'oh-fate)

Floropryl, Diisopropyl Fluorophosphate, Diflupyl

Func. class.: Miotic

Chem. class.: Cholinesterase inhibitor, irreversible

Action: Prevents breakdown of neurotransmitter acetylcholine, which then accumulates, causing enhancement, prolongation of its physiologic effects

Uses: Open-angle glaucoma, accommodative esotropia, conditions obstructing aqueous outflow

---

italics = common side effects   ***bold italic*** = life threatening reactions

Dosage and routes:
• *Adult and child:* INSTILL ¼ in strip of 0.25% oint in conjunctival sac q8-72 hr for glaucoma or qhs × 2 wk for esotropia
Available forms include: Only as ophthalmic ointment 0.25%
Side effects/adverse reactions:
CNS: Headache
CV: Hypotension, bradycardia, paradoxic tachycardia
RESP: **Bronchospasm,** dyspnea, bronchoconstriction, wheezing
EENT: Blurred vision, lacrimation, conjunctival congestion
GU: Urinary incontinence
GI: Abdominal cramps, diarrhea, increased salivation, nausea, vomiting
Contraindications: Hypersensitivity, uveal inflammation
Precautions: History of retinal detachment
NURSING CONSIDERATIONS
Administer:
• Ointment to conjunctival sac with patient supine
Teach patient/family:
• That top of tube must not come in contact with moisture; keep tube closed, dry, away from tears or cornea; to wash hands after application of ointment
• To report change in vision, blurring or loss of sight, trouble breathing, sweating, flushing
• That long-term therapy may be required
• That blurred vision will decrease with repeated use of drug
• To minimize effects of blurred vision, application should take place at bedtime
• To observe for signs/symptoms of systemic absorption (i.e., diarrhea, weakness)
• To observe eyes for irritation

• To monitor for cardiac, respiratory, or GI problems

isoniazid (INH)

(eye-soe-nye'a-zid)
Hyzyd, Isotamine,* Laniazid, Nydrazid, PMS-Isoniazid,* Rolazid, Teebaconin

Func. class.: Antitubercular
Chem. class.: Isonicotinic acid hydrazide

Action: Bactericidal interference with lipid, nucleic acid biosynthesis
Uses: Treatment, prevention of tuberculosis
Dosage and routes:
Treatment
• *Adult:* PO/IM 5 mg/kg qd as single dose for 9 mo to 2 yr, not to exceed 300 mg/day
• *Child and infants:* PO/IM 10-20 mg/kg qd as single dose for 18-24 mo, not to exceed 500 mg/day
Prevention
• *Adult* PO 300 mg qd as single dose × 12 mo
• *Child and infants:* PO/IM 10 mg/kg qd as single dose for 12 mo, not to exceed 300 mg/day
Available forms include: Tabs 50, 100, 300 mg; inj 100 mg/ml; powder
Side effects/adverse reactions:
INTEG: Dermatitis, photosensitivity
CNS: Headache, anxiety, drowsiness, tremors, **convulsions,** letnargy, depression, confusion, psychosis, aggression
EENT: Blurred vision, optic neuritis, photophobia, leukocytosis
Contraindications: Hypersensitivity, optic neuritis
Precautions: Pregnancy (C), renal disease, diabetic retinopathy, cataracts, ocular defects, child <13 yr

Pharmacokinetics:

PO: Peak 1-2 hr, duration 6-8 hr

IM: Peak 45-60 min

Metabolized in liver, excreted in urine (metabolites), crosses placenta, excreted in breast milk

Interactions/incompatibilities:

• Increased toxicity: alcohol, cycloserine, ethionamide, rifampin, carbamazepine

• Decreased absorption: aluminum antacids, benzodiazepines, MAOIs, phenytoin

NURSING CONSIDERATIONS

Assess:

• Liver studies q wk: ALT, AST, bilirubin

• Renal status: before, q mo: BUN, creatinine, output, sp gr, urinalysis

Administer:

• With meals to decrease GI symptoms

• Antiemetic if vomiting occurs

• After C&S is completed; q mo to detect resistance

Evaluate:

• Mental status often: affect, mood, behavioral changes; psychosis may occur

• Hepatic status: decreased appetite, jaundice, dark urine, fatigue

Teach patient/family:

• That compliance with dosage schedule, duration is necessary

• That scheduled appointments must be kept or relapse may occur

• Avoid alcohol while taking drug

• That, if diabetic, use Clinitest to obtain correct result

isoproterenol HCl/isoproterenol sulfate

(eye-soe-proe-ter'e-nole)

Isuprel, Proternol, Norisodrine, Vapo-Iso/Iso-Autohaler, Luf-Iso Inhalation, Medihaler-Iso, Norisodrine

Func. class.: Adrenergic

Chem. class.: Catecholamine

Action: Has β_1 and β_2 action. Relaxes bronchial smooth muscle and dilates the trachea and main bronchi, by increasing levels of cAMP, which relaxes smooth muscles; causes increased contractility and heart rate by acting on β-receptors in heart

Uses: Bronchospasm, asthma, heart block, ventricular dysrhythmias, shock

Dosage and routes:

Asthma, bronchospasm

• *Adult:* SL 10-20 mg q6-8h HCl; INH 1 puff, may repeat in 2-5 min, maintenance 1-2 puffs 4-6 × per day

• *Child:* SL 5-10 mg q6-8 HCl; INH 1 puff, may repeat in 2-5 min, maintenance 1-2 puffs 4-6× per day

Heart block/ventricular dysrhythmias

• *Adult:* IV 0.02-0.06, then 0.01-0.2 mg or 5 µg/min HCl; IM 0.2 mg, then 0.02-1 mg as needed HCl

• *Child:* IV/IM ½ of beginning adult dose

Shock

• *Adult and child:* IV INF 0.5-5 µg/min 1 mg/500 ml D₅W, titrate to B/P, CVP, and hourly urine output

Available forms include: Sol for nebulization 1:400 (0.25%), 1:200 (0.5%), 1:100 (1%); aerosol

0.25%, 0.2%; powd for INH 0.1 mg/cart; inj 1:5000 (0.2 mg/ml) IV, IM; glossets (SL) 10 mg

Side effects/adverse reactions:

CNS: Tremors, anxiety, insomnia, headache, dizziness, stimulation

CV: Palpitations, tachycardia, hypertension, *cardiac arrest*

GI: Nausea, vomiting

RESP: Bronchial irritation, edema, dryness of oropharynx

META: Hyperglycemia

Contraindications: Hypersensitivity to sympathomimetics, narrow-angle glaucoma

Precautions: Pregnancy (C), cardiac disorders, hyperthyroidism, diabetes mellitus, prostatic hypertrophy

Pharmacokinetics:

INH/SL: Onset 1-2 hr

SC: Onset 2 hr

REC: Onset 2-4 hr

Metabolized in liver, lungs, GI tract

Interactions/incompatibilities:
- Increased effects of both drugs: other sympathomimetics
- Decreased action when used with β-blockers

NURSING CONSIDERATIONS

Assess:
- Resp. function: B/P, pulse, lung sounds
- Blood studies (CBC, WBC, differential) since blood dyscrasias may occur (rare)
- I&O ratio; check for urinary retention, frequency, hesitancy

Administer:
- IV; dilute 0.2 mg/10 ml normal saline (1:50,000 sol); give over 1 min; 2 mg/500 ml of D₅W; run each 1 ml (1:250,000) sol/min; may be increased
- With meals for GI symptoms

Perform/provide:
- Storage at room temperature, do not use discolored solutions

Evaluate:
- For paresthesias and coldness of extremities, peripheral blood flow may decrease
- Injection site: tissue sloughing; if this occurs administer phentolamine mixed with NS
- Therapeutic response: increased B/P with stabilization, ease of breathing

Teach patient/family:
- To rinse mouth after use
- Use of inhaler, review package insert with patient
- To avoid getting aerosol in eyes
- To wash inhaler in warm water and dry qd
- On all aspects of drug; avoid smoking, smoke-filled rooms, persons with respiratory infections

Treatment of overdose: Administer a β-blocker

---

isosorbide

(eye-soe-sor′bide)

Ismotic

Func. class.: Miscellaneous ophthalmic agent

Action: Increases osmotic gradient between plasma and ocular fluids, which decreases intraocular pressure

Uses: Intraocular pressure from glaucoma and cataract

Dosage and routes:
- *Adult:* PO 1.5 g/kg, then increase to 1-3 g/kg bid-qid

Available forms include: Sol 45%

Side effects/adverse reactions:

CNS: Headache, lightheadedness, irritability, lethargy, syncope

GI: Nausea, vomiting, anorexia, diarrhea, cramps, thirst

INTEG: Rash

META: Hypernatremia, hyperosmolarity

Contraindications: Hypersensitivity, anuria, severe renal disease, pulmonary edema, hemorrhagic glaucoma, dehydration

Precautions: Pregnancy (C), patients on sodium restricted diet

NURSING CONSIDERATIONS
Assess:
• I&O, report decrease urinary output
• Electrolytes during treatment

Administer:
• After pouring over ice

---

isosorbide dinitrate

(eye-soe-sor′bide)

Iso-Bid, Isotrate, Isonate, Dilatrate-SR, Coronex,* Isordil, Sorbitrate

Func. class.: Antianginal

Chem. class.: Nitrate

Action: Decreases preload, afterload, which is responsible for decreasing left ventricular end-diastolic pressure, systemic vascular resistance

Uses: Chronic stable angina pectoris, prophylaxis of angina pain

Dosage and routes:
• *Adult:* PO 5-40 mg qid; SL 2.5-10 mg, may repeat q2-3h; CHEW TAB 5-10 mg prn or q2-3h as prophylaxis, sus rel 40-80 mg q8-12 h

Available forms include: Caps ext rel 40 mg; caps 40 mg; tabs 5, 10, 20, 30, 40 mg; chew tabs 5, 10 mg; tabs ext rel 40 mg; SL tabs 2.5, 5, 10 mg

Side effects/adverse reactions:
MISC: Twitching, hemolytic anemia, methemoglobinemia
CV: Postural hypotension, tachycardia, ***collapse,*** syncope
GI: Nausea, vomiting
INTEG: Pallor, sweating, rash
CNS: Vascular headache, flushing, dizziness, weakness, faintness

Contraindications: Hypersensitivity to this drug or nitrites, severe anemia, increased intracranial pressure, cerebral hemorrhage, acute MI

Precautions: Postural hypotension, pregnancy (C), lactation, children

Pharmacokinetics:
SUS ACTION: Duration 6-8 hr
PO: Onset 15-30 min, duration 4-6 hr
SL: Onset 2-5 min, duration 1-4 hr
CHEW TAB: Onset 3 min, duration ½-3 hr
Metabolized by liver, excreted in urine as metabolites (80%-100%)

Interactions/incompatibilities:
• Increased effects: β-blockers, diuretics, antihypertensives, alcohol

NURSING CONSIDERATIONS
Assess:
• B/P, pulse, respirations during beginning therapy

Administer:
• With 8 oz of water on empty stomach (oral tablet)

Evaluate:
• Pain: duration, time started, activity being performed, character
• Tolerance if taken over long period of time
• Headache, lightheadedness, decreased B/P; may indicate a need for decreased dosage

Teach patient/family:
• Leave tabs in original container
• If 3 SL tabs in 15 min does not relieve pain, go to ER
• Avoid alcohol
• May cause headache, but tolerance usually develops, taking with meals may reduce or eliminate headache
• That drug may be taken before stressful activity (exercise, sexual activity)
• That SL may sting when drug

I

---

italics = common side effects   ***bold italic*** = life threatening reactions

comes in contact with mucous membranes
• To avoid hazardous activities if dizziness occurs
• Stress patient compliance with complete medical regimen
• To make position changes slowly to prevent fainting
• Not to crush, chew SL or sus rel tabs

---

isotretinoin

(eye-soe-tret'i-noyn)
Accutane

Func. class.: Dermatologic
Chem. class.: Retinoic acid isomer, vitamin A derivative

Action: Decreases sebum secretion; improves cystic acne
Uses: Severe recalcitrant cystic acne
Dosage and routes:
• *Adult:* PO 1-2 mg/kg/day in 2 divided doses × 15-20 wk
Available forms include: Caps 10, 20, 40 mg
Side effects/adverse reactions:
INTEG: Dry skin, pruritus, cheilosis, joint muscle pain, hair loss, photosensitivity, urticaria, bruising, hirsutism
MS: Spine degeneration
CV: Chest pain
GI: Nausea, vomiting, anorexia, increased liver enzymes, regional ileus
EENT: Eye irritation, conjunctivitis, epistaxis, dry nose, mouth, contact lens intolerance
GU: Hematuria, proteinuria, hypouricemia
HEMA: Thrombocytopenia, decreased H&H, WBC, reticulocyte count
CNS: Lethargy, fatigue, headache, depression, *pseudotumor cerebri*

Contraindications: Hypersensitivity, severe renal disease, inflamed skin, pregnancy (X)
Precautions: Lactation, diabetes, photosensitivity
Pharmacokinetics:
PO: Peak 2.9-3.2 hr, half-life 10-20 hr; metabolized in liver, excreted in urine, feces
Interactions/incompatibilities:
• Additive toxic effects: vitamin A, do not use together
• Pseudotumor cerebri: minocycline or tetracycline
• Increased triglyceride levels: alcohol

NURSING CONSIDERATIONS
Assess:
• Triglyceride levels, AST, ALT, alk phosphatase; before, during treatment
• Urinalysis qwk for protein, blood
• Blood glucose in diabetics periodically
Administer:
• Whole, do not crush; give with meals
• Second course of treatment if needed after waiting 2 mo
Perform/provide:
• Storage in tight, light-resistant container
Evaluate:
• Therapeutic response: decrease in size and number of lesions
• Area of body involved, including time involved, what helps or aggravates condition
• Pseudotumor cerebri: headache, vomiting, nausea, visual disturbance; discontinue drug
Teach patient/family:
• To avoid sunlight or wear sunscreen since photosensitivity may occur
• That an increase in acne may occur during initial treatment; decrease in 4-6 wk

---

* Available in Canada only

• Not to become pregnant while taking drug
• Not to take vitamin A supplements, to take drug with meals
• Do not crush
• Minimize or eliminate alcohol consumption

Lab test interferences:
Increase: Sedimentation rate, triglyceride, liver function studies
Decrease: RBC/WBC count

---

isoxsuprine HCl
(eye-sox′syoo-preen)
Vasodilan, Voxsuprine
Func. class.: Peripheral vasodilator
Chem. class.: Nylidrin related agent

Action: α-Adrenoreceptor antagonist with β-adrenoreceptor stimulate properties; may also act directly on vascular smooth muscle; causes cardiac stimulation, uterine relaxation
Uses: Symptoms of cerebrovascular insufficiency, peripheral vascular disease including arteriosclerosis obliterans, thromboangiitis obliterans, Raynaud's disease
Dosage and routes:
• *Adult:* PO 10-20 mg tid or qid
Available forms include: Tabs 10, 20 mg
Side effects/adverse reactions:
*CV: Hypotension, **tachycardia,** palpitations, chest pain
CNS: Dizziness, weakness, tremors, anxiety
GI: Nausea, vomiting, abdominal pain, distention
INTEG: Severe rash, flushing
Contraindications: Hypersensitivity, postpartem, arterial bleeding
Precautions: Pregnancy (C), tachycardia

Pharmacokinetics:
PO: Peak 1 hr, duration 3 hr, half-life 1¼ hr; excreted in urine, crosses placenta
NURSING CONSIDERATIONS
Assess:
• B/P, pulse during treatment until stable; take B/P lying, standing; orthostatic hypotension is common
Administer:
• With meals to reduce GI upset
Perform/provide:
• Storage at room temperature
Evaluate:
• Therapeutic response: ability to walk without pain, increased pulse volume, increased temperature in extremities, orientation, long- and short-term memory
Teach patient/family:
• That medication is not cure, may need to be taken continuously depending on condition; therapeutic response may not be evident for 2-3 mo
• That it is necessary to quit smoking to prevent excessive vasoconstriction
• To avoid hazardous activities until stabilized on medication; dizziness may occur
• To make position changes slowly, or fainting will occur
• To discontinue drug, notify physician if rash develops
• To report palpitations, flushing if severe
• To avoid changes in temperature; extremities should be kept warm to promote better circulation

---

isradipine
DynaCirc
Func. class.: Calcium channel blocker
Chem. class.: Dihydropyridine

Action: Inhibits calcium ion influx

italics = common side effects   ***bold italic*** = life threatening reactions

across cell membrane during cardiac depolarization; produces relaxation of coronary vascular smooth muscle, peripheral vascular smooth muscle; dilates coronary vascular arteries; increases myocardial oxygen delivery in patients with vasospastic angina

Uses: Essential hypertension, angina

Dosage and routes:
Hypertension:
Adult: PO 1.25 mg bid, increase at 3-4 wk intervals up to 10 mg bid
Angina
Adult: PO 2.5-7.5 mg tid
Available forms include: Tabs 1.25 mg

Side effects/adverse reactions:
HEMA: ***Thrombocytopenia, leukopenia, anemia***
CV: Peripheral edema, tachycardia, hypotension, chest pain
GI: Nausea, vomiting, diarrhea, gastric upset, constipation, hepatitis
GU: Nocturia, polyuria, ***acute renal failure***
INTEG: Rash, pruritus, urticaria, photosensitivity, hair loss
CNS: Headache, fatigue, dizziness, fainting, sleep disturbances
MISC: Flushing

Contraindications: Sick sinus syndrome, 2nd or 3rd degree heart block, hypotension less than 90 mm Hg systolic, hypersensitivity

Precautions: CHF, hypotension, hepatic disease, pregnancy (C), lactation, children, renal disease, elderly

Pharmacokinetics: Metabolized in liver; metabolites are excreted in urine and feces; secreted in breast milk, peak plasma levels at 2-3 hr

Interactions/incompatibilities:
• Increased effects of: digitalis, neuromuscular blocking agents, cyclosporine
• Increased effects of isradipine: cimetidine, carbamazepine

NURSING CONSIDERATIONS
Assess:
• B/P, pulse rate, chest pain; monitor ECG periodically during therapy

Evaluate:
• Therapeutic response: decreased anginal pain, decreased B/P
• Cardiac status: B/P, pulse, respiration, ECG

Teach patient/family:
• To avoid hazardous activities until stabilized on drug, dizziness is no longer a problem
• To limit caffeine consumption
• To avoid OTC drugs unless directed by physician
• Stress patient compliance in all areas of medical regimen: diet, exercise, stress reduction, drug therapy
• To notify physician of: irregular heartbeat, shortness of breath, swelling of feet and hands, pronounced dizziness, constipation, nausea, hypotension

Treatment of overdose: Defibrillation, β-agonists, IV calcium inotropic agents, diuretics, atropine for AV block, vasopressor for hypotension

---

kanamycin sulfate
(kan-a-mye'sin)
Anamid,* Kantrex, Klebcil
Func. class.: Antibiotic
Chem. class.: Aminoglycoside

Action: Interferes with protein synthesis in bacterial cell by binding to ribosomal subunit, causing inaccurate peptide sequence to form in protein chain, causing bacterial death

Uses: Severe systemic infections of CNS, respiratory, GI, urinary tract, bone, skin, soft tissues caused by *E. coli, Enterobacter, Acinetobacter, Proteus, K. pneumoniae, S. marcescens, Staphylococcus;* also used as adjunct in hepatic coma, peritonitis, preoperatively to sterilize bowel

Dosage and routes:

Severe systemic infections

• *Adult and child:* IV INF 15 mg/kg/day in divided doses q8-12h; diluted 500 mg/200 ml of NS or D₅W given over 30-60 min, not to exceed 1.5 g/day; IM 15 mg/kg/day in divided doses q8-12h, not to exceed 1.5 g/day, irrigation not to exceed 1.5 g/day

Hepatic coma

• *Adult:* PO 8-12 g/day in divided doses

Preoperative bowel sterilization

• *Adult:* PO 1 g qlh × 4 doses, then q6h × 36-72 hr

Available forms include: Inj IM, IV 75, 500 mg/2ml, 1g/3 ml; irrigating sol 0.25%; cap 500 mg

Side effects/adverse reactions:

GU: Oliguria, hematuria, renal damage, azotemia, renal failure, nephrotoxicity

CNS: Confusion, depression, numbness, tremors, *convulsions,* muscle twitching, *neurotoxicity*

EENT: Ototoxicity, deafness, visual disturbances

HEMA: Agranulocytosis, thrombocytopenia, leukopenia, eosinophilia, anemia

GI: Nausea, vomiting, *anorexia,* increased ALT, AST, bilirubin, hepatomegaly, *hepatic necrosis,* splenomegaly

CV: Hypotension, myocarditis

INTEG: Rash, burning, urticaria, photosensitivity, dermatitis

Contraindications: Bowel obstruction, severe renal disease, hypersensitivity

Precautions: Neonates, myasthenia gravis, hearing deficits, mild renal disease, pregnancy (D), lactation

Pharmacokinetics:

IM: Onset rapid, peak 1-2 hr

IV: Onset immediate, peak 1-2 hr Plasma half-life 2-3 hr; not metabolized, excreted unchanged in urine, crosses placental barrier

Interactions/incompatibilities:

• Increased ototoxicity, neurotoxicity, nephrotoxicity: other aminoglycosides, amphotericin B, polymyxin, vancomycin, ethacrynic acid, furosemide, mannitol, methoxyflurane, cisplatin, cephalosporins

• Decreased effects of: parenteral penicillins, digoxin, vitamin B₁₂

• Do not mix in solution or syringe: carbenicillin, ticarcillin, amphotericin B, cephalothin, erythromycin, heparin

• Increased effects: nondepolarizing muscle relaxants

• Decreased effects of: oral anticoagulants

NURSING CONSIDERATIONS

Assess:

• Weight before treatment; calculation of dosage is usually done based on ideal body weight, but may be calculated on actual body weight

• I&O ratio, urinalysis daily for proteinuria, cells, casts; report sudden change in urine output

• VS during infusion, watch for hypotension, change in pulse

• IV site for thrombophlebitis including pain, redness, swelling q30 min, change site if needed; apply

K

---

italics = common side effects   ***bold italic*** = life threatening reactions

warm compresses to discontinued site
• Serum peak, drawn at 30-60 min after IV infusion or 60 min after IM injection; trough level drawn just before next dose; blood level should be 2-4 times bacteriostatic level
• Urine pH if drug is used for UTI; urine should be kept alkaline

Administer:
• IV after diluting 500 mg/100 ml of D_5W, D_5/NaCl normal saline or more, give 3-4 ml/min
• IM injection in large muscle mass, rotate injection sites
• Drug in evenly spaced doses to maintain blood level
• Bicarbonate to alkalinize urine if ordered in treating UTI, as drug is most active in alkaline environment

Perform/provide:
• Adequate fluids of 2-3 L/day unless contraindicated to prevent irritation of tubules
• Flush of IV line with NS or D_5W after infusion
• Supervised ambulation, other safety measures with vestibular dysfunction

Evaluate:
• Therapeutic effect: absence of fever, draining wounds, negative C&S after treatment
• Renal impairment by securing urine for CrCl testing, BUN, serum creatinine; lower dosage should be given in renal impairment (CrCl <80 ml/min)
• Deafness by audiometric testing, ringing, roaring in ears, vertigo; assess hearing before, during, after treatment
• Dehydration: high sp gr, decrease in skin turgor, dry mucous membranes, dark urine
• Overgrowth of infection: increased temperature, malaise, red-

ness, pain, swelling, perineal itching, diarrhea, stomatitis, change in cough, sputum
• C&S before starting treatment to identify infecting organism
• Vestibular dysfunction: nausea, vomiting, dizziness, headache; drug should be discontinued if severe
• Injection sites for redness, swelling, abscesses; use warm compresses at site

Teach patient/family:
• To report headache, dizziness, symptoms of overgrowth of infection, renal impairment
• To report loss of hearing, ringing, roaring in ears or feeling of fullness in head

Treatment of overdose: Hemodialysis, monitor serum levels of drug

---

kaolin, pectin
(kay'o-lynn)
Baropectin, Kaoparin, Kaopectate, Kapectin, Keotin, Pectokay
Func. class.: Antidiarrheal
Chem. class.: Hydrous magnesium aluminum silicate

Action: Decreases gastric motility, H_2O content of stool, adsorbent, demulcent
Uses: Diarrhea (cause undetermined)

Dosage and routes:
• *Adult:* PO 60-120 ml after each loose bowel movement
• *Child >12 yr:* PO 60 ml after each loose bowel movement
• *Child 6-12 yr:* PO 30-60 ml after each loose bowel movement
• *Child 3-6 yr:* PO 15-30 ml after each loose bowel movement
Available forms include: Susp Kaolin 0.87 g/5ml; Pectin 43 mg/5

ml; Kaolin 0.98 g/5 ml; Pectin 21.7 mg/5 ml
Side effects/adverse reactions:
GI: Constipation (chronic use)
Precautions: Pregnancy (C)
NURSING CONSIDERATIONS
Administer:
• For 48 hr only
Evaluate:
• Therapeutic response: decreased diarrhea
• Bowel pattern before; for rebound constipation
• Dehydration in children
Teach patient/family:
• Not to exceed recommended dose
• To shake well before administration

ketamine HCl

(keet'a-meen)
Ketalar
Func. class.: General anesthetic
Chem. class.: Phencyclidine derivative

Action: Acts on limbic system, cortex to provide anesthesia
Uses: Short anesthesia for diagnostic/surgical procedures
Dosage and routes:
• *Adult and child:* IV 1-4.5 mg/kg over 1 min
• *Adult and child:* IM 6.5-13 mg/kg
Available forms include: Inj IM, IV 10, 50, 100 mg/vial
Side effects/adverse reactions:
CNS: *Hallucinations, confusion, delirium, tremors, polyneuropathy, fasciculations, pseudoconvulsions*
CV: *Increased BP*, hypotension, bradycardia
EENT: *Diplopia, salivation*, small increase in intraocular pressure
INTEG: Rash, pain at injection site
Contraindications: Hypersensitivity, CVA, increased intracranial

pressure, severe hypertension, cardiac decompensation, child <2 yr
Precautions: Pregnancy (C), seizure disorders, elderly, psychiatric disorders
Pharmacokinetics:
IV: Peak 40 sec, duration 10 min
IM: Peak 3-8 min, duration 25 min
Interactions/incompatibilities:
• Increased action of ketamine: narcotics or atropine
• Respiratory depression: antihypertensives with CNS depressant effects
• Hypertension, tachycardia: thyroid hormones
• Increased action of: tubocurarine
• Do not mix with barbiturates in solution or syringe
NURSING CONSIDERATIONS
Assess:
• VS q10 min during IV administration, q30 min after IM dose
Administer:
• IV after diluting 100 mg/ml with equal parts of compatible sol; give over 1 min; may be diluted 10 ml (50 mg/ml)/500 ml of normal saline or D₅W; run at 1-2 mg/min
• Anticholinergic preoperatively to decrease solution
• Only with crash cart, resuscitative equipment nearby
• Narcotic, or diazepam to control recovery symptoms
Perform/provide:
• Quiet environment for recovery to decrease psychotic symptoms
Evaluate:
• Therapeutic response: maintenance of anesthesia
• Hallucinations, delusions, separation from environment
• Extrapyramidal reactions: dystonia, akathisia
• Increasing heart rate or decreasing B/P, notify physician at once

ketoconazole

(ke-to-con'a-zol)

Nizoral

Func. class.: Antifungal

Chem. class.: Imidazole derivative

Action: Alters cell membranes and inhibits several fungal enzymes

Uses: Systemic candidiasis, chronic mucocandidiasis, oral thrush, candiduria, coccidioidomycosis, histoplasmosis, chromomycosis, paracoccidioidomycosis

Dosage and routes:

• *Adult and child >40 kg:* PO 200 mg qd, may increase to 400 mg qd if needed

• *Child 20-40 kg:* PO 100 mg qd

• *Child <20 kg:* PO 50 mg qd

Available forms include: Tabs 200 mg; susp 100 mg/5 ml

Side effects/adverse reactions:

GU: Gynecomastia, impotence

INTEG: Pruritus, fever, chills, photophobia, rash, dermatitis, purpura, urticaria

CNS: Headache, dizziness, lethargy, anxiety, insomnia, dreams, paresthesia

SYST: Anaphylaxis

GI: Nausea, vomiting, anorexia, diarrhea, cramps, abdominal pain, constipation, flatulence, GI bleeding, *hepatotoxicity*

Contraindications: Hypersensitivity, pregnancy (C), lactation, meningitis

Precautions: Renal disease, hepatic disease, achlorhydria (drug-induced)

Pharmacokinetics:

PO: Peak 1-2 hr, half-life 2 hr, terminal 8 hr, metabolized in liver, excreted in bile, feces, requires acid pH for absorption, distributed poorly to CSF, highly protein bound

Interactions/incompatibilities:

• Hepatotoxicity: other hepatotoxic drugs

• Increased action of ketoconazole: cyclosporine

• Decreased action of: antacids, H_2-receptor antagonists, isoniazid, rifampin

• Increased anticoagulant effect, coumarin anticoagulants

• Severe hypoglycemia; oral hypoglycemics

• Disulfuram reaction: alcohol

NURSING CONSIDERATIONS

Assess:

• I&O ratio

• Liver studies (ALT, AST, bilirubin) if on long-term therapy

Administer:

• In the presence of acid products only; do not use alkaline products or antacids within 2 hr of drug; may give coffee, tea, acidic fruit juices

• With food to decrease GI symptoms

• With hydrochloric acid if achlorhydria is present

Perform/provide:

• Storage in tight containers at room temperature

Evaluate:

• Therapeutic response: decreased fever, malaise, rash, negative C&S for infecting organism

• For allergic reaction: rash, photosensitivity, urticaria, dermatitis

• For hepatotoxicity: nausea, vomiting, jaundice, clay-colored stools, fatigue

Teach patient/family:

• That long-term therapy may be needed to clear infection (1 wk-6 mo depending on infection)

• To avoid hazardous activities if dizziness occurs

• To avoid antacids, OTC medications, alkaline products

• Stress patient compliance with drug regimen
• To notify physician if GI symptoms, signs of liver dysfunction (fatigue, nausea, anorexia, vomiting, dark urine, pale stools)

ketoprofen

(ke-to-proe'fen)
Orudis
Func. class.: Nonsteroidal
Chem. class.: Propionic acid derivative

Action: Inhibits prostaglandin synthesis by decreasing enzyme needed for biosynthesis; possesses analgesic, antiinflammatory, antipyretic properties

Uses: Mild to moderate pain, osteoarthritis, rheumatoid arthritis, dysmenorrhea

Dosage and routes:
• *Adult:* PO 150-300 mg in divided doses tid-qid, not to exceed 300 mg/day
Available forms include: Caps 50, 75 mg

Side effects/adverse reactions:
GI: Nausea, anorexia, vomiting, diarrhea, jaundice, *cholestatic hepatitis,* constipation, flatulence, cramps, dry mouth, peptic ulcer
CNS: Dizziness, drowsiness, fatigue, tremors, confusion, insomnia, anxiety, depression
CV: Tachycardia, peripheral edema, palpitations, dysrhythmias
INTEG: Purpura, rash, pruritus, sweating
GU: Nephrotoxicity: dysuria, hematuria, oliguria, azotemia
HEMA: Blood dyscrasias
EENT: Tinnitus, hearing loss, blurred vision
Contraindications: Hypersensitivity, asthma, severe renal disease, severe hepatic disease

Precautions: Pregnancy (B), lactation, children, bleeding disorders, GI disorders, cardiac disorders, hypersensitivity to other antiinflammatory agents, elderly

Pharmacokinetics:
PO: Peak 2 hr, half-life 3-3½ hr, metabolized in liver, excreted in urine (metabolites), excreted in breast milk, 99% plasma protein binding

Interactions/incompatibilities:
• Increased action of: coumarin, streptokinase, probenecid

NURSING CONSIDERATIONS

Assess:
• Renal, liver, blood studies: BUN, creatinine, AST, ALT, Hgb, before treatment, periodically thereafter
• Audiometric, ophthalmic exam before, during, after treatment

Administer:
• With food to decrease GI symptoms; however, best to take on empty stomach to facilitate absorption

Perform/provide:
• Storage at room temperature

Evaluate:
• Therapeutic response: decreased pain, stiffness in joints, decreased swelling in joints, ability to move more easily
• For eye, ear problems: blurred vision, tinnitus; may indicate toxicity

Teach patient/family:
• To report blurred vision, ringing, roaring in ears; may indicate toxicity
• To avoid driving, other hazardous activities if dizziness, drowsiness occurs
• To report change in urine pattern, increased weight, edema, increased pain in joints, fever, blood in urine; indicate nephrotoxicity

K

---

italics = common side effects   ***bold italic*** = life threatening reactions

• That therapeutic effects may take up to 1 mo

---

ketorolac

(kec′toe-role-ak)
Toradol

Func. class.: Nonsteroidal antiinflammatory
Chem. class.: Pyrrole acetic acid derivative

Action: Inhibits prostaglandin synthesis by decreasing an enzyme needed for biosynthesis; possesses analgesic, antiinflammatory, antipyretic properties

Uses: Mild to moderate pain, osteoarthritis, rheumatoid arthritis

Dosage and routes:
• *Adult:* IM 10 mg qid

Available forms include: prefilled syringes 15, 30, 60 mg

Side effects/adverse reactions:
GI: Nausea, anorexia, vomiting, diarrhea, jaundice, ***cholestatic hepatitis,*** constipation, flatulence, cramps, dry mouth, peptic ulcer
CNS: Dizziness, drowsiness, fatigue, tremors, confusion, insomnia, anxiety, depression
CV: Tachycardia, peripheral edema, palpitations, dysrhythmias
INTEG: Purpura, rash, pruritus, sweating
GU: ***Nephrotoxicity: dysuria, hematuria, oliguria, azotemia***
HEMA: ***Blood dyscrasias***
EENT: Tinnitus, hearing loss, blurred vision

Contraindications: Hypersensitivity, asthma, severe renal disease, severe hepatic disease

Precautions: Pregnancy (B), lactation, children, bleeding disorders, GI disorders, cardiac disorders, hypersensitivity to other antiinflammatory agents

Pharmacokinetics:
IM: Peak 50 min, half-life 6 hr

Interactions/incompatibilities:
• Increased action of ketorolac: phenytoin, sulfonamides

NURSING CONSIDERATIONS
Assess:
• Renal, liver, blood studies: BUN, creatinine, AST, ALT, Hgb before treatment, periodically thereafter
• Audiometric, ophthalmic exam before, during, after treatment

Administer:
• With food to decrease GI symptoms; best to take on empty stomach to facilitate absorption

Perform/provide:
• Storage at room temperature

Evaluate:
• Therapeutic response: decreased pain, stiffness, swelling in joints, ability to move more easily
• For eye, ear problems: blurred vision, tinnitus (may indicate toxicity)

Teach patient/family:
• To report blurred vision or ringing, roaring in ears (may indicate toxicity)
• To avoid driving or other hazardous activities if dizziness or drowsiness occurs
• To report change in urine pattern, weight increase, edema, pain increase in joints, fever, blood in urine (indicates nephrotoxicity)
• That therapeutic effects may take up to 1 mo
• To take with a full glass of water

---

labetalol

(la-bet′a-lole)
Normodyne, Trandate

Func. class.: Antihypertensive
Chem. class.: Nonselective β-blocker

Action: Produces falls in B/P with-

---

* Available in Canada only

out reflex tachycardia or significant reduction in heart rate through mixture of α-blocking, β-blocking effects; elevated plasma renins are reduced

Uses: Mild to moderate hypertension

Dosage and routes:
Hypertension
• *Adult:* PO 100 mg bid, may be given with a diuretic, may increase to 200 mg bid after 2 days, may continue to increase q1-3 days; max 400 mg bid

Hypertensive crisis
• *Adult:* IV INF 200 mg/160 ml D₅W, run at 2 ml/min; stop infusion after desired response obtained, repeat q6-8h as needed; IV BOL 20 mg over 2 min, may repeat 40-80 mg q10 min, not to exceed 300 mg

Available forms include: Tabs 100, 200, 300 mg, inj 5 mg/ml in 20 ml amps

Side effects/adverse reactions:
*CV: Orthostatic hypotension, bradycardia, **CHF,** chest pain, **ventricular dysrhythmias,** AV block*
CNS: Dizziness, mental changes, drowsiness, fatigue, headache, catatonia, depression, anxiety, nightmares, paresthesias, lethargy
GI: Nausea, vomiting, diarrhea
INTEG: Rash, alopecia, urticaria, pruritus, fever
*HEMA: **Agranulocytosis, thrombocytopenia, purpura** (rare)*
EENT: Tinnitus, visual changes, sore throat, double vision, dry burning eyes
GU: Impotence, dysuria, ejaculatory failure
*RESP: **Bronchospasm,** dyspnea, wheezing*

Contraindications: Hypersensitivity to β-blockers, cardiogenic shock, heart block (2nd, 3rd degree), sinus bradycardia, CHF, bronchial asthma

Precautions: Major surgery, pregnancy (C), lactation, diabetes mellitus, renal disease, thyroid disease, COPD, well compensated heart failure, CAD, nonallergic bronchospasm

Pharmacokinetics:
PO: Onset 1-2 hr, peak 2-4 hr, duration 8-12 hr
IV: Peak 5 min
Half-life 6-8 hr, metabolized by liver (metabolites inactive), excreted in urine, bile, crosses placenta, excreted in breast milk

Interactions/incompatibilities:
• Increased bronchodilation: β-adrenergic agonists
• Increased hypotension: diuretics, other antihypertensives, halothane, cimetidine, nitroglycerin
• Decreased effects: sympathomimetics, lidocaine, indomethacin, theophylline, cimetidine
• Increased hypoglycemia: insulin

NURSING CONSIDERATIONS
Assess:
• I&O, weight daily
• B/P during beginning treatment, periodically thereafter, pulse q4h; note rate, rhythm, quality
• Apical/radial pulse before administration; notify physician of any significant changes
• Baselines in renal, liver function tests before therapy begins

Administer:
• IV undiluted or diluted in compatible sol; give undiluted 20 mg or less/2 min; infusion is titrated to patient response
• PO ac, hs, tablet may be crushed or swallowed whole
• Reduced dosage in renal dysfunction

italics = common side effects   ***bold italic*** = life threatening reactions

• IV, keep patient recumbent for 3 hr

Perform/provide:

• Storage in dry area at room temperature, do not freeze

Evaluate:

• Therapeutic response: decreased B/P after 1-2 wk

• Edema in feet, legs daily

• Skin turgor, dryness of mucous membranes for hydration status

Teach patient/family:

• Not to discontinue drug abruptly, taper over 2 wk, may cause precipitate angina

• Not to use OTC products containing α-adrenergic stimulants (nasal decongestants, OTC cold preparations) unless directed by physician

• To report bradycardia, dizziness, confusion, depression, fever

• To take pulse at home, advise when to notify physician

• To avoid alcohol, smoking, sodium intake

• To comply with weight control, dietary adjustments, modified exercise program

• To carry Medic Alert ID to identify drug you are taking, allergies

• To avoid hazardous activities if dizziness is present

• To report symptoms of CHF: difficult breathing, especially on exertion or when lying down, night cough, swelling of extremities

• Take medication at bedtime to prevent effect of orthostatic hypotension

• Wear support hose to minimize effects of orthostatic hypotension

Lab test interferences:

False increase: Urinary catecholamines

Treatment of overdose: Lavage, IV atropine for bradycardia, IV theophylline for bronchospasm, digitalis, O_2, diuretic for cardiac failure; hemodialysis is useful for removal, hypotension; administer vasopressor (norepinephrine)

---

lactobacillus

(lak'tyoo-ba-sill-us)

Bacid, DoFUS, Lactinex

Func. class.: Antidiarrheal

Chem. class.: Viable bacterial culture

Action: Decreases growth of organisms causing diarrhea in bowel

Uses: Diarrhea (cause undetermined), diarrhea caused by antibiotics

Dosage and routes:

• *Adult:* PO 2 caps bid-qid (Bacid), 4 tabs tid-qid (Lactinex), 1 tab qd ac (DoFUS); powder 1 pkg tid-qid (Lactinex)

Available forms include: Caps, granules 1 g/pkg, chew tabs

Side effects/adverse reactions:

GI: Flatus, fruity odor to stools with Bacid

Contraindications: Hypersensitivity, fever, child <3 yr, milk allergy

NURSING CONSIDERATIONS

Administer:

• With water, fruit juice, or milk

• For antibiotic-induced diarrhea

• Granules or tabs with cereal, food, milk, fruit juice, water

Evaluate:

• Therapeutic response: decreased diarrhea

• Bowel pattern before; for rebound constipation

• Response after 48 hr; if no response, drug should be discontinued

• Dehydration in children; do not use in infants or children <3 yr

---

Teach patient/family:
• Not to exceed recommended dose
• To store in refrigerator

---

lactulose

(lak'tyoo-lose)
Cephulac, Chronulac

Func. class.: Ammonia detoxicant
Chem. class.: Lactose synthetic derivative

Action: Prevents absorption of ammonia in colon
Uses: Constipation, portal-systemic encephalopathy in patients with hepatic disease
Dosage and routes:
Constipation
• *Adult:* PO 15-60 ml qd
Encephalopathy
• *Adult:* PO 20-30 g tid or qid until stools are soft; RET ENEMA 30-45 ml in 100 ml of fluid
Available forms include: Oral sol, rec sol 3.33 g/5 ml
Side effects/adverse reactions:
GI: Nausea, vomiting, anorexia, cramps, diarrhea, flatulence
Contraindications: Hypersensitivity, low galactose diet
Precautions: Pregnancy (C), lactation, diabetes mellitus
Pharmacokinetics: Metabolized in intestine, excreted by kidneys
Interactions/incompatibilities:
• Decreased effects of lactulose: neomycin, other oral antiinfectives
NURSING CONSIDERATIONS
Assess:
• Blood ammonia level (30-70 mg/100 ml)
• Blood, urine electrolytes if drug is used often by patient
• I&O ratio to identify fluid loss
Administer:
• With fruit juice, water, milk to increase palatability of oral form

• Retention enema by diluting 300 ml lactose/700 ml of water; administer by rectal balloon catheter
• Increase fluids to 2 L/day, do not give with other laxatives; if diarrhea occurs, reduce dosage
Evaluate:
• Therapeutic response: decreased constipation, decreased blood ammonia level
• Cause of constipation; identify whether fluids, bulk, or exercise is missing from lifestyle
• Cramping, rectal bleeding, nausea, vomiting; if these symptoms occur, drug should be discontinued
• Clearing of confusion, lethargy, restlessness, irritability
Teach patient/family:
• Not to use laxatives for long-term therapy; bowel tone will be lost

---

leucovorin calcium (citrovorum factor/folinic acid)

(loo-koe-vor'in)
Calcium Folinate, Wellcovorin

Func. class.: Vitamin/folic acid antagonist antidote
Chem. class.: Tetrahydrofolic acid derivative

Action: Needed for normal growth patterns, prevents toxicity during antineoplastic therapy by protecting normal cells
Uses: Megaloblastic or macrocytic anemia caused by folic acid deficiency, overdose of folic acid antagonist, methotrexate toxicity, toxicity caused by pyrimethamine or trimethoprim, pneumocystosis, toxoplasmosis
Dosage and routes:
Megaloblastic anemia caused by enzyme deficiency

---

italics = common side effects   ***bold italic*** = life threatening reactions

• *Adult and child:* IM 3-6 mg qd, then 1 mg PO for life
Megaloblastic anemia caused by deficiency of folate
• *Adult and child:* IM 1 mg or less qd, continued until adequate response
Methotrexate toxicity
• *Adult and child:* Given 6-36 hr after dose of methotrexate
Pyrimethamine toxicity
• *Adult and child:* PO/IM 5 mg qd
Trimethoprim toxicity
• *Adult and child:* PO IM 400 µg qd
Available forms include: Tabs 5, 25 mg; inj IM 3, 5 mg/ml; powder for inj 10 mg/ml
Side effects/adverse reactions:
RESP: Wheezing
INTEG: Rash, pruritus, erythema
Contraindications: Hypersensitivity, anemias other than megaloblastic not associated with B_{12} deficiency
Precautions: Pregnancy (C)
Interactions/incompatibilities:
• Decreased folate levels: chloramphenicol
• Increased metabolism of: phenobarbitol, hydantoins
NURSING CONSIDERATIONS
Assess:
• CrCl before leucovorin rescue and qd to detect nephrotoxicity
• I&O, watch for nausea and vomiting
Administer:
• Within 1 hr of folic acid antagonist
• After reconstituting with bacteriostatic water for inj
Perform/provide:
• Increase fluid intake if used to treat folic acid inhibitor overdose
• Protection from light and heat
Evaluate:
• Nutritional status: bran, yeast, dried beans, nuts, fruits, fresh vegetables, asparagus
• Therapeutic response: increased weight, oriented well-being, absence of fatigue
• Drugs currently taken: alcohol, hydantoins, trimethoprim may cause increased folic acid use by body
Teach patient/family:
• To take drug exactly as prescribed
• To notify physician of side effects

---

leuprolide acetate
(loo-proe'-lide)
Lupron
Func. class.: Antineoplastic hormone
Chem. class.: Gonadotropin-releasing antigen

Action: Suppresses testosterone production by stimulating FSH, then inhibiting FSH, LH; currently investigational in Canada
Uses: Metastatic prostate cancer
Dosage and routes:
• *Adult:* SC 1 mg/day
Available forms include: Inj SC 5 mg/ml
Side effects/adverse reactions:
GI: Nausea, vomiting, anorexia
GU: Edema, hot flashes, impotence, decreased libido, amenorrhea, vaginal bleeding, gynecomastia
INTEG: Rash
*CV: **Cardiac dysrhythmias, MI,** peripheral edema*
MS: Bone pain, myalgia
Contraindications: Hypersensitivity to estradiol, thromboembolic disorders, pregnancy (D)
Precautions: Edema, hepatic disease, CVA, MI, seizures, hypertension, diabetes mellitus

NURSING CONSIDERATIONS
Assess:
• Liver function tests before, during therapy (bilirubin, AST, ALT, LDH) as needed or monthly
• RBC, Hct, Hgb since these may be decreased

Perform/provide:
• Nutritious diet with iron, vitamin supplements as ordered
• Storage in tight container at room temperature

Evaluate:
• Fatigue, increased pulse, pallor, lethargy
• Food preferences; list likes, dislikes
• Edema in feet, joint, stomach pain, shaking
• Symptoms indicating severe allergic reaction: rash, pruritus, urticaria, purpuric skin lesions, itching, flushing

Teach patient/family:
• To report any complaints, side effects to nurse or physician
• How to prepare, give and rotate sites for SC injections
• To keep accurate records of dose
• How to deal with tumor flare

---

levodopa
(lee-voe-doe'pa)
Dopar, Larodopa, Levopa, Parda, Rio-Dopa
Func. class.: Antiparkinson agent
Chem. class.: Catecholamine

Action: Decarboxylation to dopamine, which increases dopamine levels in brain

Uses: Parkinsonism, carbon monoxide, chronic manganese intoxication, cerebral arteriosclerosis

Dosage and routes:
• *Adult:* PO 0.5-1 g qd divided bid-qid with meals, may increase by up to 0.75 g q3-7 days, not to exceed 8 g/day unless closely supervised
Available forms include: Caps 100, 250, 500 mg; tabs 100, 250, 500 mg

Side effects/adverse reactions:
HEMA: ***Hemolytic anemia, leukopenia, agranulocytosis***
CNS: Involuntary choreiform movements, hand tremors, fatigue, headache, anxiety, twitching, numbness, weakness, confusion, agitation, insomnia, nightmares, psychosis, hallucination, hypomania, severe depression, dizziness
GI: Nausea, vomiting, anorexia, abdominal distress, dry mouth, flatulence, dysphagia, bitter taste, diarrhea, constipation
INTEG: Rash, sweating, alopecia
CV: Orthostatic hypotension, tachycardia, hypertension, palpitation
EENT: Blurred vision, diplopia, dilated pupils
MISC: Urinary retention incontinence, weight change, dark urine

Contraindications: Hypersensitivity, narrow-angle glaucoma, undiagnosed skin lesions

Precautions: Renal disease, cardiac disease, hepatic disease, respiratory disease, MI with dysrhythmias, convulsions, peptic ulcer, pregnancy (C)

Pharmacokinetics:
PO: Peak 1-3 hr, excreted in urine (metabolites)

Interactions/incompatibilities:
• Hypertensive crisis: MAOIs, furazolidone
• Decreased effects of levodopa: anticholinergics, hydantoins, methionine, papaverine, pyridoxine, tricyclics
• Increased effects of levodopa: antacids, metoclopramide

---

italics = common side effects   ***bold italic*** = life threatening reactions

NURSING CONSIDERATIONS
Assess:
• B/P, respiration
Administer:
• Drug up until NPO before surgery
• Adjust dosage depending on patient response
• With meals; limit protein taken with drug
• Only after MAOIs have been discontinued for 2 wk
Perform/provide:
• Assistance with ambulation, during beginning therapy
• Testing for diabetes mellitus, acromegaly if on long-term therapy
Evaluate:
• Mental status: affect, mood, behavioral changes, depression, complete suicide assessment
• Therapeutic response: decrease in akathesia, increased mood
Teach patient/family:
• To change positions slowly to prevent orthostatic hypotension
• To report side effects: twitching, eye spasms; indicate overdose
• To use drug exactly as prescribed; if drug is discontinued abruptly, parkinsonian crisis may occur
• That urine, sweat may darken
• To avoid vitamin B₆ preparations, vitamin-fortified foods containing B₆; these foods can reverse effects of levodopa
Lab test interferences:
False positive: Urine ketones, urine glucose
False negative: Urine glucose (glucose oxidase)
False increase: Uric acid, urine protein
Decrease: VMA

levodopa-carbidopa
(lee-voe-doe′pa) (kar-bi-doe′pa)
Sinemet
Func. class.: Antiparkinson agent
Chem. class.: Catecholamine

Action: Decarboxylation of levodopa to periphery is inhibited by carbidopa; more levodopa is made available for transport to brain and conversion to dopamine in the brain
Uses: Parkinsonism resulting from carbon monoxide, chronic manganese intoxication, cerebral arteriosclerosis
Dosage and routes:
• *Adult:* PO 3-6 tabs of 25 mg carbidopa/250 mg levodopa qd in divided doses, not to exceed 8 tabs/day
Available forms include: Tabs 10/100, 25/100, 25 mg carbidopa/250 mg levodopa
Side effects/adverse reactions:
HEMA: **Hemolytic anemia, leukopenia, agranulocytosis**
CNS: Involuntary choreiform movements, hand tremors, fatigue, headache, anxiety, twitching, numbness, weakness, confusion, agitation, insomnia, nightmares, psychosis, hallucination, hypomania, severe depression, dizziness
GI: Nausea, vomiting, anorexia, abdominal distress, dry mouth, flatulence, dysphagia, bitter taste, diarrhea, constipation
INTEG: Rash, sweating, alopecia
CV: Orthostatic hypotension, tachycardia, hypertension, palpitation
EENT: Blurred vision, diplopia, dilated pupils
MISC: Urinary retention, incontinence, weight change, dark urine

Contraindications: Hypersensitivity, narrow-angle glaucoma, undiagnosed skin lesions
Precautions: Renal disease, cardiac disease, hepatic disease, respiratory disease, MI with dysrhythmias, convulsions, peptic ulcer, pregnancy (C)
Pharmacokinetics:
PO: Peak 1-3 hr, excreted in urine (metabolites)
Interactions/incompatibilities:
• Hypertensive crisis: MAOIs, furazolidone
• Decreased effects of levodopa: anticholinergics, hydantoins, methionine, papaverine, pyridoxine, tricyclics
• Increased effects of levodopa: antacids, metoclopramide
NURSING CONSIDERATIONS
Assess:
• B/P, respiration
Administer:
• Drug up until NPO before surgery
• Adjust dosage depending on patient response
• With meals; limit protein taken with drug
• Only after MAOIs have been discontinued for 2 wk; if previously on levodopa, discontinue for at least 8 hr before change to levodopa-carbidopa
Perform/provide:
• Assistance with ambulation during beginning therapy
• Testing for diabetes mellitus, acromegaly if on long-term therapy
Evaluate:
• Mental status: affect, mood, behavioral changes, depression, complete suicide assessment
• Therapeutic response: decrease in akathasia, increased mood
Teach patient/family:
• To change positions slowly to prevent orthostatic hypotension

• To report side effects: twitching, eye spasms; indicate overdose
• To use drug exactly as prescribed; if drug is discontinued abruptly, parkinsonian crisis may occur; MD may recommend drug-free holidays
• That urine, sweat may darken
• To use physical activities to maintain mobility and lessen spasms
• That improvement may not occur for 3-4 months
Lab test interferences:
False positive: Urine ketones
False negative: Urine glucose
False increase: Uric acid, urine protein
Decrease: VMA, BUN, creatinine

---

levorphanol tartrate
(lee-vor'fa-nole)
Levo-Dromoran

Func. class.: Narcotic analgesics
Chem. class.: Opiate, synthetic morphine derivative

Controlled Substance Schedule II
Action: Depresses pain impulse transmission at the spinal cord level by interacting with opioid receptors
Uses: Moderate to severe pain
Dosage and routes:
• *Adult:* PO/SC/IV 2-3 mg q6-8h prn
Available forms include: Inj SC/IV 2 mg/ml; tabs 2 mg
Side effects/adverse reactions:
CNS: Drowsiness, dizziness, confusion, headache, sedation, euphoria
GI: Nausea, vomiting, anorexia, constipation, cramps
GU: Increased urinary output, dysuria
INTEG: Rash, urticaria, bruising, flushing, diaphoresis, pruritus

EENT: Tinnitus, blurred vision, miosis, diplopia
CV: Palpitations, bradycardia, change in B/P
RESP: Respiratory depression
Contraindications: Hypersensitivity, addiction (narcotic)
Precautions: Addictive personality, pregnancy (B), lactation, increase intracranial pressure, MI (acute), severe heart disease, respiratory depression, hepatic disease, renal disease, child <18 yr
Pharmacokinetics:
SC: Peak 1-½ hr, duration 6-8 hr
IV: Peak 20 min, duration 6-8 hr; metabolized by liver, excreted by kidneys, crosses placenta, excreted in breast milk, half-life 11 hr
Interactions/incompatibilities:
• Effects may be increased with other CNS depressants: alcohol, narcotics, sedative/hypnotics, antipsychotics, skeletal muscle relaxants

NURSING CONSIDERATIONS
Assess:
• I&O ratio; check for decreasing output; may indicate urinary retention
Administer:
• With antiemetic if nausea, vomiting occur
• When pain is beginning to return; determine dosage interval by patient response
• IV directly over 5 min
Perform/provide:
• Storage in light-resistant area at room temperature
• Assistance with ambulation
• Safety measures: siderails, night light, call bell within easy reach
Evaluate:
• Therapeutic response: decrease in pain
• CNS changes: dizziness, drowsiness, hallucinations, euphoria, LOC, pupil reaction
• Allergic reactions: rash, urticaria
• Respiratory dysfunction: respiratory depression, character, rate, rhythm; notify physician if respirations are <10/min
• Need for pain medication, physical dependence
Teach patient/family:
• To report any symptoms of CNS changes, allergic reactions
• That physical dependency may result when used for extended periods of time
• Withdrawal symptoms may occur: nausea, vomiting, cramps, fever, faintness, anorexia
Lab test interferences:
Increase: Amylase
Treatment of overdose: Narcan 0.2-0.8 IV, O_2, IV fluids, vasopressors

---

levothyroxine sodium (T_4, L-thyroxine sodium)

(lee-voe-thye-rox′een)

Eltroxin, Levoid, Levothroid, Noroxine, Synthroid, Syroxine, Synthrox

Func. class.: Thyroid hormone
Chem. class.: Levoisomer of thyroxine

Action: Increases metabolic rates, increases cardiac output, O_2 consumption, body temperature, blood volume, growth, development at cellular level
Uses: Hypothyroidism, myxedema coma, thyroid hormone replacement, cretinism, euthyroid states, thyrotoxicosis
Dosage and routes:
• *Adult:* PO 0.025-0.1 mg qd, increased by 0.05-0.1 mg q1-4 wk

---

until desired response, maintenance dose 0.1-0.4 mg qd
• *Child:* PO 0.01-0.05 qd, may increase 0.025-0.05 mg q1-4 wk until desired response

Cretinism
• *Child:* IV 0.025-0.05 mg qd, may increase by 0.05-0.1 mg PO q2-3 wk

Myxedema coma
• *Adult:* IV 0.2-0.5 mg, may increase by 0.1-0.3 mg after 24 hr; place on oral medication as soon as possible

Available forms include: Inj IV 200, 500 µg/vial; tabs 0.025, 0.05, 0.075, 0.1, 0.125, 0.15, 0.175, 0.2, 0.3 mg

Side effects/adverse reactions:
CNS: Anxiety, insomnia, tremors, headache, *thyroid storm*
CV: Tachycardia, palpitations, angina, dysrhythmias, hypertension, *cardiac arrest*
GI: Nausea, diarrhea, increased or decreased appetite, cramps
MISC: Menstrual irregularities, weight loss, sweating, heat intolerance, fever

Contraindications: Adrenal insufficiency, myocardial infarction, thyrotoxicosis

Precautions: Elderly, angina pectoris, hypertension, ischemia, cardiac disease, pregnancy (A), lactation

Pharmacokinetics:
IV/PO: Peak 12-48 hr, half-life 6-7 days; distributed throughout body tissues

Interactions/incompatibilities:
• Decreased absorption of levothyroxine: cholestyramine
• Increased effects of: anticoagulants, sympathomimetics, tricyclic antidepressants
• Decreased effects of: digitalis drugs, insulin, hypoglycemics

• Decreased effects of levothyroxine: estrogens

NURSING CONSIDERATIONS
Assess:
• B/P, pulse before each dose
• I&O ratio
• Weight qd in same clothing, using same scale, at same time of day
• Height, growth rate if given to a child
• T_3, T_4, FTIs which are decreased, radioimmunoassay of TSH, which is increased, radio uptake, which is decreased if patient is on too low a dose of medication
• Pro-time may require decreased anticoagulant, check for bleeding, bruising

Administer:
• IV after diluting with provided diluent 0.5 mg/5 ml; shake; give through Y-tube or 3-way stopcock; give 0.1 mg or less over 1 min
• In AM if possible as a single dose to decrease sleeplessness
• At same time each day, to maintain drug level
• Only for hormone imbalances, not to be used for obesity, male infertility, menstrual conditions, lethargy
• Lowest dose that relieves symptoms

Perform/provide:
• Storage in tight, light-resistant container; solutions should be discarded if not used immediately
• Removal of medication 4 wk before RAIU test

Evaluate:
• Therapeutic response: absence of depression, increased weight loss, diuresis, pulse, appetite, absence of constipation, peripheral edema, cold intolerance, pale, cool dry skin, brittle nails, alopecia, coarse hair, menorrhagia, night blindness,

L

italics = common side effects   ***bold italic*** = life threatening reactions

paresthesias, syncope, stupor, coma, rosy cheeks
• Increased nervousness, excitability, irritability, which may indicate too high dose of medication, usually after 1-3 wk of treatment
• Cardiac status: angina, palpitation, chest pain, change in VS

Teach patient/family:
• Hair loss will occur in child, is temporary
• Report excitability, irritability, anxiety, which indicate overdose
• Not to switch brands unless approved by physician
• Drug may be discontinued after birth, thyroid panel evaluated after 1-2 mo
• That hypothyroid child will show almost immediate behavior/personality change
• That treatment drug is not to be taken to reduce weight
• To avoid OTC preparations with iodine, read labels
• To avoid iodine food, salt-iodinized, soy beans, tofu, turnips, some seafood, some bread

Lab test interferences:
Increase: CPK, LDH, AST, PBI, blood glucose
Decrease: TSH, ^{131}I uptake test, uric acid, triglycerides

---

lidocaine/lidocaine HCl (topical)

(lye'-doe-kane)
Stanacaine, Xylocaine
Func. class.: Topical anesthetic
Chem. class.: Aminoacylamide

Action: Inhibits nerve impulses from sensory nerves, which produces anesthesia
Uses: Pruritus, sunburn, toothache, sore throat, cold sores, oral pain

Dosage and routes:
• *Adult and child:* TOP apply q3-4h to affected area; INSTILL 15 ml (male) or 5 ml (female) into urethra
Available forms include: Top sol
Side effects/adverse reactions:
INTEG: Rash, irritation, sensitization
Contraindications: Hypersensitivity, application to large areas
Precautions: Sepsis, pregnancy (B), denuded skin

NURSING CONSIDERATIONS
Administer:
• After cleansing and drying of affected area
Evaluate:
• Allergy: rash, irritation, reddening, swelling
• Therapeutic response: absence of pain, itching of affected area
• Infection: if affected area is infected, do not apply
Teach patient/family:
• To report rash, irritation, redness, swelling
• How to apply ointment

---

lidocaine HCl

(lye-doe-kane)
Lido Pen Auto-Injector, Xylocaine
Func. class.: Antidysrhythmic (Class IB)
Chem. class.: Aminoacyl amide

Action: Increases electrical stimulation threshold of ventricle, his Purkinje system, which stabilizes cardiac membrane, decreases automaticity
Uses: Ventricular tachycardia, ventricular dysrhythmias during cardiac surgery, myocardial infarction, digitalis toxicity, cardiac catheterization
Dosage and routes:
• *Adult:* IV BOL 50-100 mg at 25-

---

50 mg/min, repeat q3-5 min, not to exceed 300 mg in 1 hr; begin IV INF; IV INF 20-50 µg/kg/min; IM 200-300 mg in deltoid muscle
• *Elderly, reduced liver function:* IV BOL give ½ adult dose
• *Child:* IV BOL 1 mg/kg, then IV INF; IV INF: 30 µg/kg/min
Available forms include: IV INF 0.2%, 0.4%, 0.8%; IV Ad 4%, 10%, 20%; IV Dir 1%, 2%; IM 300 mg/ml, 10%

Side effects/adverse reactions:
CNS: Headache, dizziness, involuntary movement, confusion, tremor, drowsiness, euphoria, ***convulsions***
EENT: Tinnitus, blurred vision
GI: Nausea, vomiting, anorexia
*CV: Hypotension, bradycardia, **heart block, cardiovascular collapse, arrest***
RESP: Dyspnea, ***respiratory depression***
INTEG: Rash, urticaria, edema, swelling
MISC: Febrile response, phlebitis at injection site

Contraindications: Hypersensitivity to amides, severe heart block, supraventricular dysrhythmias, Adams-Stokes syndrome, Wolff-Parkinson-White syndrome

Precautions: Pregnancy (B), lactation, children, renal disease, liver disease, CHF, respiratory depression, malignant hyperthermia

Pharmacokinetics:
IV: Onset 2 min, duration 20 min
IM: Onset 5-15 min, duration 1½ hr
Half-life 8 min, 1-2 hr (terminal), metabolized in liver excreted in urine, crosses placenta

Interactions/incompatibilities:
• Increased neuromuscular blockade of: neuromuscular blockers, tubocurarine

• Increased effects of lidocaine: cimetidine, phenytoin, propranolol, metoprolol
• Decreased effects of lidocaine: barbiturates

NURSING CONSIDERATIONS
Assess:
• ECG continuously to determine increased PR or QRS segments; if these develop, discontinue or reduce rate; watch for increased ventricular ectopic beats, may need to rebolus
• IV infusion rate using infusion pump, run at less than 4 mg/min
• Blood levels (therapeutic level: 1.5-6 µg/ml)
• B/P continuously for fluctuations
• I&O ratio, electrolytes (K, Na, Cl)

Administer:
• IV bolus undiluted; give 50 mg or less over 1 min or dilute 1 g/250-500 ml of D₅W; titrate to patient response
• IM injection in deltoid; aspirate to avoid intravascular administration; check site daily for infiltration or extravasation

Evaluate:
• Malignant hyperthermia: tachypnea, tachycardia, changes in B/P, increased temperature
• Cardiac rate, respiration: rate, rhythm, character, continuously
• Respiratory status: rate, rhythm, lung fields for rales, watch for respiratory depression
• CNS effects: dizziness, confusion, psychosis, paresthesias, convulsions; drug should be discontinued
• Lung fields, bilateral rales may occur in CHF patient
• Increased respiration, increased pulse; drug should be discontinued

Teach patient/family:
• Use of automatic lidocaine injection device if ordered

---

italics = common side effects   ***bold italic*** = life threatening reactions

Lab test interferences:
Increase: CPK
Treatment of overdose: O_2, artificial ventilation, ECG, administer dopamine for circulatory depression, administer diazepam or thiopental for convulsions

---

lidocaine HCl (local)

(lye'doe-kane)
Ardecaine, Dilocaine, Dolicaine, Nervocaine, Norocaine, Rocaine, Stanacaine, Ultracaine, Xylocaine

Func. class.: Local anesthetic
Chem. class.: Amide

Action: Competes with calcium for sites in nerve membrane that control sodium transport across cell membrane; decreases rise of depolarization phase of action potential
Uses: Peripheral nerve block, caudal anesthesia, epidural, spinal, surgical anesthesia
Dosage and routes:
Varies depending on route of anesthesia
Available forms include: Inj 0.5%, 1%, 1.5%, 2%, 4%, 5%; inj with epinephrine 0.5%, 1%, 1.5%, 2%
Side effects/adverse reactions:
CNS: Anxiety, restlessness, *convulsions, loss of consciousness,* drowsiness, disorientation, tremors, shivering
CV: Myocardial depression, cardiac arrest, dysrhythmias, bradycardia, hypotension, hypertension, fetal bradycardia
GI: Nausea, vomiting
EENT: Blurred vision, tinnitus, pupil constriction
INTEG: Rash, urticaria, allergic reactions, edema, burning, skin discoloration at injection site, tissue necrosis
RESP: Status asthmaticus, respiratory arrest, anaphylaxis
Contraindications: Hypersensitivity, child <12 yr, elderly, severe liver disease
Precautions: Elderly, severe drug allergies, pregnancy (C)
Pharmacokinetics:
Onset 4-17 min, duration 3-6 hr; metabolized by liver, excreted in urine (metabolites)
Interactions/incompatibilities:
• Dysrhythmias: epinephrine, halothane, enflurane
• Hypertension: MAOIs, tricyclic antidepressants, phenothiazines
• Decreased action of lidocaine: chloroprocaine

NURSING CONSIDERATIONS
Assess:
• B/P, pulse, respiration during treatment
• Fetal heart tones if drug is used during labor
Administer:
• Only with crash cart, resuscitative equipment nearby
• Only drugs without preservatives for epidural or caudal anesthesia
Perform/provide:
• Use of new solution, discard unused portions
Evaluate:
• Therapeutic response: anesthesia necessary for procedure
• For allergic reactions: rash, urticaria, itching
• Cardiac status: ECG for dysrhythmias, pulse, B/P during anesthesia
Treatment of overdose: Airway, O_2, vasopressor, IV fluids, anticonvulsants for seizures

---

* Available in Canada only

lidocaine HCl (topical)

(lye'doe-kane)

Xylocaine, Viscous Xylocaine

Func. class.: Anesthetic, topical, local

Chem. class.: Amide

Action: Inhibits conduction of nerve impulses from sensory nerves

Uses: Oral pain, topical anesthetic for mucous membrane

Dosage and routes:

• *Adult and child:* TOP apply q3-4h to affected area

Available forms include: Oint 5%; oral sol 2%, 5%

Side effects/adverse reactions:

EENT: Swelling, burning, stinging, tissue necrosis, irritation

INTEG: Rash, urticaria, edema

Contraindications: Hypersensitivity, secondary bacterial infections, infants

Precautions: Sepsis of affected area, pregnancy (C)

Pharmacokinetics:

TOP: Peak 2-5 min, duration ½-1 hr

NURSING CONSIDERATIONS

Administer:

• With swab to decrease chance of ointment on healthy skin

Perform/provide:

• Storage at room temperature in tight container

Evaluate:

• For redness, swelling, irritation; drug may need to be discontinued

Teach patient/family:

• Not to eat or rinse mouth for at least 1 hr after application

• Not to eat if area is anesthetized

• That burning/stinging may occur for a few doses

lincomycin HCl

(lin-koe-mye'sin)

Lincocin

Func. class.: Antibacterial

Chem. class.: Lincomycin derivative

Action: Binds to 50S subunit of bacterial ribsomes, suppresses protein synthesis

Uses: Infections caused by group A β-hemolytic streptococci, pneumococci, staphylococci (respiratory tract, skin, soft tissue, urinary tract infections, osteomyelitis, septicemia)

Dosage and routes:

• *Adult:* PO 500 mg q6-8h, not to exceed 8 g/day; IM 600 mg/day or q12h; IV 600 mg-1 g q8-12h, dilute in 100 ml IV sol, infuse over 1 hr, not to exceed 8 gm/day

• *Child >1 mo:* PO 30-60 mg/kg/day in divided doses q6-8h; IM 10 mg/kg/day q12h; IV 10-20 mg/kg/day in divided doses q6-8h; dilute to 100 ml IV sol, infuse over 1 hr

Available forms include: Caps 500 mg; caps pediatric 250 mg; inj IM, IV 300 mg/ml

Side effects/adverse reactions:

HEMA: **Leukopenia, eosinophilia, agranulocytosis, thrombocytopenia**

GI: Nausea, vomiting, abdominal pain, tenesmus, diarrhea, **pseudomembranous colitis**

GU: Increased AST, ALT, bilirubin, alk phosphatase, jaundice, *vaginitis,* urinary frequency

EENT: Rash, urticaria, pruritus, erythema, pain, abscess at injection site

Contraindications: Hypersensitivity, ulcerative colitis/enteritis, infants <1 mo

Precautions: Renal disease, liver disease, GI disease, elderly, pregnancy (C), lactation

Pharmacokinetics:

PO: Peak 45 min, duration 6 hr
IM: Peak 3 hr, duration 8-12 hr
Half-life 2½ hr, metabolized in liver, excreted in urine, bile, feces as active, inactive metabolites, crosses placenta, excreted in breast milk

Interactions/incompatibilities:

• Increased neuromuscular blockage: nondepolarizing muscle relaxants

• Decreased absorption of lincomycin: kaolin

• Decreased action of: chloramphenicol, erythromycin

NURSING CONSIDERATIONS

Assess:

• Signs of infection

• Any patient with compromised renal system; drug is excreted slowly in poor renal system function; toxicity may occur rapidly

• Liver studies: AST, ALT

• Blood studies: WBC, RBC, Hct, Hgb, platelets, serum iron, reticulocytes; drug should be discontinued if bone marrow depression occurs

• Renal studies: urinalysis, protein, blood, BUN, creatinine

• C&S before drug therapy; drug may be taken as soon as culture is taken

• Drug level in impaired hepatic, renal systems

• B/P, pulse in patient receiving drug parenterally

Administer:

• IV by infusion only; do not administer bolus dose; dilute 1g or less/100 ml or more D₅W, NS, not to exceed 100 ml/hr

• IM deep injection; rotate sites

• Orally with at least 8 oz water on empty stomach

Perform/provide:

• Storage at room temperature (capsules) and up to 2 wk (reconstituted solution)

• Adrenalin, suction, tracheostomy set, endotracheal intubation equipment on unit

• Adequate intake of fluids (2000 ml) during diarrhea episodes

Evaluate:

• Therapeutic response: decreased temperature, negative C&S

• Bowel pattern before, during treatment

• Skin eruptions, itching, dermatitis

• Respiratory status: rate, character, wheezing, tightness in chest

• Allergies before treatment, reaction of each medication; place allergies on chart, Kardex in bright red letters; notify all people giving drugs

Teach patient/family:

• To take oral drug with full glass of water; may give with food if GI symptoms occur

• Aspects of drug therapy: need to complete entire course of medication to ensure organism death (10-14 days); culture may be taken after completed course of medication

• To report sore throat, fever, fatigue; could indicate superimposed infection

• That drug must be taken in equal intervals around clock to maintain blood levels

• To notify nurse of diarrhea

Lab test interferences:

Increase: Alk phosphatase, bilirubin, CPK, AST/ALT

Treatment of hypersensitivity: Withdraw drug, maintain airway, administer epinephrine, aminophylline, O₂, IV corticosteroids

---

lindane (gamma benzene hexachloride)

(lin-dane)
gBh,* Kwell, Kwellada,* Kwildane, Scabene, G-Well

Func. class.: Scabicide
Chem. class.: Chlorinated hydrocarbon (synthetic)

Action: Stimulates nervous system of arthropods, resulting in seizures, death of organism

Uses: Scabies, lice (head/pubic), nits

Dosage and routes:
• *Adult and child:* CREAM/LOTION wash area with soap, water, remove visible crusts, apply to skin surfaces, remove with soap, water in 8-12 hr, may reapply in 1 wk if needed; SHAMPOO using 30 ml work into lather, rub for 5 min, rinse, dry with towel; comb with fine-tooth comb to remove nits

Available forms include: Lotion, shampoo, cream (1%)

Side effects/adverse reactions:
INTEG: Pruritus, rash, irritation, contact dermatitis
GI: Nausea, vomiting, diarrhea, liver damage (inhalation of vapors)
*HEMA: **Aplastic anemia** (chronic inhalation of vapors)
*CV: **Ventricular fibrillation*** (chronic inhalation of vapors)
*GU: **Kidney damage*** (chronic inhalation of vapors)
*CNS: Tremors, **convulsions,*** stimulation, dizziness (chronic inhalation of vapors)

Contraindications: Hypersensitivity, premature neonate, patients with known seizure disorders, inflammation of skin, abrasions, or breaks in skin

Precautions: Pregnancy (B), avoid contact with eyes, children <10 yr, infants, lactation

Pharmacokinetics:
Stored in body fat, metabolized in liver, excreted in urine, feces

Interactions/incompatibilities:
• Oils may enhance absorption; if an oil-based hair dressing is used, shampoo, rinse, dry hair before applying lindane shampoo

NURSING CONSIDERATIONS
Administer:
• To body areas, scalp only; do not apply to face, lips, mouth, eyes, any mucous membrane, anus, or meatus
• Topical corticosteroids as ordered to decrease contact dermatitis
• Lotions of menthol or phenol to control itching
• Topical antibiotics for infection

Perform/provide:
• Isolation until areas on skin, scalp have cleared and treatment is completed
• Removal of nits by using a fine-tooth comb rinsed in vinegar after treatment; use gloves

Evaluate:
• Area of body involved, including crusts, nits, brownish trails on skin, itching papules in skin folds

Teach patient/family:
• To wash all inhabitants' clothing, using insecticide; preventative treatment may be required of all persons living in same house, using lotion or shampoo to decrease spread of infection, use rubber gloves when applying drug
• That itching may continue for 4-6 wk
• That drug must be reapplied if accidently washed off or treatment will be ineffective
• Do not apply to face; if accidental contact with eyes occurs, flush with water

---

italics = common side effects   ***bold italic*** = life threatening reactions

• Treat sexual contacts simultaneously

Treatment of ingestion: Gastric lavage, saline laxatives, IV valium for convulsions

---

liothyronine sodium (T₃)

(lye-oh-thye'roe-neen)
Cytomel, Cyronine

Func. class.: Thyroid hormone
Chem. class.: Synthetic T_3

Action: Increases metabolic rates, increases cardiac output, O_2 consumption, body temperature, blood volume, growth, development at cellular level

Uses: Hypothyroidism, myxedema coma, thyroid hormone replacement, cretinism, nontoxic goiter, T_3 suppression test

Dosage and routes:

• *Adult:* PO 25 μg qd, increased by 12.5-25 μg q1-2 wk until desired response, maintenance dose 25-75 μg qd

Cretinism

• *Child >3 yr:* PO 50-100 μg qd

• *Child <3 yr:* PO 5 μg qd, increased by 5 μg q3-4 days titrated to response

Myxedema

• *Adult:* PO 5 μg qd, may increase by 5-10 μg q1-2 wk, maintenance dose 50-100 μg qd

Nontoxic goiter

• *Adult:* PO 5 μg qd, increased by 12.5-25 μg q1-2 wk, maintenance dose 75 μg qd

Suppression test

• *Adult:* PO 75-100 μg qd × 1 wk

Available forms include: Tabs 5, 25, 50 μg

Side effects/adverse reactions:

CNS: Insomnia, tremors, headache, *thyroid storm*

CV: Tachycardia, palpitations, an- *gina, dysrhythmias,* hypertension, cardiac arrest

GI: Nausea, diarrhea, increased or decreased appetite, cramps

MISC: Menstrual irregularities, weight loss, sweating, heat intolerance, fever

Contraindications: Adrenal insufficiency, myocardial infarction, thyrotoxicosis

Precautions: Elderly, angina pectoris, hypertension, ischemia, cardiac disease, pregnancy (A), lactation

Pharmacokinetics:

PO: Peak 12-48 hr, half-life 6-7 days

Interactions/incompatibilities:

• Decreased absorption of liothyronine: cholestyramine

• Increased effects of: anticoagulants, sympathomimetics, tricyclic antidepressants

• Decreased effects of: digitalis drugs, insulin, hypoglycemics

• Decreased effects of liothyronine: estrogens

NURSING CONSIDERATIONS

Assess:

• B/P, pulse before each dose

• I&O ratio

• Weight qd in same clothing, using same scale, at same time of day

• Height, growth rate if given to a child

• T_3, T_4, which are decreased, radioimmunoassay of TSH, which is increased, radio uptake, which is decreased if patient is on too low a dose of medication

• Pro-time may require decreased anticoagulant, check for bleeding, bruising

Administer:

• In AM if possible as a single dose to decrease sleeplessness

• At same time each day to maintain drug level

• Only for hormone imbalances, not to be used for obesity, male infertility, menstrual conditions, lethargy

• Lowest dose that relieves symptoms

Perform/provide:

• Removal of medication 4 wk before RAIU test

Evaluate:

• Therapeutic response: absence of depression, increased weight loss, diuresis, pulse, appetite, absence of constipation, peripheral edema, cold intolerance, pale, cool dry skin, brittle nails, alopecia, coarse hair, menorrhagia, night blindness, paresthesia, syncope, stupor, coma, rosy cheeks

• Increased nervousness, excitability, irritability, which may indicate too high dose of medication usually after 1-3 wk of treatment

• Cardiac status: angina, palpitation, chest pain, change in VS

Teach patient/family:

• Hair loss will occur in child, is temporary

• Report excitability, irritability, anxiety, which indicates overdose

• Not to switch brands unless approved by physician

• That hypothyroid child will show almost immediate behavior/personality change

• That treatment drug is not to be taken to reduce weight

• To avoid OTC preparations with iodine, read labels

• To avoid iodine food, salt-iodinized, soy beans, tofu, turnips, some seafood, some bread

Lab test interferences:

Increase: CPK, LDH, AST, PBI, blood glucose

Decrease: TSH, ^{131}I uptake test, uric acid, triglycerides

liotrix

(lye'oh-trix)
Euthroid, Thyrolar
Func. class.: Thyroid hormone
Chem. class.: Levothyroxine/liothyronine (synthetic T_4, T_3)

Action: Increases metabolic rates, increases cardiac output, O_2 consumption, body temperature, blood volume, growth, development at cellular level

Uses: Hypothyroidism, thyroid hormone replacement

Dosage and routes:

• *Adult and child:* PO 15-30 mg qd, increased by 15-30 mg q1-2 wk until desired response, may increase by 15-30 mg q2 wk in child

• *Geriatric:* PO 15-30 mg, double dose q6-8 wk until desired response

Available forms include: Tabs 15, 30, 60, 120, 180 mg as thyroid equivalent

Side effects/adverse reactions:

CNS: Insomnia, tremors, headache, thyroid storm

CV: Tachycardia, palpitations, angina, dysrhythmias, hypertension, cardiac arrest

GI: Nausea, diarrhea, increased or decreased appetite, cramps

MISC: Menstrual irregularities, weight loss, sweating, heat intolerance, fever

Contraindications: Adrenal insufficiency, myocardial infarction, thyrotoxicosis

Precautions: Elderly, angina pectoris, hypertension, ischemia, cardiac disease, pregnancy (A), lactation

Pharmacokinetics:

PO: Peak 12-48 hr, half-life 6-7 days

Interactions/incompatibilities:

• Decreased absorption of liotrix: cholestyramine

---

italics = common side effects   ***bold italic*** = life threatening reactions

• Increased effects of: anticoagulants, sympathomimetics, tricyclic antidepressants, catecholamines
• Decreased effects of: digitalis drugs, insulin, hypoglycemics
• Decreased effects of liotrix: estrogens

NURSING CONSIDERATIONS
Assess:
• B/P, pulse before each dose
• I&O ratio
• Weight qd in same clothing, using same scale, at same time of day
• Height, growth rate if given to a child
• T_3, T_4 FTIs that are decreased, radioimmunoassay of TSH, which is increased, radio uptake, which is decreased if patient is on too low a dose of medication
• Pro-time may require decreased anticoagulant, check for bleeding, bruising

Administer:
• In AM if possible as a single dose to decrease sleeplessness
• At same time each day to maintain drug level
• Only for hormone imbalances, not to be used for obesity, male infertility, menstrual conditions, lethargy
• Lowest dose that relieves symptoms

Perform/provide:
• Removal of medication 4 wk before RAIU test

Evaluate:
• Therapeutic response: absence of depression, increased weight loss, diuresis, pulse, appetite, absence of constipation, peripheral edema, cold intolerance, pale, cool dry skin, brittle nails, coarse hair, menorrhagia, night blindness, paresthesias, syncope, stupor, coma, rosy cheeks
• Increased nervousness, excitability, irritability, which may indicate too high dose of medication usually after 1-3 wk of treatment
• Cardiac status: angina, palpitation, chest pain, change in VS

Teach patient/family:
• Hair loss will occur in child, is temporary
• Report excitability, irritability, anxiety, which indicate overdose
• Not to switch brands unless approved by physician
• That hypothyroid child will show almost immediate behavior/personality change
• That treatment drug is not to be taken to reduce weight
• To avoid OTC preparations with iodine, read labels
• To avoid iodine food, salt-iodinized, soy beans, tofu, turnips, some seafood, some bread

Lab test interferences:
Increase: CPK, LDH, AST, PBI, blood glucose
Decrease: TSH, ^{131}I uptake test, uric acid, triglycerides

---

lisinopril

(lyse-in'oh-pril)
Prinivil, Zestril

Func. class.: Angiotensin converting enzyme (ACE) inhibitor
Chem. class.: Enalaprilat lysine analogue

Action: Selectively suppresses renin-angiotensin-aldosterone system; inhibits ACE preventing conversion of angiotensin I to angiotensin II
Uses: Mild to moderate hypertension
Dosage and routes:
• *Adult:* PO 10-40 mg qd, may increase to 80 mg qd if required
Available forms include: Tabs 5, 10, 20 mg

Side effects/adverse reactions:

GI: Nausea, vomiting, anorexia, constipation, flatulence, GI irritation

*GU: **Proteinuria, renal insufficiency,** sexual dysfunction, impotence*

INTEG: Rash, pruritus

CNS: Vertigo, depression, stroke, insomnia, paresthesias, headache, fatigue, asthenia

EENT: Blurred vision, nasal congestion

RESP: Cough, dyspnea

Contraindications: Hypersensitivity

Precautions: Pregnancy (C), lactation, renal disease, hyperkalemia

Pharmacokinetics:
Peak 6-8 hr, excreted unchanged in urine

Interactions/incompatibilities:

• Increased hypotensive effect: diuretics, other hypertensives, probenecid

• Decreased effects of lisinopril: aspirin, indomethacin

• Increased potassium levels: potassium salt substitutes, potassium-sparing diuretics, potassium supplements

• Increased effect of: antihypertensives, reserpine

• Increased effects: diuretics

• Increased hypersensitivity reactions: allopurinol

NURSING CONSIDERATIONS
Assess:

• B/P, pulse q4h; note rates rhythm, quality

• Electrolytes: potassium, sodium, chloride

• Apical/pedal pulse before administration; notify physician of any significant changes

• Baselines in renal, liver function tests before therapy begins

Evaluate:

• Edema in feet, legs daily

• Skin turgor, dryness of mucous membranes for hydration status

• Symptoms of CHF: edema, dyspnea, wet rales

Teach patient/family:

• Not to discontinue drug abruptly

• To rise slowly to sitting or standing position to minimize orthostatic hypotension

Lab test interferences:

Interfere: Glucose/insulin tolerance tests

Treatment of overdose: Lavage, IV atropine for bradycardia, IV theophylline for bronchospasm, digitalis, O_2, diuretic for cardiac failure, hemodialysis

---

lithium carbonate

(li'thee-um)

Carbolith,* Lithane, Eskalith, Lithonate, Lithotabs, Lithobid, Lithium Citrate, Lithonate-S

Func. class.: Antimanic

Chem. class.: Alkali metal ion salt

Action: May alter sodium, potassium ion transport across cell membrane in nerve, muscle cells; may balance biogenic amines of norepinephrine, serotonin in CNS areas involved in emotional responses

Uses: Manic-depressive illness (manic phase), prevention of bipolar manic depressive psychosis

Dosage and routes:

• *Adult:* PO 600 mg tid, maintenance 300 mg tid or qid; SLOW REL TABS 300 mg bid, dose should be individualized to maintain blood levels at 0.5-1.5 mEq/L

Available forms include: Caps 150, 300 mg; tabs 300 mg; tabs ext rel 300, 450 mg; oral sol 8 mEq/5 ml

---

italics = common side effects   ***bold italic*** = life threatening reactions

Side effects/adverse reactions:

CNS: Headache, drowsiness, dizziness, tremors, twitching, ataxia, seizure, slurred speech, restlessness, confusion, stupor, memory loss, clonic movements

GI: Dry mouth, anorexia, nausea, vomiting, diarrhea, incontinence, abdominal pain

*GU: **Polyuria, glycosuria, proteinuria, albuminuria,*** urinary incontinence, polydipsia, edema

CV: Hypotension, ECG changes, dysrhythmias, ***circulatory collapse***

INTEG: Drying of hair, alopecia, rash, pruritus, hyperkeratosis

*HEMA: **Leukocytosis***

EENT: Tinnitus, blurred vision

ENDO: Hyponatremia

MS: Muscle weakness

Contraindications: Hepatic disease, renal disease, brain trauma, OBS, pregnancy (D), lactation, children <12 yr, schizophrenia, severe cardiac disease, severe renal disease, severe dehydration

Precautions: Elderly, thyroid disease, seizure disorders, diabetes mellitus, systemic infection, urinary retention

Pharmacokinetics:

PO: Onset rapid, peak ½-4 hr, half-life 18-36 hr depending on age; crosses blood-brain barrier, 80% of filtered lithium is reabsorbed by the renal tubules, excreted in urine, crosses placenta, enters breast milk, well absorbed by oral method

Interactions/incompatibilities:

• Increased hypothyroid effects: antithyroid effects, calcium iodide, potassium iodide, iodinated glycerol

• Brain damage: haloperidol

• Increased effects of: neuromuscular blocking agents, phenothiazines

• Increased renal clearance: sodium bicarbonate, acetazolamide, mannitol, aminophylline

• Increased toxicity: indomethacin, diuretics, nonsteroidal antiinflammatories

• Decreased effects of lithium: theophyllines, urea, urinary alkalizers

NURSING CONSIDERATIONS

Assess:

• Weight daily, check for edema in legs, ankles, wrists; report if present

• Sodium intake; decreased sodium intake with decreased fluid intake may lead to lithium retention; increased sodium and fluids may decrease lithium retention

• Skin turgor at least daily

• Urine for albuminuria, glycosuria, uric acid during beginning treatment, q2 mo thereafter

• Neuro status: LOC, gait, motor reflexes, hand tremors

• Serum lithium levels weekly initially, then q2 mo (therapeutic level: 0.5-1.5 mEq/L)

Administer:

• With meals to avoid GI upset

• Adequate fluids (2-3 L/day) to prevent dehydration during initial treatment, 1-2 L/day during maintenance

Teach patient/family:

• Symptoms of minor toxicity: vomiting, diarrhea, poor coordination, fine motor tremors, weakness, lassitude; major toxicity: coarse tremors, severe thirst, tinnitus, dilute urine

• To monitor urine specific gravity

• That contraception is necessary since lithium may harm fetus

• Not to operate machinery until lithium levels are stable

Lab test interferences:

Increase: Potassium excretion,

urine glucose, blood glucose, protein, BUN
Decrease: VMA, T_3, T_4, PBI, ^{131}I
Treatment: Induce emesis or lavage, maintain airway, respiratory function; dialysis for severe intoxication

lomustine (CCNU)

(loe-mus'teen)
CeeNU, CCNU
Func. class.: Antineoplastic alkylating agent
Chem. class.: Nitrosourea

Action: Responsible for cross-linking DNA strands, which leads to cell death
Uses: Hodgkin's disease, lymphomas, melanomas, multiple myeloma; brain, lung, bladder, kidney, colon cancer
Dosage and routes:
• *Adult:* PO 130 mg/m^2 as a single dose q6wk; titrate dose to WBC level; do not give repeat dose unless WBCs are >4000/mm^3, platelet count >100,000/mm^3
Available forms include: Cap 10, 40, 100 mg
Side effects/adverse reactions:
*HEMA: **Thrombocytopenia, leukopenia, myelosuppression, anemia***
*GI: Nausea, vomiting, anorexia, stomatitis, **hepatotoxicity***
*GU: **Azotemia, renal failure***
INTEG: Burning at injection site
*RESP: **Fibrosis, pulmonary infiltrate***
Contraindications: Hypersensitivity, leukopenia, thrombocytopenia, pregnancy (D)
Precautions: Radiation therapy
Pharmacokinetics:
Metabolized in liver, excreted in urine; half-life 16-48 hr, 50% protein bound, crosses blood-brain barrier, appears in breast milk
Interactions/incompatibilities:
• Increased toxicity: barbiturates, phenytoin, chloral hydrate
• Increased metabolism of lomustine: phenobarbital
• Potentiation of lomustine: succinylcholine
• Increased bone marrow depression: allopurinol
NURSING CONSIDERATIONS
Assess:
• CBC, differential, platelet count weekly; withhold drug if WBC is <4000 or platelet count is <75,000; notify physician of results
• Pulmonary function tests, chest x-ray films before, during therapy; chest film should be obtained q2wk during treatment
• Renal function studies: BUN, serum uric acid, urine CrCl before, during therapy
• I&O ratio; report fall in urine output of 30 ml/hr
• Monitor temperature q4h (may indicate beginning infection); no rectal temperatures
• Liver function tests before, during therapy (bilirubin, AST, ALT, LDH) as needed or monthly
Administer:
• Antiemetic 30-60 min before giving drug to prevent vomiting
• Antibiotics for prophylaxis of infection
• Topical or systemic analgesics for pain
• Local or systemic drugs for infection
Perform/provide:
• Storage in tight container at room temperature
• Strict medical asepsis, protective isolation if WBC levels are low
• Special skin care

---

italics = common side effects   ***bold italic*** = life threatening reactions

- Deep breathing exercises with patient tid-qid; place in semi-Fowler's position
- Increase fluid intake to 2-3 L/day to prevent urate deposits, calculi formation
- Rinsing of mouth tid-qid with water, club soda; brushing of teeth bid-tid with soft brush or cotton tipped applicators for stomatitis; use unwaxed dental floss

Evaluate:

- Bleeding: hematuria, guaiac, bruising or petechiae, mucosa or orifices q8h
- Dyspnea, rales, unproductive cough, chest pain, tachypnea
- Food preferences; list likes, dislikes
- Yellowing of skin, sclera, dark urine, clay-colored stools, itchy skin, abdominal pain, fever, diarrhea
- Inflammation of mucosa, breaks in skin
- Buccal cavity q8h for dryness, sores or ulceration, white patches, oral pain, bleeding, dysphagia
- Local irritation, pain, burning, discoloration at injection site
- Symptoms indicating severe allergic reaction: rash, pruritus, urticaria, purpuric skin lesions, itching, flushing

Teach patient/family:

- Of protective isolation precautions
- To report any changes in breathing or coughing
- To avoid foods with citric acid, hot or rough texture if buccal inflammation is present
- To report any bleeding, white spots or ulcerations in mouth to physician; tell patient to examine mouth qd
- To report signs of infection: increased temperature, sore throat, flu symptoms
- To report signs of anemia: fatigue, headache, faintness, shortness of breath, irritability
- To avoid use of razors or commercial mouthwash
- To avoid use of aspirin products or ibuprofen

loperamide HCl

(loe-per'a-mide)
Imodium

Func. class.: Antidiarrheal
Chem. class.: Piperidine derivative

Action: Direct action on intestinal muscles to decrease GI peristalsis
Uses: Diarrhea (cause undetermined), chronic diarrhea, ileostomy discharge
Dosage and routes:

- *Adult:* PO 4 mg, then 2 mg after each loose stool, not to exceed 16 mg/day
- *Child 2-5 yr:* PO 5 ml tid on day 1, 0.1 mg/kg after each loose stool
- *Child 5-8 yr:* PO 10 ml bid on day 1, 0.1 mg/kg after each loose stool
- *Child 8-12 yr:* PO 10 ml tid on day 1, 0.1 mg/kg after each loose stool

Available forms include: Caps 2 mg; liq 1 mg/5 ml
Side effects/adverse reactions:
CNS: Dizziness, drowsiness, fatigue, fever
GI: Nausea, dry mouth, vomiting, constipation, abdominal pain, anorexia, *toxic megacolon*
INTEG: Rash
RESP: Respiratory depression
Contraindications: Hypersensitivity, severe ulcerative colitis, pseudomembranous colitis

---

Precautions: Pregnancy (B), lactation, children <2 yr, liver disease, dehydration, bacterial disease

Pharmacokinetics:

PO: Onset ½-1 hr, duration 4-5 hr, half-life 7-14 hr; metabolized in liver, excreted in feces as unchanged drug, small amount in urine

Interactions/incompatibilities:

• Do not mix oral solution with other solvents

NURSING CONSIDERATIONS

Assess:

• Electrolytes (K, Na, Cl) if on long-term therapy

• Skin turgor q8h if dehydration is suspected

Administer:

• For 48 hr only

Perform/provide:

• Storage in tight containers

Evaluate:

• Therapeutic response: decreased diarrhea

• Bowel pattern before; for rebound constipation

• Response after 48 hr; if no response, drug should be discontinued

• Dehydration in children

• Abdominal distention, toxic megacolon; may occur in ulcerative colitis

Teach patient/family:

• To avoid OTC products unless directed by physician

• That ostomy patient may take this drug for extended periods of time

---

loratidine

(loer-at-i-deen)
Claritin

Func. class.: Antihistamine
Chem. class.: Selective histamine-1 (Hl) receptor antagonist

Action: Binds to peripheral histamine receptors, which provides antihistamine action without sedation

Uses: Seasonal rhinitis

Dosage and routes:

• *Adult:* PO 10-40 mg qd

Available forms include: Tabs 10 mg

Side effects/adverse reactions:

CNS: Sedation (more common with increased doses)

Contraindications: Hypersensitivity, acute asthma attacks, lower respiratory tract disease

Precautions: Pregnancy (B), increased intraocular pressure, bronchial asthma

Pharmacokinetics:

Peak 1½ hr, elimination half-life 14½ hr; metabolized in liver to active metabolites, excreted in urine

NURSING CONSIDERATIONS

Perform/provide:

• Storage in tight container at room temperature

Evaluate:

• Therapeutic response: absence of running or congested nose

Teach patient/family:

• To avoid driving or other hazardous activities if drowsiness occurs

---

lorazepam

(lor-a'ze-pam)
Ativan, Novolorazem*

Func. class.: Antianxiety
Chem. class.: Benzodiazepine

Controlled Substance Schedule IV

Action: Depresses subcortical levels of CNS, including limbic system and reticular formation

Uses: Anxiety, irritability in psychiatric or organic disorders, preoperatively, insomnia, acute alcohol withdrawal symptoms, anticon-

---

vulsant, adjunct in endoscopic procedures

Dosage and routes:

Anxiety
• Adult: PO 2-6 mg/day in divided doses, not to exceed 10 mg/day

Insomnia
• Adult: PO 2-4 mg hs; only minimally effective after 2 wk continuous therapy

Preoperatively
• Adult: IM/IV 2-4 mg

Available forms include: Tabs 0.5, 1, 2 mg; IM/IV inj 2, 4 mg/ml

Side effects/adverse reactions:

CNS: Dizziness, drowsiness, confusion, headache, anxiety, tremors, stimulation, fatigue, depression, insomnia, hallucinations, weakness, unsteadiness

GI: Constipation, dry mouth, nausea, vomiting, anorexia, diarrhea

INTEG: Rash, dermatitis, itching

CV: Orthostatic hypotension, **ECG changes, tachycardia,** hypotension

EENT: Blurred vision, tinnitus, mydriasis

Contraindications: Hypersensitivity to benzodiazepines, narrow-angle glaucoma, psychosis, pregnancy (D), child <12 yr, history of drug abuse, COPD

Precautions: Elderly, debilitated, hepatic disease, renal disease

Pharmacokinetics:

PO: Peak 1-3 hr, duration 3-6 hr, metabolized by liver, excreted by kidneys, crosses placenta, breast milk, half-life 14 hr

Interactions/incompatibilities:
• Decreased effects of lorazepam: oral contraceptives, valproic acid
• Increased effects of lorazepam: CNS depressants, alcohol, disulfiram, oral contraceptives

NURSING CONSIDERATIONS

Assess:
• B/P (lying, standing), pulse; if systolic B/P drops 20 mm Hg, hold drug, notify physician; respirations q5-15 min if given IV
• Blood studies: CBC during long-term therapy, blood dyscrasias have occurred rarely
• Hepatic studies: AST, ALT, bilirubin, creatinine, LDH, alk phosphatase

Administer:
• With food or milk for GI symptoms
• Crushed if patient is unable to swallow medication whole
• Sugarless gum, hard candy, frequent sips of water for dry mouth
• IV after diluting in an equal volume of compatible sol; give through Y-tube or 3-way stopcock; give at 2 mg or less over 1 min
• Deep into large muscle mass (IM inj)

Perform/provide:
• Assistance with ambulation during beginning therapy since drowsiness/dizziness occurs
• Safety measures, including siderails
• Check to see PO medication has been swallowed

Evaluate:
• Therapeutic response: decreased anxiety, restlessness, insomnia
• Mental status: mood, sensorium, affect, sleeping pattern, drowsiness, dizziness
• Physical dependency, withdrawal symptoms: headache, nausea, vomiting, muscle pain, weakness, tremors, convulsions, after long-term, excessive use
• Suicidal tendencies

Teach patient/family:
• That drug may be taken with food
• Not to be used for everyday stress or used longer than 4 mo unless directed by physician, not to take

more than prescribed amount, may be habit forming
• Avoid OTC preparations (cough, cold, hay fever) unless approved by physician
• To avoid driving, activities that require alertness, since drowsiness may occur
• To avoid alcohol ingestion or other psychotropic medications, unless prescribed by physician
• Not to discontinue medication abruptly after long-term use
• To rise slowly or fainting may occur
• That drowsiness might worsen at beginning of treatment
• Use birth-control method if childbearing age

Lab test interferences:
Increase: AST/ALT, serum bilirubin
Decrease: RAIU
False increase: 17-OHCS

Treatment of overdose: Lavage, VS, supportive care

---

lovastatin

(lo'va-sta-tin)
Mevacor
Func. class.: Cholesterol-lowering agent
Chem. class.: Aspergillus terreus strain derivative

Action: Inhibits HMG-COA reductase enzyme, which reduces cholesterol synthesis
Uses: As an adjunct in primary hypercholesterolemia (types IIa, IIb), mixed hyperlipidemia
Dosage and routes:
(Patient should be placed on a cholesterol-lowering diet first)
• *Adult:* PO 20 mg qd with evening meal, may increase to 20-80 mg/day in single or divided doses, not

to exceed 80 mg/day; dosage adjustments should be made q month
Available forms include: Tabs 20 mg
Side effects/adverse reactions:
GI: Nausea, constipation, diarrhea, dyspepsia, flatus, abdominal pain, heartburn, **liver dysfunction**
MS: Muscle cramps, myalgia, **myositis, rhabdomyolysis**
CNS: Dizziness, headache
INTEG: Rash, pruritus
EENT: Blurred vision, dysgeusia, lens opacities
Contraindications: Pregnancy (X), lactation, active liver disease
Precautions: Past liver disease, alcoholics, severe acute infections, trauma, hypotension, uncontrolled seizure disorders, severe metabolic disorders, electrolyte imbalances
Pharmacokinetics:
PO: Peak 2-4 hr, metabolized in liver (metabolites), highly protein bound, excreted in urine, feces, crosses placenta, excreted in breast milk
Interactions/incompatibilities:
• Increased effects: bile acid sequestrants, coumadin
• Increased myalgia, myositis: cyclosporine, gemfibrozil, niacin
NURSING CONSIDERATIONS
Assess:
• Cholesterol levels periodically during treatment
• Liver function studies q 1-2 mo during the first 1½ yr of treatment; AST, ALT, liver function tests may increase
• Renal function in patients with compromised renal system: BUN, creatinine, I&O ratio
• Eyes with slit lamp before, 1 mo after treatment begins, anually, lens opacities may occur
Administer:
• In evening with meal; if dose is

---

italics = common side effects   ***bold italic*** = life threatening reactions

increased, take with breakfast and evening meal

Perform/provide:
• Storage in cool environment in tight container protected from light

Evaluate:
• Therapeutic response: decrease in cholesterol to desired level after 8 wk

Teach patient/family:
• That treatment will be ongoing for several years
• That blood work and eye exam will be necessary during treatment
• To report blurred vision, severe GI symptoms, dizziness, headache
• That previously prescribed regimen will continue: low-cholesterol diet, exercise program

Lab test interferences:
Increase: CPK, liver function tests
Note: Not all cholesterol lowering agents have been thoroughly tested. Investigate any reaction, however small, immediately.

---

loxapine succinate/ loxapine HCl

(lox'a'peen)
Loxapax,* Loxitane, Loxitane-C
Func. class.: Antipsychotic/neuroleptic
Chem. class.: Dibenzoxazepine

Action: Depresses cerebral cortex, hypothalamus, limbic system, which control activity and aggression; blocks neurotransmission produced by dopamine at synapse; exhibits strong α-adrenergic, anticholinergic blocking action; mechanism for antipsychotic effects is unclear

Uses: Psychotic disorders

Dosage and routes:
• *Adult:* PO 10 mg bid-qid initially, may be rapidly increased depending on severity of condition, maintenance 60-100 mg/day; IM 12.5-50 mg q4-6 hr or more until desired response, then start PO form

Available forms include: Caps 5, 10, 25, 50 mg; conc 25 mg/ml; inj IM 50 mg/ml

Side effects/adverse reactions:
RESP: **Laryngospasm,** dyspnea, *respiratory depression*
CNS: Extrapyramidal symptoms: pseudoparkinsonism, akathisia, dystonia, tardive dyskinesia, drowsiness, headache, seizures
HEMA: **Anemia, leukopenia, leukocytosis, agranulocytosis**
INTEG: Rash, photosensitivity, dermatitis
EENT: Blurred vision, glaucoma
GI: Dry mouth, nausea, vomiting, anorexia, constipation, diarrhea, jaundice, weight gain
GU: Urinary retention, urinary frequency, enuresis, impotence, amenorrhea, gynecomastia
CV: Orthostatic hypotension, hypertension, **cardiac arrest,** ECG changes, tachycardia

Contraindications: Hypersensitivity, blood dyscrasias, coma, child, brain damage, bone marrow depression, alcohol and barbiturate withdrawal states

Precautions: Pregnancy (C), lactation, seizure disorders, hypertension, hepatic disease, cardiac disease

Pharmacokinetics:
PO: Onset 20-30 min, peak 2-4 hr, duration 12 hr
IM: Onset 15-30 min, peak 15-20 min, duration 12 hr
Metabolized by liver, excreted in urine, crosses placenta, enters breast milk, initial half-life 5 hr, terminal half-life 19 hr

Interactions/incompatibilities:
• Toxicity: epinephrine

• Increased extrapyramidal effect: other antipsychotics
• Decreased effects: guanadrel, guanethidine

NURSING CONSIDERATIONS

Assess:
• Swallowing of PO medication; check for hoarding or giving of medication to other patients
• I&O ratio; palpate bladder if low urinary output occurs
• Bilirubin, CBC, liver function studies monthly
• Urinalysis is recommended before and during prolonged therapy

Administer:
• Antiparkinsonian agent, to be used if extrapyramidal symptoms occur
• IM injection into large muscle mass
• Concentrate mixed in orange or grapefruit juice

Perform/provide:
• Decreased noise input by dimming lights, avoiding loud noises
• Supervised ambulation until stabilized on medication; do not involve in strenuous exercise program because fainting is possible; patient should not stand still for long periods of time
• Increased fluids to prevent constipation
• Sips of water, candy, gum for dry mouth
• Storage in tight, light-resistant container

Evaluate:
• Therapeutic response: decrease in emotional excitement, hallucinations, delusions, paranoia, reorganization of patterns of thought, speech
• Affect, orientation, LOC, reflexes, gait, coordination, sleep pattern disturbances
• B/P standing and lying; take pulse and respirations q4h during initial treatment; establish baseline before starting treatment; report drops of 30 mm Hg
• Dizziness, faintness, palpitations, tachycardia on rising
• Extrapyramidal symptoms including akathisia (inability to sit still, no pattern to movements), tardive dyskinesia (bizarre movements of the jaw, mouth, tongue, extremities), pseudoparkinsonism (rigidity, tremors, pill rolling, shuffling gait)
• Skin turgor daily
• For neuroleptic malignant syndrome: muscle rigidity, increased CPK, altered mental status, hyperthermia
• Constipation, urinary retention daily; if these occur, increase bulk, water in diet

Teach patient/family:
• That orthostatic hypotension may occur and to rise from sitting or lying position gradually
• To remain lying down after IM injection for at least 30 min
• To avoid hot tubs, hot showers, or tub baths since hypotension may occur
• To avoid abrupt withdrawal of this drug or EPS may result; drug should be withdrawn slowly
• To avoid OTC preparations (cough, hayfever, cold) unless approved by physician since serious drug interactions may occur; avoid use with alcohol or CNS depressants, increased drowsiness may occur
• To avoid hazardous activities if drowsiness or dizziness occurs
• To use a sunscreen during sun exposure to prevent burns
• Regarding compliance with drug regimen; warn patient about avoiding OTC preparation

---

italics = common side effects   ***bold italic*** = life threatening reactions

• About necessity for meticulous oral hygiene since oral candidiasis may occur
• To report impaired vision, jaundice, tremors, muscle twitching
• In hot weather heat stroke may occur; take extra precautions to stay cool

Treatment of overdose: Lavage if orally ingested, provide an airway

---

lypressin

(lye-press'in)
Diapid

Func. class.: Pituitary hormone
Chem. class.: Lysine vasopressin

Action: Promotes reabsorption of water by action on renal tubular epithelium

Uses: Nonnephrogenic diabetes insipidus

Dosage and routes:
• *Adult:* INTRANASAL 1-2 sprays in one or both nostrils qid, an extra dose hs if needed

Available forms include: INTRANASAL 0.185 mg/ml

Side effects/adverse reactions:
EENT: Nasal irritation, congestion, rhinitis, conjunctivitis, rhinorrhea
CNS: Headache
GI: Nausea, heartburn, cramps
MISC: Chest tightness, cough, dyspnea

Precautions: CAD, pregnancy (B)

Pharmacokinetics:
NASAL: Onset 1 hr, duration 3-8 hr, half-life 15 min; metabolized in liver, kidneys, excreted in urine

NURSING CONSIDERATIONS
Assess:
• I&O ratio; weight daily, check for edema in extremities, if water retention is severe, diuretic may be prescribed

Perform/provide:
• Storage at room temperature
Evaluate:
• Therapeutic response: absence of severe thirst, decreased urine output, osmolality
• Water intoxication: lethargy, behavioral changes, disorientation, neuromuscular excitability
Teach patient/family:
• To clear nasal passages before using drug, not to inhale spray
• To carry drug at all times

---

mafenide acetate (topical)

(ma'fe-nide)
Sulfamylon

Func. class.: Local antiinfective
Chem. class.: Sulfonamide

Action: Interferes with bacterial cell wall synthesis

Uses: Burns (2nd, 3rd degree)

Dosage and routes:
• *Adult and child:* TOP apply $\frac{1}{16}$ in to affected area qd-bid, reapply as needed

Available forms include: Cream 85 mg/g as acetate

Side effects/adverse reactions:
INTEG: Rash, urticaria, stinging, burning, bleeding, excoriation of new skin, super infections, pruritus, blisters
OTHER: Metabolic acidosis, tachypnea, **bone marrow suppression, fatal hemolytic anemia**

Contraindications: Hypersensitivity, inhalation injury

Precautions: Pregnancy (C), impaired pulmonary function, lactation, impaired renal function

NURSING CONSIDERATIONS
Administer:
• Analgesic before application if needed

• Enough medication to completely cover burns, they must be covered at all times
• After cleansing debris from burn before each application
• Using aseptic technique to debrided areas

Perform/provide:
• Storage at room temperature in dry place

Evaluate:
• Allergic reaction: burning, stinging, swelling, redness
• Therapeutic response: appearance of granulation tissue
• Fluid loss: decreased urinary output

Teach patient/family:
• That therapy will continue until area is ready for grafting
• Signs of superimposed infection
• Changes in respiratory activity

---

magaldrate (aluminum magnesium complex)

(mag' al-drate)
Hydromagnesium, Lowsium, Riopan, Riopan Plus
Func. class.: Antacid
Chem. class.: Aluminum/magnesium hydroxide

Action: Neutralizes gastric acidity
Uses: Antacid
Dosage and routes:
• *Adult:* PO 1-2 (480-1080 mg) between meals, hs, not to exceed 20 tabs/day; CHEW TAB 1-2 (480-960 mg) between meals, hs, not to exceed 20 tabs/day; SUSP 5-10 ml (400-800 mg) with water between meals, hs, not to exceed 100 ml/day
Available forms include: Tabs 480 mg; chew tabs 480 mg; susp 540 mg/5 ml, 480 mg/5 ml, 1080 mg/5 ml

Side effects/adverse reactions:
GI: Constipation, diarrhea
META: Hypermagnesium
Contraindications: Hypersensitivity to this drug or aluminum products
Precautions: Elderly, fluid restriction, decreased GI motility, GI obstruction, dehydration, renal disease, sodium-restricted diets, pregnancy (C)
Pharmacokinetics:
PO: Duration 60 min
Interactions/incompatibilities:
• Decreased effectiveness of: tetracyclines, ketoconazole
• Decreased absorption of: anticholinergics, chlordiazepoxide, cimetidine, corticosteroids, iron salts, phenothiazines, phenytoin, salicylates

NURSING CONSIDERATIONS
Assess:
• Serum Mg^{++} levels with impaired renal function
Administer:
• Laxatives or stool softeners if constipation occurs
• After shaking, give between meals and hs
• To separate enteric-coated drugs and antacid by 1 hr
Evaluate:
• Therapeutic response: absence of pain, decreased acidity
• Constipation: increase bulk in diet if needed

---

magnesium carbonate

Func. class.: Antacid
Chem. class.: Magnesium product

Action: Neutralizes gastric acidity
Uses: Antacid, constipation
Dosage and routes:
• *Adult:* PO 0.5-2 g between meals with water

M

Laxative
• *Adult:* PO 8 g with water hs
Available forms include: Powder
Side effects/adverse reactions:
GI: Diarrhea, flatulence, cramps, belching, nausea, vomiting, impaction, *obstruction,* pain
META: Hypermagnesia: *weakness, lethargy, depression, decreased B/P, increased pulse, respiratory depression, coma*
Contraindications: Hypersensitivity
Precautions: Severe renal disease, GI bleeding, diarrhea, intestinal obstruction, pregnancy (C)
Pharmacokinetics:
PO: Excreted in urine
Interactions/incompatibilities:
• Decreased effectiveness of: tetracyclines
• Decreased absorption of: anticholinergics, chlordiazepoxide, cimetidine, corticosteroids, iron salts
NURSING CONSIDERATIONS
Administer:
• After mixing with water
Evaluate:
• Therapeutic response: absence of pain, decreased acidity
Teach patient/family:
• Not to change antacids unless directed by physician
• To store in tightly covered container
Lab test interferences:
Increase: Urinary pH, gastrin
Decrease: K⁺

---

magnesium oxide
Mag-Ox, Maox, Par-mag, Uro-mag
Func. class.: Antacid
Chem. class.: Magnesium product

Action: Neutralizes gastric acidity
Uses: Constipation, hypomagnesemia, antacid

Dosage and routes:
• *Adult:* PO 250 mg-1 g pc, hs with 4-8 oz water
Laxative
• *Adult:* PO 2-4 g with water hs
Hypomagnesemia
• *Adult:* PO 650-1.3 g qd
Available forms include: Caps 140; tabs 400, 420 mg
Side effects/adverse reactions:
GU: Renal stones
GI: Diarrhea, flatulence, cramps, belching, nausea, vomiting
META: Hypermagnesemia: *weakness, lethargy, depression, decreased B/P, increased pulse, respiratory depression, coma*
Contraindications: Hypersensitivity
Precautions: Severe renal disease, GI bleeding, diarrhea, intestinal obstruction, pregnancy (C)
Pharmacokinetics:
PO: Excreted in urine
Interactions/incompatibilities:
• Decreased effectiveness of: tetracyclines, ketoconazole
• Decreased absorption of: anticholinergics, chlordiazepoxide, cimetidine, corticosteroids, iron salts, phenothiazines, phenytoin
NURSING CONSIDERATIONS
Perform/provide:
• Storage in airtight container
Evaluate:
• Therapeutic response: absence of pain, decreased acidity
• Decreased constipation, characteristics of stools
Teach patient/family:
• Not to change antacids unless directed by physician
Lab test interferences:
Increase: Urinary pH, gastrin
Decrease: K+

---

magnesium salicylate

Analate, Arthrin, Doan's pills, Efficin, Magan, Mobidin

Func. class.: Nonnarcotic analgesic
Chem. class.: Salicylate

Action: Blocks pain impulses in CNS that occur in response to inhibition of prostaglandin synthesis; antipyretic action results from inhibition of hypothalamic heat-regulating center to produce vasodilation to allow heat dissipation

Uses: Mild to moderate pain or fever including arthritis, juvenile rheumatoid arthritis

Dosage and routes:
Arthritis
• *Adult:* PO not to exceed 4.8 g/day in divided doses
Pain/fever
• *Adult:* PO 600 mg tid or qid
Available forms include: Tabs 325, 545, 600 mg

Side effects/adverse reactions:
*HEMA: **Thrombocytopenia, agranulocytosis, leukopenia, neutropenia, hemolytic anemia,*** increased pro-time
CNS: Stimulation, drowsiness, dizziness, confusion, convulsion, headache, flushing, hallucinations, coma
*GI: **Nausea, vomiting, GI bleeding, diarrhea, heartburn,*** anorexia, ***hepatitis***
*INTEG: **Rash,*** urticaria, bruising
EENT: Tinnitus, hearing loss
CV: Rapid pulse, pulmonary edema
RESP: Wheezing, hyperpnea
ENDO: Hypoglycemia, hyponatremia, hypokalemia

Contraindications: Hypersensitivity to salicylates, GI bleeding, bleeding disorders, children < 3 yr, vitamin K deficiency

Precautions: Anemia, hepatic disease, renal disease, Hodgkin's disease, pregnancy (C), lactation

Pharmacokinetics:
PO: Onset 15-30 min, peak 1-2 hr, duration 4-6 hr, metabolized by liver, excreted by kidneys, crosses placenta, excreted in breast milk, half-life 1-3½ hr

Interactions/incompatibilities:
• Decreased effects of magnesium salicylate: antacids, steroids, urinary alkalizers
• Increased blood loss: alcohol, heparin
• Increased effects of: anticoagulants, insulin, methotrexate
• Decreased effects of: probenecid, spironolactone, sulfinpyrazone, sulfonylmides
• Toxic effects: PABA
• Decreased blood sugar levels: salicylates

NURSING CONSIDERATIONS
Assess:
• Liver function studies: AST, ALT, bilirubin, creatinine if patient is on long-term therapy
• Renal function studies: BUN, urine creatinine if patient is on long-term therapy
• Blood studies: CBC, Hct, Hgb, pro-time if patient is on long-term therapy
• I&O ratio; decreasing output may indicate renal failure (long-term therapy)
Administer:
• To patient crushed or whole; chewable tablets may be chewed
• With food or milk to decrease gastric symptoms; give 30 min before or 2 hr after meals
• With full glass of water
Evaluate:
• Hepatotoxicity: dark urine, clay-colored stools, yellowing of skin, sclera, itching, abdominal pain, fe-

M

---

italics = common side effects   ***bold italic*** = life threatening reactions

ver, diarrhea if patient is on long-term therapy

• Allergic reactions: rash, urticaria; if these occur, drug may need to be discontinued

• Renal dysfunction: decreased urine output

• Ototoxicity: tinnitus, ringing, roaring in ears; audiometric testing is needed before, after long-term therapy

• Visual changes: blurring, halos, corneal and retinal damage

• Edema in feet, ankles, legs

• Prior drug history; there are many drug interactions

Teach patient/family:

• To report any symptoms of hepatotoxicity, renal toxicity, visual changes, ototoxicity, allergic reactions (long-term therapy)

• Not to exceed recommended dosage; acute poisoning may result

• To read label on other OTC drugs; many contain aspirin

• That therapeutic response takes 2 wk (arthritis)

• To avoid alcohol ingestion; GI bleeding may occur

Lab test interferences:

Increase: Coagulation studies, liver function studies, serum uric acid, amylase, CO_2, urinary protein

Decrease: Serum potassium, PBI, cholesterol

Interfere: Urine catecholamines, pregnancy test

Treatment of overdose: Lavage, activated charcoal, monitor electrolytes, VS

---

magnesium salts

Magnesium Citrate, Magnesium Sulfate, Milk of Magnesia (MOM), Mint-O-Mag

Func. class.: Laxative, saline

Action: Increases osmotic pressure, draws fluid into colon

Uses: Constipation, bowel preparation before surgery or examination

Dosage and routes:

• *Adult:* PO 30-60 ml hs (Milk of Magnesia), 300 mg

• *Adult and child >6 yr:* PO 15 g in 8 oz of water (Magnesium Sulfate); PO 10-20 ml (Concentrated Milk of Magnesia); PO 5-10 oz hs (Magnesium Citrate)

• *Child 2-6 yr:* 5-15 ml (Milk of Magnesia)

Available forms include: Oral sol, susp 77.5 mg/g; tabs 300, 600 mg

Side effects/adverse reactions:

CNS: Muscle weakness, flushing, sweating, confusion, sedation, depressed reflexes, ***flaccid, paralysis,*** hypothermia

GI: Nausea, vomiting, anorexia, cramps

CV: Hypotension, heart block, ***circulatory collapse***

META: Electrolyte, fluid imbalances

Contraindications: Hypersensitivity, renal diseases, abdominal pain, nausea/vomiting, obstruction, acute surgical abdomen, rectal bleeding

Precautions: Pregnancy (B)

Pharmacokinetics:

PO: Peak 1-2 hr; excreted in feces

Interactions/incompatibilities:

• Increased CNS depression: CNS depressants, barbiturates, narcotics, anesthetics

NURSING CONSIDERATIONS

Assess:

• I&O ratio; check for decrease in urinary output

Administer:

• With 8 oz of water

Evaluate:

• Therapeutic response: decreased constipation

• Cause of constipation; identify

whether fluids, bulk, or exercise is missing from lifestyle

• Cramping, rectal bleeding, nausea, vomiting; if these symptoms occur, drug should be discontinued

• Magnesium toxicity: thirst, confusion, decrease in reflexes

Teach patient/family:

• Not to use laxatives for long-term therapy; bowel tone will be lost

• Chilling helps the taste of Magnesium Citrate

---

magnesium sulfate

Func. class.: Anticonvulsant
Chem. class.: Magnesium product

Action: Decreases acetylcholine in motor nerve terminals, which is responsible for anticonvulsant properties; osmotically retains fluid, which increases amount of water in feces when used as laxative; reduces SA node impulse formation, prolongs conduction time in myocardium

Uses: Hypomagnesemic seizures, control of seizures in pregnancy induced hypertension, seizures in acute nephritis

Dosage and routes:
Hypomagnesemic seizures

• *Adult:* IV 1-2 g over 15 min, then 1 g IM q4-6h, depending on response

Nephritis

• *Child:* IM 20-40 mg/kg in 20% sol, repeat as needed

Preeclampsia/eclampsia

• *Adult:* IV 4 g/250 ml D₅W and 4 g IM, then 4 g IM q4h prn; or 4 g IV loading dose, then 1-4 g IV INF hourly, not to exceed 3 ml/min

Available forms include: Inj IV, IM 10%, 50%, 12.5%, 25%; granules,

Side effects/adverse reactions:

CNS: Sweating, depressed reflexes,

flushing, drowsiness, flaccid paralysis, hypothermia, weakness, sedation

*RESP: **Paralysis***

CV: Hypotension, **circulatory collapse, heart block,** decreased cardiac function

Contraindications: Hypersensitivity, myocardial infarction, renal disease

Precaution: Pregnancy (C)

Pharmacokinetics:

IV: Onset 1-5 min, duration 30 min
IM: Onset 1 hr, duration 3-4 hr
Excreted by kidneys

Interactions/incompatibilities:

• Increased CNS depression: barbiturates, general anesthetics, narcotics, antipsychotics

• Increased effects of: neuromuscular blockers

NURSING CONSIDERATIONS
Assess:

• VS q15 min after IV dose; do not exceed 150 mg/min

• Cardiac function: monitoring, magnesium levels

• Timing of contractions, determine intensity, monitor fetal heart rate, reactivity, may decrease with this drug if using during labor

• I&O: should remain at 30 ml/hr or more; if less than this, notify physician

Administer:

• Only after calcium gluconate is available for magnesium toxicity

• IV undiluted 1.5 ml of 10% sol over 1 min; may dilute to 20% sol, infuse over 3 hr

• IV at less than 150 mg/min; circulatory collapse may occur

Perform/provide:

• Seizure precautions: placing in dark room with decreased stimuli, padded siderails

Evaluate:

• Urine output before each dose,

output should be 100 ml/4 hr or more

• Mental status: mood, sensorium, affect, memory (long, short)

• Respiratory dysfunction: respiratory depression, character, rate, rhythm; hold drug if respirations are <16/min

• Hypermagnesemia: depressed patellar reflex, flushing, polydipsia, confusion, weakness, flaccid paralysis, hypothermia, dyspnea begin to appear at blood levels of 4 mEq/L

• Respiratory rate, rhythm of newborn if drug was given 24 hr before delivery or less; check reflexes of newborn whose mother received this drug before delivery

• Reflexes: knee jerk, patellar; decrease signals Mg + + toxicity

Teach patient/family:

• Symptoms of hypermagnesemia

Treatment of overdose: Stop drug, administer calcium gluconate, monitor reflexes, magnesium levels

---

magnesium trisilicate

Trisomin

Func. class.: Antacid
Chem. class.: Magnesium product

Action: Neutralizes gastric acidity
Uses: Constipation, hypomagnesemia

Dosage and routes:

• *Adult:* PO 1-4 g qid with 4 oz of water

Available forms include: Powder, Tabs 488 mg

Side effects/adverse reactions:

GI: Diarrhea, flatulence, cramps, belching, nausea, vomiting

META: Hypermagnesemia: *weakness, lethargy, depression, de-*

creased B/P, increased pulse, *respiratory depression, coma*

Contraindications: Hypersensitivity to this drug

Precautions: Severe renal disease, pregnancy (C)

Pharmacokinetics:

PO: Excreted in urine

Interactions/incompatibilities:

• Decreased effectiveness of: tetracyclines, ketoconazole

• Decreased absorption of: anticholinergics, chlordiazepoxide, cimetidine, corticosteroids, iron salts, phenothiazines, phenytoin

NURSING CONSIDERATIONS

Administer:

• After mixing with water

Evaluate:

• Therapeutic response: absence of pain, decreased acidity

• Decreased constipation, characteristics of stools

Teach patient/family:

• Not to change antacids unless directed by physician

• Tabs must be chewed before swallowing

• Drug has a delayed reaction

• To separate doses of other drugs by 1 hr

Lab test interferences:

Increase: Urinary pH, gastrin
Decrease: K +

---

mannitol

(man'i-tole)

Osmitrol, Resectial

Func. class.: Osmotic diuretic
Chem. class.: Hexahydric alcohol

Action: Acts by increasing osmolarity of glomerular filtrate, which raises osmotic pressure of fluid in renal tubules; there is a decrease in reabsorption of water, increase in urinary output, sodium, chloride excretion

Uses: Edema, promote systemic diuresis in cerebral edema, decrease intraocular pressure, improve renal function in acute renal failure, chemical poisoning

Dosage and routes:

Oliguria, prevention
• *Adult:* IV 50-100 g of a 5%-25% sol

Oliguria, treatment
• *Adult:* IV 300-400 mg/kg of a 20%-25% sol up to 100 g of a 15%-20% sol

Intraocular pressure/intracranial pressure
• *Adult:* IV 1.5-2 g/kg of a 15%-25% sol over ½-1 hr

Renal failure
• *Adult:* IV 50-200 g/24 hr, adjusted to maintain output of 30-50 mg/hr

Diuresis in drug intoxication
• *Adult and child >12 yr:* 5%-10% sol continuously up to 200 g IV, while maintaining 100-500 ml output/hr

Available forms include: Inj IV 5%, 10%, 15%, 20%, 25%

Side effects/adverse reactions:

GU: Marked diuresis, urinary retention, thirst

CNS: Dizziness, headache, ***convulsions,*** rebound increased ICP

GI: Nausea, vomiting, dry mouth, diarrhea

CV: Edema, thrombophlebitis, hypotension, hypertension, tachycardia, angina-like chest pains, fever, chills

RESP: Pulmonary congestion

ELECT: Fluid, electrolyte imbalances, acidosis, electrolyte loss, dehydration

EENT: Loss of hearing, blurred vision, nasal congestion, decreased intraocular pressure

Contraindications: Active intracranial bleeding, hypersensitivity, anuria, severe pulmonary congestion, edema, severe dehydration

Precautions: Dehydration, pregnancy (C), severe renal disease, CHF, lactation

Pharmacokinetics:

IV: Onset 30-60 min for diuresis, ½-1 hr for intraocular pressure, 25 min for cerebrospinal fluid; duration 4-6 hr for intraocular pressure, 3-8 hr for cerebrospinal fluid; excreted in urine

Interactions/incompatibilities:
• Decreased effect: lithium
• Increased effects of: EDTA
• Incompatible with whole blood, in solution or syringe with any other drug or solution

NURSING CONSIDERATIONS

Assess:
• Weight, I&O daily to determine fluid loss; effect of drug may be decreased if used qd
• Rate, depth, rhythm of respiration, effect of exertion
• B/P lying, standing, postural hypotension may occur
• Electrolytes: potassium, sodium, chloride; include BUN, CBC, serum creatinine, blood pH, ABGs

Administer:
• IV in 15%-25% solutions with filter; give over ½-1½ hr, rapid infusion may worsen CHF
• Test dose in severe oliguria, 0.2 g/kg over 3-5 min, if no urine increase, give 2nd test dose; if no response, reassess patient

Evaluate:
• Improvement in edema of feet, legs, sacral area daily if medication is being used in CHF
• Improvement in CVP q8h
• Signs of metabolic acidosis: drowsiness, restlessness
• Signs of hypokalemia: postural

M

---

italics = common side effects   ***bold italic*** = life threatening reactions

hypotension, malaise, fatigue, tachycardia, leg cramps, weakness
• Rashes, temperature elevation qd
• Confusion, especially in elderly; take safety precautions if needed
• Hydration including skin turgor, thirst, dry mucous membranes
Teach patient/family:
• To increase fluid intake 2-3 L/day unless contraindicated; to rise slowly from lying or sitting position
Lab test interferences:
Interference: Inorganic phosphorus, ethylene glycol
Treatment of overdose: Discontinue infusion, correct fluid, electrolyte imbalances, hemodialysis, monitor hydration, CV, renal function

---

maprotiline HCl
(ma-proe'ti-leen)
Ludiomil
Func. class.: Antidepressant
Chem. class.: Tetracyclic

Action: Blocks reuptake of norepinephrine, serotonin into nerve endings, increasing action of norepinephrine, serotonin in nerve cells
Uses: Depression, dysthymic disorder, manic depressive — depressed, agitated depression
Dosage and routes:
• *Adult:* PO 75 mg/day in moderate depression, may increase to 150 mg/day; not to exceed 225 mg in hospitalized patients, severely depressed patients that are hospitalized may be given 300 mg/day
• *Elderly:* 50-75 mg/day
Available forms include: Tabs 25, 50, 75 mg
Side effects/adverse reactions:
HEMA: Agranulocytosis, thrombocytopenia, eosinophilia, leukopenia
CNS: Dizziness, drowsiness, confusion, headache, anxiety, tremors, stimulation, weakness, insomnia, nightmares, EPS (elderly), increased psychiatric symptoms, *seizures*
GI: Diarrhea, dry mouth, nausea, vomiting, *paralytic ileus,* increased appetite, cramps, epigastric distress, jaundice, *hepatitis,* stomatitis
GU: Retention, acute renal failure
INTEG: Rash, urticaria, sweating, pruritus, photosensitivity
CV: Orthostatic hypotension, ECG changes, tachycardia, hypertension, palpitations
EENT: Blurred vision, tinnitus, mydriasis
Contraindications: Hypersensitivity to tricyclic antidepressants, recovery phase of myocardial infarction, convulsive disorders, prostatic hypertrophy
Precautions: Suicidal patients, severe depression, increased intraocular pressure, narrow-angle glaucoma, urinary retention, cardiac disease, hepatic disease, hypothyroidism, hyperthyroidism, electroshock therapy, elective surgery, elderly, pregnancy (B)
Pharmacokinetics:
PO: Onset 15-30 min, peak 12 hr, duration up to 3 wk, steady state 6-10 days; metabolized by liver, excreted by kidneys, feces, crosses placenta, half-life 21-25 hr
Interactions/incompatibilities:
• Decreased effects of: guanethidine, clonidine, indirect acting sympathomimetics (ephedrine)
• Increased effects of: direct acting sympathomimetics (epinephrine), alcohol, barbiturates, benzodiazepines, CNS depressants

• Hyperpyretic crisis, convulsions, hypertensive episode: MAOI (pargyline [Eutonyl])

NURSING CONSIDERATIONS
Assess:
• B/P (lying, standing), pulse q4h; if systolic B/P drops 20 mm Hg hold drug, notify physician; take vital signs q4h in patients with cardiovascular disease
• Blood studies: CBC, leukocytes, differential, cardiac enzymes if patient is receiving long-term therapy
• Hepatic studies: AST, ALT, bilirubin, creatinine
• Weight qwk, appetite may increase with drug
• ECG for flattening of T wave, bundle branch block, AV block, dysrhythmias in cardiac patients
Administer:
• Increased fluids, bulk in diet if constipation, urinary retention occur
• With food or milk for GI symptoms
• Dosage hs if over-sedation occurs during day; may take entire dose hs; elderly may not tolerate once/day dosing
• Gum, hard candy, or frequent sips of water for dry mouth
• Concentrate with fruit juice, water, or milk to disguise taste
Perform/provide:
• Storage in tight container at room temperature, do not freeze
• Assistance with ambulation during beginning therapy since drowsiness/dizziness occurs
• Safety measures including siderails primarily in elderly
• Checking to see PO medication swallowed
Evaluate:
• EPS primarily in elderly: rigidity, dystonia, akathisia
• Mental status: mood, sensorium, affect, suicidal tendencies, increase in psychiatric symptoms: depression, panic
• Urinary retention, constipation; constipation is more likely to occur in children
• Withdrawal symptoms: headache, nausea, vomiting, muscle pain, weakness; do not usually occur unless drug was discontinued abruptly
• Alcohol consumption; if alcohol is consumed, hold dose until morning
Teach patient/family:
• That therapeutic effects may take 2-3 wk
• Use of caution in driving or other activities requiring alertness because of drowsiness, dizziness, blurred vision
• To avoid alcohol ingestion, other CNS depressants
• Not to discontinue medication quickly after long-term use, may cause nausea, headache, malaise
• To wear sunscreen or large hat since photosensitivity occurs
Lab test interferences:
Increase: Serum bilirubin, blood glucose, alk phosphatase
False increase: Urinary catecholamines
Decrease: VMA, 5-HIAA
Treatment of overdose: ECG monitoring, induce emesis, lavage, activated charcoal, administer anticonvulsant

---

mazindol
(may'zin-dole)
Mazanor, Sanorex
Func. class.: Anorexiant
Chem. class.: Imidazoisoindole derivative

Controlled Substance Schedule IV

italics = common side effects　　**bold italic** = life threatening reactions

Action: Acts on central adrenergic and dopaminergic pathways to stimulate satiety center in hypothalamic, limbic regions

Uses: Exogenous obesity

Dosage and routes:
• *Adult:* PO 1 mg ac, or 2 mg 1 hr ac lunch

Available forms include: Tabs 1, 2 mg

Side effects/adverse reactions:

HEMA: **Bone marrow depression, leukopenia, agranulocytosis**

EENT: Mydriasis, blurred vision, eye irritation

MISC: Hair loss, muscle pain, flushing, fever

CNS: *Hyperactivity, insomnia, restlessness,* dizziness, headache, stimulation, irritability, drowsiness, weakness, tremor

GI: Nausea, anorexia, dry mouth, diarrhea, constipation

GU: Impotence, change in libido, difficulty urinating

CV: Palpitations, tachycardia

INTEG: Urticaria, rash, pallor, shivering, sweating

Contraindications: Hypersensitivity to sympathomimetic amine, glaucoma, drug abuse, cardiovascular disease, children <12 yr, hypertension, hypotension, severe arteriosclerosis, agitated states

Precautions: Diabetes mellitus, pregnancy (C), lactation

Pharmacokinetics:

PO: Onset ½-1 hr, duration 8-15 hr, metabolized by liver, excreted by kidneys

Interactions/incompatibilities:
• Hypertensive crisis: MAOIs or within 14 days of MAOIs
• Increased effect of mazindol: acetazolamide, antacids, sodium bicarbonate, ascorbic acid, ammonium chloride

• Decreased effects of mazindol: tricyclics
• Decreased effects of: guanethidine, other antihypertensives
• Increased effects of: insulin

NURSING CONSIDERATIONS

Assess:
• VS, B/P since this drug may reverse antihypertensives; check patients with cardiac disease more often
• CBC, urinalysis, in diabetes: blood sugar, urine sugar; insulin changes may need to be made since eating will decrease
• Height, growth rate in children; growth rate may be decreased

Administer:
• At least 6 hr before hs to avoid sleeplessness, 1 hr ac meals
• For obesity only if patient is on weight reduction program including dietary changes, exercise; patient will develop tolerance, and weight loss won't occur without additional methods
• Gum, hard candy, frequent sips of water for dry mouth

Evaluate:
• Mental status: mood, sensorium, affect, stimulation, insomnia, aggressiveness
• Physical dependency: should not be used for extended time; dose should be discontinued gradually, tolerance will occur after long-term use
• Withdrawal symptoms: headache, nausea, vomiting, muscle pain, weakness

Teach patient/family:
• To take with meals to avoid GI symptoms
• To decrease caffeine consumption (coffee, tea, cola, chocolate), which may increase irritability, stimulation

---

* Available in Canada only

- Avoid OTC preparations unless approved by physician
- To taper off drug over several weeks, or depression, increased sleeping, lethargy may ensue
- To avoid alcohol ingestion
- To avoid hazardous activities until patient is stabilized on medication
- To get needed rest, patients will feel more tired at end of day

Treatment of overdose: Administer fluids, chlorpromazine 1 mg/kg; antihypertensive for increased B/P; ammonium Cl for increased excretion

---

measles, mumps, and rubella virus vaccine, live
M-M-R-II

Func. class.: Vaccine

Action: Produces antibodies to measles, mumps, rubella

Uses: Prevention of measles, mumps, rubella

Dosage and routes:
- *Child 1-13 yr:* SC 1000 U

Available forms include: Inj SC measles 1000 $TCID_{50}$, mumps 5000 $TCID_{50}$, rubella 1000 $TCID_{50}$

Side effects/adverse reactions:

CNS: Fever, *subacute sclerosing panencephalitis and blindness associated with optic neuritis,* paresthesias

INTEG: Urticaria, erythema

SYST: Lymphadenitis, *anaphylaxis*

MS: Osteomyelitis, arthralgia, arthritis

Contraindications: Hypersensitivity, blood dyscrasias, anemia, active infection, immunosuppression, egg, chicken allergy, pregnancy, febrile illness, neomycin allergy

Interactions/incompatibilities:
- Decreased response to: TB skin test
- Other live virus vaccines

NURSING CONSIDERATIONS

Assess:
- For skin reactions: rash, induration, erythema

Administer:
- Only with epinephrine 1:1000 on unit to treat laryngospasm
- Only SC

Perform/provide:
- Storage at 39° F (4° C), protect from heat and light; do not give within 1 month of other live virus vaccines

Evaluate:
- For history of allergies, skin conditions (eczema, psoriasis, dermatitis), reactions to vaccinations
- For anaphylaxis: inability to breathe, bronchospasm

Teach patient/family:
- That fever may occur between the 5-12th day after vaccine given
- That joint pains, tingling in extremities may occur 5-12 day after vaccine given
- That pain and inflammation may occur
- To take acetaminophen for fever

---

mebendazole
(me-ben′da-zole)
Vermox

Func. class.: Anthelmintic
Chem. class.: Carbamate

Action: Inhibits glucose uptake, degeneration of cytoplasmic microtubules in the cell; interferes with absorption, secretory function

Uses: Pinworms, roundworms, hookworms, whipworms, threadworms, pork tapeworms, dwarf

M

---

italics = common side effects   ***bold italic*** = life threatening reactions

tapeworms, beef tapeworms, hydatid cyst

Dosage and routes:
• *Adult and child >2 yr:* PO 100 mg as a single dose or bid × 3 days, depending on type of infection; course may be repeated in 3 wk if needed

Available forms include: Tabs, chewable 100 mg

Side effects/adverse reactions:
CNS: Dizziness, fever
GI: Transient diarrhea, abdominal pain

Contraindications: Hypersensitivity

Precautions: Child <2 yr, lactation, pregnancy (1st trimester) (C)

Pharmacokinetics:
PO: Peak ½-7 hr, excreted in feces primarily (metabolites), small amount in urine (unchanged), highly bound to plasma proteins

NURSING CONSIDERATIONS
Assess:
• Stools during entire treatment; specimens must be sent to lab while still warm

Administer:
• May be crushed, chewed if unable to swallow whole
• PO after meals to avoid GI symptoms since absorption is not altered by food
• Second course after 3 wk if needed; usually recommended

Perform/provide:
• Storage in tight container

Evaluate:
• For therapeutic response: expulsion of worms and 3 negative stool cultures after completion of treatment
• For allergic reaction: rash (rare)
• For diarrhea during expulsion of worms; avoid self-contamination with patient's feces
• For infection in other family members since infection from person to person is common

Teach patient/family:
• Proper hygiene after BM including handwashing technique; tell patient to avoid putting fingers in mouth
• That infected person should sleep alone; do not shake bed linen, change bed linen qd, wash in hot water
• To clean toilet qd with disinfectant (green soap solution)
• Need for compliance with dosage schedule, duration of treatment
• To wear shoes, wash all fruits and vegetables well before eating

---

mecamylamine HCl
(mek-a-mill′a-meen)
Inversine

Func. class.: Antihypertensive
Chem. class.: Ganglionic blocker

Action: Occupies receptor site, prevents acetylcholine from attaching to postsynaptic nerve ending in sympathetic ganglia

Uses: Moderate to severe hypertension, malignant hypertension

Dosage and routes:
• *Adult:* PO 2.5 mg bid, may increase in increments of 2.5 mg × 2 days until desired response, maintenance 25 mg/day in 3 divided doses

Available forms include: Tabs 2.5 mg

Side effects/adverse reactions:
CV: Postural hypotension, irregular heart rate, *CHF*
CNS: Drowsiness, sedation, headache, tremors, weakness, syncope, paresthesia, dizziness, *convulsions*
EENT: Blurred vision, nasal congestion, dry mouth, dilated pupils

GU: Impotence, urinary retention, decreased libido

GI: Anorexia, glossitis, nausea, vomiting, constipation, *paralytic ileus*

Contraindications: Hypersensitivity, myocardial infarction, coronary insufficiency, renal disease, glaucoma, organic pyloric stenosis, uremia, uncooperative patients, mild/labile hypertension

Precautions: CVA, prostatic hypertrophy, bladder neck obstruction, urethral stricture, renal dysfunction (elevated BUN), cerebral dysfunction, pregnancy (C)

Pharmacokinetics:

PO: Onset ½-2 hr, duration 6-12 hr; excreted in urine, feces, breast milk; crosses placenta

Interactions/incompatibilities:

• Increased effects: thiazide diuretics, antihypertensives, CNS depressants (alcohol, anesthetics, MAOIs), bethanechol

NURSING CONSIDERATIONS

Assess:

• B/P lying and standing, other VS throughout treatment

• Weight daily, I&O

Administer:

• Whole, do not chew or crush tablets

• After meals for better absorption; give larger dose at noon and evening, smaller dose in AM

• Gum, frequent rinsing of mouth, hard candy for dry mouth

Evaluate:

• Edema in feet, legs daily

• Skin turgor, dryness of mucous membranes for hydration status

• Tolerance to drug that occurs with prolonged use

• Constipation: number of stools, consistency, give stool softener as ordered or increase bulk in diet

Teach patient/family:

• To notify physician if tremor, seizure, or signs of paralytic ileus occur

• To avoid OTC preparations unless directed by physician

• To rise slowly from sitting or lying position, orthostatic hypotension may occur

• That impotence may occur, but is reversible after discontinuing drug

Treatment of overdose: Administer gastric lavage, discontinue drug, administer small doses of pressor amines for hypotension

---

mechlorethamine HCl (nitrogen mustard)

(me-klor-eth′a-meen)

Mustargen

Func. class.: Antineoplastic alkylating agent

Chem. class.: Nitrogen mustard

M

Action: Responsible for cross-linking DNA strands leading to cell death; rapidly degraded, a vesicant

Uses: Hodgkin's disease, lymphomas, lymphosarcoma; ovarian, breast, lung cancer; neoplastic effusions

Dosage and routes:

• *Adult:* IV 0.4 mg/kg or 10 mg/m² as 1 dose or divided doses

Neoplastic effusions

• *Adult:* INTRACAVITY 10-20 mg

Available forms include: Inj IV, intracavity 10 mg; powder for inj

Side effects/adverse reactions:

EENT: Tinnitus, hearing loss

HEMA: ***Thrombocytopenia, leukopenia, agranulocytosis,*** anemia

GI: Nausea, vomiting, diarrhea, stomatitis, weight loss, colitis, ***hepatotoxicity***

CNS: Headache, dizziness, drows-

---

italics = common side effects   ***bold italic*** = life threatening reactions

iness, paresthesia, peripheral neuropathy, **coma**

INTEG: Alopecia, pruritus, herpes zoster

Contraindications: Lactation, pregnancy (1st trimester) (D), myelosuppression, acute herpes zoster

Precautions: Radiation therapy, chronic lymphocytic leukopenia

Pharmacokinetics:

Metabolized in liver, excreted in urine

Interactions/incompatibilities:

• Increased toxicity: antineoplastics, radiation

NURSING CONSIDERATIONS
Assess:

• CBC, differential, platelet count weekly; withhold drug if WBC is <4000 or platelet count is <75,000; notify physician of results

• Renal function studies: BUN, serum uric acid, urine CrCl before, during therapy

• I&O ratio, report fall in urine output of 30 ml/hr

• Monitor temperature q4h (may indicate beginning infection), no rectal temperatures

• Liver function tests before, during therapy (bilirubin, AST, ALT, LDH) as needed or monthly

Administer:

• After using guidelines for preparation of cytotoxic drugs

• Antiemetic 30-60 min before giving drug to prevent vomiting and p.rn

• Antibiotics for prophylaxis of infection

• IV after diluting 10 mg/10 ml sterile H_2O or NaCl; leave needle in vial, shake, withdraw dose, give through Y-tube or 3-way stopcock or directly

• Slow IV infusion using 21-, 23-, 25-gauge needle, watch for infiltra-

tion. If infiltration occurs, infiltrate area with isotonic sodium thiosulfate or 1% lidocaine. Apply ice for 6-12 hrs.

• Topical or systemic analgesics for pain

• Local or systemic drugs for infection

Perform/provide:

• Storage at room temperature in dry form

• Strict medical asepsis, protective isolation if WBC levels are low

• Special skin care

• Increase fluid intake to 2-3 L/day to prevent urate deposits, calculi formation

• Diet low in purines: organ meats (kidney, liver), dried beans, peas to maintain alkaline urine

• Preparation under hood using gloves and mask

• Rinsing of mouth tid-qid with water, club soda; brushing of teeth bid-tid with soft brush or cotton tipped applicators for stomatitis; use unwaxed dental floss

• Warm compresses at injection site for inflammation

Evaluate:

• Bleeding: hematuria, guaiac, bruising or petechiae, mucosa or orifices q8h

• Food preferences; list likes, dislikes

• Yellowing of skin, sclera, dark urine, clay-colored stools, itchy skin, abdominal pain, fever, diarrhea

• Effects of alopecia on body image; discuss feelings about body changes

• Inflammation of mucosa, breaks in skin

• Buccal cavity q8h for dryness, sores, ulceration, white patches, oral pain, bleeding, dysphagia

---

*Available in Canada only

• Local irritation, pain, burning, discoloration at injection site
• Symptoms indicating severe allergic reaction: rash, pruritus, urticaria, purpuric skin lesions, itching, flushing

Teach patient/family:
• Of protective isolation precautions
• That sterility, amenorrhea can occur; reversible after discontinuing treatment
• That hair may be lost during treatment; a wig or hairpiece may make patient feel better; new hair may be different in color, texture
• To avoid foods with citric acid, hot or rough texture
• To report any bleeding, white spots, or ulcerations in mouth to physician; tell patient to examine mouth qd
• To report signs of infection: increased temperature, sore throat, flu symptoms
• To report signs of anemia: fatigue, headache, faintness, shortness of breath, irritability
• To avoid use of razors or commercial mouthwash
• To avoid use of aspirin products or ibuprofen

---

meclizine HCl

(mek'li-zeen)
Antivert, Bonamine,* Bonine, Lamine, Roclizine, Vertol
Func. class.: Antiemetic, antihistamine, anticholinergic
Chem. class.: H$_1$-receptor antagonist, piperazine derivative

Action: Acts centrally by blocking chemoreceptor trigger zone, which in turn acts on vomiting center
Uses: Dizziness, motion sickness

Dosage and routes:
• *Adult:* PO 25-100 mg qd in divided doses or 1 hr before traveling
Available forms include: Tabs 12.5, 25, 50 mg; chew tabs 25 mg; tabs film coated 25 mg

Side effects/adverse reactions:
CNS: Drowsiness, dizziness, fatigue, restlessness, headache, insomnia
GI: Nausea, anorexia
EENT: Dry mouth, blurred vision

Contraindications: Hypersensitivity to cyclizines, shock, lactation, pregnancy
Precautions: Children, narrow-angle glaucoma, glaucoma, urinary retention, lactation, prostatic hypertrophy, elderly, pregnancy (B)

Pharmacokinetics:
PO: Duration 8-24 hr, half-life 6 hr

Interactions/incompatibilities:
• Increased effect of: alcohol, tranquilizers, narcotics

NURSING CONSIDERATIONS
Assess:
• VS, B/P
Administer:
• Tablets may be swallowed whole, chewed, or allowed to dissolve
Evaluate:
• Signs of toxicity of other drugs or masking of symptoms of disease: brain tumor, intestinal obstruction
• Observe for drowsiness, dizziness, LOC
Teach patient/family:
• That a false negative result may occur with skin testing; these procedures should not be scheduled for 4 days after discontinuing use
• To avoid hazardous activities, activities requiring alertness; dizziness may occur; instruct patient to request assistance with ambulation
• Avoid alcohol, other depressants
Lab test interferences:
False negative: Allergy skin testing

italics = common side effects   ***bold italic*** = life threatening reactions

meclofenamate

(me-kloe-fen-am′ate)
Meclamen
Func. class.: Nonsteroidal antiinflammatory
Chem. class.: Anthranilic acid derivative

Action: Inhibits prostaglandin synthesis by decreasing an enzyme needed for biosynthesis; possesses analgesic, antiinflammatory, antipyretic properties

Uses: Mild to moderate pain, osteoarthritis, rheumatoid arthritis

Dosage and routes:
• *Adult:* PO 200-400 mg/day in divided doses tid-qid

Available forms include: Caps 50, 100 mg

Side effects/adverse reactions:
GI: Nausea, anorexia, vomiting, diarrhea, jaundice, *cholestatic hepatitis,* constipation, flatulence, cramps, dry mouth, peptic ulcer
CNS: Dizziness, drowsiness, fatigue, tremors, confusion, insomnia, anxiety, depression
CV: Tachycardia, peripheral edema, palpitations, dysrhythmias
INTEG: Purpura, rash, pruritus, sweating
GU: Nephrotoxicity: dysuria, hematuria, oliguria, azotemia
HEMA: Blood dyscrasias
EENT: Tinnitus, hearing loss, blurred vision

Contraindications: Hypersensitivity, asthma, severe renal disease, severe hepatic disease

Precautions: Pregnancy (B), lactation, children, bleeding disorders, GI disorders, cardiac disorders, hypersensitivity to other antiinflammatory agents

Pharmacokinetics:
PO: Peak 2 hr, half-life 3-3½ hr;

metabolized in liver, excreted in urine (metabolites), excreted in breast milk

Interactions/incompatibilities:
• Increased action of: coumarin, phenytoin, sulfonamides

NURSING CONSIDERATIONS
Assess:
• Renal, liver, blood studies: BUN, creatinine, AST, ALT, Hgb, Hct before treatment, periodically thereafter
• Audiometric and ophthalmic exam before, during, after treatment
• For history of peptic ulcer disease

Administer:
• With food to decrease GI symptoms; best to take on empty stomach to facilitate absorption

Perform/provide:
• Storage at room temperature

Evaluate:
• Therapeutic response: decreased pain, stiffness, swelling in joints, ability to move more easily
• For eye, ear problems: blurred vision, tinnitus (may indicate toxicity)

Teach patient/family:
• To report increased GI symptoms; dose may need to be reduced
• To report blurred vision, ringing, roaring in ears (may indicate toxicity)
• To avoid driving or other hazardous activities if dizziness or drowsiness occurs
• To report change in urine pattern, weight increase, edema, pain increase in joints, fever, blood in urine (indicates nephrotoxicity)
• That therapeutic effects may take up to 1 mo

medium-chain triglycerides
MCT Oil
Func. class.: Caloric

Action: Needed for energy in body; more rapidly hydrolyzed than fat

Uses: Inadequate dietary fat intake or absorption

Dosage and routes:
• *Adult:* PO 15 ml tid-qid, not to exceed 100 ml/day

Available forms include: Oil (115 calories/15 ml)

Side effects/adverse reactions:
CNS: Loss of consciousness (reversible)
GI: Nausea, vomiting, anorexia, cramps, diarrhea, distention

Contraindications: Hypersensitivity, severe hepatic disease, lipoproteinemia

Precautions: Portacaval shunts, pregnancy (C), pancreatis, hyperlipemia

NURSING CONSIDERATIONS
Assess:
• Triglycerides, free fatty acid levels, platelet counts daily to prevent fat overload, thrombocytopenia
• Liver function: AST, ALT

Evaluate:
• Therapeutic response: increased weight
• Nutritional status: calorie count by dietician

Teach patient/family:
• Reason for use of lipids
• Methods of incorporating drug in food or beverages (salad dressings, chilled fruit juices)

medroxyprogesterone acetate
(me-drox'ee-proe-jess'te-rone)
Amen, Curretab, Depo-Provera, Provera
Func. class.: Progestogen
Chem. class.: Progesterone derivative

Action: Inhibits secretion of pituitary gonadotropins, which prevents follicular maturation and ovulation, stimulates growth of mammary tissue, antineoplastic action against endometrial cancer

Uses: Uterine bleeding (abnormal), secondary amenorrhea, endometrial cancer, renal cancer

Dosage and routes:
Secondary amenorrhea
• *Adult:* PO 5-10 mg qd × 5-10 days

Endometrial/renal cancer
• *Adult:* 1M 400-1000 mg/wk

Uterine bleeding
• *Adult:* PO 5-10 mg qd × 5-10 days starting on 16th day of menstrual cycle

Available forms include: Tabs 2.5, 10 mg; inj susp 100, 400 mg/ml

Side effects/adverse reactions:
CNS: Dizziness, headache, migraines, depression, fatigue
CV: Hypotension, thrombophlebitis, edema, ***thromboembolism, stroke, pulmonary embolism, myocardial infarction***
GI: Nausea, vomiting, anorexia, cramps, increased weight, ***cholestatic jaundice***
EENT: Diplopia
GU: Amenorrhea, cervical erosion, breakthrough bleeding, dysmenorrhea, vaginal candidiasis, breast changes, ***gynecomastia, testicular***

M

atrophy, impotence, endometriosis, ***spontaneous abortion***
INTEG: Rash, urticaria, acne, hirsutism, alopecia, oily skin, seborrhea, purpura, melasma, photosensitivity
META: Hyperglycemia
Contraindications: Breast cancer, hypersensitivity, thromboembolic disorders, reproductive cancer, genital bleeding (abnormal, undiagnosed), pregnancy (X)
Precautions: Lactation, hypertension, asthma, blood dyscrasias, gallbladder disease, CHF, diabetes mellitus, bone disease, depression, migraine headache, convulsive disorders, hepatic disease, renal disease, family history of cancer of breast or reproductive tract
Pharmacokinetics:
PO: Duration 24 hr, excreted in urine and feces, metabolized in liver

NURSING CONSIDERATIONS
Assess:
• Weight daily, notify physician of weekly weight gain >5 lb
• B/P at beginning of treatment and periodically
• I&O ratio; be alert for decreasing urinary output, increasing edema
• Liver function studies: ALT, AST, bilirubin, periodically during long-term therapy
Administer:
• Titrated dose, use lowest effective dose
• Oil solution deeply in large muscle mass (IM), rotate sites
• In one dose in AM
• With food or milk to decrease GI symptoms
• After warming to dissolve crystals
Perform/provide:
• Storage in dark area

Evaluate:
• Therapeutic response: decreased abnormal uterine bleeding, absence of amenorrhea
• Edema, hypertension, cardiac symptoms, jaundice
• Mental status: affect, mood, behavioral changes, depression
• Hypercalcemia
Teach patient/family:
• To avoid sunlight or use sunscreen; photosensitivity can occur
• About cushingoid symptoms
• To report breast lumps, vaginal bleeding, edema, jaundice, dark urine, clay colored stools, dyspnea, headache, blurred vision, abdominal pain, numbness or stiffness in legs, chest pain; male to report impotence or gynecomastia
• To report suspected pregnancy
Lab test interferences:
Increase: Alk phosphatase, nitrogen (urine), pregnanediol, amino acids
Decrease: GTT, HDL

---

mefenamic acid
(me-fe-nam'-ik)
Ponstan, Ponstel
Func. class.: Nonsteroidal antiinflammatory
Chem. class.: Anthranilic acid derivative

Action: Inhibits prostaglandin synthesis by decreasing an enzyme needed for biosynthesis and interferes with prostaglandins at receptor sites; possesses analgesic, antiinflammatory, antipyretic properties
Uses: Mild to moderate pain, dysmenorrhea, inflammatory disease
Dosage and routes:
• *Adult and child >14 yr:* PO 500

mg, then 250 mg q4h, use not to exceed 1 wk

Available forms include: Caps 250 mg

Side effects/adverse reactions:

GI: Nausea, anorexia, vomiting, diarrhea, jaundice, ***cholestatic hepatitis,*** constipation, flatulence, cramps, dry mouth, peptic ulcer

CNS: Dizziness, drowsiness, fatigue, tremors, confusion, insomnia, anxiety, depression

CV: Tachycardia, peripheral edema, palpitations, dysrhythmias

INTEG: Purpura, rash, pruritus, sweating

GU: ***Nephrotoxicity: dysuria, hematuria, oliguria, azotemia***

HEMA: ***Blood dyscrasias***

EENT: Tinnitus, hearing loss, blurred vision

Contraindications: Hypersensitivity, asthma, severe renal disease, severe hepatic disease

Precautions: Pregnancy (C), lactation, children, bleeding disorders, GI disorders, cardiac disorders, hypersensitivity to other antiinflammatory agents

Pharmacokinetics:

PO: Peak 2 hr, half-life 3-3½ hr; metabolized in liver, excreted in urine (metabolites), excreted in breast milk, extensive protein binding

Interactions/incompatibilities:

• Increased action of: coumarin, phenytoin, sulfonamides

NURSING CONSIDERATIONS

Assess:

• Renal, liver, blood studies: BUN, creatinine, AST, ALT, Hgb before treatment, periodically thereafter

• Audiometric, ophthalmic exam before, during, after treatment

Administer:

• With food to decrease GI symptoms; best to take on empty stomach to facilitate absorption

Perform/provide:

• Storage at room temperature

Evaluate:

• Therapeutic response: decreased pain, stiffness, swelling in joints, ability to move more easily

• For eye, ear problems: blurred vision, tinnitus (may indicate toxicity)

Teach patient/family:

• To report blurred vision, or ringing, roaring in ears (may indicate toxicity)

• To avoid driving or other hazardous activities if dizziness or drowsiness occurs

• To report change in urine pattern, weight increase, edema, pain increase in joints, fever, blood in urine (indicates nephrotoxicity)

• That therapeutic effects may take up to 1 mo

• To report diarrhea or skin rash: drug may be discontinued

• To take with full glass of water

---

mefloquine HCl

(me-flow'quine)

Lariam

Func. class.: Antimalarial

Chem. class.: Analog of quinine

Action: Exact mechanism not known; blood schizonticide

Uses: Treatment and prevention of *Plasmodium falciparum* malaria, *P. vivax*

Dosage and routes:

• *Adult:* PO 1250 mg as a single dose (treatment); 250 mg q wk × 4 wk, then 250 mg q other wk (prevention)

Available forms include: Tabs 250 mg

---

italics = common side effects   ***bold italic*** = life threatening reactions

Side effects/adverse reactions:
CV: Bradycardia, extrasystole
CNS: Dizziness, headache, syncope, *neuropsychiatric disturbances: disorientation, hallucinations, coma, convulsions*
GI: Nausea, vomiting, loss of appetite, diarrhea, abdominal pain
INTEG: Itching, rash
MISC: Myalgia
Contraindications: Hypersensitivity, pregnancy (X)
Precautions: Cardiac dysrhythmias, neurologic disease, lactation, children
Pharmacokinetics:
Protein binding 98%, excreted in breast milk and urine, half-life 21 days (adults)
Interactions/incompatibilities:
• Increased ECG abnormalities, possible cardiac arrest: beta blockers, quinine, quinidine
• Increased potential for convulsions: chloroquine, valproic acids
NURSING CONSIDERATIONS
Assess:
• B/P, pulse, watch for bradycardia
• Neuropsychiatric symptoms: disorientation, hallucinations; drug should be discontinued
• Liver studies weekly: ALT, AST, bilirubin
Administer:
• On empty stomach with at least 8 oz of water
Perform/provide:
• Storage in tight, light-resistant container
Teach patient/family:
• To take drug on an empty stomach with full glass of water

megestrol acetate

(me-jess'trole)
Megace, Pallace
Func. class.: Antineoplastic
Chem. class.: Hormone, progestin

Action: Affects endometrium by antiluteinizing effect; this is thought to bring about cell death
Uses: Breast, endometrial cancer, renal cell cancer
Dosage and routes:
• *Adult:* PO 40-320 mg/day in divided doses
Available forms include: Tabs 20, 40 mg
Side effects/adverse reactions:
GI: Nausea, vomiting, anorexia, diarrhea, abdominal cramps
GU: Gynecomastia, fluid retention, *hypercalcemia*
CV: Thrombophlebitis
INTEG: Alopecia, rash, pruritus, purpura, itching
CNS: Mood swings
Contraindications: Hypersensitivity, pregnancy (X)
Pharmacokinetics:
PO: Duration 1-3 days, half-life 60 min, metabolized in liver, excreted in feces, breast milk
NURSING CONSIDERATIONS
Assess:
• I&O ratio weights
• Serum Ca levels
• Homan's sign
Administer:
• Antispasmodic
• Diuretics for increased fluids
Perform/provide:
• Increase fluid intake to 2-3 L/day to prevent dehydration and maintain normal Ca
• Nutritious diet with iron, vitamin supplements as ordered
• Limitation of calcium (dairy products)

---

*Available in Canada only

- Storage in tight container at room temperature

Evaluate:
- Food preferences; list likes, dislikes
- Effects of alopecia on body image; discuss feelings about body changes
- Symptoms indicating severe allergic reaction: rash, pruritus, urticaria, purpuric skin lesions, itching, flushing
- Frequency of stools, characteristics: cramping, acidosis, signs of dehydration (rapid respirations, poor skin turgor, decreased urine output, dry skin, restlessness, weakness)
- Mood swings
- Anorexia, nausea, vomiting, constipation, weakness, loss of muscle tone

Teach patient/family:
- To report any complaints or side effects to nurse or physician
- That gynecomastia can occur; reversible after discontinuing treatment
- To recognize and report signs of fluid retention, thromboemboli, hepatotoxicity

Lab test interferences:
Increase: Alk phosphatase, urinary nitrogen, urinary pregnanediol, plasma amino acids
False positive: Urine glucose
Decrease: HDL, glucose tolerance test

---

melphalan
(mel'fa-lan)
Alkeran
Func. class.: Antineoplastic alkylating agent
Chem. class.: Nitrogen mustard

Action: Responsible for cross-linking DNA strands leading to cell death

Uses: Multiple myeloma, breast cancer, reticulum cell sarcoma, testicular seminoma, malignant melanoma, advanced ovarian cancer

Dosage and routes:
- *Adult:* PO 6 mg qd × 2-3 wk, stop drug for 4 wk or until WBC level begins to rise; do not administer if WBC <3000/mm³ or platelets <100,000/mm³; may be given 0.15 mg/kg/day × 7 days; wait until platelets and WBCs rise, then 0.05 mg/kg/day

Available forms include: Tabs 2 mg

Side effects/adverse reactions:
HEMA: **Thrombocytopenia, neutropenia, myelosuppression,** anemia
GI: *Nausea, vomiting,* stomatitis
GU: Amenorrhea, hyperuricemia
INTEG: Rash, urticaria
RESP: **Fibrosis, dysplasia**

Contraindications: Lactation, pregnancy (D)

Precautions: Radiation therapy, bone marrow depression

Pharmacokinetics:
Metabolized in liver, excreted in urine, half-life 1½ hr

Interactions/incompatibilities:
- Increased toxicity: antineoplastics, radiation

NURSING CONSIDERATIONS
Assess:
- CBC, differential, platelet count weekly; withhold drug if WBC is <4000 or platelet count is <75,000; notify physician of results
- Renal function studies: BUN, serum uric acid, urine CrCl before, during therapy
- I&O ratio; report fall in urine output of 30 ml/hr
- Monitor temperature q4h (may

M

---

italics = common side effects   ***bold italic*** = life threatening reactions

indicate beginning infection), no rectal temperatures
• Liver function tests before, during therapy (bilirubin, AST, ALT, LDH) as needed or monthly

Administer:
• Antiemetic 30-60 min before giving drug to prevent vomiting
• Antibiotics for prophylaxis of infection
• Topical or systemic analgesics for pain
• Local or systemic drugs for infection

Perform/provide:
• Storage in tight, light-resistant container
• Strict medical asepsis, protective isolation if WBC levels are low
• Special skin care
• Increase fluid intake to 2-3 L/day to prevent urate deposits, calculi formation
• Diet low in purines: organ meats (kidney, liver), dried beans, peas to maintain alkaline urine
• Rinsing of mouth tid-qid with water, club soda; brushing of teeth bid-tid with soft brush or cotton tipped applicators for stomatitis; use unwaxed dental floss
• Warm compresses at injection site for inflammation

Evaluate:
• Bleeding: hematuria, guaiac, bruising or petechiae, mucosa or orifices q8hr
• Food preferences; list likes, dislikes
• Yellowing of skin, sclera, dark urine, clay-colored stools, itchy skin, abdominal pain, fever, diarrhea
• Inflammation of mucosa, breaks in skin
• Buccal cavity q8h for dryness, sores, ulceration, white patches, oral pain, bleeding, dysphagia

• Local irritation, pain, burning, discoloration at injection site
• Symptoms indicating severe allergic reaction: rash, pruritus, urticaria, purpuric skin lesions, itching, flushing

Teach patient/family:
• Of protective isolation precautions
• That sterility, amenorrhea can occur; reversible after discontinuing treatment
• To avoid foods with citric acid, hot or rough texture
• To report any bleeding, white spots, or ulcerations in mouth to physician; tell patient to examine mouth qd
• To report signs of infection: increased temperature, sore throat, flu symptoms
• To report signs of anemia: fatigue, headache, faintness, shortness of breath, irritability
• To avoid use of razors or commercial mouthwash
• To avoid use of aspirin products or ibuprofen

---

menadione/menadiol sodium diphosphate (vitamin K₃)

(men-a-dye'one)
Synkavite,* Synkayvite
Func. class.: Vitamin, fat soluble

Action: Needed for adequate blood clotting (factors II, VII, IX, X)
Uses: Vitamin K malabsorption, hypoprothrombinemia

Dosage and routes:
• *Adult:* PO 2-10 mg (menadione)
• *Adult:* PO/IM 5-15 mg (menadiol sodium diphosphate)

Available forms include: Tabs 5 mg; inj 5, 10, 37.5 mg/ml

Side effects/adverse reactions:
CNS: Headache, ***brain damage*** (large doses)
GI: Nausea, decreased liver function tests
*HEMA: **Hemolytic anemia, hemoglobinuria, hyperbilirubinemia***
INTEG: Rash, urticaria.
Contraindications: Hypersensitivity, severe hepatic disease, last few weeks of pregnancy (X)
Precautions: Neonates
Pharmacokinetics: Metabolized, crosses placenta
Interactions/incompatibilities:
• Decreased action of menadione: oral antibiotics, cholestyramine, mineral oil
• Decreased action of: oral anticoagulants

NURSING CONSIDERATIONS
Assess:
• Pro-time during treatment (2 sec deviation from control time, bleeding time, and clotting time)
Administer:
• Deep IM, IV slowly over 7 min
Evaluate:
• Therapeutic response: decreased bleeding tendencies, decreased pro-time, decreased clotting time
• Nutritional status: liver (beef), spinach, tomatoes, coffee, asparagus, broccoli, cabbage, lettuce, greens
Teach patient/family:
• Not to take other supplements, unless directed by physician
• Necessary foods to be included in diet
• Avoid use of mineral oil

---

menotropin
(men-oh-troe'pin)
Pergonal
Func. class.: Gonadotropin
Chem. class.: Exogenous gonadotropin

Action: In women, increases follicular growth, maturation; in men, when given with HCG, stimulates spermatogenesis
Uses: Infertility, anovulation
Dosage and routes:
Infertility
• *Adult (men):* IM 1 amp 3 × wk with HCG 2000 U 2 × wk × 4 mo
• *Adult (women):* IM 75 IU of FSH, LH qd × 9-12 days, then 10,000 U HCG 1 day after these drugs; repeat × 2 menstrual cycles; then increase to 150 IU of FSH, LH qd × 9-12 days, then 10,000 U HCG 1 day after these drugs × 2 menstrual cycles
Anovulation
• *Adult (women):* IM 75 IU FSH, LH qd × 9-12 days, then 10,000 U HCG 1 day after last dose of these drugs; repeat × 1-3 menstrual cycles
Available forms include: Powder for inj 17 IU/amp
Side effects/adverse reactions:
CNS: Fever
CV: Hypovolemia
GI: Nausea, vomiting, diarrhea, anorexia
GU: Ovarian enlargement, abdominal distention/pain, multiple births, ovarian hyperstimulation: sudden ovarian enlargement, ascites with or without pain, pleural effusion
*HEMA: **Hemoperitoneum***
Contraindications: Primary anovulation, thyroid/adrenal dysfunction, organic intracranial lesion, ovarian cysts, primary testicular failure
Precautions: Pregnancy (C)

NURSING CONSIDERATIONS
Assess:
• Weight qd; notify physician if weight gain increases rapidly
• Estrogen excretion level; if >100

M

μg/24 hr, drug is withheld, hyperstimulation syndrome may occur
• I&O ratio; be alert for decreasing urinary output

Administer:
• After reconstituting with 1-2 ml sterile saline injection; use immediately

Evaluate:
• Ovarian enlargement, abdominal distention/pain; report symptoms immediately

Teach patient/family:
• That multiple births are possible. If pregnancy occurs, it usually occurs in 4-6 wk after start of treatment
• To keep appointment during treatment qd × 2 wk
• That daily intercourse is necessary from day preceding administration of gonadotropin until ovulation occurs

---

mepenzolate bromide

(me-pen'zoe'late)
Cantil

Func. class.: Gastrointestinal anticholinergic
Chem. class.: Synthetic quaternary ammonium antimuscarinic

Action: Inhibits muscarinic actions of acetylcholine at postganglionic parasympathetic neuroeffector sites
Uses: Treatment of peptic ulcer disease, irritable bowel syndrome in combination with other drugs; for other GI disorders

Dosage and routes:
• *Adult:* PO 25-50 mg qid with meals, hs, titrate to patient response
Available forms include: Tabs 25 mg
Side effects/adverse reactions:
CNS: Confusion, stimulation in el-

derly, headache, insomnia, dizziness, drowsiness, anxiety, weakness, hallucination
*GI: Dry mouth, constipation, **paralytic ileus,** heartburn, nausea,* vomiting, dysphagia, absence of taste
GU: Hesitancy, retention, impotence
CV: Palpitations, tachycardia
EENT: Blurred vision, photophobia, mydriasis, cycloplegia, increased ocular tension
INTEG: Urticaria, rash, pruritus, anhidrosis, fever, allergic reactions
Contraindications: Hypersensitivity to anticholinergics, narrow-angle glaucoma, GI obstruction, myasthenia gravis, paralytic ileus, GI atony, toxic megacolon
Precautions: Hyperthyroidism, coronary artery disease, dysrhythmias, CHF, ulcerative colitis, hypertension, hiatal hernia, hepatic disease, renal disease, pregnancy (C), elderly, urinary retention, prostatic hypertrophy
Pharmacokinetics:
PO: Onset 1 hr, duration 3-4 hr; metabolized by liver, excreted in urine
Interactions/incompatibilities:
• Increased anticholinergic effect: amantadine, tricyclic antidepressants, MAOIs
• Decreased effect of: phenothiazines, levodopa, ketoconazole
NURSING CONSIDERATIONS
Assess:
• VS, cardiac status: checking for dysrhythmias, increased rate, palpitations
• I&O ratio; check for urinary retention or hesitancy
Administer:
• ½-1 hr ac for better absorption
• Decreased dose to elderly patients; their metabolism may be slowed

---

• Gum, hard candy, frequent rinsing of mouth for dryness of oral cavity

Perform/provide:

• Storage in tight container protected from light

• Increased fluids, bulk, exercise to patient's lifestyle to decrease constipation

Evaluate:

• Therapeutic response: absence of epigastric pain, bleeding, nausea, vomiting

• GI complaints: pain, bleeding (frank or occult), nausea, vomiting, anorexia

Teach patient/family:

• Avoid driving or other hazardous activities until stabilized on medication

• Avoid alcohol or other CNS depressants; will enhance sedating properties of this drug

• To avoid hot environments, stroke may occur, drug suppresses perspiration

• Use sunglasses when outside to prevent photophobia, may cause blurred vision

• To drink plenty fluids

• To report dysphagia

---

meperidine HCl

(me-per′i-deen)

Demerol

Func. class.: Narcotic analgesics
Chem. class.: Opiate, phenylpiperidine derivative

Controlled Substance Schedule II

Action: Depresses pain impulse transmission at the spinal cord level by interacting with opioid receptors

Uses: Moderate to severe pain, preoperatively

Dosage and routes:

Pain

• *Adult:* PO/SC/IM 50-150 mg q3-4h prn, dose should be decreased if given IV

• *Child:* PO/SC/IM 1 mg/kg q4-6h prn, not to exceed 100 mg q4h

Preoperatively

• *Adult:* IM/SC 50-100 mg q30-90 min before surgery, dose should be reduced if given IV

• *Child:* IM/SC 1-2.2 mg/kg 30-90 min before surgery

Available forms include: Inj SC, IM, IV 25, 50, 75, 100 mg/ml; tabs 50, 100 mg; syr 50 mg/5 ml

Side effects/adverse reactions:

CNS: Drowsiness, dizziness, confusion, headache, sedation, euphoria, increased intracranial pressure

GI: Nausea, vomiting, anorexia, constipation, cramps

GU: Increased urinary output, dysuria, urinary retention

INTEG: Rash, urticaria, bruising, flushing, diaphoresis, pruritus

EENT: Tinnitus, blurred vision, miosis, diplopia, depressed corneal reflex

CV: Palpitations, bradycardia, change in B/P, tachycardia (IV)

RESP: Respiratory depression

Contraindications: Hypersensitivity, addiction (narcotic)

Precautions: Addictive personality, pregnancy (B), lactation, increased intracranial pressure, MI (acute), severe heart disease, respiratory depression, hepatic disease, renal disease, child <18 yr

Pharmacokinetics:

PO: Onset 15 min, peak 1 hr, duration 4-5 hr

SC/IM: Onset 10 min, peak 1 hr, duration 2-4 hr

IV: Onset 5 min, duration 2 hr

Metabolized by liver (to active/inactive metabolites), excreted by

---

italics = common side effects   ***bold italic*** = life threatening reactions

kidneys, crosses placenta, excreted in breast milk, half-life 3-4 hr

Interactions/incompatibilities:
• Increased effects with other CNS depressants: alcohol, narcotics, sedative/hypnotics, antipsychotics, skeletal muscle relaxants, MAO inhibitors, chlorpromazine

NURSING CONSIDERATIONS
Assess:
• I&O ratio; check for decreasing output; may indicate urinary retention
• Need for drug

Administer:
• IV after diluting with 5 ml or more sterile H_2O or NS, give directly over 4-5 min; may be further diluted in solutions to 1 mg/ml during anesthesia
• With antiemetic if nausea, vomiting occur
• When pain is beginning to return; determine dosage interval by patient response

Perform/provide:
• Storage in light-resistant area at room temperature
• Assistance with ambulation
• Safety measures: siderails, night light, call bell within easy reach

Evaluate:
• Therapeutic response: decrease in pain
• CNS changes: dizziness, drowsiness, hallucinations, euphoria, LOC, pupil reaction
• Allergic reactions: rash, urticaria
• Respiratory dysfunction: respiratory depression, character, rate, rhythm; notify physician if respirations are <12/min
• Need for pain medication, physical dependence

Teach patient/family:
• To report any symptoms of CNS changes, allergic reactions
• That physical dependency may

result when used for extended periods of time
• Withdrawal symptoms may occur: nausea, vomiting, cramps, fever, faintness, anorexia

Lab test interferences:
Increase: Amylase

Treatment of overdose: Narcan 0.2-0.8 IV, O_2, IV fluids, vasopressors

---

mephentermine sulfate
(me-fen'ter-meen)
Wyamine

Func. class.: Adrenergic, direct and indirect acting
Chem. class.: Substituted phenylethylamine

Action: Causes increased contractility and heart rate by acting on β-receptors in heart; also, acts on α-receptors, causing vasoconstriction in blood vessels, cardiac output is elevated and systolic and diastolic pressures are increased

Uses: Shock and hypotension following variety of procedures

Dosage and routes:
Hypotension
• *Adult:* IV 15-45 mg depending on procedure
Hypotension/shock
• *Adult:* IV 0.5 mg/kg
• *Child:* IV 0.4 mg/kg

Available forms include: Inj IV 15, 30 mg/ml

Side effects/adverse reactions:
CV: Palpitations, tachycardia, hypertension
CNS: Tremors, drowsiness, confusion, incoherence

Contraindications: Hypersensitivity to sympathomimetics

Precautions: Pregnancy (B), cardiac disorders, hyperthyroidism, diabetes mellitus, prostatic hypertrophy

Pharmacokinetics:
IV: Onset immediate, duration ½-1 hr; metabolized in liver, excreted in urine

Interactions/incompatibilities:
• Do not use with MAOIs or tricyclic antidepressants; hypertensive crisis may occur
• Decreased effect of mephentermine: methyldopa, urinary acidifiers, rauwolfia alkaloids
• Increased effect of mephentermine: urinary alkalizers
• Dysrhythmias: halothane, cyclopropaine, digitalis

NURSING CONSIDERATIONS
Assess:
• I&O ratio, notify MD if output is < 30 cc/hr
• ECG during administration continuously; if B/P increases, drug is decreased
• B/P, pulse q5 min after parenteral route
• CVP or PWP during infusion if possible

Administer:
• Plasma expanders for hypovolemia
• IV undiluted 30 mg or less/1 min, or diluted 600 mg/500 ml D₅W, titrate to patient response, check site for extravasation; use an infusion pump

Perform/provide:
• Storage of reconstituted solution if refrigerated for no longer than 24 hr
• Do not use discolored solutions

Evaluate:
• Therapeutic response: increased B/P with stabilization

Teach patient/family:
• Reason for drug administration

mephenytoin
(me-fen′i-toyn)
Mesantoin
Func. class.: Anticonvulsant
Chem. class.: Hydantoin derivative

Action: Reduces electrical discharges in motor cortex, reducing seizures; increases AV conduction velocity, prolongs refractory period

Uses: Generalized tonic-clonic, complex-partial seizures

Dosage and routes:
• *Adult:* PO 50-100 mg/day, may increase by 50-100 mg q7 days, up to 200 mg tid
• *Child:* PO 50-100 mg/day or 100-450 mg/m²/day in 3 divided doses, initially; then increase 50-100 mg q7 days, up to 200 mg tid in divided doses q8h

Available forms include: Tabs 100 mg

Side effects/adverse reactions:
*HEMA: **Agranulocytosis, leukopenia, neutropenia, pancytopenia, eosinophilia, lymphadenopathy***
CNS: Drowsiness, dizziness, fatigue, irritability, tremors, insomnia, depression
GI: Nausea, vomiting
INTEG: Rash, exfoliative dermatitis
EENT: Photophobia, conjunctivitis, nystagmus, diplopia
*RESP: **Pulmonary fibrosis***

Contraindications: Hypersensitivity to hydantoins, sinus bradycardia, heart block, Adams-Stokes syndrome

Precautions: Alcoholism, hepatic disease, renal disease, blood dyscrasias, CHF, elderly, pregnancy (C), respiratory depression, diabetes mellitus

Pharmacokinetics:
PO: Onset 30 min, duration 24-48

M

---

italics = common side effects   ***bold italic*** = life threatening reactions

hr, metabolized by liver, excreted by kidneys, half-life 144 hr

Interactions/incompatibilities:

• Decreased effects: rifampin, chronic alcohol use, barbiturates, antihistamines, antacids, other anticonvulsants antineoplastics, calcium products, folic acid, oxacillin

• Increased effects: benzodiazepines, cimetidine, salicylates, sulfonamide, pyrazolones, phenothiazines, estrogens, disulfiram, chloramphenicol, anticoagulants

• Seizures: valproic acid

• Myocardial depression: lidocaine, propanolol, sympathomimetics

NURSING CONSIDERATIONS
Assess:

• Blood studies: CBC, platelets q2 wk until stabilized, then q mo × 12, then q3 mo; discontinue drug if neutrophils are <1600/mm³, liver function tests with long-term use

• Drug level: therapeutic level 25-40 μg/ml

Evaluate:

• Therapeutic response: decreased seizure activity

• Mental status: mood, sensorium, affect, behavioral changes; if mental status changes, notify physician

• Eye problems: need for ophthalmic examinations before, during, after treatment (slit lamp, fundoscopy, tonometry)

• Allergic reaction: red raised rash; if this occurs, drug should be discontinued

• Blood dyscrasias: fever, sore throat, bruising, rash, jaundice

• Toxicity: bone marrow depression, nausea, vomiting, ataxia, diplopia, cardiovascular collapse, Stevens-Johnson syndrome

Teach patient/family:

• Not to discontinue drug quickly; should be tapered

• To avoid activities that require alertness if drowsiness or dizziness occur

• Use of alcohol may decrease effects of drug

---

mephobarbital

(me-foe-bar'bi-tal)

Mebaral, Mentabal, Mephoral

Func. class.: Anticonvulsant
Chem. class.: Barbiturate

Controlled Substance Schedule IV

Action: Depresses sensory cortex, motor activity; inhibits ascending conduction in reticular formation of thalamus

Uses: Generalized tonic-clonic (grand mal), absence (petit mal) seizures

Dosage and routes:

• *Adult:* PO 400-600 mg/day or in divided doses

• *Child:* PO 6-12 mg/kg/day in divided doses q6-8h

Available forms include: Tabs 32, 50, 100, 200 mg

Side effects/adverse reactions:

HEMA: ***Thrombocytopenia, agranulocytosis, megaloblastic anemia***

CNS: Dizziness, headache, hangover, paradoxic stimulation, drowsiness, increased pain

GI: Nausea, vomiting, epigastric pain

INTEG: Rash, urticaria, purpara, erythema multiforme, facial edema

EENT: Tinnitus, hearing loss

CV: Hypotension, bradycardia

RESP: Wheezing, hyperpnea

ENDO: Hypoglycemia, hyponatremia, hypokalemia

Contraindications: Hypersensitivity to barbiturates, pregnancy (D)

Precautions: Hepatic disease, renal disease, lactation, alcoholism, drug abuse, hyperthyroidism

Pharmacokinetics:

PO: Onset 20-60 min, duration 6-8 hr

REC: Onset slow, duration 4-6 hr
Metabolized by liver, excreted by kidneys, half-life 34 hr

Interactions/incompatibilities:

• Increased effects: CNS depressants, chloramphenicol, valproic acid, disulfiram, nondepolarizing skeletal muscle relaxants, sulfonamides

• Increased orthostatic hypotension: furosemide

NURSING CONSIDERATIONS

Assess:

• Drug level, CBC, BUN, creatinine

Perform/provide:

• Storage in light-resistant container

Evaluate:

• Mental status: mood, sensorium, affect, memory (long, short)

• Respiratory depression: respiration <10/min, shallow

• Blood dyscrasias: fever, sore throat, bruising, rash, jaundice

Teach patient/family:

• Never withdraw drug abruptly; notify physician if side effects occur

• Avoid hazardous activities until stabilized on drug

• Dreaming may increase when drug is discontinued

Treatment of overdose: Administer calcium gluconate IV

---

mepivacaine HCl

(meep-ee-va-kane)
Carbocaine, Cavacaine, Isocaine
Func. class.: Local anesthetic
Chem. class.: Amide

Action: Competes with calcium for sites in nerve membrane that control sodium transport across cell membrane; decreases rise of depolarization phase of action potential

Uses: Nerve block, caudal anesthesia, epidural, pain relief, paracervical block, transvaginal block or infiltration

Dosage and routes:

Varies depending on route of anesthesia

Available forms include: Inj 1%, 1.5%, 2%, 3%

Side effects/adverse reactions:

CNS: Anxiety, restlessness, *convulsions, loss of consciousness,* drowsiness, disorientation, tremors, shivering

CV: Myocardial depression, cardiac arrest, dysrhythmias, bradycardia, hypotension, hypertension, fetal bradycardia

GI: Nausea, vomiting

EENT: Blurred vision, tinnitus, pupil constriction

INTEG: Rash, urticaria, allergic reactions, edema, burning, skin discoloration at injection site, tissue necrosis

RESP: Status asthmaticus, respiratory arrest, anaphylaxis

Contraindications: Hypersensitivity, child <12 yr, elderly, severe liver disease

Precautions: Elderly, severe drug allergies, pregnancy (C)

Pharmacokinetics:

Onset 15 min, duration 3 hr; metabolized by liver, excreted in urine (metabolites)

Interactions/incompatibilities:

• Dysrhythmias: epinephrine, halothane, enflurane

• Hypertension: MAOIs, tricyclic antidepressants, phenothiazines

• Decreased action of mepivacaine: chloroprocaine

---

italics = common side effects   ***bold italic*** = life threatening reactions

NURSING CONSIDERATIONS
Assess:
• B/P, pulse, respiration during treatment
• Fetal heart tones if drug is used during labor
Administer:
• Only with crash cart, resuscitative equipment nearby
• Only drugs without preservatives for epidural or caudal anesthesia
Perform/provide:
• Use of new solution, discard unused portions
Evaluate:
• Therapeutic response: anesthesia necessary for procedure
• Allergic reactions: rash, urticaria, itching
• Cardiac status: ECG for dysrhythmias, pulse, B/P during anesthesia
Treatment of overdose: Airway, O₂, vasopressor, IV fluids, anticonvulsants for seizures

---

meprobamate

(me-proe-ba'mate)
Arcoban, Equanil, Kalmm, Meditran,* Meprocon, Meprotabs, Meribam, Miltown, Neo-Tran,* Novomepro,* Saronil, Tranmep

Func. class.: Sedative/hypnotic
Chem. class.: Propanediol carbamate derivative

Controlled Substance Schedule IV

Action: Blocks impulses from cortex to thalamus in CNS
Uses: Anxiety
Dosage and routes:
• *Adult:* PO 1.2-1.6 g in 2-3 divided doses, not to exceed 2.4 g/day
• *Child 6-12 yr:* PO 100-200 mg bid-tid

Available forms include: Tabs 200, 400, 600 mg; caps 400 mg sust rel caps 200, 400 mg
Side effects/adverse reactions:
HEMA: **Thrombocytopenia, leukopenia, eosinophilia**
CNS: Dizziness, drowsiness, headache, **convulsions**
GI: Nausea, vomiting, anorexia, diarrhea, stomatitis
INTEG: Urticaria, pruritus, maculopapular rash
CV: Hypotension, tachycardia, palpitations, **hyperthermia**
EENT: Blurred vision, tinnitus, mydriasis, slurred speech
Contraindications: Hypersensitivity, renal failure, porphyria, pregnancy (D), history of drug abuse or dependence
Precautions: Suicidal patients, severe depression, renal disease, hepatic disease, elderly
Pharmacokinetics:
PO: Onset 1 hr, metabolized by liver, excreted by kidneys, in feces, crosses placenta, breast milk, half-life 6-16 hr
Interactions/incompatibilities:
• Increased effects of meprobamate: CNS depressants, alcohol, tricyclic antidepressants
NURSING CONSIDERATIONS
Assess:
• B/P (lying, standing), pulse; if systolic B/P drops 20 mm Hg, hold drug, notify physician; respirations q5-15 min if given IV
• Blood studies: CBC during long-term therapy, blood dyscrasias have occurred rarely
• Hepatic studies: AST, ALT, bilirubin, creatinine, LDH, alk phosphatase
Administer:
• With food or milk for GI symptoms

- Crushed tabs if patient is unable to swallow medication whole
- Sugarless gum, hard candy, frequent sips of water for dry mouth

Perform/provide

- Assistance with ambulation during beginning therapy since drowsiness/dizziness occurs
- Safety measures, including siderails
- Check to see PO medication has been swallowed

Evaluate:

- Therapeutic response: decreased anxiety, restlessness, insomnia
- Mental status: mood, sensorium, affect, sleeping pattern, drowsiness, dizziness
- Physical dependency, withdrawal symptoms: headache, nausea, vomiting, muscle pain, weakness, hyperthermia, death, convulsions after long-term use
- Suicidal tendencies

Teach patient/family:

- That drug may be taken with food
- Not to be used for everyday stress or used longer than 4 months, unless directed by physician, not to take more than prescribed amount, may be habit forming
- Avoid OTC preparations (alcohol, cold, hay fever) unless approved by physician
- To avoid driving, activities that require alertness, since drowsiness may occur
- To avoid alcohol ingestion or other psychotropic medications, unless prescribed by physician
- Not to discontinue medication abruptly after long-term use
- To rise slowly or fainting may occur
- That drowsiness might worsen at beginning of treatment

Lab test interferences:

False increase: 17-OHCS

False positive: Phentolamine test

Treatment of overdose: Lavage, VS, supportive care

merbromin

Mercurochrome

Func. class.: Disinfectant

Chem. class.: Polychlorinated phenol derivative

Action: Inhibits growth of gram-positive bacteria

Uses: Surgical scrub, bacteriostatic skin cleanser, gram-positive infection when other treatment has been ineffective

Dosage and routes:

- *Adult and child:* Use prn

Available forms include: Top soap, emul

Side effects/adverse reactions:

INTEG: Irritation, dryness, dermatitis, scaling

Contraindications: Hypersensitivity, occlusive dressings, infants, burns

M

NURSING CONSIDERATIONS

Administer:

- To body areas only; do not apply to face, lips, mouth, eyes, mucous membrane, anus, meatus
- Only to adults; repeated use may lead to systemic absorption

Evaluate:

- Area of the body involved: irritation, rash, breaks, dryness, scales

Teach patient/family:

- To report itching, irritation, dizziness, headache, confusion, discontinue drug immediately

Treatment of ingestion: Gastric lavage, administer vegetable oil, saline laxative, supportive treatment

---

italics = common side effects   ***bold italic*** = life threatening reactions

mercaptopurine (6-MP)

(mer-kap-toe-pyoor'een)
Purinethol

Func. class.: Antineoplastic-antimetabolite
Chem. class.: Purine analog

Action: Inhibits purine metabolism at multiple sites, which inhibits DNA and RNA synthesis

Uses: Chronic myelocytic leukemia, acute lymphoblastic leukemia in children, acute myelogenous leukemia

Dosage and routes:
• *Adult and child:* PO 2.5 mg/kg/day, not to exceed 5 mg/kg/day; maintenance 1.5-2.5 mg/kg/day
• *Child:* 70 mg/m²/day
Available forms include: Tabs 50 mg

Side effects/adverse reactions:
CNS: Fever, headache, weakness
*HEMA: **Thrombocytopenia, leukopenia, myelosuppression, anemia***
*GI: Nausea, vomiting, anorexia, diarrhea, stomatitis, **hepatotoxicity*** (with high doses), jaundice, gastritis
*GU: **Renal failure,** hyperuricemia, **oliguria,** crystalluria, **hematuria***
INTEG: Rash, dry skin, urticaria

Contraindications: Patients with prior drug resistance, leukopenia (<2500/mm³), thrombocytopenia (<100,000/mm³), anemia, pregnancy (D)

Precautions: Renal disease

Pharmacokinetics: Incompletely absorbed when taken orally, metabolized in liver, excreted in urine

Interactions/incompatibilities:
• Increased toxicity: radiation or other antineoplastics
• Increased bone marrow depression: allopurinol

• Reversal of neuromuscular blockade: nondepolarizing muscle relaxants

NURSING CONSIDERATIONS
Assess:
• CBC, differential, platelet count weekly; withhold drug if WBC is <3500 or platelet count is <100,000; notify physician of these results; drug should be discontinued
• Renal function studies: BUN, serum uric acid, urine CrCl, electrolytes before, during therapy
• I&O ratio; report fall in urine output to <30 ml/hr
• Monitor temperature q4h; fever may indicate beginning infection; no rectal temperatures
• Liver function tests before, during therapy: bilirubin, alk phosphatase, AST, ALT, q wk during beginning therapy
Administer:
• Antacid before oral agent; give drug after evening meal before bedtime
• Allopurinol or sodium bicarbonate to maintain uric acid levels, alkalinization of urine
• Antibiotics for prophylaxis of infection
• Topical or systemic analgesics for pain
• Transfusion for anemia
Perform/provide:
• Strict medical asepsis, protective isolation if WBC levels are low
• Increase fluid intake to 2-3 L/day to prevent urate deposits, calculi formation, unless contraindicated
• Diet low in purines: absence of organ meats (kidney, liver), dried beans, peas to maintain alkaline urine
• Rinsing of mouth tid-qid with water, club soda; brushing of teeth bid-tid with soft brush or cotton-

tipped applicators for stomatitis; use unwaxed dental floss
• Nutritious diet with iron, vitamin supplements as ordered
• Storage in tightly closed container in cool environment

Evaluate:
• Bleeding: hematuria, guaiac, bruising, petechiae, mucosa or orifices q8h
• Food preferences; list likes, dislikes
• Inflammation of mucosa, breaks in skin
• Buccal cavity q8h for dryness, sores, ulceration, white patches, oral pain, bleeding, dysphagia
• Symptoms indicating severe allergic reaction: rash, urticaria, itching, flushing

Teach patient/family:
• To avoid foods with citric acid, hot or rough texture if stomatitis is present
• To report stomatitis: any bleeding, white spots, ulcerations in mouth; tell patient to examine mouth qd, report symptoms
• Contraceptive measures are recommended during therapy
• To drink 10-12 glasses of fluid/day
• Notify physician of fever, chills, sore throat, nausea, vomiting, anorexia, diarrhea, bleeding, bruising, which may indicate blood dyscrasias
• To report signs of infection: increased temperature, sore throat, flu symptoms
• To report signs of anemia: fatigue, headache, faintness, shortness of breath, irritability
• To report bleeding: avoid use of razors or commercial mouthwash
• To avoid use of aspirin products or ibuprofen

mesalamine

(mez-al'a-meen)
Rowasa
Func. class.: GI antiinflammatory

Action: May diminish inflammation by blocking cyclooxygenase, inhibiting prostaglandin production in colon

Uses: Mild to moderate active distal ulcerative colitis, proctosigmoiditis, proctitis

Dosage and routes:
• *Adult:* REC 60 ml (4 g) hs, retained for 8 hr

Available forms include: Rec susp 4 g/60 ml

Side effects/adverse reactions:
GI: Cramps, gas, nausea, diarrhea, rectal pain, constipation
CNS: Headache, fever, dizziness, insomnia, asthenia, weakness, fatigue
INTEG: Rash, itching, alopecia
SYST: Flu, malaise, back pain, peripheral edema
EENT: Sore throat

Contraindications: Hypersensitivity

Precautions: Renal disease, pregnancy (B), lactation, children, sulfite sensitivity

Pharmacokinetics:
REC: Primarily excreted in feces but some in urine as metabolite; half-life 1 hr, metabolite half-life 5-10 hr

NURSING CONSIDERATIONS
Assess:
• GI symptoms: cramps, gas, nausea, diarrhea, rectal pain; if severe the drug should be discontinued
Administer:
• Rectally only, drug should be given hs, retained until morning
Perform/provide:
• Storage at room temperature

---

italics = common side effects   ***bold italic*** = life threatening reactions

Evaluate:
• Therapeutic response: absence of pain, bleeding from GI tract, decrease in number of diarrhea stools

Teach patient/family:
• Usual course of therapy is 3-6 wk
• Shake bottle well
• Method of rectal administration
• To inform physician of GI symptoms

---

mesoridazine besylate

(mez-oh-rid′a-zeen)
Serentil

Func. class.: Antipsychotic/neuroleptic
Chem. class.: Phenothiazine, piperidine

Action: Depresses cerebral corex, hypothalamus, limbic system, which control activity, aggression; blocks neurotransmission produced by dopamine at synapse; exhibits strong α-adrenergic, anticholinergic blocking action; mechanism for antipsychotic effects is unclear

Uses: Psychotic disorders, schizophrenia, anxiety, alcoholism, behavioral problems in mental deficiency, chronic brain syndrome

Dosage and routes:
Schizophrenia
• *Adult:* PO 50 mg tid, optimum dose 100-400 mg/day; IM 25 mg may repeat ½-1 hr; dosage range 25-200 mg/day
Behavior problems
• *Adult:* PO 25 mg tid; optimum dose 75-300 mg/day;
Alcoholism
• *Adult:* PO 25 mg bid; optimum dose 50-200 mg/day
Schizoaffective disorders
• *Adult:* PO 10 mg tid; optimum dose 30-150 mg/day
Available forms include: Tabs 10, 25, 50, 100 mg; conc 25 mg/ml; inj IM 25 mg/ml

Side effects/adverse reactions:
*RESP: **Laryngospasm,** dyspnea, **respiratory depression***
CNS: Extrapyramidal symptoms: pseudoparkinsonism, akathisia, dystonia, tardive dyskinesia, drowsiness, headache,
*HEMA: **Anemia, leukopenia, leukocytosis, agranulocytosis***
INTEG: Rash, photosensitivity, dermatitis
EENT: Blurred vision, glaucoma
GI: Dry mouth, nausea, vomiting, anorexia, constipation, diarrhea, jaundice, weight gain
GU: Urinary retention, urinary frequency, enuresis, impotence, amenorrhea, gynecomastia
CV: Orthostatic hypotension, hypertension, **cardiac arrest,** ECG changes, tachycardia

Contraindications: Hypersensitivity, circulatory collapse, liver damage, cerebral arteriosclerosis, coronary disease, severe hypertension/hypotension, blood dyscrasias, coma, brain damage, bone marrow depression

Precautions: Pregnancy (C), lactation, seizure disorders, hypertension, hepatic disease, cardiac disease

Pharmacokinetics:
PO: Onset erratic, peak 2 hr, duration 4-6 hr
IM: Onset 15-30 min, peak 30 min, duration 6-8 hr
Metabolized by liver, excreted in urine, crosses placenta, enters breast milk

Interactions/incompatibilities:
• Oversedation: other CNS depressants, alcohol, barbiturate anesthetics
• Toxicity: epinephrine
• Decreased absorption: aluminum

---

hydroxide or magnesium hydroxide antacids
• Decreased effects of: lithium, levodopa
• Increased effects of both drugs: β-adrenergic blockers, alcohol
• Increased anticholinergic effects: anticholinergics

NURSING CONSIDERATIONS

Assess:
• Swallowing of PO medication; check for hoarding or giving of medication to other patients
• I&O ratio; palpate bladder if low urinary output occurs
• Bilirubin, CBC, liver function studies monthly
• Urinalysis is recommended before, during prolonged therapy

Administer:
• Antiparkinsonian agent, after securing order from physician to be used if extrapyramidal symptoms occur
• Concentrate mixed in distilled water, orange, grape juice; do not prepare, store bulk dilutions
• IM injection into large muscle mass

Perform/provide:
• Decreased noise input by dimming lights, avoiding loud noises
• Supervised ambulation until stabilized on medication; do not involve in strenuous exercise program because fainting is possible; patient should not stand still for long periods of time
• Increased fluids to prevent constipation
• Sips of water, candy, gum for dry mouth
• Storage in tight, light-resistant container

Evaluate:
• Therapeutic response: decrease in emotional excitement, hallucinations, delusions, paranoia, and re-organization of patterns of thought, speech
• Affect, orientation, LOC, reflexes, gait, coordination, sleep pattern disturbances
• B/P standing and lying; also include pulse and respirations; take these q4h during initial treatment; establish baseline before starting treatment; report drops of 30 mm Hg
• Dizziness, faintness, palpitations, tachycardia on rising
• Extrapyramidal symptoms including akathisia (inability to sit still, no pattern to movements), tardive dyskinesia (bizarre movements of jaw, mouth, tongue, extremities), pseudoparkinsonism (rigidity, tremors, pill rolling, shuffling gait)
• For neuroleptic malignant syndrome: hyperthermia, altered mental status, muscle rigidity, increased CPK
• Skin turgor daily
• Constipation, urinary retention daily; if these occur increase bulk, water in diet

Teach patient/family:
• That orthostatic hypotension occurs frequently, and to rise from sitting or lying position gradually
• To remain lying down after IM injection for at least 30 min
• To avoid hot tubs, hot showers, or tub baths since hypotension may occur
• To avoid abrupt withdrawal of mesoridazine or extrapypramidal symptoms may result; drugs should be withdrawn slowly
• To avoid OTC preparations (cough, hayfever, cold) unless approved by physician since serious drug interactions may occur; avoid use with alcohol or CNS depres-

M

---

italics = common side effects   ***bold italic*** = life threatening reactions

sants, increased drowsiness may occur
• To use sunscreen during sun exposure to prevent burns
• Regarding compliance with drug regimen
• About necessity for meticulous oral hygiene since oral candidiasis may occur
• To report sore throat, malaise, fever, bleeding, mouth sores; if these occur, a CBC should be drawn and drug discontinued
• In hot weather heat stroke may occur; take extra precautions to stay cool

Lab test interferences:
Increase: Liver function tests, cardiac enzymes, cholesterol, blood glucose, prolactin, bilirubin, PBI, cholinesterase, ^{131}I
Decrease: Hormones (blood, urine)
False positive: Pregnancy tests, PKU
False negative: Urinary steroids, 17-OHCS

Treatment of overdose: Lavage if orally injested, provide an airway; *do not induce vomiting*

---

metaproterenol sulfate

(met-a-proe-ter'e-nole)
Alupent, Metaprel
Func. class.: Selective β_2-agonist

Action: Relaxes bronchial smooth muscle by direct action on β_2-adrenergic receptors

Uses: Bronchial asthma, bronchospasm

Dosage and routes:
• *Adult and child>12 yr:* INH 2-3 puffs, may repeat q 3-4h, not to exceed 12 puffs/day
Asthma/bronchospasm
• *Adult:* PO 20 mg q6-8h

• *Child >9 yr or >27 kg:* PO 20 mg q6-8h or 0.4-0.9 mg/kg/dose tid
• *Child 6-9 yr or <27 kg:* PO 10 mg q6-8h or 0.4-0.9 mg/kg/dose tid

Available forms include: Tabs 10, 20 mg; aerosol 0.65 mg/dose; syrup 10 mg/5 ml; sol nebulizer 0.6%, 5%

Side effects/adverse reactions:
CNS: Tremors, anxiety, insomnia, headache, dizziness, stimulation
CV: Palpitations, tachycardia, hypertension, *cardiac arrest*
GI: Nausea
RESP: Dyspnea

Contraindications: Hypersensitivity to sympathomimetics, narrow-angle glaucoma

Precautions: Pregnancy (C), cardiac disorders, hyperthyroidism, diabetes mellitus, prostatic hypertrophy

Pharmacokinetics:
PO: Onset 15-30 min, peak 1 hr, duration 4 hr, excreted in urine as metabolites

Interactions/incompatibilities:
• Increased effects of both drugs: other sympathomimetics
• Decreased action of: β-blockers

NURSING CONSIDERATIONS
Assess:
• Respiratory function: vital capacity, forced expiratory volume, ABGs

Administer:
• 2 hr before hs to avoid sleeplessness

Perform/provide:
• Storage at room temperature, do not use discolored solutions

Evaluate:
• Therapeutic response: absence of dyspnea, wheezing
• Tolerance over long-term ther-

---

apy, dose may need to be increased or changed

Teach patient/family:
• Not to use OTC medications, extra stimulation may occur
• Use of inhaler, review package insert with patient
• To avoid getting aerosol in eyes
• To wash inhaler in warm water and dry qd
• On all aspects of drug; avoid smoking, smoke-filled rooms, persons with respiratory infections

---

methadone HCl

(meth'a-done)
Dolophine, Methadone HCl Oral Solution
Func. class.: Narcotic analgesics
Chem. class.: Opiate, synthetic diphenylheptane derivative

Controlled Substance Schedule II
Action: Depresses pain impulse transmission at the spinal cord level by interacting with opioid receptors
Uses: Severe pain, narcotic withdrawal

Dosage and routes:
Pain
• *Adult:* PO/SC/IM 2.5-10 mg q4-12h prn
Narcotic withdrawal
• *Adult:* PO 15-40 mg/day individualized initially, then 20-120 mg/day titrated to patient response
Available forms include: Inj SC, IM 10 mg/ml; tabs 5, 10 mg; oral sol 5, 10 mg/5 ml; dispersible tabs 40 mg

Side effects/adverse reactions:
CNS: Drowsiness, dizziness, confusion, headache, sedation, euphoria
GI: Nausea, vomiting, anorexia, constipation, cramps, biliary tract spasm

GU: Increased urinary output, dysuria, urinary retention
INTEG: Rash, urticaria, bruising, flushing, diaphoresis, pruritus
EENT: Tinnitus, blurred vision, miosis, diplopia
CV: Palpitations, bradycardia, change in B/P
RESP: Respiratory depression
Contraindications: Hypersensitivity, addiction (narcotic)
Precautions: Addictive personality, pregnancy (B), lactation, increased intracranial pressure, MI (acute), severe heart disease, respiratory depression, hepatic disease, renal disease, child <18 yr
Pharmacokinetics:
PO: Onset 30-60 min, duration 6-8 hr, cumulative 22-48 hr
SC/IM: Onset 10-20 min, peak 1 hr, duration 6-8 hr, cumulative 22-48 hr
Metabolized by liver, excreted by kidneys, crosses placenta, excreted in breast milk, half-life 1-1½ days, 90% bound to plasma proteins
Interactions/incompatibilities:
• Increased effects with other CNS depressants: alcohol, narcotics, sedative/hypnotics, antipsychotics, skeletal muscle relaxants, rifampin, phenytoin
NURSING CONSIDERATIONS
Assess:
• I&O ratio; check for decreasing output; may indicate urinary retention
Administer:
• With antiemetic if nausea, vomiting occurs
• When pain is beginning to return; determine dosage interval by patient response
• Rotating injection sites
Perform/provide:
• Storage in light-resistant area at room temperature

M

---

italics = common side effects   ***bold italic*** = life threatening reactions

- Assistance with ambulation
- Safety measures: siderails, night light, call bell within easy reach

Evaluate:
- Therapeutic response: decrease in pain
- CNS changes: dizziness, drowsiness, hallucinations, euphoria, LOC, pupil reaction
- Allergic reactions: rash, urticaria
- Respiratory dysfunction: respiratory depression, character, rate, rhythm; notify physician if respirations are <10/min
- Need for pain medication, physical dependence

Teach patient/family:
- To report any symptoms of CNS changes, allergic reactions
- That physical dependency may result when used for extended periods of time
- Withdrawal symptoms may occur: nausea, vomiting, cramps, fever, faintness, anorexia

Lab test interferences:
Increase: Amylase

Treatment of overdose: Narcan 0.2-0.8 IV, O_2, IV fluids, vasopressors

---

methamphetamine HCl

(meth-am-fet′a-meen)
Desoxyn Gradumey

Func. class.: Cerebral stimulants
Chem. class.: Amphetamine

Controlled Substance Schedule II
Action: Increases release of norepinephrine and dopamine in cerebral cortex to reticular activating system
Uses: Exogenous obesity, minimal brain dysfunction, attention deficit disorder with hyperactivity
Dosage and routes:
Attention deficit disorder

- *Child >6 yr:* 2.5-5 mg qd or bid increasing by 5 mg/wk
Obesity
- *Adult:* PO 5 mg, 30 min ac or 10-15 mg long-acting tab qd in AM

Available forms include: Tabs 5; tabs long-acting 5, 10, 15 mg
Side effects/adverse reactions:
CNS: Hyperactivity, insomnia, restlessness, talkativeness, dizziness, headache, chills, stimulation, dysphoria, irritability, aggressiveness, tremor
GI: Anorexia, dry mouth, diarrhea, constipation, weight loss, metallic taste, cramps
GU: Impotence, change in libido
CV: Palpitations, tachycardia, hypertension, decreased heart rate, dysrhythmia
INTEG: Urticaria
Contraindications: Hypersensitivity to sympathomimetic amines, hyperthyroidism, hypertension, glaucoma hypertrophy, severe arteriosclerosis, drug abuse, cardiovascular disease, anxiety
Precautions: Gilles de la Tourette's disorder, pregnancy (C), lactation, child <3 years
Pharmacokinetics:
PO: Duration 3-6 hr, metabolized by liver, excreted by kidneys, crosses blood-brain barrier
Interactions/incompatibilities:
- Hypertensive crisis: MAOIs or within 14 days of MAOIs
- Increased effect of methamphetamine: acetazolamide, antacids, sodium bicarbonate
- Decreased effects of methamphetamine: barbiturates, tricyclics, ascorbic acid, ammonium chloride
- Decreased effects of: guanethidine

NURSING CONSIDERATIONS
Assess:
- VS, B/P since this drug may re-

verse antihypertensives; check patients with cardiac disease more often

• CBC, urinalysis, in diabetes: blood sugar, urine sugar; insulin changes may need to be made since eating will decrease

• Height, growth rate in children; growth rate may be decreased

Administer:

• At least 6 hr before hs to avoid sleeplessness

• For obesity only if patient is on weight reduction program including dietary changes, exercise; patient will develop tolerance, loss of weight won't occur without additional methods give 2 hr before meals

• Gum, hard candy or frequent sips of water for dry mouth

Evaluate:

• Mental status: mood, sensorium, affect, stimulation, insomnia, aggressiveness

• Physical dependency: should not be used for extended time; dose should be discontinued gradually, tolerance will occur after long-term use

• Withdrawal symptoms: headache, nausea, vomiting, muscle pain, weakness

Teach patient/family:

• To decrease caffeine consumption (coffee, tea, cola, chocolate), which may increase irritability, stimulation

• Avoid OTC preparations unless approved by physician

• To taper off drug over several weeks, or depression, increased sleeping, lethargy may ensue

• To avoid alcohol ingestion

• To avoid hazardous activities until patient is stabilized on medication

• To get needed rest; patients will feel more tired at end of day

• Not to chew or crush sus rel forms

Treatment of overdose: Administer fluids, hemodialysis or peritoneal dialysis; antihypertensive for increased B/P; ammonium Cl for increased excretion.

---

methantheline bromide

(meth-an′tha-leen)

Banthine

Func. class.: Gastrointestinal anticholinergic

Chem. class.: Synthetic quaternary ammonium antimuscarinic

Action: Inhibits muscarinic actions of acetylcholine at postganglionic parasympathetic neuroeffector sites

Uses: Treatment of peptic ulcer disease, irritable bowel syndrome, pancreatitis, gastritis, biliary dyskinesia, pylorospasm, reflex neurogenic bladder in children

Dosage and routes:

• *Adult:* PO 50-100 mg q6h

• *Child >1 yr:* PO 12.5-50 mg qid

• *Child <1 yr:* PO 12.5-25 mg qid

• *Neonate:* PO 12.5 mg bid-tid

Available forms include: Tabs 50 mg

Side effects/adverse reactions:

CNS: Confusion, stimulation in elderly, headache, insomnia, dizziness, drowsiness, anxiety, weakness, hallucination

GI: Dry mouth, constipation, paralytic ileus, heartburn, nausea, vomiting, dysphagia, absence of taste

GU: Hesitancy, retention, impotence

CV: Palpitations, tachycardia

EENT: Blurred vision, photophobia, mydriasis, cycloplegia, increased ocular tension

M

---

italics = common side effects   ***bold italic*** = life threatening reactions

INTEG: Urticaria, rash, pruritus, anhidrosis, fever, allergic reactions

Contraindications: Hypersensitivity to anticholinergics, narrow-angle glaucoma, GI obstruction, myasthenia gravis, paralytic ileus, GI atony, toxic megacolon

Precautions: Hyperthyroidism, coronary artery disease, dysrhythmias, CHF, ulcerative colitis, hypertension, hiatal hernia, hepatic disease, renal disease, pregnancy (C), urinary retention, prostatic hypertrophy

Pharmacokinetics:

PO: Onset 30-45 min, duration 4-6 hr; metabolized by liver, excreted in urine, bile

Interactions/incompatibilities:
• Increased anticholinergic effect: amantadine, tricyclic antidepressants, MAOIs, H₁ antihistamines
• Increased effect of: nitrofurantoin
• Decreased effect of: phenothiazines, levodopa

NURSING CONSIDERATIONS
Assess:
• VS, cardiac status: checking for dysrhythmias, increased rate, palpitations
• I&O ratio; check for urinary retention, hesitancy

Administer:
• ½-1 hr ac for better absorption
• Decreased dose to elderly patients; their metabolism may be slowed
• Gum, hard candy, frequent rinsing of mouth for dryness of oral cavity

Perform/provide:
• Storage in tight container protected from light
• Increased fluids, bulk, exercise to patient's lifestyle to decrease constipation

Evaluate:
• Therapeutic response: absence of

epigastric pain, bleeding, nausea, vomiting
• GI complaints: pain, bleeding (frank or occult), nausea, vomiting, anorexia

Teach patient/family:
• Avoid driving or other hazardous activities until stabilized on medication
• Avoid alcohol or other CNS depressants; will enhance sedating properties of this drug
• May cause blurred vision

---

methazolamide

(meth-a-zoe′la-mide)
Neptazane

Func. class.: Carbonic anhydrase inhibitor diuretic
Chem. class.: Sulfonamide derivative

Action: Decreases production of aqueous humor in eye, which lowers intraocular pressure

Uses: Open-angle glaucoma or preoperatively in narrow-angle glaucoma

Dosage and routes:
• *Adult:* PO 50-100 mg bid or tid
Available forms include: Tabs 50 mg

Side effects/adverse reactions:
GU: Frequency, hypokalemia, polyuria, uremia, ***glucosuria, hematuria,*** dysuria
CNS: Drowsiness, paresthesia, anxiety, depression, headache, dizziness, confusion, stimulation, fatigue, ***convulsions,*** sedation, nervousness
GI: Nausea, vomiting, anorexia, constipation, diarrhea, melena, weight loss, hepatic insufficiency
EENT: Myopia, tinnitus
INTEG: Rash, pruritus, urticaria, fe-

ver, photosensitivity, Stevens-
Johnson syndrome
ENDO: Hyperglycemia
HEMA: **Aplastic anemia, hemolytic
anemia, leukopenia, agranulocytosis, thrombocytopenia, purpura,
pancytopenia**
Contraindications: Hypersensitivity to sulfonamides, severe renal
disease, severe hepatic disease,
electrolyte imbalances (hyponatremia, hypokalemia), hyperchloremic acidosis, Addison's disease,
COPD
Precautions: Hypercalciuria, pregnancy (C)
Pharmacokinetics:
PO: Onset 2-4 hr, peak 6-8 hr, duration 10-18 hr; excreted in urine,
crosses placenta
Interactions/incompatibilities:
• Increased action of: amphetamines, procainamide, quinidine,
flecainide, ephedrine, pseudoephedrine
• Hypokalemia: with other diuretics, corticosteroids, amphotericin B
• Toxicity: salicylates

NURSING CONSIDERATIONS
Assess:
• Weight, I&O daily to determine
fluid loss; effect of drug may be
decreased if used qd
• Rate, depth, rhythm of respiration, effect of exertion
• B/P lying, standing; postural hypotension may occur
• Electrolytes: potassium, sodium,
chloride; include BUN, blood
sugar, CBC, serum creatinine,
blood pH, ABGs, liver function
tests
Administer:
• In AM to avoid interference with
sleep if using drug as a diuretic
• Potassium replacement if potassium is less than 3.0

• With food, if nausea occurs, absorption may be decreased slightly
Evaluate:
• Therapeutic response: improvement in edema of feet, legs, sacral
area daily if medication is being
used in CHF; or decrease in
aqueous humor if medication is
being used in glaucoma
• Improvement in CVP q8h
• Signs of metabolic acidosis:
drowsiness, restlessness
• Signs of hypokalemia: postural
hypotension, malaise, fatigue,
tachycardia, leg cramps, weakness
• Rashes, temperature elevation qd
• Confusion, especially in elderly;
take safety precautions if needed
Teach patient/family:
• To increase fluid intake 2-3 L/
day unless contraindicated; to rise
slowly from lying or sitting position
• To notify physician if sore throat,
unusual bleeding, bruising, paresthesias, tremors, flank pain, or skin
rash occurs
• To avoid hazardous activities if
drowsiness occurs
Lab test interferences:
False positive: Urinary protein
Treatment of overdose: Lavage if
taken orally, monitor electrolytes,
administer dextrose in saline, monitor hydration, CV, renal status

---

methenamine hippu-
rate/methenamine
mandelate

(meth-en'a-meen) (hip'yoo-rate)
Hiprex, Hip-Rex,* Urex/Mandel-
amine

Func. class.: Urinary antiinfective
Chem. class.: Methenamine, man-
delic acid

Action: In acid urine, it is hydrolyzed to ammonia, formaldehyde, which are bactericidal

Uses: Urinary tract infections caused by *E. coli, Klebsiella, Enterobacter, P. mirabilis, P. morganii, Serratia, Citrobacter*

Dosage and routes:
• *Adult and child >12 yr:* PO 1 g q12h, maximum: 4 g/24 hr
• *Child 6-12 yr:* PO 500 mg-1g q12h

Neurogenic bladder
• *Adult:* PO 1 g qid pc
• *Child 6-12 yr:* PO 500 mg qid pc
• *Child <6 yr:* PO 50 mg/kg in 4 divided doses pc

Available forms include: Tabs 500 mg, 1 g; oral sol 500 mg, 1 g; susp 250, 500 mg/5 ml; tabs, enteric-coated 250, 500 mg, g; tabs, film-coated 500 mg, 1g

Side effects/adverse reactions:
CNS: Headache
INTEG: Pruritus, rash, urticaria
GI: Nausea, vomiting, anorexia, abdominal pain, increase AST, ALT
GU: Dysuria, bladder irritation, *albuminuria, hematuria,* crystalluria
EENT: Tinnitus, stomatitis

Contraindications: Hypersensitivity, severe dehydration, renal insufficiency

Precautions: Renal disease, pregnancy (C), lactation

Pharmacokinetics:
PO: Excreted in urine, half-life 4 hr

Interactions/incompatibilities:
• Insoluble precipitate in urine: sulfonamides
• Do not use with silver, iron, mercury salts

NURSING CONSIDERATIONS
Assess:
• I&O ratio, urine pH <5.5 is ideal, monitor for hematuria indicating crystalluria

• Periodic liver function test: AST, ALT, alk phosphatase
• C&S before treatment, after completion

Administer:
• After clean-catch urine is obtained for C&S
• Two daily doses if urine output is high or if patient has diabetes
• Up to 12 g of Vitamin C if needed to acidify urine; cranberry, prune juice may be used

Perform/provide:
• Storage protected from high temperature
• Limited intake of alkaline foods or drugs: milk, dairy products, peanuts, vegetables, alkaline antacids, sodium bicarbonate

Evaluate:
• Therapeutic response: decreased pain, frequency, urgency, negative C&S, absence of infection
• Allergy: fever, flushing, rash, urticaria, pruritus

Teach patient/family:
• Keep urine acidic by eating food that acidifies urine (meats, eggs, fish, gelatin products, prunes, plums, cranberries)
• Fluids must be increased to 3 L/day to avoid crystallization in kidneys
• Complete full course of drug therapy; take drug at evenly spaced intervals around clock for best results

Lab test interferences:
Interfere: VMA, urinary catecholamines
False decrease: Urine estriol, 5HIAA
False increase: 17-OHCS

---

* Available in Canada only

methicillin sodium

(meth-i-sill'in)
Celbenin, Staphcillin
Func. class.: Broad-spectrum antibiotic
Chem. class.: Penicillinase-resistant penicillin

Action: Interferes with cell wall replication of susceptible organisms; osmotically unstable cell wall swells, bursts from osmotic pressure

Uses: Effective for gram-positive cocci *(S. aureus, S. pyogenes, S. viridans, S. faecalis, S. bovis, S. pneumoniae)*, infections caused by penicillinase-producing *Staphylococcus*

Dosage and routes:
• *Adult:* IM/IV 4-12 g/day in divided doses q4-6h
• *Child:* IM/IV 50-300 mg/kg/day in divided doses q4-12h

Available forms include: Powder for inj IM, IV 1, 4, 6, 10 g; IV INF only 1 g

Side effects/adverse reactions:
HEMA: Anemia, increased bleeding time, *bone marrow depression, granulocytopenia*
GI: Nausea, vomiting, diarrhea, increased AST, ALT, abdominal pain, glossitis, colitis
GU: Oliguria, *proteinuria, hematuria, vaginitis, moniliasis, glomerulonephritis*
CNS: Lethargy, hallucinations, anxiety, depression, twitching, *coma, convulsions*

Contraindications: Hypersensitivity to penicillins
Precautions: Pregnancy (B), hypersensitivity to cephalosporins, neonates

Pharmacokinetics:
IM: Peak ½-1 hr, duration 4 hr

IV: Peak 15 min, duration 2 hr
Metabolized in liver, excreted in urine, bile, breast milk, crosses placenta

Interactions/incompatibilities:
• Decreased antimicrobial effectiveness of methicillin: tetracyclines, erythromycins
• Increased methicillin concentrations: aspirin, probenecid

NURSING CONSIDERATIONS
Assess:
• I&O ratio; report hematuria, oliguria since penicillin in high doses is nephrotoxic
• Any patient with compromised renal system since drug is excreted slowly in poor renal system function; toxicity may occur rapidly
• Liver studies: AST, ALT
• Blood studies: WBC, RBC, H&H, bleeding time
• Renal studies: urinalysis, protein, blood
• C&S before drug therapy; drug may be taken as soon as culture is taken

Administer:
• IV after diluting 1 g/1.8 ml sterile H₂O, further dilute each 500 mg/25 ml or more NaCl; give directly over 1 min or more or by inf over ½-8 hr
• Drug after C&S has been completed

Perform/provide:
• Adrenalin, suction, tracheostomy set, endotracheal intubation equipment
• Adequate fluid intake (2000 ml) during diarrhea episodes
• Scratch test to assess allergy after securing order from physician; usually done when penicillin is only drug of choice
• Storage at room temperature; reconstituted solution is stable for 8 hr

italics = common side effects   ***bold italic*** = life threatening reactions

Evaluate:
• Therapeutic effectiveness: absence of fever, draining wounds
• Bowel pattern before, during treatment
• Skin eruptions after administration of penicillin to 1 wk after discontinuing drug
• Respiratory status: rate, character, wheezing, tightness in chest
• Allergies before initiation of treatment, reaction of each medication; highlight allergies on chart, Kardex

Teach patient/family:
• Culture may be taken after completed course of medication
• To report sore throat, fever, fatigue (could indicate superimposed infection)
• To wear or carry Medic Alert ID if allergic to penicillins
• To notify nurse of diarrhea

Lab test interferences:
False positive: Urine glucose, urine protein

Treatment of overdose: Withdraw drug, maintain airway, administer epinephrine, aminophylline, O_2, IV corticosteroids for anaphylaxis

---

methimazole

(meth-im′a-zole)
Tapazole
Func. class.: Antithyroid hormone
Chem. class.: Thioamide

Action: Inhibits synthesis of thyroid hormones by decreasing iodine use in manufacture of thyroglobin and iodothyronine; does not affect already formed hormones
Uses: Hyperthyroidism, preparation for thyroidectomy, thyrotoxic crisis, thyroid storm
Dosage and routes:
Hyperthyroidism

• *Adult:* PO 5-20 mg tid depending on severity of condition, continue until euthyroid, maintenance dose 5 mg qd-tid, maximal dose 150 mg qd
• *Child:* PO 0.4 mg/kg/day in divided doses q8h, continue until euthyroid maintenance dose 0.2 mg/kg/day in divided doses q8h
Preparation for thyroidectomy
• *Adult and child:* PO same as above; iodine may be added × 10 days before surgery
Thyrotoxic crisis
• *Adult and child:* PO same as hyperthyroidism with iodine and propranolol
Available forms include: Tabs 5, 10 mg
Side effects/adverse reactions:
ENDO: Enlarged thyroid
INTEG: Rash, urticaria, pruritus, alopecia, hyperpigmentation, lupus-like syndrome
GU: Nephritis
CNS: Drowsiness, headache, vertigo, fever, paresthesias, neuritis
HEMA: Agranulocytosis, leukopenia, thrombocytopenia, hypothrombinemia, lymphadenopathy, bleeding, vasculitis
GI: Nausea, diarrhea, vomiting, jaundice, hepatitis, loss of taste
MS: Myalgia, arthralgia, nocturnal muscle cramps
Contraindications: Hypersensitivity, pregnancy (3rd trimester) (D), lactation
Precautions: Infection, bone marrow depression, hepatic disease, pregnancy (1st, 2nd trimester)
Pharmacokinetics:
PO: Onset 30-40 min, duration 2-4 hr, half-life 1-2 hr, excreted in urine, bile, breast milk, crosses placenta

NURSING CONSIDERATIONS
Assess:
• Pulse, B/P, temperature

- I&O ratio, check for edema: puffy hands, feet, periorbits; indicate hypothyroidism
- Weight qd; same clothing, scale, time of day
- T$_3$, T$_4$, which are increased; serum TSH, which is decreased; free thyroxine index, which is increased if dosage is too low; discontinue drug 3-4 wk before RAIU
- Blood work: CBC for blood dyscrasias: leukopenia, thrombocytopenia, agranulocytosis; LFTs

Administer:
- With meals to decrease GI upset
- At same time each day, to maintain drug level
- Lowest dose that relieves symptoms, discontinue before RAI

Perform/provide:
- Storage in light-resistant container
- Fluids to 3-4 L/day, unless contraindicated

Evaluate:
- Therapeutic effect: weight gain, decreased pulse, decreased T$_4$, B/P
- Overdose: peripheral edema, heat intolerance, diaphoresis, palpitations, dysrhythmias, severe tachycardia, increased temperature, delirium, CNS irritability
- Hypersensitivity: rash, enlarged cervical lymph nodes; drug may need to be discontinued
- Hypoprothrombinemia: bleeding, petechiae, ecchymosis
- Clinical response: after 3 wk should include increased weight, pulse; decreased T$_4$
- Bone marrow depression: sore throat, fever, fatigue

Teach patient/family:
- To abstain from breast feeding after delivery
- To take pulse daily
- Report redness, swelling, sore throat, mouth lesions, which indicate blood dyscrasias
- To keep graph of weight, pulse, mood
- Avoid OTC products that contain iodine
- That seafood, other iodine products may be restricted
- Not to discontinue this medication abruptly; thyroid crisis may occur; stress patient response
- That response may take several months if thyroid is large
- Symptoms/signs of overdose: periorbital edema, cold intolerance, mental depression
- Symptoms of inadequate dose: tachycardia, diarrhea, fever, irritability

Lab test interferences:
Increase: Pro-time, AST/ALT, alk phosphatase

M

methocarbamol
(meth-oh-kar′ba-mole)
Delaxin, Forbaxin, Robamol, Robaxin, Romethocarb, Spenaxin, Tresortil*
Func. class.: Skeletal muscle relaxant
Chem. class.: Carbamate derivative

Action: Depresses multisynaptic pathways in the spinal cord
Uses: Adjunct for relief of spasm and pain in musculoskeletal conditions, tetanus management
Dosage and routes:
Pain
- *Adult:* PO 1.5 g × 2-3 days, then 1 g qid; IM 500 mg in each gluteal region, may repeat q8h; IV BOL 1-3 g/day at 3 ml/min; IV INF 1 gm/250 ml D$_5$W or NS, not to exceed 3 g/day
Tetanus

---

italics = common side effects   ***bold italic*** = life threatening reactions

- *Adult:* IV INF 1-3 g/L of solution q6h; IV BOL 1-2 g injected into running IV
- *Child:* IV 15 mg/kg q6h

Available forms include: Tabs 500, 750 mg; inj IM, IV 100 mg/ml

Side effects/adverse reactions:

CNS: Dizziness, weakness, drowsiness, headache, tremor, depression, insomnia, *seizures*

HEMA: Hemolysis, increased hemoglobin (IV only)

EENT: Diplopia, temporary loss of vision, blurred vision, nystagmus

CV: Postural hypotension, bradycardia

GI: Nausea, vomiting, hiccups, anorexia, metallic taste

GU: Brown, black, green urine

INTEG: Rash, pruritus, fever, facial flushing, urticaria

Contraindications: Hypersensitivity, child <12 yr, intermittent porphyria

Precautions: Renal disease, hepatic disease, addictive personalities, pregnancy (C), myasthenia gravis, epilepsy

Pharmacokinetics:

PO: Onset ½ hr, peak 1-2 hr, half-life 1-2 hr, metabolized in liver, excreted in urine (unchanged), crosses placenta

Interactions/incompatibilities:

- Increased CNS depression: alcohol, tricylic antidepressants, narcotics, barbiturates, sedatives, hypnotics

NURSING CONSIDERATIONS

Assess:

- Blood studies: CBC, WBC, differential; blood dyscrasias may occur
- During and after injection: CNS effects, rash, conjunctivitis, and nasal congestion may occur
- Liver function studies: AST, ALT, alk phosphatase; hepatitis may occur
- ECG in epileptic patients; poor seizure control has occurred with patients taking this drug

Administer:

- With meals for GI symptoms
- IV undiluted over 1 min or more, give 300 mg or less/1 min or longer; may be diluted in 250 ml or less compatible sol
- By slow IV to prevent phlebitis; keep recumbent for 15 min to prevent orthostatic hypotension; check for extravasation
- IM deeply in large muscle mass; rotate sites

Perform/provide:

- Storage in tight container at room temperature
- Assistance with ambulation if dizziness, drowsiness occurs

Evaluate:

- Therapeutic response: decreased pain, spasticity
- Allergic reactions: rash, fever, respiratory distress
- Severe weakness, numbness in extremities
- Psychologic dependency: increased need for medication, more frequent requests for medication, increased pain
- CNS depression: dizziness, drowsiness, psychiatric symptoms

Teach patient/family:

- Not to discontinue medication quickly; insomnia, nausea, headache, spasticity, tachycardia will occur, drug should be tapered off over 1-2 wk
- That urine may turn green, black or brown
- Not to take with alcohol, other CNS depressants
- To avoid altering activities while taking this drug

• To avoid hazardous activities if drowsiness, dizziness occurs
• To avoid using OTC medication: cough preparations, antihistamines, unless directed by physician
Lab test interferences:
False increase: VMA, urinary 5-HIAA
Treatment of overdose: Induce emesis of conscious patient, lavage, dialysis; have epinephrine, antihistamines, and corticosteroids available

methohexital sodium
(meth-oh-hex′i-tal)
Brevital Sodium, Brietal Sodium*
Func. class.: General anesthetic
Chem. class.: Barbiturate

Controlled Substance Schedule IV
Action: Acts in reticular-activating system to produce anesthesia
Uses: General anesthesia, for electroshock therapy, reduction of fractures
Dosage and routes:
• *Adult and child:* IV 50-100 mg given 1 ml/5 sec
Maintenance
• *Adult and child:* IV 20-40 mg q4-7 min of a 0.1% solution; CONT IV 1 gtt/sec of a 0.2% solution
Available forms include: Inj IV 500 mg, 2.5, 5g
Side effects/adverse reactions:
RESP: Respiratory depression, bronchospasm
CNS: Retrograde amnesia, prolonged somnolence
CV: Tachycardia, hypotension, *myocardial depression, dysrhythmias*
EENT: Sneezing, coughing
INTEG: Chills, *shivering*, necrosis, pain at injection site

MS: Muscle irritability
Contraindications: Hypersensitivity, status asthmaticus, hepatic/intermittent porphyrias, pregnancy (D)
Precautions: Severe cardiovascular disease, renal disease, hypotension, liver disease, myxedema, myasthenia gravis, asthma, increased intracranial pressure
Pharmacokinetics:
IV: Onset 30-40 sec; half-life 11.5 hr, crosses placenta
Interactions/incompatibilities:
• Increased action: CNS depressants
• Do not mix with atropine or silicone in solution or syringe
NURSING CONSIDERATIONS
Assess:
• VS q3-5 min during IV administration, after dose, q4 hr postoperatively
Administer:
• After preparation with sterile water of 0.9% or 5% dextrose
• Only with crash cart, resuscitative equipment nearby
• IV slowly only by qualified persons
Evaluate:
• Extravasation, if it occurs use nitroprusside or chloroprocaine to decrease pain, increase circulation
• Dysrhythmias or myocardial depression

methotrexate/methotrexate sodium (amethopterin, MTX)
(meth-oh-trex′ate)
Folex, Mexate
Func. class.: Antineoplastic-antimetabolite
Chem. class.: Folic acid antagonist

Action: Inhibits an enzyme that reduces folic acid, which is needed for nucleic acid synthesis in all cells

Uses: Acute lymphocytic leukemia, in combination for breast, lung, head, neck cancer, lymphosarcoma, psoriasis, gestational choriocarcinoma, hydatidiform mole

Dosage and routes:

Leukemia

• *Adult and child:* PO 3.3 mg/m²/day, maintenance 30 mg/m²/day 2 × /wk; IV 2.5 mg/kg q2 wk

Choriocarcinoma

• *Adult and child:* PO 15-30 mg/m² qd × 5 days, then off 1 wk; may repeat

Available forms include: Tabs, 2.5 mg; inj IV 25 mg/ml; powder for inj IV 20, 25, 50, 100, 250 mg; sodium inj IV 2.5, 25 mg/ml

Side effects/adverse reactions:

*HEMA: **Leukopenia, thrombocytopenia, myelosuppression, anemia***

*GI: Nausea, vomiting, anorexia, diarrhea, stomatitis, **hepatotoxicity,** cramps, ulcer, gastritis, **GI hemorrhage,** abdominal pain, hematemesis*

*GU: Urinary retention, **renal failure,** menstrual irregularities, defective spermatogenesis, **hematuria, azotemia, uric acid nephropathy***

INTEG: Rash, alopecia, dry skin, urticaria, photosensitivity, folliculitis, vasculitis, petechiae, ecchymosis, acne, alopecia

*CNS: Dizziness, **convulsions,** headache, confusion, hemiparesis, malaise, fatigue, chills, fever*

Contraindications: Hypersensitivity, leukopenia (<2500/mm³), thrombocytopenia (<100,000/mm³), anemia, psoriatic patients with severe renal/hepatic disease, pregnancy (D)

Precautions: Renal disease, lactation

Pharmacokinetics:

PO: Readily absorbed when taken orally, peak 1-4 hr

IV/IM: Peak ½-2 hr

Not metabolized, excreted in urine (unchanged), crosses placenta, blood-brain barrier, 50% plasma protein bound

Interactions/incompatibilities:

• Increased toxicity: aspirin, sulfa drugs, other antineoplastics, radiation, alcohol, probenecid, phenytoin, phenylbutazone, pyrimethamine

• Decreased effect of: oral digoxin

• Increased hypoprothrombinemia: oral anticoagulants

• Decreased effect of methotrexate: folic acid supplements

• Possible fatal interactions: nonsteroidal antiinflammatory drugs

NURSING CONSIDERATIONS

Assess:

• CBC, differential, platelet count weekly; withhold drug if WBC is <3500/mm³ or platelet count is <100,000/mm³; notify physician of these results; drug should be discontinued

• Renal function studies: BUN, serum uric acid, urine CrCl, electrolytes before, during therapy

• I&O ratio; report fall in urine output to <30 ml/hr

• Monitor temperature q4h; fever may indicate beginning infection, no rectal temperatures

• Liver function tests before and during therapy: bilirubin, alk phosphatase, AST, ALT; liver biopsy should be done before start of therapy (psoriasis patients)

• Bleeding time, coagulation time during treatment

Administer:

• IV after diluting 5 mg/2 ml of sterile H₂O for inj; give through Y-

---

* Available in Canada only

tube or 3-way stopcock at 10 mg or less/min
• Antacid before oral agent; give drug after evening meal before bedtime
• Antiemetic 30-60 min before giving drug to prevent vomiting
• Allopurinol or sodium bicarbonate to maintain uric acid levels, alkalinization of urine, adequate fluids
• Leucovorin calcium within 12 hr of this drug to prevent tissue damage, check agency policy
• Antibiotics for prophylaxis of infection
• Topical or systemic analgesics for pain
• Transfusion for anemia

Perform/provide:
• Strict medical asepsis and protective isolation if WBC levels are low
• Liquid diet: carbonated beverage, Jello; dry toast, crackers may be added when patient is not nauseated or vomiting
• Increased fluid intake to 2-3 L/day to prevent urate deposits, calculi formation, unless contraindicated
• Diet low in purines: absence of organ meats (kidney, liver), dried beans, peas to maintain alkaline urine
• Rinsing of mouth tid-qid with water, club soda; brushing of teeth bid-tid with soft brush or cotton-tipped applicators for stomatitis; use unwaxed dental floss
• Nutritious diet with iron, vitamin supplements
• Storage in tightly closed container in cool environment; store injection, powder for injection in dark, dry area

Evaluate:
• Bleeding: hematuria, guaiac, bruising or petechiae, mucosa or orifices q8h
• Food preferences; list likes, dislikes
• Effects of alopecia on body image; discuss feelings about body changes
• **Hepatotoxicity:** yellowing of skin, sclera, dark urine, clay-colored stools, pruritus, abdominal pain, fever, diarrhea
• Buccal cavity q8h for dryness, sores, ulceration, white patches, oral pain, bleeding, dysphagia
• Symptoms indicating severe allergic reaction: rash, urticaria, itching, flushing

Teach patient/family:
• Why protective isolation precautions are needed
• To report any complaints, side effects to nurse or physician: black tarry stools, chills, fever, sore throat, bleeding, bruising, cough, shortness of breath, dark or bloody urine
• That hair may be lost during treatment and wig or hairpiece may make patient feel better; tell patient that new hair may be different in color, texture (alopecia is rare)
• To avoid foods with citric acid, hot or rough texture if stomatitis is present
• To report stomatitis: any bleeding, white spots, ulcerations in mouth to physician; tell patient to examine mouth qd, report symptoms to nurse
• That contraceptive measures are recommended during therapy for at least 8 wk following cessation of therapy
• To drink 10-12 glasses of fluid/day
• To avoid alcohol, salicylates
• To avoid use of razors or commercial mouthwash

M

methotrimeprazine HCl

(meth-oh-trye-mep'ra-zeen)
Levoprome, Nozinan*

Func. class.: Analgesic
Chem. class.: Aliphatic (propyl-amine-phenothiazine derivative)

Action: Depresses cerebral cortex, hypothalamus, limbic system; blocks neurotransmission produced by dopamine at synapse; exhibits strong α-adrenergic, anticholinergic blocking action, antihistamine

Uses: Sedation, analgesia, preoperative and postoperative analgesia, obstetric analgesia

Dosage and routes:

Analgesia/sedation

• *Adult and child >12 yr:* IM 10-20 mg q4-6h prn

• *Elderly:* IM 5-10 mg q4-6h

Preoperative medication

• *Adult and child >12 yr:* IM 2-20 mg 45 min to 3 hr before surgery

Postoperative medication

• *Adult and child >12 yr:* IM 2.5-7.5 mg q4-6h titrated to patient's needs

Available forms include: Inj IM 20 mg/ml

Side effects/adverse reactions:

*HEMA: **Thrombocytopenia, agranulocytosis, leukopenia, neutropenia, hemolytic anemia*** (long-term, high dose)

CNS: Weakness, dizziness, drowsiness, confusion, delirium, euphoria, headache, sedation, EPS

GI: Nausea, vomiting, abdominal pain, dry mouth, jaundice (long-term use)

*GU: **Hematuria,*** dysuria, hesitancy, retention, uterine inertia (rare)

INTEG: Pain, edema at injection site, fever, chills

EENT: Nasal congestion, blurred vision, slurred speech

CV: Orthostatic hypotension, palpitations, tachycardia, bradycardia

Contraindications: Hypersensitivity to this drug, phenothiazines, bisulfite; seizures; severe hepatic disease; severe renal disease; severe cardiac disease; coma

Precautions: Elderly, pregnancy (C)

Pharmacokinetics:

IM: Onset 20-30 min, peak 1-2 hr, duration 4 hr; metabolized by liver, excreted by kidneys and in feces, crosses placenta, excreted in breast milk

Interactions/incompatibilities:

• Mix only with scopolamine or atropine; not to be mixed in syringe or solution with any other drugs

• Increased sedation: CNS depressants, alcohol, barbiturates, reserpine, narcotics, general anesthetics, meprobamate

NURSING CONSIDERATIONS

Assess:

• Blood studies: CBC, ALT, AST, bilirubin

• VS q10 min for 30 min; watch for decreasing B/P with increased pulse that may occur 10-30 min after injection; continue to closely monitor for 6-12 hr after several injections

• Effect on uterine contractions, fetal heart tones if using for labor

Administer:

• After removal of cigarettes, to prevent fires

• IM injection in deep large muscle mass to prevent tissue sloughing, rotate sites

• Lowest dose, then gradually increase; lower doses are required after general anesthesia

Perform/provide:

• Bedrest for several hours after injection if orthostatic hypotension occurs

• Safety measure: siderails, nightlight, callbell within easy reach

• Storage in darkness, expires after 5 yr

• Assistance with ambulation for 6 hr after injection

Evaluate:

• Therapeutic response: decrease in pain, grimacing, absence of change in VS, ability to cough and breathe deep after surgery

Teach patient/family:

• To avoid ambulation without assistance for 6 hr after drug is given

Treatment of overdose: Lavage, activated charcoal, monitor electrolytes, vital signs

---

methoxsalen

(meth-ox'a-len)
Oxsoralen, Oxsoralen-Ultra 8-MOP, UltraMOP

Func. class.: Pigmenting agent
Chem. class.: Psoralen derivative

Action: Decreases cell turnover by combining with epidermal cell DNA, causing photo damage when used with ultraviolet rays

Uses: Vitiligo, psoriasis

Dosage and routes:

Vitiligo

• *Adult and child >12 yr:* PO 20 mg qd 2-4 hr before exposure to therapeutic ultraviolet rays; TOP apply 1-2 hr before exposure to UVA light, administered on an alternate-day schedule

Psoriasis

Adult PO: Dosage individualized according to weight; taken 2 hr before exposure to therapeutic ultraviolet rays

Available forms include: Lotion

1%; hard caps 10 mg; soft caps 10 mg; contains tartrazine

Side effects/adverse reactions:

CNS: Headache, depression, restlessness, anxiety, nervousness, vertigo, insomnia, malaise

GI: Nausea

INTEG: Rash, pruritus, burning, peeling, erythema, edema, urticaria, hypopigmentation

MISC: Leg cramps, hypotension, herpes simplex

Contraindications: Hypersensitivity, melanoma, LE, albinism, sunburn, cataracts, squamous cell cancer, child ≤12 yr, diseases associated with photosensitivity

Precautions: Hepatic disease, cardiac disease, children, lactation, pregnancy (C); contains tartrazine (FD & C #5)

Pharmacokinetics:

PO: Duration 8 hr, half-life 2 hr, metabolized in liver, excreted in urine

Interactions/incompatibilities:

• Increased effects of methoxsalen: other photosensitizing agents, phenothiazines, thiazides, tetracyclines, griseofulvin, halogenated salicylamides, sulfonamides, coal tar derivatives

NURSING CONSIDERATIONS

Assess:

• Hepatic test (AST, ALT, bilirubin), renal test (BUN, protein), antinuclear antibodies during treatment

Administer:

• With food or milk to prevent GI upset

• To prevent extensive phototoxicity, qod

• Lotion to small areas, use systemic treatment for large areas

Perform/provide:

• Protection to eyes, lips during treatment

---

italics = common side effects   ***bold italic*** = life threatening reactions

• Use of finger cot or gloves to apply lotion

Evaluate:

• Therapeutic response: increased pigmentation in vitiligo, decreased psoriatic areas

Teach patient/family:

• To avoid UVA exposure for at least 24 hr after topical application, and 8 hr after PO dose

• Sunscreen may be used if exposure to sunlight occurs after treatment

• Repigmentation may require 6-9 months

---

methscopolamine bromide

(meth-skoe-pol′a-meen)

Pamine

Func. class.: Gastrointestinal anticholinergic

Chem. class.: Synthetic quaternary ammonium antimuscarinic

Action: Inhibits muscarinic actions of acetylcholine at postganglionic parasympathetic neuroeffector sites

Uses: Treatment of peptic ulcer disease

Dosage and routes:

• *Adult:* PO 2.5-5 mg ½ hr ac, hs

Available forms include: Tabs 2.5 mg

Side effects/adverse reactions:

CNS: Confusion, stimulation in elderly, headache, insomnia, dizziness, drowsiness, anxiety, weakness, hallucination

*GI: Dry mouth, constipation, **paralytic ileus,*** heartburn, nausea, vomiting, dysphagia, absence of taste

GU: Hesitancy, retention, impotence

CV: Palpitations, tachycardia

EENT: Blurred vision, photophobia, mydriasis, cycloplegia, increased ocular tension

INTEG: Urticaria, rash, pruritus, anhidrosis, fever, allergic reactions

Contraindications: Hypersensitivity to anticholinergics, narrow-angle glaucoma, GI obstruction, myasthenia gravis, paralytic ileus, GI atony, toxic megacolon

Precautions: Hyperthyroidism, coronary artery disease, dysrhythmias, CHF, ulcerative colitis, hypertension, hiatal hernia, hepatic disease, renal disease, pregnancy (C), urinary retention, prostatic hypertrophy

Pharmacokinetics:

PO: Onset 1 hr, duration 6-8 hr; metabolized by liver, excreted in urine

Interactions/incompatibilities:

• Increased anticholinergic effect: amantadine, tricyclic antidepressants, MAOIs, H₁ antihistamines

• Decreased effect of: phenothiazines, levodopa, ketoconazole

NURSING CONSIDERATIONS

Assess:

• VS, cardiac status: checking for dysrhythmias, increased rate, palpitations

• I&O ratio; check for urinary retention or hesitancy

Administer:

• ½-1 hr ac for better absorption

• Decreased dose to elderly patients; their metabolism may be slowed

• Gum, hard candy, frequent rinsing of mouth for dryness of oral cavity

Perform/provide:

• Storage in tight container protected from light

• Increased fluids, bulk, exercise to patient's lifestyle to decrease constipation

Evaluate:

• Therapeutic response: absence of

---

epigastric pain, bleeding, nausea, vomiting
• GI complaints: pain, bleeding (frank or occult), nausea, vomiting, anorexia
Teach patient/family:
• To avoid driving or other hazardous activities until stabilized on medication
• To avoid alcohol or other CNS depressants; will enhance sedating properties of this drug
• To drink plenty of fluids
• To report dysphagia
• May cause blurred vision

---

methsuximide

(meth-sux'i-mide)
Celontin
Func. class.: Anticonvulsant
Chem. class.: Succinimide

Action: Inhibits spike, wave formation in absence seizures (petit mal), decreases amplitude, frequency, duration, spread of discharge in minor motor seizures
Uses: Refractory absence seizures (petit mal)
Dosage and routes:
• *Adult and child:* PO 300 mg/day; may increase by 300 mg/wk, not to exceed 1.2 g/day in divided doses
Available forms include: Caps, half-strength 150 mg; caps 300 mg
Side effects/adverse reactions:
*HEMA: **Agranulocytosis, aplastic anemia, thrombocytopenia, leukocytosis,** eosinophilia, **pancytopenia***
CNS: Drowsiness, dizziness, fatigue, euphoria, lethargy, irritability, depression, insomnia, anxiety, aggressiveness, ataxia, headache, confusion
GI: Nausea, vomiting, heartburn,

anorexia, diarrhea, abdominal pain, cramps, constipation, gum hypertrophy, tongue swelling
GU: Vaginal bleeding, **hematuria, renal damage**
INTEG: Urticaria, pruritic erythema, hirsutism, **Stevens-Johnson syndrome**
EENT: Myopia, blurred vision
Contraindications: Hypersensitivity to succinimide derivatives
Precautions: Hepatic disease, renal disease, pregnancy (C), lactation
Pharmacokinetics:
PO: Onset 15-30 min, peak 1-2 hr, duration 4-6 hr
REC: Onset slow, duration 4-6 hr
Metabolized by liver, excreted by kidneys, half-life 2⅖-4 hr
Interactions/incompatibilities:
• Antagonist effect: tricyclic antidepressants
• Decreased effects of: estrogens, oral contraceptives
NURSING CONSIDERATIONS
Assess:
• Renal studies: urinalysis, BUN, urine creatinine
• Blood studies: CBC, Hct, Hgb, reticulocyte counts q wk for 4 wk then q mo
• Hepatic studies: ALT, AST, bilirubin, creatinine
• Drug levels during initial treatment, therapeutic range (40-80 µg/ml)
Administer:
• With food, milk to decrease GI symptoms
Perform/provide:
• Hard candy, frequent rinsing of mouth, gum for dry mouth
• Assistance with ambulation during early part of treatment; dizziness occurs
Evaluate:
• Therapeutic response: decreased

M

---

italics = common side effects   **bold italic** = life threatening reactions

seizure activity, document on patient's chart

• Mental status: mood, sensorium, affect, behavioral changes; if mental status changes notify physician

• Eye problems; need for ophthalmic exams before, during, after treatment (slit lamp, fundoscopy, tonometry)

• Allergic reaction: red raised rash; if this occurs, drug should be discontinued

• Blood dyscrasias: fever, sore throat, bruising, rash, jaundice

• Toxicity: bone marrow depression, nausea, vomiting, ataxia, diplopia

Teach patient/family:

• To avoid driving, other activities that require alertness

• To avoid alcohol ingestion, CNS depressants; increased sedation may occur

• Not to discontinue medication quickly after long-term use

• To call physician promptly if lupuslike syndrome occurs (enlarged lymph nodes, fever, bruising, sore throat)

• That drug may change urine to pink or brown

Lab test interferences:

Increase: Coombs' test

Treatment of overdose: Lavage, activated charcoal, monitor electrolytes, VS

---

methylcellulose

(meth-ill-sell'yoo-lose)

Cellothyl, Citrucel, Cologel, Hydrolose, Syncelose,

Func. class.: Laxative, bulk

Chem. class.: Hydrophilic semisynthetic cellulose derivative

Action: Attracts water, expands in intestine to increase peristalsis; also absorbs excess water in stool; decreases diarrhea

Uses: Constipation

Dosage and routes:

• *Adult:* PO 5-20 ml tid with 8 oz of water

• *Child:* PO 5-10 ml qd or bid with water or 500 mg tid with 8 oz of water

Available forms include: Powder 105 mg/g; sol 450 mg/5 ml; tab 500 mg

Side effects/adverse reactions:

GI: Obstruction, abdominal distention

Contraindications: Hypersensitivity, GI obstruction, hepatitis

Pharmacokinetics:

PO: Onset 12-24 hr, peak 1-3 days

Interactions/incompatibilities:

• Decreased absorption: antibiotics, digitalis, nitrofurantoin, salicylates, tetracyclines, oral anticoagulants

NURSING CONSIDERATIONS

Assess:

• Blood, urine electrolytes if drug is used often by patient

• I&O ratio to identify fluid loss

Administer:

• Alone for better absorption; do not take within 1 hr of other drugs

• In morning or evening (oral dose)

Evaluate:

• Therapeutic response: decrease in constipation

• Cause of constipation; identify whether fluids, bulk, or exercise is missing from lifestyle

• Cramping, rectal bleeding, nausea, vomiting; if these symptoms occur, drug should be discontinued

Teach patient/family:

• Swallow tabs whole; do not chew

• That normal bowel movements do not always occur daily

• Do not use in presence of abdominal pain, nausea, vomiting

• Notify physician if constipation unrelieved or if symptoms of electrolyte imbalance occur: muscle cramps, pain, weakness, dizziness, excessive thirst

methyldopa/methyldopate

(meth-ill-doe′pa)

Aldomet, Dopamet,* Medimet,* Novomedopa*

Func. class.: Antihypertensive

Chem. class.: Centrally-acting adrenergic inhibitor

Action: Stimulates central inhibitory α-adrenergic receptors or acts as false transmitter, resulting in reduction of arterial pressure

Uses: Hypertension

Dosage and routes:

• *Adult:* PO 250 mg bid or tid, then adjusted q2 days as needed, 0.5-3 g qd in 2-4 divided doses (maintenance), not to exceed 3 g day; IV 250 mg-500 mg in 100 ml D₅W q6h, run over 30-60 min, not to exceed 1 g q6h

• *Child:* PO 10 mg/kg/day in 2-4 divided doses, not to exceed 65 mg/kg or 3 g/day, whichever is less; IV 20-40 mg/kg/day in 4 divided doses, not to exceed 65 mg/kg

Available forms include: Tabs 125, 250, 500 mg; oral susp 250 mg/5ml; inj IV 50 mg/ml

Side effects/adverse reactions:

GI: Nausea, vomiting, diarrhea, constipation, hepatic dysfunction

CV: Bradycardia, myocarditis, orthostatic hypotension, angina, edema, weight gain

CNS: Drowsiness, weakness, dizziness, weakness, sedation, headache, depression, psychosis

EENT: Nasal congestion, eczema

HEMA: Leukopenia, thrombocytopenia, anemia, positive Coombs' test

INTEG: Lupus-like syndrome

GU: Impotence, failure to ejaculate

Contraindications: Active hepatic disease, hypersensitivity, blood dyscrasias

Precautions: Pregnancy (C), liver disease, eclampsia, severe cardiac disease

Pharmacokinetics:

PO: Peak 2-4 hr, duration 12-24 hr

IV: Peak 2 hr, duration 10-16 hr

Metabolized by liver, excreted in urine

Interactions/incompatibilities:

• Increased hypoglycemia: talbutal

• Increased pressor effect: sympathomimetic amines (norepinephrine, phenylpropanolamine)

• Increased hypotension: levodopa

• Increased sedation: haloperidol

• Increased action of: anesthetics

NURSING CONSIDERATIONS

Assess:

• Blood studies: neutrophils, decreased platelets

• Renal studies: protein, BUN, creatinine, watch for increased levels, may indicate nephrotic syndrome

• Baselines in renal, liver function tests before therapy begins

• K levels, although hyperkalemia rarely occurs

• B/P during beginning treatment, periodically thereafter

Administer:

• IV after diluting with 100 mg of compatible sol run over ½-1 hr

Perform/provide:

• Storage of tablets in tight containers

Evaluate:

• Therapeutic response: decrease in B/P in hypertension

• Allergic reaction: rash, fever, pruritus, urticaria; drug should be

italics = common side effects   ***bold italic*** = life threatening reactions

discontinued if antihistamines fail to help

• Symptoms of CHF: edema, dyspnea, wet rales, B/P
• Renal symptoms: polyuria, oliguria, frequency

Teach patient/family:

• To avoid hazardous activities
• Administer 1 hr before meals
• Not to discontinue drug abruptly or withdrawal symptoms may occur: anxiety, increased B/P, headache, insomnia, increased pulse, tremors, nausea, sweating
• Not to use OTC (cough, cold, allergy) products unless directed by physician
• Tell patient to avoid sunlight or wear sunscreen if in sunlight, photosensitivity may occur
• Stress patient compliance with dosage schedule even if feeling better
• To rise slowly to sitting or standing position to minimize orthostatic hypotension
• Notify physician of: mouth sores, sore throat, fever, swelling of hands or feet, irregular heartbeat, chest pain, signs of angioedema
• Excessive perspiration, dehydration, vomiting, diarrhea may lead to fall in blood pressure; consult physician if these occur
• Dizziness, fainting, light-headedness may occur during 1st few days of therapy
• That compliance is necessary, not to skip or stop drug unless directed by physician
• May cause skin rash or impaired perspiration

methylene blue

(meth'i-leen)
MG-Blue, Urolene Blue, Wright's Stain
Func. class.: Urinary tract antiseptic
Chem. class.: Antiseptic dye

Action: Oxidation-reduction; has opposite action on hemoglobin depending on concentration; with increased concentration, converts ferrous ion of reduced hemoglobin to ferric form, methemoglobin is thus produced; prolonged administration accelerates destruction of erythrocytes

Uses: Oxalate urinary tract calculi; urinary tract infections caused by *E. coli, Klebsiella, Enterobacter, P. mirabilis, P. vulgaris, P. morganii, Serratia, Citrobacter*

Dosage and routes:

• *Adult:* PO 65-130 mg pc with full glass of water

Cyanide poisoning/methemoglobinemia

• *Adult and child:* IV 1-2 mg/kg of 1% sol, inject slowly over 5 min or more

Available forms include: Tabs 65 mg, inj 10 mg/ml

Side effects/adverse reactions:

CV: Cyanosis, CV abnormalities
INTEG: Pruritus, rash, urticaria, photosensitivity, profuse sweating
CNS: Dizziness, headache, drowsiness, mental confusion, fever with large doses
GI: Nausea, vomiting, abdominal pain, diarrhea
GU: Bladder irritation

Contraindications: Hypersensitivity to this drug, renal insufficiency

Precautions: Anemia, renal disease, hepatic disease, G-6-PD deficiency, pregnancy (C)

Pharmacokinetics:
PO/IV: Excreted in urine, bile, feces

NURSING CONSIDERATIONS
Assess:
• For cyanosis
• I&O ratio, urine pH <5.5 is ideal
• Hct, Hgb

Administer:
• After clean-catch urine is obtained for C&S
• Two daily doses if urine output is high or if patient has diabetes

Perform/provide:
• Limited intake of alkaline foods, drugs: milk, dairy products, peanuts, vegetables, alkaline antacids, sodium bicarbonate

Evaluate:
• Therapeutic response: decreased pain, frequency, urgency, C&S absence of infection
• CNS symptoms: insomnia, headache, drowsiness, confusion
• Allergic reactions: fever, flushing, rash, urticaria, pruritus

Teach patient/family:
• Instruct patient that anemia may result with continued administration
• Instruct patient that drug turns urine, sometimes stool, blue green
• If symptoms do not improve, or become worse, notify physician
• Notify physician of any sign/symptoms of side effects or adverse reactions

---

methylergonovine maleate

(meth-ill-er-goe-noe′veen)
Methergine, Methylergobasine*
Func. class.: Oxytocic
Chem. class.: Ergot alkaloid

Action: Stimulates uterine contractions, decreases bleeding

Uses: Treatment of hemorrhage associated with postpartum or post-abortion

Dosage and routes:
• *Adult:* IM 0.2 mg q2-5h, not to exceed 5 doses; IV 0.2 mg given over 1 min; PO 0.2-0.4 mg q6-12h × 2-7 days after initial IM or IV dose

Available forms include: Inj IM, IV 0.2 mg/ml; tabs 0.2 mg

Side effects/adverse reactions:
CNS: Headache, dizziness
GI: Nausea, vomiting
CV: Chest pain, palpitation, hypertension
EENT: Tinnitus
INTEG: Sweating, rash

Contraindications: Hypersensitivity to ergot preparations, indication of labor, before delivery of placenta, hypertension, PID, respiratory disease, cardiac disease, peripheral vascular disease

Precautions: Pregnancy (C), severe hepatic disease, severe renal disease, jaundice, diabetes mellitus, convulsive disorders

Pharmacokinetics:
PO: Onset 5-25 min, duration 3 hr
IM: Onset 2-5 min, duration 3 hr
IV: Onset immediate, duration 45 min
Metabolized in liver, excreted in urine

NURSING CONSIDERATIONS
Assess:
• B/P, pulse, character and amount of vaginal bleeding; watch for changes that may indicate hemorrhage
• Respiratory rate, rhythm, depth; notify physician of abnormalities

Administer:
• IV undiluted through Y-tube or 3-way stopcock; give 0.2 mg or less/min
• Only during fourth stage of labor,

M

---

italics = common side effects   ***bold italic*** = life threatening reactions

not to be used to augment labor
• IM in deep muscle mass; rotate injection sites if additional doses are given
• After having crash cart available on unit, IV route used only in emergencies
Evaluate:
• For uterine relaxation, observe for severe cramping
• Ergot toxicity: tinnitus, hypertension, palpitations, chest pain
Teach patient/family:
• To report increased blood loss, severe abdominal cramps, increased temperature or foul-smelling lochia

---

methylphenidate HCl

(meth-ill-fen′i-date)
Methidate, Ritalin, Ritalin SR
Func. class.: Cerebral stimulant
Chem. class.: Piperidine derivative

Controlled Substance Schedule II
Action: Increases release of norepinephrine, dopamine in cerebral cortex to reticular activating system; exact action not known
Uses: Attention deficit disorder with hyperactivity, narcolepsy
Dosage and routes:
Attention deficit disorder
• *Child >6 yr:* 5 mg before breakfast and lunch, increasing by 5-10 mg/wk, not to exceed 60 mg/day
Narcolepsy
• *Adult:* PO 10 mg bid-tid, 30-45 min before meals, may increase up to 40-60 mg/day
Available forms include: Tabs 5, 10, 20 mg; tabs sus rel 20 mg
Side effects/adverse reactions:
CNS: Hyperactivity, insomnia, restlessness, talkativeness, dizziness, headache, akathisia, dyskinesia, Tourette's disease

GI: Nausea, anorexia, dry mouth, diarrhea, constipation, weight loss, abdominal pain
CV: Palpitations, tachycardia, B/P changes, angina, dysrhythmias
INTEG: Exfoliative dermatitis, urticaria, rash, erythema-multiforme
ENDO: Growth retardation
GU: Uremia
HEMA: Thrombocytopenia
Contraindications: Hypersensitivity, anxiety, history of Tourette's disorder; with history of seizures
Precautions: Hypertension, depression, pregnancy (C), seizures, lactation, drug abuse
Pharmacokinetics:
PO: Onset ½-1 hr, duration 4-6 hr, metabolized by liver, excreted by kidneys
Interactions/incompatibilities:
• Hypertensive crisis: MAOIs or within 14 days of MAOIs
• Decreased effects of: guanethidine, other antihypertensives
NURSING CONSIDERATIONS
Assess:
• VS, B/P since this drug may reverse antihypertensives; check patients with cardiac disease more often
• CBC, urinalysis, in diabetes: blood sugar, urine sugar; insulin changes may need to be made since eating will decrease
• Height, growth rate in children; growth rate may be decreased
Administer:
• At least 6 hr before hs to avoid sleeplessness
• For obesity only if patient is on weight reduction program including dietary changes, exercise; patient will develop tolerance, and weight loss won't occur without additional methods, give 30-45 min before meals

---

* Available in Canada only

• Gum, hard candy, frequent sips of water for dry mouth

Evaluate:

• Mental status: mood, sensorium, affect, stimulation, insomnia, aggressiveness

• Physical dependency: should not be used for extended time; dose should be discontinued gradually, tolerance occurs after long-term use

• Withdrawal symptoms: headache, nausea, vomiting, muscle pain, weakness

Teach patient/family:

• To decrease caffeine consumption (coffee, tea, cola, chocolate); may increase irritability, stimulation

• Avoid OTC preparations unless approved by physician

• To taper off drug over several weeks, or depression, increased sleeping, lethargy will ensue

• To avoid alcohol ingestion

• To avoid hazardous activities until patient is stabilized on medication

• To get needed rest; patients will feel more tired at end of day

Treatment of overdose: Administer fluids, hemodialysis or peritoneal dialysis; antihypertensive for increased B/P, administer short-acting barbiturate before lavage

---

methylprednisolone/ methylprednisolone acetate/methylprednisolone sodium succinate

(meth-ill-pred-niss′oh-lone)
Medrol/Depo-Medrol, Duralone, Medralone, Rep-Pred/A-Meth-apred, Solu-Medrol

Func. class.: Corticosteroid
Chem. class.: Glucocorticoid, immediate acting

Action: Decreases inflammation by suppression of migration of polymorphonuclear leukocytes, fibroblasts, reversal of increased capillary permeability and lysosomal stabilization

Uses: Severe inflammation, shock, adrenal insufficiency, collagen disorders

Dosage and routes:

Adrenal insufficiency/inflammation

• *Adult:* PO 2-60 mg in 4 divided doses; IM 40-80 mg (acetate); IM/IV 10-250 mg (succinate); INTRA-ARTICULAR: 4-30 mg (acetate)

• *Child:* IV 117 µg-1.66 mg/kg in 3-4 divided doses (succinate)

Shock

• *Adult:* IV 100-250 mg q2-6h, (succinate)

Available forms include: Tabs 2, 4, 6, 8, 16, 24, 32 mg; inj 20, 40, 80 mg/ml acetate; inj 40, 125, 500, 1000 mg/vial succinate

Side effects/adverse reactions:

INTEG: Acne, poor wound healing, ecchymosis, petechiae

CNS: Depression, flushing, sweating, headache, mood changes

*CV: Hypertension, **circulatory collapse, thrombophlebitis, embolism**,* tachycardia

*HEMA: **Thrombocytopenia***

MS: Fractures, osteoporosis, weakness

*GI: Diarrhea, nausea, abdominal distention, **GI hemorrhage**, increased appetite, **pancreatitis***

EENT: Fungal infections, increased intraocular pressure, blurred vision

Contraindications: Psychosis, hypersensitivity, idiopathic thrombocytopenia, acute glomerulonephritis, amebiasis, fungal infections, nonasthmatic bronchial disease, child <2 yr, *AIDS*, TB

Precautions: Pregnancy (C), diabetes mellitus, glaucoma, osteo-

M

porosis, seizure disorders, ulcerative colitis, CHF, myasthenia gravis, renal disease, esophagitis, peptic ulcer

Pharmacokinetics:

PO: Peak 1-2 hr, duration 1½ day

IM: Peak 4-8 days, duration 1-4 wk

INTRAARTICULAR: Peak 1 wk

Half-life >3½ hr

Interactions/incompatibilities:

• Decreased action of methylprednisolone: cholestyramine, colestipol, barbiturates, rifampin, ephedrine, phenytoin, theophylline

• Decreased effects of: anticoagulants, anticonvulsants, antidiabetics, ambenonium, neostigmine, isoniazid, toxoids, vaccines

• Increased side effects: alcohol, salicylates, indomethacin, amphotericin B, digitalis preparations

• Increased action of methylprednisolone: salicylates, estrogens, indomethacin

NURSING CONSIDERATIONS

Assess:

• Potassium, blood sugar, urine glucose while on long-term therapy; hypokalemia and hyperglycemia

• Weight daily, notify physician of weekly gain >5 lb

• B/P q4h, pulse, notify physician if chest pain occurs

• I&O ratio, be alert for decreasing urinary output and increasing edema

• Plasma cortisol levels during long-term therapy (normal level: 138-635 nmol/L SI units when drawn at 8 AM)

Administer:

• IV after diluting with diluent provided, agitate slowly, give 500 mg or less/1 min or longer; may be given as IV infusion

• After shaking suspension (parenteral)

• Titrated dose, use lowest effective dose

• IM inj deeply in large mass, rotate sites, avoid deltoid, use 21G needle

• In one dose in AM to prevent adrenal suppression, avoid SC administration, damage may be done to tissue

• With food or milk to decrease GI symptoms

Perform/provide:

• Assistance with ambulation in patient with bone tissue disease to prevent fractures

Evaluate:

• Therapeutic response: ease of respirations, decreased inflammation

• Infection: increased temperature, WBC, even after withdrawal of medication; drug masks symptoms of infection

• Potassium depletion: paresthesias, fatigue, nausea, vomiting, depression, polyuria, dysrhythmias, weakness

• Edema, hypertension, cardiac symptoms

• Mental status: affect, mood, behavioral changes, aggression

Teach patient/family:

• That ID as steroid user should be carried

• To notify physician if therapeutic response decreases; dosage adjustment may be needed

• Not to discontinue this medication abruptly or adrenal crisis can result

• To avoid OTC products: salicylates, alcohol in cough products, cold preparations unless directed by physician

• About cushingoid symptoms

• Symptoms of adrenal insufficiency: nausea, anorexia, fatigue, dizziness, dyspnea, weakness, joint pain

---

* Available in Canada only

Lab test interferences:
Increase: Cholesterol, sodium, blood glucose, uric acid, calcium, urine glucose
Decrease: Calcium, potassium, T_4, T_3, thyroid ^{131}I uptake test, urine 17-OHCS, 17-KS, PBI
False negative: Skin allergy tests

---

methylprednisolone acetate

(meth-ill-pred-niss'oh-lone)
Medrol
Func. class.: Topical corticosteroid
Chem. class.: Synthetic nonfluorinated agent, group VI potency

Action: Possesses antipruritic, antiinflammatory actions
Uses: Psoriasis, eczema, contact dermatitis, pruritus
Dosage and routes:
• *Adult and child:* Apply to affected area qd-qid
Available forms include: Oint 0.25%, 1%
Side effects/adverse reactions:
INTEG: Burning, dryness, itching, irritation, acne, folliculitis, hypertrichosis, perioral dermatitis, hypopigmentation, atrophy, striae, miliaria, allergic contact dermatitis, secondary infection
Contraindications: Hypersensitivity to corticosteroids, fungal infections
Precautions: Pregnancy (C), lactation, viral or bacterial infections
NURSING CONSIDERATIONS
Assess:
• Temperature; if fever develops, drug should be discontinued
Administer:
• Only to affected areas; do not get in eyes
• Medication, then cover with occlusive dressing (only if pre-

scribed), seal to normal skin, change q12h, systemic absorption may occur, use gloves for application
• Only to dermatoses; do not use on weeping, denuded, or infected area
Perform/provide:
• Cleansing before application of drug
• Treatment for a few days after area has cleared
• Storage at room temperature
Evaluate:
• Therapeutic response: absence of severe itching, patches on skin, flaking
• For systemic absorption: increased temperature, inflammation, irritation
Teach patient/family:
• To avoid sunlight on affected area, burns may occur

---

methyprylon

(meth-i-prye'lon)
Noludar
Func. class.: Sedative-hypnotic
Chem. class.: Piperidine derivative

Controlled Substance Schedule III (USA), Schedule F (Canada)
Action: Acts at level of thalamus to produce CNS mood alterations by interfering with nerve impulse transmission in sensory cortex by increasing threshold of arousal centers
Uses: Insomnia
Dosage and routes:
• *Adult:* PO 200-400 mg 15-30 min before hs
• *Child >12 yrs:* PO 50 mg hs, may increase to 200 mg
Available forms include: Caps 300 mg, tabs 50, 200 mg
Side effects/adverse reactions:
CNS: Residual sedation, dizziness,

ataxia, stimulation, headache, pyrexia, nightmares, depression

GI: Nausea, vomiting, diarrhea, esophagitis, constipation

INTEG: Rash, pruritus

Contraindications: Hypersensitivity to piperidine derivatives, severe pain, severe renal or hepatic disease, porphyria

Precautions: Depression, suicidal individuals, drug abuse, cardiac dysrhythmias, narrow-angle glaucoma, prostatic hypertrophy, stenosed peptic ulcer, pyloroduodenal/bladder neck obstruction, pregnancy (B)

Pharmacokinetics:

PO: Onset 45 min, peak 1-2 hr, duration 5-8 hr; metabolized by the liver, excreted by the kidneys, crosses placenta, excreted in breast milk; half-life 3-6 hr

Interactions/incompatibilities:

• Increased CNS depression: alcohol, barbiturates, narcotics and other CNS depressants

NURSING CONSIDERATIONS

Assess:

• Blood studies: Hct, Hgb, RBCs (long-term therapy)

• Hepatic studies: AST, ALT, bilirubin (long-term therapy)

Administer:

• After removal of cigarettes to prevent fires

• After trying conservative measures for insomnia

• ½-1 hr before hs for sleeplessness

• On empty stomach for fast onset, but may be taken with food if GI symptoms occur

• Overdosing symptoms: respiratory depression, hypotension, confusion, coma, constricted pupils

Perform/provide:

• Assistance with ambulation after receiving dose

• Safety measures: siderails, nightlight, callbell within easy reach

• Checking to see PO medication has been swallowed, watch depressed, drug-dependent patients for hoarding, self-overdosing

• Storage in tight, light-resistant container in cool environment

Evaluate:

• Therapeutic response: ability to sleep at night, decreased amount of early morning awakening if taking drug for insomnia

• Mental status: mood, sensorium, affect, memory (long, short)

• Type of sleep problem: falling asleep, staying asleep

• Physical dependency including more frequent requests for medication, shakes, anxiety

• Withdrawal: nausea, vomiting, anxiety, hallucinations, insomnia, tachycardia, fever, cramps, tremors, seizures

• Allergic reaction: rash; discontinue drug if rash occurs

Teach patient/family:

• To avoid driving or other activities requiring alertness until drug stabilized

• To avoid alcohol ingestion or CNS depressants; serious CNS depression may result

• Not to discontinue medication quickly after long-term use; drug should be tapered over 1-2 wk

• That effects may take 2 nights for benefits to be noticed

• Alternate measures to improve sleep: reading, exercise several hours before hs, warm bath, warm milk, TV, self-hypnosis, deep breathing

• That hangover is common in elderly, but less common than with barbiturates

Treatment of overdose: Lavage, activated charcoal, monitor electrolytes, vital signs

---

* Available in Canada only

methysergide maleate

(meth-i-ser'jide)

Sansert

Func. class.: Serotonin antagonist
Chem. class.: Ergot derivative

Action: Competitively blocks serotonin HT receptors in CNS and periphery; potent vasoconstrictor
Uses: Prophylaxsis for migraine and other vascular headaches
Dosage and routes:
• *Adult:* PO 2 mg bid with meals
Available forms include: Tabs 2 mg
Side effects/adverse reactions:
CNS: Tremors, anxiety, insomnia, headache, dizziness, euphoria, confusion, depersonalization, hallucination, paresthesias, drowsiness
CV: Retroperitoneal fibrosis, valvular thickening, palpitations, tachycardia, postural hypertension, angina, thrombophlebitis, ECG changes, *cardiac fibrosis*
GI: Nausea, vomiting, weight gain
MS: Arthralgia, myalgia
INTEG: Flushing, rash, alopecia
HEMA: Blood dyscrasias
Contraindications: Hypersensitivity to ergot, tartrazine, pregnancy, occlusion (peripheral, vascular), CAD, hepatic disease, renal disease, peptic ulcer, hypertension, connective tissue disease, fibrotic pulmonary disease
Precautions: Pregnancy (C), lactation, children
Pharmacokinetics:
PO: Half-life 10 hr, metabolized by liver, excreted in urine (metabolites/unchanged drug)
Interactions/incompatibilities:
• Increased vasoconstriction: beta blockers

• Decreased effect of: narcotic analgesics
NURSING CONSIDERATIONS
Assess:
• Weight daily, check for peripheral edema in feet, legs, B/P
Administer:
• At beginning of headache, dose must be titrated to patient response
• Give with meals or after meals to avoid GI symptoms
• Only to women who are not pregnant, harm to fetus may occur
Perform/provide:
• Storage in dark area
• Quiet, calm environment with decreased stimulation for noise, bright light, or excessive talking
Evaluate:
• Therapeutic response: decrease in frequency, severity of headache
• For stress level, activity, recreation, coping mechanisms of patient
• Neurological status: LOC, blurring vision, nausea, vomiting, tingling in extremities that occur preceding headache
• Ingestion of tyramine foods (pickled products, beer, wine, aged cheese), food additives, preservatives, colorings, artificial sweeteners, chocolate, caffeine; may precipitate these types of headaches
Teach patient/family:
• Not to use OTC medications, serious drug interactions may occur
• To maintain dose at approved level, not to increase even if drug does not relieve headache
• To report side effects: increased vasoconstriction starting with cold extremities, then paresthesia, weakness
• That an increase in headaches may occur when this drug is discontinued after long-term use

M

---

italics = common side effects   ***bold italic*** = life threatening reactions

- To keep drug out of reach of children, death may occur
- To report at once: dyspnea, paresthesias, urinary problems, pain in abdomen, chest, back, legs
- To use drug for less than 6 months
- That drug may cause drowsiness

metipranolol HCl

(met-ee-pran′oh-lole)
Betamet
Func. class.: I-isomer

Action: Reduces production of aqueous humor by unknown mechanism
Uses: Ocular hypertension, chronic open-angle glaucoma, secondary glaucoma, aphakic glaucoma
Dosage and routes:
- *Adult:* Instill bid
Available forms include: Sol 0.6%
Side effects/adverse reactions:
CNS: Weakness, fatigue, depression, anxiety, headache, confusion
GI: Nausea, anorexia, dyspepsia
EENT: Eye irritation, conjunctivitis, keratitis
INTEG: Rash, urticaria
Contraindications: Hypersensitivity, asthma, 2nd-3rd degree heart block, right ventricular failure, congenital glaucoma (infants)
Pharmacokinetics:
INSTILL: Onset 15-30 min, peak 1-2 h, duration 24 hr
Interactions/incompatibilities:
- Increased effect: propranolol, metoprolol
NURSING CONSIDERATIONS
Teach patient/family:
- To report change in vision (blurring or loss of sight), trouble breathing, sweating, flushing
- Method of instillation, including pressure on lacrimal sac for 1 min, and not to touch dropper to eye

- That long-term therapy may be required
- That blurred vision will decrease with continued use of drug

metoclopramide HCl

(met-oh-kloe-pra′ mide)
Maxeran,* Reglan
Func. class.: Cholinergic
Chem. class.: Central dopamine receptor antagonist

Action: Enhances response to acetylcholine of tissue in upper GI tract, which causes contraction of gastric muscle, relaxes pyloric, duodenal segments, increases peristalsis without stimulating secretions
Uses: Prevention of nausea, vomiting induced by chemotherapy, radiation, delayed gastric emptying, gastroesophageal reflux
Dosage and routes:
Nausea/vomiting
- *Adult:* IV 2 mg/kg q2h × 5 doses 30 min before administration of chemotherapy
Delayed gastric emptying
- *Adult:* PO 10 mg 30 min ac, hs × 2-8 wk
Gastroesophageal reflux
- *Adult:* PO 10-15 mg qid 30 min ac
Available forms include: Tabs 5, 10 mg; syr 5 mg/5 ml; inj IV 5 mg/ml
Side effects/adverse reactions:
CNS: Sedation, fatigue, restlessness, headache, sleeplessness, dystonia, dizziness, drowsiness
GI: Dry mouth, constipation, nausea, anorexia, vomiting
GU: Decreased libido, prolactin secretion, amenorrhea, galactorrhea
CV: Hypotension, supraventricular tachycardia

---

* Available in Canada only

INTEG: Urticaria, rash

Contraindications: Hypersensitivity to this drug or procaine or procainamide, seizure disorder, pheochromocytoma, breast cancer, GI obstruction

Precautions: Pregnancy (B), lactation, GI hemorrhage, CHF

Pharmacokinetics:

IV: Onset 1-3 min, duration 1-2 hr
PO: Onset ½-1 hr, duration 1-2 hr
IM: Onset 10-15 min, duration 1-2 hr
Metabolized by liver, excreted in urine, half-life 4 hr

Interactions/incompatibilities:
• Decreased action of metoclopramide: anticholinergics, opiates
• Increased sedation: alcohol, other CNS depressants

NURSING CONSIDERATIONS
Administer:
• IV undiluted if dose is <10 mg; give over 2 min; 10 mg or more may be diluted in 50 ml or more compatible sol and given over 15 min
• ½-1 hr before meals for better absorption
• Gum, hard candy, frequent rinsing of mouth for dryness of oral cavity

Perform/provide:
• Protect from light with aluminum foil during infusion
• Discard open ampules

Evaluate:
• Therapeutic response: absence of nausea, vomiting, anorexia, fullness
• GI complaints: nausea, vomiting, anorexia, constipation

Teach patient/family:
• To avoid driving or other hazardous activities until patient is stabilized on this medication
• To avoid alcohol or other CNS depressants that will enhance sedating properties of this drug

Lab test interferences:
Increase: Prolactin, aldosterone, thyrotropin

metocurine iodide

(met-oh-kyoo′reen)
Metubine Iodide
Func. class.: Neuromuscular blocker (nondepolarizing)
Chem. class.: Methyl analog of tubocurarine

Action: Inhibits transmission of nerve impulses by binding with cholinergic receptor sites, antagonizing action of acetylcholine

Uses: Facilitation of endotracheal intubation, skeletal muscle relaxation during mechanical ventilation, surgery, or general anesthesia, reduction of fractures/dislocations

Dosage and routes:
• *Adult:* IV 2-4 mg if given cyclopropane as an anesthetic; 1.5-3 mg if given ether as an anesthetic; 4-7 mg if given nitrous oxide

Available forms include: Inj IV 2 mg/ml

Side effects/adverse reactions:
CV: Bradycardia, tachycardia, increased, decreased B/P
RESP: **Prolonged apnea, bronchospasm, cyanosis, respiratory depression**
EENT: Increased secretions
INTEG: Rash, flushing, pruritus, urticaria

Contraindications: Hypersensitivity to iodides

Precautions: Pregnancy (C), cardiac disease, hepatic disease, renal disease, lactation, children <2 yr, electrolyte imbalances, dehydration, neuromuscular disease (myasthenia gravis), respiratory dis-

M

italics = common side effects   ***bold italic*** = life threatening reactions

ease, or when histamine release is a definite hazard (e.g. asthma)

Pharmacokinetics:
IV: Peak 3-5 min, duration 35-90 min; half-life 3½ hr, excreted in urine, bile (½ unchanged), crosses placenta

Interactions/incompatibilities:
• Increased neuromuscular blockade: aminoglycosides, clindamycin, lincomycin, quinidine, local anesthetics, polymyxin antibiotics, lithium, narcotic analgesics, thiazides, enflurane, isoflurane
• Dysrhythmias: theophylline
• Do not mix with barbiturates in solution or syringe

NURSING CONSIDERATIONS
Assess:
• For electrolyte imbalances (K, Mg), may lead to increased action of this drug
• Vital signs (B/P, pulse, respirations, airway) until fully recovered; rate, depth, pattern of respirations (keep airway clear), strength of hand grip
• I&O ratio, check for urinary retention, frequency, hesitancy

Administer:
• Using nerve stimulator by anesthesiologist to determine neuromuscular blockade
• Anticholinesterase to reverse neuromuscular blockade
• By slow IV over 1-2 min (only by qualified person, usually an anesthesiologist)
• Only slightly discolored solution

Perform/provide:
• Storage in light-resistant, cool area
• Reassurance if communication is difficult during recovery from neuromuscular blockade

Evaluate:
• Therapeutic response: paralysis

of jaw, eyelid, head, neck, rest of body
• Recovery: decreased paralysis of face, diaphragm, leg, arm, rest of body
• Allergic reactions: rash, fever, respiratory distress, pruritus; drug should be discontinued

Treatment of overdose: Edrophonium or neostigmine, atropine, monitor VS; may require mechanical ventilation

Teach patient/family: That postoperative stiffness is normal and will subside

---

metolazone
(me-tole'a-zone)
Diulo, Zaroxolyn
Func. class.: Diuretic
Chem. class.: Thiazide-like; quinazoline derivative

Action: Acts on distal tubule by increasing excretion of water, sodium, chloride, potassium
Uses: Edema, hypertension, CHF
Dosage and routes:
Edema
• *Adult:* PO 5-20 mg/day
Hypertension
• *Adult:* PO 2.5-5 mg/day
Available forms include: Tabs 0.5, 2.5, 5, 10 mg
Side effects/adverse reactions:
GU: Frequency, polyuria, *uremia, glucosuria*
CNS: Drowsiness, paresthesia, anxiety, depression, headache, *dizziness, fatigue, weakness*
GI: Nausea, vomiting, anorexia, constipation, diarrhea, cramps, pancreatitis, GI irration, *hepatitis*
EENT: Blurred vision
INTEG: Rash, urticaria, purpura, photosensitivity, fever
META: Hyperglycemia, hyperuri-

cemia, increased creatinine, BUN
*HEMA: **Aplastic anemia, hemolytic anemia, leukopenia, agranulocytosis, thrombocytopenia,** neutropenia*
CV: Irregular pulse, orthostatic hypotension, palpitations, volume depletion
ELECT: Hypokalemia, hypomagnesia, hypercalcemia, hyponatremia, hypochloremia
Contraindications: Hypersensitivity to thiazides or sulfonamides, anuria, pregnancy (D)
Precautions: Hypokalemia, renal disease, hepatic disease, gout, COPD, lupus erythematosus, diabetes mellitus
Pharmacokinetics:
PO: Onset 1 hr, peak 2 hr, duration 12-24 hr; excreted unchanged by kidneys, crosses placenta, enters breast milk, half-life 8 hr
Interactions/incompatibilities:
• Synergism: furosemide
• Increased toxicity of: lithium, nondepolarizing skeletal muscle relaxants
• Decreased effects of: antidiabetics
• Decreased absorption of: thiazides, cholestyramine, colestipol
• Decreased hypotensive response: indomethacin
• Hyperglycemia, hyperuricemia, hypotension: diazoxide
• Hypoglycemia: sulfonylureas
NURSING CONSIDERATIONS
Assess:
• Weight, I&O daily to determine fluid loss; effect of drug may be decreased if used qd
• Rate, depth, rhythm of respiration, effect of exertion
• B/P lying, standing, postural hypotension may occur
• Electrolytes: potassium, magnesium, sodium, chloride; include

BUN, blood sugar, CBC, serum creatinine, blood pH, ABGs, uric acid, calcium
• Glucose in urine if patient is diabetic
Administer:
• In AM to avoid interference with sleep if using drug as a diuretic
• Potassium replacement if potassium is less than 3.0
• With food, if nausea occurs, absorption may be decreased slightly
Evaluate:
• Improvement in edema of feet, legs, sacral area daily if medication is being used in CHF
• Improvement in CVP q8h
• Signs of metabolic alkalosis: drowsiness, restlessness
• Signs of hypokalemia: postural hypotension, malaise, fatigue, tachycardia, leg cramps, weakness
• Rashes, temperature elevation qd
• Confusion, especially in elderly; take safety precautions if needed
Teach patient/family:
• To increase fluid intake 2-3 L/day unless contraindicated, to rise slowly from lying or sitting position
• To notify physician of muscle weakness, cramps, nausea, dizziness
• That drug may be taken with food or milk
• That blood sugar may be increased in diabetics
• Take early in day to avoid nocturia
Lab test interferences:
Increase: BSP retention, calcium, amylase, parathyroid test
Decrease: PBI, PSP
Treatment of overdose: Lavage if taken orally, monitor electrolytes, administer dextrose in saline, monitor hydration, CV, renal status

M

---

italics = common side effects   ***bold italic*** = life threatening reactions

metoprolol tartrate

(met-oh'proe-lole)
Betaloc,* Lopresor,* Lopressor
Func. class.: Antihypertensive
Chem. class.: β₁-blocker

Action: Produces falls in B/P without reflex tachycardia or significant reduction in heart rate through β-blocking effects; elevated plasma renins are reduced; blocks β₂-adrenergic receptors in bronchial, vascular smooth muscle only at high doses (decreases rate of SA node)

Uses: Mild to moderate hypertension, acute myocardial infarction to reduce cardiovascular mortality, angina pectoris

Dosage and routes:

Hypertension
• *Adult:* PO 50 mg bid, or 100 mg qd, may give up to 200-450 mg in divided doses

Myocardial infarction
• *Adult:* (Early treatment) IV BOL 5 mg q 2 min × 3, then 50 mg PO 15 min after last dose and q6h × 48 hr; (late treatment) PO maintenance 100 mg bid for 3 mo

Available forms include: Tabs 50, 100 mg; inj IV 1 mg/ml

Side effects/adverse reactions:

CV: Hypotension, *bradycardia, CHF: Palpitations,* dysrhythmias, *cardiac arrest, AV block*

CNS: Insomnia, *dizziness,* mental changes, hallucinations, *depression,* anxiety, headaches, nightmares, confusion, fatigue

GI: Nausea, vomiting, colitis, cramps, *diarrhea,* constipation, flatulence, dry mouth, *hiccups*

INTEG: Rash, purpura, alopecia, dry skin, urticaria, pruritus

HEMA: Agranulocytosis, eosino-philia, thrombocytopenia, purpura

EENT: Sore throat, dry burning eyes

GU: Impotence

RESP: Bronchospasm, dyspnea, wheezing

Contraindications: Hypersensitivity to β-blockers, cardiogenic shock, heart block (2nd, 3rd degree), sinus bradycardia, CHF, bronchial asthma

Precautions: Major surgery, pregnancy (C), lactation, diabetes mellitus, renal disease, thyroid disease, COPD, heart failure, CAD, non-allergic bronchospasm, hepatic disease

Pharmacokinetics:

PO: Peak 2-4 hr, duration 13-19 hr; half-life 3-4 hr, metabolized in liver (metabolites), excreted in urine, crosses placenta, enters breast milk

Interactions/incompatibilities:
• Increased hypotension, bradycardia: reserpine, hydralazine, methyldopa, prazosin, anticholinergics
• Decreased antihypertensive effects: indomethacin, sympathomimetics
• Increased hypoglycemic effects: insulin
• Decreased bronchodilation: theophyllines

NURSING CONSIDERATIONS

Assess:
• ECG, directly when giving IV during initial treatment
• I&O, weight daily
• B/P during initial treatment, periodically thereafter; pulse q4h; note rate, rhythm, quality
• Apical/radial pulse before administration; notify physician of any significant changes
• Baselines in renal, liver function tests before therapy begins

Administer:
• PO ac, hs, tablet may be crushed or swallowed whole

* Available in Canada only

- Reduced dosage in renal dysfunction
- IV, undiluted, give over 1 min, keep patient recumbent for 3 hr

Perform/provide:
- Storage in dry area at room temperature, do not freeze

Evaluate:
- Therapeutic response: decreased B/P after 1-2 wk
- Edema in feet, legs daily
- Skin turgor, dryness of mucous membranes for hydration status

Teach patient/family:
- To take with or immediately after meals
- Not to discontinue drug abruptly, taper over 2 wk, may cause precipitate angina
- Not to use OTC products containing α-adrenergic stimulants (nasal decongestants, OTC cold preparations) unless directed by physician
- To report bradycardia, dizziness, confusion, depression, fever, sore throat, shortness of breath to physician
- To take pulse at home, advise when to notify physician
- To avoid alcohol, smoking, sodium intake
- To comply with weight control, dietary adjustments, modified exercise program
- To carry Medic Alert ID to identify drug you are taking, allergies
- To avoid hazardous activities if dizziness is present
- To report symptoms of CHF: difficult breathing, especially on exertion or when lying down, night cough, swelling of extremities
- To take medication hs to prevent effect of orthostatic hypotension
- To wear support hose to minimize effects of orthostatic hypotension

Lab test interferences:
Increase: Liver function tests, renal function tests
Treatment of overdose: Lavage, IV atropine for bradycardia, IV theophylline for bronchospasm, digitalis, O_2, diuretic for cardiac failure, hemodialysis, hypotension administer vasopressor (norepinephrine)

---

metronidazole/metronidazole HCl

(me-troe-ni'da-zole)
Apo-Metronidazole,* Flagyl, Metryl, Neo-Tric,* Novonidazole,* PMS-Metronidazole,* Satric, Trikacide,* Flagyl IV, Flagyl IV RTU, Metro IV, Femazole, Metizol, Metronid, Protostat
Func. class.: Trichomonacide, amebicide
Chem. class.: Nitroimidazole derivative

Action: Direct-acting amebicide/trichomonacide binds, degrades DNA in organism
Uses: Intestinal amebiasis, amebic abscess, trichomoniasis, refractory trichomoniasis, bacterial anaerobic infections, giardiasis
Dosage and routes:
Trichomoniasis
- *Adult:* PO 250 mg tid × 7 days, or 2 g in single dose; do not repeat treatment for 2-3 wk
Refractory trichomoniasis
- *Adult:* PO 250 mg bid × 10 days
Amebic abscess
- *Adult:* PO 500-750 mg tid × 5-10 days
- *Child:* PO 35-50 mg/kg/day in 3 divided doses × 10 days
Intestinal amebiasis
- *Adult:* PO 750 mg tid × 5-10 days

italics = common side effects   **bold italic** = life threatening reactions

• *Child:* PO 35-50 mg/kg/day in 3 divided doses × 10 days; then give oral iodoquinol

Anerobic bacterial infections

• *Adult:* IV INF 15 mg/kg over 1 hr, then 7.5 mg/kg IV or PO q6h, not to exceed 4 g/day

Giardiasis

• *Adult:* PO 250 mg tid × 5 days
• *Child:* PO 5 mg/kg tid × 5 days

Available forms include: Tabs 250, 500 mg; film-coated tabs 250, 1500 mg; inj IV 5 mg/vial; HCl inj IV 500 mg

Side effects/adverse reactions:

CV: Flat T waves

HEMA: **Leukopenia, bone marrow aplasia**

INTEG: Rash, pruritus, urticaria, flushing

CNS: Headache, dizziness, confusion, depression, fatigue, drowsiness, insomnia, paresthesia, peripheal neuropathy, *convulsions,* incoordination, depression

EENT: Blurred vision, sore throat, retinal edema, dry mouth, bitter taste, furry tongue, glossitis, stomatitis

GI: Nausea, vomiting, diarrhea, epigastric distress, anorexia, constipation, abdominal cramps, metallic taste, *pseudomembranous colitis*

GU: Polyuria, *albuminuria,* dysuria, cystitis, decreased libido, *nephrotoxicity,* incontinence, dyspareunia

Contraindications: Hypersensitivity to this drug, renal disease, hepatic disease, contracted visual or color fields, blood dyscrasias, pregnancy (1st trimester), lactation, CNS disorders

Precautions: *Candida* infections, pregnancy (2nd, 3rd trimesters) (B)

Pharmacokinetics:

IV/PO: Peak 1-2 hr, half-life 6⅓-11½ hr, crosses placenta, excreted in feces

Interactions/incompatibilities:

• Disulfiram reaction: alcohol
• May increase action of: warfarin
• Psychosis: disulfiram
• Decreased action of metronidazole: phenobarbital

NURSING CONSIDERATIONS
Assess:

• Stools during entire treatment; should be clear at end of therapy, stools should be free of parasites for 1 yr before patient is considered cured (amebiasis)

• Vision by ophthalmalogic exam during, after therapy; vision problems occur often

• I&O, stools for number, frequency, character

Administer:

• IV is prediluted, Flagyl IV; dilute with 4.4 ml sterile H_2O or 0.9% sodium chloride; must be diluted further with 8 mg/ml or more compatible sol, must neutralize with 5 mEq of Na_2CO_3/500 mg; may need to vent, run over 1 hr; primary IV must be discontinued; may be given as continuous infusion

• PO after meals to avoid GI symptoms, metallic taste

Perform/provide:

• Storage in light-resistant container

Evaluate:

• Neurotoxicity: peripheral neuropathy, seizures, dizziness, incoordination, pruritus, joint pains; may be discontinued

• Allergic reaction: fever, rash, itching, chills; drug should be discontinued if these occur

• Superimposed infection: fever, monilial growth, fatigue, malaise

• Renal and reproductive dysfunction: dysuria, polyuria, impotence, dyspareunia, decreased libido

---

Teach patient family:
• That urine may turn dark reddish brown
• Proper hygiene after BM: handwashing technique
• Need for compliance with dosage schedule, duration of treatment
• To use condoms if treatment for trichomoniasis or cross contamination may occur
• That treatment of both partners is necessary
• Not to drink alcohol
Lab test interferences:
Decrease: AST, ALT

---

metyrosine

(me-tye′roe-seen)
Demser
Func. class.: Antihypertensive
Chem. class.: Adrenergic blocker

Action: Inhibits enzyme tyrosine hydroxylase, resulting in decreased levels of catecholamines
Uses: Pheochromocytoma
Dosage and routes:
• *Adult and child >12 yr:* PO 250 mg qid, may increase by 250-500 mg qd to a max of 4 g/day in divided doses
Available forms include: Caps 250 mg
Side effects/adverse reactions:
CNS: Sedation, drowsiness, dizziness, headache, depression, EPS, hallucinations, psychosis, agitation
INTEG: Rash, urticaria
EENT: Dry mouth
GU: Dysuria, *oliguria, hematuria,* enuresis, impotence
GI: Nausea, vomiting, anorexia, diarrhea, abdominal pain
MISC: Breast swelling, nasal stuffiness
Contraindications: Hypersensitiv-

ity, essential hypertension, children <12 yr
Precautions: Pregnancy (C), lactation, hepatic disease, renal disease
Pharmacokinetics:
PO: Onset 2 days, duration 3-4 days; half-life 3.4-3.7 hr, excreted in urine
Interactions/incompatibilities:
• Increased sedation: CNS depressants: alcohol, barbiturates, antipsychotics
• Decreased effects of: levodopa
• Extrapyramidal effects: phenothiazines, haloperidol

NURSING CONSIDERATIONS
Assess:
• Electrolytes: K, Na, Cl, CO_2
• Renal function studies: catecholamines, BUN, creatinine
• Hepatic function studies: AST, ALT, alk phosphatase
• ECG, BMR
• B/P, other VS throughout treatment
• Weight daily, I&O
Administer:
• Antiemetic or antidiarrheals for vomiting, diarrhea
Perform/provide:
• Fluids to 2 L/day to prevent crystallization by kidneys
Evaluate:
• Change in behavior or personality: psychosis, anxiety, hallucinations, EPS
• Nausea, vomiting, diarrhea
• Edema in feet, legs daily
• Skin turgor, dryness of mucous membranes for hydration status
Teach patient/family:
• To take each dose with a full glass of water; maintain sufficient daily intake
• Not to drive or perform hazardous tasks if behavioral changes, dizziness, or drowsiness occurs

M

---

italics = common side effects   ***bold italic*** = life threatening reactions

- To avoid alcohol or other CNS depressants
- To notify physician if any of following occur: jaw stiffness, drooling, speech difficulty, tremors, disorientation, diarrhea, painful urination

Lab test interferences:
False increase: Urinary catecholamines

Treatment of overdose: Administer vasopressors, discontinue drug

mexiletine HCl
(mex-il'e-teen)
Mexitil
Func. class.: Antidysrhythmic (Class IB)
Chem. class.: Lidocaine analog

Action: Increases electrical stimulation threshold of ventricle, His Purkinje system, which stabilizes cardiac membrane

Uses: Ventricular tachycardia, ventricular dysrhythmias during cardiac surgery, myocardial infarction

Dosage and routes:
- *Adult:* PO 200-400 mg q8h
Available forms include: Caps 150, 200, 250 mg

Side effects/adverse reactions:
CNS: Headache, dizziness, confusion, **convulsions,** tremors, psychosis, nervousness, paresthesias, weakness, fatigue, coordination difficulties, change in sleep habits
EENT: Blurred vision, hearing loss, tinnitus
GI: Nausea, vomiting, anorexia, diarrhea, abdominal pain, **hepatitis,** dry mouth, peptic ulcer, altered taste, GI bleeding
CV: Hypotension, bradycardia, angina, PVCs, **heart block, cardiovascular collapse, arrest,** sinus node slowing, **left ventricular failure,** syncope, **cardiogenic shock**
RESP: Dyspnea, **fibrosis, embolism,** pneumonia
INTEG: Rash, alopecia, dry skin
HEMA: **Thrombocytopenia, leukopenia, agranulocytosis, hypoplastic anemia,** SLE syndrome
GU: Urinary hesitancy, decreased libido
MISC: Edema, arthralgia, fever

Contraindications: Hypersensitivity to amides, cardiogenic shock, blood dyscrasias, severe heart block

Precautions: Pregnancy (C), lactation, children, renal disease, liver disease, CHF, respiratory depression, myasthenia gravis

Pharmacokinetics:
PO: Peak 2-3 hr; half-life 12 hr, metabolized by liver, excreted unchanged by kidneys (10%), excreted in breast milk

Interactions/incompatibilities:
- Increased effects: cimetidine
- Decreased levels of mexiletine: phenytoin, phenobarbital, rifampin

NURSING CONSIDERATIONS
Assess:
- ECG continuously to determine increased PR or QRS segments; if these develop, discontinue or reduce rate; watch for increased ventricular ectopic beats, may need to rebolus
- Blood levels (therapeutic level 0.5-2 μg/ml)
- B/P continuously for fluctuations
- I&O ratio, electrolytes (K, Na, Cl), liver enzymes

Evaluate:
- Malignant hyperthermia: tachypnea, tachycardia, changes in B/P, increased temperature
- Cardiac rate, respiration: rate, rhythm, character

• Respiratory status: rate, rhythm, lung fields for rales, watch for respiratory depression
• CNS effects: dizziness, confusion, psychosis, paresthesias, convulsions; drug should be discontinued
• Lung fields, bilateral rales may occur in CHF patient
• Increased respiration, increased pulse, drug should be discontinued
Lab test interferences:
Increase: CPK

Treatment of overdose: O₂, artificial ventilation, ECG, administer dopamine for circulatory depression, administer diazepam or thiopental for convulsions

---

mezlocillin sodium

(mez-loe-sill′in)
Mezlin
Func. class.: Broad-spectrum antibiotic
Chem. class.: Extended-spectrum penicillin

Action: Interferes with cell wall replication of susceptible organisms; osmotically unstable cell wall swells, bursts from osmotic pressure

Uses: Effective for gram-positive cocci (*S. aureus, S. viridans, S. faecalis, S. pneumoniae*), gram-negative cocci *(N. gonorrhoeae)*, gram-positive bacilli, *C. perfringens, C. tetani,* gram-negative bacilli (*Bacteroides, E. coli, H. influenzae, Klebsiella, P. mirabilis, Peptococcus, Peptostreptococcus, M. morganii, Enterobacter, Serratia, Pseudomonas, P. vulgaris, P. rettgeri, Shigella, Citrobacter, Veillonella*)

Dosage and routes:
• *Adult:* IM/IV 200-300 mg/kg/ day in divided doses q4-6h, may give up to 24 g/day for severe infections
• *Child:* IM/IV 50 mg/kg q4-6h
• *Infants >8 days; >2000 g:* 75 mg/kg q6h; <2000 g: 75 mg/kg q8h
• *Infants <8 days:* 75 mg/kg q12h
Available forms include: Powder for inj IM, IV 1, 2, 3, 4 g; IV INF 2, 3, 4 g

Side effects/adverse reactions:
HEMA: Anemia, increased bleeding time, *bone marrow depression, granulocytopenia*
GI: Nausea, vomiting, diarrhea, increased AST, ALT, abdominal pain, glossitis, colitis
GU: Oliguria, proteinuria, hematuria, (vaginitis, moniliasis), *glomerulonephritis*
CNS: Lethargy, hallucinations, anxiety, depression, twitching, *coma, convulsions*
META: Hyperkalemia, hypokalemia, alkalosis, hypernatremia

Contraindications: Hypersensitivity to penicillins
Precautions: Pregnancy (B), hypersensitivity to cephalosporins, neonates

Pharmacokinetics:
IM: Peak 45 min
IV: Peak 5 min
Half-life 50-55 min, partially metabolized in liver, excreted in urine, bile, breast milk (small amount), crosses placenta

Interactions/incompatibilities:
• Decreased effectiveness of: aminoglycosides
• Decreased antimicrobial effectiveness of mezlocillin: tetracyclines, erythromycins
• Increased mezlocillin concentrations: aspirin, probenecid

NURSING CONSIDERATIONS
Assess:
• I&O ratio; report hematuria, oli-

---

guria since penicillin in high doses is nephrotoxic

• Any patient with compromised renal system since drug is excreted slowly in poor renal system function; toxicity may occur rapidly

• Liver studies: AST, ALT

• Blood studies: WBC, RBC, H&H, bleeding time

• Renal studies: urinalysis, protein, blood

• C&S before drug therapy; drug may be taken as soon as culture is taken

Administer:

• IV after diluting 1g or less/ 10 ml of sterile H_2O, D_5, or 0.9% NaCl for inj, shake, dilute further with D_5W or 0.45 NaCl and give over 3-5 min; may be given by intermittent INF over ½ hr

• Drug after C&S has been completed

Perform/provide:

• Adrenalin, suction, tracheostomy set, endotracheal intubation equipment

• Adequate fluid intake (2000 ml) during diarrhea episodes

• Scratch test to assess allergy, after securing order from physician; usually done when penicillin is only drug of choice

• Storage at room temperature; reconstituted solution is stable for 24 hr refrigerated

Evaluate:

• Therapeutic effectiveness: absence of fever, draining wounds

• Bowel pattern before and during treatment

• Skin eruptions after administration of penicillin to 1 wk after discontinuing drug

• Respiratory status: rate, character, wheezing, and tightness in chest

• Allergies before initiation of

treatment, and reaction of each medication; highlight allergies on chart, Kardex

Teach patient/family:

• That culture may be taken after completed course of medication

• To report sore throat, fever, fatigue (could indicate superimposed infection)

• To wear or carry Medic Alert ID if allergic to penicillins

• To notify nurse of diarrhea

Lab test interferences:

False positive: Urine glucose, urine protein

Treatment of overdose: Withdraw drug, maintain airway, administer epinephrine, aminophylline, O_2, IV corticosteroids for anaphylaxis

---

miconazole

(mi-kon'a-zole)
Monistat, Monistat IV
Func. class.: Antifungal
Chem. class.: Imidazole

Action: Alters cell membranes and inhibits fungal enzymes

Uses: Coccidioidomycosis, candidiasis, cryptococcosis, paracoccidioidomycosis, chronic mucocutaneous candidiasis, fungal meningitis; IV used for severe infections only

Dosage and routes:

• *Adult:* IV INF 200-3600 mg/day; may be divided in 3 infusions 200-1200 mg/infusion; may need to repeat course; INTRATHECAL 20 mg given simultaneously with IV for fungal meningitis q3-7 days

• *Adult:* TOP apply to affected areas bid; VAG CREAM apply × 1 wk qhs or × 3 days (Monistat 3 vs Monistat 7)

• *Child:* IV 20-40 mg/kg/day, not to exceed 15 mg/kg/inf

Available forms include: Inj IV 10 mg/ml; aerosol 2%; cream, lotion, powder, vaginal cream (2%); supp, vaginal 100, 200 mg

Side effects/adverse reactions:

CV: Tachycardia, dysrhythmias (rapid IV)

INTEG: Pruritus, rash, fever, flushing, **anaphylaxis,** hives

CNS: Drowsiness, headache

GU: Vulvovaginal burning, itching, hyponatremia, pelvic cramps (topical forms)

GI: Nausea, vomiting, anorexia, diarrhea, cramps

HEMA: Decreased Hct, **thrombocytopenia,** hyperlipidemia

Contraindications: Hypersensitivity

Precautions: Renal disease, hepatic disease, pregnancy (B)

Pharmacokinetics:

IV: Half-life triphasic 0.4, 2.1, 24.1 hr, metabolized in liver, excreted in feces, urine (inactive metabolites), >90% protein binding

Interactions/incompatibilities:

• Increased action of: anticoagulants

• Decreased action of both drugs: amphotericin

NURSING CONSIDERATIONS
Assess:

• Cardiac system: B/P, pulse, ECG; watch for increasing pulse, cardiac dysrhythmias; drug should be discontinued if these occur

• Blood studies: Hct, Ca, cholesterol, triglycerides, platelets, sodium

Administer:

• After C&S is obtained to identify causative organism

• Antiemetic for nausea and vomiting as ordered

• After test dose of 200 mg is given by physician; watch for allergic reactions

• IV over ½-1 hr, dilute in 200 ml isotonic saline or D_5W

• IV after diluting with NS if hyponatremia has occurred

• Topical by rubbing into affected area

Evaluate:

• Therapeutic response: decreased fever, malaise, rash, negative C&S for infecting organism

• For phlebitis, pruritus; may need benadryl IV, continue unless reaction is severe

• Allergic reaction after test dose; have epinephrine available

Perform/provide:

• Storage of diluted preparations at room temperature for 24 hr

Teach patient/family:

• That long-term therapy may be needed to clear infection (1 wk-1 mo)

• Proper hygiene: handwashing techniques, nail care

• To report vaginitis; use light-day pad for vaginal dose

• To avoid contact with eyes, nose

• To avoid sexual contact during treatment; reinfection may occur

• To avoid use of occlusive dressings

miconazole nitrate (topical)
(mi-kon'a-zole)

Micatin, Monistat-Derm, Monistat

Func. class.: Local antiinfective
Chem. class.: Antifungal

Action: Interferes with fungal cell membrane, which increases permeability, leaking of nutrients

Uses: Tinea pedis, tinea cruris, tinea corporis, tinea versicolor, vaginal or vulvae *Candida albicans*

Dosage and routes:

• *Adult and child:* TOP apply to affected area bid × 2-4 wk

---

italics = common side effects **bold italic** = life threatening reactions

• *Adult:* INTRA VAG give 1 applicator or suppository ×7 days hs
Available forms include: Cream, lotion, powder, spray 2%; vag cream 2%; vag supp 100, 200 mg
Side effects/adverse reactions:
GU: Vulvovaginal burning, itching, pelvic cramps
INTEG: Rash, urticaria, stinging, burning, contact dermatitis
Contraindications: Hypersensitivity
Precautions: Child <2 yr, pregnancy (B), lactation
NURSING CONSIDERATIONS
Administer:
• Enough medication to completely cover lesions
• After cleansing with soap, water before each application, dry well
Perform/provide:
• Storage at room temperature in dry place
Evaluate:
• Allergic reaction: burning, stinging, swelling, redness
• Therapeutic response: decrease in size, number of lesions
Teach patient/family:
• To apply with glove to prevent further infection
• To avoid use of OTC creams, ointments, lotions unless directed by physician
• To use medical asepsis (hand washing) before, after each application
• To avoid contact with eyes
• To avoid use of occlusive dressings
• To notify physician if no improvement in condition

microfibrillar collagen hemostat
Avitene, MCH
Func. class.: Hemostatic
Chem. class.: Purified cattle collagen

Action: Platelets adhere to hemostat, cause aggregation to and formation of thrombi
Uses: For hemostasis in surgery when ligature is ineffective/impractical
Dosage and routes:
• *Adult and child:* TOP apply to bleeding area after drying with sponge, compress for 1-5 min, may reapply if needed
• *Available forms include:* Fibrous form, non-woven web form
Side effects/adverse reactions:
INTEG: Rash, abscess, allergic reactions, infection
HEMA: Hematoma
Contraindications: Hypersensitivity, closure of skin incision
Precautions: Pregnancy (C)
NURSING CONSIDERATIONS
Administer:
• Dry, do not moisten
• Using gloves with forceps; area must be dry for drug to work
• Only new product; do not resterilize
Evaluate:
• Possible infection: hematoma, abscess
• Allergy: rash, itching

midazolam HCl
(mid'-az-zoe-lam)
Versed
Func. class.: General anesthetic
Chem. class.: Benzodiazepine, short-acting

Controlled Substance Schedule IV
Action: Depresses subcortical

levels in CNS; may act on limbic system, reticular formation; may potentiate γ-aminobenzoic acid (GABA) by binding to specific benzodiazepine receptors

Uses: Preoperative sedation, general anesthesia induction, sedation for diagnostic endoscopic procedures, intubation

Dosage and routes:

Preoperative sedation

Adult: IM 0.07-0.08 mg/kg ½-1 hr before general anesthesia

Induction of general anesthesia

Adult: IV (unpremedicated patients) 0.3-0.35 mg/kg over 30 sec, wait 2 min, follow with 25% of initial dose if needed; (premedicated patients) 0.15-0.35 mg/kg over 20-30 sec, allow 2 min for effect

Available forms include: Inj 1, 5 mg/ml

Side effects/adverse reactions:

CNS: Retrograde amnesia, euphoria, confusion, headache, anxiety, insomnia, slurred speech, paresthesia, euphoria, tremors, weakness, chills

RESP: Coughing, ***apnea, bronchospasm, laryngospasm,*** dyspnea

CV: Hypotension, PVCs, tachycardia, bigeminy, nodal rhythm

EENT: Blurred vision, nystagmus, diplopia, blocked ears, loss of balance

GI: Nausea, vomiting, increased salivation, hiccups

INTEG: Urticaria, pain, swelling at injection site, rash, pruritus

Contraindications: Pregnancy (D), hypersensitivity to benzodiazepines, shock, coma, alcohol intoxication, acute narrow-angle glaucoma

Precautions: COPD, CHF, chronic renal failure, chills, elderly, debilitated

Pharmacokinetics:

IM: Onset: 15 min, peak ½-1 hr

IV: Onset: 3-5 min, onset of anesthesia 1½-2½ min, protein binding 97%, half-life 1.2-12.3 hr, metabolized in liver, metabolites excreted in urine, crosses placenta, blood-brain barrier

Interactions/incompatibilities:

• Prolonged respiratory depression: other CNS depressants, alcohol, barbiturates

• Increased hypnotic effect: fentanyl, narcotic agonists, analgesics, droperidol

NURSING CONSIDERATIONS

Assess:

• Injection site for redness, pain, swelling

• Degree of amnesia in elderly; may be increased

Administer:

• IV after diluting with D_5W or 0.9% NaCl to a concentration of 0.25 mg/ml; give over 2 min (conscious sedation) or over 30 sec (anesthesia induction)

• IM deep into large muscle mass

Perform/provide:

• Assistance with ambulation until drowsy period relieved

• Storage at room temperature

Evaluate:

• Therapeutic response: induction of sedation, general anesthesia

• Anterograde amnesia

• Vital signs for recovery period in obese patient, since half-life may be extended

Teach patient/family:

• To avoid hazardous activities until drowsiness, weakness subsides

• That amnesia occurs, events may not be remembered

Treatment of overdose: O_2, vasopressors, physostigmine, resuscitation

M

---

italics = common side effects   ***bold italic*** = life threatening reactions

mineral oil

Agoral Plain, Fleet Mineral Oil Enema, Kondremul, Milkinol, Neo-Cultol, Petrogalar Plain, Zymenol

Func. class.: Laxative
Chem. class.: Petroleum hydrocarbon

Action: Eases passage of stool by decreasing water absorption from feces, acts as lubricant
Uses: Constipation, preparation for bowel surgery or examination
Dosage and routes:
• *Adult:* PO 15-30 ml hs; ENEMA 4 oz
• *Child:* PO 5-15 ml hs; ENEMA 1-2 oz
Available forms include: Oil, enema; jelly 55%; susp 1.4, 2.5, 2.75 mg/5 ml
Side effects/adverse reactions:
CNS: Muscle weakness
GI: Nausea, vomiting, anorexia, diarrhea, pruritus ani, hepatic infiltration
*META: **Hypoprothrombinemia***
RESP: Lipoid pneumonia
Contraindications: Hypersensitivity, intestinal obstruction, abdominal pain, nausea/vomiting
Precautions: Pregnancy (C)
Pharmacokinetics: Excreted in feces
Interactions/incompatibilities:
• Increased effect of: oral anticoagulants
• Decreased absorption: fat-soluble vitamins (A, D, E, K) if used for prolonged time
NURSING CONSIDERATIONS
Assess:
• Blood, urine electrolytes if drug is used often by patient
• I&O ratio to identify fluid loss

Administer:
• Alone for better absorption
• In morning or evening (oral dose)
• Cautiously in elderly to prevent aspiration
Evaluate:
• Therapeutic response: decrease in constipation
• Cause of constipation; identify whether fluids, bulk, or exercise is missing from lifestyle
• Cramping, rectal bleeding, nausea, vomiting; if these symptoms occur, drug should be discontinued
Teach patient/family:
• Not to use laxatives for long-term therapy; bowel tone will be lost
• That normal bowel movements do not always occur daily
• Not to use in presence of abdominal pain, nausea, vomiting
• To notify physician if constipation unrelieved or if symptoms of electrolyte imbalance occur: muscle cramps, pain, weakness, dizziness, excessive thirst

minocycline HCl

(mi-noe-sye'kleen)
Minocin, Vectrin, Minocin IV

Func. class.: Broad spectrum antibiotic
Chem. class.: Tetracycline

Action: Inhibits protein synthesis, phosphorylation in microorganisms by binding to 30S ribosomal subunits, reversibly binding to 50S ribosomal subunits
Uses: Syphilis, chlamydia trachomatis, gonorrhea, lymphogranuloma venereum, rickettsial infections, inflammatory acne, *Mycobacterium marinum, Neisseria* meningitis carriers
Dosage and routes:
• *Adult:* PO/IV 200 mg, then 100 mg q12h or 50 mg q6h

• *Child >8 yr:* PO/IV 4 mg/kg then 4 mg/kg/day PO in divided doses q12h
Gonorrhea
• *Adult:* PO 200 mg, then 100 mg q12h × 4 days
Chlamydia trachomatis
• *Adult:* PO 100 mg bid × 7 days
Syphilis
• *Adult:* PO 200 mg, then 100 mg q12h × 10-15 days
Available forms include: Tabs 50, 100 mg; oral susp 50 mg/5 ml; powder for inj IV 100 mg/vial
Side effects/adverse reactions:
CNS: Dizziness, fever, headache, paresthesia
HEMA: Eosinophilia, neutropenia, thrombocytopenia, leukocytosis, hemolytic anemia
EENT: Dysphagia, glossitis, decreased calcification of deciduous teeth, abdominal pain, oral candidiasis
GI: Nausea, vomiting, diarrhea, anorexia, enterocolitis, *hepatotoxicity,* flatulence, abdominal cramps, epigastric burning, stomatitis, *pseudomembranous colitis*
CV: Pericarditis
GU: Increased BUN, polyuria, polydipsia, *renal failure, nephrotoxicity*
INTEG: Rash, urticaria, photosensitivity, increased pigmentation, exfoliative dermatitis, pruritus, angioedema
Contraindications: Hypersensitivity to tetracyclines, children <8 yr, pregnancy (D)
Precautions: Hepatic disease, lactation
Pharmacokinetics:
PO: Peak 2-3 hr half-life 11-17 hr; excreted in urine, feces, crosses placenta, excreted in breast milk, 55%-88% protein bound

Interactions/incompatibilities:
• Decreased effect of minocycline: antacids, NaHCO₃, alkali products, iron, kaolin/pectin
• Increased effect of: anticoagulants
• Decreased effect of: penicillins, oral contraceptives
• Nephrotoxicity: methoxyflurane
• Do not mix with other drugs
NURSING CONSIDERATIONS
Assess:
• I&O ratio
• Blood studies: PT, CBC, AST, ALT, BUN, creatinine
• Signs of anemia: Hct, Hgb, fatigue
Administer:
• IV after diluting 100 mg/5 ml sterile H₂O for inj; further dilute in 500-1000 ml of compatible sol; run 100 mg/6 hr
• After C&S obtained
• 2 hr before or after laxative or ferrous products; 3 hr after antacid or kaolin-pectin product
Perform/provide:
• Storage in tight, light-resistant container at room temperature
Evaluate:
• Therapeutic response: decreased temperature, absence of lesions, negative C&S
• Allergic reactions: rash, itching, pruritus, angioedema
• Nausea, vomiting, diarrhea; administer antiemetic, antacids as ordered
• Overgrowth of infection: increased temperature, malaise, redness, pain, swelling, drainage, perineal itching, diarrhea, changes in cough or sputum
Teach patient/family:
• To avoid sun exposure since burns may occur; sunscreen does not seem to decrease photosensitivity

M

---

italics = common side effects   ***bold italic*** = life threatening reactions

• Of diabetic to avoid use of Clinistix, Diastix, or Tes-Tape for urine glucose testing
• That all prescribed medication must be taken to prevent superimposed infection
• To take with a full glass of water; may take with food or milk if GI symptoms occur

Lab test interferences:
False negative: Urine glucose with Clinistix or Tes-Tape

---

minoxidil
(mi-nox-i-dill)
Loniten

Func. class.: Antihypertensive
Chem. class.: Vasodilator—peripheral

Action: Directly relaxes arteriolar smooth muscle, causing vasodilation

Uses: Severe hypertension not responsive to other therapy; use with diuretic, topically to treat alopecia

Dosage and routes:
• *Adult:* PO 5 mg/day not to exceed 100 mg daily, usual range 10-40 mg/day in single doses
• *Child <12 yr:* (Initial) 0.2 mg/kg/day; (effective range) 0.25-1 mg/kg/day; (max) 50 mg/day

Alopecia
• *Adult:* Apply topically, rub into scalp daily

Available forms include: Tabs 2.5, 10 mg, top 2%

Side effects/adverse reactions:
CV: Severe rebound hypertension, tachycardia, angina, increased T wave, **CHF, pulmonary edema, pericardial effusion,** edema, sodium, water retention
CNS: Drowsiness, dizziness, sedation, headache, depression
GI: Nausea, vomiting

GU: Gynecomastia, breast tenderness
INTEG: Pruritus, **Stevens-Johnson syndrome,** rash, hirsutism

Contraindications: Acute myocardial infarction, dissecting aortic aneurysm, hypersensitivity, pheochromocytoma

Precautions: Pregnancy (C), lactation, children, renal disease, CAD, CHF

Pharmacokinetics:
PO: Onset 30 min, peak 2-3 hr, duration 75 hr; half-life 4.2 hr, metabolized in liver, metabolites, excreted in urine, feces

Interactions/incompatibilities:
• Orthostatic hypotension: guanethidine

NURSING CONSIDERATIONS
Monitor:
• Electrolytes: K, Na, Cl, CO_2
• Renal function studies: catecholamines, BUN, creatinine
• Hepatic function studies: AST, ALT, alk phosphatase
• B/P, pulse
• Weight daily, I&O

Administer:
• With meals for better absorption, to decrease GI symptoms
• With β-blocker and/or diuretic

Evaluate:
• Therapeutic response: decreased B/P or increased hair growth
• Nausea
• Edema in feet, legs daily
• Skin turgor, dryness of mucous membranes for hydration status
• Rales, dyspnea, orthopnea

Teach patient/family:
• That body hair will increase but is reversible after discontinuing treatment
• Not to discontinue drug abruptly
• To report pitting edema, dizziness, weight gain >5 lb, shortness of breath, bruising or bleeding,

---

heart rate >20 beats/min over normal, severe indigestion, dizziness, light-headedness, panting, new or aggravated symptoms of angina
• To take drug exactly as prescribed or serious side effects may occur

Lab test interferences:
Increase: Renal function studies
Decrease: Hgb/Hct/RBC

Treatment of overdose: Administer normal saline IV, phenylephrine, angiotensin II, vasopressor, dopamine may reverse hypotension

---

misoprostol

(mye-soe-prost′ ole)
Cytotec
Func. class.: Gastric mucosa protectant
Chem. class.: Prostaglandin E_1 analog

Action: Inhibits gastric acid secretion, may protect gastric mucosa; can increase bicarbonate, mucus production

Uses: Prevention of nonsteroidal antiinflammatory drug-induced gastric ulcers

Dosage and routes:
• *Adult:* PO 200 μg qid with food for duration of nonsteroidal antiinflammatory therapy; if 200 μg is not tolerated, 100 μg may be given
Available forms include: Tabs 200 μg

Side effects/adverse reactions:
GI: Diarrhea, nausea, vomiting, flatulence, constipation, dyspepsia, abdominal pain
GU: Spotting, cramps, hypermenorrhea, menstrual disorders

Contraindications: Hypersensitivity, pregnancy (X)

Precautions: Lactation, children, elderly, renal disease

Pharmacokinetics:
PO: Peak 12 min, plasma steady state achieved within 2 days, excreted in urine

NURSING CONSIDERATIONS
Assess:
• Gastric pH (>5 should be maintained)
• I&O ratio, BUN, creatinine

Perform/provide:
• Storage at room temperature

Evaluate:
• Therapeutic response: absence of pain or GI complaints

Teach patient/family:
• To take only as directed
• Not to take if pregnant (can cause miscarriage) and do not become pregnant while taking this medication; if pregnancy occurs during therapy, discontinue drug, notify physician
• Not to give drug to anyone else or take for more than 4 wk unless directed by physician

M

---

mitomycin

(mye-toe-mye′sin)
Mutamycin
Func. class.: Antineoplastic, antibiotic

Action: Inhibits DNA synthesis, primarily; derived from *Streptomyces caespitosus;* appears to cause cross-linking of DNA, a vesicant

Uses: Pancreas, stomach cancer, head and neck or breast cancer

Dosage and routes:
• *Adult:* IV 2 mg/m²/day × 5 days, stop drug for 2 days, then repeat cycle; or 10-20 mg/m² as a single dose, repeat cycle in 6-8 wk; stop drug if platelets are <75,000/mm³ or WBC is <3000/mm³
Available forms include: Inj IV

---

italics = common side effects   ***bold italic*** = life threatening reactions

Side effects/adverse reactions:

HEMA: **Thrombocytopenia, leukopenia, anemia**

GI: Nausea, vomiting, anorexia, stomatitis, **hepatotoxicity,** diarrhea

GU: Urinary retention, **renal failure,** edema

INTEG: Rash, alopecia, **extravasation**

RESP: **Fibrosis, pulmonary infiltrate,** dyspnea

CNS: Fever, headache, confusion, drowsiness, syncope, fatigue

EENT: Blurred vision, drowsiness, syncope

Contraindications: Hypersensitivity, pregnancy (1st trimester) (D), as a single agent, thrombocytopenia, coagulation disorders

Precautions: Renal disease, bone marrow depression

Pharmacokinetics: Half-life 17 min, metabolized in liver, 10% excreted in urine (unchanged)

Interactions/incompatibilities:

• Increased toxicity: other antineoplastics (vinca alkaloids) or radiation

NURSING CONSIDERATIONS
Assess:

• CBC, differential, platelet count weekly; withhold drug if WBC is <4000/mm³ or platelet count is <75,000/mm³; notify physician of these results

• Pulmonary function tests, chest x-ray before, during therapy; chest x-ray should be obtained q2 wk during treatment

• Renal function studies: BUN, serum uric acid, urine CrCl, electrolytes before, during therapy

• I&O ratio; report fall in urine output to <30 ml/hr

• Monitor temperature q4h; fever may indicate beginning infection

• Liver function tests before, during therapy: bilirubin, AST, ALT, alk phosphatase as needed or monthly

Administer:

• Sodium thiosulfate for extravasation, apply ice compress

• Antiemetic 30-60 min before giving drug to prevent vomiting

• IV after diluting 5 mg/10 ml sterile H₂O for inj; allow to stand, give through Y-tube or 3-way stopcock; give over 5-10 min

• Transfusion for anemia

• Antispasmodic for GI symptoms

Perform/provide:

• Liquid diet: carbonated beverages, gelatin may be added if patient is not nauseated or vomiting

• Rinsing of mouth tid-qid with water; brushing of teeth with baking soda bid-tid with soft brush or cotton-tipped applicators for stomatitis; use unwaxed dental floss

• Storage at room temperature for 1 wk after reconstituting or 2 wk refrigerated

Evaluate:

• Alkalosis if severe vomiting is present

• Bleeding: hematuria, guaiac, bruising, petechiae, mucosa or orifices q8h

• Dyspnea, rales, unproductive cough, chest pain, tachypnea, fatigue, increased pulse, pallor, lethargy

• Food preferences; list likes, dislikes

• Effects of alopecia on body image; discuss feelings about body changes

• Inflammation of mucosa, breaks in skin

• Yellowing of skin, sclera, dark urine, clay-colored stools, itchy skin, abdominal pain, fever, diarrhea

• Buccal cavity q8h for dryness,

sores, ulceration, white patches, oral pain, bleeding, dysphagia
• Local irritation, pain, burning at injection site
• GI symptoms: frequency of stools, cramping
• Acidosis, signs of dehydration: rapid respirations, poor skin turgor, decreased urine output, dry skin, restlessness, weakness
Teach patient/family:
• To report any complaints, side effects to nurse or physician
• That hair may be lost during treatment and wig or hairpiece may make the patient feel better; tell patient that new hair may be different in color, texture
• To avoid foods with citric acid, hot or rough texture
• To report any bleeding, white spots, ulcerations in mouth; tell patient to examine mouth qd
• To avoid crowds, people with infections if granulocyte count is low

mitotane
(mye'toe-tane)
Lysodren
Func. class.: Antineoplastic
Chem. class.: Hormone, adrenal cytotoxic agent

Action: Acts on adrenal cortex to suppress activity; a cytotoxic agent that suppresses activity and causes cell death
Uses: Adrenocortical carcinoma
Dosage and routes:
• *Adult:* PO 9-10 g/day in divided doses tid or qid; may need to decrease dose if severe reactions occur
Available forms include: Tabs 500 mg
Side effects/adverse reactions:
GI: Nausea, vomiting, anorexia, diarrhea

*GU: **Proteinuria, hematuria***
INTEG: Rash
*RESP: **Fibrosis, pulmonary infiltrate***
CV: Hypertension, orthostatic hypotension
CNS: Lightheadedness, flushing, sedation, vertigo
EENT: Lethargy, blurring, retinopathy
Contraindications: Hypersensitivity
Precautions: Lactation, hepatic disease, pregnancy (C)
Pharmacokinetics: Adequately absorbed orally (40%), excreted in urine, bile
Interactions/incompatibilities:
• Decreased effects of: corticosteroids
NURSING CONSIDERATIONS
Assess:
• Adrenal insufficiency: fatigue, orthostatic hypotension, weight loss, weakness, nausea, vomiting, diarrhea
• Pulmonary function tests, chest x-ray films before, during therapy; chest film should be obtained q2wk during treatment
• Renal function studies: BUN, serum uric acid, urine CrCl electrolytes before, during therapy
• I&O ratio
• Urinary 17-OHCS before, during treatment
Administer:
• Antacid before oral agent, give drug after evening meal, before bedtime
• Antiemetic 30-60 min before giving drug to prevent vomiting
• Antispasmodic
Perform/provide:
• Increase fluid intake to 2-3 L/day to prevent dehydration
• HOB increased to facilitate breathing

italics = common side effects **bold italic** = life threatening reactions

• Increased fluid intake to 2000 ml/day if not contraindicated
• Nutritious diet with iron, vitamin supplements as ordered
• Storage in tight, light-resistant container

Evaluate:
• Dyspnea, chest pain, tachypnea, fatigue, increased pulse, pallor, lethargy
• Food preferences; list likes, dislikes
• Muscular weakness, fatigue, oliguria, hypoglycemia
• Frequency of stools, characteristics: cramping, acidosis, signs of dehydration (rapid respirations, poor skin turgor, decreased urine output, dry skin, restlessness, weakness)
• Symptoms indicating severe allergic reactions: rash, pruritus, itching, flushing
• Signs of infection: increased temperature, cough, fatigue, malaise

Teach patient/family:
• To report any complaints, side effects to nurse or physician
• To report any changes in breathing, coughing
• To avoid driving or other activities requiring alertness

Lab test interferences:
Decrease: PBI, urinary 17-OHCS

---

mitoxantrone

(mye-toe-zan'trone)
Novantrone
Func. class.: Antineoplastic
Chem. class.: Synthetic anthraquinone

Action: DNA reactive agent, cytocidal effect on both proliferating and nonproliferating cells suggesting lack of cell cycle phase specificity

Uses: Acute nonlymphocytic leukemia (adult)

Dosage and routes:
• *Adult:* IV inf 12 mg/m²/day on days 1-3, and 100 mg/m² cytosine arabinoside × 7 days
Available forms include: Inj 2 mg/ml

Side effects/adverse reactions:
*GI: Nausea, vomiting, diarrhea, anorexia, mucositis, **hepatotoxicity***
*HEMA: **Thrombocytopenia, leukopenia, myelosuppression, anemia***
INTEG: Rash, necrosis at injection site, dermatitis, thrombophlebitis at injection site, alopecia
*CV: **CHF, cardiopathy,** dysrhythmias*
MISC: Fever
RESP: Cough, dyspnea

Contraindications: Hypersensitivity

Precautions: Myelosuppression, lactation, cardiac disease, children, pregnancy (D), renal, hepatic disease, gout

Pharmacokinetics:
Highly bound to plasma proteins, metabolized in liver, excreted via renal, hepatobiliary systems; half-life 24-72 hr

Interactions/incompatibilities:
• Do not mix with heparin, precipitate will form

NURSING CONSIDERATIONS
Assess:
• CBC, differential, platelet count weekly, withhold drug if WBC is <4000/mm³ or platelet count is <75,000/mm³, notify physician of these results
• Liver function test before, during therapy: bilirubin, AST, ALT, alk phosphatase prn or monthly
• Renal function studies: BUN, serum uric acid, urine CrCl, electrolytes before, during therapy

---

Administer:

• Medications by oral route if possible, avoid IM, SC, IV routes to prevent infections

• Antiemetic 30-60 min before giving drug to prevent vomiting

• IV after diluting with 50 ml or more normal saline or D$_5$W; give over 3-5 min running IV of D$_5$W or NS; may be diluted further in compatible sol and run over 15-30 min; check for extravasation

Perform/provide:

• Liquid diet: carbonated beverages, Jell-O; dry toast, crackers may be added if patient is not nauseated or vomiting

• Rinsing of mouth tid-qid with water, club soda, brushing of teeth bid-qid with soft brush or cotton-tipped applicators for stomatitis; use unwaxed dental floss

Evaluate:

• Bleeding, hematuria, guaiac, bruising or petechiae, mucosa or orifices q8h

• Food preferences; list likes, dislikes

• Yellowing of skin, sclera, dark urine, clay-colored stools, itchy skin, abdominal pain, fever, diarrhea

• Acidosis, signs of dehydration: rapid respirations, poor skin turgor, decreased urine output, dry skin, restlessness, weakness

Teach patient/family:

• To report side effects to nurse or physician

• To avoid foods with citric acid, rough texture, or hot

• To report any bleeding, white spots, ulcerations in mouth; tell patient to examine mouth daily

molindone HCl

(moe-lin′done)

Moban

Func. class.: Antipsychotic/neuroleptic

Chem. class.: Dihydroindolone

Action: Depresses cerebral cortex, hypothalamus, limbic system, which control activity, aggression; blocks neurotransmission produced by dopamine at synapse; exhibits strong α-adrenergic, anticholinergic blocking action; mechanism for antipsychotic effects is unclear

Uses: Psychotic disorders

Dosage and routes:

• *Adult:* PO 50-75 mg/day increasing to 225 mg/day if needed

Available forms include: Tabs 5, 10, 25, 50, 100 mg; conc 20 mg/ml

Side effects/adverse reactions:

RESP: **Laryngospasm,** dyspnea, **respiratory depression**

CNS: Extrapyramidal symptoms: pseudoparkinsonism, akathisia, dystonia, tardive dyskinesia, drowsiness, headache, seizures

HEMA: **Anemia, leukopenia, leukocytosis, agranulocytosis**

INTEG: Rash, photosensitivity, dermatitis

EENT: Blurred vision, glaucoma

GI: Dry mouth, nausea, vomiting, anorexia, constipation, diarrhea, jaundice, weight gain

GU: Urinary retention, urinary frequency, enuresis, impotence, amenorrhea, gynecomastia

CV: Orthostatic hypotension, hypertension, **cardiac arrest,** ECG changes, **tachycardia**

Contraindications: Hypersensitivity, coma, child

Precautions: Pregnancy (C), lac-

M

---

tation, hypertension, hepatic disease, cardiac disease, Parkinson's disease, brain tumor, glaucoma, urinary retention

Pharmacokinetics:

PO: Onset erratic, peak 1½ hr, duration 24-36 hr; metabolized by liver, excreted in urine and feces, may cross placenta, enters breast milk, half-life 1½ hr

Interactions/incompatibilities:

• Increased sedation: other CNS depressants

• Increased EPS: other antipsychotics, lithium

NURSING CONSIDERATIONS
Assess:

• Swallowing of PO medication; check for hoarding or giving of medication to other patients

• I&O ratio; palpate bladder if low urinary output occurs

• Bilirubin, CBC, liver function studies monthly

• Urinalysis is recommended before, during prolonged therapy

Administer:

• Antiparkinsonian agent, after securing order from physician, to be used if extrapyramidal symptoms occur

• IM injection into large muscle mass

• Concentrate mixed in orange or grapefruit juice

Perform/provide:

• Decreased noise input by dimming lights, avoiding loud noises

• Supervised ambulation until stabilized on medication; do not involve in strenuous exercise program because fainting is possible; patient should not stand still for long periods of time

• Increased fluids to prevent constipation

• Sips of water, candy, gum for dry mouth

• Storage in tight, light-resistant container

Evaluate:

• Therapeutic response: decrease in emotional excitement, hallucinations, delusions, paranoia, reorganization of patterns of thought, speech

• Affect, orientation, LOC, reflexes, gait, coordination, sleep pattern disturbances

• B/P standing and lying; also include pulse, respirations; take these q4h during initial treatment; establish baseline before starting treatment; report drops of 30 mm Hg, watch for ECG changes

• Dizziness, faintness, palpitations, tachycardia on rising

• Extrapyramidal symptoms including akathisia (inability to sit still, no pattern to movements), tardive dyskinesia (bizarre movements of the jaw, mouth, tongue, extremities), pseudoparkinsonism (rigidity, tremors, pill rolling, shuffling gait)

• For neuroleptic malignant syndrome: hyperthermia, increased CPK, altered mental status, muscle rigidity

• Skin turgor daily

• Constipation, urinary retention daily; if these occur, increase bulk and water in diet

Teach patient/family:

• That orthostatic hypotension may occur and to rise from sitting or lying position gradually

• To avoid hot tubs, hot showers, or tub baths since hypotension may occur

• To avoid abrupt withdrawal of this drug or EPS may result; drugs should be withdrawn slowly

• To avoid OTC preparations (cough, hayfever, cold) unless approved by physician since serious

drug interactions may occur; avoid use with alcohol or CNS depressants, increased drowsiness may occur
• To avoid hazardous activities if drowsiness or dizziness occurs
• To use sunscreen during sun exposure to prevent burns
• Regarding compliance with drug regimen
• About necessity for meticulous oral hygiene since oral candidiasis may occur
• To report impaired vision, jaundice, tremors, muscle twitching
• In hot weather, that heat stroke may occur; take extra precautions to stay cool

Lab test interferences:
Alterations in: BUN, RBC, serum glucose, WBC
Increase: Serum prolactin levels
Treatment of overdose: Lavage if orally injested, provide an airway; *do not induce vomiting*

---

moricizine

(mor iss' i-zeen)
Ethmozine
Func. class.: Antidysrhythmic, type I
Chem. class.: Phenothiazine

Action: Decreased rate of rise of action potential, prolonging refractory period and shortening the action potential duration; depression of inward influx if sodium mediates the effects; drug may slow atrial and AV nodal conduction
Uses: Symptomatic vertricular and life-threatening dysrhythmias
Dosage and routes:
Adult: PO 10-15 mg/kg/day in 2-3 divided doses
Available forms include: Film-coated tabs 200, 250, 300 mg

italics = common side effects

Side effects/adverse reactions:
GI: Nausea, abdominal pain, vomiting, diarrhea
CNS: (Dizziness, headache, fatigue, perioral numbness, euphoria) nervousness, sleep disorders, depression, tinnitus, fatigue
RESP: Dyspnea, hyperventilation, *apnea,* asthma, pharyngitis, cough
GU: Sexual dysfunction, difficult urination, dysuria, incontinence
CV: Palpitations, chest pain, *CHF,* hypertension, syncope, dysrythmias, bradycardia, *MI,* thrombophlebitis
MISC: Sweating, musculoskeletal pain
Contraindications: 2-3 degree AV block, right bundle branch block, cardiogenic shock, hypersensitivity
Precautions: CHF, hypokalemia, hyperkalemia, sick sinus syndrome, pregnancy (B), lactation, children, impaired hepatic and renal function, cardiac dysfunction
Pharmacokinetics: Half-life 1.5-3.5 hr; peak 0.5-2.2 hr; metabolized by the liver; metabolites are excreted in feces and urine, protein binding >90%
Interactions/incompatibilities:
• Increased plasma levels of moricizine: ametadine
• Digoxin or propranolol may enhance some of cardiac effects of moricizine; moricizine may decrease effects of theophylline
NURSING CONSIDERATIONS
Assess:
• GI status: bowel pattern, number of stools
• Cardiac status: rate, rhythm, quality
• Chest x-ray, pulmonary function test during treatment
• I&O ratio: check for decreasing output
• B/P for fluctuations

bold italic = life threatening reactions

• Lung fields: bilateral rales may occur in CHF patient
• Increased respiration, increased pulse; drug should be discontinued
Evaluate:
• Therapeutic response: absence of dysrhythmias
• Toxicity: fine tremors, dizziness
• Cardiac rate: respiration, rate, rhythm, character continuously
Lab test interferences:
Increase: CPK
Treatment of overdose: O_2 artificial ventilitation, ECG, administer dopamine for circulatory depression, administer diazepam or thiopental for convulsions

---

morphine sulfate

(mor'feen)
Duramorph PF, MS Contin, RMS, Roxanol, Roxanol SR
Func. class.: Narcotic analgesics
Chem. class.: Opiate

Controlled Substance Schedule II
Action: Depresses pain impulse transmission at the spinal cord level by interacting with opioid receptors
Uses: Severe pain
Dosage and routes:
• *Adult:* SC/IM 4-15 mg q4h prn; PO 10-30 mg q4h prn; EXT REL q8-12h; REC 10-20 mg q4h prn; IV 4-10 mg diluted in 4-5 ml of water for injection, over 5 min
• *Child:* SC 0.1-0.2 mg/kg, not to exceed 15 mg
Available forms include: Inj SC, IM, IV 2, 4, 5, 8, 10, 15 mg/ml; sol tabs 10, 15, 30 mg; oral sol 10, 20 mg/5 ml, 20 mg/10 ml, 20 mg/ml; oral tabs 15, 30 mg; rec supp 5, 10, 20 mg; ext rel tabs 300 mg
Side effects/adverse reactions:
CNS: Drowsiness, dizziness, con-fusion, headache, sedation, euphoria
GI: Nausea, vomiting, anorexia, constipation, cramps, biliary tract pressure
GU: Increased urinary output, dysuria, urinary retention
INTEG: Rash, urticaria, bruising, flushing, diaphoresis, pruritus
EENT: Tinnitus, blurred vision, miosis, diplopia
CV: Palpitations, bradycardia, change in B/P
RESP: Respiratory depression
Contraindications: Hypersensitivity, addiction (narcotic), hemorrhage, bronchial asthma, increased intracranial pressure
Precautions: Addictive personality, pregnancy (B), lactation, MI (acute), severe heart disease, respiratory depression, hepatic disease, renal disease, child <18 yr
Pharmacokinetics:
PO: Onset variable, peak variable, duration variable
SC: Onset 15-30 min, peak 50-90 min, duration 3-5 hrs
IV: Peak 20 min
Metabolized by liver, excreted by kidneys, crosses placenta, excreted in breast milk, half-life 2½-3 hr
Interactions/incompatibilities:
• Increased effects with other CNS depressants: alcohol, narcotics, sedative/hypnotics, antipsychotics, skeletal muscle relaxants

NURSING CONSIDERATIONS
Assess:
• I&O ratio; check for decreasing output; may indicate urinary retention
Administer:
• IV after diluting with 5 ml of compatible sol; give 15 mg or less over 4-5 min; give through Y-tube or 3-way stopcock; may be added to IV sol

- With antiemetic if nausea, vomiting occur
- When pain is beginning to return; determine dosage interval by patient response

Perform/provide:
- Storage in light-resistant area at room temperature
- Assistance with ambulation
- Safety measures: siderails, night light, call bell within easy reach

Evaluate:
- Therapeutic response: decrease in pain
- CNS changes: dizziness, drowsiness, hallucinations, euphoria, LOC, pupil reaction
- Allergic reactions: rash, urticaria
- Respiratory dysfunction: respiratory depression, character, rate, rhythm; notify physician if respirations are <10/min
- Need for pain medication, physical dependence

Teach patient/family:
- To report any symptoms of CNS changes, allergic reactions
- That physical dependency may result when used for extended periods of time
- Withdrawal symptoms may occur: nausea, vomiting, cramps, fever, faintness, anorexia

Lab test interferences:
Increase: Amylase

Treatment of overdose: Narcan 0.2-0.8 IV, O_2, IV fluids, vasopressors

---

moxalactam disodium
(mox'a-lak-tam)
Moxam

Func. class.: Antibiotic, broad-spectrum

Chem. class.: Cephalosporin (3rd generation)

Action: Inhibits bacterial cell wall synthesis, rendering cell wall osmotically unstable

Uses: Gram-negative organisms: *H. influenzae, E. coli, P. mirabilis, Klebsiella, Citrobacter, Salmonella, Shigella, Serratia;* gram-positive organisms: *S. pneumoniae, S. pyogenes, S. aureus;* serious lower respiratory tract, urinary tract, skin, bone infections, septicemia, meningitis, intraabdominal infections

Dosage and routes:
- *Adult:* IM/IV 2-4 g q8-12h

Mild infections
- *Adult:* IM/IV 250-500 mg q8-12h

Severe infections
- *Adult:* IM/IV 2-6 g q8h
- *Child:* IM/IV 50 mg/kg q6-8h
- Dosage reduction indicated even for mild renal impairment (CrCl < 80 ml/min)

Available forms include: Powder for inj IM, IV 1, 2, 10 g

Side effects/adverse reactions:
CNS: Headache, dizziness, weakness, paresthesia, fever, chills

GI: Nausea, *vomiting, diarrhea, anorexia,* pain, glossitis, bleeding, increased AST, ALT, bilirubin, LDH, alk phosphatase, abdominal pain

GU: **Proteinuria,** vaginitis, pruritus, candidiasis, increased BUN, **nephrotoxicity, renal failure**

HEMA: **Leukopenia, thrombocytopenia, agranulocytosis, anemia, neutropenia, lymphocytosis, eosinophilia, pancytopenia, hemolytic anemia, bleeding, hypoprothrombinemia**

INTEG: Rash, urticaria, dermatitis, **anaphylaxis**

RESP: Dyspnea

Contraindications: Hypersensitivity to cephalosporins

Precautions: Hypersensitivity to

---

italics = common side effects   **bold italic** = life threatening reactions

penicillins, pregnancy (C), lactation, renal disease

Pharmacokinetics:

IV: Peak 5 min

IM: Peak ½-2 hr

Half-life 1½-2½ hr, 25% bound by plasma proteins, 60-97% eliminated unchanged in urine in 24 hr, crosses placenta, blood-brain barrier, excreted in breast milk, not metabolized

Interactions/incompatibilities:

• Do not mix with tetracyclines, erythromycins, aminoglycosides in same parenteral fluid

• Decreased effects of: tetracyclines, erythromycins

• Increased toxicity: aminoglycosides, furosemide, probenecid, sulfinpyrazone, colistin, ethacrynic acid, vancomycin, agents affecting platelet function

• Disulfiram reaction: ethanol

NURSING CONSIDERATIONS

Assess:

• Nephrotoxicity: increased BUN, creatinine

• I&O daily

• Blood studies: AST, ALT, CBC, Hct, bilirubin, LDH, alk phosphatase, Coombs' test pro-time monthly if patient is on long-term therapy

• Electrolytes: potassium, sodium, chloride monthly if patient is on long-term therapy

• Bowel pattern qd; if severe diarrhea occurs, drug should be discontinued; may indicate pseudomembranous colitis

• IV site for extravasation, phlebitis; change site q72h

Administer:

• For 10-14 days to ensure organism death, prevent superimposed infection

• IV after diluting 1 g/10 ml sterile H_2O, D_5, 0.9% NaCl; give through Y-tube over 3-5 min; may be further diluted 1 g/20 ml in compatible sol, give over ½ hr; may be added 500-1000, give over 6-24 hr

• Vitamin K for bleeding (10 mg/wk)

• After C&S

Evaluate:

• Therapeutic response: decreased fever, malaise, chills

• Urine output: if decreasing, notify physician; may indicate nephrotoxicity

• Allergic reactions: rash, urticaria, pruritus, chills, fever, joint pain, angioedema; may occur few days after therapy begins

• Bleeding: ecchymosis, bleeding gums, hematuria, stool guaiac daily

• Overgrowth of infection: perineal itching, fever, malaise, redness, pain, swelling, drainage, rash, diarrhea, change in cough, sputum

Teach patient/family:

• To report sore throat, bruising, bleeding, joint pain; may indicate blood dyscrasias (rare)

• Not to drink alcohol while taking this drug

Lab test interferences:

Increase (false): Urinary 17-KS

False positive: Urinary protein, direct Coombs', urine glucose

Interference: Cross-matching

Treatment of overdose: Epinephrine, antihistamines, resuscitate if needed (anaphylaxis)

---

multivitamins

Many brands

Func. class.: Vitamin

Action: Needed for adequate metabolism

Uses: Prevention and treatment of vitamin deficiencies

Dosage and routes:
• *Adult and child:* PO depends on brand
Available forms include: Many forms available
Side effects/adverse reactions: None known
Precautions: Pregnancy (A)
Interactions/incompatibilities:
• Check each vitamin for specific interactions
NURSING CONSIDERATIONS
Evaluate:
• Therapeutic response: check each individual vitamin for guidelines
• Vitamin deficiency: usually more than one vitamin is deficient
Teach patient/family:
• That adequate nutrition must be maintained to prevent further deficiencies
• Drug interaction that should be avoided
• Stress compliance with regimen
• To avoid using flavored multivitamins as candy; child may overdose
• Store out of children's reach

---

mupirocin

(meew-per'-o-sen)
Bactroban

Func. class.: Topical antiinfective
Chem. class.: Pseudomonic acid A

Action: Inhibits bacterial protein synthesis, shows no cross resistance to most antibiotics
Uses: Impetigo caused by *S. aureus,* β-hemolytic *Streptococcus, S. pyogenes*
Dosage and routes:
Apply small amount to affected area tid
Available forms include: Oint 2% (20 mg/g)

Side effects/adverse reactions:
INTEG: Burning, stinging, itching, rash, dry skin, swelling, contact dermatitis, erythema, tenderness
Contraindications: Hypersensitivity
Precautions: Pregnancy (B), lactation
NURSING CONSIDERATIONS
Assess:
• Affected area for continuing infection: increased size, amount of lesions
Administer:
• Then cover with 2 in × 2 in gauze if needed
Perform/provide:
• Storage at room temperature
• Isolation (wound) for hospitalized child (2-5 days)
• Washing of hands after applying ointment
Evaluate:
• Therapeutic response: reduction in size, amount of lesions
Teach patient/family:
• To wash hands after applying ointment
• To trim fingernails to prevent scratching
• To report irritation, worsening of condition

---

muromonab-CD3

(mur-oo-mone'ab)
Orthoclone OKT3

Func. class.: Immunosuppressive
Chem. class.: Murine monoclonal antibody

Action: Reverses graft rejection by blocking T cell function
Uses: Acute allograft rejection in renal transplant patients
Dosage and routes:
• *Adult:* IV BOL 5 mg/day × 10-14 days; usually methylpredniso-

lone sodium succinate, 1 mg/kg IV is given before muromonab-CD3, 100 mg IV hydrocortisone sodium succinate is given ½ hr after muromonab-CD3

Available forms include: Inj 5 mg/ 5 ml

Side effects/adverse reactions:

CNS: Pyrexia, chills, tremors

RESP: Dyspnea, wheezing, pulmonary edema

CV: Chest pain

GI: Vomiting, nausea, diarrhea

MISC: Infection

Contraindications:

Hypersensitivity to murine origin, fluid overload

Precautions: Pregnancy (C), child <2 yr, fever

Pharmacokinetics:

Trough level steady state 3-14 days

NURSING CONSIDERATIONS

Assess:

• Blood studies: Hgb, WBC, platelets during treatment monthly; if leukocytes are <3000/mm³ drug should be discontinued

• Liver function studies: alk phosphatase, AST, ALT, bilirubin

Administer:

• IV undiluted, withdraw with a 0.2-0.22 low protein-binding micron filter, discard and use new needle for administration; give over 1 min

• For several days before transplant surgery

• All medications PO if possible, avoid IM injection since infection may occur

Evaluate:

• Hepatotoxicity: dark urine, jaundice, itching, light-colored stools; drug should be discontinued

Teach patient/family:

• To report fever, chills, sore throat, fatigue since serious infection may occur

• To use contraceptive measures during treatment, for 12 wk after ending therapy

---

nadolol

(nay-doe'-lole)

Corgard

Func. class.: Antihypertensive, antianginal

Chem. class.: β-adrenergic receptor blocker

Action: Long-acting, nonselective β-adrenergic receptor blocking agent; mechanism is similar to propranolol

Uses: Chronic stable angina pectoris, mild to moderate hypertension

Dosage and routes:

• *Adult:* PO 40 mg qd, increase by 40-80 mg q3-7 days; maintenance 40-240 mg/day for angina, 40-320 mg/day for hypertension

Available forms include: Oral tabs 20, 40, 80, 120, 160 mg

Side effects/adverse reactions:

RESP: Dyspnea, respiratory dysfunction, ***bronchospasm,*** cough, wheezing, nasal stuffiness, pharyngitis, ***laryngospasm***

*CV: Bradycardia, hypotension, **CHF,*** palpitations, AV block

*HEMA: **Agranulocytosis, thrombocytopenia,*** chest pain, peripheral ischemia, flushing, edema, vasodilation, conduction disturbances

GI: Nausea, vomiting, diarrhea, colitis, constipation, cramps, dry mouth, flatulence, hepatomegaly, pancreatitis, taste distortion

INTEG: Rash, pruritus, fever

CNS: Depression, hallucinations, dizziness, fatigue, lethargy, paresthesias, headache

EENT: Sore throat

Contraindications: Hypersensitiv-

---

ity to this drug, cardiac failure, cardiogenic shock, 2nd or 3rd degree heart block, bronchospastic disease, sinus bradycardia, CHF, COPD

Precautions: Diabetes mellitus, pregnancy (C), renal disease, lactation, hyperthyroidism, peripheral vascular disease, myasthenia gravis

Pharmacokinetics:

PO: Onset variable, peak 3-4 hr, duration 17-24 hr; half-life 16-20 hr, not metabolized, excreted in urine (unchanged), bile, breast milk

Interactions/incompatibilities:

• Increased effects of: reserpine, digitalis, ergots, neuromuscular blocking agents, calcium channel blockers

• Decreased effects of: norepinephrine, xanthines, isoproterenol, thyroid, nonsteroidals, salicylates

NURSING CONSIDERATIONS
Assess:

• B/P, pulse, respirations during beginning therapy

• Weight qd, report gain of 5 lb

• I&O ratio, CrCl if kidney damage is diagnosed

• qd, note need to be administered more often

Administer:

• With 8 oz water

Evaluate:

• Pain: duration, time started, activity being performed, character

• Tolerance if taken over long period of time

• Headache, lightheadedness, decreased B/P; may indicate a need for decreased dosage

Teach patient/family:

• Drug may mask signs of hypoglycemia or alter blood glucose in diabetics

• Not to discontinue abruptly

• To avoid OTC drugs unless physician approves

• To avoid hazardous activities if dizziness occurs

• Stress patient compliance with complete medical regimen

Lab test interferences:

Increase: Serum potassium, serum uric acid, ALT/AST, alk phosphatase, LDH

Decrease: Blood glucose

---

nafarelin acetate
Synarel

Func. class.: Gonadotropin
Chem. class.: Analog of gonadotropin-releasing hormone

Action: Stimulates the release of LH and FSH, which increases ovarian steroid production; repeated dosing prevents stimulation of the pituitary gland

Uses: Endometriosis

Doses and routes: 400 μg/day as one spray (200 μg) into one nostril in morning and one spray into other nostril in evening; start treatment between days 2 and 4 of menstrual cycle; may increase to 800 μg/day (one spray into each nostril twice a day); recommended duration of treatment is 6 months

Available forms include: Nasal sol 2 mg/ml

Side effects/adverse reactions:

GU: Decreased libido, vaginal dryness, breast tenderness

CNS: Headache, flushing, depression, insomnia, emotional lability

INTEG: Nasal irritation, acne

Contraindications: Hypersensitivity, pregnancy (X), lactation, undiagnosed abnormal vaginal bleeding

Precautions: Children

Pharmacokinetics: Rapidly absorbed, peak 10-40 min, half-life 3 hr, 80% bound to plasma proteins

N

---

italics = common side effects   ***bold italic*** = life threatening reactions

NURSING CONSIDERATIONS
Assess:
• Test results: pituitary/hypothalamus dysfunction (decreased LH); postmenopausal (increased LH)
Administer:
• Repeated doses may be necessary to elevate pituitary gonadotropin reserve
Perform/provide:
• Storage at room temperature; protect from light

---

nafcillin sodium

(naf-sill′-in)
Nafcil, Nallpen, Unipen
Func. class.: Broad-spectrum antibiotic
Chem. class.: Penicillinase-resistant penicillin

Action: Interferes with cell wall replication of susceptible organisms; osmotically unstable cell wall swells, bursts from osmotic pressure
Uses: Effective for gram-positive cocci *(S. aureus, S. viridans, S. pneumoniae)*, infections caused by penicillinase-producing *Staphylococcus*
Dosage and routes:
• *Adult:* IM/IV 2-6 g/day in divided doses q4-6h; PO 2-6 g/day in divided doses q4-6h
• *Child:* IM 25 mg/kg q12h; PO 25-50 mg/kg/day in divided doses q6h
• *Neonates* IM 10 mg/kg bid
Available forms include: Caps 250 mg; tabs 500 mg; powder for oral susp 250 mg/5 ml; powder for inj IM, IV 500 mg, 1, 2, 10 g; IV 1, 1.5, 2, 4 g
Side effects/adverse reactions:
HEMA: Anemia, increased bleeding time, *bone marrow depression, granulocytopenia*
GI: Nausea, vomiting, diarrhea, increased AST, ALT, abdominal pain, glossitis, colitis
GU: Oliguria, *proteinuria, hematuria, vaginitis, moniliasis, glomerulonephritis*
CNS: Lethargy, hallucinations, anxiety, depression, twitching, *coma, convulsions*
Contraindications: Hypersensitivity to penicillins
Precautions: Pregnancy (B), hypersensitivity to cephalosporins, neonates
Pharmacokinetics:
IM/PO: Peak 30-60 min, duration 4-6 hr, half-life 1 hr, metabolized by the liver, excreted in bile, urine
Interactions/incompatibilities:
• Decreased antimicrobial effectiveness of nafcillin: tetracyclines, erythromycins
• Increased nafcillin concentrations: aspirin, probenecid
NURSING CONSIDERATIONS
Assess:
• I&O ratio; report hematuria, oliguria since penicillin in high doses is nephrotoxic
• Any patient with compromised renal system since drug is excreted slowly in poor renal system function; toxicity may occur rapidly
• Liver studies: AST, ALT
• Blood studies: WBC, RBC, H&H, bleeding time
• Renal studies: urinalysis, protein, blood
• C&S before drug therapy; drug may be taken as soon as culture is taken
Administer:
• IV after diluting 500 mg/1.7 ml of sterile H_2O for inj; further dilute each 500 mg/15-30 ml of compatible sol; give through Y-tube or

stopcock 500 mg or less/5-10 min; may be further diluted and run over 24 hr
• Drug after C&S has been completed
• Divided doses on empty stomach before meals

Perform/provide:
• Adrenalin, suction, tracheostomy set, endotracheal intubation equipment
• Adequate fluid intake (2000 ml) during diarrhea episodes
• Scratch test to assess allergy, after securing order from physician; usually done when penicillin is only drug of choice
• Storage in tight container; refrigerate reconstituted solution

Evaluate:
• Therapeutic effectiveness: absence of fever, draining wounds
• Bowel pattern before and during treatment
• Skin eruptions after administration of penicillin to 1 wk after discontinuing drug
• Respiratory status: rate, character, wheezing, and tightness in chest
• Allergies before initiation of treatment, and reaction of each medication; highlight allergies on chart, Kardex

Teach patient/family:
• Aspects of drug therapy, including need to complete course of medication to ensure organism death (10-14 days); culture may be taken after completed course
• To report sore throat, fever, fatigue (could indicate superimposed infection)
• To wear or carry Medic Alert ID if allergic to penicillins
• To notify nurse of diarrhea

Lab test interferences:
False positive: Urine glucose, urine protein

Treatment of overdose: Withdraw drug, maintain airway, administer epinephrine, aminophylline, O_2, IV corticosteroids for anaphylaxis

---

naftifine HCl

(naf-tee-fin)
Naftin
Func. class.: Topical antifungal
Chem. class.: Synthetic allylamine derivative

Action: Interferes with cell membrane permeability in fungi such as *T. rubrum, T. mentagrophytes, T. tonsurans, E. floccosum, M. canis, M. audouinii, M. gypseum, Candida sp.,* broad-spectrum antifungal

Uses: Tinea cruris, tinea corporis

Dosage and routes:
Massage into affected area, surrounding area bid, continue for 7-14 days

Available forms include: Cream 1%

Side effects/adverse reactions:
INTEG: Burning, stinging, dryness, itching, local irritation

Contraindications: Hypersensitivity

Precautions: Pregnancy (B), lactation, children

NURSING CONSIDERATIONS
Assess:
• For continuing infection: increased size, amount of lesions

Administer:
• To affected area, surrounding area; do not cover with occlusive dressings

Perform/provide:
• Storage below 30° C (86° F)

Evaluate:
• Therapeutic response: decrease in size, amount of lesions

N

---

italics = common side effects   **bold italic** = life threatening reactions

Teach patient/family:
• To wear cotton clothing
• To use clean towel, dry well
• To keep away from mucous membranes

---

nalbuphine HCl

(nal'byoo-feen)
Nubain

Func. class.: Nonnarcotic analgesics

Chem. class.: Synthetic opiate

Controlled Substance Schedule II

Action: Depresses pain impulse transmission at the spinal cord level by interacting with opioid receptors

Uses: Moderate to severe pain

Dosage and routes:
• *Adult:* SC/IM/IV 10-20 mg q3-6h prn, not to exceed 160 mg/day

Available forms include: Inj SC, IM, IV 10, 20 mg/ml

Side effects/adverse reactions:

CNS: Drowsiness, dizziness, confusion, headache, sedation, euphoria, dysphoria (high doses)

GI: Nausea, vomiting, anorexia, constipation, cramps

GU: Increased urinary output, dysuria, urinary retention

INTEG: Rash, urticaria, bruising, flushing, diaphoresis, pruritus

EENT: Tinnitus, blurred vision, miosis, diplopia

CV: Palpitations, bradycardia, change in B/P

RESP: Respiratory depression

Contraindications: Hypersensitivity, addiction (narcotic)

Precautions: Addictive personality, pregnancy (B), lactation, increased intracranial pressure, MI (acute), severe heart disease, respiratory depression, hepatic disease, renal disease

Pharmacokinetics:

SC/IM/IV: Duration 3-6 h; metabolized by liver, excreted by kidneys, half-life 5 hr

Interactions/incompatibilities:
• Increased effects with other CNS depressants: alcohol, narcotics, sedative/hypnotics, antipsychotics, skeletal muscle relaxants

NURSING CONSIDERATIONS

Assess:
• I&O ratio; check for decreasing output; may indicate urinary retention
• For withdrawal reactions in narcotic-dependent individuals: pulmonary embolus, vascular occlusion; abscesses, ulcerations, nausea, vomiting, convulsions

Administer:
• IV undiluted 10 mg or less over 3-5 min
• With antiemetic if nausea, vomiting occur
• When pain is beginning to return; determine dosage interval by patient response

Perform/provide:
• Storage in light-resistant area at room temperature
• Assistance with ambulation
• Safety measures: siderails, night light, call bell within easy reach

Evaluate:
• Therapeutic response: decrease in pain
• CNS changes: dizziness, drowsiness, hallucinations, euphoria, LOC, pupil reaction
• Allergic reactions: rash, urticaria
• Respiratory dysfunction: respiratory depression, character, rate, rhythm; notify physician if respirations are <10/min
• Need for pain medication, physical dependence

Teach patient/family:
• To report any symptoms of CNS changes, allergic reactions

• That physical dependency may result when used for extended periods of time

• Withdrawal symptoms may occur: nausea, vomiting, cramps, fever, faintness, anorexia

Lab test interferences:
Increase: Amylase

Treatment of overdose: Narcan 0.2-0.8 IV, O_2, IV fluids, vasopressors

---

nalidixic acid

(nal-i-dix'ik)

NegGram, Nogram, Cybis, Wintomylon

Func. class.: Urinary tract anti-infective

Chem. class.: Synthetic naphthyridine derivative

Action: Appears to inhibit DNA polymerization, primary target being single-stranded DNA precursors in late stages of chromosomal replication

Uses: Urinary tract infections (acute/chronic) caused by *E. coli, Klebsiella, Enterobacter, P. mirabilis, P. vulgaris, P. morganii*

Dosage and routes:
• *Adult:* PO 1 g qid × 1-2 wk, 2 g/day for long-term treatment
• *Child >3 months:* PO 55 mg/kg/day in 4 divided doses for 1-2 wk; 33 mg/kg/day in 4 divided doses for long-term treatment

Available forms include: Tabs 100, 250, 500 mg, 1 g susp 250 mg/5 ml

Side effects/adverse reactions:
INTEG: Pruritus, rash, urticaria, photosensitivity
CNS: Dizziness, headache, drowsiness, insomnia, ***convulsions***
GI: Nausea, vomiting, abdominal pain, diarrhea

EENT: Sensitivity to light, blurred vision, change in color perception

Contraindications: Hypersensitivity, CNS damage, liver disease, liver failure, infants <3 months

Precautions: Elderly, renal disease, hepatic disease, pregnancy (B)

Pharmacokinetics:
PO: Peak 1-2 hr, metabolized in liver, excreted in urine (unchange/conjugates), crosses placenta, enters breast milk

Interactions/incompatibilities:
• Increased effects of: oral coagulants
• Decreased effects of: antacids

NURSING CONSIDERATIONS

Assess:
• Blood count for patients on chronic therapy
• I&O ratio, urine pH <5.5 is ideal
• Renal, hepatic function
• Photosensitivity: if present, drug should be discontinued

Administer:
• After clean-catch urine is obtained for C&S
• Two daily doses if urine output is high or if patient has diabetes

Perform/provide:
• Limited intake of alkaline foods, drugs: milk, dairy products, peanuts, vegetables, alkaline antacids, sodium bicarbonate
• Protection from freezing

Evaluate:
• CNS symptoms: insomnia, vertigo, headache, drowsiness, convulsions
• Allergy: fever, flushing, rash, urticaria, pruritus

Teach patient/family:
• That photosensitivity occurs; that patient should avoid sunlight or use sunscreen to prevent burns
• Take medication with food or milk to decrease GI irritation

N

---

italics = common side effects   ***bold italic*** = life threatening reactions

• Instruct client to protect suspension from freezing, shake well before taking

• May cause drowsiness; instruct client to seek aid in walking, other activities; advise client not to drive or operate machinery while on medication

• Instruct clients with diabetes that Clinitest may prove false positive for glucose; therefore Tes-Tape or Clinistix should be used

Lab test interferences:
False positive: Urinary glucose
False increase: 17-OHCS, VMA

---

naloxone HCl
Narcan

Func. class.: Narcotic antagonist
Chem. class.: Thebaine derivative

Action: Competes with narcotics at narcotic receptor sites

Uses: Respiratory depression induced by narcotics, pentazocine, propoxyphene

Dosage and routes:
Narcotic-induced respiratory depression
• *Adult:* IV/SC/IM 0.4-2 mg; repeat q2-3 min, if needed
Postoperative respiratory depression
• *Adult:* IV 0.1-0.2 mg q2-3 min prn
• *Child:* IV/IM/SC 0.01 mg/kg q2-3 min prn
Asphyxia neonatorum
• *Neonates:* IV 0.01 mg/kg given into umbilical vein after delivery, may repeat in q2-3 min × 3 doses
Available forms include: Inj IV, IM, SC 0.02, 0.4, 1 mg/ml
Side effects/adverse reactions:
CNS: Drowsiness, nervousness
GI: Nausea, vomiting

CV: Rapid pulse, increased systolic B/P high doses
RESP: Hyperpnea
Contraindications: Hypersensitivity, respiratory depression
Precautions: Pregnancy (B), children
Pharmacokinetics:
Metabolized by liver, excreted by kidneys, crosses placenta, excreted in breast milk, half-life 1 hr, onset 1-2 min (IV)

NURSING CONSIDERATIONS
Assess:
• VS q3-5 min
• ABGs including PO_2, PCO_2
Administer:
• IV undiluted, diluted with sterile H_2O for inj, may be further diluted with NS or D_5 and given as an INF; give 0.4 mg or less over 15 sec or titrate INF to response
• Only if resuscitative equipment is nearby
• Only solutions prepared within 24 hrs
Perform/provide:
• Storage at room temperature in darkness
Evaluate:
• Signs of withdrawal in drug-dependent individuals
• Cardiac status: tachycardia, hypertension
• Respiratory dysfunction: respiratory depression, character, rate, rhythm; if respirations are <10/min, administer Narcan, it is probably due to narcotic overdose not Narcan
Lab test interferences:
Interfere: Urine VMA, 5-HIAA, urine glucose

naltrexone HCl

(nal-trex'one)
Trexan
Func. class.: Narcotic antagonist
Chem. class.: Thebaine derivative

Action: Competes with narcotics at narcotic receptor sites
Uses: Blockage of opioid analgesics, used in treatment of opiate addiction
Dosage and routes:
• *Adult:* PO 25 mg, may give 25 mg after 1 hr if there are no withdrawal symptoms; 50-150 mg may be given qd depending on patient need, maintenance 50 mg q24h
Available forms include: Tabs 50 mg
Side effects/adverse reactions:
*HEMA: **Thrombocytopenia, agranulocytosis, leukopenia, neutropenia, hemolytic anemia,*** increased pro-time
CNS: Stimulation, drowsiness, dizziness, confusion, convulsion, headache, flushing, hallucinations
GI: Nausea, vomiting, diarrhea, heartburn, anorexia, ***hepatitis***
INTEG: Rash, urticaria, bruising
EENT: Tinnitus, hearing loss
CV: Rapid pulse, pulmonary edema, hypertension
RESP: Wheezing, hyperpnea
Contraindications: Hypersensitivity, opioid dependence, hepatic failure, hepatitis
Precautions: Pregnancy (C)
Pharmacokinetics:
PO: Onset 15-30 min, peak 1-2 hr, duration is dose dependent
Metabolized by liver, excreted by kidneys, crosses placenta, excreted in breast milk, half-life 4 hr, extensive first-pass metabolism

NURSING CONSIDERATIONS
Assess:
• VS q3-5 min
• ABGs including PO_2, PCO_2
Administer:
• Only if resuscitative equipment is nearby
Perform/provide:
• Storage in tight container
Evaluate:
• Signs of withdrawal in drug-dependent individuals
• Cardiac status: tachycardia, hypertension
• Respiratory dysfunction: respiratory depression, character, rate, rhythm; if respirations are <10/min, respiratory stimulant should be administered

nandrolone decanoate/nandrolone phenpropionate

(nan'droe-lone)
Androlone-50, Androlone-D 50, Deca-Durabolin, Hybolin Decanoate, Anabolin, Anorolone, Durabolin, Hybolin Improved, Nandrobolic, Nandrolin
Func. class.: Androgenic anabolic steroid
Chem. class.: Halogenated testosterone derivative

Action: Increases weight by building body tissue, increases potassium, phosphorus, chloride, nitrogen levels, increases bone development
Uses: Tissue building, severe disease, refractory anemias, metastatic breast cancer
Dosage and routes:
Tissue building (possibly effective)
• *Adult:* IM 50-100 mg q3-4 wk (decanoate)

N

- *Child 2-13 yr:* IM 25-50 mg q3-4 wk (decanoate)

Severe disease/refractory anemias
- *Adult:* IM 100-200 mg q wk (decanoate)

Breast cancer
- *Adult:* IM 50-100 mg q wk (phenpropionate)

Available forms include: Phenpropionate inj IM 25, 50 mg/ml; decanoate inj IM 50, 100, 200 mg/ml

Side effects/adverse reactions:

INTEG: Rash, acneiform lesions, oily hair, skin, flushing, sweating, acne vulgaris, alopecia, hirsutism

CNS: Dizziness, headache, fatigue, tremors, paresthesias, flushing, sweating, anxiety, lability, insomnia

MS: Cramps, spasms

CV: Increased B/P

GU: Hematuria, amenorrhea, vaginitis, decreased libido, decreased breast size, clitoral hypertrophy, testicular atrophy

GI: Nausea, vomiting, constipation, weight gain, *cholestatic jaundice*

EENT: Carpal tunnel syndrome, conjunctival edema, nasal congestion

ENDO: Abnormal GTT

Contraindications: Severe renal disease, severe cardiac disease, severe hepatic disease, hypersensitivity, pregnancy (X), lactation, abnormal genital bleeding, males with CA of breast, prostate

Precautions: Diabetes mellitus, CV disease, MI

Pharmacokinetics:

IM: Metabolized in liver, excreted in urine, crosses placenta, excreted in the breast milk

Interactions/incompatibilities:
- Increased effects of: oral antidiabetics, oxyphenbutazone
- Increased PT: anticoagulants

- Edema: ACTH, adrenal steroids
- Decreased effects of: insulin

NURSING CONSIDERATIONS

Assess:
- Weight daily, notify physician if weekly weight gain is >5 lb
- B/P q4h
- I&O ratio; be alert for decreasing urinary output, increasing edema
- Growth rate in children since growth rate may be uneven (linear/bone growth) when used for extended periods of time
- Electrolytes: K, Na, Cl, Ca; cholesterol
- Liver function studies: ALT, AST, bilirubin

Administer:
- Titrated dose, use lowest effective dose

Perform/provide:
- Diet with increased calories, protein; decrease sodium if edema occurs

Evaluate:
- Therapeutic response: increased appetite, increased stamina
- Edema, hypertension, cardiac symptoms, jaundice
- Mental status: affect, mood, behavioral changes, aggression
- Signs of masculinization in female: increased libido, deepening of voice, breast tissue, enlarged clitoris, menstrual irregularities; male: gynecomastia, impotence, testicular atrophy
- Hypercalcemia: lethargy, polyuria, polydipsia, nausea, vomiting, constipation, drug may need to be decreased
- Hypoglycemia in diabetics; since oral anticoagulant action is decreased

Teach patient/family:
- That drug needs to be combined with complete health plan: diet, rest, exercise

---

*Available in Canada only

- To notify physician if therapeutic response decreases
- Not to discontinue medication abruptly
- About changes in sex characteristics
- Females to report menstrual irregularities
- That 1-3 mo course is necessary for response in breast cancer
- Procedure for use of buccal tablets: requires 30-60 min to dissolve, change absorption site with each dose; do not eat, drink, chew, or smoke while tablet is in place

Lab test interferences:

Increase: Serum cholesterol, blood glucose, urine glucose

Decrease: Serum calcium, serum potassium, T_4, T_3, thyroid ^{131}I uptake test, urine 17-OHCS, 17-KS, PBI, BSP

---

naphazoline HCl

(naf-az'oh-leen)
Privine

Func. class.: Nasal decongestant
Chem. class.: Sympathomimetic amine

Action: Produces vasoconstriction (rapid, long-acting) of arterioles thereby decreasing fluid exudation, mucosal engorgement

Uses: Nasal congestion

Dosage and routes:

- *Adult:* INSTILL 2 gtts or sprays to nasal mucosa q3-4h
- *Child 6-12 yr:* INSTILL 1-2 gtts or sprays, repeat q3-4h prn, not to exceed 5 days

Available forms include: Sol 0.025, 0.05%

Side effects/adverse reactions:

GI: Nausea, vomiting, anorexia
EENT: Irritation, burning, sneez-

ing, stinging, dryness, rebound congestion

INTEG: Contact dermatitis

CNS: Anxiety, restlessness, tremors, weakness, insomnia, dizziness, fever, headache

Contraindications: Hypersensitivity to sympathomimetic amines

Precautions: Child <6 yr, elderly, diabetes, cardiovascular disease, hypertension, hyperthyroidism, increased ICP, prostatic hypertrophy, pregnancy (C), glaucoma

Interactions/incompatibilities:

- Hypertension: MAOIs, β-adrenergic blockers
- Hypotension: methyldopa, mecamylamine, reserpine

NURSING CONSIDERATIONS

Administer:

- No more than q4h
- For <4 consecutive days

Perform/provide:

- Environmental humidification to decrease nasal congestion, dryness
- Storage in light-resistant containers; do not expose to high temperatures

Evaluate:

- Redness, swelling, pain in nasal passages

Teach patient/family:

- That stinging may occur for several applications; drying of mucosa may be decreased by environmental humidification
- To notify physician if irregular pulse, insomnia, dizziness, or tremors occur
- Proper administration to avoid systemic absorption

N

---

naphazoline HCl

(naf-az'oh-leen)

Allerest Eye Drops, AK-Con Ophthalmic, Albalon, Clear Eyes, Muro's Opcon, Nafazair, Naphcon, Vasocon

Func. class.: Ophthalmic vasoconstrictor

Chem. class.: Direct imidazoline derivative

Action: Vasoconstriction of eye arterioles; decreases eye engorgement by stimulation of α-adrenergic receptors

Uses: Relieves hyperemia, irritation in superficial corneal vascularity

Dosage and routes:
• *Adult:* INSTILL 1-2 gtts q3-4h

Available forms include: Sol 0.1%, 0.02%, 0.025%, 0.05%, 0.03%, 0.012%

Side effects/adverse reactions:

CNS: Headache, dizziness, sedation, anxiety, weakness, sweating (systemic absorption)

CV: Hypertension, dysrhythmias, tachycardia, *CV collapse* (systemic absorption)

EENT: Pupil dilation, increased intraocular pressure, photophobia

Contraindications: Hypersensitivity, glaucoma (narrow-angle)

Precautions: Hypertension, hyperthyroidism, elderly, severe arteriosclerosis, cardiac disease, pregnancy (C)

Pharmacokinetics:

INSTILL: Duration 2-3 hr

Interactions/incompatibilities:
• Increased pressor effects: MAOIs, tricyclic antidepressants

NURSING CONSIDERATIONS

Perform/provide:
• Storage in tight, light-resistant container

Teach patient/family:
• To report change in vision, blurring, or loss of sight; breathing trouble, sweating, flushing, anxiety, weakness
• Method of instillation; tilt head backward, hold dropper over eye, drop medication inside lower lid, using pressure on inside corner of eye hold 1 min, do not touch dropper to eye
• That blurred vision will decrease with repeated use of drug
• To notify physician if headache, spots, redness, pain occur; discontinue use

naproxen/naproxen sodium

(na-prox'en)

Naprosyn/Anaprox

Func. class.: Nonsteroidal antiinflammatory

Chem. class.: Propionic acid derivative

Action: Inhibits prostaglandin synthesis by decreasing an enzyme needed for biosynthesis; possesses analgesic, antiinflammatory, antipyretic properties

Uses: Mild to moderate pain, osteoarthritis, rheumatoid, gouty arthritis

Dosage and routes:
• *Adult:* PO 250-500 mg bid, not to exceed 1 g/day (base); 525 mg, then 275 mg q6-8h prn, not to exceed 1475 mg (sodium)

Available forms include: Tabs 250, 275, 375, 500 mg; susp 125 mg/5 ml

Side effects/adverse reactions:

GI: Nausea, anorexia, vomiting, diarrhea, jaundice, *cholestatic hepatitis,* constipation, flatulence, cramps, dry mouth, peptic ulcer

CNS: Dizziness, drowsiness, fatigue, tremors, confusion, insomnia, anxiety, depression
CV: Tachycardia, peripheral edema, palpitations, dysrhythmias
INTEG: Purpura, rash, pruritus, sweating
GU: **Nephrotoxicity: dysuria, hematuria, oliguria, azotemia**
HEMA: **Blood dyscrasias**
EENT: Tinnitus, hearing loss, blurred vision
Contraindications: Hypersensitivity, asthma, severe renal disease, severe hepatic disease
Precautions: Pregnancy (B), lactation, children, bleeding disorders, GI disorders, cardiac disorders, hypersensitivity to other antiinflammatory agents, elderly
Pharmacokinetics:
PO: Peak 2-4 hr, half-life 3-3½ hr; metabolized in liver, excreted in urine (metabolites), excreted in breast milk, 99% protein binding
Interactions/incompatibilities:
• May increase action of: heparin
• Increased lithium toxicity: lithium
NURSING CONSIDERATIONS
Assess:
• Renal, liver, blood studies: BUN, creatinine, AST, ALT, Hgb before treatment, periodically thereafter
• Audiometric, ophthalmic exam before, during, after treatment
Administer:
• With food to decrease GI symptoms; best to take on empty stomach to facilitate absorption
Perform/provide:
• Storage at room temperature
Evaluate:
• Therapeutic response: decreased pain, stiffness, swelling in joints, ability to move more easily
• For eye, ear problems: blurred vi-

sion, tinnitus (may indicate toxicity)
Teach patient/family:
• To report blurred vision, ringing, roaring in ears (may indicate toxicity)
• To avoid driving or other hazardous activities if dizziness or drowsiness occurs
• To report change in urine pattern, weight increase, edema (face, lower extremities), pain increase in joints, fever, blood in urine (indicates nephrotoxicity)
• That therapeutic effects may take up to 1 mo
Laboratory test interferences:
Increase: BUN, alk phosphatase
False increase: 5-HIAA, 17KGS

---

natamycin (ophthalmic)

(na-ta-mye′sin)
Natacyn
Func. class.: Antiinfective/antifungal
Chem. class.: Tetraene polyene compound

N

Action: Inhibits transport functions and cell permeability in organism
Uses: Eye infection, fungal blepharitis, conjunctivitis, keratitis
Dosage and routes:
• *Adult and child:* INSTILL 1 gtt q1-2h × 3-4 days, then decrease to 1 gtt 8×/day, duration of therapy, 14-21 days
Available forms include: Susp 5%
Side effects/adverse reactions:
EENT: Temporary visual haze, overgrowth of nonsusceptible organisms
Contraindications: Hypersensitivity
Precautions: Antibiotic hypersensitivity, pregnancy (C); failure of keratitis to improve after 7-10 days

---

italics = common side effects   ***bold italic*** = life threatening reactions

suggests infection not caused by susceptible organism

NURSING CONSIDERATIONS

Administer:

• After washing hands, cleanse crusts or discharge from eye before application

Perform/provide:

• Storage at room temperature

Evaluate:

• Therapeutic response: absence of redness, inflammation, tearing, photophobia

• Allergy: itching, lacrimation, redness, swelling, eye pain

Teach patient/family:

• To use drug exactly as prescribed, shake well before using

• Not to use eye makeup, towels, washcloths, eye medication of others; reinfection may occur

• That drug container tip should not be touched to eye

• To report itching, increased redness, burning, stinging, swelling; drug should be discontinued

---

neomycin sulfate

(nee-oh-mye′sin)

Mycifradin Sulfate, Neobiotic

Func. class.: Antibiotic

Chem. class.: Aminoglycoside

Action: Inferferes with protein synthesis in bacterial cell by binding to ribosomal subunit causing inaccurate peptide sequence to form in protein chain, causing bacterial death

Uses: Severe systemic infections of CNS, respiratory, GI, urinary tract, eye, bone, skin, soft tissues caused by *P. aeruginosa, E. coli, Enterobacter, K. pneumoniae, P. vulgaris;* also used for hepatic coma, preoperatively to sterilize bowel,

infectious diarrhea caused by enteropathogenic *E. coli*

Dosage and routes:

Severe systemic infections

• *Adult:* IM 15 mg/kg/day in 4 divided doses, not to exceed 1 g/day

Hepatic coma

• *Adult:* PO 4-12 g/day in divided doses × 5-6 days; REC 200 ml of 1% or 100 ml of 2% retained for ½-1 hr

• *Child:* 50-100 mg/kg/day in divided doses

Preoperative bowel sterilization

• *Adult:* PO 1 g qlh × 4 doses, then q4h × balance of 24 hr; give saline cathartic before giving this drug

Available forms include: Tabs 500 mg; top, inj IM 500 mg; ophth oint, oral sol 125 mg/5 ml

Side effects/adverse reactions:

GU: Oliguria, hematuria, renal damage, azotemia, renal failure, nephrotoxicity

CNS: Confusion, depression, numbness, tremors, *convulsions,* muscle twitching, *neurotoxicity*

EENT: Ototoxicity, deafness, visual disturbances

HEMA: Agranulocytosis, thrombocytopenia, leukopenia, eosinophilia, anemia

GI: Nausea, vomiting, anorexia, increased ALT, AST, bilirubin, hepatomegaly, *hepatic necrosis,* splenomegaly

CV: Hypotension, myocarditis

INTEG: Rash, burning, urticaria, photosensitivity, dermatitis

Contraindications: Bowel obstruction (oral use), severe renal disease, hypersensitivity

Precautions: Neonates, mild renal disease, pregnancy (C), hearing deficits, lactation, myasthenia gravis

Pharmacokinetics:

PO: Onset rapid, peak 1-2 hr

REC: Onset immediate, peak 1-2 hr Plasma half-life 1-3 hr; not metabolized, excreted unchanged in urine, crosses placental barrier

Interactions/incompatibilities:
• Increased ototoxicity, neurotoxicity, nephrotoxicity: other aminoglycosides, amphotericin B, polymyxin, vancomycin, ethacrynic acid, furosemide, mannitol, methoxyflurane, cisplatin, cephalosporins
• Decreased effects of: parenteral penicillins, vitamin B$_{12}$
• Do not mix in solution or syringe: carbenicillin, ticarcillin, amphotericin B, cephalothin, erythromycin, heparin
• Increased effects: nondepolarizing muscle relaxants, oral anticoagulants when given with oral neomycin
• Decreased effects of: digoxin when given with oral neomycin

NURSING CONSIDERATIONS
Assess:
• Weight before treatment; calculation of dosage is usually done based on ideal body weight, but may be calculated on actual body weight
• I&O ratio, urinalysis daily for proteinuria, cells, casts; report sudden change in urine output
• Urine pH if drug is used for UTI; urine should be kept alkaline

Administer:
• IM injection in large muscle mass, rotate injection sites
• Drug in evenly spaced doses to maintain blood level
• Bicarbonate to alkalinize urine if ordered in treating UTI, as drug is most active in alkaline environment

Perform/provide:
• Adequate fluids of 2-3 L/day unless contraindicated to prevent irritation of tubules

• Supervised ambulation, other safety measures with vestibular dysfunction

Evaluate:
• Therapeutic effect: absence of fever, draining wounds, negative C&S after treatment
• Renal impairment by securing urine for CrCl testing, BUN, serum creatinine; lower dosage should be given in renal impairment (CrCl <80 ml/min)
• Deafness by audiometric testing, ringing, roaring in ears, vertigo; assess hearing before, during, after treatment
• Dehydration: high sp gr, decrease in skin turgor, dry mucous membranes, dark urine
• Overgrowth of infection: increased temperature, malaise, redness, pain, swelling, perineal itching, diarrhea, stomatitis, change in cough, sputum
• C&S before starting treatment to identify infecting organism
• Vestibular dysfunction: nausea, vomiting, dizziness, headache; drug should be discontinued if severe
• Injection sites for redness, swelling, abscesses; use warm compresses at site

Teach patient/family:
• To report headache, dizziness, symptoms of overgrowth of infection, renal impairment
• To report loss of hearing, ringing, roaring in ears or a feeling of fullness in head

Treatment of overdose: Hemodialysis, monitor serum levels of drug

N

---

italics = common side effects   ***bold italic*** = life threatening reactions

neomycin sulfate

(nee-oh-mye'sin)

Drotic, Otocort

Func. class.: Otic, antibiotic
Chem. class.: Aminoglycoside

Action: Inhibits protein synthesis in susceptible microorganisms

Uses: Ear infection (external), short-term use

Dosage and routes:
• *Adult and child:* INSTILL 2-5 gtts tid-qid

Available forms include: Otic sol in combination with neomycin, hydrocortisone 0.25%, 0.5%

Side effects/adverse reactions:
EENT: Itching, irritation in ear
INTEG: Rash, urticaria

Contraindications: Hypersensitivity, perforated eardrum

Precautions: Pregnancy (C)

NURSING CONSIDERATIONS
Administer:
• After removing impacted cerumen by irrigation
• After cleaning stopper with alcohol
• After restraining child if necessary
• Warming solution

Evaluate:
• Therapeutic response: decreased ear pain
• For redness, swelling, fever, pain in ear, which indicates superimposed infection

Teach patient/family:
• Method of instillation using aseptic technique, including not touching dropper to ear
• That dizziness may occur after instillation

neomycin sulfate (topical)

(nee-oh-mye'sin)

Myciguent

Func. class.: Local antibacterial
Chem. class.: Aminoglycoside

Action: Interferes with bacterial protein synthesis

Uses: Skin infections

Dosage and routes:
• *Adult and child:* TOP rub into affected area bid-tid

Available forms include: Oint, cream 0.5%

Side effects/adverse reactions:
INTEG: Rash, urticaria, scaling, redness

Contraindications: Hypersensitivity, large areas, burns, ulcerations

Precautions: Pregnancy (C), lactation, impaired renal function, external ear of perforated eardrum

NURSING CONSIDERATIONS
Administer:
• Enough medication to completely cover lesions
• After cleansing with soap, water before each application, dry well
• To less than 20% of body surface area

Perform/provide:
• Storage at room temperature in dry place

Evaluate:
• Allergic reaction: burning, stinging, swelling, redness
• Therapeutic response: decrease in size, number of lesions
• For signs of nephrotoxicity or ototoxicity

Teach patient/family:
• To apply with glove to prevent further infection
• To avoid use of OTC creams, ointments, lotions unless directed by physician

---

* Available in Canada only

• To use medical asepsis (hand washing) before, after each application

• To notify physician if condition worsens

---

neostigmine bromide/ neostigmine methylsulfate

(nee-oh-stig′meen)
Prostigmin Bromide/Prostigmin
Func. class.: Cholinergic stimulant
Chem. class.: Quaternary compound

Action: Inhibits destruction of acetylcholine, which increases concentration at sites where acetylcholine is released; this facilitates transmission of impulses across myoneural junction

Uses: Myasthenia gravis, nondepolarizing neuromuscular blocker, antagonist, bladder distention, postoperative ileus

Dosage and routes:
Myasthenia gravis
• *Adult:* PO 15-375 mg/day; IM/IV 0.5-2 mg q1-3h
• *Child:* PO 2 mg/kg/day q3-4h
Tubocurarine antagonist
• *Adult:* IV 0.5-2 mg slowly, may repeat if needed (give 0.6-1.2 mg atropine before this drug)
Abdominal distention/postoperative ileus
• *Adult:* IM/SC 0.25-1 mg q4-6h depending on condition
Available forms include: Tabs 15 mg; inj IM, SC, IV 1:1000, 1:2000, 1:4000

Side effects/adverse reactions:
INTEG: Rash, urticaria, flushing
CNS: Dizziness, headache, sweating, confusion, weakness, *convulsions,* incoordination, *paralysis*

GI: Nausea, diarrhea, vomiting, cramps
CV: Tachycardia, dysrhythmias, bradycardia, hypotension, AV block, ECG changes, *cardiac arrest*
GU: Frequency, incontinence
RESP: Respiratory depression, bronchospasm, constriction, laryngospasm, respiratory arrest
EENT: Miosis, blurred vision, lacrimation

Contraindications: Obstruction of intestine, renal system, pregnancy (C), bromide sensitivity

Precautions: Bradycardia, hypotension, seizure disorders, bronchial asthma, coronary occlusion, hyperthyroidism, dysrhythmias, peptic ulcer, megacolon, poor GI motility, lactation, children

Pharmacokinetics:
PO: Onset 45-75 min, duration 2½-4 hr
IM/SC: Onset 10-30 min, duration 2½-4 hr
IV onset 4-8 min; duration 2-4 hr
Metabolized in liver, excreted in urine

Interactions/incompatibilities:
• Decreased action of: gallamine, metocurine, pancuronium, tubocurarine, atropine
• Increased action of: decamethonium, succinylcholine
• Decreased action of neostigmine: aminoglycosides, anesthetics, procainamide, quinidine, mecamylamine, polymyxin, magnesium

NURSING CONSIDERATIONS
Assess:
• VS, respiration q8h
• I&O ratio; check for urinary retention or incontinence
Administer:
• IV undiluted, give through Y-tube or 3-way stopcock; give 0.5 mg or less over 1 min

---

italics = common side effects   ***bold italic*** = life threatening reactions

- Only with atropine sulfate available for cholinergic crisis
- Only after all other cholinergics have been discontinued
- Increased doses if tolerance occurs
- Larger doses after exercise or fatigue
- With food or milk to decrease GI symptoms
- On empty stomach for better absorption

Perform/provide:

- Storage at room temperature

Evaluate:

- Therapeutic response: increased muscle strength, hand grasp, improved gait, absence of labored breathing (if severe)
- Bradycardia, hypotension, bronchospasm, headache, dizziness, convulsions, respiratory depression; drug should be discontinued if toxicity occurs

Teach patient/family:

- That drug is not a cure, it only relieves symptoms
- To wear Medic Alert ID specifying myasthenia gravis, drugs taken

Treatment of overdose:

Respiratory support, atropine 1-4 mg (IV)

---

netilmicin sulfate

(ne-til-mye′sin)

Netromycin

Func. class.: Antibiotic
Chem. class.: Aminoglycoside

Action: Interferes with protein synthesis in bacterial cell by binding to ribosomal subunit, causing inaccurate peptide sequence to form in protein chain, causing bacterial death

Uses: Severe systemic infections of CNS, respiratory, GI, urinary tract, bone, skin, soft tissues caused by *P. aeruginosa, E. coli, Enterobacter, Providencia, Citrobacter, Staphylococcus, K. pneumoniae, P. mirabilis, Serratia*

Dosage and routes:
Normal renal function

- *Adult and child >12 yr:* IM/IV 3-6.5 mg/kg/day; may give q8-12h for severe infections
- *Child and infant 6 wk-12 yr:* IM/IV 5.5-8 mg/kg/day in divided doses q8-12h
- *Neonate <6 wk:* IM/IV 4-6.5 mg/kg/day in divided doses q12h

Available forms include: Inj IM, IV 10, 25, 100 mg/ml

Side effects/adverse reactions:

GU: Oliguria, hematuria, renal damage, azotemia, renal failure, nephrotoxicity

CNS: Confusion, depression, numbness, tremors, *convulsions,* muscle twitching, *neurotoxicity*

EENT: Ototoxicity, deafness, visual disturbances

HEMA: Agranulocytosis, thrombocytopenia, leukopenia, eosinophilia, anemia

GI: Nausea, vomiting, anorexia, increased ALT, AST, bilirubin, hepatomegaly, *hepatic necrosis,* splenomegaly

CV: Hypotension, myocarditis

INTEG: Rash, burning, urticaria, photosensitivity, dermatitis

Contraindications: Severe renal disease, hypersensitivity

Precautions: Neonates, mild renal disease, pregnancy (D), children <12 yr, lactation, myasthenia gravis, hearing deficit

Pharmacokinetics:

IM: Onset rapid, peak 1-2 hr
IV: Onset immediate, peak 1-2 hr
Plasma half-life 2-3 hr, not metab-

---

olized, excreted unchanged in urine, crosses placental barrier

Interactions/incompatibilities:

• Increased ototoxicity, neurotoxicity, nephrotoxicity: other aminoglycosides, amphotericin B, polymyxin, vancomycin, ethacrynic acid, furosemide, mannitol, methoxyflurane, cisplatin, cephalosporins

• Decreased effects: parenteral penicillins

• Do not mix in solution or syringe: carbenicillin, ticarcillin, amphotericin B, cephalothin, erythromycin, heparin

• Increased effects: nondepolarizing muscle relaxants

NURSING CONSIDERATIONS

Assess:

• Weight before treatment; calculation of dosage is usually done based on ideal body weight, but may be calculated on actual body weight

• Daily I&O ratio, urinalysis for proteinuria, cells, casts; report sudden change in urine output

• VS during infusion, watch for hypotension, change in pulse

• IV site for thrombophlebitis including pain, redness, swelling q30 min, change site if needed; apply warm compresses to discontinued site

• Serum peak, drawn at 30-60 min after IV infusion or 60 min after IM injection; trough level drawn just before next dose; blood level should be 2-4 times bacteriostatic level

• Urine pH if drug is used for UTI; urine should be kept alkaline

Administer:

• IM injection in large muscle mass, rotate injection sites

• Drug in evenly spaced doses to maintain blood level

• Bicarbonate to alkalinize urine if ordered in treating UTI, as drug is most active in alkaline environment

• IV diluted in 50-200 ml IV sol, infuse over ½-2 hr

Perform/provide:

• Adequate fluids of 2-3 L/day unless contraindicated to prevent irritation of tubules

• Flush of IV line with NS or D_5W after infusion

• Supervised ambulation, other safety measures with vestibular dysfuncton

Evaluate:

• Therapeutic effect: absence of fever, draining wounds, negative C&S after treatment

• Renal impairment by securing urine for CrCl testing, BUN, serum creatinine; a lower dosage should be given in renal impairment (CrCl <80 ml/min)

• Deafness by audiometric testing, ringing, roaring in ears, vertigo; assess hearing before, during, after treatment

• Dehydration: high sp gr, decrease in skin turgor, dry mucous membranes, dark urine

• Overgrowth of infection· increased temperature, malaise, redness, pain, swelling, perineal itching, diarrhea, stomatitis, change in cough or sputum

• C&S before starting treatment to identify infecting organism

• Vestibular dysfunction: nausea, vomiting, dizziness, headache; drug should be discontinued if severe

• Injection sites for redness, swelling, abscesses; use warm compresses at site

Teach patient/family:

• To report headache, dizziness, symptoms of overgrowth of infection, renal impairment

---

italics = common side effects   ***bold italic*** = life threatening reactions

• To report loss of hearing, ringing, roaring in ears or feeling of fullness in head

Treatment of overdose: Hemodialysis, monitor serum levels of drug

---

niacin (vitamin B₃/ nicotinic acid)/niacin-amide (nicotinamide)

(nye'a-sin) (nye-a-sin'a-mide)

Niac, Nico-400, Nicobid, Nicolar, Nico-Span, Novoniacin*

Func. class.: Vitamin B₃

Chem. class.: Water-soluble vitamin

Action: Needed for conversion of fats, protein, carbohydrates, by oxidation reduction; acts directly on vascular smooth muscle causing vasodilation; high doses decrease serum lipids

Uses: Pellagra, hyperlipidemias, (niacin) peripheral vascular disease (niacin)

Dosage and routes:

Adjunct in hyperlipidemia

• *Adult:* PO 1.5-3 g qd in 3 divided doses after meals, may be increased to 6 g/day

Pellagra

• *Adult:* IM/SC/PO/IV INF 10-20 mg, not to exceed 500 mg total dose

• *Child:* IM/SC/PO/IV INF 300 mg until desired response

Peripheral vascular disease

• *Adult:* PO 250-800 mg qd in divided doses

Available forms include: Nicotinic acid—tabs 20, 25, 50, 100, 500 mg; caps timed released 125, 250, 300, 400, 500 mg; tabs time released 150 mg; elix 50 mg/5 ml; inj 100 mg/ml; nicotinamide—tabs 50, 100, 500 mg; tabs timed release 1000 mg; inj IV, IM, SC 100 mg/ml

Side effects/adverse reactions:

CNS: Paresthesias, headache, dizziness, anxiety

GI: Nausea, vomiting, anorexia, flatulence, xerostomia, *jaundice,* diarrhea, peptic ulcer

GU: Hyperuricemia, *glycosuria, hypoalbuminemia*

CV: Postural hypotension, vasovagal attacks, dysrhythmias, vasodilation

EENT: Blurred vision, ptosis

INTEG: Flushing, dry skin, rash, pruritus

RESP: Wheezing

Contraindications: Hypersensitivity, peptic ulcer, hepatic disease, lactation, hemorrhage, severe hypotension

Precautions: Glaucoma, cardiovascular disease, CAD, diabetes mellitus, gout, schizophrenia, pregnancy (A)

Pharmacokinetics:

PO: Peak 30-70 min, half-life 45 min, metabolized in liver, 30% excreted unchanged in urine

Interactions/incompatibilities:

• Increased action of: ganglionic blockers

NURSING CONSIDERATIONS

Assess:

• Liver function studies: AST, ALT, bilirubin, alk phosphatase; blood glucose before and during treatment

• Niacin levels while taking this drug

Administer:

• With meals for GI symptoms

Evaluate:

• Therapeutic response: decreased lipids, warm extremities, absence of numbness in extremities

• Nutritional status: liver, yeast, legumes, organ meat, lean poultry

• Liver dysfunction: clay colored stools, itching, dark urine, jaundice

---

* Available in Canada only

• CNS symptoms: headache, paresthesias, blurred vision

Teach patient/family:

• That flushing and increase in feelings of warmth will occur several hours after taking drug (PO) or immediately (IM/IV/SC); time-release product will minimize flushing

• To remain recumbent if postural hypotension occurs

• To abstain from alcohol if drug is prescribed for hyperlipidemia

• To avoid sunlight if skin lesions are present

Lab test interferences:

Increase: Bilirubin, alk phosphatase, liver enzymes, LDH, uric acid

Decrease: Cholesterol

False increase: Urinary catecholamines

False positive: Urine glucose

---

nicardipine

(nye-card'i-peen)
Cardene

Func. class.: Calcium channel blocker

Chem. class.: Dihydropyridine

Action: Inhibits calcium ion influx across cell membrane during cardiac depolarization; produces relaxation of coronary vascular smooth muscle, peripheral vascular smooth muscle; dilates coronary vascular arteries; increases myocardial oxygen delivery in patients with vasospastic angina

Uses: Chronic stable angina pectoris, hypertension

Dosage and routes:

Angina

Adult: PO 20 mg tid initially, may increase after 3 days (range 20-40 mg tid)

Hypertension

Adult: PO 20 mg tid initially, then increase after 3 days (range 20-40 mg tid)

Available forms include: Caps 20, 30 mg

Side effects/adverse reactions:

CV: Dysrythmia, edema, CHF, bradycardia, hypotension, palpitations, *MI, pulmonary edema*

GI: Nausea, vomiting, diarrhea, gastric upset, constipation, *hepatitis,* abdominal cramps

GU: Nocturia, polyuria, *acute renal failure*

INTEG: Rash, pruritus, urticaria, photosensitivity, hair loss

CNS: Headache, fatigue, drowsiness, dizziness, anxiety, depression, weakness, insomnia, confusion, paresthesia, somnolence

OTHER: Blurred vision, flushing, nasal congestion, sweating, shortness of breath, gynecomastia, hyperglycemia, sexual difficulties

Contraindications: Sick sinus syndrome, 2nd or 3rd degree heart block, hypotension less than 90 mm Hg systolic, hypersensitivity

Precautions: CHF, hypotension, hepatic injury, pregnancy (C), lactation, children, renal disease, elderly

Pharmacokinetics:

PO: Onset 10 min, peak 1-2 hr, half-life 2-5 hr; metabolized by liver, excreted in urine (98% as metabolites)

Interactions/incompatibilities:

• Increased effects of: digitalis, neuromuscular blocking agents, theophylline

• Increased effects of: nicardipine, cimetidine

NURSING CONSIDERATIONS

Administer:

• ac, hs

---

italics = common side effects   ***bold italic*** = life threatening reactions

Evaluate:
• Therapeutic response: decreased anginal pain, decreased B/P
• Cardiac status: B/P, pulse, respiration, ECG
Teach patient/family:
• To avoid hazardous activities until stabilized on drug, dizziness is no longer a problem
• To limit caffeine consumption
• To avoid OTC drugs unless directed by physician
• Stress patient compliance in all areas of medical regimen: diet, exercise, stress reduction, drug therapy
• To notify physician of: irregular heart beat, shortness of breath, swelling of feet and hands, pronounced dizziness, constipation, nausea, hypotension
Treatment of overdose: Defibrillation, β-agonists, IV calcium inotropic agents, diuretics, atropine for AV block, vasopressor for hypotension

---

niclosamide

(ni-kloe′sa-mide)
Niclocide
Func. class.: Anthelmintic
Chem. class.: Salicylanilide derivative

Action: Inhibits synthesis of ATP in mitochondria; leads to destruction in intestine where worm may be digested, removed in feces; not effective for ova or larval stage
Uses: Regular, dwarf tapeworms
Dosage and routes:
• *Adult:* PO 2 g chewed as a single dose for *T saginata* and *D latum*; 2g × 7 days for *Hymenolepis nana*
• *Child >34 kg:* PO 1.5 g chewed as a single dose for *T saginata* and *D latum*; 1.5 g as single dose on day 1 followed by 1 g × 6 days for *Hymenolepis nana*
• *Child <34 kg:* PO 1 g chewed as a single dose for *T saginata* and *D latum*; 1 g on day 1, then 0.5 g × 6 days for *Hymenolepis nana*
Available forms include: Tabs, chewable 500 mg
Side effects/adverse reactions:
INTEG: Rash, pruritus, pruritus ani, alopecia
CNS: Dizziness, headache, drowsiness, restlessness, sweating, fever
EENT: Bad taste, oral irritation
GI: Nausea, vomiting, anorexia, diarrhea, constipation, rectal bleeding
Contraindications: Hypersensitivity
Precautions: Child <2 yr, pregnancy (B), lactation

NURSING CONSIDERATIONS
Assess:
• Stools during entire treatment, 1, 3 mo after treatment; specimens must be sent to lab while still warm
Administer:
• May be crushed, mixed with water if unable to swallow whole
• Laxatives if constipated; not needed for drug to work
• After breakfast, tab must be chewed, not swallowed
Perform/provide:
• Storage in tight, light-resistant container in cool environment: do not freeze
Evaluate:
• Therapeutic response: expulsion of worms, 3 negative stool cultures after completion of treatment
• For allergic reaction: rash, itching in anal area
• For diarrhea during expulsion of worms
• For infection in other family members since infection from person to person is common

---

*Available in Canada only

Teach patient/family:
• Proper hygiene after BM including handwashing technique; tell patient to avoid putting fingers in mouth
• That infected person should sleep alone; do not shake bed linen, change bed linen qd, wash in hot water
• To clean toilet qd with disinfectant (green soap solution)
• Need for compliance with dosage schedule, duration of treatment
• To drink fruit juice to remove mucus that intestinal tapeworms burrow in, aids in explusion of worms (dwarf tapeworms only)
Treatment of overdose: Enemas, laxatives; do not induce vomiting

---

nicotine resin complex

(nik′o-teen)
Nicorette, Nicotine Pola Crile
Func. class.: Smoking deterrent
Chem. class.: Ganglionic cholinergic agonist

Action: Agonist at nicotinic receptors in the peripheral and central nervous system; acts at sympathetic ganglia; on chemoreceptors of the aorta and carotid bodies; also affects adrenal-releasing catecholamines
Uses: Deter cigarette smoking
Dosage and routes:
• *Adult:* GUM 1 piece chewed × ½ hr as needed to abstain from smoking, not to exceed 30/day
Available forms include: Gum 2 mg/piece of gum
Side effects/adverse reactions:
RESP: Breathing difficulty, cough, hoarseness, sneezing, wheezing
EENT: Jaw ache, irritation in buccal cavity
CNS: Dizziness, vertigo, insomnia,
headache, confusion, convulsions, depression, euphoria, numbness, tinnitus
GI: Nausea, vomiting, anorexia, indigestion, diarrhea, abdominal pain, constipation, eructation
CV: Dysrhythmias, tachycardia, palpitations
Contraindications: Hypersensitivity, immediate post MI recovery period, severe angina pectoris, pregnancy (X)
Precautions: Vasospastic disease, dysrhythmias, diabetes mellitus, children, hyperthyroidism, pheochromocytoma, coronary disease, esophagitis, peptic ulcer
Pharmacokinetics:
Onset 15-30 min, metabolized in liver, excreted in urine, half-life 2-3 hr, 30-120 hr, (terminal)
Interactions/incompatibilities:
• Smoking cessation increases diuretic effects of; furosemide
• Increased blood levels with cessation of smoking: caffeine, theophylline, petazocine, impramine
NURSING CONSIDERATIONS
Assess:
• Adverse reaction: irritation of buccal cavity, dislike of taste, jaw ache
Evaluate:
• Therapeutic response: decrease in urge to smoke, decreased need for gum after 3-6 mo
Teach patient/family:
• To chew gum slowly for 30 min to promote buccal absorption of the drug; do not chew over 45 min
• To begin drug withdrawal after 3 mo use; not to exceed 6 mo
• All aspects of drug; give package insert to patient and explain
• That gum will not stick to dentures, dental appliances
• That gum is as toxic as cigarette;

N

---

italics = common side effects   ***bold italic*** = life threatening reactions

it is to be used only to deter smoking
• Not to use during pregnancy; birth defects may occur

---

nifedipine

(nye-fed'i-peen)
Adalat,* Procardia
Func. class.: Calcium channel blocker
Chem. class.: Dihydropyridine

Action: Inhibits calcium ion influx across cell membrane during cardiac depolarization; produces relaxation of coronary vascular smooth muscle, dilates coronary arteries; increases myocardial oxygen delivery in patients with vasospastic angina; dilates peripheral arteries

Uses: Chronic stable angina pectoris, vasospastic angina, hypertension (sustained release only)

Dosage and routes:
• *Adult:* PO Immediate release: 10 mg tid, increase in 10 mg increments q4-6h, not to exceed 180 mg or single dose of 30 mg
• *Adult:* PO sus rel: 30-60 mg qd, may increase q7-14days, doses >120 mg not recommended

Available forms include: Caps 10, 20 mg, tabs sus rel 30, 60, 90 mg

Side effects/adverse reactions:
CV: Dysrhythmia, edema, CHF, hypotension, palpitations, *MI,* pulmonary edema, tachycardia
GI: Nausea, vomiting, diarrhea, gastric upset, constipation, increased liver function studies, dry mouth
GU: Nocturia, polyuria
INTEG: Rash, pruritus, flushing, photosensitivity, hair loss
MISC: Flushing, sexual difficulties, cough, fever, chills

CNS: Headache, fatigue, drowsiness, dizziness, anxiety, depression, weakness, insomnia, light-headedness, paresthesia, tinnitus, blurred vision

Contraindications: Hypersensitivity

Precautions: CHF, hypotension, sick sinus syndrome, 2nd or 3rd degree heart block, hypotension less than 90 mm Hg systolic, hepatic injury, pregnancy (C), lactation, children, renal disease

Pharmacokinetics:
PO: Onset 20 min, peak 0.5-6 hr, half-life 2-5 hr; metabolized by liver, excreted in urine (98% as metabolites)

Interactions/incompatibilities:
• Increased effects of: theophylline, beta-blockers, antihypertensives, digitalis
• Increased nifedipine level: cimetidine
• Decreased effects: quinidine

NURSING CONSIDERATIONS

Administer:
• Before meals, hs

Evaluate:
• Therapeutic response: decreased anginal pain, B/P
• Cardiac status: B/P, pulse, respiration, ECG

Teach patient/family:
• To avoid hazardous activities until stabilized on drug, dizziness is no longer a problem
• To limit caffeine consumption
• To avoid OTC drugs unless directed by a physician
• Stress patient compliance to all areas of medical regimen: diet, exercise, stress reduction, drug therapy
• Do not chew, divide, or crush sus rel tabs

Treatment of overdose: Defibril-

---

lation, atropine for AV block, vasopressor for hypotension

---

nitrofurantoin/nitrofurantoin macrocrystals

(nye-troe-fyoor'an-toyn)
Furadantin, Furalan, Furantoin, J-Dantin, Nephronex,* Nitrex, Novofuran,* Sarodant

Func. class.: Urinary tract antiinfective
Chem. class.: Synthetic nitrofuran derivative

Action: Appears to inhibit bacterial enzymes

Uses: Urinary tract infections caused by *E. coli, Klebsiella, Pseudomonas, P. vulgaris, P. morganii, Serratia, Citrobacter, S. aureus*

Dosage and routes:
• *Adult and child >12 yr:* PO 50-100 mg qid pc or 50-100 mg hs for long-term treatment
• *Child 1 mo-3 yr:* PO 5-7 mg/kg/day in 4 divided doses; 1-3 mg/kg/day for long-term treatment

Available forms include: Caps 25, 50, 100 mg; tabs 50, 100 mg; susp 25 mg/5 ml

Side effects/adverse reactions:
INTEG: Pruritus, rash, urticaria, angioedema, alopecia, tooth staining
CNS: Dizziness, headache, drowsiness, peripheral neuropathy
GI: Nausea, vomiting, abdominal pain, diarrhea, **cholestatic jaundice**

Contraindications: Hypersensitivity, anuria, severe renal disease

Precautions: Pregnancy (B), lactation

Pharmacokinetics:
PO: Half-life 20-60 min, crosses blood-brain barrier, placenta, enters breast milk, excreted as inactive metabolites in liver

Interactions/incompatibilities:
• Increased levels of nitrofurantoin: probenecid
• Antagonistic effect: nalidixic acid
• Decreased absorption of: magnesium trisilicate antacid

NURSING CONSIDERATIONS
Assess:
• Blood count for patients on chronic therapy
• I&O ratio, urine pH <5.5 is ideal
• Renal and hepatic function

Administer:
• After clean-catch urine is obtained for C&S
• Two daily doses if urine output is high or if patient has diabetes

Evaluate:
• CNS symptoms: insomnia, vertigo, headache, drowsiness, convulsions
• Allergy: fever, flushing, rash, urticaria, pruritus

Teach patient/family:
• To take medication with food or milk
• Instruct client to protect susp from freezing and shake well before taking
• May cause drowsiness; instruct client to seek aid in walking and other activities; advise client not to drive or operate machinery while on medication
• Instruct clients with diabetes that Clinitest may prove false-positive for glucose; and therefore Tes-Tape or Clinistix should be used
• May turn urine rust-yellow to brown

N

---

italics = common side effects   ***bold italic*** = life threatening reactions

nitrofurazone (topical)

(nye-troe-fyoor′a-zone)

Furacin

Func. class.: Local antibacterial

Chem. class.: Synthetic nitrofuran

Action: Unknown antibacterial action

Uses: Burns (2nd, 3rd degree)

Dosage and routes:

• *Adult and child:* TOP apply to affected area qd or qod

Available forms include: Sol, oint (soluble dressing), cream 0.2%

Side effects/adverse reactions:

INTEG: Rash, urticaria, stinging, burning, superinfections, photosensitivity

Contraindications: Hypersensitivity, G-6-PD deficiency

Precautions: Pregnancy (C), lactation; superinfection may result in bacterial or fungal overgrowth

NURSING CONSIDERATIONS

Administer:

• Analgesic before application if needed

• Enough medication to completely cover burns

• After cleansing debris from area before each application

• Using sterile technique

Perform/provide:

• Storage at room temperature in dry place

Evaluate:

• Allergic reaction: burning, stinging, swelling, redness

• Therapeutic response: development of granulation tissue

Teach patient/family:

• That drug may be used until grafting is possible

• To avoid sunlight or ultraviolet light

nitroglycerin

(nye-troe-gli′ser-in)

Nitro-Bid, Nitrocap, Nitrodisc, Nitro-Dur, Nitrolingual, Nitrol, Nitrospan, Nitrostat, Tridil, Nitrogard, Nitrone, Nitroglyn, Nitrone, Deponit, Transderm Nitro

Func. class.: Vasodilatory coronary

Chem. class.: Nitrate

Action: Decreases preload, afterload, which is responsible for decreasing left ventricular end-diastolic pressure, systemic vascular resistance

Uses: Chronic stable angina pectoris, prophylaxis of angina pain, CHF associated with acute MI, controlled hypotension in surgical procedures

Dosage and routes:

• *Adult:* SL dissolve tablet under tongue when pain begins; may repeat q5min until relief occurs; take no more than 3 tabs/15 min; use 1 tab prophylactically 5-10 min before activities; SUS CAP q6-12h on empty stomach; TOP 1-2 in q8h, increase to 4 in q4h as needed; IV 5 μg/min, then increase by 5 μg/min q3-5 min; if no response after 20 μg/min, increase by 10-20 μg/min until desired response; TRANS apply a pad qd to a site free of hair

Available forms include: Buccal tabs 1, 2, 3 mg; aero 0.4 mg/meter spray; caps 2.5, 6.5, 9 mg; tabs ext rel 2.6, 6.5, 9 mg; inj 0.5, 0.8, 5, 10 mg/ml; SL tabs 0.15, 0.3, 0.4, 0.6 mg; top oint 2%; trans derm syst 2.5, 5, 7.5, 10, 15 mg/24 hr

Side effects/adverse reactions:

CV: Postural hypotension, tachycardia, *collapse,* syncope

GI: Nausea, vomiting

INTEG: Pallor, sweating, rash

CNS: Headache, flushing, dizziness

Contraindications: Hypersensitivity to this drug or nitrites, severe anemia, increased intracranial pressure, cerebral hemorrhage

Precautions: Postural hypotension, pregnancy (C), lactation

Pharmacokinetics:

SUS REL: Onset 20-45 min, duration 3-8 hr

SL: Onset 1-3 min, duration 30 min

TRANS DER: Onset ½-1 hr, duration 12-24 hr

IV: Onset immediately, duration variable

TRANSMUC: Onset 3 min, duration 10-30 min

AEROSOL: Onset 2 min, duration 30-60 min

TOP OINT: Onset 30-60 min, duration 2-12 hr

Metabolized by liver, excreted in urine

Interactions/incompatibilities:

• Increased effects: β-blockers, diuretics, antihypertensives, anticoagulants, alcohol

• Decreased heparin: IV nitroglycerin

NURSING CONSIDERATIONS

Assess:

• B/P, pulse, respirations during beginning therapy

Administer:

• IV diluted in amount specified D₅ or NS for infusion; use glass infusion bottles, nonpolyvinyl chloride infusion tubing; titrate to patient response

• With 8 oz of water on empty stomach (oral tablet)

Evaluate:

• Pain: duration, time started, activity being performed, character

• Tolerance if taken over long period of time

• Headache, lightheadedness, decreased B/P; may indicate a need for decreased dosage

Teach patient/family:

• Place buccal tab between lip and gum above incisors or between cheek and gum; sus rel must be swallowed whole, do not chew; SL should be dissolved under tongue, do not swallow; aerosol should be sprayed under tongue, do not inhale

• To keep tabs in original container

• If 3 SL tabs in 15 min do not relieve pain, to go to emergency room

• To avoid alcohol

• May cause headache, tolerance usually develops, use nonnarcotic analgesic

• That drug may be taken before stressful activity: exercise, sexual activity

• That SL may sting when drug comes in contact with mucous membranes

• To avoid hazardous activities if dizziness occurs

• Stress patient compliance with complete medical regimen

• To make position changes slowly to prevent fainting

---

nitroprusside sodium

(nye-troe-pruss'ide)

Nipride, Nitropress

Func. class.: Antihypertensive

Chem. class.: Peripheral vasodilator

Action: Directly relaxes arteriolar, venous smooth muscle; resulting in reduction in cardiac preload, afterload

Uses: Hypertensive crisis, to decrease bleeding by creating hypotension during surgery

---

italics = common side effects   ***bold italic*** = life threatening reactions

Dosage and routes:
• *Adult:* IV INF dissolve 50 mg in 2-3 ml of D_5W, then dilute in 250-1000 ml of D_5W; run at 0.5-8 µg/kg/min
Available forms include: Inj IV 50 mg
Side effects/adverse reactions:
GI: Nausea, vomiting, abdominal pain
CNS: Dizziness, headache, agitation, twitching, decreased reflexes, *loss of consciousness,* restlessness
EENT: Tinnitus, blurred vision
GU: Impotence
INTEG: Pain, irritation at injection site, sweating
Contraindications: Hypersensitivity, hypertension (compensatory)
Precautions: Pregnancy (C), lactation, children, fluid, electrolyte imbalances, hepatic disease, renal disease, hypothyroidism, elderly
Pharmacokinetics:
IV: Onset 1-2 min, duration 1-10 min after IV done, half-life 4 days in patients with abnormal renal function; metabolized in liver, excreted in urine
Interactions/incompatibilities:
• Severe hypotension: ganglionic blockers, volatile liquid anesthetics, halothane, enflurane, circulatory depressants
• Do not mix with any drug in syringe or solution
NURSING CONSIDERATIONS
Assess:
• Electrolytes: K, Na, Cl, CO_2
• Renal function studies: catecholamines, BUN, creatinine
• Hepatic function studies: AST, ALT, alk phosphatase
• B/P by direct means if possible, check ECG continuously
• Weight daily, I&O
• Thiocyanate levels qd if on long-term treatment

Administer:
• Depending on B/P reading q15 min
• IV after diluting 50 mg/2-3 ml of D_5W, further dilute in 250 ml of D_5W; use an infusion pump only, wrap bottle with aluminum foil to protect from light; observe for color change in the infusion, discard if highly discolored (blue, green, dark red), titrate to patient response
Evaluate:
• Therapeutic response: decreased B/P, absence of bleeding
• Nausea, vomiting, diarrhea
• Edema in feet, legs daily
• Skin turgor, dryness of mucous membranes for hydration status
• Rales, dyspnea, orthopnea q30 min
Treatment of overdose: Administer amyl nitrite inhalation until 3% sodium nitrate solution can be prepared for IV administration, then inject sodium thiosulfate IV, correct drop in BP with vasopressor

norepinephrine injection
(nor-ep-i-nef'rin)
Levophed
Func. class.: Adrenergic
Chem. class.: Catecholamine

Action: Causes increased contractility and heart rate by acting on β-receptors in heart; also, acts on α-receptors, causing vasoconstriction in blood vessels; B/P is elevated, coronary blood flow improves, cardiac output increases, B/P elevates
Uses: Acute hypotension
Dosage and routes:
• *Adult:* IV INF 8-12 µg/min titrated to B/P

Available forms include: Inj IV 1 mg/ml

Side effects/adverse reactions:

CNS: Headache, anxiety, dizziness, insomnia, restlessness, tremor

CV: Palpitations, tachycardia, hypertension, ectopic beats, angina

GI: Nausea, vomiting

INTEG: Necrosis, tissue sloughing with extravasation, **gangrene**

RESP: Dyspnea

GU: Decreased urine output

Contraindications: Hypersensitivity, ventricular fibrillation, tachydysrhythmias, pheochromocytoma, pregnancy (D)

Precautions: Lactation, arterial embolism, peripheral vascular disease, hypertension, hyperthyroidism, elderly, heart disease

Pharmacokinetics:

IV: Onset 1-2 min, metabolized in liver, excreted in urine (inactive metabolites), crosses placenta

Interactions/incompatibilities:

• Do not use within 2 wk of MAOIs, or hypertensive crisis may result

• Dysrhythmias: general anesthetics

• Decreased action of norepinephrine: α-blockers

• Increased B/P: oxytocics

• Increased pressor effect: tricyclic antidepressant, MAOIs

• Incompatible with alkaline solutions: Na, HCO_3

NURSING CONSIDERATIONS

Assess:

• I&O ratio, notify MD if output < 30 cc/hr

• ECG during administration continuously, if B/P increases, drug is decreased

• B/P and pulse q5 min after parenteral route

• CVP or PWP during infusion if possible

Administer:

• Plasma expanders for hypovolemia

• IV after diluting 500-1000 ml D_5W or NS, give as infusion 2-3 ml/min; titrate to patient response

• Using 2 bottle set up so drug may be discontinued while IV is still running, use infusion pump

Perform/provide:

• Storage of reconstituted solution if refrigerated for no longer than 24 hr

• Do not use discolored solutions

Evaluate:

• For paresthesias and coldness of extremities, peripheral blood flow may decrease

• Injection site: tissue sloughing; if this occurs, administer phentolamine mixed with NS

• Therapeutic response: increased B/P with stabilization

Teach patient/family:

• Reason for drug administration

Treatment of overdose: Administer fluids, electrolyte replacement

N

---

norethindrone

(nor-eth-in′drone)

Micronor, Norlutin, Nor-QD

Func. class.: Progestogen

Chem. class.: Progesterone derivative

Action: Inhibits secretion of pituitary gonadotropins, which prevents follicular maturation, ovulation, stimulates growth of mammary tissue, antineoplastic action against endometrial cancer

Uses: Uterine bleeding (abnormal), amenorrhea, endometriosis

Dosage and routes:

• Adult: PO 5-20 mg qd days 5-25 of menstrual cycle

Endometriosis

---

italics = common side effects   ***bold italic*** = life threatening reactions

• Adult: PO 10 mg qd × 2 wk, then increased by 5 mg qd × 2 wk, up to 30 mg qd

Available forms include: Tabs 5 mg

Side effects/adverse reactions:

CNS: Dizziness, headache, migraines, depression, fatigue

CV: Hypotension, thrombophlebitis, edema, ***thromboembolism, stroke, pulmonary embolism, myocardial infarction***

GI: Nausea, vomiting, anorexia, cramps, increased weight, ***cholestatic jaundice***

EENT: Diplopia

GU: Amenorrhea, cervical erosion, breakthrough bleeding, dysmenorrhea, vaginal candidiasis, breast changes, (gynecomastia, testicular atrophy, impotence), endometriosis, ***spontaneous abortion***

INTEG: Rash, urticaria, acne, hirsutism, alopecia, oily skin, seborrhea, purpura, melasma

META: Hyperglycemia

Contraindications: Breast cancer, hypersensitivity, thromboembolic disorders, reproductive cancer, genital bleeding (abnormal, undiagnosed), pregnancy (X)

Precautions: Lactation, hypertension, asthma, blood dyscrasias, gallbladder disease, CHF, diabetes mellitus, bone disease, depression, migraine headache, convulsive disorders, hepatic disease, renal disease, family history of breast or reproductive tract cancer

Pharmacokinetics:

PO: Duration 24 hr, excreted in urine, feces, metabolized in liver

NURSING CONSIDERATIONS

Assess:

• Weight daily: notify physician of weekly weight gain >5 lb

• B/P at beginning of treatment and periodically

• I&O ratio; be alert for decreasing urinary output, increasing edema

• Liver function studies: ALT, AST, bilirubin, periodically during long-term therapy

Administer:

• Titrated dose, use lowest effective dose

• Oil solution deeply in large muscle mass (IM), rotate sites

• In one dose in AM

• With food or milk to decrease GI symptoms

• After warming to dissolve crystals

Perform/provide:

• Storage in dark area

Evaluate:

• Therapeutic response: decreased abnormal uterine bleeding, absence of amenorrhea

• Edema, hypertension, cardiac symptoms, jaundice

• Mental status: affect, mood, behavioral changes, depression

• Hypercalcemia

Teach patient/family:

• About cushingoid symptoms

• To report breast lumps, vaginal bleeding, edema, jaundice, dark urine, clay-colored stools, dyspnea, headache, blurred vision, abdominal pain, numbness or stiffness in legs, chest pain; male to report impotence or gynecomastia

• To report suspected pregnancy

Lab test interferences:

Increase: Alk phosphatase, nitrogen (urine), pregnanediol, amino acids, factors VII, VIII, IX, X

Decrease: GTT, HDL

---

* Available in Canada only

norethindrone acetate

(nor-eth-in′drone)
Aygestin, Norlutate
Func. class.: Progestogen
Chem. class.: Progesterone derivative

Action: Inhibits secretion of pituitary gonadotropins, which prevents follicular maturation, ovulation, stimulates growth of mammary tissue, antineoplastic action against endometrial cancer

Uses: Uterine bleeding (abnormal), amenorrhea, endometriosis

Dosage and routes:
• *Adult:* PO 2.5-10 mg qd days 5-25 of menstrual cycle

Endometriosis
• *Adult:* PO 5 mg qd × 2 wk, then increased by 2.5 mg qd × 2 wk, up to 15 mg qd

Available forms include: Tabs 5 mg

Side effects/adverse reactions:
CNS: Dizziness, headache, migraines, depression, fatigue
CV: Hypotension, thrombophlebitis, edema, ***thromboembolism, stroke, pulmonary embolism, myocardial infarction***
GI: Nausea, vomiting, anorexia, cramps, increased weight, ***cholestatic jaundice***
EENT: Diplopia
GU: Amenorrhea, cervical erosion, breakthrough bleeding, dysmenorrhea, vaginal candidiasis, breast changes, *gynecomastia, testicular atrophy, impotence,* endometriosis, ***spontaneous abortion***
INTEG: Rash, urticaria, acne, hirsutism, alopecia, oily skin, seborrhea, purpura, melasma
META: Hyperglycemia

Contraindications: Breast cancer, hypersensitivity, thromboembolic disorders, reproductive cancer, genital bleeding (abnormal, undiagnosed), cerebral hemorrhage, pregnancy (X)

Precautions: Lactation, hypertension, asthma, blood dyscrasias, gallbladder disease, CHF, diabetes mellitus, bone disease, depression, migraine headache, convulsive disorders, hepatic disease, renal disease, family history of breast or reproductive tract cancer

Pharmacokinetics:
PO: Duration 24 hr, excreted in urine, feces, metabolized in liver

NURSING CONSIDERATIONS

Assess:
• Weight daily; notify physician of weekly weight gain >5 lb
• B/P at beginning of treatment and periodically
• I&O ratio; be alert for decreasing urinary output, increasing edema
• Liver function studies: ALT, AST, bilirubin, periodically during long-term therapy

Administer:
• Titrated dose, use lowest effective dose
• Oil solution deeply in large muscle mass (IM), rotate sites
• In one dose in AM
• With food or milk to decrease GI symptoms
• After warming to dissolve crystals

Perform/provide:
• Storage in dark area

Evaluate:
• Therapeutic response: decreased abnormal uterine bleeding, absence of amenorrhea
• Edema, hypertension, cardiac symptoms, jaundice
• Mental status: affect, mood, behavioral changes, depression
• Hypercalcemia

N

---

italics = common side effects   ***bold italic*** = life threatening reactions

Teach patient/family:
• About cushingoid symptoms
• To report breast lumps, vaginal bleeding, edema, jaundice, dark urine, clay-colored stools, dyspnea, headache, blurred vision, abdominal pain, numbness or stiffness in legs, chest pain; male to report impotence or gynecomastia
• To monitor blood sugar, if diabetic
• To report suspected pregnancy

Lab test interferences:
Increase: Alk phosphatase, nitrogen (urine), pregnanediol, amino acids, factors VII, VIII, IX, X
Decrease: GTT, HDL

---

norfloxacin

(nor-flox′-a-sin)
Noroxin

Func. class.: Urinary antiinfective
Chem. class.: Fluoroquinolone antibacterial

Action: Interferes with conversion of intermediate DNA fragments into high-molecular-weight DNA in bacteria
Uses: Adult urinary tract infections (including complicated) caused by *E. coli, E. cloacae, P. mirabilis, K. pneumoniae,* group D strep, indole-positive *Proteus* sp., *C. freundii, S. aureus*

Dosage and routes:
Uncomplicated
• *Adult:* 400 mg bid × 7-10 days 1 hr before or 2 hr after meals
Complicated
• *Adult:* 400 mg bid × 10-21 days; 400 mg qd × 7-10 days in impaired renal function
Available forms include: Tabs 400 mg

Side effects/adverse reactions:
CNS: Headache, dizziness, fatigue, somnolence, depression, insomnia
GI: Nausea, constipation, increased ALT, AST, flatulence, heartburn, vomiting, diarrhea, dry mouth
INTEG: Rash
EENT: Visual disturbances
Contraindications: Hypersensitivity to quinolones
Precautions: Pregnancy (C), lactation, children, renal disease, seizure disorders
Pharmacokinetics:
Peak 1 hr, half-life 3-4 hr; steady state 2 days; excreted in urine as active drug, metabolites

NURSING CONSIDERATIONS
Assess:
• Kidney, liver function studies: BUN, creatinine, AST, ALT
• I&O ratio, urine pH; <5.5 is ideal
Administer:
• After clean-catch urine is obtained for C&S
• Two daily doses if urine output is high or if patient has diabetes
Perform/provide:
• Limited intake of alkaline foods, drugs: milk, dairy products, peanuts, vegetables, alkaline antacids, sodium bicarbonate
Evaluate:
• Therapeutic response: decreased pain, frequency, urgency, C&S, absence of infection
• CNS symptoms: insomnia, vertigo, headache, agitation, confusion
• Allergic reactions: fever, flushing, rash, urticaria, pruritus
Teach patient/family:
• Fluids must be increased to 3 L/day to avoid crystallization in kidneys
• If dizziness occurs, to ambulate, perform activities with assistance
• Complete full course of drug therapy

• To contact physician if adverse reaction occurs
• To take 1 hr before or 2 hr after meals; not to take antacids with or within 2 hr of this drug, use sips of water or hard candy for dry mouth
Lab test interferences:
Increase: AST, ALT, BUN, creatinine, alk phosphatase

norgestrel

(nor-jess'trel)
Ovrette, Ovral*
Func. class.: Progestogen
Chem. class.: Progesterone derivative

Action: Inhibits secretion of pituitary gonadotropins, which prevents follicular maturation, ovulation, stimulates growth of mammary tissue, antineoplastic action against endometrial cancer
Uses: Female contraception
Dosage and routes:
• *Adult:* PO 1 tablet qd
Available forms include: Tabs 0.35, 0.075 mg
Side effects/adverse reactions:
CNS: Dizziness, headache, migraines, depression, fatigue
CV: Hypotension, thrombophlebitis, edema, *thromboembolism, stroke, pulmonary embolism, myocardial infarction*
GI: Nausea, vomiting, anorexia, cramps, increased weight, *cholestatic jaundice*
EENT: Diplopia
GU: Amenorrhea, cervical erosion, breakthrough bleeding, dysmenorrhea, vaginal candidiasis, breast changes, *gynecomastia, testicular atrophy, impotence,* endometriosis, *spontaneous abortion*
INTEG: Rash, urticaria, acne, hir-

sutism, alopecia, oily skin, seborrhea, purpura, melasma
META: Hyperglycemia
Contraindications: Breast cancer, hypersensitivity, thromboembolic disorders, reproductive cancer, genital bleeding (abnormal, undiagnosed), cerebral hemorrhage, pregnancy (X)
Precautions: Lactation, hypertension, asthma, blood dyscrasias, gallbladder disease, CHF, diabetes mellitus, bone disease, depression, migraine headache, convulsive disorders, hepatic disease, renal disease, family history of breast or reproductive tract cancer
Pharmacokinetics:
PO: Duration 24 hr, excreted in urine and feces, metabolized in liver
NURSING CONSIDERATIONS
Assess:
• Weight daily; notify physician of weekly weight gain >5 lb
• B/P at beginning of treatment and periodically
• I&O ratio; be alert for decreasing urinary output, increasing edema
• Liver function studies: ALT, AST, bilirubin, periodically during long-term therapy
Administer:
• Titrated dose; use lowest effective dose
• Oil solution deeply in large muscle mass (IM), rotate sites
• In one dose in AM
• With food or milk to decrease GI symptoms
• After warming to dissolve crystals
Perform/provide:
• Storage in dark area
Evaluate:
• Therapeutic response: absence of pregnancy

N

italics = common side effects   ***bold italic*** = life threatening reactions

- Edema, hypertension, cardiac symptoms, jaundice
- Mental status: affect, mood, behavioral changes, depression
- Hypercalcemia

Teach patient/family:

- About cushingoid symptoms
- To report breast lumps, vaginal bleeding, edema, jaundice, dark urine, clay-colored stools, dyspnea, headache, blurred vision, abdominal pain, numbness or stiffness in legs, chest pain
- To report suspected pregnancy
- To monitor blood sugar, if diabetic

Lab test interferences:

Increase: Alk phosphatase, nitrogen (urine), pregnanediol, amino acids, factors VII, VIII, IX, X

Decrease: GTT, HDL

---

nortriptyline HCl

(nor-trip′ti-leen)

Aventyl, Pamelor

Func. class.: Antidepressant—tricyclic

Chem. class.: Dibenzocycloheptene—secondary amine

Action: Blocks reuptake of norepinephrine, serotonin into nerve endings, increasing action of norepinephrine, serotonin in nerve cells

Uses: Major depression

Dosage and routes:

- *Adult:* PO 25 mg tid or qid, may increase to 150 mg/day; may give daily dose hs

Available forms include: Caps 10, 25, 75 mg; sol 10 mg/5 ml

Side effects/adverse reactions:

HEMA: Agranulocytosis, thrombocytopenia, eosinophilia, leukopenia

CNS: Dizziness, drowsiness, con-

fusion, headache, anxiety, tremors, stimulation, weakness, insomnia, nightmares, EPS (elderly), increased psychiatric symptoms

GI: Constipation, dry mouth, nausea, vomiting, *paralytic ileus,* increased appetite, cramps, epigastric distress, jaundice, *hepatitis,* stomatitis

GU: Retention, acute renal failure

INTEG: Rash, urticaria, sweating, pruritus, photosensitivity

CV: Orthostatic hypotension, ECG changes, tachycardia, hypertension, palpitations

EENT: Blurred vision, tinnitus, mydriasis

Contraindications: Hypersensitivity to tricyclic antidepressants, recovery phase of myocardial infarction, convulsive disorders, prostatic hypertrophy

Precautions: Suicidal patients, severe depression, increased intraocular pressure, narrow-angle glaucoma, urinary retention, cardiac disease, hepatic disease, hyperthyroidism, electroshock therapy, elective surgery, pregnancy (C)

Pharmacokinetics:

PO: Steady state 4-19 days; metabolized by liver, excreted by kidneys, crosses placenta, excreted in breast milk, half-life 18-28 hr

Interactions/incompatibilities:

- Decreased effects of: guanethidine, clonidine, indirect acting sympathomimetics (ephedrine)
- Increased effects of: direct acting sympathomimetics (epinephrine), alcohol, barbiturates, benzodiazepines, CNS depressants
- Hyperpyretic crisis, convulsions, hypertensive episode: MAOI

NURSING CONSIDERATIONS

Assess:

- B/P (lying, standing), pulse q4h; if systolic B/P drops 20 mm Hg

hold drug, notify physician; take vital signs q4h in patients with cardiovascular disease
• Blood studies: CBC, leukocytes, differential, cardiac enzymes if patient is receiving long-term therapy
• Hepatic studies: AST, ALT, bilirubin, creatinine
• Weight qwk, appetite may increase with drug
• ECG for flattening of T wave, bundle branch block, AV block, dysrhythmias in cardiac patients

Administer:
• Increased fluids, bulk in diet if constipation, urinary retention occur
• With food or milk for GI symptoms
• Dosage hs if over-sedation occurs during day; may take entire dose hs; elderly may not tolerate once/day dosing
• Gum, hard candy, or frequent sips of water for dry mouth
• Concentrate with fruit juice, water, or milk to disguise taste

Perform/provide:
• Storage in tight, light-resistant container at room temperature
• Assistance with ambulation during beginning therapy since drowsiness/dizziness occurs
• Safety measures including siderails primarily in elderly
• Checking to see PO medication swallowed

Evaluate:
• EPS primarily in elderly: rigidity, dystonia, akathisia
• Mental status: mood, sensorium, affect, suicidal tendencies, increase in psychiatric symptoms: depression, panic
• Urinary retention, constipation; constipation is more likely to occur in children
• Withdrawal symptoms: headache, nausea, vomiting, muscle pain, weakness; do not usually occur unless drug was discontinued abruptly
• Alcohol consumption; if alcohol is consumed, hold dose until morning

Teach patient/family:
• That therapeutic effects may take 2-3 wk
• To use caution in driving or other activities requiring alertness because of drowsiness, dizziness, blurred vision
• To avoid alcohol ingestion, other CNS depressants
• Not to discontinue medication quickly after long-term use, may cause nausea, headache, malaise
• To wear sunscreen or large hat since photosensitivity occurs

Lab test interferences:
Increase: Serum bilirubin, blood glucose, alk phosphatase
False increase: Urinary catecholamines
Decrease: VMA, 5-HIAA

Treatment of overdose: ECG monitoring, induce emesis, lavage, activated charcoal, administer anticonvulsant

---

nylidrin HCl
(nye'li-drin)
Arlidin, Rolidrin, Adrin
Func. class.: Peripheral vasodilator, β-adrenergic agonist
Chem. class.: β-Adrenergic agonist-phenylisopropylamine

Action: Acts on β-adrenergic receptors to dilate arterioles in skeletal muscles; increases cardiac output, may have direct vasodilatory effect on vascular smooth muscle
Uses: Arteriosclerosis obliterans, thromboangiitis obliterans, dia-

betic vascular disease, night leg cramps, Raynaud's disease, ischemic ulcer, frostbite, acrocyanosis, acroparesthesia, thrombophlebitis, primary cochlear cell ischemia, cochlear stria ischemia, muscular or ampullar ischemia, other disturbances from labyrinth artery spasm or obstruction

Dosage and routes:
• *Adult:* PO 3-12 mg tid or qid
Available forms include: Tabs 6, 12 mg

Side effects/adverse reactions:
CV: Postural hypotension, palpitations
CNS: Dizziness, anxiety, tremors, weakness, nervousness
GI: Nausea, vomiting
INTEG: Flushing

Contraindications: Hypersensitivity, paroxysmal tachycardia, progressive angina pectoris, thyrotoxicosis, myocardial infarction

Precautions: CHF, pregnancy (C)

Pharmacokinetics:
PO: Onset 10 min, peak 30 min, duration 2 hr; slowly metabolized in liver, excreted in urine, therapeutic effect may take several weeks

Interactions/incompatibilities:
• Increased hypotension: phenothiazines, other vasodilators, antihypertensives

NURSING CONSIDERATIONS
Assess:
• B/P, pulse during treatment until stable; take B/P lying, standing; orthostatic hypotension is common

Administer:
• With meals to reduce GI upset

Perform/provide:
• Storage at room temperature

Evaluate:
• Therapeutic response: ability to walk without pain, increased pulse volume, increased temperature in

extremities or orientation, long- and short-term memory

Teach patient/family:
• That medication is not cure, may need to be taken continuously depending on condition; therapeutic response may not be evident for 2-3 mo
• That it is necessary to quit smoking to prevent excessive vasoconstriction
• To avoid hazardous activities until stabilized on medication; dizziness may occur
• That palpitations should subside as therapy continues

---

nystatin

(nye-stat'in)
Mycostatin, Nadostine,* Nilstat, O-V Statin
Func. class.: Antifungal
Chem. class.: Amphoteric polyene

Action: Interferes with fungal DNA replication; binds sterols in fungal cell membrane, which increases permeability, leaking of cell nutrients

Uses: *Candida* species causing oral, vaginal, intestinal infections

Dosage and routes:
Oral infection
• *Adult:* SUSP 400,000-600,000 U qid
• *Child and infants >3 mo:* SUSP 250,000-500,000 U qid
• *Newborn and premature infants:* SUSP 100,000 U qid
GI infection
• *Adult:* PO 500,000-1,000,000 U tid
Vaginal infection
• *Adult:* VAG TAB 100,000 U inserted high into vagina qd-bid × 2 wk

Available forms include: Tabs

500,000 U; vag tabs 100,000 U; powder 50 mill, 150 mill, 500 mill, 1 bill, 2 bill, 5 bill U; susp 100,000 U; top cream, oint, powder 100,000 U

Side effects/adverse reactions:

INTEG: Rash, urticaria (rare)

GI: Nausea, vomiting, anorexia, diarrhea, cramps

Contraindications: Hypersensitivity

Precautions: Pregnancy (B)

Pharmacokinetics:

PO: Little absorption, excreted in feces

NURSING CONSIDERATIONS

Administer:

• Oral suspension dose by placing ½ in each cheek, then swallow

• Topical dose after cleansing area; mouth may be swabbed

Perform/provide:

• Storage in refrigerator, oral susp, tabs in tight, light-resistant containers at room temperature

Evaluate:

• For allergic reaction: rash, urticaria; drug may need to be discontinued

• For predisposing factors: antibiotic therapy, pregnancy, diabetes mellitus, sexual partner infection (vaginal infections)

Teach patient/family:

• That long-term therapy may be needed to clear infection; to complete entire course of medication

• Proper hygiene: changing socks if feet are infected, using no commercial mouthwashes for mouth infection

• To avoid getting preparation on hands

• To wear light-day pad for vaginal preparations

• To avoid tight shoes, bandages when using for feet infection

• To avoid sexual contact during

treatment to minimize reinfection

• To notify physician if irritation occurs; drug may need to be discontinued

• That relief from itching may occur after 24-72 hr

---

nystatin (topical)

(nye-stat'in)

Mycostatin, Nystex, Nilstat, Mykinac

Func. class.: Local antiinfective

Chem. class.: Antifungal

Action: Interferes with fungal DNA replication; binds sterols in fungal cell membrane, which increases permeability, leaking of cell nutrients

Uses: Cutaneous vulvovaginal candidiasis, mucocutaneous fungal infections

Dosage and routes:

• *Adult and child:* TOP apply to affected area bid-tid × 14 days; VAG 1-2 tabs (100,000 U each) inserted into vagina

Available forms include: Cream, oint, powder, spray, vag tabs 100,000 U

Side effects/adverse reactions:

INTEG: Rash, urticaria, stinging, burning

Contraindications: Hypersensitivity

Precautions: Pregnancy (B), lactation

NURSING CONSIDERATIONS

Administer:

• To moist lesions with powder

• Vaginal tablets by inserting high into vagina

• Enough medication to completely cover lesions

• After cleansing with soap, water before each application, dry well

italics = common side effects   ***bold italic*** = life threatening reactions

Perform/provide:
• Storage at room temperature in dry place, protect from light, air, heat

Evaluate:
• Allergic reaction: burning, stinging, swelling, redness
• Therapeutic response: decrease in size, number of lesions, decreased itching, white patches on vulvae

Teach patient/family:
• To discontinue use and notify physician if irritation occurs
• To apply with glove to prevent further infection
• To avoid use of OTC creams, ointments, lotions unless directed by physician
• To use medical asepsis (hand washing) before, after each application

---

olsalazine sodium

Dipentum

Func. class.: Antiinflammatory
Chem. class.: Salicylate derivative

Action: Bioconverted to 5-aminosalicylic acid, which decreases inflammation

Uses: Maintenance of remission of ulcerative colitis in patients intolerant to sulfasalazine

Dosage and routes:
Adult: PO 1 g/day in 2 divided doses

Available forms include: Tabs 250 mg

Side effects/adverse reactions:
SYST: Anaphylaxis
GI: Nausea, vomiting, abdominal pain, stomatitis, hepatitis, pancreatitis, diarrhea, bloating
CNS: Headache, insomnia, hallucinations, depression, vertigo, fatigue, drug fever, chills, dizziness, drowsiness, tremors

HEMA: Leukopenia, neutropenia, thrombocytopenia, agranulocytosis, anemia
INTEG: Rash, dermatitis, urticaria, *Stevens-Johnson syndrome,* erythema, photosensitivity, alopecia
GU: Frequency, dysuria, hematuria, impotence
CV: Allergic myocarditis, 2nd degree heart block, hypertension, peripheral edema, chest pain, palpitations
RESP: Bronchospasm, shortness of breath

Contraindications: Hypersensitivity to salicylates, child <14 yr

Precautions: Pregnancy (C), lactation, impaired hepatic function, severe allergy, bronchial asthma

Pharmacokinetics:
PO: Partially absorbed, peak 1½ hr, half-life 5-10 hr, excreted in urine as 5-aminosalicylic acid and metabolites, crosses placenta

NURSING CONSIDERATIONS
Assess:
• I&O ratio: note color, character, pH of urine if drug is administered for urinary tract infections; output should be 800 ml less than intake; if urine is highly acidic, alkalization may be needed
• Kidney function studies: BUN, creatinine, urinalysis if on long-term therapy

Administer:
• With food in evenly divided doses
• Medication after C&S; repeat C&S after full course of medication completed
• With resuscitative equipment available; severe allergic reactions may occur
• Total daily dose in evenly spaced doses to help minimize GI intolerance

Perform/provide:
• Storage in tight, light-resistant containers at room temperature

---

*Available in Canada only

Evaluate:
• Therapeutic effectiveness: absence of fever, mucus in stools
• Blood dyscrasias: skin rash, fever, sore throat, bruising, bleeding, fatigue, joint pain
• Allergic reaction: rash, dermatitis, urticaria, pruritus, dyspnea, bronchospasm

Lab test interferences:
False positive: Urinary glucose test

---

omeprazole

(om-ee-pray-zole)
Prilosec

Func. class.: Antisecretory compound
Chem. class.: Benzimidazole

Action: Suppresses gastric secretion by inhibiting hydrogen/potassium ATPase enzyme system in the gastric parietal cell; characterized as a gastric acid pump inhibitor, since it blocks the final step of acid production

Uses: Gastroesophageal reflux disease (GERD), severe erosive esophagitis, poorly responsive systemic GERD, pathologic hypersecretory conditions (Zollinger-Ellison syndrome, systemic mastocytosis, multiple endocrine adenomas); possibly effective for treatment of duodenal ulcers

Dosage and routes:
Severe erosine esophagitis/poorly responsive gastroesophageal reflux disease
• *Adult:* PO 20 mg gd × 4-8 wk
Pathological hypersecretory conditions
• *Adult:* PO 60 mg/day, may increase to 120 mg tid; daily doses >80 mg should be given in divided doses

Available forms include: Cap, sus rel 20 mg

Side effects/adverse reactions
CNS: Headache, dizziness, asthenia
GI: Diarrhea, abdominal pain, vomiting, nausea, constipation, flatulence, acid regurgitation, abdominal swelling, anorexia, irritable colon, esophageal candidiasis, dry mouth
RESP: Upper respiratory infections, cough, epistaxis
INTEG: Rash, dry skin, urticaria, pruritus, alopecia
META: Hypoglycemia, increased hepatic enzymes, weight gain
EENT: Tinnitus, taste perversion
CV: Chest pain, angina, tachycardia, bradycardia, palpitations, peripheral edema
GU: Urinary tract infection, frequency, increased creatinine, ***proteinuria, hematuria,*** testicular pain, glycosuria
*HEMA: **Pancytopenia, thrombocytopenia, neutropenia, leukocytosis,*** anemia
*MISC: **Back pain,*** fever, fatigue, malaise

Contraindications: Hypersensitivity

Precautions: Pregnancy (C), lactation, children

Pharmacokinetics:
Peak: ½-3½ hr, ½ life−½-1 hr, protein binding 95%, eliminated in urine as metabolites and in feces; in the elderly the elimination rate is decreased, bioavailability is increased

Interactions/incompatibilities:
• Increased serum levels: diazepam, phenytoin
• Possible increased bleeding: warfarin

NURSING CONSIDERATIONS
Assess:
• GI system: bowel sounds q8h,

abdomen for pain, swelling, anorexia

• Hepatic enzymes: AST, ALT during treatment

Administer:

• Before eating; swallow capsule whole; do not open, chew, or crush

Evaluate:

• Therapeutic response: absence of epigastric pain, swelling, fullness

Teach patient/family:

• To report severe diarrhea; drug may need to be discontinued

• That the diabetic patient should be aware that hypoglycemia may occur

---

opium tincture/ camphorated opium tincture

(oh'pee-um)

Paregoric, Paregorique*

Func. class.: Antidiarrheal

Chem. class.: Opium/opium and morphine

Controlled Substance Schedule III/II (depending on amount of opium)

Action: Antiperistaltic activity

Uses: Diarrhea (cause undetermined); to treat withdrawal symptoms in infants born to addicted mothers

Dosage and routes:

• *Adult:* PO 0.3-1 ml qid, not to exceed 6 ml/day (tincture) or 5-10 ml bid-qid (camphorated)

• *Child:* PO 0.25-0.5 ml/kg qd-qid (camphorated)

Withdrawal

• *Neonates:* PO 1:25 dilution, 3-6 gtt q3-6 hr (tincture), dosage adjustment is made to control symptoms

Available forms include: Liq 2 mg morphine equivalent per 5 ml

Side effects/adverse reactions:

CNS: Dizziness, drowsiness, fainting, flushing, physical dependency

CNS depression

GI: Nausea, vomiting, constipation, abdominal pain

Contraindications: Hypersensitivity

Precautions: Liver disease, addiction-prone individuals, prostatic hypertrophy (severe), pregnancy (B)

Pharmacokinetics:

PO: Duration 4 hr, half-life 2-3 hr; metabolized in liver, excreted in urine

Interactions/incompatibilities:

• Increased action of both drugs: other CNS depressants

• Increased CNS toxicity: cimetidine

NURSING CONSIDERATIONS

Assess:

• Electrolytes (K, Na, Cl) if on long-term therapy

• Skin turgor q8h if dehydration is suspected

Administer:

• Undiluted with water

• For 48 hr only

Evaluate:

• Therapeutic response: decreased diarrhea

• Bowel pattern before; for rebound constipation

• Response after 48 hr; if no response, drug should be discontinued

• Dehydration in children

• Abdominal distention; toxic megacolon may occur in ulcerative colitis

Teach patient/family:

• To avoid OTC products (cough, cold, hay fever preparations) unless directed by physician

• Not to exceed recommended dose

• May be habit-forming

---

*Available in Canada only

oral contraceptives

Func. class.: Hormone
Chem. class.: Estrogen/progestin combinations

Action: Prevents ovulation by suppressing follicle stimulating, luteinizing hormone
Uses: To prevent pregnancy, endometriosis, hypermenorrhea
Dosage and routes:
• *Adult:* PO 1 qd starting on day 5 of menstrual cycle; day 1 is 1st day of period
20/21 tablet packs
• *Adult:* PO 1 qd starting on day 7 of menstrual cycle; day 1 is 1st day of period, then on 20 or 21 days, off 7 days
28 tablet packs
• *Adult:* PO 1 qd continuously
Biphasic
• *Adult:* 1 qd × 10 days, then next color 1 qd × 11 days
Triphasic
• *Adult:* 1 qd; check package insert for each new brand
Endometriosis
• *Adult:* PO 1 qd × 20 days from day 5 to 24 of cycle
• *Adult:* PO 1 qd; check package insert for specific instructions
Available forms include: Check specific brand
Side effects/adverse reactions:
GI: Nausea, vomiting, cramps, diarrhea, bloating, constipation, change in appetite, *cholestatic jaundice*
INTEG: Chloasma, melasma, acne, rash, urticaria, erythema, pruritus, hirsutism, alopecia, photosensitivity
CV: Increased B/P, thromboembolic conditions, fluid retention, edema
ENDO: Decreased glucose tolerance, increased TBG, PBI, T_4, T_3
GU: Breakthrough bleeding, amenorrhea, spotting, dysmenorrhea, galactorrhea, endocervical hyperplasia, vaginitis, cystitis-like syndrome, breast change
CNS: Depression, fatigue, dizziness, nervousness, anxiety, headache
EENT: Optic neuritis, retinal thrombosis, cataracts
HEMA: Increased fibrinogen, clotting factor
Contraindications: Pregnancy (X), lactation, reproductive cancer, thrombophlebitis, MI, hepatic tumors, hepatic disease, CAD, women 40 and over, CVA
Precautions: Depression, hypertension, renal disease, seizure disorders, lupus erythematosus, rheumatic disease, migraine headache, amenorrhea, irregular menses, breast cancer (fibrocystic), gallbladder disease, diabetes mellitus, heavy smoking, acute mononucleosis, sickle cell disease
Pharmacokinetics: Excreted in breast milk
Interactions/incompatibilities:
• Decreased effectiveness of oral contraceptives: anticonvulsants, rifampin, analgesics, antibiotics, antihistamines, chenodiol, griseofulvin
• Decreased action of: oral anticoagulants
• Increased clotting: aminocaproic acid
NURSING CONSIDERATIONS
Assess:
• Glucose, thyroid function, liver function tests
Evaluate:
• Therapeutic response: absence of pregnancy, endometriosis, hypermenorrhea
• Reproductive changes: change in

---

italics = common side effects   ***bold italic*** = life threatening reactions

breasts, tumors, positive Pap smear; drug should be discontinued if changes occur

Teach patient/family:
• Detection of clots using Homan's sign
• To use sunscreen or avoid sunlight; photosensitivity can occur
• To take at same time each day to ensure equal drug level
• To report GI symptoms that occur after 4 mo
• To use another birth control method during 1st week of oral contraceptive use
• To take another tablet as soon as possible if one is missed
• That after drug is discontinued, pregnancy may not occur for several months
• To report abdominal pain, change in vision, shortness of breath, change in menstrual flow, spotting, breakthrough bleeding, breast lumps, swelling, headache, severe leg pain
• That continuing medical care is needed: PAP smear and gynecologic examinations q6 mo
• To notify MD and dentist of oral contraceptive use

Lab test interferences:
Increase: Pro-time, clotting factors VII, VIII, IX, X, TBG, PBI, T_4, platelet aggregability, BSP, triglycerides, bilirubin, AST, ALT
Decrease: T_3, antithrombin III, folate, metyrapone test, GTT, 17-OHCS

orphenadrine citrate

(or-fen'a-dreen)
Banflex, Flexon, Myolin, Norflex, Ro-Orphena, X-Otag

Func. class.: Skeletal muscle relaxant, central acting; anticholinergics
Chem. class.: Tertiary amine

Action: Acts centrally on skeletal muscle to relax, inhibit muscle spasm
Uses: Pain in musculoskeletal conditions
Dosage and routes:
• *Adult:* PO 100 mg bid; IM/IV 60 mg q12h
Available forms include: Tabs 100 mg; tabs sus rel 100 mg; inj IM, IV 30 mg/ml
Side effects/adverse reactions:
*HEMA: **Aplastic anemia***
CNS: Dizziness, weakness, fatigue, drowsiness, headache, disorientation, insomnia, stimulation, hallucination, agitation
EENT: Nasal congestion, blurred vision, increased intraocular pressure, mydriasis
CV: Orthostatic hypotension, tachycardia
GI: Nausea, vomiting, constipation, dry mouth
GU: Urinary frequency, hesitancy, retention
INTEG: Rash, pruritus, urticaria
Contraindications: Hypersensitivity, narrow-angle glaucoma, GI obstruction, myasthenia gravis, stenosing peptic ulcer, bladder neck obstruction, cardiospasm
Precautions: Pregnancy (C), children, cardiac disease, tachycardia
Pharmacokinetics:
PO: Peak 2 hr, duration 4-6 hr, half-life 14 hr, metabolized in liver, excreted in urine (unchanged)

Interactions/incompatibilities:
• Increased CNS effects: propoxyphene, other anticholinergics, oral contraceptives

NURSING CONSIDERATIONS
Assess:
• Monitor vital signs q10-15 min during administration
• Blood studies: CBC, WBC, differential; blood dyscrasias may occur (rare)
• I&O ratio; check for urinary retention, frequency, hesitancy
• Dosage. Even slight overdose can cause toxicity

Administer:
• With meals for GI symptoms
• IV undiluted, or diluted in 5-10 ml sterile H₂O for inj; give 60 mg or less over 5 min
• When giving IV may cause paradoxical initial bradycardia; usually disappears in 2 min

Perform/provide:
• Assistance with ambulation if dizziness, drowsiness occurs

Evaluate:
• Therapeutic response: decreased rigidity, spasms
• Allergic reactions: rash, fever, respiratory distress
• Blood dyscrasias: temperature, bleeding, fatigue (rare)
• CNS symptoms: dizziness, drowsiness, psychiatric symptoms

Teach patient/family:
• Not to discontinue medication quickly; insomnia, nausea, headache will occur
• Not to take with alcohol, other CNS depressants
• To avoid altering activities while taking this drug
• To avoid hazardous activities if drowsiness, dizziness occurs
• To avoid using OTC medication: cough preparations, antihistamines, unless directed by physician

• To use gum, frequent sips of water for dry mouth

---

oxacillin sodium
(ox-a-sill′in)
Bactocill, Prostaphilin
Func. class.: Broad-spectrum antibiotic
Chem. class.: Penicillinase-resistant penicillin

Action: Interferes with cell wall replication of susceptible organisms; osmotically unstable cell wall swells, bursts from osmotic pressure

Uses: Effective for gram-positive cocci *(S. aureus, S. pneumoniae)*, infections caused by penicillinase-producing *Staphylococcus*

Dosage and routes:
• *Adult:* PO 2-6 g/day in divided doses q4-6h; IM/IV 2-12 g/day in divided doses q4-6h
• *Child:* PO 50-100 mg/kg/day in divided doses q6h; IM/IV 50-100 mg/kg/day in divided doses q4-6h
Available forms include: Caps 250, 500 mg; powder for oral susp 250 mg/5 ml; powder for inj IM, IV 250, 500 mg, 1, 2, 4, 10 g; IV INF 1, 2 g

Side effects/adverse reactions:
HEMA: Anemia, increased bleeding time, *bone marrow depression, granulocytopenia*
GI: Nausea, vomiting, diarrhea, increased AST, ALT, abdominal pain, glossitis, colitis
GU: Oliguria, proteinuria, hematuria, vaginitis, moniliasis, glomerulonephritis
CNS: Lethargy, hallucinations, anxiety, depression, twitching, *coma, convulsions*
Contraindications: Hypersensitivity to penicillins

---

italics = common side effects   ***bold italic*** = life threatening reactions

Precautions: Pregnancy (B), hypersensitivity to cephalosporins, neonates

Pharmacokinetics:

PO/IM: Peak 30-60 min, duration 4-6 hr

IV: Peak 5 min, duration 4-6 hr, half-life 30-60 min, metabolized in the liver, excreted in urine, bile, breast milk, crosses placenta

Interactions/incompatibilities:

• Decreased antimicrobial effectiveness of oxacillin: tetracyclines, erythromycins

• Increased oxacillin concentrations: aspirin, probenecid

NURSING CONSIDERATIONS

Assess:

• I&O ratio; report hematuria, oliguria since penicillin in high doses is nephrotoxic

• Any patient with compromised renal system since drug is excreted slowly in poor renal system function; toxicity may occur rapidly

• Liver studies: AST, ALT

• Blood studies: WBC, RBC, Hct/Hgb, bleeding time

• Renal studies: urinalysis, protein, blood

• C&S before drug therapy; drug may be taken as soon as culture is taken

Administer:

• IV after diluting 500 mg or less/5 ml sterile H_2O or NaCl for inj; may dilute further in compatible sol and give 1 g/10 min; may be given as infusion over 6 hr

• Drug after C&S has been completed

Perform/provide:

• Adrenalin, suction, tracheostomy set, endotracheal intubation equipment

• Scratch test to assess allergy, after securing order from physician; usually done when penicillin is only drug of choice

• Storage in tight container; refrigerate reconstituted solution up to 2 wk

Evaluate:

• Therapeutic effectiveness: absence of fever, draining wounds

• Bowel pattern before and during treatment

• Skin eruptions after administration of penicillin to 1 wk after discontinuing drug

• Respiratory status: rate, character, wheezing, tightness in chest

• Allergies before initiation of treatment, and reaction of each medication; highlight allergies on chart, Kardex

Teach patient/family:

• Aspects of drug therapy including need to complete course of medication to ensure organism death (10-14 days); culture may be taken after completed course

• To report sore throat, fever, fatigue; (could indicate superimposed infection)

• To wear or carry Medic Alert ID if allergic to penicillins

• To take on empty stomach with a full glass of water

Lab test interferences:

False positive: Urine glucose, urine protein

Treatment of overdose: Withdraw drug, maintain airway, administer epinephrine, aminophylline, O_2, IV corticosteroids for anaphylaxis

---

oxamniquine

(ox-am'ni-kwin)

Vansil

Func. class.: Anthelmintic

Chem. class.: Tetrahydroquinone derivative

Action: Causes paralysis, contraction, leading to dislodgement of suckers; they are carried to liver where phagocytosis takes place

Uses: Schistosomiasis

Dosage and routes:
• *Adult and child >30 kg:* PO 12-15 mg/kg as single dose
• *Child <30 kg:* PO 20 mg/kg in 2 divided doses q2-8h

Available forms include: Caps 250 mg

Side effects/adverse reactions:
INTEG: Rash, pruritus, urticaria
CNS: Dizziness, headache, drowsiness, insomnia, **convulsions,** hallucination, personality changes, stimulation
EENT: Bad taste, oral irritation
GI: Nausea, vomiting, anorexia, abdominal pain
HEMA: Increased sed rate, reticulocyte count, increase or decrease in leukocytes

Contraindications: Hypersensitivity

Precautions: Pregnancy (C), lactation, seizure disorders

Pharmacokinetics:
PO: Peak 1-1½ hr, half-life 1-2½ hr, excreted in urine, (unchanged/metabolites)

NURSING CONSIDERATIONS
Assess:
• Stools during entire treatment, 1, 3 mo after treatment; specimens must be sent to lab while still warm

Administer:
• PO after meals to avoid GI symptoms

Perform/provide:
• Storage in tight container, cool environment

Evaluate:
• Therapeutic response: expulsion of worms, 3 negative stool cultures after completion of treatment
• For allergic reaction: rash, itching, urticaria

• For infection in other family members since infection from person to person is common

Teach patient/family:
• Proper hygiene after BM including handwashing technique; tell patient to avoid putting fingers in mouth
• That infected person should sleep alone; do not shake bed linen; change bed linen daily, wash in hot water
• To clean toilet qd with disinfectant (green soap solution)
• Need for compliance with dosage schedule, duration of treatment
• That urine may turn orange or red
• To avoid hazardous activities since drowsiness occurs
• That seizures may recur in patient who is controlled on medication

Lab test interferences:
Interferes: Urinalysis

---

oxandrolone
(ox-an′droe-lone)
Anavar
Func. class.: Androgenic anabolic steroid
Chem. class.: Halogenated testosterone derivative

Action: Increases weight by building body tissue, increases potassium, phosphorus, chloride, nitrogen levels, increases bone development

Uses: Tissue building after steroid therapy, osteoporosis, prolonged immobility

Dosage and routes:
• *Adult:* PO 2.5 mg bid-qid, not to exceed 20 mg qd × 2-3 wk
• *Child:* PO 0.25 mg/kg/day × 2-4 wk, not to exceed 3 mo

Available forms include: Tabs 2.5 mg

---

italics = common side effects   **bold italic** = life threatening reactions

Side effects/adverse reactions:
INTEG: Rash, acneiform lesions, oily hair, skin, flushing, sweating, acne vulgaris, alopecia, hirsutism
CNS: Dizziness, headache, fatigue, tremors, paresthesias, flushing, sweating, anxiety, lability, insomnia
MS: Cramps, spasms
CV: Increased B/P
GU: **Hematuria,** amenorrhea, vaginitis, decrease libido, decreased breast size, clitoral hypertrophy, testicular atrophy
GI: Nausea, vomiting, constipation, weight gain, **cholestatic jaundice**
EENT: Carpal tunnel syndrome, conjunctival edema, nasal congestion
ENDO: Abnormal GTT
Contraindications: Severe renal disease, severe cardiac disease, severe hepatic disease, hypersensitivity, pregnancy (X), lactation, genital bleeding (abnormal)
Precautions: Diabetes mellitus, CV disease, MI
Pharmacokinetics:
PO: Metabolized in liver, excreted in urine, crosses placenta, excreted in breast milk
Interactions/incompatibilities:
• Increased effects of: oral antidiabetics, oxyphenbutazone
• Increased PT: anticoagulants
• Edema: ACTH, adrenal steroids
• Decreased effects of: insulin
NURSING CONSIDERATIONS
Assess:
• Weight daily, notify physician if weekly weight gain is >5 lb
• B/P q4h
• I&O ratio; be alert for decreasing urinary output, increasing edema
• Growth rate in children since growth rate may be uneven (linear/ bone browth) when used for extended time
• Electrolytes: K, Na, Cl, Ca; cholesterol
• Liver function studies: ALT, AST, bilirubin
Administer:
• Titrated dose, use lowest effective dose
Perform/provide:
• Diet with increased calories and protein; decrease sodium if edema occurs
• Supportive drug of enemia
Evaluate:
• Therapeutic response: occurs in 4-6 wk in osteoporosis
• Edema, hypertension, cardiac symptoms, jaundice
• Mental status: affect, mood, behavioral changes, aggression
• Signs of masculinization in female: increased libido, deepening of voice, breast tissue, enlarged clitoris, menstrual irregularities; male: gynecomastia, impotence, testicular atrophy
• Hypercalcemia: lethargy, polyuria, polydipsia, nausea, vomiting, constipation; drug may need to be decreased
• Hypoglycemia in diabetics, since oral anticoagulant action is decreased
Teach patient/family:
• That drug needs to be combined with complete health plan: diet, rest, exercise
• To notify physician if therapeutic response decreases
• Not to discontinue this medication abruptly
• About change in sex characteristics
• Women to report menstrual irregularities
• That 1-3 mo course is necessary for response in breast cancer

---

• Procedure for use of buccal tablets (requires 30-60 min to dissolve, change absorption site with each dose; do not eat, drink, chew, or smoke while tablet is in place)

Lab test interferences:
Increase: Serum cholesterol, blood glucose, urine glucose
Decrease: Serum calcium, serum potassium, T_4, T_3, thyroid ^{131}I uptake test, urine 17-OHCS, 17-KS, PBI, BSP

---

oxazepam

(ox-a'ze-pam)
Apo-Oxazepam,* Novoxapam,* Serax

Func. class.: Antianxiety
Chem. class.: Benzodiazepine

Controlled Substance Schedule IV

Action: Depresses subcortical levels of CNS, including limbic system and reticular formation

Uses: Anxiety, alcohol withdrawal

Dosage and routes:
Anxiety
• *Adult:* PO 10-30 mg tid-qid
Alcohol withdrawal
• *Adult:* PO 15-30 mg tid-qid

Available forms include: Caps 10, 15, 30 mg, tabs 15 mg

Side effects/adverse reactions:
CNS: Dizziness, drowsiness, confusion, headache, anxiety, tremors, fatigue, depression, insomnia, hallucinations, paradoxical excitement, transient amnesia
GI: Nausea, vomiting, anorexia
INTEG: Rash, dermatitis, itching
*CV: Orthostatic hypotension, **ECG changes, tachycardia,*** hypotension
EENT: Blurred vision, tinnitus, mydriasis

Contraindications: Hypersensitivity to benzodiazepines, narrowangle glaucoma, psychosis, pregnancy (D), child <12 yr

Precautions: Elderly, debilitated, hepatic disease, renal disease

Pharmacokinetics:
PO: Peak 2-4 hr, metabolized by liver, excreted by kidneys, half-life 5-15 hr

Interactions/incompatibilities:
• Decreased effects of oxazepam: oral contraceptives, valproic acid
• Increased effects of oxazepam: CNS depressants, alcohol, disulfiram, oral contraceptives

NURSING CONSIDERATIONS
Assess:
• B/P (lying, standing), pulse; if systolic B/P drops 20 mm Hg, hold drug, notify physician; respirations q5-15 min if given IV
• Blood studies: CBC during longterm therapy, blood dyscrasias have occurred rarely
• Hepatic studies: AST, ALT, bilirubin, creatinine, LDH, alk phosphatase

Administer:
• With food or milk for GI symptoms
• Sugarless gum, hard candy, frequent sips of water for dry mouth

Perform/provide:
• Assistance with ambulation during beginning therapy; drowsiness/dizziness occurs
• Safety measures, including siderails
• Check to see PO medication has been swallowed

Evaluate:
• Therapeutic response: decreased anxiety, restlessness, insomnia
• Mental status: mood, sensorium, affect, sleeping pattern, drowsiness, dizziness
• Physical dependency, withdrawal symptoms: headache, nausea,

---

italics = common side effects   ***bold italic*** = life threatening reactions

vomiting, muscle pain, weakness, tremors, *convulsions* after long-term use
• Suicidal tendencies

Teach patient/family:
• That drug may be taken with food
• Not to be used for everyday stress or used longer than 4 mo, unless directed by physician; not to take more than prescribed dose, may be habit forming
• Avoid OTC preparations (cough, cold, hay fever) unless approved by physician
• To avoid driving, activities that require alertness, since drowsiness may ocur
• To avoid alcohol ingestion or other psychotropic medications unless prescribed by physician
• Not to discontinue medication abruptly after long-term use
• To rise slowly or fainting may occur
• That drowsiness might worsen at beginning of treatment

Lab test interferences:
Increase: AST/ALT, serum bilirubin
Decrease: RAIU
False increase: 17-OHCS
Treatment of overdose: Lavage, VS, supportive care

---

oxidized cellulose

Oxycel, Surgicel
Func. class.: Hemostatic
Chem. class.: Cellulose product

Action: Absorbs blood, acts like an artificial clot
Uses: Hemostasis in surgery, oral surgery, exodontia
Dosage and routes:
Adult and child: TOP apply using sterile technique as needed, remove

after bleeding stops, if possible, or leave in place if needed
Available forms include: TOP knitted fabric

Side effects/adverse reactions:
EENT: Sneezing, burning in epistaxis
INTEG: Burning, stinging, encapsulation of fluid, foreign bodies
CNS: Headache in epistaxis
Contraindications: Hypersensitivity, large artery hemorrhage, oozing surfaces, implantation in bone deficit, placement around optic nerve, and chiasm

NURSING CONSIDERATIONS
Administer:
• Dry, use only amount needed to control bleeding
• Loosely, remove excess before closure in surgery; irrigate first, then remove using sterile technique
• Using sterile technique
Evaluate:
• Allergy: fever, rash, itching, burning, stinging

---

oxtriphylline

(ox-trye'fi-lin)
Choledyl, Novotriphyl,* Theophyllinate, Theophylline Choline
Func. class.: Bronchodilator, spasmolytic
Chem. class.: Choline salt of theophylline

Action: Relaxes smooth muscle of respiratory system by blocking phosphodiesterase, which increases cyclic AMP; 64% theophylline
Uses: Acute bronchial asthma, reversible bronchospasm in chronic bronchitis and COPD
Dosage and routes:
• *Adult and child >12 yr:* PO 200 mg qid

• *Child 2-12 yr:* PO 4 mg/kg q6h; may be increased to desired response, therapeutic level
Available forms include: Elix 100 mg/5 ml; syr 50 mg/5 ml; tabs 100, 200, 400, 600 mg
Side effects/adverse reactions:
*CNS: Anxiety, restlessness, insomnia, dizziness, **convulsions,** headache, light-headedness*
CV: Palpitations, sinus tachycardia, hypotension
GI: Nausea, vomiting, anorexia, diarrhea, bitter taste, dyspepsia
RESP: Increased rate
INTEG: Flushing, urticaria
Contraindications: Hypersensitivity to xanthines, tachydysrhythmias
Precautions: Elderly, CHF, cor pulmonale, hepatic disease, active peptic ulcer disease, diabetes mellitus, hyperthyroidism, hypertension, children, pregnancy (C), glaucoma, prostatic hypertrophy
Pharmacokinetics:
SOL: Peak 1 hr, metabolized in liver, excreted in urine, breast milk, crosses placenta
Interactions/incompatibilities:
• Increased action of oxtriphylline: cimetidine, erythromycin, troleandomycin
• May increase effects of: anticoagulants, coffee
• Cardiotoxicity: beta blockers
• Decreased effect of: lithium
NURSING CONSIDERATIONS
Assess:
• Therapeutic blood levels; toxicity may occur with small increase above therapeutic level
• Therapeutic theophylline levels: 11-20
• Smoking reduces effects of theophyllines, requiring larger doses
Administer:
• PO after meals to decrease GI symptoms; absorption may be affected
• After meals, hs
Perform/provide:
• Storage in closed container, away from heat, protect elixir from light
Evaluate:
• Therapeutic response: absence of dyspnea, wheezing
• Respiratory rate, rhythm, depth; auscultate lung fields bilaterally; notify physician of abnormalities
• Allergic reactions: rash, urticaria; if these occur, drug should be discontinued
Teach patient/family:
• To check OTC medications, current prescription medications for ephedrine, which will increase stimulation
• To avoid hazardous activities; dizziness may occur
• If GI upset occurs, to take drug with 8 oz water; avoid food; absorption may be decreased
• To notify physician of toxicity: nausea, vomiting, anxiety, convulsions, insomnia, rapid pulse
• To notify physician of change in smoking habit; may need to change dose

oxybutynin chloride
(ox-i-byoo'ti-nin)
Ditropan
Func. class.: Spasmolytic
Chem. class.: Synthetic tertiary amine

Action: Relaxes smooth muscles in urinary tract
Uses: Antispasmodic for neurogenic bladder
Dosage and routes:
• *Adult:* PO 5 mg bid-tid, not to exceed 5 mg qid

• *Child >5 yr:* PO 5 mg bid, not to exceed 5 mg tid

Available forms include: Sol 5 mg/ 5 ml; tabs 5 mg

Side effects/adverse reactions:

*HEMA: **Leukopenia, eosinophilia***

*CNS: Anxiety, restlessness, dizziness, **convulsions**, headache, drowsiness, confusion*

CV: Palpitations, sinus tachycardia, hypotension

GI: Nausea, vomiting, anorexia, abdominal pain, constipation

GU: Dysuria, retention, hesitancy

INTEG: Urticaria, dermatitis

EENT: Blurred vision, increased intraocular tension, dry mouth, throat

Contraindications: Hypersensitivity, GI obstruction, GI hemorrhage, GU obstruction, glaucoma, severe colitis, myasthenia gravis, unstable CV status in acute hemorrhage

Precautions: Pregnancy (C), lactation, suspected glaucoma, children <12 yr

Pharmacokinetics: Onset ½-1 hr, peak 3-4 hr, duration 6-10 hr, metabolized by liver, excreted in urine

NURSING CONSIDERATIONS

Evaluate:

• Urinary status: dysuria, frequency, nocturia, incontinence

• Allergic reactions: rash, urticaria; if these occur, drug should be discontinued

Teach patient/family

• To avoid hazardous activities; dizziness may occur

---

oxycodone HCl

(ox-i-koe'done)

Supeudol*; Combinations—Codoxy, Percocet,* Percocet-Demi, Percodan, Tylox

Func. class.: Narcotic analgesics

Chem. class.: Opiate, semisynthetic derivative

Controlled Substance Schedule II

Action: Inhibits ascending pain pathways in CNS, increases pain threshold, alters pain perception

Uses: Moderate to severe pain

Dosage and routes:

• *Adult:* REC 1-3 supp/day prn (Supeubol)

• *Child:* PO ¼-½ tab q6h prn (Percodan-Demi)

• *Adult:* PO 1-2 tab q6h prn (Combinations)

Available forms include: Tabs 5 mg; sol 5 mg/5ml

Side effects/adverse reactions:

CNS: Drowsiness, dizziness, confusion, headache, sedation, euphoria

GI: Nausea, vomiting, anorexia, constipation, cramps

GU: Increased urinary output, dysuria, urinary retention

INTEG: Rash, urticaria, bruising, flushing, diaphoresis, pruritus

EENT: Tinnitus, blurred vision, miosis, diplopia

CV: Palpitations, bradycardia, change in B/P

*RESP: **Respiratory depression***

Contraindications: Hypersensitivity, addiction (narcotic)

Precautions: Addictive personality, pregnancy (B), lactation, increased intracranial pressure, MI (acute), severe heart disease, respiratory depression, hepatic disease, renal disease, child <18 yr

Pharmacokinetics:

PO: Onset 10-15 min, peak ½-1 hr, duration 4-5 hr; detoxified by liver, excreted in urine, crosses placenta, excreted in breast milk

Interactions/incompatibilities:

• Increased effects with other CNS depressants: alcohol, narcotics, sedative/hypnotics, antipsychotics, skeletal muscle relaxants

NURSING CONSIDERATIONS

Assess:

• I&O ratio; check for decreasing

output; may indicate urinary retention

Administer:
• With antiemetic if nausea, vomiting occur
• When pain is beginning to return; determine dosage interval by patient response

Perform/provide:
• Storage in light-resistant area at room temperature
• Assistance with ambulation
• Safety measures: siderails, night light, call bell within easy reach

Evaluate:
• Therapeutic response: decrease in pain
• CNS changes: dizziness, drowsiness, hallucinations, euphoria, LOC, pupil reaction
• Allergic reactions: rash, urticaria
• Respiratory dysfunction: respiratory depression, character, rash, rhythm; notify physician if respirations are <10/min
• Need for pain medication, physical dependence

Teach patient/family:
• To report any symptoms of CNS changes, allergic reactions
• That physical dependency may result when used for extended periods of time
• That withdrawal symptoms may occur: nausea, vomiting, cramps, fever, faintness, anorexia

Lab test interferences:
Increase: Amylase

Treatment of overdose: Narcan 0.2-0.8 IV, O_2, IV fluids, vasopressors

oxymetazoline HCl (nasal)

(ox-i-met-az'oh-leen)

Afrin, Afrin Pediatric Nose Drops, Dristan Long-Lasting, Duramist, Duration, Nafrine,* Nostrilla, NTZ Long-Acting, Sinex Long-Lasting, St. Joseph's Decongestant for Children

Func. class.: Nasal decongestant
Chem. class.: Sympathomimetic amine

Action: Produces vasoconstriction (rapid, long-acting) of arterioles, thereby decreasing fluid exudation, mucosal engorgement

Uses: Nasal congestion

Dosage and routes:
• *Adult and child >6 yr:* INSTILL 2-3 gtts or sprays to each nostril bid
• *Child 2-6 yr:* INSTILL 2-3 gtts or sprays .025% sol bid, not to exceed 5 days

Available forms include: Sol 0.025%, 0.05%

Side effects/adverse reactions:
GI: Nausea, vomiting, anorexia
EENT: Irritation, burning, sneezing, stinging, dryness, rebound congestion
INTEG: Contact dermatitis
CNS: Anxiety, restlessness, tremors, weakness, insomnia, dizziness, fever, headache

Contraindications: Hypersensitivity to sympathomimetic amines

Precautions: Child <6 yr, elderly, diabetes, cardiovascular disease, hypertension, hyperthyroidism, increased ICP, prostatic hypertrophy, pregnancy (C), glaucoma

Interactions/incompatibilities:
• Hypertension: MAOIs, β-adrenergic blockers
• Hypotension: methyldopa, mecamylamine, reserpine

O

---

italics = common side effects   ***bold italic*** = life threatening reactions

NURSING CONSIDERATIONS
Administer:
- No more than q4h
- For <4 consecutive days

Perform/provide:
- Environmental humidification to decrease nasal congestion, dryness
- Storage in light-resistant containers; do not expose to high temperatures

Evaluate:
- For redness, swelling, pain in nasal passages

Teach patient/family:
- Stinging may occur for a few applications; drying of mucosa may be decreased by environmental humidification
- To notify physician if irregular pulse, insomnia, dizziness, or tremors occur
- Proper administration to avoid systemic absorption

---

oxymetholone
(ox-i-meth'oh-lone)
Adroyd, Anadrol-50, Anapolon 50*

Func. class.: Androgenic anabolic steroid
Chem. class.: Halogenated testosterone derivative

Action: Increases weight by building body tissue, increases potassium, phosphorus, chloride, and nitrogen levels, increases bone development

Uses: Tissue building after steroid therapy, osteoporosis, aplastic anemia, anemias caused by deficient RBC production

Dosage and routes:
Aplastic anemia
- *Adult and child:* PO 1-5 mg/kg/day, titrated to patient response, not to exceed 3 months

Osteoporosis/tissue building (possible indication)
- *Adult:* PO 5-15 mg/day, not to exceed 30 mg/day or 3 mo
- *Child >6 yr:* PO up to 10 mg/day, not to exceed 1 mo
- *Child <6 yr:* PO 1.25 mg qd-qid, not to exceed 1 mo

Available forms include: Tabs 50 mg

Side effects/adverse reactions:
INTEG: Rash, acneiform lesions, oily hair, skin, flushing, sweating, acne vulgaris, alopecia, hirsutism
CNS: Dizziness, headache, fatigue, tremors, paresthesias, flushing, sweating, anxiety, lability, insomnia
MS: Cramps, spasms
CV: Increased B/P
GU: **Hematuria,** amenorrhea, vaginitis, decreased libido, decreased breast size, clitoral hypertrophy, testicular atrophy
GI: Nausea, vomiting, constipation, weight gain, **cholestatic jaundice**
EENT: Carpal tunnel syndrome, conjunctival edema, nasal congestion
ENDO: Abnormal GTT

Contraindications: Severe renal disease, severe cardiac disease, severe hepatic disease, hypersensitivity, pregnancy (X), lactation, genital bleeding (abnormal)

Precautions: Diabetes mellitus, CV disease, MI

Pharmacokinetics:
PO: Metabolized in liver, excreted in urine, crosses placenta, excreted in breast milk

Interactions/incompatibilities:
- Increased effects of: oral antidiabetics, oxyphenbutazone
- Increased PT: anticoagulants
- Edema: ACTH, adrenal steroids
- Decreased effects of: insulin

NURSING CONSIDERATIONS
Assess:
• Weight daily, notify physician if weekly weight gain is >5 lb
• B/P q4h
• I&O ratio; be alert for decreasing urinary output, increasing edema
• Growth rate in children since growth rate may be uneven (linear/bone browth) when used for extended period
• Electrolytes: K, Na, Cl, Ca; cholesterol
• Liver function studies: ALT, AST, bilirubin
Administer:
• Titrated dose, use lowest effective dose
Perform/provide:
• Diet with increased calories and protein; decrease sodium if edema occurs
• Supportive drug of anemia
Evaluate:
• Therapeutic response: occurs in 4-6 wk in osteoporosis
• Edema, hypertension, cardiac symptoms, jaundice
• Mental status: affect, mood, behavioral changes, aggression
• Signs of masculinization in female: increased libido, deepening of voice, breast tissue, enlarged clitoris, menstrual irregularities; male: gynecomastia, impotence, testicular atrophy
• Hypercalcemia: lethargy, polyuria, polydipsia, nausea, vomiting, constipation; drug may need to be decreased
• Hypoglycemia in diabetics, since oral anticoagulant action is decreased
Teach patient/family:
• Drug needs to be combined with complete health plan: diet, rest, exercise
• To notify physician if therapeutic response decreases
• Not to discontinue this medication abruptly
• About changes in sex characteristics
• Women to report menstrual irregularities
• That 1-3 mo course is necessary for response in breast cancer
• Procedure for use of buccal tablets (requires 30-60 min to dissolve, change absorption site with each dose; do not eat, drink, chew, or smoke while tablet is in place)
Lab test interferences:
Increase: Serum cholesterol, blood glucose, urine glucose
Decrease: Serum calcium, serum potassium, T_4, T_3, thyroid ^{131}I uptake test, urine 17-OHCS, 17-KS, PBI, BSP

---

oxymorphone HCl
(ox-i-mor-fone)
Numorphan
Func. class.: Narcotic analgesics
Chem. class.: Opiate, semisynthetic phenanthrene derivative

Controlled Substance Schedule II
Action: Inhibits ascending pain pathways in CNS, increases pain threshold, alters pain perception
Uses: Moderate to severe pain
Dosage and routes:
• *Adult:* IM/SC 1-1.5 mg q4-6h prn; IV 0.5 mg q4-6h prn; REC 2.5-5 mg q4-6h prn
Available forms include: Inj SC, IM, IV 1, 1.5 mg/ml; supp 5 mg
Side effects/adverse reactions:
CNS: Drowsiness, dizziness, confusion, headache, sedation, euphoria
GI: Nausea, vomiting, anorexia, constipation, cramps

---

italics = common side effects   ***bold italic*** = life threatening reactions

GU: Increased urinary output, dysuria, urinary retention

INTEG: Rash, urticaria, bruising, flushing, diaphoresis, pruritus

EENT: Tinnitus, blurred vision, miosis, diplopia

CV: Palpitations, bradycardia, change in B/P

RESP: Respiratory depression

Contraindications: Hypersensitivity, addiction (narcotic)

Precautions: Addictive personality, pregnancy (B), lactation, increased intracranial pressure, MI (acute), severe heart disease, respiratory depression, hepatic disease, renal disease, child <18 yr

Pharmacokinetics:

SC/IM: Onset 10-15 min, peak 1-½ hr, duration 2-6 hr

IV: Onset 5-10 min, peak 1-½ hr, duration 3-6 hr

REC: Onset 15-30 min, duration 3-6 hr

Metabolized by liver, excreted in urine, crosses placenta

Interactions/incompatibilities:

• Increased effects with other CNS depressants: alcohol, narcotics, sedative/hypnotics, antipsychotics, skeletal muscle relaxants

NURSING CONSIDERATIONS

Assess:

• I&O ratio; check for decreasing output; may indicate urinary retention

Administer:

• IV after diluting with 5 ml sterile H₂O or NS for inj; give over 5 min through Y-tube or 3-way stopcock

• With antiemetic if nausea, vomiting occur

• When pain is beginning to return; determine dosage interval by patient response

Perform/provide:

• Storage in light-resistant area at room temperature

• Assistance with ambulation

• Safety measures: siderails, night light, call bell within easy reach

Evaluate:

• Therapeutic response: decrease in pain

• CNS changes: dizziness, drowsiness, hallucinations, euphoria, LOC, pupil reaction

• Allergic reactions: rash, urticaria

• Respiratory dysfunction: respiratory depression, character, rate, rhythm; notify physician if respirations are <10/min

• Need for pain medication, physical dependence

Teach patient/family:

• To report any symptoms of CNS changes, allergic reactions

• That physical dependency may result when used for extended periods of time

• That withdrawal symptoms may occur: nausea, vomiting, cramps, fever, faintness, anorexia

Lab test interferences:

Increase: Amylase

Treatment of overdose: Narcan 0.2-0.8 IV, O₂, IV fluids, vasopressors

oxyphenbutazone

(ox-i-fen-byoo'ta-zone)

Oxalid, Oxybutazone*

Func. class.: Nonsteroidal

Chem. class.: Pyrazolone derivative

Action: Inhibits prostaglandin synthesis by decreasing an enzyme needed for biosynthesis; possesses analgesic, antiinflammatory, antipyretic properties

Uses: Mild to moderate pain, osteoarthritis, rheumatoid arthritis

Dosage and routes:

Pain

*Available in Canada only

• *Adult:* PO 100-200 mg tid-qid
Acute arthritis
• *Adult:* PO 400 mg, then 100 mg q4h × 4 days or until desired response
Available forms include: Tabs 100 mg
Side effects/adverse reactions:
GI: Nausea, anorexia, vomiting, diarrhea, jaundice, *cholestatic hepatitis,* constipation, flatulence, cramps, dry mouth, peptic ulcer
CNS: Dizziness, drowsiness, fatigue, tremors, confusion, insomnia, anxiety, depression
CV: Tachycardia, peripheral edema, palpitations, dysrhythmias
INTEG: Purpura, rash, pruritus, sweating
GU: Nephrotoxicity: dysuria, hematuria, oliguria, azotemia
HEMA: Blood dyscrasias
EENT: Tinnitus, hearing loss, blurred vision
Contraindications: Hypersensitivity, asthma, severe renal disease, severe hepatic disease, pregnancy (D)
Precautions: Lactation, children, bleeding disorders, GI disorders, cardiac disorders, hypersensitivity to other antiinflammatory agents
Pharmacokinetics:
PO: Peak 2 hr, half-life 3-3½ hr; metabolized in liver, excreted in urine (metabolites), excreted in breast milk
Interactions/incompatibilities:
• Increased action of: coumarin, phenytoin, sulfonamides
NURSING CONSIDERATIONS
Assess:
• Renal, liver, blood studies: BUN, creatinine, AST, ALT, Hgb before treatment, periodically thereafter
• Audiometric, ophthalmic exam before, during, after treatment

Administer:
• With food to decrease GI symptoms; best to take on empty stomach to facilitate absorption
Perform/provide:
• Storage at room temperature
Evaluate:
• Therapeutic response: decreased pain, stiffness, swelling in joints, ability to move more easily
• For eye, ear problems: blurred vision, tinnitus (may indicate toxicity)
Teach patient/family:
• To report blurred vision, or ringing, roaring in ears (may indicate toxicity)
• To avoid driving or other hazardous activities if dizziness or drowsiness occurs
• To report change in urine pattern, weight increase, edema, pain increase in joints, fever, blood in urine (indicates nephrotoxicity)
• That therapeutic effects may take up to 1 mo

---

oxytetracycline HCl
(ox-i-tet-ra-sye′kleen)
Dalimycin, Oxlopar, Oxytetraclor, Terramycin, Uri-tet, E.P. mycin
Func. class.: Broad spectrum antibiotic/antiinfective
Chem. class.: Tetracycline

Action: Inhibits protein synthesis, phosphorylation in microorganisms by binding to 30S ribosomal subunits, reversibly binding to 50S ribosomal subunits
Uses: Syphilis, chlamydia trachomatis, gonorrhea, lymphogranuloma venereum, uncommon gram positive/negative organisms, rickettsial infections
Dosage and routes:
• *Adult:* PO 250 mg q6h; IM 100

mg q8h or 150 mg q12h IV 250-500 mg q12h

• *Child >8 yr:* PO 25-50 mg/kg/day in divided doses q6h; IM 15-25 mg/kg/day in divided doses q8-12h; IV 10-20 mg/kg/day in divided doses q12h

Gonorrhea

• *Adult:* PO 1.5 g, then 500 mg qid for a total of 9 g

Chlamydia trachomatis

• *Adult:* PO 100 mg bid × 7 days

Syphilis

• *Adult:* PO 2-3 g in divided doses × 10-15 days up to 30-40 g total

• Dosage adjustment necessary in renal impairment

Available forms include: Tabs 250 mg; caps 125, 250 mg; powder for inj IV 250, 500 mg; inj IM 50, 125 mg/ml

Side effects/adverse reactions:

CNS: Fever, headache, paresthesia

HEMA: Eosinophilia, neutropenia, thrombocytopenia, leukocytosis, hemolytic anemia

EENT: Dysphagia, glossitis, decreased calcification of deciduous teeth, abdominal pain, oral candidiasis

GI: Nausea, vomiting, diarrhea, anorexia, enterocolitis, *hepatotoxicity,* flatulence, abdominal cramps, epigastric burning, stomatitis, *pseudomembranous colitis*

CV: Pericarditis

GU: Increased BUN, polyuria, polydipsia, *renal failure, nephrotoxicity*

INTEG: Rash, urticaria, photosensitivity, increased pigmentation, exfoliative dermatitis, pruritus, angioedema, pain at injection site

Contraindications: Hypersensitivity to tetracyclines, children <8 yr, pregnancy (D)

Precautions: Renal disease, hepatic disease, lactation, cross sensitivity with "caine-type" local anesthetics

Pharmacokinetics:

PO: Peak 2-4 hr, half-life 6-9 hr; excreted in urine, bile, feces, in active form, crosses placenta 10%-40% protein bound

Interactions/incompatibilities:

• Decreased effect of oxytetracycline: antacids, $NaHCO_3$, dairy products, alkali products, iron, kaolin/pectin

• Increased effect: anticoagulants

• Decreased effect: penicillins

• Nephrotoxicity: methoxyflurane

• Do not mix with other drugs

NURSING CONSIDERATIONS

Assess:

• I&O ratio

• Blood studies: PT, CBC, AST, ALT, BUN, creatinine

• Signs of anemia: Hct, Hgb, fatigue

Administer:

• PO with a full glass of water

• IM, deep only

• IV after diluting 250 mg or less/10 ml of sterile H_2O for inj; further dilute with at least 100 ml of D_5W or NS for inj; give 100 mg or less/5 min or more; use within 12 hr, decrease rate or increase volume of diluent if vein irritation occurs. Do not give SC

• After C&S obtained

• 2 hr before or after laxative or ferrous products, 3 hr after antacid

Perform/provide:

• Storage in tight, light-resistant container at room temperature

Evaluate:

• Therapeutic response: decreased temperature, absence of lesions, negative C&S

• Allergic reactions: rash, itching, pruritus, angioedema

• Nausea, vomiting, diarrhea; administer antiemetic, antacids as ordered

• Overgrowth of infection: increased temperature, malaise, redness, pain, swelling, drainage, perineal itching, diarrhea, changes in cough or sputum

Teach patient/family:

• To avoid sun exposure since burns may occur; sunscreen does not seem to decrease photosensitivity

• If diabetic to avoid use of Clinistix, Diastix, or Tes-Tape for urine glucose testing

• That all prescribed medication must be taken to prevent superimposed infection

• To avoid milk products, to take with a full glass of water

Lab test interferences:

False negative: Urine glucose with Clinistix or Tes-Tape

False increase: Urinary catecholamines

---

oxytocin, synthetic injection

(ox-i-toe′sin)

Pitocin, Syntocinon, Uteracon

Func. class.: Oxytocic

Chem. class.: Hormone

Action: Acts directly on myofibrils producing uterine contraction, stimulates milk ejection by the breast

Uses: Stimulation of labor, induction; missed or incomplete abortion; postpartum bleeding

Dosage and routes:

Stimulation of labor

• *Adult:* IV INF 1 ml/1000 ml D₅W or 0.9% NaCl over 1-2 milli U/min; may increase q15-30 min, not to exceed 20 milli U/min

Incomplete abortion

• *Adult:* IV INF 10 U/500 ml D₅W or 0.9% NaCl given at 20-40 milli U/min

Postpartum bleeding

• *Adult:* IV INF 10-40 U/1000 ml D₅W or 0.9% NaCl given at 20-40 milli U/min

Available forms include: Inj IV 10 U/ml

Side effects/adverse reactions:

CNS: Hypertension, convulsions, tetanic contractions

GI: Nausea, vomiting, constipation

CV: Hypotension, dysrhythmias, increased pulse

GU: Abruptio placentae, decreased uterine blood flow

INTEG: Rash

HEMA: Increased hyperbilirubimia

CV: Bradycardia, tachycardia, PVC

RESP: Anorexia, asphyxia

*FETUS: **Dysrhythmias, jaundice, hypoxia, intracranial hemorrhage***

Contraindications: Hypersensitivity, serum toxemia, cephalopelvic disproportion, fetal distress, hypertonic uterus

Precautions: Cervical/uterine surgery, sepsis (uterine), primipara >35, 1st, 2nd stage of labor

Pharmacokinetics:

IM: Onset 3-7 min, duration 1 hr, half-life 12-17 min

IV: Onset 1 min, duration 30 min, half-life 12-17 min

Interactions/incompatibilities:

• Hypertension: vasopressors

NURSING CONSIDERATIONS

Assess:

• I&O ratio

• Contraction FHT, B/P, pulse, respiration

• B/P, pulse; watch for changes that may indicate hemorrhage

• Respiratory rate, rhythm, depth; notify physician of abnormalities

Administer:

• IV after diluting 10 U/L of 0.9%

---

italics = common side effects   ***bold italic*** = life threatening reactions

NS or D_5 NS run at 1-2 mU/min; increase by 1-2 mU/min at 15-30 min intervals to begin normal labor; dilute 10-40 U/L of solution, run 10-20 mU/min, titrate to control pp bleeding; dilute 10 U/500 ml of solution, run 10 U-20 mU/ml, administer by only one route at a time, use infusion pump
• After having crash cart available on unit (Mg^+, SO_4 at bedside)
Evaluate:
• Length, intensity, duration of contraction; notify physician of contractions lasting over 1 min or absence of contractions, turn patient on her side
• FHTs, fetal distress, watch for acceleration, deceleration, notify physician if problems occur
• For signs and symptoms of water intoxication
Teach patient/family:
• To report increased blood loss, abdominal cramps, increased temperature or foul-smelling lochia

---

oxytocin, synthetic nasal

(ox-i-toe′sin)

Func. class.: Oxytocic hormone

Action: Acts directly on myofibrils producing uterine contraction, stimulates milk ejection by the breast
Uses: Postpartum breast engorgement, initial milk let-down
Dosage and routes:
• *Adult:* NAS SPRAY 1 spray into one or both nostrils q2-3 min before breast feeding; NAS DROPS 3 gtts into one or both nostrils q2-3 min before breast feeding
Available forms include: Nas spray 40 U/ml; nas drops
Side effects/adverse reactions: None

Pharmacokinetics:
Onset 5-10 min, half-life 1 min
Interactions/incompatibilities:
• Hypertension: vasopressors
NURSING CONSIDERATIONS
Assess:
• I&O ratio
• Environment conducive to let-down reflex
Teach patient/family:
• To blow nose before administering
• To rinse dropper with warm water after each use
• Not to over use

---

pancreatin

(pan′kree-a-tin)

Elzyme 303 enseals

Func. class.: Digestant
Chem. class.: Pancreatic enzyme concentrate—bovine/porcine

Action: Pancreatic enzyme needed for proper pancreatic functioning
Uses: Exocrine pancreatic secretion insufficiency, cystic fibrosis (digestive aid)
Dosage and routes:
• *Adult:* PO 8000-24,000 USP U with meals
Available forms include: Tab 650, 2000, 12,000 U
Side effects/adverse reactions:
GI: Anorexia, nausea, vomiting, diarrhea, glossitis, anal soreness
GU: Hyperuricuria, hyperuricemia
INTEG: Rash, hypersensitivity
EENT: Buccal soreness
Contraindications: Hypersensitivity to pork
Precautions: Pregnancy (C), lactation
Interactions/incompatibilities:
• Decreased absorption: cimetidine, antacids, oral iron

NURSING CONSIDERATIONS
Assess:
• I&O ratio, watch for increasing urinary output
• Fecal fat, nitrogen, pro-time, calcium during treatment
Administer:
• After antacid or H$_2$ blockers; decreased pH inactivates drug
• Whole, not to be crushed, chewed (enteric coated)
• Low fat diet to decrease GI symptoms
Perform/provide:
• Storage in tight container at room temperature
Evaluate:
• For allergy to pork
• For polyuria, polydipsia, polyphagia (may indicate diabetes mellitus)

---

pancrelipase

(pan-kre-li′pase)
Cotazym, Cotazyme-S, Ilozyme, Ku-Zyme HP, Pancrease, Viokase
Func. class.: Digestant
Chem. class.: Pancreatic enzyme—bovine/porcine

Action: Pancreatic enzyme needed for proper pancreatic functioning
Uses: Exocrine pancreatic secretion insufficiency, cystic fibrosis (digestive aid), steatorrhea, pancreatic enzyme deficiency
Dosage and routes:
• *Adult and child:* PO 1-3 caps/tabs ac or with meals, or 1 caps/tab with snack or 1-2 pdr pkt ac
Available forms include: Tab 8000, 11,000, 30,000 U; caps 8000, 30,000 U; enteric coated caps 4000, 5000, 20,000, 25,000 U; powd 16,800 U
Side effects/adverse reactions:
GI: Anorexia, nausea, vomiting, diarrhea

GU: Hyperuricuria, hyperuricemia
Contraindications: Allergy to pork
Precautions: Pregnancy (C)
Interactions/incompatibilities:
• Decreased absorption: cimetidine, antacids, oral iron
NURSING CONSIDERATIONS
Assess:
• I&O ratio, watch for increasing urinary output
• Fecal fat, nitrogen, pro-time during treatment
Administer:
• After antacid or cimetidine; decreased pH inactivates drug
• Powder mixed in prepared fruit for infants, children
• Whole, not crushed or chewed (enteric coated)
• Low fat diet to decrease GI symptoms
• Powder mixed with pureed fruit, take tabs with or before food
Perform/provide:
• Storage in tight container at room temperature
Evaluate:
• For allergy to pork
• For polyuria, polydipsia, polyphagia (may indicate diabetes mellitus)

---

pancuronium bromide

(pan-kyoo-roe′nee-um)
Pavulon
Func. class.: Neuromuscular blocker (nondepolarizing)
Chem. class.: Synthetic curariform

Action: Inhibits transmission of nerve impulses by binding with cholinergic receptor sites, antagonizing action of acetylcholine
Uses: Facilitation of endotracheal intubation, skeletal muscle relaxa-

P

---

italics = common side effects   ***bold italic*** = life threatening reactions

tion during mechanical ventilation, surgery, or general anesthesia

Dosage and routes:
- *Adult:* IV 0.04-0.1 mg/kg, then 0.01 mg/kg q ½-1 hr
- *Child >10 yr:* IV 0.04-0.1 mg/kg, then ⅕ initial dose q ½-1 hr

Available forms include: Inj IV, IM, 1, 2 mg/ml

Side effects/adverse reactions:
CV: Bradycardia, tachycardia, increased, decreased B/P, ventricular extra systoles
*RESP: **Prolonged apnea, bronchospasm, cyanosis, respiratory depression***
EENT: Increased secretions
MS: Weakness to prolonged skeletal muscle relaxation
INTEG: Rash, flushing, pruritus, urticaria, sweating, salivation

Contraindications: Hypersensitivity to bromide ion

Precautions: Pregnancy (C), renal disease, cardiac disease, lactation, children <2 yr, electrolyte imbalances, dehydration, neuromuscular disease, respiratory disease

Pharmacokinetics:
IV: Onset 30-45 sec, peak 3-5 min; metabolized (small amounts), excreted in urine (unchanged), crosses placenta

Interactions/incompatibilities:
- Increased neuromuscular blockade: aminoglycosides, clindamycin, lincomycin, quinidine, local anesthetics, polymyxin antibiotics, lithium, narcotic analgesics, thiazides, enflurane, isoflurane
- Dysrhythmias: theophylline
- Do not mix with barbiturates in solution or syringe

NURSING CONSIDERATIONS
Assess:
- For electrolyte imbalances (K, Mg), may lead to increased action of this drug

- Vital signs (B/P, pulse, respirations, airway) until fully recovered; rate, depth, pattern of respirations, strength of hand grip
- I&O ratio; check for urinary retention, frequency, hesitancy

Administer:
- With diazepam or morphine when used for therapeutic paralysis; this drug provides no sedation alone
- Using nerve stimulator by anesthesiologist to determine neuromuscular blockade
- Atropine to counteract muscarinic effects
- After succinylcholine effects subside
- Anticholinesterase to reverse neuromuscular blockade
- IV undiluted, give over 1-2 min (only by qualified persons)

Perform/provide:
- Storage in refrigerator; do not store in plastic containers or syringes; use only fresh solutions
- Reassurance if communication is difficult during recovery from neuromuscular blockade
- Frequent (q2h) instillation of artificial tears and covering eyes to prevent drying of cornea

Evaluate:
- Therapeutic response: paralysis of jaw, eyelid, head, neck, rest of body
- Recovery: decreased paralysis of face, diaphragm, leg, arm, rest of body, allow to recover fully before completing a neuro assessment
- Allergic reactions: rash, fever, respiratory distress, pruritus; drug should be discontinued

Treatment of overdose: Edrophonium or neostigmine, atropine, monitor VS; may require mechanical ventilation

Lab test interferences:
Decrease: Cholinesterase

---

papaverine HCl
(pa-pav'er-een)

Cerebid, Cerespan, Lapav, Myobid, Pavabid, Pavacen, Pavadel, Pavasule, Ro-Papav, Vasal, Vasocap, Vasospan, Vazosan

Func. class.: Peripheral vasodilator

Chem. class.: Opium alkaloid (no narcotic activity)

Action: Relaxes all smooth muscle, inhibits cyclic nucleotide phosphodiesterase, which increases intracellular cAMP, causing vasodilation

Uses: Arterial spasm resulting in cerebral and peripheral ischemia; myocardial ischemia, associated with vascular spasm; or dysrhythmias; angina pectoris, peripheral, pulmonary embolism; visceral spasm; as in ureteral, biliary, GI colic PVD

Dosage and routes:
• *Adult:* PO 100-300 mg 3-5 times day; SUS REL 150-300 mg q8-12 h; IM/IV 30-120 mg q3h prn
Available forms include: Cap timerelease 150, 200, 300 mg; tabs 30, 60, 100, 150, 200, 300 mg; inj IM/IV 30 mg/ml

Side effects/adverse reactions:
*CV: **Tachycardia,*** increased B/P
RESP: Increased depth of respirations
CNS: Headache, dizziness, drowsiness, sedation, vertigo, malaise
GI: Nausea, anorexia, abdominal pain, constipation, diarrhea, jaundice, altered liver enzymes, ***hepatotoxicity***
INTEG: Flushing, sweating, rash

Contraindications: Hypersensitivity, complete AV heart block
Precautions: Cardiac dysrhythmias, glaucoma, pregnancy (C), lactation, drug dependency, children

Pharmacokinetics:
PO: Onset 30 sec, peak 1-2 hr, duration 3-4 hr
SUS REL: Onset erratic
90% bound to plasma proteins, metabolized in liver, excreted in urine (inactive metabolites)

Interactions/incompatibilities:
• Decreased effect of: levodopa
• Increased hypotension: antihypertensives, vasodilators, diazoxide, alcohol
• Do not add to LR solution, precipitation will occur

NURSING CONSIDERATIONS
Assess:
• B/P, pulse, respiratory rate, rhythm, character during treatment until stable; take B/P lying, standing; orthostatic hypotension is common
• Hepatic tests: AST, ALT, bilirubin; liver enzymes may increase

Administer:
• With meals to reduce GI upset
• An ordered analgesic if headache develops
• IV undiluted or diluted in equal amount of sterile H_2O, give 30 mg or less/2 min through Y-tube or stopcock

Perform/provide:
• Storage at room temperature

Evaluate:
• Therapeutic response: ability to walk without pain, increased pulse volume, increased temperature in extremities or orientation, long- and short-term memory
• Hepatic hypersensitivity reaction: nausea, vomiting, jaundice;

P

---

italics = common side effects   ***bold italic*** = life threatening reactions

drug should be discontinued if this occurs

Teach patient/family:
• That medication is not cure, may need to be taken continuously depending on condition; therapeutic response may not be evident for 2-3 mo
• That it is necessary to quit smoking to prevent excessive vasoconstriction
• To avoid hazardous activities until stabilized on medication; dizziness may occur
• To notify physician if nausea, flushing, sweating, headache, or jaundice occur

Treatment of overdose: Discontinue medication

---

paraldehyde
(par-al'de-hyde)
Paral

Func. class.: Anticonvulsant
Chem. class.: Cyclic ether

Controlled Substance Schedule IV

Action: CNS depressant; exact mechanism of action is unknown

Uses: Refractory seizures, status epilepticus, sedation, insomnia, alcohol withdrawal, tetanus, eclampsia

Dosage and routes:
Seizures
• *Adult:* IM 5-10 ml, divide 10 ml into 2 inj; IV 0.2-0.4 ml/kg in NS inj
• *Child:* IM 0.15 ml/kg; REC 0.3 ml/kg q4-6h or 1 ml/yr of age, not to exceed 5 ml, may repeat in 1 hr prn; IV 5 ml/90 ml NS inj, begin infusion at 5 ml/hr, titrate to patient response

Alcohol withdrawal
• *Adult:* PO/REC 5-10 ml, not to exceed 60 ml; IM 5 ml q4-6h × 24 hr, then q6h on following days, not to exceed 30 ml

Sedation
• *Adult:* PO/REC 4-10 ml; IM 5 ml; IV 3-5 ml to be used in emergency only
• *Child:* PO/REC/IM 0.15 ml/kg

Tetanus
• *Adult:* IV 4-5 ml or 12 ml by gastric tube q4h diluted with water; IM 5-10 ml prn

Available forms include: Inj IM, IV; oral and rectal liquid

Side effects/adverse reactions:
*HEMA: **Thrombocytopenia, agranulocytosis, leukopenia, neutropenia, hemolytic anemia,*** increased pro-time

CNS: Stimulation, drowsiness, dizziness, confusion, **convulsion,** headache, flushing, hallucinations, coma

GI: Foul breath, irritation

GU: Nephrosis

INTEG: Rash, erythema, local pain, sloughing fat necrosis

CV: Pulmonary edema, **pulmonary hemorrhage, circulatory collapse, respiratory depression**

Contraindications: Hypersensitivity, gastroenteritis with ulceration

Precautions: Asthma, hepatic disease, pulmonary disease, pregnancy (C)

Pharmacokinetics:
PO: Onset 10-15 min, peak 1-2 hr, duration 6-8 hr
REC: Onset slow, duration 4-6 hr
Metabolized by liver, excreted by kidneys, lungs, crosses placenta, half-life 7.5 hr

Interactions/incompatibilities:
• Increased blood levels of paraldehyde: alcohol, CNS depressants, general anesthetics, disulfiram

---

• Increase crystallization in kidneys: sulfonamides

NURSING CONSIDERATIONS
Assess:

• VS q30 min after parenteral route
• Blood studies: Hct, Hgb, RBCs, serum folate, vitamin D if on long-term therapy
• Hepatic studies: AST, ALT, bilirubin, creatinine, failure

Administer:

• IM injection in deep large muscle mass, use Z-track method to prevent tissue sloughing, maximum of 5 ml at any one site
• After conservative measures have been tried for insomnia
• Rectal after diluting in cottonseed oil or olive oil as retention enema or 200 ml NS for enema
• Keep patient's room well ventilated to remove exhaled drug
• Oral with juice or milk to cover taste/smell, decrease GI symptoms
• Use fresh supply; don't expose to air, don't use if brown or odor is vinegary or if container opened >24 h
• Using glass container only, reacts with plastic

Perform/provide:

• Ventilation of room

Evaluate:

• Mental status: mood, sensorium, affect, memory (long, short)
• Respiratory dysfunction; respiratory depression, character, rate, rhythm; hold drug if respirations are >10/min or if pupils are dilated

Teach patient/family:

• That physical dependency may result when used for extended periods of time
• To avoid driving, other activities that require alertness
• Not to discontinue medication

quickly after long-term use, taper over several weeks

Lab test interferences:

False positive: Ketones (serum)(urine), interference, 17-OHCS

---

paramethadione

(par-a-meth-a-dye'one)
Paradione
Func. class.: Anticonvulsant
Chem. class.: Oxazolidinedione

Action: Increases seizure threshold in cortex and basal ganglia; decreases synaptic stimulation to low-frequency impulses

Uses: Refractory absence (petit mal) seizures

Dosage and routes:

• *Adult:* PO 300 mg tid, may increase by 300 mg/wk, not to exceed 600 mg qid
• *Child >6 yr:* PO 0.9 g/day in divided doses tid or qid
• *Child 2-6 yr:* PO 0.6 g/day in divided doses tid or qid
• *Child <2 yr:* PO 0.3 g/day in divided doses tid or qid

Available forms include: Caps 150, 300 mg; sol 300 mg/ml

Side effects/adverse reactions:

HEMA: **Thrombocytopenia, agranulocytosis, leukopenia, neutropenia, hemolytic anemia,** increased pro-time

CNS: Drowsiness, dizziness, fatigue, paresthesia, irritability, headache

GU/GYN: Vaginal bleeding, albuminuria, nephrosis

GI: Nausea, vomiting, abdominal pain, weight loss, bleeding gums, abnormal liver function tests

---

italics = common side effects   ***bold italic*** = life threatening reactions

INTEG: Exfoliative dermatitis, rash, alopecia, petechiae, erythema
EENT: Photophobia, diplopia, epistaxis, retinal hemorrhage
CV: Hypertension, hypotension
Contraindications: Hypersensitivity, blood dyscrasias, pregnancy (D)
Precautions: Hepatic disease, renal disease, retinal or optic nerve damage
Pharmacokinetics:
PO: Onset 15-30 min, peak 1-2 hr, duration 4-6 hr
REC: Onset slow, duration 4-6 hr, metabolized by the liver, excreted by the kidneys, crosses placenta, excreted in breast milk, half-life 1-3½ hr
NURSING CONSIDERATIONS
Assess:
• Blood studies: Hct, Hgb, RBCs, serum folate, vitamin D if on long-term therapy; discontinue drug if neutrophil count falls below 2500/mm³
• Hepatic studies: ALT, AST, bilirubin, creatinine, failure
• Skin: If rash occurs withhold drug
Administer:
• After diluting oral solution with water
• Oral with juice or milk to cover taste-smell to decrease GI symptoms
Perform/provide:
• Ventilation of room
Evaluate:
• Mental status: mood, sensorium, affect, memory (long, short)
Teach patient/family:
• To avoid driving, other activities that require alertness
• Not to discontinue medication quickly after long-term use; convulsions may result

• To obtain liver function tests and urinalysis monthly
• To notify physician if sore throat, fever, malaise, bruises, petechiae, or epistaxis occurs
• To wear dark glasses if photosensitivity occurs
• To take drug with food, milk to decrease GI symptoms

---

paramethasone acetate
(par-a-meth′a-sone)
Haldrone

Func. class.: Corticosteroid
Chem. class.: Glucocorticoid, long acting

Action: Decreases inflammation by suppression of migration of polymorphonuclear leukocytes, fibroblasts, reversal to increase capillary permeability and lysosomal stabilization
Uses: Severe inflammation, collagen disorders, respiratory, dermatologic disorders, adrenal insufficiency
Dosage and routes:
• *Adult:* PO 0.5-6 mg tid-qid
• *Child:* PO 58-800 µg/kg/day in divided doses tid-qid
Available forms include: Tabs 2 mg
Side effects/adverse reactions:
INTEG: Acne, poor wound healing, ecchymosis, petechiae
CNS: Depression, flushing, sweating, headache, mood changes
CV: Hypertension, **circulatory collapse, thrombophlebitis, embolism,** tachycardia, edema
HEMA: Thrombocytopenia
MS: Fractures, osteoporosis, weakness
GI: Diarrhea, nausea, abdominal distention, *GI hemorrhage,* increased appetite, *pancreatitis*
EENT: Fungal infections, increased

intraocular pressure, blurred vision

Contraindications: Psychosis, hypersensitivity, idiopathic thrombocytopenia, acute glomerulonephritis, amebiasis, fungal infections, nonasthmatic bronchial disease, child <2 yr, AIDS, TB

Precautions: Pregnancy (C), diabetes mellitus, glaucoma, osteoporosis, seizure disorders, ulcerative colitis, CHF, myasthenia gravis, renal disease, esophagitis, peptic ulcer

Pharmacokinetics:
PO: Peak 1-2 hr, duration 2 days
IM: Peak 3-45 hr

Interactions/incompatibilities:
• Decreased action of paramethasone: cholestyramine, colestipol, barbiturates, rifampin, ephedrine, phenytoin, theophylline
• Decreased effects of: anticoagulants, anticonvulsants, antidiabetics, ambenonium, neostigmine, isoniazid, toxoids, vaccines
• Increased side effects: alcohol, salicylates, indomethacin, amphotericin B, digitalis preparations
• Increased action of paramethasone: salicylates, estrogens, indomethacin

NURSING CONSIDERATIONS
Assess:
• Potassium, blood sugar, urine glucose while on long-term therapy; hypokalemia and hyperglycemia
• Weight daily, notify physician of weekly gain >5 lb
• B/P q4h, pulse, notify physician if chest pain occurs
• I&O ratio, be alert for decreasing urinary output and increasing edema
• Plasma cortisol levels during long-term therapy (normal level: 138-635 nmol/L SI units when drawn at 8 AM)

Administer:
• Titrated dose, use lowest effective dose
• In one dose in AM to prevent adrenal suppression, avoid SC administration, damage may be done to tissue
• With food or milk to decrease GI symptoms

Perform/provide:
• Assistance with ambulation in patient with bone tissue disease to prevent fractures

Evaluate:
• Therapeutic response: ease of respirations, decreased inflammation
• Infection: increased temperature, WBC, even after withdrawal of medication; drug masks symptoms of infection
• Potassium depletion: paresthesias, fatigue, nausea, vomiting, depression, polyuria, dysrhythmias, weakness
• Edema, hypertension, cardiac symptoms
• Mental status: affect, mood, behavioral changes, aggression

Teach patient/family:
• That ID as steroid user should be carried
• To notify physician if therapeutic response decreases; dosage adjustment may be needed
• Not to discontinue this medication abruptly or adrenal crisis can result
• To avoid OTC products: salicylates, alcohol in cough products, cold preparations unless directed by physician
• About cushingoid symptoms
• Symptoms of adrenal insufficiency: nausea, anorexia, fatigue,

P

---

italics = common side effects   ***bold italic*** = life threatening reactions

dizziness, dyspnea, weakness, joint pain
Lab test interferences:
Increase: Cholesterol, sodium, blood glucose, uric acid, calcium, urine glucose
Decrease: Calcium, potassium, T_4, T_3, thyroid ^{131}I uptake test, urine 17-OHCS, 17-KS, PBI
False negative: Skin allergy tests

---

pargyline HCl
(par′gi-leen)
Eutonyl
Func. class.: Antihypertensive
Chem. class.: MAOI

Action: Inhibits monoamine oxidase, decreasing B/P
Uses: Moderate to severe hypertension
Dosage and routes:
• *Adult:* PO 25 mg daily, increase by 10 mg q7 days, not to exceed 200 mg; maintenance dosage: 25-50 mg daily
Available forms include: Tabs 10, 25, 50 mg
Side effects/adverse reactions:
CV: Orthostatic hypotension, tachycardia, chest pain, bradycardia, fluid retention, *CHF*
CNS: Drowsiness, dizziness, sedation, headache, depression, insomnia, weakness, fatigue, confusion, blurred vision, EPS
GI: Nausea, vomiting, anorexia, constipation, weight gain
EENT: Dry mouth
GU: Impotence
MS: Arthralgia
MISC: Sweating, increased appetite, hypoglycemia
Contraindications: Hypersensitivity, malignant hypertension, paranoid schizophrenia, severe pulmonary failure, pheochromocytoma,

hyperthyroidism, advanced renal failure, children <12 yr
Precautions: Pregnancy (C), lactation, impaired renal function, liver disease, CAD, parkinsonism, diabetes mellitus
Pharmacokinetics:
Excreted in urine, therapeutic response may take 4 days-3 weeks
Interactions/incompatibilities:
• Hypertensive crisis: amphetamine, cyclopent-amide, ephedrine, pseudoephedrine, metaraminol, methylphenidate, phenylpropanolamine, levodopa, methyldopa, reserpine, tryptamine, tyramine foods
• Hypotension and increased sedation: barbiturates, alcohol, narcotics, CNS depressants, antihypertensive agents
• May potentiate effects: doxapram, narcotics, phenothiazines, other psychotropic agents, tricyclic antidepressants
NURSING CONSIDERATIONS
Assess:
• Electrolytes: K, Na, Cl, CO_2
• Renal function studies: catecholamines, BUN, creatinine
• Hepatic function studies: AST, ALT, alk phosphatase
• Weight daily, I&O
• B/P lying, standing before starting treatment
Administer:
• Gum, frequent rinsing of mouth or hard candy for dry mouth
Teach patient/family:
• To report dizziness, palpitations, fainting
• To change position slowly or fainting may occur
• To take drug exactly as prescribed
• Not to eat tyramine-rich foods: beer, wine, pickled products, yeast

products, aged cheeses, avocados, chocolate
• May cause drowsiness
• To avoid all OTC products unless directed by physician
Evaluate:
• Therapeutic response: decreased B/P
• Nausea, vomiting, diarrhea
• Edema in feet, legs daily
• Skin turgor, dryness of mucous membranes for hydration status
Treatment of overdose: Induce emesis or gastric lavage, support respiration, severe hypertension—administer α-blocker, treat CNS stimulation with IV diazepam, maintain fluid or electrolyte balance

---

paromomycin sulfate
(par-oh-moe-mye′sin)
Humatin
Func. class.: Amebicide
Chem. class.: Aminoglycoside antibiotic

Action: Direct action in intestinal lumen
Uses: Intestinal amebiasis, tapeworms
Dosage and routes:
Intestinal amebiasis
• *Adult and child:* PO 25-35 mg/kg/day in 3 divided doses × 5-10 days pc
Tapeworms
• *Adult:* PO 1 g q15 min × 4 doses
• *Child:* PO 11 mg/kg q15 min × 4 doses
Available forms include: Caps 250 mg
Side effects/adverse reactions:
HEMA: **Eosinophilia**
INTEG: Rash
CNS: Headache, dizziness
EENT: Ototoxicity

GI: Nausea, vomiting, diarrhea, epigastric distress, anorexia, steatorrhea, pruritus ani, hypocholesterolemia
GU: **Nephrotoxicity, hematuria**
Contraindications: Hypersensitivity, renal disease, GI obstruction
Precautions: GI ulcerations, pregnancy (C)
Pharmacokinetics:
PO: Excreted in feces, urine, slowly

NURSING CONSIDERATIONS
Assess:
• Stools during entire treatment; should be clear at end of therapy, stools should be free of parasite for 1 yr before patient is considered cured
• I&O, stools for number, frequency, character
Administer:
• Cleansing enema if ordered before beginning treatment
• PO after meals to avoid GI symptoms
Perform/provide:
• Storage in tight container
Evaluate:
• Allergic reaction: rash, itching; drug should be discontinued if these occur
• Diarrhea for 2-3 days
Teach patient/family:
• Proper hygiene after BM: handwashing technique
• Avoid contact of drug with eyes, mouth, nose, other mucous membranes
• Need for compliance with dosage schedule, duration of treatment
Lab test interferences:
Decrease: Serum cholesterol

---

italics = common side effects   **bold italic** = life threatening reactions

pemoline

(pem'oh-leen)
Cylert
Func. class.: Cerebral stimulant
Chem. class.: Oxazolidinone derivative

Controlled Substance Schedule IV

Action: Exact mechanism unknown; may act through dopaminergic mechanisms

Uses: Attention deficit disorder with hyperactivity

Dosage and routes:
• *Child >6 yr:* 37.5 mg in AM, increasing by 18.75 mg/wk, not to exceed 112.5 mg/day

Available forms include: Tabs 18.75, 37.5, 75 mg; chewable tabs 37.5 mg

Side effects/adverse reactions:
MISC: Rashes, growth suppression in children

CNS: Hyperactivity, insomnia, restlessness, dizziness, depression, headache, stimulation, irritability, aggressiveness, hallucination seizures, Gilles de la Tourette's disorder, drowsiness, dyskinetic movements

GI: Nausea, anorexia, diarrhea, abdominal pain, increased liver enzymes, hepatitis, jaundice

Contraindications: Hypersensitivity, hepatic insufficiency

Precautions: Renal disease, pregnancy (B), lactation, drug abuse, child <6

Pharmacokinetics:
PO: Peak 2-4 hr, duration 8 hr, metabolized by liver, excreted by kidneys, half-life 12 hr

NURSING CONSIDERATIONS
Assess:
• Hepatic function studies: ALT, AST, bilirubin, creatinine

• Child for height, growth rate, since growth retardation occurs

Administer:
• At least 6 hr before hs
• Gum, hard candy, frequent sips of water for dry mouth

Evaluate:
• Mental status: mood, sensorium, affect, stimulation, insomnia, aggressiveness

Teach patient/family:
• To decrease caffeine consumption (coffee, tea, cola, chocolate), which may increase irritability, stimulation
• To avoid OTC preparations unless approved by physician
• To taper off drug over several weeks
• To avoid alcohol ingestion
• To avoid hazardous activities until patient is stabilized on medication
• That therapeutic effect may take 2-4 wk

penicillin G benzathine

(pen-i-sill'in)
Bicillin L-A, Megacillin,* Permapen
Func. class.: Broad-spectrum antibiotic
Chem. class.: Natural penicillin

Action: Interferes with cell wall replication of susceptible organisms; osmotically unstable cell wall swells, bursts from osmotic pressure

Uses: Respiratory infections, scarlet fever, erysipelas, otitis media, pneumonia, skin and soft tissue infections, gonorrhea; effective for gram-positive cocci *(Staphylococcus, S. pyogenes, S. viridans, S. faecalis, S. bovis, S. pneumoniae),* gram-negative cocci *(N. gonorrhoeae),* gram-positive bacilli *(B.*

anthracis, C. perfringens, C. tetani, C. diphtheriae, L. monocytogenes), gram-negative bacilli *(E. coli, P. mirabilis, Salmonella, Shigella, Enterobacter, S. moniliformis),* spirochetes *(T. pallidum),* Actinomyces

Dosage and routes:
Early syphilis
• *Adult:* IM 2.4 million U in single dose
Congenital syphilis
• *Child <2 yr:* IM 50,000 U/kg in single dose
Prophylaxis of rheumatic fever, glomerulonephritis
• *Adult and child >60 lb:* IM 1.2 million U in single dose q month or 600,000 U q 2 wk
• *Child <60 lb:* IM 600,000 U in single dose
Upper respiratory infections (group A streptococcal)
• *Adult:* IM 1.2 million U in single dose, PO 400,000-600,000 U q4-6h
• *Child >27 kg:* IM 900,000 U in single dose
• *Child <27 kg:* IM 50,000 U/kg in single dose
Available forms include: Inj IM 300,000, 600,000 U/ml; tabs 200,000 U

Side effects/adverse reactions:
HEMA: Anemia, increased bleeding time, ***bone marrow depression, granulocytopenia***
GI: Nausea, vomiting, diarrhea, increased AST, ALT, abdominal pain, glossitis, colitis
*GU: **Oliguria, proteinuria, hematuria,** vaginitis, moniliasis, **glomerulonephritis***
CNS: Lethargy, hallucinations, anxiety, depression, twitching, ***coma, convulsions***
META: Hyperkalemia, hypokalemia, alkalosis, hypernatremia

Contraindications: Hypersensitivity to penicillins; neonates
Precautions: Hypersensitivity to cephalosporins, pregnancy (B)
Pharmacokinetics:
IM: Very slow absorption, duration 21-28 days, half-life 30-60 min, excreted in urine, feces, breast milk, crosses placenta
Interactions/incompatibilities:
• Decreased antimicrobial effect of penicillin: tetracyclines, erythromycins
• Increased penicillin concentrations: aspirin, probenecid

NURSING CONSIDERATIONS
Assess:
• I&O ratio; report hematuria, oliguria since penicillin in high doses is nephrotoxic
• Any patient with compromised renal system since drug is excreted slowly in poor renal system function; toxicity may occur rapidly
• Liver studies: AST, ALT
• Blood studies: WBC, RBC, H&H, bleeding time
• Renal studies: urinalysis, protein, blood
• C&S before drug therapy; drug may be taken as soon as culture is taken
Administer:
• On an empty stomach for best absorption
• Drug after C&S has been completed
• After shaking well, deep IM inj in large muscle masses; avoid intravascular inj, aspirate
Perform/provide:
• Adrenalin, suction, tracheostomy set, endotracheal intubation equipment
• Adequate fluid intake (2000 ml) during diarrhea episodes
• Scratch test to assess allergy, after securing order from physician;

P

---

italics = common side effects   ***bold italic*** = life threatening reactions

usually done when penicillin is only drug of choice

• Storage in tight container; refrigerate injection

Evaluate:

• Therapeutic response: absence of fever, purulent drainage, redness, inflammation

• Bowel pattern before and during treatment

• Skin eruptions after administration of penicillin to 1 wk after discontinuing drug

• Respiratory status: rate, character, wheezing, tightness in chest

• Allergies before initiation of treatment, reaction of each medication; highlight allergies on chart, Kardex

Teach patient/family:

• To take oral penicillin on empty stomach with full glass of water

• Culture may be taken after completed course of medication

• To report sore throat, fever, fatigue; (could indicate superimposed infection)

• To wear or carry Medic Alert ID if allergic to penicillins

• To notify nurse of diarrhea

Lab test interferences:

False positive: Urine glucose, urine protein

Treatment of hypersensitivity: Withdraw drug, maintain airway, administer epinephrine, aminophylline, O_2, IV corticosteroids for anaphylaxis

---

penicillin G potassium

Acrocillin, Burcillin-G, Deltapen, Megacillin,* Novopen G,* Pentids, Pfizerpen

Func. class.: Broad-spectrum antibiotic-penicillin

Chem. class.: Natural penicillin

Action: Interferes with cell wall replication of susceptible organisms; osmotically unstable cell wall swells, bursts from osmotic pressure

Uses: Empyema, gangrene, anthrax, gonorrhea, mastoiditis, meningitis, osteomyelitis, pneumonia, tetanus, urinary tract infections, prophylactically in rheumatic fever; effective for gram-positive cocci *(S. aureus, S. pyogenes, S. viridans, S. faecalis, S. bovis, S. pneumoniae),* gram-negative cocci *(N. gonorrhoeae, N. meningitidis),* gram-positive bacilli *(B. anthracis, C. perfringens, C. tetani, C. diphtheriae, L. monocytogenes),* gram-negative bacilli *(Bacteroides, F. nucleatum, P. multocida, S. minor, S. moniliformis),* Spirochetes *(T. pallidum, T. pertenue, B. recurrentis, L. icterohaemorrhagiae),* Actinomyces

Dosage and routes:

Pneumococcal/streptococcal infections (mild-moderate)

• *Adult:* PO 400,000-500,000 U q6-8h × 10 days (streptococcal infections) or afebrile × 2 days (pneumococcal infections)

• *Child <12 yr:* PO 25,000-90,000 U/kg/day in 3-6 divided doses

Prevention of recurrence of rheumatic fever

• *Adult:* PO 200,000-250,000 U bid continuously

• *Child <12 yr:* PO 25,000-90,000 U/kg/day in 3-6 divided doses

Vincent's gingivitis/pharyngitis

• *Adult:* PO 400,000-500,000 U q6-8h

Available forms include: Tabs 200,000, 250,000, 400,000, 500,000, 800,000 U; powder for oral sol 200,000, 400,000 U/5 ml

Side effects/adverse reactions:

HEMA: Anemia, increased bleeding

---

time, *bone marrow depression, granulocytopenia*
GI: Nausea, vomiting, diarrhea, increased AST, ALT, abdominal pain, glossitis, colitis
GU: Oliguria, proteinuria, hematuria, vaginitis, moniliasis, glomerulonephritis
CNS: Lethargy, hallucinations, anxiety, depression, twitching, *coma, convulsions*
META: Hyperkalemia, hypokalemia, alkalosis, hypernatremia
Contraindications: Hypersensitivity to penicillins; neonates
Precautions: Hypersensitivity to cephalosporins, pregnancy (B)
Pharmacokinetics:
PO: Duration 6 hr, peak 1 hr
Excreted in urine unchanged, breast milk, crosses placenta
Interactions/incompatibilities:
• Decreased antimicrobial effectiveness of penicillin: tetracyclines, erythromycins
• Decreased absorption: cholestyramine, colestipol
• Increased penicillin concentrations: aspirin, probenecid
NURSING CONSIDERATIONS
Assess:
• I&O ratio; report hematuria, oliguria since penicillin in high doses is nephrotoxic
• Any patient with compromised renal system since drug is excreted slowly in poor renal system function; toxicity may occur rapidly
• Liver studies: AST, ALT
• Blood studies: WBC, RBC, H&H, bleeding time
• Renal studies: urinalysis, protein, blood
• C&S before drug therapy; drug may be taken as soon as culture is taken
Administer:
• On an empty stomach for best absorption

• Drug after C&S has been completed
Perform/provide:
• Adrenalin, suction, tracheostomy set, endotracheal intubation equipment
• Adequate fluid intake (2000 ml) during diarrhea episodes
• Scratch test to assess allergy, after securing order from physician; usually done when penicillin is only drug of choice
• Storage in dry, tight container; oral susp refrigerated 2 wk, 1 wk at room temperature
Evaluate:
• Therapeutic effectiveness: absence of fever, draining wounds
• Bowel pattern before and during treatment
• Skin eruptions after administration of penicillin to 1 wk after discontinuing drug
• Respiratory status: rate, character, wheezing, tightness in chest
• Allergies before initiation of treatment, reaction of each medication; highlight allergies on chart, Kardex
Teach patient/family:
• Aspects of drug therapy, including need to complete course of medication to ensure organism death (10-14 days); culture may be taken after completed course
• To report sore throat, fever, fatigue; (could indicate superimposed infection)
• To wear or carry Medic Alert ID if allergic to penicillins
• To notify nurse of diarrhea
Lab test interferences:
Decrease: Uric acid
False positive: Urine glucose, urine protein
Treatment of overdose: Withdraw drug, maintain airway, administer

---

italics = common side effects   ***bold italic*** = life threatening reactions

epinephrine, aminophylline, O_2, IV corticosteroids for anaphylaxis

---

penicillin G procaine

Crysticillin A.S., Duracillin A.S., Wycillin, Pfizerpen-AS

Func. class.: Broad-spectrum long-acting antibiotic

Chem. class.: Natural penicillin

Action: Interferes with cell wall replication of susceptible organisms; osmotically unstable cell wall swells, bursts from osmotic pressure

Uses: Empyema, gangrene, anthrax, gonorrhea, mastoiditis, meningitis, osteomyelitis, pneumonia, tetanus, urinary tract infections, prophylactically in rheumatic fever; effective for gram-positive cocci *(S. aureus, S. pyogenes, S. viridans, S. faecalis, S. bovis, S. pneumoniae),* gram-negative cocci *(N. gonorrhoeae, N. meningitidis),* gram-positive bacilli *(B. anthracis, C. perfringens, C. tetani, C. diphtheriae, L. monocytogenes),* gram-negative bacilli *(Bacteroides, F. nucleatum, P. multocida, S. minor, S. moniliformis),* Spirochetes *(T. pallidum, T. pertenue, B. recurrentis, L. icterohaemorrhagiae),* Actinomyces

Dosage and routes:
Moderate to severe infections
• *Adult and child:* IM 600,000-1.2 million U in one or two doses/day for 10 days to 2 weeks
• *Newborn:* 50,000 U/kg IM once daily
Gonorrhea
• *Adult and child >12 yr:* IM 4.8 million units in two injections given 30 mins after probenecid 1 gm.

Pneumonia (pneumococcal)
• *Adult and child >12 yr:* IM 300,000-600,000 U q6-12h
Available forms include: Inj IM 300,000, 500,000, 600,000 U/ml, 600,000 U/1.2 ml, 1,200,000 U/dose, 2,400,000 U/dose
Side effects/adverse reactions:
HEMA: Anemia, increased bleeding time, *bone marrow depression, granulocytopenia*
GI: Nausea, vomiting, diarrhea, increased AST, ALT, abdominal pain, glossitis, colitis
GU: Oliguria, proteinuria, hematuria, vaginitis, moniliasis, glomerulonephritis
CNS: Lethargy, hallucinations, anxiety, depression, twitching, *coma, convulsions*
META: Hyperkalemia, hypokalemia, alkalosis, hypernatremia
Contraindications: Hypersensitivity to penicillins, procaine; neonates
Precautions: Hypersensitivity to cephalosporins, pregnancy (B)
Pharmacokinetics:
IM: Peak 1-4 hr, duration 15 hr, excreted in urine
Interactions/incompatibilities:
• Decreased antimicrobial effect of penicillin: tetracyclines, erythromycins
• Increased penicillin concentrations: aspirin, probenecid
NURSING CONSIDERATIONS
Assess:
• I&O ratio; report hematuria, oliguria since penicillin in high doses is nephrotoxic
• Any patient with compromised renal system since drug is excreted slowly in poor renal system function; toxicity may occur rapidly
• Liver studies: AST, ALT
• Blood studies: WBC, RBC, H&H, bleeding time

---

* Available in Canada only

• Renal studies: urinalysis, protein, blood

• C&S before drug therapy; drug may be taken as soon as culture is taken

Administer:

• Drug after C&S has been completed

• Deep IM, avoid intravascular inj, aspirate

Perform/provide:

• Adrenalin, suction, tracheostomy set, endotracheal intubation equipment

• Adequate fluid intake (2000 ml) during diarrhea episodes

• Scratch test to assess allergy, after securing order from physician; usually done when penicillin is only drug of choice

• Storage in refrigerator

Evaluate:

• Therapeutic response: absence of fever, purulent drainage, redness, inflammation

• Bowel pattern before and during treatment

• Skin eruptions after administration of penicillin to 1 wk after discontinuing drug

• Respiratory status: rate, character, wheezing, tightness in chest

• Allergies before initiation of treatment, reaction of each medication; highlight allergies on chart, Kardex

Teach patient/family:

• That culture may be taken after completed course of medication

• To report sore throat, fever, fatigue; (could indicate superimposed infection)

• To wear or carry Medic Alert ID if allergic to penicillins

• To notify nurse of diarrhea

Lab test interferences:

False positive: Urine glucose, urine protein

Treatment of hypersensitivity: Withdraw drug, maintain airway, administer epinephrine, aminophylline, O_2, IV corticosteroids for anaphylaxis

penicillin G sodium

Crystapen,* Pfizerpen

Func. class.: Broad-spectrum antibiotic

Chem. class.: Natural penicillin

Action: Acts by interfering with cell wall replication of susceptible organisms; osmotically unstable cell wall swells and bursts from osmotic pressure

Uses: Empyema, gangrene, anthrax, gonorrhea, mastoiditis, meningitis, osteomyelitis, pneumonia, tetanus, urinary tract infections, prophylactically in rheumatic fever; effective for gram-positive cocci *(S. aureus, S. pyogenes, S. viridans, S. faecalis, S. bovis, S. pneumoniae),* gram-negative cocci *(N. gonorrhoeae, N. meningitidis),* gram-positive bacilli *(B. anthracis, C. perfringens, C. tetani, C. diphtheriae, L. monocytogenes),* gram-negative bacilli *(Bacteroides, E. nucleatum, P. multocida, S. minor, S. moniliformis),* Spirochetes *(T. pallidum, T. pertenue, B. recurrentis, L. icterohaemorrhagiae),* Actinomyces

Dosage and routes:

Moderate to severe infections

• *Adult:* IM/IV 12-30 million U/day in divided doses q4h

• *Child:* IM/IV 25,000-300,000 U/day in divided doses q4-12h

Dental surgery prophylaxis for endocarditis

• *Adult:* IM/IV 2 million units ½-1 hr before procedure, then 1 million 6 hr after procedure

P

Available forms include: Inj IM, IV 1 million, 5 million, 20 million units

Side effects/adverse reactions:

HEMA: Anemia, increased bleeding time, *bone marrow depression, granulocytopenia*

GI:Nausea, vomiting, diarrhea, increased AST, ALT, abdominal pain, glossitis, colitis

GU: Oliguria, proteinuria, hematuria, vaginitis, moniliasis, *glomerulonephritis*

CNS: Lethargy, hallucinations, anxiety, depression, twitching, *convulsions*

META: Hyperkalemia, hypokalemia, alkalosis, hypernatremia

Contraindications: Hypersensitivity to penicillins; neonates

Precautions: CHF caused by sodium content, pregnancy (B)

Pharmacokinetics:

IM: Peak 1-3 hr, duration 6 hr; excreted in urine

Interactions/incompatibilities:

• Decreased antimicrobial effect of penicillin: tetracyclines, erythromycins

• Increased penicillin concentrations: aspirin, probenecid

NURSING CONSIDERATIONS

Assess:

• I&O ratio; report hematuria, oliguria since penicillin in high doses is nephrotoxic

• Any patient with a compromised renal system since drug is excreted slowly in poor renal system function; toxicity may occur rapidly

• Liver studies: AST, ALT

• Blood studies: WBC, RBC, H&H, bleeding time

• Renal studies: urinalysis, protein, blood

• C&S before drug therapy; drug may be taken as soon as culture is taken

Administer:

• IV after diluting with sterile H_2O, shake, follow manufacturers' instructions for dilution; give by continuous INF, usually over 12 hr

• Drug after C&S has been completed

Perform/provide:

• Adrenalin, suction, tracheostomy set, endotracheal intubation equipment

• Adequate fluid intake (2000 ml) during diarrhea episodes

• Scratch test to assess allergy, after securing order from physician; usually done when penicillin is only drug of choice

• Storage of sterile sol in refrigerator for 1 wk, IV sol at room temperature for 24 hr

Evaluate:

• Therapeutic response: absence of fever, purulent drainage, redness, inflammation

• Bowel pattern before, during treatment

• Skin eruptions after administration of penicillin to 1 wk after discontinuing drug

• Respiratory status: rate, character, wheezing, tightness in chest

• Allergies before initiation of treatment, reaction of each medication; highlight allergies on chart, Kardex

Teach patient family:

• That culture may be taken after completed course of medication

• To report sore throat, fever, fatigue; (could indicate superimposed infection)

• To wear or carry Medic Alert ID if allergic to penicillins

• To notify nurse of diarrhea

Lab test interferences:

False positive: Urine glucose, urine protein

Treatment of overdose: Withdraw drug, maintain airway, administer epinephrine, aminophylline, O₂, IV corticosteroids for anaphylaxis

penicillin V potassium

Pen-Vee K*, Deltapen-VK, V-Cillin K, Veetids, PVFK,* Apo-Pen-VK,* No-vopen-VK,* Ledercillin-VK, Uticillin-VK, Betapen-VK, Penapar-VK, Robi-cillin-VK

Func. class.: Broad-spectrum anti-biotic
Chem. class.: Natural penicillin

Action: Interferes with cell wall replication of susceptible organisms; osmotically unstable cell wall swells, bursts from osmotic pressure.
Uses: Effective for gram-positive cocci *(S. aureus, S. pyogenes, S. viridans, S. faecalis, S. bovis, S. pneumoniae)*, gram-negative cocci *(N. gonorrhoeae, N. meningitidis)*, gram-positive bacilli *(B. anthracis, C. perfringens, C. tetani, C. diphtheriae, L. monocytogenes)*, gram-negative bacilli *(S. moniliformis)*, spirochetes *(T. pallidum)*, Actinomyces

Dosage and routes:
Pneumococcal/staphylococcal infections
• *Adult:* PO 250-500 mg q6h
• *Child <12 yr:* PO 25,000-90,000 U/kg/day in 3-6 divided doses (125 mg = 200,000 U)
Streptococcal infections
• *Adult:* PO 125-250 mg q6-8h × 10 days
Prevention of recurrence of rheumatic fever/chorea
• *Adult:* PO 125-250 mg bid continuously
Vincent's infection of oropharynx

• *Adult:* PO 500 mg q6h
Available forms include: Tabs 125, 250, 500 mg; film-coated tabs 250, 500 mg; powder for oral susp 125, 250 mg/5 ml
Side effects/adverse reactions:
HEMA: Anemia, increased bleeding time, *bone marrow depression, granulocytopenia*
GI: Nausea, vomiting, diarrhea, increased AST, ALT, abdominal pain, glossitis, colitis
GU: Oliguria, proteinuria, hematuria, vaginitis, moniliasis, glomerulonephritis
CNS: Lethargy, hallucinations, anxiety, *depression,* twitching, *coma, convulsions*
META: Hyperkalemia, hypokalemia, alkalosis
Contraindications: Hypersensitivity to penicillins; neonates
Precautions: Hypersensitivity to cephalosporins, pregnancy (B)
Pharmacokinetics:
PO: Peak 30-60 min, duration 6-8 hr, half-life 30 min, excreted in urine, breast milk
Interactions/incompatibilities:
• Decreased antimicrobial effectiveness of penicillin: tetracyclines, erythromycins
• Increased penicillin concentrations: aspirin, probenecid
NURSING CONSIDERATIONS
Assess:
• I&O ratio; report hematuria, oliguria since penicillin in high doses is nephrotoxic
• Any patient with compromised renal system since drug is excreted slowly in poor renal system function; toxicity may occur rapidly
• Liver studies: AST, ALT
• Blood studies: WBC, RBC, H&H, bleeding time
• Renal studies: urinalysis, protein, blood

italics = common side effects   ***bold italic*** = life threatening reactions

- C&S before drug therapy; drug may be taken as soon as culture is taken

Administer:
- On an empty stomach for best absorption
- Drug after C&S has been completed

Perform/provide:
- Adrenalin, suction, tracheostomy set, endotracheal intubation equipment
- Adequate fluid intake (2000 ml) during diarrhea episodes
- Scratch test to assess allergy, after securing order from physician; usually done when penicillin is only drug of choice
- Storage in tight container; after reconstituting, refrigerate for up to 2 wk

Evaluate:
- Therapeutic effectiveness: absence of fever, draining wounds
- Bowel pattern before and during treatment
- Skin eruptions after administration of penicillin to 1 wk after discontinuing drug
- Respiratory status: rate, character, wheezing, tightness in chest
- Allergies before initiation of treatment, reaction of each medication; highlight allergies on chart, Kardex

Teach patient/family:
- Aspects of drug therapy, including need to complete entire course of medication to ensure organism death (10-14 days); culture may be taken after completed course
- To report sore throat, fever, fatigue; (could indicate superimposed infection)
- To wear or carry Medic Alert ID if allergic to penicillins
- To notify nurse of diarrhea

Lab test interferences:
False positive: Urine glucose, urine protein

Treatment of overdose: Withdraw drug, maintain airway, administer epinephrine, aminophylline, O_2, IV corticosteroids for anaphylaxis

---

pentaerythritol tetranitrate

(pen-ta-er-ith'ri-tole)
Desatrate, Duotrate, Nitrin, PETN, Pentraspan, Naptrate, Pentylan, Peritrate, Vasolate

Func. class.: Vasodilatory, coronary

Chem. class.: Nitrate

Action: Decreases preload, afterload; which is responsible for decreasing left ventricular end-diastolic pressure, systemic vascular resistance

Uses: Chronic stable angina pectoris, prophylaxis of angina pain

Dosage and routes:
- *Adult:* PO 10-20 mg tid or qid, max 40 mg qid; SUS REL 30-80 mg q12h

Available forms include: Caps ext rel 30, 45, 80 mg; tabs 10, 20, 40, 80 mg; tabs ext rel 80 mg

Side effects/adverse reactions:
CV: Postural hypotension, palpitations, tachycardia, *collapse*, syncope

GI: Nausea, vomiting, abdominal pain

INTEG: Pallor, sweating, rash

CNS: Headache, flushing, dizziness, restlessness, weakness, faintness

MISC: Muscle twitching, *hemolytic anemia, methemoglobinemia*

Contraindications: Hypersensitivity to this drug or nitrites, severe anemia, increased intracranial pres-

---

sure, cerebral hemorrhage, acute MI

Precautions: Postural hypotension, pregnancy (C), lactation, children

Pharmacokinetics:

PO: Onset 30 min, duration 4-5 hr

SUS REL: Onset 30 min, duration 12 hr

Metabolized by liver, excreted in urine, half-life 10 min

Interactions/incompatibilities:

• Increased effects: β-blockers, diuretics, antihypertensives, alcohol

NURSING CONSIDERATIONS

Assess:

• B/P, pulse, respirations during beginning therapy

Administer:

• With 8 oz of water on empty stomach

Evaluate:

• Pain: duration, time started, activity being performed, character

• Tolerance if taken over long period of time

• Headache, lightheadedness, decreased B/P; may indicate a need for decreased dosage

Teach patient/family:

• To keep tabs in original container; do not crush or chew sus rel preparations

• To avoid alcohol

• May cause headache, tolerance usually develops

• That drug may be taken before stressful activity: exercise, sexual activity

• To avoid hazardous activities if dizziness occurs

• Stress patient compliance with complete medical regimen

• To make position changes slowly to prevent fainting

---

pentamidine isethionate

(pen-tam'i-deen)

Pentam 300, Pentacarinat,* Nebu Pent

Func. class.: Antiprotozoal

Chem. class.: Aromatic diamide derivative

Action: Interferes with DNA/RNA synthesis in protozoa

Uses: *Pneumocystis carinii* infections

Dosage and routes:

• *Adult and child:* IV/IM 4 mg/kg/day × 2 wk

Available forms include: Inj IV, IM 300 mg/vial

Side effects/adverse reactions:

CV: Hypotension, ventricular tachycardia, ECG abnormalities

HEMA: Anemia, ***leukopenia, thrombocytopenia***

INTEG: Sterile abscess, pain at injection site, pruritus, urticaria, rash

GU: ***Acute renal failure***

GI: Nausea, vomiting, anorexia, increased AST, ALT, ***acute pancreatitis***

CNS: Disorientation, hallucinations, dizziness

META: Hyperkalemia, hypocalcemia, hypoglycemia

Precautions: Blood dyscrasias, hepatic disease, renal disease, diabetes mellitus, cardiac disease, hypocalcemia, pregnancy (C)

Pharmacokinetics: Excreted unchanged in urine (66%)

Interactions/incompatibilities

• Nephrotoxicity: aminoglycosides, amphotercin B, colistin, cisplatin, methoxyflurane, polymyxin B, vancomycin

NURSING CONSIDERATIONS

Assess:

• Blood studies, blood glucose, CBC, platelets

- I&O ratio; report hematuria, oliguria
- ECG for cardiac dysrhythmias, check B/P
- Any patient with compromised renal system; drug is excreted slowly in poor renal system function; toxicity may occur rapidly
- Liver studies: AST, ALT
- Renal studies: urinalysis, BUN, creatinine; nephrotoxicity may occur
- Signs of infection, anemia

Administer:
- IV by intermittent INF over 60 min
- Inhalation through nebulizer over 30-45 min until chamber is empty
- IM diluted in 3 ml sterile H_2O; give deep IM; painful by this route

Perform/provide:
- Storage in refrigerator protected from light

Evaluate:
- Therapeutic response: decreased temperature, ability to breath
- Bowel pattern before, during treatment
- Sterile abscess, pain at injection site
- Respiratory status: rate, character, wheezing, dyspnea
- Dizziness, confusion, hallucination
- Allergies before treatment, reaction of each medication; place allergies on chart, Kardex in bright red letters; notify all people giving drugs

Teach patient/family:
- To report sore throat, fever, fatigue, could indicate superimposed infection

pentazocine HCl/ pentazocine lactate

(pen-taz′oh-seen)
Talwin
Func. class.: Narcotic analgesic, antagonist
Chem. class.: Synthetic benzomorphan

Controlled Substance Schedule IV
Action: Inhibits ascending pain pathways in CNS, increases pain threshold, alters pain perception
Uses: Moderate to severe pain
Dosage and routes:
- *Adult:* PO 50-100 mg q3-4h prn, not to exceed 600 mg/day; IV/IM/SC 30 mg q3-4h prn, not to exceed 360 mg/day

Available forms include: SC, IM, IV 30 mg/ml; tabs 50 mg
Side effects/adverse reactions:
CNS: Drowsiness, dizziness, confusion, headache, sedation, euphoria, hallucinations
GI: Nausea, vomiting, anorexia, constipation, cramps
GU: Increased urinary output, dysuria
INTEG: Rash, urticaria, bruising, flushing, diaphoresis, pruritus
EENT: Tinnitus, blurred vision, miosis, diplopia
CV: Palpitations, bradycardia, change in B/P, tachycardia, increased B/P (high doses)
RESP: Respiratory depression
Contraindications: Hypersensitivity, addiction (narcotic)
Precautions: Addictive personality, pregnancy (B), lactation, increased intracranial pressure, MI (acute), severe heart disease, respiratory depression, hepatic disease, renal disease, child <18 yr

Pharmacokinetics:
SC/IM: Onset 15-30 min, peak 1-2 hr, duration 2-4 hr
IV: Onset 2-3 min, duration 4-6 hr
Metabolized by liver, excreted by kidneys, crosses placenta, half-life 2-3 hr, extensive first-pass metabolism with less than 20% entering circulation

Interactions/incompatibilities:
• Increased effects: CNS depressants; alcohol, sedative/hypnotics, antipsychotics, skeletal muscle relaxants
• Decreased effects: narcotics
• Do not mix in solutions or syringe with barbiturates

NURSING CONSIDERATIONS
Assess:
• I&O ratio; check for decreasing output; may indicate urinary retention
• For withdrawal symptoms in narcotic-dependent patients
• Pulmonary embolism, abscesses, ulcerations, vascular occlusion

Administer:
• IV undiluted or diluted 5 mg/ml of sterile H_2O for inj; give 5 mg or less over 1 min
• With antiemetic if nausea, vomiting occur
• When pain is beginning to return; determine dosage interval by patient response

Perform/provide:
• Storage in light-resistant area at room temperature
• Assistance with ambulation
• Safety measures: siderails, night light, call bell within easy reach

Evaluate:
• Therapeutic response: decrease in pain
• CNS changes: dizziness, drowsiness, hallucinations, euphoria, LOC, pupil reaction
• Allergic reactions: rash, urticaria

• Respiratory dysfunction: respiratory depression, character, rate, rhythm; notify physician if respirations are <10/min
• Need for pain medication, physical dependence

Teach patient/family:
• To report any symptoms of CNS changes, allergic reactions
• That physical dependency may result when used for extended periods of time
• That withdrawal symptoms may occur: nausea, vomiting, cramps, fever, faintness, anorexia

Lab test interferences:
Increase: Amylase

Treatment of overdose: Narcan 0.2-0.8 IV, O_2, IV fluids, vasopressors

---

pentobarbital/pentobarbital sodium

(pen-toe-bar′bi-tal)
Nebralin/Nembutal sodium, Nova-Rectal,* Penital, Pentogen*
Func. class.: Sedative/hypnotic-barbiturate
Chem. class.: Barbitone, short acting

P

Controlled Substance Schedule II (USA), Schedule G (Canada)
Action: Depresses activity in brain cells primarily in reticular activating system in brainstem; selectively depresses neurons in posterior hypothalamus, limbic structures
Uses: Insomnia, sedation, preoperative medication, increased intracranial pressure, dental anesthetic
Dosage and routes:
• *Adult:* PO 100-200 mg hs; IM 150-200 mg hs; IV 100 mg initially, then up to 500 mg; REC 120-200 mg hs

---

italics = common side effects   ***bold italic*** = life threatening reactions

- *Child:* IM 3-5 mg, not to exceed 100 mg
- *Child 2 mo-1 yr:* REC 30 mg
- *Child 1-4 yr:* REC 30-60 mg
- *Child 5-12 yr:* REC 60 mg
- *Child 12-14 yr:* REC 60-120 mg

Available forms include: Caps 50, 100 mg; elix 18.2 mg/5 ml; powder, rec supp 30, 60, 120, 200 mg; inj IM, IV 50 mg/ml

Side effects/adverse reactions:

CNS: Lethargy, drowsiness, hangover, dizziness, paradoxical stimulation in elderly and children, lightheadedness, dependence, *CNS depression,* mental depression, slurred speech

GI: Nausea, vomiting, diarrhea, constipation

INTEG: Rash, urticaria, pain, abscesses at injection site, angioedema, thrombophlebitis, *Stevens-Johnson syndrome*

CV: Hypotension, bradycardia

RESP: Depression, apnea, laryngospasm, bronchospasm

HEMA: Agranulocytosis, thrombocytopenia, megaloblastic anemia (long-term treatment)

Contraindications: Hypersensitivity to barbiturates, respiratory depression, addiction to barbiturates, severe liver, renal impairment, porphyria, uncontrolled pain

Precautions: Anemia, pregnancy (D), lactation, hepatic disease, renal disease, hypertension, elderly, acute/chronic pain

Pharmacokinetics:

PO: Onset 15-30 min, duration 4-6 hr

REC: Onset slow, duration 4-6 hr Metabolized by liver, excreted by kidneys (metabolites); half-life 15-48 hr

Interactions/incompatibilities:

- Do not mix with other drugs in solution or syringe

- Increased CNS depression: alcohol, MAOIs, sedative, narcotics
- Decreased effect of: oral anticoagulants, corticosteroids, griseofulvin, quinidine
- Increased half-life of: doxycycline

NURSING CONSIDERATIONS
Assess:

- VS q 30 min after parenteral route for 2 hr
- Blood studies: Hct, Hgb, RBCs, serum folate, vitamin D (if on long-term therapy); pro-time in patients receiving anticoagulants
- Hepatic studies: AST, ALT, bilirubin; if increased, drug is usually discontinued

Administer:

- After removal of cigarettes, to prevent fires
- IM injection in deep large muscle mass to prevent tissue sloughing and abscesses; do not inject more than 5 ml in one site
- After trying conservative measures for insomnia
- After mixing with sterile water for injection, inject within 30 min of preparation
- IV undiluted or dilute in sterile H_2O, LR, NaCl, give 50 mg or less/min; titrate to patient response; don't use cloudy sol; avoid extravasation
- IV only with resuscitative equipment available, administer at <100 mg/min (only by qualified personnel)
- ½-1 hr before hs for sleeplessness
- On empty stomach for best absorption
- For <14 days since not effective after that; tolerance develops
- Crushed or whole
- Alone, do not mix with other drugs or inject if there is precipitate

---

Perform/provide:
• Assistance with ambulation after receiving dose
• Safety measure: siderails, nightlight, callbell within easy reach
• Checking to see PO medication has been swallowed
• Storage of suppositories in refrigerator; do not use aqueous solutions that contain precipitate

Evaluate:
• Therapeutic response: ability to sleep at night, decreased amount of early morning awakening if taking drug for insomnia, or decrease in number, severity of seizures if taking drug for seizure disorder
• Mental status: mood, sensorium, affect, memory (long, short)
• Physical dependency: more frequent requests for medication, shakes, anxiety
• Barbiturate toxicity: hypotension; pupillary constriction; cold, clammy skin; cyanosis of lips; insomnia; nausea; vomiting; hallucinations; delirium; weakness; coma; mild symptoms may occur in 8-12 hr without drug
• Respiratory dysfunction: respiratory depression, character, rate, rhythm; hold drug if respirations are <10/min or if pupils are dilated
• Blood dyscrasias: fever, sore throat, bruising, rash, jaundice, epistaxis

Teach patient/family:
• That morning hangover is common
• That drug is indicated only for short-term treatment of insomnia and is probably ineffective after 2 wk
• That physical dependency may result when used for extended periods of time (45-90 days depending on dose)

• To avoid driving or other activities requiring alertness
• To avoid alcohol ingestion or CNS depressants; serious CNS depression may result
• Not to discontinue medication quickly after long-term use; drug should be tapered over 1-2 wk
• To tell all prescribers that a barbiturate is being taken
• That withdrawal insomnia may occur after short-term use; do not start using drug again; insomnia will improve in 1-3 nights
• That effects may take 2 nights for benefits to be noticed
• Alternate measures to improve sleep (reading, exercise several hours before hs, warm bath, warm milk, TV, self-hypnosis, deep breathing)

Lab test interferences:
False increase: Sulfobromophthalein

Treatment of overdose: Lavage, activated charcoal, warming blanket, vital signs, hemodialysis, I&O ratio

---

pentoxifylline

(pen-tox-i'fi-leen)
Trental

Func. class.: Hemorheologic agent
Chem. class.: Dimethylxanthine derivative

Action: Decreases blood viscosity, increases blood flow by increasing flexibility of RBCs; decreases RBC hyperaggregation; reduces platelet aggregation, decreases fibrinogin concentration

Uses: Intermittent claudication related to chronic occlusive vascular disease

Dosage and routes:
• *Adult:* PO 400 mg tid with meals

---

italics = common side effects   ***bold italic*** = life threatening reactions

Available forms include: Tabs, controlled-release 400 mg

Side effects/adverse reactions:

MISC: Epistaxis, flulike symptoms, laryngitis, nasal congestion, leukopenia, malaise, weight changes

EENT: Blurred vision, earache, increased salivation, sore throat, conjunctivitis

CNS: Headache, anxiety, tremors, confusion, dizziness

GI: Nausea, vomiting, anorexia, bloating, belching, constipation, dyspepsia, cholecystitis, dry mouth, thirst

INTEG: Rash, pruritus, urticaria, brittle fingernails

CV: Angina, dysrhythmias, palpitation, hypotension, chest pain

Contraindications: Hypersensitivity to this drug or xanthines

Precautions: Pregnancy (C), angina pectoris, cardiac disease, lactation, children, impaired renal function

Pharmacokinetics:

PO: Peak 2-4 hr, half-life ½-1 hr, degradation in liver, excreted in urine

NURSING CONSIDERATIONS

Assess:

• B/P, respirations of patient taking antihypertensives also

Administer:

• With meals

Evaluate:

• Therapeutic response: decreased pain, cramping, increased ambulation

Teach patient/family:

• That therapeutic response may take 2-4 wk

• That decreased fats, increased cholesterol, increased exercise, decreased smoking are necessary to correct condition

• To observe feet for arterial insufficiency

• To use cotton socks, well-fitted shoes; not to go barefoot

• To watch for bleeding, bruises, petechiae, epistaxis

---

permethrin

(per-meth′ren)

Nix

Func. class.: Pediculicide

Chem. class.: Synthetic pyrethroid

Action: Acts by disrupting sodium channel current in parasite's nerve cell; delayed repolarization, paralysis of lice

Uses: Lice, nits, ticks, flea nits

Dosage and routes:

• *Adult and child:* Wash hair, towel dry—apply liberally to hair, leave on 10 min, rinse with water

Available forms include: Liq 1%

Side effects/adverse reactions:

INTEG: Pruritus, burning, stinging, rash, tingling, numbness, edema

Contraindications: Hypersensitivity

Precautions: Head rash, children, lactation

Pharmacokinetics:

Metabolized in liver to inactive metabolites, excreted in urine

NURSING CONSIDERATIONS

Administer:

• To body area, scalp only; do not apply to face, lips, mouth, eyes, any mucous membranes, anus, or meatus

• Topical corticosteroids as ordered to decrease contact dermatitis

• Lotions of menthol or phenol to control itching

• Topical antibiotics for infection

Perform/provide:

• Isolation until areas on skin, scalp have cleared and treatment is completed

• Removal of nits by using a fine-

---

tooth comb rinsed in vinegar after treatment

Evaluate:

• Area of body involved, including crusts, nits, itching papules in skin folds

Teach patient/family:

• To wash all inhabitants' clothing, bed-linen using insecticide; preventative treatment may be required of all persons living in same house, using lotion or shampoo to decrease spread of infection

• That itching may continue for 4-6 wk

• That drug must be reapplied if accidently washed off or treatment will be ineffective

• Do not apply to face, apply from neck down for body lice

• Treat sexual contact simultaneously

Treatment of ingestion: Gastric lavage, saline laxatives, IV valium for convulsions

---

perphenazine

(per-fen'a-zeen)

Trilafon

Func. class.: Antipsychotic/neuroleptic

Chem. class.: Phenothiazine-piperidine

Action: Depresses cerebral cortex, hypothalamus, limbic system, which control activity, aggression; blocks neurotransmission produced by dopamine at synapse; exhibits strong α-adrenergic, anticholinergic blocking action; as antiemetic inhibits medullary chemoreceptor trigger zone; mechanism for antipsychotic effects is unclear

Uses: Psychotic disorders, schizophrenia, alcoholism, nausea, vomiting

Dosage and routes:

Nausea/vomiting/alcoholism

• *Adult and child >12 yr:* IM 5-10 mg prn, max 15 mg in ambulatory patients, 30 mg in hospitalized patients; PO 8-16 mg/day in divided doses, up to 24 mg; IV not to exceed 5 mg, give diluted or slow IV drip

Psychiatric use in hospitalized patients

• *Adults:* PO 8-16 mg bid-qid, gradually increased to desired dose, not to exceed 64 mg/day; IM 5 mg q6h, not to exceed 30 mg/day

• *Child >12 yr:* PO 6-12 mg in divided doses

Nonhospitalized patients

• *Adult:* PO 4-8 mg tid or 8-32 mg repeat-action bid; IM 5 mg q6h

Available forms include: Tabs 2, 4, 8, 16 mg; sol 16 mg/5ml; inj IM 5 mg/ml; sus rel tabs 8 mg

Side effects/adverse reactions:

RESP: **Laryngospasm,** dyspnea, *respiratory depression*

*CNS: Extrapyramidal symptoms: pseudoparkinsonism, akathisia, dystonia, tardive dyskinesia, **seizures,** headache*

HEMA: Anemia, **leukopenia, leukocytosis, agranulocytosis**

INTEG: Rash, photosensitivity, dermatitis

EENT: Blurred vision, glaucoma

GI: Dry mouth, nausea, vomiting, anorexia, constipation, diarrhea, jaundice, weight gain

GU: Urinary retention, urinary frequency, enuresis, impotence, amenorrhea, gynecomastia

CV: Orthostatic hypotension, hypertension, **cardiac arrest,** ECG changes, **tachycardia**

Contraindications: Hypersensitivity, blood dyscrasias, coma, child <12 yr, brain damage, bone marrow depression

---

italics = common side effects   ***bold italic*** = life threatening reactions

P

Precautions: Pregnancy (C), lactation, seizure disorders, hypertension, hepatic disease, cardiac disease

Pharmacokinetics:
PO: Onset erratic, peak 2-4 hr
IM: Onset 10 min, peak 1-2 hr, duration 6 hr, occasionally 12-24 hr
Metabolized by liver, excreted in urine, crosses placenta, enters breast milk

Interactions/incompatibilities:
• Oversedation: other CNS depressants, alcohol, barbiturate anesthetics
• Toxicity: epinephrine
• Decreased absorption: aluminum hydroxide or magnesium hydroxide antacids
• Decreased effects of: lithium, levodopa
• Increased effects of both drugs: β-adrenergic blockers, alcohol
• Increased anticholinergic effects: anticholinergics

NURSING CONSIDERATIONS
Assess:
• Swallowing of PO medication; check for hoarding or giving of medication to other patients
• I&O ratio; palpate bladder if low urinary output occurs
• Bilirubin, CBC, liver function studies monthly
• Urinalysis is recommended before and during prolonged therapy

Administer:
• Antiparkinsonian agent, after securing order from physician to be used if extrapyramidal symptoms occur
• Concentrate mixed in water, orange, pineapple, apricot, prune, tomato, grapefruit juice; do not mix with caffeine beverages (coffee, cola), tannics (tea), or pectinates (apple juice) since incompatibility

may result; use 60 ml diluent for each 5 ml of concentrate
• Repeat-action tablets whole; do not crush or chew
• IM injection into a large muscle mass

Perform/provide:
• Decreased noise input by dimming lights, avoiding loud noises
• Supervised ambulation until stabilized on medication; do not involve in strenuous exercise program because fainting is possible; patient should not stand still for long periods of time
• Increased fluids to prevent constipation
• Sips of water, candy, gum for dry mouth
• Storage in tight, light-resistant container

Evaluate:
• Therapeutic response: decrease in emotional excitement, hallucinations, delusions, paranoia, reorganization of patterns of thought, speech
• Affect, orientation, LOC, reflexes, gait, coordination, sleep pattern disturbances
• B/P standing and lying; also include pulse, respirations q4h during initial treatment; establish baseline before starting treatment; report drops of 30 mm Hg
• Dizziness, faintness, palpitations, tachycardia on rising
• Extrapyramidal symptoms including akathisia (inability to sit still, no pattern to movements), tardive dyskinesia (bizarre movements of jaw, mouth, tongue, extremities), pseudoparkinsonism (rigidity, tremors, pill rolling, shuffling gait)
• Skin turgor daily
• For neuroleptic malignant syndrome; hyperthermia, altered men-

tal status, increased CPK, muscle rigidity

• Constipation, urinary retention daily; if these occur, increase bulk, water in diet

Teach patient/family:

• That orthostatic hypotension occurs frequently, and to rise from sitting or lying position gradually

• To remain lying down after IM injection for at least 30 min

• To avoid hot tubs, hot showers, or tub baths since hypotension may occur

• To avoid abrupt withdrawal of this drug or extrapyramidal symptoms may result; drugs should be withdrawn slowly

• To avoid OTC preparations (cough, hayfever, cold) unless approved by physician since serious drug interactions may occur; avoid use with alcohol or CNS depressants, increased drowsiness may occur

• To use a sunscreen during sun exposure to prevent burns

• Regarding compliance with drug regimen

• About necessity for meticulous oral hygiene since oral candidiasis may occur

• To report sore throat, malaise, fever, bleeding, mouth sores; if these occur, CBC should be drawn and drug discontinued

• In hot weather, that heat stroke may occur; take extra precautions to stay cool

Lab test interferences:

Increase: Liver function tests, cardiac enzymes, cholesterol, blood glucose, prolactin, bilirubin, PBI, cholinesterase, ^{131}I

Decrease: Hormones (blood, urine)

False positive: Pregnancy tests, PKU

False negative: Urinary steroids, 17-OHCS

Treatment of overdose: Lavage if orally injested, provide an airway; *do not induce vomiting*

---

phenacemide

(fe-nass'e-mide)

Phenurone

Func. class.: Anticonvulsant

Chem. class.: Hydantoin

Action: Increases seizure threshold in cortex

Uses: Refractory, generalized tonic-clonic, (grand mal) complex-partial, (psychomotor) absence, (petit mal) atypical seizures

Dosage and routes:

• *Adult:* PO 500 mg tid, may increase by 500 mg/wk, not to exceed 5 g/day

• *Child 5-10 yr:* PO 250 mg tid, may increase by 250 mg/wk, not to exceed 1.5 g/day prn

Available forms include: Tabs 500 mg

Side effects/adverse reactions:

*HEMA: **Agranulocytosis, leukopenia, aplastic anemia***

CNS: Drowsiness, dizziness, insomnia, paresthesias, depression, suicidal tendencies, aggression, headache

GI: Anorexia, weight loss, ***hepatitis***, jaundice, nausea

GU: Nephritis, ***albuminuria***

INTEG: Rash

Contraindications: Hypersensitivity, psychiatric disease, pregnancy (D)

Precautions: Allergies, hepatic disease, renal disease

Pharmacokinetics:

PO: Duration 5 hr, metabolized by liver, excreted by kidneys

P

---

italics = common side effects   ***bold italic*** = life threatening reactions

NURSING CONSIDERATIONS
Assess:
• Blood, liver function, renal function studies
• Drug level: drug is extremely toxic
Administer:
• With food to decrease GI symptoms
Evaluate:
• Mental status: mood, sensorium, affect, memory (long, short); psychosis is common
• Respiratory depression: respirations <10/min, shallow
• Blood dyscrasias: fever, sore throat, bruising, rash, jaundice
Teach patient/family:
• To notify physician if sore throat, fever, rash, fatigue, bleeding, bruising occur (blood dyscrasia)
• To notify physician if dark urine, jaundice, yellow sclerae, itching occur (liver dysfunction)
• To avoid hazardous activities until stabilized on drug
• Never to withdraw abruptly
• Have family report personality changes

---

phenazopyridine HCl
(fen-az-eh-peer'i-deen)
Baridium, Di-Azo, Diridone, Phenazo,* Phenazodine, Pyridiate, Pyridium, Urodine
Func. class.: Nonnarcotic analgesic
Chem. class.: Azodye

Action: Exerts analgesic, anesthetic action on the urinary tract mucosa; exact mechanism of action unknown
Uses: Urinary tract irritation, infection
Dosage and routes:
• *Adult:* PO 100-200 mg tid

• *Child 6-12 yr:* PO 12 mg/kg/24 hr in divided doses
Available forms include: Tabs 100, 200 mg
Side effects/adverse reactions:
HEMA: ***Thrombocytopenia, agranulocytosis, leukopenia, neutropenia, hemolytic anemia, methemoglobinemia***
CNS: Headache, vertigo
GI: Nausea, vomiting, GI bleeding, diarrhea, heartburn, anorexia, ***hepatic toxicity***
INTEG: Rash, urticaria, skin pigmentation
GU: ***Renal toxicity,*** orange-red urine
Contraindications: Hypersensitivity, hepatic disease
Precautions: Pregnancy (B), renal disease
Pharmacokinetics: Metabolized by liver, excreted by kidneys, crosses placenta, duration 6-8 hr
NURSING CONSIDERATIONS
Assess:
• Liver function studies: AST, ALT, bilirubin if patient is on long-term therapy
Administer:
• To patient crushed or whole; chewable tablets may be chewed
• With food or milk to decrease gastric symptoms
Evaluate:
• Therapeutic response: decrease in pain
• Hepatotoxicity: dark urine, clay-colored stools, yellowing of skin, sclera, itching, abdominal pain, fever, diarrhea if patient is on long-term therapy
• Allergic reactions: rash, urticaria; if these occur, drug may need to be discontinued
Teach patient/family:
• To report any symptoms of hepatotoxicity

---

*Available in Canada only

• Not to exceed recommended dosage, and to take with meals
• To read label on other OTC drugs; many contain aspirin
• Urine may turn red-orange

Lab test interferences:

Interference: Bilirubin, urinary glucose tests, urinalysis, PSP excretion, urinary ketones, steroids, proteins

Treatment of overdose: Methylene blue 1-2 mg/kg IV or 100-200 mg vitamin C PO

---

phendimetrazine tartrate

(fen-dye-me′tra-zeen)

Adipost, Anorex, Bacarate, Bontril, Delcozine, Di-Ap-Trol, Metra Obalan, Obeval, Obezine, Phenzine, Plegine, SPRX 1, SPRX-105, Statobex, Trimstat, Trimtabs, Melfiat, Weightrol, Weh-less, Trimcaps, Adphen, Dyrexan-OD, Prel-2

Func. class.: Anorexiant
Chem. class.: Morpholine derivative

Controlled Substance Schedule III

Action: Increases release of norepinephrine, dopamine in cerebral cortex to reticular activating system

Uses: Exogenous obesity

Dosage and routes:

Adult: PO 35 mg bid-tid 1 hr ac, not to exceed 70 mg tid, sus rel 105 mg qd ac AM

Available forms include: Tabs 35 mg, caps 35 mg, sus rel cap 105 mg

Side effects/adverse reactions:

CNS: Hyperactivity, insomnia, restlessness, dizziness, tremor headache

INTEG: Urticaria

GI: Nausea, anorexia, dry mouth, diarrhea, constipation, cramps

GU: Dysuria

CV: Palpitations, tachycardia, hypertension

EENT: Blurred vision

Contraindications: Hypersensitivity, hyperthyroidism, hypertension, glaucoma, severe arteriosclerosis, severe cardiovascular disease, children <12 yr, agitated states

Precautions: Drug abuse, anxiety, pregnancy (C), lactation

Pharmacokinetics:

PO: Onset 30 min, peak 1-3 hr, duration 4-20 hr, metabolized by liver, excreted by kidneys, crosses placenta, excreted in breast milk, half-life 2-10 hr

Interactions/incompatibilities:

• Hypertensive crisis: MAOIs or within 14 days of MAOIs
• Increased effect of phendimetrazine: acetazolamide, antacids, sodium bicarbonate, ascorbic acid, ammonium chloride
• Decreased effect of phendimetrazine: tricyclics
• Decreased effect of: guanethidine, other antihypertensives

NURSING CONSIDERATIONS

Assess:

• VS, B/P since this drug may reverse antihypertensives; check patients with cardiac disease more often
• CBC, urinalysis, in diabetes: blood sugar, urine sugar; insulin changes may need to be made since eating will decrease
• Height, growth rate in children; growth rate may decrease

Administer:

• At least 6 hr before hs to avoid sleeplessness
• For obesity only if patient is on weight reduction program, includ-

---

italics = common side effects   ***bold italic*** = life threatening reactions

ing dietary changes, exercise; patient will develop tolerance, loss of weight won't occur without additional methods, give 1 hr before meals
• Gum, hard candy, frequent sips of water for dry mouth
Teach patient/family:
• Not to crush or chew sus rel preps
• To decrease caffeine consumption (coffee, tea, cola, chocolate) which may increase irritability, stimulation
• To avoid OTC preparations unless approved by physician
• To taper off drug over several weeks, or depression, increased sleeping, lethargy will ensue
• To avoid alcohol ingestion
• To avoid hazardous activities until patient is stabilized on medication
• To get needed rest; patients will feel more tired at end of day
Treatment of overdose: Administer fluids, hemodialysis or peritoneal dialysis; antihypertensive for increased B/P; ammonium Cl for increase excretion

---

phenelzine sulfate

(fen'el-zeen)
Nardil
Func. class.: Antidepressant MAOI
Chem. class.: Hydrazine

Action: Increases concentrations of endogenous epinephrine, norepinephrine, serotonin, dopamine in storage sites in CNS by inhibition of MAO; increased concentration reduces depression
Uses: Depression, when uncontrolled by other means
Dosage and routes:
• *Adult:* PO 45 mg/day in divided

doses, may increase to 60 mg/day, dose should be reduced to 15 mg/day, not to exceed 90 mg/day
Available forms include: Tabs 15 mg
Side effects/adverse reactions:
HEMA: Anemia
CNS: Dizziness, drowsiness, confusion, headache, anxiety, tremors, stimulation, weakness, hyperreflexia, mania, insomnia, fatigue, weight gain
GI: Constipation, dry mouth, nausea, vomiting, *anorexia,* diarrhea, weight gain
GU: Change in libido, frequency
INTEG: Rash, flushing, increased perspiration
CV: Orthostatic hypotension, hypertension, dysrhythmias, hypertensive crisis
EENT: Blurred vision
ENDO: SIADH-like syndrome
Contraindications: Hypersensitivity to MAOIs, elderly, hypertension, CHF, severe hepatic disease, pheochromocytoma, severe renal disease, severe cardiac disease
Precautions: Suicidal patients, convulsive disorders, severe depression, schizophrenia, hyperactivity, diabetes mellitus, pregnancy (C)
Pharmacokinetics:
Metabolized by liver, excreted by kidneys
Interactions/incompatibilities:
• Increased pressor effects: guanethidine, clonidine, indirect acting sympathomimetics (ephedrine)
• Increased effects of: direct acting sympathomimetics (epinephrine), alcohol, barbiturates, benzodiazepines, CNS depressants, levodopa
• Hyperpyretic crisis, convulsions, hypertensive episode: tricyclic antidepressants, meperidine

---

* Available in Canada only

• Increased hypoglycemic effect: insulin

NURSING CONSIDERATIONS
Assess:

• B/P (lying, standing), pulse; if systolic B/P drops 20 mm Hg hold drug, notify physician
• Blood studies: CBC, leukocytes, cardiac enzymes if patient is receiving long-term therapy
• Hepatic studies: ALT, AST, bilirubin, creatinine; hepatotoxicity may occur

Administer:

• Increased fluids, bulk in diet if constipation, urinary retention occur
• With food or milk or GI symptoms
• Crushed if patient is unable to swallow medication whole
• Dosage hs if over-sedation occurs during day
• Gum, hard candy, or frequent sips of water for dry mouth
• Phentolamine for severe hypertension

Perform/provide:

• Storage in tight container in cool environment
• Assistance with ambulation during beginning therapy since drowsiness/dizziness occurs
• Safety measures including siderails
• Checking to see PO medication swallowed

Evaluate:

• Toxicity: increased headache, palpitation, discontinue drug immediately; prodromal signs of hypertensive crisis
• Mental status: mood, sensorium, affect, memory (long, short); increase in psychiatric symptoms
• Urinary retention, constipation, edema, take weight weekly
• Withdrawal symptoms: headache, nausea, vomiting, muscle pain, weakness

Teach patient/family:

• That therapeutic effects may take 1-4 wk
• To avoid driving or other activities requiring alertness
• To avoid alcohol ingestion, CNS depressants or OTC medications: cold, weight, hay fever, cough syrup
• Not to discontinue medication quickly after long-term use
• To avoid high tyramine foods: cheese (aged), sour cream, beer, wine, pickled products, liver, raisins, bananas, figs, avocados, meat tenderizers, chocolate, yogurt; increase caffeine
• To report headache, palpitation, neck stiffness

Treatment of overdose: Lavage, activated charcoal, monitor electrolytes, vital signs, diazepam IV, NaHCO₃

---

phenmetrazine HCl

(fen-met'ra-zeen)
Preludin

Func. class.: Anorexiant
Chem. class.: Morpholine

Controlled Substance Schedule II
Action: Increases release of norepinephrine, dopamine in cerebral cortex to reticular activating system
Uses: Exogenous obesity
Dosage and routes:

• *Adult:* EXT REL 50-75 mg qd in AM

Available forms include: Tabs ext rel 75 mg
Side effects/adverse reactions:

CNS: Hyperactivity, insomnia, restlessness, dizziness, headache
GI: Nausea, anorexia, dry mouth, constipation, abdominal pain

---

italics = common side effects   ***bold italic*** = life threatening reactions

GU: Impotence, change in libido
CV: Palpitations, tachycardia, hypertension, hypotension
INTEG: Urticaria
EENT: Blurred vision

Contraindications: Hypersensitivity, hyperthyroidism, hypertension, glaucoma, severe arteriosclerosis, angina pectoris, drug abuse, cardiovascular disease, agitation

Precautions: Anxiety, pregnancy (C), lactation

Pharmacokinetics:
EXT REL: Duration 12 hr, metabolized by liver, excreted by kidneys

Interactions/incompatibilities:
• Hypertensive crisis: MAOIs or within 14 days of MAOIs
• Increased effect of phenmetrazine: acetazolamide, antacids, sodium bicarbonate, ascorbic acid, ammonium chloride
• Decreased effect of phenmetrazine: tricyclics
• Decreased effect of: guanethidine, other antihypertensives

NURSING CONSIDERATIONS
Assess:
• VS, B/P since this drug may reverse antihypertensives; check patients with cardiac disease more often
• CBC, urinalysis, in diabetes: blood sugar, urine sugar; insulin changes may need to be made since eating will decrease
• Height, growth rate in children; growth rate may be decreased

Administer:
• At least 6 hr before hs to avoid sleeplessness
• For obesity only if patient is on weight reduction program including dietary changes, exercise; patient will develop tolerance, loss of weight won't occur without additional methods, give 1 hr before meals

• Gum, hard candy, frequent sips of water for dry mouth

Evaluate:
• Mental status: mood, sensorium, affect, stimulation, insomnia, aggressiveness
• Physical dependency: should not be used for extended time; dose should be discontinued gradually, tolerance occurs with long-term use
• Withdrawal symptoms: headache, nausea, vomiting, muscle pain, weakness

Teach patient/family:
• Not to crush or chew sus rel preps
• To decrease caffeine consumption (coffee, tea, cola, chocolate), which may increase irritability, stimulation
• To avoid OTC preparations unless approved by physician
• To taper off drug over several weeks, or depression, increased sleeping, lethargy may ensue
• To avoid alcohol ingestion
• To avoid hazardous activities until patient is stabilized on medication
• To get needed rest; patients will feel more tired at end of day

Treatment of overdose: Administer fluids, hemodialysis or peritoneal dialysis; antihypertensive for increased B/P; ammonium Cl for increased excretion

---

phenobarbital, phenobarbital sodium

(fee-noe-bar'bi-tal)
Bar, Barbita, Eskabarb, Floramine, Luminal, Orpine, SoluBarb, Stental, Luminal sodium

Func. class.: Anticonvulsant
Chem. class.: Barbiturate

Controlled Substance Schedule IV

Action: Decreases impulse transmission, increases seizure threshold at cerebral cortex level

Uses: All forms of epilepsy, status epilepticus, febrile seizures in children, sedation, insomnia, hyperbilirubinemia, chronic cholestasis

Dosage and routes:

Seizures
• *Adult:* PO 100-200 mg/day in divided doses tid or total dose hs
• *Child:* PO 4-6 mg/kg/day in divided doses q12h, may be given as single dose

Status epilepticus
• *Adult:* IV INF 10 mg/kg, run no faster than 50 mg/min, may give up to 20 mg/kg
• *Child:* IV INF 5-10 mg/kg, may repeat q10-15 min, up to 20 mg/kg, run no faster than 50 mg/min

Insomnia
• *Adult:* PO/IM 100-320 mg
• *Child:* PO/IM 3-6 mg/kg

Sedation
• *Adult:* PO 30-120 mg/day in 2-3 divided doses
• *Child:* PO 6 mg/kg/day in 3 divided doses

Preoperative sedation
• *Adult:* IM 100-200 mg 1-1½ hr before surgery
• *Child:* IM 16-100 mg 1-1½ hr before surgery

Hyperbilirubinemia
• *Neonate:* PO 7 mg/kg/day from days 1-5 after birth
IM 5 mg/kg/day on day 1, then PO on days 2-7 after birth

Chronic cholestasis
• *Adult:* PO 90-180 mg/day in 2-3 divided doses
• *Child <12 yr:* PO 3-12 mg/kg/day in 2-3 divided doses

Available forms include: Caps 16 mg; elix 15, 20 mg/5 ml; tabs 8, 15, 16, 30, 32, 60, 65, 100 mg; inj 30, 60, 65, 130 mg/ml

Side effects/adverse reactions:

CNS: Paradoxical excitement (elderly), *drowsiness,* lethargy, hangover headache, flushing, hallucinations, coma

GI: Nausea, vomiting

INTEG: Rash, urticaria, **Stevens-Johnson syndrome, angioedema,** local pain, swelling, necrosis, thrombophlebitis

Contraindications: Hypersensitivity to barbiturates, porphyria, hepatic disease, respiratory disease, nephritis, hyperthyroidism, diabetes mellitus, elderly, lactation, pregnancy (D)

Precautions: Anemia

Pharmacokinetics:

PO: Onset 20-60 min, peak 8-12 hr, duration 6-10 hr, metabolized by liver, excreted by kidneys, crosses placenta, excreted in breast milk, half-life 53-118 hr

Interactions/incompatibilities:
• Increased effects: CNS depressants, alcohol, chloramphenicol, valproic acid, disulfiram, nondepolarizing skeletal muscle relaxants, sulfonamides
• Increased orthostatic hypotension: furosemide

NURSING CONSIDERATIONS

Assess:
• Blood studies, liver function tests during long-term treatment
• Therapeutic level 15-40 mg/ml

Administer:
• IV after slow dilution with at least 10 ml sterile H_2O for inj; give 65 mg or less/min; titrate to patient response
• Give IM inj deeply into large muscle mass to prevent tissue sloughing

Evaluate:
• Mental status: mood, sensorium, affect, memory (long, short)
• Respiratory depression

P

---

italics = common side effects   ***bold italic*** = life threatening reactions

• Blood dyscrasias: fever, sore throat, bruising, rash, jaundice
Teach patient/family:
• To avoid hazardous activities until stabilized on drug
• Never to withdraw drug abruptly
• Therapeutic effects (PO) may not be seen for 2-3 wk
Treatment of overdose: Administer calcium gluconate IV

---

phenolphthalein

(fee-nol-thay'leen)
Alophen, Espotabs, Evac-U-Gen, Evac-U-Lax, Ex-Lax, Feen-A-Mint, Phenolax, Prulet

Func. class.: Laxative, stimulant/irritant
Chem. class.: Diphenylmethane

Action: Directly acts on intestinal smooth muscle by increasing motor activity; thought to irritate colonic intramural plexus
Uses: Constipation, preparation for bowel surgery or examination
Dosage and routes:
• *Adult:* PO 60-270 mg hs
• *Child >6 yr:* 30-60 mg/day
• *Child 2-5 yr:* 15-20 mg/day
Available forms include: Tabs 60 mg; chew tab 60, 64.8, 80, 90, 97.2 mg; chew gum 97.2 mg; susp 22 mg/5 ml
Side effects/adverse reactions:
INTEG: Rash, urticaria, ***Stevens-Johnson syndrome***
GI: Nausea, vomiting, anorexia, diarrhea
META: Hypokalemia, electrolyte, fluid imbalances
Contraindications: Hypersensitivity, GI obstructions, abdominal pain, nausea/vomiting, fecal impaction
Pharmacokinetics:
PO: Onset 6-8 hr; excreted in feces

NURSING CONSIDERATIONS
Assess:
• Blood, urine electrolytes if drug is used often by patient
• I&O ratio to identify fluid loss
Administer:
• Alone for better absorption
• In morning or evening (oral dose)
Evaluate:
• Therapeutic response: decrease in constipation
• Cause of constipation; identify whether fluids, bulk, or exercise is missing from lifestyle
• Cramping, rectal bleeding, nausea, vomiting; if these symptoms occur, drug should be discontinued
Teach patient/family:
• Keep out of children's reach, some is fruit or chocolate flavored
• Swallow tabs whole; do not chew
• Not to use laxatives for long-term therapy; bowel tone will be lost
• That normal bowel movements do not always occur daily
• Do not use in presence of abdominal pain, nausea, vomiting
• Notify physician if constipation unrelieved or if symptoms of electrolyte imbalance occur: muscle cramps, pain, weakness, dizziness
• Urine, feces may turn pink to yellow-brown
Lab test interferences:
BSP test

---

phenoxybenzamine HCl

(fen-ox-ee-ben'za-meen)
Dibenzyline

Func. class.: Antihypertensive
Chem. class.: α-Adrenergic blocker

Action: α-Adrenergic blocker, which binds to α-adrenergic receptors, dilating peripheral blood vessels, lowers peripheral resistance, lowers blood pressure

Uses: Pheochromocytoma

Dosage and routes:

• *Adult:* PO 10 mg bid, increase by 10 mg qod, not to exceed 60 mg/ day; usual range: 20-40 mg bid-tid

Available forms include: Caps 10 mg

Side effects/adverse reactions:

GI: Dry mouth, nausea, vomiting, diarrhea

CV: Postural hypotension, tachycardia, palpitations

CNS: Dizziness, flushing, drowsiness, sedation, weakness, confusion, headache, malaise

GU: Inhibition of ejaculation

EENT: Nasal congestion, dry mouth, miosis

INTEG: Allergic contact dermatitis

Contraindications: Hypersensitivity, CHF, angina, cerebral vascular insufficiency, coronary arteriosclerosis

Precautions: Severe renal disease, severe pulmonary disease, pregnancy (C)

Pharmacokinetics:

PO: Onset 2 hr, peak 4-6 hr, duration 3-4 days; half-life 24 hr, metabolized in liver, excreted in urine, bile

Interactions/incompatibilities:

• Hypotensive response: epinephrine, antihypertensives

NURSING CONSIDERATIONS

Assess:

• Electrolytes: K, Na, Cl, CO_2

• Weight daily, I&O

• B/P lying, standing before starting treatment, q4h after

Administer:

• Starting with low dose, gradually increasing to prevent side effects

• Gum, frequent rinsing of mouth or hard candy for dry mouth

• With food or milk for GI symptoms

Evaluate:

• Therapeutic response: decreased B/P, increased peripheral pulses

• Nausea, vomiting, diarrhea

• Skin turgor, dryness of mucous membranes for hydration status

Teach patient/family:

• Avoid alcoholic beverages

• To report dizziness, palpitations, fainting

• To change position slowly or fainting may occur

• To take drug exactly as prescribed

• To avoid all OTC products: cough, cold, allergy, unless directed by physician

Treatment of overdose: Administer IV saline, norepinephrine, elevate legs, discontinue drug

---

phensuximide

(fen-sux′i-mide)

Milontin

Func. class.: Anticonvulsant

Chem. class.: Succinimide

Action: Inhibits spike, wave formation in absence seizures (petit mal), decreases amplitude, frequency, duration

Uses: Absence (petit mal) seizures

Dosage and routes:

• *Adult and child:* PO 500 mg-1 g bid or tid

Available forms include: Caps 500 mg

Side effects/adverse reactions:

HEMA: Agranulocytosis, aplastic anemia, thrombocytopenia, leukocytosis, eosinophilia, pancytopenia

CNS: Drowsiness, dizziness, fatigue, euphoria, lethargy, anxiety, depression, irritability, insomnia,

---

italics = common side effects   ***bold italic*** = life threatening reactions

aggressiveness, weakness, headache

GI: Nausea, vomiting, heartburn, anorexia, diarrhea, abdominal pain, cramps, constipation

GU: Vaginal bleeding, *hematuria, renal damage,* urinary frequency

INTEG: Urticaria, pruritic erythema, hirsutism, *Stevens-Johnson syndrome*

EENT: Myopia, gum hypertrophy, tongue swelling, blurred vision

Contraindications: Hypersensitivity to succinimide derivatives

Precautions: Lactation, hepatic disease, pregnancy (D), renal disease

Pharmacokinetics:

PO: Peak 1-4 hr, metabolized by liver, excreted by kidneys, half-life 5-12 hr

Interactions/incompatibilities:

• Antagonist effect: tricyclic antidepressants (imipramine, doxepin)

• Decreased effects of: estrogens, oral contraceptives

NURSING CONSIDERATIONS

Assess:

• Renal studies: urinalysis, BUN, urine creatinine, q6 mo

• Blood studies: CBC, Hct, Hgb, reticulocyte counts q3 mo

• Hepatic studies: AST, ALT, bilirubin, creatinine q6 mo

• Drug levels during initial treatment, therapeutic range (40-80 μg/ml)

Administer:

• With food, milk to decrease GI symptoms

Perform/provide:

• Hard candy, frequent rinsing of mouth, gum for dry mouth

• Assistance with ambulation during early part of treatment; dizziness occurs

Evaluate:

• Mental status: mood, sensorium, affect, behavioral changes; if mental status changes, notify physician

• Eye problems; need for ophthalmic exam before, during, after treatment (slit lamp, fundoscopy, tonometry)

• Allergic reaction: red raised rash; if this occurs, drug should be discontinued

• Blood dyscrasias: fever, sore throat, bruising, rash, jaundice

• Toxicity: bone marrow depression, nausea, vomiting, ataxia, diplopia

Teach patient/family:

• To carry ID card or Medic-Alert bracelet stating drugs taken, condition, physician's name, phone number

• To avoid driving, other activities that require alertness

• To avoid alcohol ingestion, CNS depressants; increased sedation may occur

• Not to discontinue medication quickly after long-term use

• To call physician if sore throat, fever, malaise, bruises, epistaxis occur

• May color urine pink or red

Lab test interferences:

Increase: Coombs' test

Treatment of overdose: Lavage, activated charcoal, monitor electrolytes, VS

---

phentermine HCl

(fen'ter-meen)

Anoxine, Fastin, Ionamin, Obe-Nix, Adipex-P, Dapex, Obephen, Obermine, Parmine, Phentrol, Rolaphent, Wilpowr

Func. class.: Cerebral stimulant

Chem. class.: Sympathomimetic amine

Controlled Substance Schedule IV

Action: Stimulates satiety center by action on adrenergic pathways
Uses: Exogenous obesity
Dosage and routes:
• *Adult:* PO 8 mg tid 30 min before meals or 15-37.5 mg qd
Available forms include: Tabs 8, 30, 37.5 mg; caps 15, 18.75, 30, 37.5 mg; caps time rel 30 mg
Side effects/adverse reactions:
CNS: Hyperactivity, insomnia, restlessness, dizziness, tremor, headache
GI: Nausea, anorexia, dry mouth, constipation, unpleasant taste
GU: Impotence, change in libido
CV: Palpitations, tachycardia, hypertension
INTEG: Urticaria
EENT: Blurred vision
Contraindications: Hypersensitivity, hyperthyroidism, hypertension, glaucoma, severe arteriosclerosis, angina pectoris, cardiovascular disease, pregnancy (C), child <12 yr
Precautions: Pregnancy (C), lactation, drug abuse, anxiety
Pharmacokinetics:
CON REL: Duration 10-14 hr; metabolized by liver, excreted by kidneys
Interactions/incompatibilities:
• Hypertensive crisis: MAOIs or within 14 days of MAOIs
• Increased effect of phentermine: acetazolamide, antacids, sodium bicarbonate, ascorbic acid, ammonium chloride
• Decreased effect of phentermine: tricyclics
• Decreased effect of: guanethidine, other antihypertensives
• Decreased insulin requirements: diabetes mellitus

NURSING CONSIDERATIONS
Assess:
• VS, B/P since this drug may re-

verse antihypertensives check patients with cardiac disease more often
• CBC, urinalysis, in diabetes: blood sugar, urine sugar; insulin changes may need to be made since eating will decrease
• Height and growth rate in children; growth rate may be decreased
Administer:
• At least 6 hr before hs to avoid sleeplessness
• For obesity only if patient is on weight reduction program including dietary changes, exercise; patient will develop tolerance, and loss of weight won't occur without additional methods, give 30 mins before meals
• Gum, hard candy, frequent sips of water for dry mouth
Perform/provide:
• Check to see PO medication has been swallowed
Evaluate:
• Mental status: mood, sensorium, affect, stimulation, insomnia, aggressiveness
• Physical dependency: should not be used for extended periods of time; dose should be discontinued gradually, tolerance occurs with long-term use
• Withdrawal symptoms: headache, nausea, vomiting, muscle pain, weakness
Teach patient/family:
• To decrease caffeine consumption (coffee, tea, cola, chocolate), which may increase irritability, stimulation
• Avoid OTC preparations unless approved by physician
• To taper off drug over several weeks, or depression, increased sleeping, lethargy may ensue
• To avoid alcohol ingestion
• To avoid hazardous activities un-

P

italics = common side effects   ***bold italic*** = life threatening reactions

til patient is stabilized on medication

• To get needed rest; patients will feel more tired at end of day

Treatment of overdose: Administer fluids, hemodialysis or peritoneal dialysis; antihypertensive for increased B/P; ammonium Cl for increase excretion

---

phentolamine mesylate

(fen-tole'a-meen)
Regitine, Rogitine*

Func. class.: Antihypertensive
Chem. class.: α-Adrenergic blocker

Action: α-Adrenergic blocker, binds to α-adrenergic receptors, dilating peripheral blood vessels, lowering peripheral resistances, lowering blood pressure

Uses: Hypertension, pheochromocytoma, prevention, treatment of dermal necrosis following extravasation of norepinephrine or dopamine

Dosage and routes:
Treatment of hypertensive episodes in pheochromocytoma
• *Adult:* 5 mg IV/IM, repeat if necessary
• *Child:* 1 mg IV/IM, repeat if necessary
• *Adult:* 2.5 mg IV, if negative repeat with 5 mg IV
• *Child:* 0.5 mg IV, if negative repeat with 1 mg IV
Prevention, treatment of necrosis
• *Adult:* 5-10 mg/10 ml NS injected into area of norepinephrine extravasation within 12 hr; 10 mg/1000 ml norepinephrine solution is preventive dose

Available forms include: Inj IM, IV 5 mg/ml; tabs 25, 50 mg (only injectable form available in US)

Side effects/adverse reactions:
GI: Dry mouth, nausea, vomiting, diarrhea, abdominal pain
CV: Hypotension, tachycardia, angina, dysrhythmias, myocardial infarction
CNS: Dizziness, flushing, weakness
EENT: Nasal congestion

Contraindications: Hypersensitivity, myocardial infarction, coronary insufficiency, angina

Precautions: Pregnancy (C), lactation

Pharmacokinetics:
IV: Peak 2 min, duration 10-15 min
IM: Peak 15-20 min, duration 3-4 hr
Metabolized in liver, excreted in urine

Interactions/incompatibilities:
• Increased effects of: epinephrine, antihypertensives
• Not to be mixed in solution or syringe with any drug except levarterenol

NURSING CONSIDERATIONS
Assess:
• Electrolytes: K, Na, Cl, CO_2
• Weight daily, I&O
• B/P lying, standing before starting treatment, q4h after

Administer:
• IV after diluting 5 mg/1 ml sterile H_2O for inj; may be further diluted with 5-10 ml sterile H_2O for inj; give 5 mg or less/min
• Gum, frequent rinsing of mouth or hard candy for dry mouth
• After having vasopressor nearby
• After discontinuing all medication for 24 hr

Evaluate:
• Nausea, vomiting, diarrhea
• Edema in feet, daily
• Skin turgor, dryness of mucous membranes for hydration status
• Postural hypotension
• Cardiac system: pulse, ECG

---

* Available in Canada only

Teach patient/family:
• That bedrest is required during treatment, 1 hr after
Treatment of overdose: Administer norepinephrine, discontinue drug

---

phenylbutazone

(fen-ill-byoo'-ta-zone)
Algoverine, Azolid, Butagesic, Butazolidin, Intrabutazone, Malgesic, Neo-Zoline
Func. class.: Nonsteroidal antiinflammatory
Chem. class.: Pyrazolone derivative

Action: Inhibits prostaglandin synthesis by decreasing an enzyme needed for biosynthesis; possesses analgesic, antiinflammatory, antipyretic properties
Uses: Mild to moderate pain, osteoarthritis, rheumatoid arthritis
Dosage and routes:
Pain
• *Adult:* PO 100-200 mg tid-qid, then after desired response 100 mg tid-qid, not to exceed 600 mg/day
Acute Arthritis
• *Adult:* PO 400 mg, then 100 mg q4h × 4 days or until desired response
Available forms include: Tabs 100 mg; caps 100 mg
Side effects/adverse reactions:
GI: Nausea, anorexia, vomiting, diarrhea, jaundice, ***cholestatic hepatitis,*** constipation, flatulence, cramps, dry mouth, peptic ulcer
CNS: Dizziness, drowsiness, fatigue, tremors, confusion, insomnia, anxiety, depression
CV: Tachycardia, peripheral edema, palpitations, dysrhythmias
INTEG: Purpura, rash, pruritus, sweating

*GU: **Nephrotoxicity: dysuria, hematuria, oliguria, azotemia***
*HEMA: **Bone marrow suppression***
EENT: Tinnitus, hearing loss, blurred vision
Contraindications: Hypersensitivity, asthma, severe renal disease, severe hepatic disease, pregnancy (D)
Precautions: Lactation, children, bleeding disorders, GI disorders, cardiac disorders, hypersensitivity to other antiinflammatory agents
Pharmacokinetics:
PO: Peak 2 hr, half-life 3-3½ hr; metabolized in liver, excreted in urine (metabolites) excreted in breast milk, 98% protein binding
Interactions/incompatibilities:
• Increased action of: coumarin, phenytoin, sulfonamides when used with this drug
NURSING CONSIDERATIONS
Assess:
• Renal, liver, blood studies: BUN, creatinine, AST, ALT, Hgb, before treatment, periodically thereafter
• Audiometric, ophthalmic exam before, during, after treatment
• For past history of peptic ulcer disease
Administer:
• With food to decrease GI symptoms; best to take on empty stomach to facilitate absorption
Perform/provide:
• Storage at room temperature
Evaluate:
• Therapeutic response: decreased pain, stiffness, swelling in joints, ability to move more easily
• For eye, ear problems: blurred vision, tinnitus (may indicate toxicity)
Teach patient/family:
• To report blurred vision or ringing, roaring in ears (may indicate toxicity)

---

italics = common side effects   ***bold italic*** = life threatening reactions

- To avoid driving or other hazardous activities if dizziness or drowsiness occurs
- To report change in urine pattern, weight increase, edema, pain increase in joints, fever, blood in urine (indicates nephrotoxicity)
- That therapeutic effects may take up to 1 mo
- To report black, tarry stools
- To take with full glass of water

---

phenylephrine HCl

(fen-ill-ef′rin)

Neo-Synephrine

Func. class.: Adrenergic, direct acting

Chem. class.: Substituted phenylethylamine

Action: Powerful and selective (α_1) receptor agonist causing contraction of blood vessels

Uses: Hypotension, paroxysmal supraventricular tachycardia, shock

Dosage and routes:

Hypotension

- *Adult:* SC/IM 2-5 mg, may repeat q10-15 min if needed IV 0.1-0.5 mg, may repeat q10-15 min if needed

PVCs

- *Adult:* IV BOL 0.5 mg given rapidly, not to exceed prior dose by >0.1 mg total dose >1 mg

Shock

- *Adult:* IV INF 10 mg/500 ml D_5W given 100-180 gtts/min, then 40-60 gtts/min titrated to B/P

Available forms include: Inj IV, SC, IM, 1% (10 mg/ml)

Side effects/adverse reactions:

CNS: Headache, anxiety, tremor, insomnia, dizziness

CV: Palpitations, tachycardia, hypertension, ectopic beats, angina

GI: Nausea, vomiting

INTEG: Necrosis, tissue sloughing with extravasation, *gangrene*

Contraindications: Hypersensitivity, ventricular fibrillation, tachydysrhythmias, pheochromocytoma

Precautions: Pregnancy (C), lactation, arterial embolism, peripheral vascular disease

Pharmacokinetics:

IV: Duration 20-30 min

IM/SC: Duration 45-60 min

Interactions/incompatibilities:

- Do not use within 2 wk of MAOIs, or hypertensive crisis may result
- Dysrhythmias: general anesthetics
- Decreased action of phenylephrine: α-blockers
- Increase in B/P: oxytocics
- Increased pressor effect: tricyclic antidepressant, MAOIs
- Incompatible with alkaline solutions: Na HCO_3

NURSING CONSIDERATIONS

Assess:

- I&O ratio, notify MD if output <30 cc/hr
- ECG during administration continuously; if B/P increases, drug is decreased
- B/P and pulse q5 min after parenteral route
- CVP or PWP during infusion if possible

Administer:

- Plasma expanders for hypovolemia
- IV after diluting 1 mg/9 ml sterile H_2O for inj; give dose over ½-1 min; may be diluted 10 mg/500 ml of D_5W or NS; titrate to patient response, check for extravastion, check site for infiltration, use infusion pump

Perform/provide:

- To store reconstituted solution if

---

refrigerated for no longer than 24 hr
• Not to use discolored solutions
Evaluate:
• For paresthesias and coldness of extremities, peripheral blood flow may decrease
• For therapeutic response: increase B/P with stabilization
Teach patient/family:
• The reason for drug administration
• To report pain at infusion site immediately
Treatment of overdose: Administer an α-blocker

---

phenylephrine HCl (nasal)

(fen-ill-ef'rin)

Alconefrin, Coricidin Nasal Mist, Coryzine, Ephrine, Neo-Synephrine, Sinarest Nasal Spray, Sinophen Intranasal, Vacon

Func. class.: Nasal decongestant
Chem. class.: Sympathomimetic amine

Action: Produces vasoconstriction (rapid, long-acting) of arterioles, thereby decreasing fluid exudation, mucosal engorgement
Uses: Nasal congestion
Dosage and routes:
• *Adult:* INSTILL 2-3 gtts or sprays to nasal mucosa bid (0.25%-1%); TOP apply to nasal mucosa q3-4h prn
• *Child 6-12 yr:* INSTILL 1-2 gtts or sprays (0.25%) q3-4h prn
• *Child <6 yr:* INSTILL 2-3 gtts or sprays (0.125%) q3-4h prn
Available forms include: Sol 0.125%, 0.16%, 0.2%, 0.25%, 0.5%, 1%; jelly 0.5%
Side effects/adverse reactions:
GI: Nausea, vomiting, anorexia

EENT: Irritation, burning, sneezing, stinging, dryness, rebound congestion
INTEG: Contact dermatitis
CNS: Anxiety, restlessness, tremors, weakness, insomnia, dizziness, fever, headache
Contraindications: Hypersensitivity to sympathomimetic amines
Precautions: Child <6 yr, elderly, diabetes, cardiovascular disease, hypertension, hyperthyroidism, increased ICP, prostatic hypertrophy, pregnancy (C), glaucoma
Interactions/incompatibilities:
• Hypertension: MAOIs, β-adrenergic blockers
• Hypotension: methyldopa, mecamylamine, reserpine
NURSING CONSIDERATIONS
Administer:
• No more than q4h
• For <4 consecutive days
Perform/provide:
• Environmental humidification to decrease nasal congestion, dryness
• Storage in light-resistant containers; do not expose to high temperatures
Evaluate:
• Redness, swelling, pain in nasal passages
Teach patient/family:
• Stinging may occur for a few applications; drying of mucosa may be decreased by environmental humidification
• To notify physician if irregular pulse, insomnia, dizziness, or tremors occur
• Proper administration to avoid systemic absorption

P

---

italics = common side effects   **bold italic** = life threatening reactions

phenylephrine HCl (optic)

(fen-ill-ef'rin)

AK-Dilate, Isopto Frin, Neo-Synephrine 10% Plain, Neo-Synephrine Viscous, Prefrin

Func. class.: Ophthalmic vasoconstrictor

Chem. class.: Direct sympathomimetic amine (α-agonist)

Action: Vasoconstriction of eye arterioles; decreases eye engorgement by stimulation of α-adrenergic receptors

Uses: Topical ocular vasoconstrictor

Dosage and routes:

Eye irritation

• *Adult:* INSTILL 2 gtts of a 0.12% sol; may repeat q3-4h

Uveitis/glaucoma/surgery

• *Adult and child:* INSTILL 1 gtt of a 2.5% or 10% sol in upper surface of cornea

Available forms include: Sol 10%, 2.5%, 0.12%

Side effects/adverse reactions:

CNS: Headache, dizziness, weakness

CV: Bradycardia, hypertension, dysrhythmias, *tachycardia, CV collapse,* palpitation

EENT: Stinging, lacrimation, blurred vision, conjunctival allergy

Contraindications: Hypersensitivity, glaucoma (narrow-angle)

Precautions: Severe hypertension, diabetes, hyperthyroidism, elderly, severe arteriosclerosis, cardiac disease, infants, pregnancy (C)

Pharmacokinetics:

INSTILL: Peak 1 hr, duration 0.5-7 hr depending on strength

Interactions/incompatibilities:

• Increased pressor effects: MAOIs, tricyclic antidepressants, H_1 antihistamines, guanethidine

NURSING CONSIDERATIONS

Assess:

• B/P, pulse, systemic absorption does occur

Perform/provide:

• Storage in tight, light-resistant container, do not use discolored solutions

Teach patient/family:

• To report change in vision, blurring, loss of sight; breathing trouble, sweating, flushing

• Method of instillation, tilt head backward, hold dropper over eye, drop medication inside lower lid, using pressure on inside corner of eye hold 1 min, do not touch dropper to eye

• That blurred vision will decrease with repeated use of drug

• To notify physician if headache, spots, redness, pain occurs; discontinue use

• To use sunglasses if photophobia occurs

• To use exactly as prescribed

phenytoin sodium/ phenytoin sodium extended/phenytoin sodium prompt

(fen'i-toy-in)

Dilantin, Dilantin Capsules, Di-Phen, Diphenylan

Func. class.: Anticonvulsant

Chem. class.: Hydantoin

Action: Inhibits spread of seizure activity in motor cortex

Uses: Generalized tonic-clonic (grand-mal) seizures, status epilepticus, nonepileptic seizures associated with Reye's syndrome or after head trauma, migraines, trigeminal neuralgia, Bell's palsy, ventricular dysrhythmias uncontrolled by antidysrhythmics

Dosage and routes:

Seizures

• *Adult:* IV loading dose of 900 mg-1.5 g run at 50 mg/min; if patient has received phenytoin, then 100-300 mg run at 50 mg/min; PO loading dose of 900 mg-1.5 g divided tid, then 300 mg/day (extended) or divided tid (extended/prompt)

• *Child:* IV loading dose of 15 mg/kg run at 50 mg/min; if patient has received phenytoin, then 5-7 mg/kg run at 50 mg/min, may repeat in 30 min; PO loading dose of 15 mg/kg divided q8-12h, then 5-7 mg/kg in divided doses q12h

Neuritic pain

• *Adult:* PO 200-400 mg/day

Ventricular dysrhythmias

• *Adult:* PO loading dose 1 g divided over 24 hr, then 500 mg/day × 2 days; IV 250 mg given over 5 min, until dysrhythmias subside or 1 g is given, or 100 mg q15 min until dysrhythmias subside or 1 g is given

• *Child:* PO 3-8 mg/kg or 250 mg/m²/day as single dose or divided in 2 doses; IV 3-8 mg/kg given over several min, or 250 mg/m²/day as single dose or divided in 2 doses

Available forms include: Susp 30, 125 mg/5 ml; tabs, chewable 50 mg; inj 50 mg/ml; caps ext 30, 100 mg; caps prompt 30, 100 mg

Side effects/adverse reactions:

*HEMA: **Agranulocytosis, leukopenia, aplastic anemia, thrombocytopenia, megloblastic anemia***

CV: Hypotension, ventricular fibrillation

CNS: Drowsiness, dizziness, insomnia, paresthesias, depression, suicidal tendencies, aggression, headache, confusion, slurred speech

GI: Nausea, vomiting, constipation, anorexia, weight loss, ***hepatitis,*** jaundice, ***gingival hyperplasia***

GU: Nephritis, albuminuria

INTEG: Rash, lupus erythematosis, ***Stevens-Johnson syndrome,*** hirsutism

EENT: Nystagmus, diplopia, blurred vision

Contraindications: Hypersensitivity, psychiatric disease, pregnancy (D), bradycardia, SA and AV block, Stokes-Adams syndrome

Precautions: Allergies, hepatic disease, renal disease

Pharmacokinetics:

PO: Duration 5 hr, metabolized by liver, excreted by kidneys

Interactions/incompatibilities:

• Decreased effects of phenytoin: alcohol (chronic use), antihistamines, antacids, antineoplastics, CNS depressants, rifampin, folic acid

NURSING CONSIDERATIONS

Assess:

• Drug level: toxic level 30-50 µg/ml

• Blood studies: CBC, platelets q2 wk until stabilized, then q mo × 12, then q3 mo; discontinue drug if neutrophils are <1600/mm³

Administer:

• After diluting with normal saline, never water; inject slowly <50 mg/min, clear IV tubing first with NS sol, use in-line filter, discard 4 hr after preparation; inject into larger veins to prevent purple glove syndrome

• PO doses divided with or after meals to decrease adverse effects

Evaluate:

• Therapeutic response: decrease in

P

---

italics = common side effects   **bold italic** = life threatening reactions

severity of seizures, or ventricular dysrhythmias

• Mental status: mood, sensorium, affect, memory (long, short)

• Respiratory depression

• Blood dyscrasias: fever, sore throat, bruising, rash, jaundice

Teach patient/family:

• That urine may turn pink

• Not to discontinue drug abruptly, seizures may occur

• Proper brushing of teeth using a soft toothbrush, flossing to prevent gingival hyperplasia

• To avoid hazardous activities until stabilized on drug

• To carry Medic-Alert ID stating drug use

• That heavy use of alcohol may diminish effect of drug

• Not to change brands or forms once stabilized on therapy

Lab test interferences:

Decrease: Dexamethasone, metyrapone test, PBI, urinary steroids

Increase: Glucose, alk phosphatase, BSP

---

physostigmine salicylate/physostigmine sulfate

(fi-zoe-stig'meen)

Isopto Eserine Solution/Eserine Sulfate Ointment, Fisostin, Antilirium, Geneserine

Func. class.: Miotic

Chem. class.: Cholinesterase inhibitor

Action: Increases concentration of acetylcholine at cholinergic transmission sites, thus causing prolonged, exaggerated action; produces constriction of ciliary muscles, iris sphincter, causing iris to be pulled away from anterior chamber angle, aiding in aqueous humor drainage

Uses: Used in treatment of wide-angle glaucoma reversal of anticholinergic or antidepressant poisoning

Dosage and routes:

• *Adult and child:* INSTILL OINT ¼ inch strip of 0.25% oint in conjunctival sac; INSTILL SOL 1-2 gtts of a 0.25%-0.5% sol in conjunctival sac qd-qid

Available forms include: Oint 0.25% (sulfate); sol 0.25% (salicylate)

Side effects/adverse reactions:

CNS: Convulsions, headache

CV: Hypertension, hypotension, bradycardia, irregular pulse

GI: Nausea, vomiting, abdominal cramps

RESP: Bronchospasm, dyspnea, *pulmonary edema*

EENT: Blurred vision, conjunctivitis, allergic reactions, rhinorrhea, salivation, eye, brow pain, lacrimation, twitching of eyelids

Contraindications: Asthma, bronchitis, diabetes mellitus, CV disease, inflammatory disease of iris or ciliary body

Precautions: Epilepsy, parkinsonism, bradycardia, pregnancy (C)

Interactions/incompatibilities:

• Benzalkonium chloride in solution or syringe

NURSING CONSIDERATIONS

Administer:

• Topically to conjunctival sac

• Immediately after reconstituting; discard unused portion

Perform/provide:

• Only clear solutions, never pink or brown

Teach patient/family:

• To report change in vision, blurring or loss of sight, trouble breathing, sweating, flushing

• Method of instillation, including

---

*Available in Canada only

pressure on lacrimal sac for 1 min, not to touch dropper to eye
• That long-term therapy may be required
• That blurred vision will decrease with repeated use of drug
• That drug is often irritating to eye, rarely tolerated for prolonged periods
• That drug may be prescribed for bedtime use to prevent nocturnal rise in ocular tension
• That maximal effect of topical application is reached in 30 min, may last 12-36 hr
• To observe eyes for irritation, development of cataracts

---

physostigmine salicylate

(fi-zoe-stig′meen)
Antilirium
Func. class.: Antidote, reversible anticholinesterase
Chem. class.: Tertiary amine

Action: Increases acetylcholine at cholinergic nerve terminals, reverses central, peripheral anticholinergic effects
Uses: To reverse CNS effects of diazepam; anticholinergic, tricyclic antidepressant, Alzheimer's disease, hereditary ataxia
Dosage and routes:
Overdose of anticholinergics
• *Adult:* IM/IV 2 mg, give no more than 1 mg/min; may repeat
• *Pediatric:* IM/IV inj 0.02 mg/kg, not more than 0.5 mg/min; may repeat at 5-10 min intervals until max dose of 2 mg
Postanesthesia
• *Adult:* IM/IV 0.5-1 mg, give no more than 1 mg/min (IV); can repeat at 10 to 30 min intervals
Available forms include: Inj IM, IV 1 mg/ml

Side effects/adverse reactions:
INTEG: Rash, urticaria
CNS: Dizziness, headache, sweating, confusion, weakness, ***convulsions,*** incoordination, ***paralysis,*** hallucination, delirium
GI: Nausea, diarrhea, vomiting, cramps
CV: Bradycardia, hypotension
GU: Frequency, incontinence
*RESP: **Respiratory depression, bronchospasm, constriction***
EENT: Miosis, blurred vision, lacrimation
Contraindications: Hypotension, obstruction of intestine, renal system, asthma, gangrene, CV disease, choline esters, depolarizing neuromuscular blocking agents
Precautions: Seizure disorders, bronchial asthma, coronary occlusion, hyperthyroidism, dysrhythmias, peptic ulcer, megacolon, poor GI motility, pregnancy (C), Parkinson's disease, bradycardia, lactation
Pharmacokinetics:
IM/IV: Onset 5 min, duration 45-60 min; crosses blood-brain barrier, excreted in urine
Interactions/incompatibilities:
• Decreased action of: gallamine, metocurine, pancuronium, tubocurarine, atropine
• Increased action of: decamethonium, succinylcholine
• Decreased action of physostigmine: aminoglycosides, anesthetics, procainamide, quinidine
NURSING CONSIDERATIONS
Assess:
• VS; respiration q8h
• I&O ratio; check for urinary retention or incontinence
Administer:
• IV undiluted, give through Y-tube or 3-way stopcock; give 1 mg or less/1-3 min

P

---

italics = common side effects   ***bold italic*** = life threatening reactions

• Only with atropine sulfate available for cholinergic crisis
• Only after all other cholinergics have been discontinued
• Increased doses if tolerance occurs

Perform/provide:
• Storage at room temperature

Evaluate:
• Therapeutic response: LOC—alert
• Drug should be discontinued if toxicity occurs

Treatment of overdose: Can cause cholinergic crisis; atropine is an antagonist

---

phytonadione (vitamin K₁)

(fye-toe-na-dye'one)
AquaMEPHYTON, Konakion, Mephyton
Func. class.: Vitamin K₁, fat-soluble vitamin

Action: Needed for adequate blood clotting (factors II, VII, IX, X)
Uses: Vitamin K malabsorption, hypoprothrombinemia, prevention of hypoprothrombinemia caused by oral anticoagulants

Dosage and routes:
Hypoprothrombinemia caused by vitamin K malabsorption
• *Adult:* PO/IM 2-25 mg may repeat or increase to 50 mg
• *Child:* PO/IM 5-10 mg
• *Infants:* PO/IM 2 mg
Prevention of hemorrhagic disease of the newborn
• *Neonate:* SC/IM 0.5-1 mg after birth, repeat in 6-8 hrs if required
Hypoprothrombinemia caused by oral anticoagulants
• *Adult:* PO/SC/IM 2.5-10 mg, may repeat 12-48 hr after PO dose

or 6-8 hr after SC/IM dose, based on PT
Available forms include: Tabs 5 mg; inj aqueous colloidal IM, IV; inj aqueous dispersion 2, 10 mg/ml, IM only

Side effects/adverse reactions:
CNS: Headache, *brain damage* (large doses)
GI: Nausea, decrease liver function tests
HEMA: Hemolytic anemia, hemoglobinuria, hyperbilirubinemia
INTEG: Rash, urticaria

Contraindications: Hypersensitivity, severe hepatic disease, last few weeks of pregnancy
Precautions: Pregnancy (C), neonates
Pharmacokinetics:
PO/INJ: Metabolized, crosses placenta

Interactions/incompatibilities:
• Decreased action of phytonadione: cholestyramine, mineral oil
• Decreased action of: oral anticoagulants

NURSING CONSIDERATIONS
Assess:
• Pro-time during treatment (2 sec deviation from control time, bleeding time, and clotting time)

Administer:
• IV after diluting with D₅ NS or NS 10 ml or more; give 1 mg/min or more
• IV only when other routes not possible (deaths have occurred)

Perform/provide
• Storage in tight, light-resistant container

Evaluate:
• Therapeutic response: decreased bleeding tendencies, decreased pro-time, decreased clotting time
• Nutritional status: liver (beef), spinach, tomatoes, coffee, aspara-

---

gus, broccoli, cabbage, lettuce, greens

Teach patient/family
• Not to take other supplements, unless directed by physician
• Necessary foods to be included in diet

---

pilocarpine HCl/pilocarpine nitrate

(pye-loe-kar′peen)
Adsorbocarpine, Akarpine, Almocarpine, Isopto Carpine, Miocarpine,* Ocusert Pilo, Pilocar, Pilocel, Pilomiotin, P.V. Carpine Liquifilm
Func. class.: Miotic, direct-acting
Chem. class.: Cholinergic agonist

Action: Directly acts on cholinergic receptor sites, induces miosis, spasm of accommodation, fall in intraocular pressure, caused by stimulation of ciliary, pupillary sphincter muscles which leads to pulling away of iris from filtration angle, resulting in increased outflow of aqueous humor

Uses: Primary glaucoma, early stages of wide-angle glaucoma (less useful in advanced stages), chronic open-angle glaucoma, acute narrow-angle glaucoma before emergency surgery; also used to neutralize mydriatics used during eye exam; may be used alternately with mydriatics to break adhesions between iris and lens

Dosage and routes:
• *Adult and child:* INSTILL SOL 1-2 gtts of 1% or 2% solution in eye q6-8h; INSTILL 20-40 μg/hr (Ocusert) in cul-de-sac of eye
Available forms include: 0.25% to 10% sol; Ocusert Pilo 20, 40
Side effects/adverse reactions:
CV: Hypotension, tachycardia
RESP: **Bronchospasm**

GI: Nausea, vomiting, abdominal cramps, diarrhea
EENT: Blurred vision, browache, twitching of eyelids, eye pain with change in focus
Contraindications: Bradycardia, hyperthyroidism, coronary artery disease, obstruction of GI/urinary tracts (or if strength of walls of these structures in question, peptic ulcers), epilepsy, parkinsonism, asthma
Precautions: Bronchial asthma, hypertension, pregnancy (C)
NURSING CONSIDERATIONS
Assess:
• Heart rate, respiratory status, B/P
• Replacement of ocular systems q wk; check system each hs, AM
Administer:
• After shaking vial to mix drug to clear solution, push stopper to mix sterile water with powder
• After cleaning stopper with alcohol
• Excess solution must be wiped away promptly to prevent its flow into lacrimal system, producing systemic symptoms
• Atropine should be readily available as antidote
• Immediately after reconstituting; discard unused portion
Perform/provide:
• Protect solution from light
• Store Ocusert systems between 2° and 8° C
Teach patient/family:
• To report change in vision, blurring or loss of sight, trouble breathing, sweating, flushing
• Method of instillation, including pressure on lacrimal sac for 1 min, not to touch dropper to eye
• That long-term therapy may be required

---

italics = common side effects   ***bold italic*** = life threatening reactions

• That blurred vision will decrease with repeated use of drug
• To discontinue use if local hypersensitivity reaction occurs
• That acuity in dim light will be reduced
• Not to drive while using drug

---

pinacidil

(pye-na'di-dil)
Pindac

Func. class.: Antihypertensive
Chem. class.: Vasodilator—peripheral

Action: Directly relaxes arteriolar smooth muscle, causing vasodilation
Uses: Severe hypertension not responsive to other therapy; topically to treat alopecia
Dosage and routes:
• *Adult:* PO 12.5-25 mg bid
Available forms include: Tabs 12.5, 25 mg
Side effects/adverse reactions:
CV: Severe rebound hypertension, tachycardia, angina, increased T wave, *CHF*, pulmonary edema, edema, sodium, water retention
CNS: Drowsiness, dizziness, sedation, headache, depression
GI: Nausea, vomiting, diarrhea, constipation, dry mouth
GU: Gynecomastia, breast tenderness
INTEG: Pruritus, *Stevens-Johnson syndrome*, rash, hirsutism
Contraindications: Acute myocardial infarction, dissecting aortic aneurysm, hypersensitivity, pheochromocytoma
Precautions: Pregnancy (C), lactation, children, renal disease, CAD, post MI
Pharmacokinetics:
Peak 1 hr, 60% protein bound, metabolized in the liver, excreted in urine/feces (active metabolites), half-life 1½-3 hr
Interactions/incompatibilities:
• Orthostatic hypotension: guanethidine
• Reduced effect of pinacidil: nonsteroidal antiinflammatory drugs
NURSING CONSIDERATIONS
Assess:
• Electrolytes: K, Na, Cl, CO_2
• Renal function studies: AST, ALT, alk phosphatase
• B/P, pulse
• Weight daily, I&O, nausea
Administer:
• With meals for better absorption, to decrease GI symptoms
• With β-blocker and/or diuretic
Evaluate:
• Therapeutic response: decreased B/P or increased hair growth
• Edema in feet, legs daily
• Skin turgor, dryness of mucous membranes for hydration status
• Rales, dyspnea, orthopnea
Teach patient/family:
• That body hair will increase, but is reversible after treatment is discontinued
• Not to discontinue drug abruptly
• To report pitting edema, dizziness, weight gain >5 lb, shortness of breath, bruising or bleeding, heart rate >20 beats/min over normal, severe indigestion, dizziness, light-headedness, panting, new or aggravated symptoms of angina
• To take drug exactly as prescribed or serious side effects may occur
Lab test interferences:
Increase: renal function studies
Decrease: Hgb/Hct/RBC
Treatment of overdose: Administer normal saline IV, phenylephrine, angiotensin II, vasopressor, dopamine may reverse hypotension

---

pindolol

(pin'doe-lole)

Visken

Func. class.: Antihypertensive

Chem. class.: Nonselective β-blocker

Action: Competitively blocks stimulation of β-adrenergic receptor within vascular smooth muscle; produces chronotropic, inotropic activity (decreases rate of SA node discharge, increases recovery time), slows conduction of AV node, decreases heart rate, which decreases O_2 consumption in myocardium; also, decreases renin-aldosterone-angiotensin system, at high doses inhibits β-2 receptors in bronchial system

Uses: Mild to moderate hypertension

Dosage and routes:

• *Adult:* PO 5 mg bid, usual dose 15 mg/day (5 mg tid), may increase by 10 mg/day q3-4 wk to a max of 60 mg/day

Available forms include: Tabs 5, 10 mg

Side effects/adverse reactions:

CV: Hypotension, bradycardia, **CHF,** edema, chest pain, palpitation, claudication, tachycardia, *AV block*

CNS: Insomnia, dizziness, hallucinations, anxiety, fatigue

GI: Nausea, vomiting, *ischemic colitis,* diarrhea, *abdominal pain, mesenteric arterial thrombosis*

INTEG: Rash, alopecia, pruritus, fever

*HEMA: **Agranulocytosis, thrombocytopenia, purpura***

EENT: Visual changes, sore throat, *double vision,* dry burning eyes

GU: Impotence, frequency

*RESP: **Bronchospasm,** dyspnea,* cough, rales

MISC: Joint pain, muscle pain

Contraindications: Hypersensitivity to β-blockers, cardiogenic shock, heart block (2nd, 3rd degree), sinus bradycardia, CHF, cardiac failure, bronchial asthma

Precautions: Major surgery, pregnancy (B), lactation, diabetes mellitus, renal disease, thyroid disease, COPD, well compensated heart failure, CAD, nonallergic bronchospasm

Pharmacokinetics:

PO: Peak 2-4 hr; half-life 3-4 hr, excreted 30%-45% unchanged, 60%-65% is metabolized by liver, excreted in breast milk

Interactions/incompatibilities:

• Increased hypotension, bradycardia: reserpine, hydralazine, methyldopa, prazosin, anticholinergics

• Decreased antihypertensive effects: indomethacin, sympathomimetics

• Increased hypoglycemic effect: insulin

• Decreased bronchodilation: theophyllines

NURSING CONSIDERATIONS

Assess:

• I&O, weight daily

• B/P during initial treatment, periodically thereafter; pulse q4h, note rate, rhythm, quality

• Apical/radial pulse before administration; notify physician of any significant changes

• Baselines in renal, liver function tests before therapy begins

Adminster:

• PO ac, hs, tablet may be crushed or swallowed whole

• Reduced dosage in renal dysfunction

Perform/provide:

• Storage in dry area at room temperature, do not freeze

P

---

italics = common side effects　　　**bold italic** = life threatening reactions

Evaluate:

• Therapeutic response: decreased B/P after 1-2 wk

• Edema in feet, legs daily

• Skin turgor, dryness of mucous membranes for hydration status

Teach patient/family:

• To take with or immediately after meals

• Not to discontinue drug abruptly, taper over 2 wk, may cause precipitate angina

• Not to use OTC products containing α-adrenergic stimulants (nasal decongestants, OTC cold preparations) unless directed by physician

• To report bradycardia, dizziness, confusion, depression, fever, sore throat, shortness of breath to physician

• To take pulse at home, advise when to notify physician

• To avoid alcohol, smoking, sodium intake

• To comply with weight control, dietary adjustments, modified exercise program

• To carry Medic Alert ID to identify drug you are taking, allergies

• To avoid hazardous activities if dizziness if present

• To report symptoms of CHF: difficult breathing, especially on exertion or when lying down, night cough, swelling of extremities

• To take medication at bedtime to prevent orthostatic hypotension

• To wear support hose to minimize effects of orthostatic hypotension

Lab test interferences:

Increase: Liver function tests, renal function tests

Treatment of overdose: Lavage, IV atropine for bradycardia, IV theophylline for bronchospasm, digitalis, O_2, diuretic for cardiac failure, hemodialysis, hypotension; give vasopressor (norepinephrine)

---

pipecuronium bromide
Arduran

Func. class.: Neuromuscular blocker (nondepolarizing)

Chem. class.: Synthetic curariform

Action: Inhibits transmission of nerve impulses by binding with cholinergic receptor sites, antagonizing action of acetylcholine

Uses: Facilitation of endotracheal intubation, skeletal muscle relaxation during mechanical ventilation, surgery, or general anesthesia

Dosage and routes: Dosage is individualized; in patients with normal renal function who are not obese, initial dose is 70-85 µg/kg; maintenance dose ranges from 10-15 µg/kg

Available forms include: inj IV 10-mg vials

Side effects/adverse reactions:

CV: Bradycardia, tachycardia, increased or decreased B/P, ventricular extrasystole, *myocardial ischemia, cardiovascular accident, thrombosis, atrial fibrillation*

RESP: Prolonged apnea, bronchospasm, cyanosis, respiratory depression

GU: Anuria

EENT: Increased secretions

CNS: Hypesthesia, CNS depression

MS: Weakness to prolonged skeletal muscle relaxation

INTEG: Rash, urticaria

METABOLIC: Hypoglycemia, hyperkalemia, increased creatinine

Contraindications: Hypersensitivity to bromide ion

Precautions: Pregnancy (C), renal disease, cardiac disease, lactation, children <3 mo, fluid and electrolyte imbalances, neuromuscular diseases, respiratory disease, obesity

Pharmacokinetics:

IV: Onset 30-45 sec, peak 3-5 min: metabolized (small amounts), excreted in urine (unchanged), crosses placenta

Interactions/incompatibilities:

• Increased neuromuscular blockade: aminoglycosides, quinidine, local anesthetics, polymyxin antibiotics, enflurane, isoflurane, tetracyclines, halothane, magnesium, colistin

NURSING CONSIDERATIONS

Assess:

• For electrolyte imbalances (K, Mg); may lead to increased action of this drug

• Vital signs (B/P, pulse, respirations, airway) until fully recovered: rate, depth, pattern of respirations, strength of hand grip

• I&O ratio; check for urinary retention, frequency, hesitancy

d**Administer:**

• Using nerve stimulator by anesthesiologist to determine neuromuscular blockade

• Atropine to counteract muscarinic effects

• After succinylcholine effects subside

• Anticholinesterase to reverse neuromuscular blockade

• By slow IV over 1-2 min (only by qualified persons, usually an anesthesiologist)

• Only fresh solution

Perform/provide:

• Storage in refrigerator; do not store in plastic containers or syringes

• Reassurance if communication is difficult during recovery from neuromuscular blockade

• Use reconstituted solution within 24 hr

• Frequent (q2h) instillation of artificial tears and covering eyes to prevent drying of cornea

Evaluate:

• Therapeutic response: paralysis of jaw, eyelid, head, neck, rest of body

• Recovery: decreased paralysis of face, diaphragm, leg, arm, rest of body

• Allergic reactions: rash, fever, respiratory distress, pruritus; drug should be discontinued

Treatment of overdose: Neostigmine, atropine, monitor VS; may require mechanical ventilation

---

piperacillin sodium

(pi-per'a-sill-in)

Pipracil*

Func. class.: Broad-spectrum antibiotic

Chem. class.: Extended-spectrum penicillin

Action: Interferes with cell wall replication of susceptible organisms; osmotically unstable cell wall swells and bursts from osmotic pressure

Uses: Respiratory, skin, urinary tract, bone infections, gonorrhea, pneumonia; effective for gram-positive cocci *(S. aureus, S. pyogenes, S. viridans, S. faecalis, S. bovis, S. pneumoniae)*, gram-negative cocci *(N. gonorrhoeae, N. meningitidis)*, gram-positive bacilli, *C. perfringens, C. tetani,* gram-negative bacilli *(Bacteroides, F. nucleatum, E. coli, Klebsiella, P. mirabilis, M. morganii, P. vulgaris, P. rehgesii, Enterobacter, Citrobacter, P. aeruginosa, Ser-*

ratia, Acinetobacter, Peptococcus, Peptostreptococcus, Eubacterium)

Dosage and routes:
Systemic infections
• *Adult and child >12 yr:* IM/IV 100-300 mg/kg/day in divided doses q4-6h

Prophylaxis of surgical infections
• *Adult:* IV 2g ½-1 hr before procedure, may be repeated during surgery or after surgery

Available forms include: Inj IM, IV 2, 3, 4, 40 g; IV INF 2, 3, 4 g

Side effects/adverse reactions:
HEMA: Anemia, increased bleeding time, *bone marrow depression*
GI: Nausea, vomiting, diarrhea, increased AST, ALT, abdominal pain, glossitis, colitis
GU: Oliguria, proteinuria, hematuria, vaginitis, moniliasis, *glomerulonephritis*
CNS: Lethargy, hallucinations, anxiety, depression, twitching, *coma, convulsions*
META: Hypokalemia, hypernatremia

Contraindications: Hypersensitivity to penicillins; neonates
Precautions: Pregnancy (B), hypersensitivity to cephalosporins, CHF

Pharmacokinetics:
IM: Peak 30-50 min
IV: Peak 20-30 min
Half-life 0.7-1.33 hr, excreted in urine, bile, breast milk, crosses placenta

Interactions/incompatibilities:
• Decreased antimicrobial effect of piperacillin: tetracyclines, erythromycins, aminoglycosides IV
• Increased piperacillin concentrations: aspirin, probenecid

NURSING CONSIDERATIONS
Assess:
• I&O ratio; report hematuria, oliguria since penicillin in high doses is nephrotoxic
• Any patient with compromised renal system since drug is excreted slowly in poor renal system function; toxicity may occur rapidly
• Liver studies: AST, ALT
• Blood studies: WBC, RBC, H&H, bleeding time
• Renal studies: urinalysis, protein, blood
• C&S before drug therapy; drug may be taken as soon as culture is taken

Administer:
• IV after diluting 1 g/5 ml or more sterile H_2O or 0.9% NaCl, shake, give dose over 3-5 min; may further dilute with D_5W, 0.9% NS, and give over ½ hr; discontinue primary IV
• Drug after C&S has been completed

Perform/provide:
• Adrenalin, suction, tracheostomy set, endotracheal intubation equipment on unit
• Adequate intake of fluids (2000 ml) during diarrhea episodes
• Scratch test to assess allergy, after securing order from physician; usually done when penicillin is only drug of choice
• Storage at room temperature, reconstituted solution for 24 hr or 7 days refrigerated

Evaluate:
• Therapeutic response: absence of fever, purulent drainage, redness, inflammation
• Bowel pattern before and during treatment
• Skin eruptions after administration of penicillin to 1 wk after discontinuing drug
• Respiratory status: rate, character, wheezing, tightness in chest

• Allergies before initiation of treatment, reaction of each medication; highlight allergies on chart, Kardex

Teach patient/family:

• That culture may be taken after completed course of medication

• To report sore throat, fever, fatigue; (could indicate superimposed infection)

• To wear or carry Medic Alert ID if allergic to penicillins

• To notify nurse of diarrhea

Lab test interferences:

False positive: Urine glucose, urine protein, Coombs'

Treatment of overdose: Withdraw drug, maintain airway, administer epinephrine, aminophylline, O₂, IV corticosteroids for anaphylaxis

---

piperazine adipate/ piperazine citrate

(pi′per-a-zeen)

Antepar, Bryrol, Entacyl,* Pin-Tega Tabs, Ta-Verm, Vermizine

Func. class.: Anthelmintic

Action: Causes paralysis in worm, leading to expulsion

Uses: Pinworm, roundworm

Dosage and routes:

Pinworm

• *Adult and child:* PO 65 mg/kg × 7-8 days, not to exceed 2.5 g/day

Roundworm

• *Adult:* PO 3.5 g in single dose × 2 days

• *Child:* PO 75 mg/kg/day in a single dose × 2 days

Available forms include: Tabs 250, 500 mg; syr 500 mg/5 ml; powder, oral sol 500 mg

Side effects/adverse reactions:

HEMA: Hemolytic anemia

INTEG: Rash, uriticaria, photosensitivity

RESP: Bronchospasm

CNS: Dizziness, headache, paresthesia, convulsions, fever

EENT: Blurred vision, nystagmus, strabismus, cataracts, rhinorrhea

GI: Nausea, vomiting, anorexia, diarrhea, abdominal cramps

Contraindications: Hypersensitivity, renal disease, hepatic disease, seizures

Precautions: Severe malnutrition, seizure disorders, anemia, pregnancy (B)

Pharmacokinetics:

PO: Excreted in urine (unchanged)

Interactions/incompatibilities:

• Increased extrapyramidal symptoms: phenothiazines

NURSING CONSIDERATIONS

Assess:

• Stools during entire treatment, 1, 3 mo after treatment; specimens must be sent to lab while still warm

Administer:

• May be crushed or chewed if unable to swallow whole

• Laxatives if constipated; not needed for drug to work

• Second course after 1 wk off drug, if infection is severe

Perform/provide:

• Storage in tight container at room temperature

Evaluate:

• Therapeutic response: expulsion of worms, 3 negative stool cultures after completion of treatment

• For allergic reaction: rash, itching, urticaria

• For infection in other family members since infection from person to person is common

Teach patient/family:

• Proper hygiene after BM including handwashing technique, tell patient to avoid putting fingers in mouth

• That infected person should sleep

---

italics = common side effects   ***bold italic*** = life threatening reactions

alone; do not shake bed linen; change bed linen daily, wash in hot water
• To clean toilet qd with disinfectant (green soap solution)
• Need for compliance with dosage schedule and duration of treatment
• That urine may turn orange or red
• To avoid hazardous activities since drowsiness occurs
• That seizures may recur in patient who is controlled on medication

Lab test interferences:
Decrease: Serum uric acid

---

pirbuterol acetate
(purr-byoo′-ter-ole)
Maxair
Func. class.: Bronchodilator
Chem. class.: β-Adrenergic agonist

Action: Causes bronchodilation with little effect on heart rate by action on β receptors, causing increased cAMP and relaxation of smooth muscle

Uses: Reversible bronchospasm (prevention, treatment) including asthma; may be given with theophylline or steroids

Dosage and routes:
• *Adult and child >12 yr:* Aerosol 1-2 inh (0.4 mg) q4-6h; do not exceed 12 inh/day
*Available forms include:*Aerosol delivers 0.2 mg pirbuterol/actuation

Side effects/adverse reactions:
CNS: Tremors, anxiety, insomnia, headache, dizziness, stimulation, restlessness, hallucinations, drowsiness, irritability
EENT: Dry nose, irritation of nose, throat
CV: Palpitations, tachycardia, hy-

pertension, angina, hypotension, dysrhythmias
GI: Heartburn, nausea, vomiting, anorexia
MS: Muscle cramps
RESP: **Bronchospasm,** dyspnea, coughing

Contraindications: Hypersensitivity to sympathomimetics, tachycardia

Precautions: Lactation, pregnancy (C), cardiac disorders, hyperthyroidism, diabetes mellitus, prostatic hypertrophy

Pharmacokinetics:
INH: Onset 3 min, peak ½-1 hr, duration 5 hr

Interactions/incompatibilities:
• Increased action of: other aerosol bronchodilators
• Increased action of pirbuterol: tricyclic antidepressants, antihistamines, sodium levothyroxine
• Decreased action of pirbuterol: β-blockers
• Increased dysrhythmias: halogenated hydrocarbon anesthetics

NURSING CONSIDERATIONS
Assess:
• Respiratory function: vital capacity, forced expiratory volume, ABGs, B/P
Administer:
• After shaking, exhale, place mouthpiece in mouth, inhale slowly, hold breath, remove, exhale slowly
• Gum, sips of water for dry mouth
Perform/provide:
• Storage in light-resistant container, do not expose to temperatures over 86° F
Evaluate:
Therapeutic response: absence of dyspnea, wheezing over 1 hr
Teach patient/family:
• Not to use OTC medications; extra stimulation may occur

• Use of inhaler, review package insert with patient
• To avoid getting aerosol in eyes
• To wash inhaler in warm water and dry qd, rinse mouth after use; if used with inhalers containing glucocorticosteroids, wait 5 min before using steroid inhaler
• On all aspects of drug; avoid smoking, smoke-filled rooms, persons with respiratory infections
• To keep fluid intake >2 L/day to liquefy thick secretions

Treatment of overdose: Administer a β-adrenergic blocker

---

piroxicam

(peer-ox′i-kam)
Feldene

Func. class.: Nonsteroidal antiinflammatory
Chem. class.: Oxicam derivative

Action: Inhibits prostaglandin synthesis by decreasing an enzyme needed for biosynthesis; possesses analgesic, antiinflammatory, antipyretic properties

Uses: Mild to moderate pain, osteoarthritis, rheumatoid arthritis

Dosage and routes:
• *Adult:* PO 20 qd or 10 mg bid
Available forms include: Caps 10, 20 mg

Side effects/adverse reactions:
GI: Nausea, anorexia, vomiting, diarrhea, jaundice, ***cholestatic hepatitis,*** constipation, flatulence, cramps, dry mouth, peptic ulcer
CNS: Dizziness, drowsiness, fatigue, tremors, confusion, insomnia, anxiety, depression
CV: Tachycardia, peripheral edema, palpitations, dysrhythmias
INTEG: Purpura, rash, pruritus, sweating

*GU: **Nephrotoxicity: dysuria, hematuria, oliguria, azotemia***
*HEMA: **Blood dyscrasias***
EENT: Tinnitus, hearing loss, blurred vision

Contraindications: Hypersensitivity, asthma, severe renal disease, severe hepatic disease

Precautions: Pregnancy (C), lactation, children, bleeding disorders, GI disorders, cardiac disorders, hypersensitivity to other antiinflammatory agents

Pharmacokinetics:
PO: Peak 2 hr, half-life 3-3½ hr; metabolized in liver, excreted in urine (metabolites) excreted in breast milk; 99% protein binding

Interactions/incompatibilities:
• Increased action of: coumarin, phenytoin, sulfonamides

NURSING CONSIDERATIONS

Assess:
• Renal, liver, blood studies: BUN, creatinine, AST, ALT, Hgb, before treatment, periodically thereafter
• Audiometric, ophthalmic exam before, during, after treatment

Administer:
• With food to decrease GI symptoms; best to take on empty stomach to facilitate absorption

Perform/provide:
• Storage at room temperature

Evaluate:
• Therapeutic response: decreased pain, stiffness, swelling in joints, ability to move more easily
• For eye, ear problems: blurred vision, tinnitus (may indicate toxicity)

Teach patient/family:
• To report blurred vision or ringing, roaring in ears (may indicate toxicity)
• To avoid driving or other hazardous activities if dizziness or drowsiness occurs

---

italics = common side effects   ***bold italic*** = life threatening reactions

• To report change in urine pattern, weight increase, edema, pain increase in joints, fever, blood in urine (indicates nephrotoxicity)
• That therapeutic effects may take up to 1 mo

---

plasma protein fraction

Plasmanate, Plasma Plex, Plasmatein, PPF Protenate

Func. class.: Blood derivative
Chem. class.: Human plasma in NaCl

Action: Exerts similar oncotic pressure as human plasma, expands blood volume
Uses: Hypovolemic, shock, hypoproteinemia
Dosage and routes:
Shock
• *Adult:* IV INF 250-500 ml (12.5-25 g protein), not to exceed 10 ml/min
• *Child:* IV INF 22-33 ml/kg at 5-10 ml/min
Hypoproteinemia
• *Adult:* IV INF 1000-1500 ml qd, not to exceed 8 ml/min
Available forms include: Inj IV 50 mg/ml
Side effects/adverse reactions:
GI: Nausea, vomiting, increased salivation
INTEG: Rash, urticaria, cyanosis
CNS: Fever, chills, headache, paresthesias, flushing
RESP: Altered respirations, dyspnea, pulmonary edema
CV: Fluid overload, hypotension, erratic pulse
Contraindications: Hypersensitivity, congestive heart failure, severe anemia
Precautions: Decreased salt intake, decreased cardiac reserve, lack of albumin deficiency, hepatic disease, renal disease, pregnancy (C)
Pharmacokinetics:
Metabolized as a protein/energy source
Interactions/incompatibilities:
• Incompatible with solution containing alcohol or norepinephrine
NURSING CONSIDERATIONS
Assess:
• Blood studies: Hct, Hgb; if serum protein declines, dyspnea, hypoxemia can result
• B/P (decreased), pulse (erratic), respiration
• I&O ratio; urinary output may decrease
• CVP, pulmonary wedge pressure (increases if overload occurs)
Administer:
• No dilution required; use infusion pump
• Within 4 hr of opening
Perform/provide:
• Adequate hydration before administration
• Storage—check type of albumin, date; may need to refrigerate
Evaluate:
• Therapeutic repsonse: increased B/P, decrease edema, increased serum albumin
• Allergy: fever, rash, itching, chills, flushing, urticaria, nausea, vomiting, or hypotension requires discontinuation of infusion; use new lot if therapy reinstituted
• Increased CVP reading: distended neck veins indicate circulatory overload; SOB, anxiety, insomnia, expiratory rales, frothy blood-tinged cough, cyanosis indicate pulmonary overload
Lab test interferences:
False increase: Alk phosphatase

---

*Available in Canada only

plicamycin
(mithramycin)
(plik-a-mi'cin)
Mithracin
Func. class.: Antineoplastic, antibiotic
Chem. class.: Crystalline aglycone

Action: Inhibits DNA, RNA, protein synthesis; derived from *Streptomyces plicatus;* replication is decreased by binding to DNA; demonstrates calcium-lowering effect not related to its tumoricidal activity; also acts on osteoclasts and blocks action of parathyroid hormone; a vesicant

Uses: Testicular cancer, hypercalcemia, hypercalciuria, symptomatic treatment of advanced neoplasms

Dosage and routes:
Testicular tumors
• *Adult:* IV 25-30 µg/kg/day × 8-10 days, not to exceed 30 µg/kg/day
Hypercalcemia/hypercalciuria
• *Adult:* IV 25 µg/kg/day × 3-4 days, repeat at intervals of 1 wk
Available forms include: Inj IV 2.5 mg

Side effects/adverse reactions:
META: Decreased serum calcium, phosphorous, potassium
HEMA: **Hemorrhage, thrombocytopenia,** decreased pro-time, WBC count
GI: Nausea, vomiting, anorexia, diarrhea, stomatitis, increased liver enzymes
GU: Increased BUN, creatinine, *proteinuria*
INTEG: Rash, cellulitis, *extravasation,* facial flushing
CNS: Drowsiness, weakness, lethargy, headache, flushing, fever, depression

Contraindications: Hypersensitivity, thrombocytopenia, bone marrow depression, bleeding disorders, pregnancy (X)
Precautions: Renal disease, hepatic disease, electrolyte imbalances
Pharmacokinetics: Crosses blood-brain barrier, excreted in urine; little known about pharmacokinetics
Interactions/incompatibilities:
• Increased toxicity: other antineoplastics or radiation

NURSING CONSIDERATIONS
Assess:
• CBC, differential, platelet count weekly; withhold drug if WBC is <4000/mm³ or platelet count is <50,000/mm³; notify physician of results
• Renal function studies: BUN, serum uric acid, urine CrCl, electrolytes before, during therapy
• I&O ratio; report fall in urine output to <30 ml/hr
• Monitor temperature q4h; fever may indicate beginning infection
• Liver function tests before, during therapy: bilirubin, AST, ALT, alk phosphatase prn or monthly
Administer:
• IV dilute 2.5 mg/4.9 ml of sterile H₂O; dilute single dose in 1000 ml of D₅W run over 4-6 hr
• EDTA for extravasation, apply ice compress
• Antiemetic 30-60 min before giving drug and 4-10 hr after treatment to prevent vomiting
• Slow IV infusion using 20-, 21-gauge needle
• Transfusion for anemia
• Antispasmodic for diarrhea, phenothiazine for nausea and vomiting
Perform/provide:
• Liquid diet: carbonated beverages, gelatin may be added if patient is not nauseated or vomiting

P

---

italics = common side effects   ***bold italic*** = life threatening reactions

- Rinsing of mouth tid-qid with water; brushing of teeth with baking soda bid-tid with soft brush or cotton-tipped applicators for stomatitis; use unwaxed dental floss
- Usage immediately after mixing

Evaluate:
- Alkalosis if severe vomiting is present
- Toxicity: facial flushing, epistaxis, increased pro-time, thrombocytopenia; drug should be discontinued
- Bleeding: hematuria, guaiac stools, bruising or petechiae, mucosa or orifices q8h
- Food preferences; list likes, dislikes
- Inflammation of mucosa, breaks in skin
- Yellowing of skin, sclera, dark urine, clay-colored stools, itchy skin, abdominal pain, fever, diarrhea
- Buccal cavity q8h for dryness, sores, ulceration, white patches, oral pain, bleeding, dysphagia
- Local irritation, pain, burning at injection site
- Frequency of stools, characteristics, cramping
- Acidosis, signs of dehydration: rapid respirations, poor skin turgor, decreased urine output, dry skin, restlessness, weakness

Teach patient/family:
- To report any complaints or side effects to nurse or physician
- To avoid foods with citric acid, hot or rough texture
- To report to physician any bleeding, white spots, ulcerations in the mouth; tell patient to examine mouth qd
- To avoid driving or activities requiring alertness; drowsiness may occur
- To report leg cramps, tingling of

fingertips, weakness; may indicate hypocalcemia
- To avoid crowds or persons with infections when granulocyte count is low

---

podophyllum resin
(poe-doe-fil' um)
Podoben, Podofilm*
Func. class.: Keratolytic
Chem. class.: Podophyllum derivative

Action: Arrests mitosis by binding to tubulin, protein subunit of spindle microtubules; also interferes with movements of chromosomes
Uses: Venereal warts, keratoses, multiple superficial, epitheliomatoses
Dosage and routes:
Warts
- *Adult:* TOP cover wart, cover with wax paper, bandage for 4-6 hr, wash, may repeat q wk if needed
Keratoses/epitheliomatoses
- *Adult:* TOP apply qd with applicator, let dry, remove tissue, may reapply if needed
Available forms include: Sol 11.5%, 25%
Side effects/adverse reactions:
HEMA: **Thrombocytopenia, leukopenia**
INTEG: Irritation of unaffected areas
CNS: Peripheral neuropathy
Contraindications: Hypersensitivity, pregnancy (X)
Interactions/incompatibilities:
- Necrosis of skin: when used with other keratolytic
NURSING CONSIDERATIONS
Assess:
- Platelets, WBC if systemic absorption occurs

Administer:
- Only to affected area, cover normal skin with petrolatum for protection, do not apply to broken or inflamed skin
- Only to small areas or for short periods of time or absorption (systemic) may occur

Evaluate:
- Therapeutic response: decrease in size and amount of lesions
- Allergic reactions: irritation, redness, itching, stinging, burning; drug should be discontinued
- Blood dyscrasias if systemic absorption is suspected: decrease platelets
- CNS toxicity: peripheral neuropathy; drug should be discontinued

Teach patient/family:
- That discomfort will begin after 24 hr, subside in 2-4 days
- To use soap and water to clean area and remove drug

---

poliovirus vaccine, live, oral, trivalent
Orimune

Func. class.: Vaccine

Action: Produces specific antibodies for poliomyelitis

Uses: Prevention of polio

Dosage and routes:
- *Adult and child >2 yr:* PO 0.5 ml, given q8 wk × 2 doses, then 0.5 ml ½-1 yr after dose 2
- *Infant:* PO 0.5 ml at 2, 4, 18 mo

Available forms include: Oral vaccine

Side effects/adverse reactions:
*SYST: **Paralysis***

Contraindications: Hypersensitivity, active infection, allergy to neomycin/streptomycin, immunosuppression, vomiting or diarrhea

Precautions: Pregnancy

Interactions/incompatibilities:
- Do not use TB skin test or other live virus vaccines within 6 wk of vaccine
- Do not use within 3 mo of transfusion of whole blood, plasma, or use with immune serum globulin

NURSING CONSIDERATIONS

Administer:
- Only PO
- Do not administer within 1 mo of other live virus vaccines

Perform/Provide:
- Storage at 7°F (−13°C)

Evaluate:
- For history of allergies, skin conditions (eczema, psoriasis, dermatitis), reactions to vaccinations
- For anaphylaxis: inability to breathe, bronchospasm

---

polymyxin B sulfate
(pol-i-mix'in)
Aerosporin

Func. class.: Antibacterial
Chem. class.: Polymyxin

Action: Interferes with phospholipids, penetrates cell wall; changes occur immediately in bacterial membrane causing leakage of essential metabolites

Uses: Serious *P. aeruginosa, E. aerogenes, K. pneumoniae, E. coli, H. influenzae* infections or when other antibiotics cannot be used

Dosage and routes:
- *Adult and child:* IV INF 15,000-25,000 U/kg/day in divided doses q12h, or 25,000 U/kg/day in divided doses q4-8h

P. aeruginosa/H. influenzae
- *Adult and child >2 yr:* INTRATHECAL 50,000 U/day × 3-4 days, then 50,000 U/qod × 2

---

wk after CSF negative, glucose normal

• *Child <2 yr:* INTRATHECAL 20,000 U/day × 3-4 days, then 25,000 U qod × 2 wk after CSF negative

Available forms include: Inj IV, intrathecal, 500,000 U

Side effects/adverse reactions:

INTEG: Urticaria

CNS: Dizziness, confusion, weakness, drowsiness, paresthesia, slurred speech, *coma, seizures,* headache, stiff neck

RESP: Paralysis

GU: Proteinuria, hematuria, azotemia, leukocyturia

Contraindications: Hypersensitivity, severe renal disease

Precautions: Pregnancy (B)

Pharmacokinetics:

IM: Peak 2 hr, half-life 4½-6 hr, excreted in urine unchanged (60%)

IV: Data not available

Interactions/incompatibilities:

• Increased skeletal muscle relaxation: anesthetics, neuromuscular blockers (tubocurarine decamethonium, succinylcholine, gallamine)

• Increased nephrotoxicity, neurotoxicity: aminoglycosides

NURSING CONSIDERATIONS

Assess:

• I&O ratio; report hematuria, oliguria

• Any patient with compromised renal system; drug is excreted slowly in poor renal system function; toxicity may occur rapidly; monitor BUN, creatinine

• Renal studies: urinalysis, protein, blood

• C&S before drug therapy; drug may be taken as soon as culture is taken; C&S may be done after completion of therapy

Administer:

• IV after diluting 500,000 U/5 ml sterile H_2O or NS for inj; then dilute each dose with 300-500 ml D_5W given over 60-90 min

• Intrathecal after reconstituting with 10 ml NS to yield 50,000 U/ml

Perform/provide:

• Storage in dark area at room temperature

• Do not use procaine HCl in intrathecal injection

• Adrenalin, suction, tracheostomy set, endotracheal intubation equipment on unit

Evaluate:

• Therapeutic response: absence of fever, purulent drainage, C&S negative

• Skin eruptions, itching; drug should be discontinued

• Respiratory status: rate, character, dyspnea, symptoms of neuromuscular blockade, tightness in chest; discontinue drug if these occur

• Allergies before initiation of treatment, reaction of each medication; place allergies on chart, Kardex in bright red letters; notify all people giving drugs

• For flushing of face, dizziness, disorientation, weakness, paresthesia, blurred vision, slurred speech, restlessness, irritability; indicate neurotoxicity

• For headache, fever, stiff neck; after intrathecal administration, indicate meningeal irritation

Teach patient/family:

• To report sore throat, fever, fatigue; could indicate superimposed infection

Treatment of overdose: Withdraw drug, maintain airway, administer epinephrine, aminophylline, O_2, IV corticosteroids

---

* Available in Canada only

polymyxin B sulfate (ophthalmic)

(pol-ee-mix′in)

Func. class.: Antiinfective (ophthalmic)

Action: Inhibits cell wall permeability in susceptible organism
Uses: Superficial external ocular infections
Dosage and routes:
• *Adult and child:* INSTILL 1-2 gtts bid-qid × 7-10 days
Available forms include: Powder for sol; 500,000 U
Side effects/adverse reactions:
EENT: Poor corneal wound healing, temporary visual haze, overgrowth of nonsusceptible organisms
Contraindications: Hypersensitivity
Precautions: Antibiotic hypersensitivity, pregnancy (B)
NURSING CONSIDERATIONS
Administer:
• After washing hands, cleanse crusts or discharge from eye before application
Perform/provide:
• Storage in refrigerator
Evaluate:
• Therapeutic response: absence of redness, inflammation, tearing
• Allergy: itching, lacrimation, redness, swelling
Teach patient/family:
• To use drug exactly as prescribed
• Not to use eye makeup, towels, washcloths, eye medication of others; reinfection may occur
• That drug container tip should not be touched to eye
• To report itching, increased redness, burning, stinging, swelling; drug should be discontinued

posterior pituitary

Pituitrin

Func. class.: Pituitary hormone

Action: Stimulates contraction of smooth muscle
Uses: Postoperative ileus, diabetes insipidus, surgical hemostasis
Dosage and routes:
• *Adult:* IM/SC 5-20 units
Available forms include: Inj IM, SC 10, 20 U/ml
Side effects/adverse reactions:
INTEG: Facial pallor
GU: Uterine cramps
EENT: Tinnitus, mydriasis, blurred vision
GI: Increased GI motility, diarrhea
Contraindications: Hypersensitivity, toxemia, hypertension, seizure disorders, advanced arteriosclerosis, cardiac disease
Precautions: Pregnancy (C)
Interactions/incompatibilities:
• Decreased action: lithium, demeclocycline
• Increased action: chlorpropamide
NURSING CONSIDERATIONS
Administer:
• IM if possible
Evaluate:
• Allergic reaction: rash, urticaria, wheezing, fever, nausea, vomiting; drug should be discontinued, administer epinephrine 1:1000

potassium bicarbonate/ potassium acetate/ potassium chloride/ potassium gluconate/ potassium phosphate

Micro-K/K-Lyte, K-Lor, Kaon, Kay Ciel, Slow-K/Klorvess, Kolyum, Ka-ochlor, Klotrix

Func. class.: Electrolyte
Chem. class.: Potassium

Action: Needed for adequate trans-

---

mission of nerve impulses and cardiac contraction, renal function intracellular ion maintenance

Uses: Prevention and treatment of hypokalemia

Dosage and routes:

Potassium bicarbonate
• *Adult:* PO dissolve 25-50 mEq in water qd-qid

Potassium acetate—hypokalemia
• *Adult and child:* PO 40-100 mEq/day in divided doses 2-4 days

Hypokalemia (prevention)
• *Adult and child:* PO 20 mEq/day in 2-4 divided doses

Potassium chloride
• *Adult:* PO 40-100 mEq in divided doses tid-qid; IV 20 mEq/hr when diluted as 40 mEq/1000 ml, not to exceed 150 mEq/day

Potassium gluconate
• *Adult:* PO 40-100 mEq in divided doses tid-qid

Potassium phosphate
• *Adult:* IV 1 mEq/hr in sol of 60 mEq/L, not to exceed 150 mEq/day; PO 40-100 mEq/day in divided doses

Available forms include: Tabs for sol 6.5, 25 mEq/inj for prep of IV 2, 4 mEq/caps ext rel 8, 10 mEq; powder for sol 3.3, 5, 6.7, 10, 13.3 mEq/5 ml; tabs 4, 13.4 mEq; tabs ext rel 6.7, 8, 10 mEq; inj for prep of IV 1.5, 2, 2.4, 3, 3.2 mEq/ml; elix 6.7 mEq/5 ml; tabs 2, 5 mEq; oral sol 2.375 mEq/5 ml; inj for prep of IV 4.4, 4.7 mEq/ml

Side effects/adverse reactions:

CNS: Confusion

CV: Bradycardia, *cardiac depression, dysrhythmias, arrest, peaking T waves, lowered R and depressed RST, prolonged P-R interval, widened QRS complex*

GI: Nausea, vomiting, cramps, pain, diarrhea, ulceration of small bowel

GU: Oliguria

INTEG: Cold extremities, rash

Contraindications: Renal disease (severe), severe hemolytic disease, Addison's disease, hyperkalemia, acute dehydration, extensive tissue breakdown

Precautions: Cardiac disease, potassium sparing diuretic therapy, systemic acidosis, pregnancy (A)

Interactions/incompatibilities:
• Hyperkalemia: potassium phosphate IV and products containing calcium or magnesium; potassium sparing, diuretic, or other potassium products

Pharmacokinetics:

PO: Excreted by kidneys and in feces; onset of action $\approx$ 30 min

IV: Immediate onset of action

NURSING CONSIDERATIONS

Assess:
• ECG for peaking T waves, lowered R, depressed RST, prolonged P-R interval, widening QRS complex, hyperkalemia; drug should be reduced or discontinued
• Potassium level during treatment (3.5-5.0 mg/dl is normal level)
• I&O ratio; watch for decreased urinary output, notify physician immediately

Administer:
• Through large-bore needle, to decrease vein inflammation, check for extravasation
• In large vein, avoiding scalp vein in child (IV)
• Slowly by IV, INF to prevent toxicity, never give IV bolus or IM

Perform/provide:
• Storage at room temperature

Evaluate:
• Therapeutic response: absence of fatigue, muscle weakness, and decreased thirst and urinary output, cardiac changes
• Cardiac status: rate, rhythm,

---

*Available in Canada only

CVP, PWP, PAWP, if being monitored directly

Teach patient/family:

• To add potassium-rich foods to diet: bananas, orange juice, avocados; whole grains, broccoli, carrots, prunes, cocoa after this medication is discontinued

• To avoid OTC products: antacids, salt substitutes, analgesics, vitamin preparations, unless specifically directed by physician

• To report hyperkalemia symptoms (lethargy, confusion, diarrhea, nausea, vomiting, fainting, decreased output) or continued hypokalemia symptoms (fatigue, weakness, polyuria, polydipsia, cardiac changes)

• Take capsules with full glass of liquid

• To completely dissolve powder or tablet in at least 120 ml water or juice

• Not to chew time release or extended release preparations

---

potassium iodide

Iostat, Potassium Iodide Solution, Strong Iodine Solution, Lugol's Solution, Thyro-Block

Func. class.: Thyroid hormone antagonist

Chem. class.: Iodine product

Action: Inhibits secretion of thyroid hormone, fosters colloid accumulation in thyroid follicles, decreases vascularity of gland

Uses: Preparation for thyroidectomy, thyrotoxic crisis, thyroid storm

Dosage and routes:

Thyrotoxic crisis

• *Adult and child:* PO 1 ml in water tid after meals; IV 2 g as adjunct

Preparation for thyroidectomy

• *Adult and child:* PO 0.1-0.3 ml tid (Strong Iodine Solution) or 5 gtts in water tid pc × 2-3 wk before surgery (Potassium Iodide Solution)

Available forms include: Solution 5%, 10%, 21 mg/gtt; tabs 130, 300 mg; inj IV 10%, 20%

Side effects/adverse reactions:

ENDO: Hypothyroidism, hyperthyroid adenoma

INTEG: Rash, urticaria, *angineurotic edema,* acne, mucosal hemorrhage, fever

CNS: Headache, confusion, paresthesias

GI: Nausea, diarrhea, vomiting, small bowel lesions, upper gastric pain

MS: Myalgia, arthralgia, weakness

EENT: Metallic taste, stomatitis, salivation, periorbital edema, sore teeth and gums, cold symptoms

Contraindications: Hypersensitivity to iodine, pulmonary edema, pulmonary TB, pregnancy (D)

Precautions: Lactation, children

Pharmacokinetics:

PO: Onset 24-48 hr, peak 10-15 days after continuous therapy, uptake by thyroid gland or excreted in urine; crosses placenta

Interactions/incompatibilities:

• Hypothyroidism: lithium, other antithyroid agents

NURSING CONSIDERATIONS

Assess:

• Pulse, B/P, temperature

• I&O ratio; check for edema: puffy hands, feet, periorbit; indicate hypothyroidism

• Weight qd; same clothing, scale, time of day

• T_3, T_4, which is increased; serum TSH, which is decreased; free thyroxine index, which is increased if dosage is too low; discontinue drug 3-4 wk before RAIU

---

italics = common side effects   ***bold italic*** = life threatening reactions

Administer:
• Strong iodine solution after diluting with water or juice to improve taste
• Through straw to prevent tooth discoloration
• With meals to decrease GI upset
• At same time each day, to maintain drug level
• Lowest dose that relieves symptoms, discontinue before RAI

Perform/provide:
• Fluids to 3-4 L/day, unless contraindicated

Evaluate:
• Therapeutic effect: weight gain, decreased pulse, decreased T₄
• Overdose: peripheral edema, heat intolerance, diaphoresis, palpitations, dysrhythmias, severe tachycardia, increased temperature delirium, CNS irritability
• Hypersensitivity: rash, enlarged cervical lymph nodes may indicate drug may need to be discontinued
• Hypoprothrombinemia: bleeding, petechiae, ecchymosis
• Clinical response: after 3 wk should include increased weight, pulse; decreased T₄

Teach patient/family:
• To abstain from breast feeding after delivery
• To take pulse daily
• To keep graph of weight, pulse, mood
• To avoid OTC products that contain iodine
• That seafood, other iodine products may be restricted
• Not to discontinue this medication abruptly; thyroid crisis may occur; stress patient response
• That response may take several months if thyroid is large
• Discontinue drug, notify physician if fever, rash, metallic taste, swelling of throat, burning of mouth, throat, sore gums, teeth, severe GI distress, enlargement of thyroid, cold symptoms occur

Lab test interferences:
Interferes: Urinary 17-OHCS

---

potassium iodide (SSKI)
Pima, Iosat, Thyro-Block
Func. class.: Expectorant

Action: Increases respiratory tract fluid by decreasing surface tension, adhesiveness, which increases removal of mucus

Uses: Bronchial asthma, emphysema, bronchitis, nuclear radiation protection

Dosage and routes:
• *Adult:* PO 0.3-0.6 ml q4-6h
• *Child:* PO 0.25-1 ml saturated sol bid-qid

Radiation protection:
• *Adult:* PO 0.13 ml SSKI before or after initial exposure
• *Infant <1 yr:* Half adult dose

Available forms include: Sol 1 g/ml

Side effects/adverse reactions:
EENT: Burning mouth, throat, eye irritation, swelling of eyelids
GI: Gastric irritation
ENDO: Iodism, goiter, myxedema
RESP: **Pulmonary edema**
INTEG: **Angioedema,** rash
CNS: Frontal headache, **CNS depression,** fever, parkinsonism

Contraindications: Hypersensitivity to iodides, pulmonary TB, pregnancy (D), hyperthyroidism, hyperkalemia, acute bronchitis

Precautions: Hypothyroidism, cystic fibrosis, lactation

Pharmacokinetics: Excreted in urine

Interactions/incompatibilities:
• Increased hypothyroid effects: lithium, antithyroid drugs

• Dysrhythmias, hyperkalemia: potassium-sparing diuretics, potassium-containing medication

NURSING CONSIDERATIONS
Administer:
• Decreased dose to elderly patients; their excretion may be slowed
• Diluted water or fruit juice to improve taste, decrease nausea

Perform/provide:
• Storage at room temperature in tight containers
• Increased fluids to liquefy secretions

Evaluate:
• Therapeutic response: absence of cough
• Cough: type, frequency, character including sputum

Teach patient/family:
• Not to use if pregnant
• Symptoms of iodism: eruptions, burning of oral cavity, eye irritation
• Symptoms of hyperthyroidism: CNS depression, fever, glomerulonephritis
• To discontinue, notify physician if fever, rash, metallic taste occur

---

povidone-iodine

(poe'vi-done)
ACU-dyne, Aerodine, Betadine, Efo-dine, Mallisol, Proviodine*
Func. class.: Disinfectant
Chem. class.: Iodophor

Action: Destroys a wide variety of microorganisms by local irritation, germicidal action
Uses: Cleansing wounds, disinfection, preoperative skin preparation removal

Dosage and routes:
• *Adult and child:* SOL Use as needed, topical only

Available forms include: Top sol 1.5%, 3%
Side effects/adverse reactions:
GU: **Renal damage**
META: Metabolic acidosis
INTEG: Irritation
Contraindications: Hypersensitivity to iodine, pregnancy (vaginal antiseptic) (D)
Precautions: Extensive burns
Interactions/incompatibilities:
• Do not use with alcohol or hydrogen peroxide

NURSING CONSIDERATIONS
Assess:
• For allergies to seafood, drug should not be used

Perform/provide:
• Storage in tight, light-resistant container
• Bandaging of areas if needed

Evaluate:
• Area of the body involved: irritation, rash, breaks, dryness, scales

Teach patient/family:
• To discontinue use if rash, irritation, or redness occurs

---

pralidoxime chloride

P

(pra-li-dox'eem)
Protopam chloride, PAM
Func. class.: Cholinesterase reactivator
Chem. class.: Quaternary ammonium oxide

Action: Reactivated enzyme metabolizes and inactivates acetylcholine at both muscarinic and nicotinic sites in the periphery
Uses: Cholinergic crisis in myasthenia gravis, organophosphate poisoning antidote, paralysis of respiratory muscles; used as an adjunct to systemic atropine administration

---

italics = common side effects   **bold italic** = life threatening reactions

Dosage and routes:

Anticholinesterase overdosage

• *Adult:* IV 1-2 g, then 250 mg q5 min until desired response

Organophosphate poisoning

• *Adult:* IV INF 1-2 g/100 ml NS over 15-30 min, may repeat in 1 hr; PO 1-3 g q5h

• *Child:* IV INF 20-40 mg/kg/dose diluted in 100 ml NS over 15-30 min

Available forms include: Inj IV 600 mg/2 ml; tabs 500 mg; emergency kit 1 g/20-ml vial

Side effects/adverse reactions:

CNS: Dizziness, headache, drowsiness, blurred vision, diplopia, impaired accommodation

GI: Nausea

MS: Weakness, muscle rigidity

CV: Tachycardia

RESP: Hyperventilation, *laryngospasm*

Contraindications: Hypersensitivity, carbamate insecticide poisoning

Precautions: Myasthenia gravis, pregnancy (C), renal insufficiency, children, lactation

Pharmacokinetics:

PO: 2-3 hr

IV: Peak 5-15 min

IM: Peak 10-20 min

Half-life 1½ hr, metabolized in liver, excreted in urine (unchanged)

Interactions/incompatibilities:

• Avoid use with aminophylline, morphine, phenothiazines, reserpine, succinylcholine, theophylline in organophosphate poisoning

NURSING CONSIDERATIONS

Assess:

• For 48-72 hr after poisoning

• B/P, VS, I&O ratio; observe for decreased urinary output for 48-72 hr after poisoning to determine atropine toxicity from poisoning effects

Administer:

• Only with emergency equipment available

• As soon as possible after poisoning; within 4 hr

• IV after diluting 1 g/20 ml sterile H_2O for inj; further dilute/100 ml NS and give 1 g/15-30 min

• Slowly (IV) after dilution with sterile water

• Concurrent atropine 2-4 mg IV or IM if cyanosis is present, to block accumulated acetylcholine in respiratory center; repeat q5-10 min until toxicity occurs: dry mouth, flushing, tachycardia, delirium, hallucinations

• Only with edrophonium (Tensilon) on unit for myasthenia gravis patient

Evaluate:

• Airway, need for assistance with respiration

• Respiratory status: rate, rhythm, characteristics

---

pramoxine HCl (topical)

(pra-mox'-een)

ProctoFoam, Tronolane, Tronothane

Func. class.: Topical anesthetic

Action: Inhibits nerve impulses from sensory nerves, which produces anesthesia

Uses: Pruritus, sunburn, toothache, sore throat, cold sores, oral pain, rectal pain and irritation

Dosage and routes:

• *Adult and child:* TOP apply q3-4h; REC apply 1 full applicator bid-tid and after each BM

Available forms include: Aero, cream, gel, lotion 1%; rec oint 1%; rec or top aero, cream 1%

Side effects/adverse reactions:

INTEG: Rash, irritation, sensitization

Contraindications: Hypersensitivity, infants <1 yr, application to large areas

Precautions: Child <6 yr, sepsis, pregnancy (C), denuded skin

NURSING CONSIDERATIONS

Administer:
• After cleansing and drying of affected area
• Rectal aerosol using applicator or tissue
• Directly using gauze

Evaluate:
• Allergy: rash, irritation, reddening, swelling
• Therapeutic response: absence of pain, itching of affected area
• Infection: if affected area is infected, do not apply

Teach patient/family:
• To report rash, irritation, redness, swelling
• How to apply
• Not for long-term use, consult MD after 4 wks of use

---

prazepam

(pra′ze-pam)

Centrax

Func. class.: Antianxiety
Chem. class.: Benzodiazepine

Controlled Substance Schedule IV

Action: Depresses subcortical levels of CNS, including limbic system and reticular formation

Uses: Anxiety

Dosage and routes:
• *Adult:* PO 30 mg in divided doses or at hs

Available forms include: Caps 5, 10, 20 mg; tabs 10 mg

Side effects/adverse reactions:

CNS: Dizziness, drowsiness, confusion, headache, anxiety, tremors, stimulation, fatigue, insomnia, weakness

GI: Constipation, dry mouth, nausea, vomiting, anorexia, diarrhea

INTEG: Rash, dermatitis, itching

*CV: Orthostatic hypotension, **ECG changes, tachycardia,** hypotension, palpitations, syncope

EENT: Blurred vision, tinnitus, mydriasis

Contraindications: Hypersensitivity to benzodiazepines, narrow-angle glaucoma, psychosis, pregnancy (D), child <18 yr

Precautions: Elderly, debilitated, hepatic disease, renal disease

Pharmacokinetics:

PO: Peak 6 hr, duration up to 48 hr, metabolized by liver, excreted by kidneys, crosses placenta, breast milk, half-life 30-100 hr

Interactions/incompatibilities:
• Decreased effects of prazepam: oral contraceptives, valproic acid
• Increased effects of prazepam: CNS depressants, alcohol, disulfiram, oral contraceptives

NURSING CONSIDERATIONS

Assess:
• B/P (lying, standing), pulse; if systolic B/P drops 20 mm Hg, hold drug, notify physician
• Blood studies: CBC
• Hepatic studies: AST, ALT, bilirubin, CrCl

Administer:
• With food or milk for GI symptoms
• Crushed if patient is unable to swallow medication whole
• Gum, hard candy, frequent sips of water for dry mouth

Perform/provide:
• Assistance with ambulation during beginning therapy, since drowsiness/dizziness occurs
• Safety measure including side-rails

---

italics = common side effects **bold italic** = life threatening reactions

Evaluate:
• Mental status: mood, sensorium, affect
• Physical dependency, withdrawal symptoms: headache, nausea, vomiting, muscle pain, weakness, tremors, *convulsions* after long-term use
• Check to see PO medication has been swallowed

Teach patient/family:
• Not to be used for everyday stress or used longer than 4 mo; not to use more than prescribed amount, may be habit forming
• Avoid OTC preparations (cough, cold, hay fever) unless approved by physician
• To avoid driving or other activities that require alertness
• To avoid alcohol ingestion or other psychotropic medications
• Not to discontinue medication quickly after long-term use

Lab test interferences:
Increase: AST, ALT, serum bilirubin, LDH
Decrease: RAIU
False increase: 17-OHCS

Treatment of overdose: Lavage, VS, supportive care

---

praziquantel

(pray-zi-kwon'tel)
Biltricide

Func. class.: Anthelmintic
Chem. class.: Pyrazinoisoquiolone derivative

Action: Causes contraction, paralysis, leading to dislodgement of suckers; they are carried to liver where phagocytosis takes place
Uses: Schistosomiasis, liver flukes, lung flukes, intestinal flukes, tapeworms

Dosage and routes:
• *Adult and child >4 yr:* PO 20 mg/kg q4-6h × 1 day
Available forms include: Tabs 600 mg

Side effects/adverse reactions:
INTEG: Rash, pruritus, urticaria, internal hypertension
CNS: Dizziness, headache, drowsiness, malaise, increased seizure activity, fever, sweating
GI: Nausea, vomiting, anorexia, diarrhea, abdominal pain, increased liver enzymes

Contraindications: Hypersensitivity, lactation
Precautions: Child <4 yr, seizure disorders, pregnancy (B)

Pharmacokinetics:
PO: Peak 1-3 hr, half-life 48-90 min, metabolized by liver (metabolites), excreted in urine, breast milk, CSF

NURSING CONSIDERATIONS
Assess:
• Liver function test: AST, ALT; watch for increase
• Stools during entire treatment, 1, 3 mo after treatment; specimens must be sent to lab while still warm

Administer:
• Corticosteroids as ordered to reduce CNS effects (cerebral cysticerosis)
• Laxatives before treatment to cleanse bowel
• Po with liquids during meals to avoid GI symptoms, not to be chewed

Perform/provide:
• Storage in tight container in cool environment
• To avoid driving or hazardous activities on day of, day after treatment

Evaluate:
• For therapeutic response: expulsion of worms, 3 negative stool cul-

tures after completion of treatment
• For allergic reaction: rash, urticaria, pruritus
• For diarrhea during expulsion of
worms
• For CSF reaction: headache, high
fever; if these occur, drug should
be discontinued, physician notified
Teach patient/family:
• Proper hygiene after BM including handwashing technique, tell patient to avoid putting fingers in
mouth
• Need for compliance with dosage
schedule, duration of treatment
• To refrain from breast feeding on
day of treatment, 72 hr after
Treatment of overdose: Fast-act-
ing laxative

---

prazosin HCl

(pra'zoe-sin)
Minipress
Func. class.: Antihypertensive
Chem. class.: α-Adrenergic
blocker

Action: Peripheral blood vessels
are dilated, peripheral resistance
lowered, reduction in blood pressure results from α-adrenergic receptors being blocked
Uses: Hypertension, refractory
CHF, Raynaud's vasospasm
Dosage and routes:
• *Adult:* PO 1 mg bid or tid, increasing to 20 mg qd in divided
doses if required, usual range 6-15
mg/day, not to exceed 1 mg initially
Available forms include: Caps 1,
2, 5 mg
Side effects/adverse reactions:
CV: Palpitations, orthostatic hypotension, tachycardia, edema, rebound hypertension
CNS: Dizziness, headache, drows-

iness, anxiety, depression, vertigo,
weakness, fatigue
GI: Nausea, vomiting, diarrhea,
constipation, abdominal pain
GU: Urinary frequency, inconti-
nence, impotence, priapism
EENT: Blurred vision, epistaxis,
tinnitus, dry mouth, red sclera
Contraindications: Hypersensitiv-
ity
Precautions: Pregnancy (C), chil-
dren
Pharmacokinetics:
PO: Onset 2 hr, peak 1-3 hr, du-
ration 6-12 hr; half-life 2-3 hr, me-
tabolized in liver, excreted via bile,
feces (>90%), in urine (<10%)
Interactions/incompatibilities:
• Increased hypotensive effects: β-
blockers, nitroglycerin
• Decreased effect: indomethacin
NURSING CONSIDERATIONS
Assess:
• B/P during initial treatment, pe-
riodically thereafter
• Pulse, jugular venous distention
q4h
• BUN, uric acid if on long-term
therapy
• Weight daily, I&O
Perform/provide:
• Storage in tight containers in cool
environment
Evaluate:
• Edema in feet, legs daily
• Skin turgor, dryness of mucous
membranes for hydration status
• Rales, dyspnea, orthopnea q30
min
Teach patient/family:
• Fainting occasionally occurs after
1st dose; do not drive or operate
machinery for 4 hr after 1st dose or
take 1st dose at bedtime
Lab test interferences:
Increased: Urinary norepinephrine,
VMA
Treatment of overdose: Admin-

P

ister volume expanders or vaso-pressors, discontinue drug, place in supine position

---

prednisolone/predniso-lone acetate/predniso-lone phosphate/pred-nisolone tebutate

(pred-niss'oh-lone)

Cortalone, Delta-Cortef, Ferniso-lone-P/Predoxine/Savacort/Hy-deltrasol, PSP-IV/Hydeltra-TBA, Metalone-TBA

Func. class.: Corticosteroid

Chem. class.: Glucocorticoid, im-mediate acting

Action: Decreases inflammation by suppression of migration of poly-morphonuclear leukocytes, fibro-blasts, reversal to increase capillary permeability and lysosomal stabi-lization

Uses: Severe inflammation, im-munosuppression, neoplasms

Dosage and routes:

• *Adult:* PO 2.5-15 mg bid-qid; IM 2-30 mg (acetate, phosphate) q12h; IV 2-30 mg (phosphate) q12h, 2-30 mg in joint or soft tissue (phos-phate), 4-40 mg in joint of lesion (tebutate), 0.25-1 ml q wk in joints (acetate-phosphate)

Available forms include: Tabs 5 mg; inj 25, 50, 100 mg/ml acetate; inj 20 mg/ml terbutate; inj 20 mg/ml phosphate; inj 80 mg/ml ace-tate/phosphate

Side effects/adverse reactions:

INTEG: Acne, poor wound healing, ecchymosis, petechiae

CNS: **Depression,** flushing, sweat-ing, headache, mood changes

CV: Hypertension, **circulatory col-lapse, thrombophlebitis, embo-lism,** tachycardia

HEMA: **Thrombocytopenia**

MS: Fractures, osteoporosis, weak-ness

GI: Diarrhea, nausea, abdominal distention, **GI hemorrhage,** in-creased appetite, *pancreatitis*

EENT: Fungal infections, increased intraocular pressure, blurred vision

Contraindications: Psychosis, hy-persensitivity, idiopathic thrombo-cytopenia, acute glomerulonephri-tis, amebiasis, fungal infections, nonasthmatic bronchial disease, child <2 yr

Precautions: Pregnancy (C), dia-betes mellitus, glaucoma, osteo-porosis, seizure disorders, ulcer-ative colitis, CHF, myasthenia gravis

Pharmacokinetics:

PO: Peak 1-2 hr, duration 2 days

IM: Peak 3-45 hr

Interactions/incompatibilities:

• Decreased action of predniso-lone: cholestyramine, colestipol, barbiturates, rifampin, ephedrine, phenytoin, theophylline

• Decreased effects of: anticoagu-lants, anticonvulsants, antidiabet-ics, ambenonium, neostigmine, isoniazid, toxoids, vaccines

• Increased side effects: alcohol, salicylates, indomethacin, ampho-tericin B, digitalis preparations

• Increased action of prednisolone: salicylates, estrogens, indometha-cin

NURSING CONSIDERATIONS

Assess:

• Potassium, blood sugar, urine glucose while on long-term ther-apy; hypokalemia and hypergly-cemia

• Weight daily, notify physician if weekly gain of >5 lb

• B/P q4h, pulse, notify physician if chest pain occurs

• I&O ratio, be alert for decreasing

---

urinary output and increasing edema

• Plasma cortisol levels during long-term therapy (normal level: 138-635 nmol/L SI units when drawn at 8 AM)

Administer:

• IV undiluted or added to NaCl or D$_5$ and given by IV INF; give 10 mg or less/1 min

• After shaking suspension (parenteral)

• Titrated dose, use lowest effective dose

• IM inj deeply in large mass, rotate sites, avoid deltoid, use 21G needle

• In one dose in AM to prevent adrenal suppression, avoid SC administration, damage may be done to tissue

• With food or milk to decrease GI symptoms

Perform/provide:

• Assistance with ambulation in patient with bone tissue disease to prevent fractures

Evaluate:

• Therapeutic response: ease of respirations, decreased inflammation

• Infection: increased temperature, WBC, even after withdrawal of medication; drug masks symptoms of infection

• Potassium depletion: paresthesias, fatigue, nausea, vomiting, depression, polyuria, dysrhythmias, weakness

• Edema, hypertension, cardiac symptoms

• Mental status: affect, mood, behavioral changes, aggression

Teach patient/family:

• That ID as steroid user should be carried

• To notify physician if therapeutic response decreases; dosage adjustment may be needed

• Not to discontinue this medication abruptly or adrenal crisis can result

• To avoid OTC products: salicylates, alcohol in cough products, cold preparations unless directed by physician

• About cushingoid symptoms

• Symptoms of adrenal insufficiency: nausea, anorexia, fatigue, dizziness, dyspnea, weakness, joint pain

Lab test interferences:

Increase: Cholesterol, sodium, blood glucose, uric acid, calcium, urine glucose

Decrease: Calcium, potassium, T$_4$, T$_3$, thyroid ^{131}I uptake test, urine 17-OHCS, 17-KS, PBI

False negative: Skin allergy tests

---

prednisolone acetate (suspension)/prednisolone sodium phosphate (solution)

(pred-niss'oh-lone)

Econopred, Pred-Forte, Pred Mild, Predulose Ophthalmic/Ak-Pred, Hydelthrasol, Inflamase Forte, Inflamase Ophthalmic, Metreton Ophthalmic

Func. class.: Ophthalmic antiinflammatory

Chem. class.: Analog of hydrocortisone

Action: Decreases inflammation, resulting in decreases in pain, photophobia, hyperemia, cellular infiltration

Uses: Inflammation of eye, lids, conjunctiva, cornea, uveitis, iridocyclitis, allergic condition, burns, foreign bodies

Dosage and routes:

• *Adult and child:* Instill 1-2 gtts

into conjunctival sac q1h × 2 days, if needed, then bid-qid

Available forms include: Susp 0.12%, 0.125%, 1%; sol 0.125%, 0.5%, 1%

Side effects/adverse reactions:

EENT: Increased intraocular pressure, poor corneal wound healing, increased possibility of corneal infections, glaucoma exacerbation, *optic nerve damage,* decreased acuity, visual field

Contraindications: Hypersensitivity, acute superficial herpes simplex, fungal/viral diseases of eye or conjunctiva, active diabetes mellitus, ocular TB, infections of the eye

Precautions: Corneal abrasions, glaucoma, pregnancy (C)

NURSING CONSIDERATIONS
Evaluate:

• Therapeutic response: absence of swelling, redness, exudate

Administer:

• After shaking

Perform/provide:

• Storage in tight, light-resistant container

Teach patient/family:

• Instillation method: pressure on lacrimal sac for 1 min

• Not to share eye medications with others

• Not to use if purulent drainage is present

• Not to discontinue abruptly, taper over 1-2 wk

---

prednisone

(pred-ni-sone)

Deltasone, Meticorten, Orasone

Func. class.: Corticosteroid

Chem. class.: Glucocorticoid, intermediate acting

Action: Decreases inflammation by suppression of migration of polymorphonuclear leukocytes, fibroblasts, reversal to increase capillary permeability, and lysosomal stabilization

Uses: Severe inflammation, immunosuppression, neoplasms, multiple sclerosis, collagen disorders, dermatologic disorders

Dosage and routes:

• *Adult:* PO 2.5-15 mg bid-qid, then qd or qod maintenance up to 250 mg/day

Nephrosis

• *Child:* 18 mo-4 yr 7.5-10 mg qid initially

• *Child:* 4 yr-10 yr 15 mg qid initially

• *Child:* >10 yr 20 mg qid initially

Multiple sclerosis

• *Adult:* PO 200 mg/day × 1 wk, then 80 mg qod × 1 mo

Available forms include: Tabs 1, 2.5, 5, 10, 20, 25, 50 mg; oral sol 5 mg/5 ml; syr 5 mg/5 ml

Side effects/adverse reactions:

INTEG: Acne, poor wound healing, ecchymosis, petechiae

CNS: Depression, flushing, sweating, headache, mood changes

CV: Hypertension, circulatory collapse, thrombophlebitis, embolism, tachycardia

HEMA: Thrombocytopenia

MS: Fractures, osteoporosis, weakness

GI: Diarrhea, nausea, abdominal distention, GI hemorrhage, increased appetite, *pancreatitis*

EENT: Fungal infections, increased intraocular pressure, blurred vision

Contraindications: Psychosis, hypersensitivity, idiopathic thrombocytopenia, acute glomerulonephritis, amebiasis, fungal infections, nonasthmatic bronchial disease, child <2 yr, AIDS, TB

Precautions: Pregnancy (C), diabetes mellitus, glaucoma, osteoporosis, seizure disorders, ulcerative colitis, CHF, myasthenia gravis, renal disease, esophagitis, peptic ulcer

Pharmacokinetics:

PO: Peak 1-2 hr, duration 1-1½ days, half-life 3½-4 hr

Interactions/incompatibilities:

• Decreased action of prednisone: cholestyramine, colestipol, barbiturates, rifampin, ephedrine, phenytoin, theophylline

• Decreased effects of: anticoagulants, anticonvulsants, antidiabetics, ambenonium, neostigmine, isoniazid, toxoids, vaccines

• Increased side effects: alcohol, salicylates, indomethacin, amphotericin B, digitalis preparations

• Increased action of prednisone: salicylates, estrogens, indomethacin

NURSING CONSIDERATIONS

Assess:

• Potassium, blood sugar, urine glucose while on long-term therapy; hypokalemia and hyperglycemia

• Weight daily, notify physician of weekly gain >5 lb

• B/P q4h, pulse, notify physician if chest pain occurs

• I&O ratio, be alert for decreasing urinary output and increasing edema

• Plasma cortisol levels during long-term therapy (normal level: 138-635 nmol/L SI units when drawn at 8 AM)

Administer:

• Titrated dose, use lowest effective dose

• With food or milk to decrease GI symptoms

Perform/provide:

• Assistance with ambulation in pa-

tient with bone tissue disease to prevent fractures

Evaluate:

• Therapeutic response: ease of respirations, decreased inflammation

• Infection: increased temperature, WBC, even after withdrawal of medication; drug masks symptoms of infection

• Potassium depletion: paresthesias, fatigue, nausea, vomiting, depression, polyuria, dysrhythmias, weakness

• Edema, hypertension, cardiac symptoms

• Mental status: affect, mood, behavioral changes, aggression

Teach patient/family:

• That ID as steroid user should be carried

• To notify physician if therapeutic response decreases; dosage adjustment may be needed

• Not to discontinue this medication abruptly or adrenal crisis can result

• To avoid OTC products: salicylates, alcohol in cough products, cold preparations unless directed by physician

• About cushingoid symptoms

• Symptoms of adrenal insufficiency: nausea, anorexia, fatigue, dizziness, dyspnea, weakness, joint pain

Lab test interferences:

Increase: Cholesterol, sodium, blood glucose, uric acid, calcium, urine glucose

Decrease: Calcium, potassium, T_4, T_3, thyroid ^{131}I uptake test, urine 17-OHCS, 17-KS, PBI

False negative: Skin allergy tests

P

---

italics = common side effects   ***bold italic*** = life threatening reactions

primaquine phosphate

(prim'a-kween)

Func. class.: Antimalarial
Chem. class.: Synthetic 8-amino-quinolone

Action: Action is unknown; thought to destroy exoerythrocytic forms by gametocidal action
Uses: Malaria caused by *Plasmodium vivax*
Dosage and routes:
• *Adult:* PO 15 mg qd × 2 wk
• *Child:* PO 0.3 mg/kg × 2 wk
Available forms include: Tabs 26.3 mg
Side effects/adverse reactions:
INTEG: Pruritus, skin eruptions
CNS: Headache
EENT: Blurred vision, difficulty focusing
GI: Nausea, vomiting, anorexia, cramps
CV: Hypertension
*HEMA: **Agranulocytosis, granulocytopenia, leukopenia, hemolytic anemia, leukocytosis,** mild anemia, **methemoglobinemia***
Contraindications: Hypersensitivity, anemia, lupus erythematosus, methemoglobinemia, porphyria, rheumatoid arthritis, methemoglobin reductase deficiency, G-6-PD deficiency
Precautions: Pregnancy (C)
Pharmacokinetics:
PO: Metabolized by liver (metabolites), half-life 3.7-9.6 hr
Interactions/incompatibilities:
• Toxicity: quinacrine
NURSING CONSIDERATIONS
Assess:
• Ophthalmic test if long-term treatment or drug dosage >150 mg/day
• Liver studies q wk: AST, ALT, bilirubin, if on long-term therapy
• Blood studies: CBC, since blood dyscrasias occur
Administer:
• Before or after meals at same time each day to maintain drug level
Evaluate:
• Allergic reactions: pruritus, rash, urticaria
• Blood dyscrasias: malaise, fever, bruising, bleeding (rare)
• For renal status: dark urine, hematuria, decreased output
• For hemolytic reaction: chills, fever, chest pain, cyanosis; drug should be discontinued immediately
Teach patient/family:
• To report visual problems, fever, fatigue, dark urine, bruising, bleeding; may indicate blood dyscrasias

primidone

(pri'mi-done)

Mysoline, Sertan*

Func. class.: Anticonvulsant
Chem. class.: Barbiturate derivative

Action: Raises seizure threshold by conversion of drug to phenobarbital
Uses: Generalized tonic-clonic (grand mal), complex-partial psychomotor seizures
Dosage and routes:
• *Adult and child >8 yr:* PO 250 mg/day, may increase by 250 mg/wk, not to exceed 2 g/day in divided doses qid
• *Child <8 yr:* PO 125 mg/day, may increase by 125 mg/wk, not to exceed 1 g/day in divided doses qid
Available forms include: Tabs 50, 250 mg; susp 250 mg/5 ml

Side effects/adverse reactions:
*HEMA: **Thrombocytopenia, leukopenia, neutropenia, eosinophilia, megaloblastic anemia,** serum folate level, lymphadenopathy
*CNS: **Stimulation, drowsiness,** dizziness, confusion, sedation, headache, flushing, hallucinations, coma, psychosis, ataxia vertigo
*GI: **Nausea, vomiting, anorexia**
*INTEG: **Rash,** edema, alopecia, lupuslike syndrome
EENT: Diplopia, nystagmus, edema of eyelids
GU: Impotence, polyuria
Contraindications: Hypersensitivity, porphyria, pregnancy (D)
Precautions: COPD, hepatic disease, renal disease, hyperactive children
Pharmacokinetics:
PO: Peak 4 hr, excreted by kidneys, excreted in breast milk, half-life 3-24 hr
Interactions/incompatibilities:
• Increased blood levels: alcohol, heparin, CNS depressants, isoniazid, phenytoin, phenobarbital
NURSING CONSIDERATIONS
Assess:
• Drug level: therapeutic level 5-10 μg/ml; CBC should be done q6 mo
Administer:
• Shake liquid susp well
Evaluate:
• Mental status: mood, sensorium, affect, memory (long, short)
• Respiratory depression
• Blood dyscrasias: fever, sore throat, bruising, rash, jaundice
Teach patient/family:
• Not to withdraw drug quickly, withdrawal symptoms may occur
• To avoid hazardous activities until stabilized on drug

probenecid
(proe-ben'e-sid)
Benemid, Benn, Benuryl,* Probalan, Probenimead, Robenecid
Func. class.: Uricosuric
Chem. class.: Sulfonamide derivative

Action: Inhibits tubular reabsorption of urates, with increased excretion of uric acids
Uses: Gonorrhea, hyperuricemia in gout, gouty arthritis, adjunct to cephalosporin or penicillin treatment
Dosage and routes:
Gonorrhea
• *Adult:* PO 1 g with 3.5 g ampicillin or 1 g ½ hr before 4.8 mill U of aqueous penicillin G procaine injected into 2 sites IM
Gout/gouty arthritis
• *Adult:* PO 250 mg bid for 1 wk, then 500 mg bid, not to exceed 2 g/day; maintenance: 500 mg/day × 6 mos
Adjunct in penicillin/cephalosporin treatment
• *Adult and child >50 kg:* PO 500 mg qid
• *Child <50 kg:* PO 25 mg/kg, then 40 mg/kg in divided doses qid
Available forms include: Tabs 0.5 g
Side effects/adverse reactions:
CNS: Drowsiness, headache
CV: Bradycardia
GU: Glycosuria, thirst, frequency, **nephrotic syndrome**
*GI: Gastric irritation, nausea, vomiting, anorexia, **hepatic necrosis**
INTEG: Rash, dermatitis, pruritus, fever
META: Acidosis, hypokalemia, hyperchloremia, hyperglycemia
*RESP: **Apnea,** irregular respirations

P

Contraindications: Hypersensitivity, severe hepatic disease, blood dyscrasias, severe renal disease, CrC <50 mg/min, history of uric acid calculus

Precautions: Pregnancy (B), severe respiratory disease, lactation, cardiac edema, child <2 yr

Pharmacokinetics:

PO: Peak 2-4 hr, duration 8 hr, half-life 8-10 hr; metabolized by liver, excreted in urine, crosses placenta

Interactions/incompatibilities:

• Increased activity of: oral anticoagulants

• Increased toxicity: sulfa drugs, dapsone, clofibrate, PAS, indomethacin, rifampin, naproxen, methotrexate, pantothenic acid, oral hypoglycemics

• Decreased action of probenecid: alcohol, salicylates, nitrofurantoin, diazoxides, diuretics

• Decreased action of: oral hypoglycemics

NURSING CONSIDERATIONS

Assess:

• Uric acid levels (3-7 mg/dl)

• Respiratory rate, rhythm, depth; notify physician of abnormalities

• Electrolytes, CO_2 before, during treatment

• Urine pH, output, glucose during beginning treatment

Administer:

• After meals or with milk if GI symptoms occur

• Increase fluid intake 2-3 L/day to prevent urinary calculi

Perform/provide:

• Low purine diet restricting: organ meats, anchovies, sardines, meat gravy, dried beans, meat extracts

Evaluate:

• Therapeutic response: absence of pain, stiffness in joints

• For CNS symptoms: confusion, twitching, hyperreflexia, stimula-

tion, headache; may indicate overdose

Teach patient/family

• To avoid high purine foods, alcohol, urinary calculi may form

• To avoid OTC preparations (aspirin) unless directed by physician

Lab test interferences:

False positive: Urine glucose with copper sulfate test (Clinitest)

False positive: theophylline levels

Increase: BSP/urinary PSP

Decrease: Urinary 17-KS

---

probucol

(proe'byoo-kole)

Lorelco

Func. class.: Antilipemic

Action: Increases bile acid excretion, catabolism of LDL-cholesterol; increases HDL reverse cholesterol transport and blocks oxidation of LDL-cholesterol

Uses: Severe hypercholesterolemia when other treatment unsuccessful

Dosage and routes:

Adult: PO 500 mg bid with breakfast, supper

Available forms include: Tabs 250, 500 mg

Side effects/adverse reactions:

GI: Nausea, vomiting, diarrhea, flatulence, anorexia

CV: Palpitations, dysrhythmias, *myocardial infarction,* prolonged QT interval

EENT: Visual disturbances, ptosis, tinnitus

CNS: Insomnia, dizziness, palpitations, paresthesias, syncope

Contraindications: Hypersensitivity

Precautions: Dysrhythmias, pregnancy (B), lactation, children

---

Pharmacokinetics:
PO: Excreted in bile/feces
Interactions/incompatibilities:
• Do not use with clofibrate
NURSING CONSIDERATIONS
Assess:
• Hepatic function if patient is on long-term therapy
Administer:
• Drug with meals if GI symptoms occur
Evaluate:
• Therapeutic response: decreased cholesterol levels, (hyperlipidemia), diarrhea, pruritus (excess bile area)
• Bowel pattern daily; increase bulk, water in diet if constipation develops
Teach patient/family:
• That compliance is needed since toxicity may result if doses are missed
• That risk factors should be decreased: high fat diet, smoking, alcohol consumption, absence of exercise
• Birth control should be practiced while on this drug
Lab test interferences:
Increase: Liver function studies, CPK, blood glucose, uric acid, BUN
Note: Not all cholesterol lowering agents have been thoroughly tested. Investigate any reaction, however small, immediately

---

procainamide HCl

(proe-kane-a'mide)
Procan SR, Promine, Pronestyl, Sub-Quin, Rhythmin
Func. class.: Antidysrhythmic (Class IA)
Chem. class.: Procaine HCl amide analog

Action: Depresses excitability of cardiac muscle to electrical stimulation and slows conduction in atrium, bundle of His, and ventricle
Uses: PVCs, atrial fibrillation, PAT, ventricular tachycardia, atrial dysrhythmias, ventricular tachycardia
Dosage and routes:
Atrial fibrillation/PAT
• *Adult:* PO 1-1.25 g, may give another 750 mg if needed, if no response then 500 mg-1g q2h until desired response; maintenance 50 mg/kg in divided doses q6h
Ventricular tachycardia
• *Adult:* PO 1g; maintenance 50 mg/kg/day given in 3 hr intervals; SUS REL TABS 500 mg-1.25 g q6h
Other dysrhythmias
• *Adult:* IV BOL 100 mg q5 min, given 25-50 mg/min, not to exceed 500 mg; then IV INF 2-6 mg/min
Available forms include: Caps 250, 375, 500 mg; tabs 250, 375, 500 mg; tabs sus rel 250, 500, 750, 1000 mg; inj IV 100, 500 mg/ml
Side effects/adverse reactions:
CNS: Headache, dizziness, confusion, psychosis, restlessness, irritability, weakness
GI: Nausea, vomiting, anorexia, diarrhea, hepatomegaly
*CV: Hypotension, **heart block, cardiovascular collapse, arrest***
HEMA: SLE syndrome, ***agranulocytosis, thrombocytopenia, neutropenia, hemolytic anemia***
INTEG: Rash, urticaria, edema, swelling (rare), pruritus
Contraindications: Hypersensitivity, myasthenia gravis, severe heart block
Precautions: Pregnancy (C), lactation, children, renal disease, liver disease, CHF, respiratory depression
Pharmacokinetics:
PO: Peak 1-2 hr, duration 3 hr (8 hr extended)

---

italics = common side effects   ***bold italic*** = life threatening reactions

IM: Peak 10-60 min, duration 3 hr
Half-life 3 hr, metabolized in liver to active metabolites, excreted unchanged by kidneys (60%)

Interactions/incompatibilities:
• Increased effects of: neuromuscular blockers, anticholinergics, antihypertensives
• Increased effects: cimetidine
• Decreased effects of procainamide: barbiturates
• Increased toxicity: other antidysrhythmics

NURSING CONSIDERATIONS
Assess:
• ECG continuously to determine increased PR or QRS segments; if these develop, discontinue immediately; watch for increased ventricular ectopic beats, maximum need to rebolus
• Blood levels, 3-10 mg/ml
• B/P continuously for fluctuations
• I&O ratio, electrolytes (K, Na, Cl)

Administer:
• IV after diluting 100 mg/ml of D₅W or sterile H₂O for inject, give 20 mg or less/1 min; may dilute 1 g/250-500 ml D₅W, run at 2-6 mg/min
• IM injection in deltoid; aspirate to avoid intravascular administration; check IV site q8h for infiltration or extravasation

Evaluate:
• Malignant hyperthermia: tachypnea, tachycardia, changes in B/P, increased temperature
• Cardiac rate, respiration: rate, rhythm, character
• Respiratory status: rate, rhythm, lung fields, watch for respiratory depression
• CNS effects: dizziness, confusion, psychosis, paresthesias, convulsions; drug should be discontinued

• Lung fields, bilateral rales may occur in CHF patient
• Increased respiration, increased pulse; drug should be discontinued

procaine HCl

(proe'-kane)
Novocain, Unicaine
Func. class.: Local anesthetic
Chem. class.: Ester

Action: Competes with calcium for sites in nerve membrane that control sodium transport across cell membrane; decreases rise of depolarization phase of action potential

Uses: Spinal anesthesia, epidural, peripheral nerve block, perineum, lower extremities, infiltration

Dosage and routes:
Varies depending on route of anesthesia

Available forms include: Inj 1%, 2%, 10%

Side effects/adverse reactions:
CNS: Anxiety, restlessness, **convulsions, loss of consciousness,** drowsiness, disorientation, tremors, shivering
CV: **Myocardial depression, cardiac arrest, dysrhythmias,** bradycardia, hypotension, hypertension, fetal bradycardia
GI: Nausea, vomiting
EENT: Blurred vision, tinnitus, pupil constriction
INTEG: Rash, urticaria, allergic reactions, edema, burning, skin discoloration at injection site, tissue necrosis
RESP: **Status asthmaticus, respiratory arrest, anaphylaxis**
Contraindications: Hypersensitivity, child <12 yr, elderly, severe liver disease

Precautions: Elderly, severe drug allergies, pregnancy (C)

Pharmacokinetics:
Onset 2-5 min, duration 1 hr; metabolized by liver, excreted in urine (metabolites)

Interactions/incompatibilities:
• Dysrhythmias: epinephrine, halothane, enflurane
• Hypertension: MAOIs, tricyclic antidepressants, phenothiazines
• Decreased action of procaine: chloroprocaine

NURSING CONSIDERATIONS
Assess:
• B/P, pulse, respiration during treatment
• Fetal heart tones if drug is used during labor

Administer:
• Only drugs that are not cloudy, do not contain precipitate
• Only with crash cart, resuscitative equipment nearby
• Only drugs without preservatives for epidural or caudal anesthesia

Perform/provide:
• Use of new solution, discard unused portions

Evaluate:
• Therapeutic response: anesthesia necessary for procedure
• Allergic reactions: rash, urticaria, itching
• Cardiac status: ECG for dysrhythmias, pulse, B/P during anesthesia

Treatment of overdose: Airway, O₂, vasopressor, IV fluids, anticonvulsants for seizures

---

procarbazine HCl
(proe-kar'ba-zeen)
Matulane, Natulan*
Func. class.: Antineoplastic, miscellaneous
Chem. class.: Hydrazine derivative

Action: Inhibits DNA, RNA, protein synthesis; has multiple sites of action; a nonvesicant

Uses: Lymphoma, Hodgkin's disease, cancers resistant to other therapy

Dosage and routes:
• *Adult:* PO 2-4 mg/kg/day for first wk; maintain dosage of 4-6 mg/kg/day until platelets and WBC fall; after recovery, 1-2 mg/kg/day
• *Child:* PO 50 mg/day for 7 days, then 100 mg/m² until desired response, leukopenia, or thrombocytopenia occurs; 50 mg/day is maintenance after bone marrow recovery

Available forms include: Caps 50 mg

Side effects/adverse reactions:
*HEMA: **Thrombocytopenia, anemia, leukopenia, myelosuppression, bleeding tendencies,*** purpura, petechiae, epistaxis
GI: Nausea, vomiting, anorexia, diarrhea, constipation, dry mouth, stomatitis
EENT: Retinal hemorrhage, nystagmus, photophobia, diplopia
INTEG: Rash, pruritus, dermatitis, alopecia, herpes, hyperpigmentation
CNS: Headache, dizziness, insomnia, hallucinations, confusion, coma, pain, chills, fever, sweating, paresthesias
RESP: Cough, pneumonitis
MS: Arthralgias, myalgias
GU: Azospermia, cessation of menses

Contraindications: Hypersensitivity, thrombocytopenia, bone marrow depression

Precautions: Renal disease, hepatic disease, pregnancy (D), radiation therapy

Pharmacokinetics: Half-life 1 hr; concentrates in liver, kidney, skin;

---

italics = common side effects   ***bold italic*** = life threatening reactions

metabolized in liver, excreted in urine

Interactions/incompatibilities:

• Increased CNS depression: barbiturates, antihistamines, narcotics, hypotensive agents, phenothiazines

• Disulfiram-like reaction: ethyl alcohol, MAOIs, tricyclic antidepressants, tyramine foods, sympathomimetic drugs

• Hypertension: guanethidine, levodopa, methyldopa, reserpine

• Increased hypoglycemia: insulin, oral hypoglycemics

NURSING CONSIDERATIONS
Assess:

• CBC, differential, platelet count weekly; withhold drug if WBC is <4000/mm³ or platelet count is <100,000/mm³; notify physician of these results

• Renal function studies: BUN, serum uric acid, urine CrCl, electrolytes before, during therapy

• I&O ratio, report fall in urine output to <30 ml/hr

• Monitor temperature q4h; fever may indicate beginning infection

• Liver function tests before, during therapy: bilirubin, AST, ALT, alk phosphatase prn or monthly

• CNS changes: confusion, paresthesias, neuropathies, drug should be discontinued

Administer:

• In divided doses and at hs to minimize nausea and vomiting

• Nonphenothiazine antiemetic 30-60 min before giving drug and 4-10 hr after treatment to prevent vomiting

• Transfusion for anemia

• Antispasmodic for GI symptoms

Perform/provide:

• Liquid diet: carbonated beverages, gelatin may be added if patient is not nauseated or vomiting

• Storage in tight, light-resistant container in cool environment

Evaluate:

• Toxicity: facial flushing, epistaxis, increased pro-time, thrombocytopenia; drug should be discontinued

• Bleeding: hematuria, guaiac stools, bruising or petechiae, mucosa or orifices q8h

• Food preferences; list likes, dislikes

• Effects of alopecia on body image; discuss feelings about body changes

• Inflammation of mucosa, breaks in skin

• Yellowing of skin, sclera, dark urine, clay-colored stools, itchy skin, abdominal pain, fever, diarrhea

• Buccal cavity q8h for dryness, sores or ulceration, white patches, oral pain, bleeding, dysphagia

• Alkalosis if vomiting is severe

• GI symptoms: frequency of stools, cramping

• Acidosis, signs of dehydration: rapid respirations, poor skin turgor, decreased urine output, dry skin, restlessness, weakness

Teach patient/family:

• To report any complaints, side effects to nurse or physician: cough, shortness of breath, fever, chills, sore throat, bleeding, bruising, vomiting blood, black tarry stools

• That hair may be lost during treatment and wig or hairpiece may make patient feel better; tell patient that new hair may be different in color, texture

• To avoid foods with citric acid, hot or rough texture

• To report any bleeding, white spots, ulcerations in mouth to physician; tell patient to examine mouth qd

---

* Available in Canada only

- To avoid driving or activities requiring alertness; dizziness may occur
- That contraceptive measures are recommended during therapy
- To avoid ingestion of alcohol, tyramine-containing foods; cold, hayfever, or weight-reducing products may cause serious drug interactions
- To avoid crowds or persons with infections if granulocytes are low

prochlorperazine edisylate/prochlorperazine maleate

(proe-klor-per'a-zeen)

Chlorazine, Compazine, Stemetil*

Func. class.: Antiemetic

Chem. class.: Phenothiazine, piperazine derivative

Action: Acts centrally by blocking chemoreceptor trigger zone, which in turn acts on vomiting center

Uses: Nausea, vomiting

Dosage and routes:

Postoperative nausea/vomiting

- *Adult:* IM 5-10 mg 1-2 hr before anesthesia; may repeat in 30 min; IV 5-10 mg 15-30 min before anesthesia; IV INF 20 mg/L D₅W or NS 15-30 min before anesthesia, not to exceed 40 mg/day

Severe nausea/vomiting

- *Adult:* PO 5-10 mg tid-qid; SUS REL 15 mg qd in AM or 10 mg q12h; REC 25 mg/bid; IM 5-10 mg; may repeat q4h, not to exceed 40 mg/day
- *Child 18-39 kg:* PO 2.5 mg tid or 5 mg bid; do not exceed 15 mg/day; IM 0.132 mg/kg
- *Child 14-17 kg:* PO/REC 2.5 mg bid-tid, not to exceed 10 mg/day; IM 0.132 mg/kg

- *Child 9-13 kg:* PO/REC 2.5 mg qd-bid, not to exceed 7.5 mg/day; IM 0.132 mg/kg

Available forms include: Oral sol 5 mg/ml; inj 5 mg/ml; tabs 5, 10, 25 mg; caps ext rel 10, 15, 30 mg

Side effects/adverse reactions:

CNS: Euphoria, depression, extrapyramidal symptoms, restlessness, tremor, dizziness

GI: Nausea, vomiting, anorexia, dry mouth, diarrhea, constipation, weight loss, metallic taste, cramps

CV: Circulatory failure, tachycardia

RESP: Respiratory depression

Contraindications: Hypersensitivity to phenothiazines, coma, seizure, encephalopathy, bone marrow depression

Precautions: Children <2 yr, pregnancy (C), elderly

Pharmacokinetics:

PO: Onset 30-40 min, duration 3-4 hr

EX REL: Onset 30-40 min, duration 10-12 hr

REC: Onset 60 min, duration 3-4 hr

IM: Onset 10-20 min, duration 12 hr, metabolized by liver, excreted by kidneys, crosses placenta, excreted in breast milk

Interactions/incompatibilities:

- Decreased effect of prochlorperazine: barbiturates, antacids
- Increased anticholinergic action: anticholinergics, antiparkinson drugs, antidepressants
- Do not mix with other drug in syringe or solution

NURSING CONSIDERATIONS

Assess:

- VS, B/P; check patients with cardiac disease more often

Administer:

- IM injection in large muscle mass; aspirate to avoid IV administration

P

---

italics = common side effects   ***bold italic*** = life threatening reactions

• IV after diluting 5 mg/9 ml of NaCl for inj, give 5 mg or less/min; may dilute 10-20 mg/1000 ml NaCl and give as infusion

Evaluate:

• Therapeutic response: absence of nausea, vomiting

• Respiratory status before, during, after administration of emetic; check rate, rhythm, character; respiratory depression can occur rapidly with elderly or debilitated patients

Teach patient/family:

• Avoid hazardous activities, activities requiring alertness; dizziness may occur

---

procyclidine HCl

(proe-sye'kli-deen)

Kemadrin, Procyclid*

Func. class.: Cholinergic blocker
Chem. class.: Tertiary amine

Action: Centrally acting anticholinergic

Uses: Parkinson symptoms

Dosage and routes:

• *Adult:* PO 2.5 mg tid pc, titrated to patient response

Available forms include: Tabs 5 mg

Side effects/adverse reactions:

MS: Weakness, cramping

INTEG: Rash, urticaria, dermatoses

MISC: Increased temperature, flushing, decreased sweating, hyperthermia, heat stroke, numbness of fingers

CNS: Confusion, anxiety, restlessness, irritability, delusions, hallucinations, headache, sedation, depression, incoherence, dizziness, lightheadedness, memory loss

EENT: Blurred vision, photopho-

bia, dilated pupils, difficulty swallowing, mydriasis

CV: Palpitations, tachycardia, postural hypotension, bradycardia

GI: Dryness of mouth, constipation, nausea, vomiting, abdominal distress, paralytic ileus, *epigastric distress*

GU: Hesitancy, retention

Contraindications: Hypersensitivity, narrow-angle glaucoma, myasthenia gravis, GI/GU obstruction, child <3 yr, megacolon, stenosing peptic ulcer

Precautions: Pregnancy (C), elderly, lactation, tachycardia, prostatic hypertrophy, children, kidney, liver disease, drug abuse, hypotension, hypertension, psychiatric patients

Pharmacokinetics:

PO: Onset 30-45 mins, duration 4-6 hr

Interactions/incompatibilities:

• Decreased action of: haloperidol, levodopa

• Increased anticholinergic effect: antihistamines, MAOIs, phenothiazines

NURSING CONSIDERATIONS

Assess:

• I&O ratio; retention commonly causes decreased urinary output

• Heart rate, rhythm, B/P

Administer:

• With or after meals for GI upset; may give with fluids other than water

• At hs to avoid daytime drowsiness in patient with parkinsonism

Perform/provide:

• Storage at room temperature in tight container

• Hard candy, frequent drinks, sugarless gum to relieve dry mouth

Evaluate:

• Parkinsonism: shuffling gait, muscle rigidity, involuntary move-

---

* Available in Canada only

ments
• Urinary hesitancy, retention; palpate bladder if retention occurs
• Constipation; increase fluids, bulk, exercise if this occurs, palpate abdomen
• For tolerance over long-term therapy; dose may need to be increased or changed
• Mental status: affect, mood, CNS depression, worsening of mental symptoms during early therapy

Teach patient/family:
• Not to discontinue this drug abruptly; to taper off over 1 wk
• To avoid driving or other hazardous activities; drowsiness may occur
• To avoid OTC medication: cough, cold preparations with alcohol, antihistamines unless directed by physician
• To avoid alcohol

---

progesterone

(proe-jess′ter-one)
Femotrone, Profac-O, Progelan, Progest-50, Progestaject-50, Progestasert
Func. class.: Progestogen
Chem. class.: Progesterone derivative

Action: Inhibits secretion of pituitary gonadotropins, which prevents follicular maturation, ovulation, stimulates growth of mammary tissue, antineoplastic action against endometrial cancer

Uses: Contraception, amenorrhea, premenstrual syndrome, abnormal uterine bleeding

Dosage and routes:
Amenorrhea/uterine bleeding
• Adult: IM 5-10 mg qd × 6-8 doses
Contraception

• Adult: INSERT 1 placed in uterine cavity, active for 1 yr
PMS
• Adult: REC SUPP/VAG SUPP 200-400 mg
Available forms include: Inj IM 25, 50, 100 mg/ml; IU system 38 mg, rec supp, vag supp

Side effects/adverse reactions:
CNS: Dizziness, headache, migraines, depression, fatigue
CV: Hypotension, thrombophlebitis, edema, ***thromboembolism, stroke, pulmonary embolism, myocardial infarction***
GI: Nausea, vomiting, anorexia, cramps, increased weight, ***cholestatic jaundice***
EENT: Diplopia
GU: Amenorrhea, cervical erosion, breakthrough bleeding, dysmenorrhea, vaginal candidiasis, breast changes, ***gynecomastia, testicular atrophy, impotence,*** endometriosis, ***spontaneous abortion***
INTEG: Rash, urticaria, acne, hirsutism, alopecia, oily skin, seborrhea, purpura, melasma
META: Hyperglycemia

Contraindications: Breast cancer, hypersensitivity, thromboembolic disorders, reproductive cancer, genital bleeding (abnormal, undiagnosed), cerebral hemorrhage, pregnancy (X)

Precautions: Lactation, hypertension, asthma, blood dyscrasias, gallbladder disease, CHF, diabetes mellitus, bone disease, depression, migraine headache, convulsive disorders, hepatic disease, renal disease, family history of breast or reproductive tract cancer

Pharmacokinetics:
IM: Duration 24 hr
Excreted in urine, feces, metabolized in liver

P

---

italics = common side effects   ***bold italic*** = life threatening reactions

NURSING CONSIDERATIONS
Assess:
- Weight daily; notify physician of weekly weight gain >5 lb
- B/P at beginning of treatment and periodically
- I&O ratio; be alert for decreasing urinary output, increasing edema
- Liver function studies: ALT, AST, bilirubin periodically during long-term therapy

Administer:
- Titrated dose; use lowest effective dose
- Oil solution deeply in large muscle mass IM, rotate sites
- In one dose in AM
- With food or milk to decrease GI symptoms
- After warming to dissolve crystals

Perform/provide:
- Storage in dark area

Evaluate:
- Therapeutic response: decrease abnormal uterine bleeding, absence of amenorrhea
- Edema, hypertension, cardiac symptoms, jaundice
- Mental status: affect, mood, behavioral changes, depression
- Hypercalcemia

Teach patient/family:
- About cushingoid symptoms
- To report breast lumps, vaginal bleeding, edema, jaundice, dark urine, clay-colored stools, dyspnea, headache, blurred vision, abdominal pain, numbness or stiffness in legs, chest pain
- To report suspected pregnancy
- To monitor blood sugar, if diabetic

Lab test interferences:
Increase: Alk phosphatase, nitrogen (urine), pregnanediol, amino acids, factors VII, VIII, IX, X
Decrease: GTT, HDL

promazine HCl
(proe'ma-zeen)
Promanyl,* Prozine, Sparine
Func. class.: Antipsychotic/neuroleptic
Chem. class.: Phenothiazine, aliphatic

Action: Depresses cerebral cortex, hypothalamus, limbic system, which control activity, aggression; blocks neurotransmission produced by dopamine at synapse; exhibits a strong α-adrenergic, anticholinergic blocking action; as antiemetic, inhibits medullary chemoreceptor trigger zone; mechanism for antipsychotic effects is unclear

Uses: Psychotic disorders, schizophrenia, nausea, vomiting, alcohol withdrawal

Dosage and routes:
Psychosis
- *Adult:* PO 10-200 mg q4-6h, max dose 1000 mg/day; IM 50-150 mg, followed in 30 min with additional dose up to a total dose of 300 mg
- *Child >12 yr:* PO 10-25 mg q4-6h

Nausea/vomiting
- *Adult:* PO 25-50 mg q4-6h; IM 50 mg; IV not recommended, but may use in concentrations of <25 mg/ml

Available forms include: Tabs 25, 50, 100 mg; syr 10 mg/5ml; inj IV, IM 25, 50 mg/ml

Side effects/adverse reactions:
*RESP: **Laryngospasm**, dyspnea, **respiratory depression***
*CNS: Extrapyramidal symptoms: pseudoparkinsonism, akathisia, dystonia, tardive dyskinesia, drowsiness, headache, **seizures***
*HEMA: Anemia, **leukopenia, leukocytosis, agranulocytosis***

INTEG: Rash, photosensitivity, dermatitis

EENT: Blurred vision, glaucoma

GI: Dry mouth, nausea, vomiting, anorexia, constipation, diarrhea, jaundice, weight gain

GU: Urinary retention, urinary frequency, enuresis, impotence, amenorrhea, gynecomastia

CV: Orthostatic hypotension, hypertension, ***cardiac arrest,*** ECG changes, ***tachycardia***

Contraindications: Hypersensitivity, blood dyscrasias, coma, child <12 yr, brain damage, bone marrow depression

Precautions: Pregnancy (C), lactation, seizure disorders, hypertension, hepatic disease, cardiac disease

Pharmacokinetics:

PO: Onset erratic, peak 2-4 hr

IM: Onset 15 min, peak 1 hr, duration 4-6 hr

Metabolized by liver, excreted in urine, crosses placenta, enters breast milk

Interactions/incompatibilities:

• Oversedation: other CNS depressants, alcohol, barbiturate anesthetics

• Toxicity: epinephrine

• Decreased absorption: aluminum hydroxide or magnesium hydroxide antacids

• Decreased effects of: lithium, levodopa

• Increased effects of both drugs: β-adrenergic blockers, alcohol

• Increased anticholinergic effects: anticholinergics

NURSING CONSIDERATIONS

Assess:

• Swallowing of PO medication; check for hoarding or giving of medication to other patients

• I&O ratio; palpate bladder if low urinary output occurs

• Bilirubin, CBC, liver function studies monthly

• Urinalysis is recommended before and during prolonged therapy

Administer:

• IV undiluted, give at 25 mg/min or less over 1 min; may dilute 25-60 mg/9 ml NaCl for inj

• Antiparkinsonian agent, after securing order from physician to be used if EPS occur

• Syrup mixed in citrus- or chocolate-flavored drinks

• IM injection into large muscle mass

Perform/provide:

• Decreased noise input by dimming lights, avoiding loud noises

• Supervised ambulation until stabilized on medication; do not involve in strenuous exercise program because fainting is possible; patient should not stand still for long periods of time

• Increased fluids to prevent constipation

• Sips of water, candy, gum for dry mouth

• Storage in tight, light-resistant container

Evaluate:

• Therapeutic response: decrease in emotional excitement, hallucinations, delusions, paranoia, reorganization of patterns of thought, speech

• Affect, orientation, LOC, reflexes, gait, coordination, sleep pattern disturbances

• B/P standing and lying; also include pulse, respirations, q4h during initial treatment; establish baseline before starting treatment; report drops of 30 mm Hg

• Dizziness, faintness, palpitations, tachycardia on rising

• Extrapyramidal symptoms including akathisia (inability to sit

P

---

italics = common side effects   ***bold italic*** = life threatening reactions

still, no pattern to movements), tardive dyskinesia (bizarre movements of jaw, mouth, tongue, extremities), pseudoparkinsonism (rigidity, tremors, pill rolling, shuffling gait)
• For neuroleptic malignant syndrome: muscle rigidity, altered mental status, hyperthermia, increased CPK
• Skin turgor daily
• Constipation, urinary retention daily, if these occur increase bulk and water in diet

Teach patient/family:
• That orthostatic hypotension occurs frequently, and to rise from sitting or lying position gradually
• To remain lying down after IM injection for at least 30 min
• To avoid hot tubs, hot showers, or tub baths since hypotension may occur
• To avoid abrupt withdrawal of this drug or extrapyramidal symptoms may result; drugs should be withdrawn slowly
• To avoid OTC preparations (cough, hayfever, cold) unless approved by physician since serious drug interactions may occur; avoid use with alcohol or CNS depressants, increased drowsiness may occur
• To use a sunscreen during sun exposure to prevent burns
• Regarding compliance with drug regimen
• About extrapyramidal symptoms and necessity for meticulous oral hygiene since oral candidiasis may occur
• To report sore throat, malaise, fever, bleeding, mouth sores; if these occur, CBC should be drawn and drug discontinued
• In hot weather, heat stroke may occur; take extra precautions to stay cool

Lab test interferences:
Increase: Liver function tests, cardiac enzymes, cholesterol, blood glucose, prolactin, bilirubin, PBI, cholinesterase, ^{131}I
Decrease: Hormones (blood and urine)
False positive: Pregnancy tests, PKU
False negative: Urinary steroids, 17-OHCS
Treatment of overdose: Lavage if orally injested, provide an airway; *do not induce vomiting*

---

promethazine HCl
(proe-meth'a-zeen)
Ganphen, Methazine, Pentazine, Phencen-50, Phenergan, Prorex, Provigan, Remsed, Rolamethazine, Sigazine

Func. class.: Antihistamine, H$_1$-receptor antagonist
Chem. class.: Phenothiazine derivative

Action: Acts on blood vessels, GI, respiratory system by competing with histamine for H$_1$-receptor site; decreases allergic response by blocking histamine
Uses: Motion sickness, rhinitis, allergy symptoms, sedation, nausea, preoperative, postoperative sedation

Dosage and routes:
Nausea
• *Adult:* PO/IM 25 mg, may repeat 12.5-25 mg q4-6h
• *Child:* PO/IM 0.5 mg/lb q4-6h
Motion sickness
• *Adult:* PO 25 mg bid
• *Child:* PO/IM/REC 12.5-25 mg bid
Allergy/rhinitis

• *Adult:* PO 12.5 mg qid, or 25 mg hs
• *Child:* PO 6.25-12.5 mg tid or 25 mg hs
Sedation
• *Adult:* PO/IM 25-50 mg hs
• *Child:* PO/IM/REC 12.5-25 mg hs
Sedation (preoperative/postoperative)
• *Adult:* PO/IM/IV 25-50 mg
• *Child:* PO/IM/IV 12.5-25 mg
Available forms include: Tabs 12.5, 25, 50 mg; syr 6.25, 25 mg/5 ml; supp 12.5, 25, 50 mg; inj 25, 50 mg/ml

Side effects/adverse reactions:
CNS: Dizziness, drowsiness, poor coordination, fatigue, anxiety, euphoria, confusion, paresthesia, neuritis
CV: Hypotension, palpitations, tachycardia
RESP: Increased thick secretions, wheezing, chest tightness
HEMA: Thrombocytopenia, agranulocytosis, hemolytic anemia
GI: Constipation, dry mouth, nausea, vomiting, anorexia, diarrhea
INTEG: Rash, urticaria, photosensitivity
GU: Retention, dysuria, frequency
EENT: Blurred vision, dilated pupils, tinnitus, nasal stuffiness, dry nose, throat, mouth, photosensitivity

Contraindications: Hypersensitivity to H_1-receptor antagonist, acute asthma attack, lower respiratory tract disease

Precautions: Increased intraocular pressure, renal disease, cardiac disease, hypertension, bronchial asthma, seizure disorder, stenosed peptic ulcers, hyperthyroidism, prostatic hypertrophy, bladder neck obstruction, pregnancy (C)

Pharmacokinetics:
PO: Onset 20 min, duration 4-6 hr, metabolized in liver, excreted by kidneys, GI tract (inactive metabolites)

Interactions/incompatibilities:
• Increased CNS depression: barbiturates, narcotics, hypnotics, tricyclic antidepressants, alcohol
• Decreased effect of: oral anticoagulants, heparin
• Increased effect of promethazine: MAOIs

NURSING CONSIDERATIONS
Assess:
• I&O ratio; be alert for urinary retention, frequency, dysuria; drug should be discontinued if these occur
• CBC during long-term therapy
Administer:
• IV after diluting 25-50 mg/9 ml of NaCl for inj; give 25 mg or less/2 min
• With meals if GI symptoms occur, absorption may slightly decrease
• Deep IM in large muscle; rotate site
• When used for motion sickness, 30 min before travel
Perform/provide:
• Hard candy, gum, frequent rinsing of mouth for dryness
• Storage in tight, light-resistant container
Evaluate:
• Therapeutic response: absence of running, congested nose, rashes, absence of motion sickness, nausea; sedation
• Respiratory status: rate, rhythm, increase in bronchial secretions, wheezing, chest tightness
• Cardiac status: palpitations, increased pulse, hypotension
Teach patient/family:
• That drug may cause photosen-

P

italics = common side effects   ***bold italic*** = life threatening reactions

sitivity; to avoid prolonged sunlight
• To notify physician if confusion, sedation, hypotension occurs
• To avoid driving or other hazardous activity if drowsiness occurs
• To avoid concurrent use of alcohol or other CNS depressants

Lab test interferences:
False negative: Skin allergy tests
False positive: Urine pregnancy test

Treatment of overdose: Administer ipecac syrup or lavage, diazepam, vasopressors, barbiturates (short-acting)

---

propafenone
(proe-pa-fen′one)
Rythmol
Func. class.: Antidysrhythmic, (Class CI)

Action: Able to slow conduction velocity; reduces membrane responsiveness, inhibits automaticity, increases ratio of effective refractory period to action potential duration, β-blocking activity

Uses: Life-threatening dysrhythmias, sustained ventricular tachycardia

Dosage and routes:
• *Adult:* PO 300-900 mg/day in divided doses, allow a 3-4 day interval before increasing dose
Available forms include: Tabs 150, 300 mg

Side effects/adverse reactions:
INTEG: Rash
CV: Dysrhythmias, palpitations, AV block, intraventricular conduction delay, AV dissociation, CHF, *sudden death,* atrial flutter
*HEMA: **Leukopenia, agranulocytosis, granulocytopenia, thrombocytopenia,** anemia*
CNS: Headache, dizziness, abnor-

mal dreams, syncope, confusion, *seizures*
GI: Nausea, vomiting, constipation, dyspepsia, cholestasis, ***hepatitis,*** abnormal liver function studies, dry mouth
RESP: Dyspnea
EENT: Blurred vision, altered taste, tinnitus

Contraindications: 2nd-3rd degree AV block, right bundle branch block, cardiogenic shock, hypersensitivity, bradycardia, uncontrolled CHF, sick-sinus node syndrome, marked hypotension, bronchospastic disorders

Precautions: CHF, hypokalemia, hyperkalemia, recent MI, nonallergic branchospasm, pregnancy (C), lactation, children, hepatic or renal disease

Pharmacokinetics:
Peak 3-5 hr, half-life 2-10 hr, metabolized in liver, excreted in urine (metabolite)

Interactions/incompatibilities:
• Increased effect of propafenone: cimetidine, quinidine
• Increased anticoagulation: warfarin
• Increased digoxin level: digoxin
• Increased β-blocker effect: propranolol, metoprolol

NURSING CONSIDERATIONS
Assess:
• GI status: bowel pattern, number of stools
• Cardiac status: rate, rhythm, quality
• Chest x-ray, pulmonary function test during treatment
• I&O ratio; check for decreasing output
• B/P for fluctuations
• Lung fields; bilateral rales may occur in CHF patient
• Increased respiration, increased pulse; drug should be discontinued

---

* Available in Canada only

Evaluate:
- Therapeutic response: absence of dysrhythmias
- Toxicity: fine tremors, dizziness
- Cardiac rate: respiration, rate, rhythm, character continuously

Lab test interferences:
Increase: CPK

Treatment of overdose: O$_2$, artificial ventilation, ECG, administer dopamine for circulatory depression, administer diazepam or thiopental for convulsions

---

propantheline bromide
(proe-pan'the-leen)
Banlin,* Norpanth, Pro-Banthine, Propanthel*

Func. class.: Gastrointestinal anticholinergic
Chem. class.: Synthetic quarternary ammonium compound

Action: Inhibits muscarinic actions of acetylcholine at postganglionic parasympathetic neuroeffector sites

Uses: Treatment of peptic ulcer disease, irritable bowel syndrome, duodenography, urinary incontinence

Dosage and routes:
- *Adult:* PO 15 mg tid ac, 30 mg hs
- *Elderly:* PO 7.5 mg tid ac

Available forms include: Tabs 7.5, 15 mg

Side effects/adverse reactions:
CNS: Confusion, stimulation in elderly, headache, insomnia, dizziness, drowsiness, anxiety, weakness, hallucinations
GI: Dry mouth, constipation, paralytic ileus, heartburn, nausea, vomiting, dysphagia, absence of taste
GU: Hesitancy, retention, impotence

CV: Palpitations, tachycardia
EENT: Blurred vision, photophobia, mydriasis, cycloplegia, increased ocular tension
INTEG: Urticaria, rash, pruritus, anhidrosis, fever, allergic reactions

Contraindications: Hypersensitivity to anticholinergics, narrowangle glaucoma, GI obstruction, myasthenia gravis, paralytic ileus, GI atony, toxic megacolon

Precautions: Hyperthyroidism, coronary artery disease, dysrhythmias, CHF, ulcerative colitis, hypertension, hiatal hernia, hepatic disease, renal disease, pregnancy (C), urinary retention, prostatic hypertrophy

Pharmacokinetics:
PO: Onset 30-45 min, duration 6 hr; metabolized by liver, GI system, excreted in urine, bile

Interactions/incompatibilities:
- Increased anticholinergic effect: amantadine, tricyclic antidepressants, MAOIs, H$_1$ antihistamines
- Decreased effect of: phenothiazines, levodopa, ketoconazole

NURSING CONSIDERATIONS
Assess:
- VS, cardiac status: checking for dysrhythmias, increased rate, palpitations
- I&O ratio; check for urinary retention or hesitancy

Administer:
- ½-1 hr ac for better absorption
- Decreased dose to elderly patients; their metabolism may be slowed
- Gum, hard candy, frequent rinsing of mouth for dryness of oral cavity

Perform/provide:
- Storage in tight container protected from light
- Increased fluids, bulk, exercise to

---

italics = common side effects   ***bold italic*** = life threatening reactions

patient's lifestyle to decrease constipation

Evaluate:
• Therapeutic response: absence of epigastric pain, bleeding, nausea, vomiting
• GI complaints: pain, bleeding (frank or occult), nausea, vomiting, anorexia

Teach patient/family:
• To avoid driving or other hazardous activities until stabilized on medication, may cause blurred vision
• To avoid alcohol or other CNS depressants; will enhance sedating properties of this drug
• To drink plenty of fluids
• To report dysphagia

---

propofol

(proe-po'foel)
Diprivan
Func. class.: General anesthetic

Controlled Substance Schedule II

Action: Inhibits ascending pain pathways in CNS, increases pain threshold, alters pain perception

Uses: Induction or maintenance of anesthesia, as part of balanced anesthetic technique

Dosage and routes:
Induction
• *Adult:* IV 2-2.5 mg/kg, approximately 40 mg q10 sec until inducton onset
• *Elderly:* 1-1.5 mg/kg, approximately 20 mg q10 sec until induction onset
Maintenance
• *Adult:* 0.1-0.2 mg/kg/min (6-12 mg/kg/hr)
• *Elderly:* 0.05-0.1 mg/kg/min (3-6 mg/kg/hr)
Intermittent bolus

• *Adult:* Increments of 25-50 mg as needed

Available forms include: Inj 10 mg/ml in 20 ml amp

Side effects/adverse reactions:

CNS: Movement, headache, jerking, fever, dizziness, shivering, tremor, confusion, somnolence, paresthesia, agitation, abnormal dreams, euphoria, fatigue

GI: Nausea, vomiting, abdominal cramping, dry mouth, swallowing, hypersalivation

MS: Myalgia

GU: Urine retention, green urine

EENT: Blurred vision, tinnitus, eye pain, strange taste

CV: Bradycardia, hypotension, hypertension, PVC, PAC, tachycardia, abnormal ECG, ST segment depression

RESP: **Apnea,** *cough, hiccups,* dyspnea, hypoventilation, sneezing, wheezing, tachypnea, hypoxia

INTEG: Flushing, phlebitis, hives, burning/stinging at injection site

Contraindications: Hypersensitivity

Precautions: Elderly, respiratory depression, severe respiratory disorders, cardiac dysrhythmias, pregnancy (B), labor and delivery, lactation, children

Pharmacokinetics:
Onset 40 sec, rapid distribution, half-life 1-8 min, terminal elimination half-life 5-10 hr, 70% excreted in urine, metabolized in liver by conjugation to inactivate metabolites

Interactions/incompatibilities:
• Increased CNS depression: alcohol, narcotics, sedative/hypnotics, antipsychotics, skeletal muscle relaxants, inhalational anesthetics

NURSING CONSIDERATIONS

Assess:
• Injection site: phlebitis, burning/stinging

---

* Available in Canada only

- ECG for changes: PVC, PAC, S-T segment changes

Administer:
- After diluting with D_5W, use only glass containers when mixing, not stable in plastic
- By injection (IV only)
- Alone, do not mix with other agents before using
- Only with resuscitative equipment available
- Only by qualified persons trained in anesthesia

Perform/provide:
- Storage in light-resistant area at room temperature
- Coughing, turning, deep breathing for postoperative patients
- Safety measures: siderails, night light, call bell within reach

Evaluate:
- CNS changes: movement, jerking, tremors, dizziness, LOC, pupil reaction
- Allergic reactions: hives
- Respiratory dysfunction: respiratory depression, character, rate, rhythm; notify physician if respirations are <10/min

Treatment of overdose: discontinue drug, artificial ventilation, administer vasopressor agents or anticholinergics

---

propoxyphene HCl/ propoxyphene napsylate
(proe-pox'i-feen)
Darvon, Dolene, Doraphen, Myospaz, Pargesic-65, Proxagesic, Ropoxy 642*/Darvocet-N, Darvon-N

Func. class.: Narcotic analgesics
Chem. class.: Synthetic opiate

Controlled Substance Schedule IV

italics = common side effects

Action: Depresses pain impulse transmission at the spinal cord level by interacting with opioid receptors

Uses: Mild to moderate pain

Dosage and routes:
- *Adult:* PO 65 mg q4h prn (HCl)
- *Adult:* PO 100 mg q4h prn (Napsylate)

Available forms include: HCl-tabs 32, 65 mg; napsylate-tabs 100 mg; susp 10 mg/ml

Side effects/adverse reactions:
CNS: Drowsiness, dizziness, confusion, headache, sedation, euphoria, convulsions, hyperthermia
GI: Nausea, vomiting, anorexia, constipation, cramps
GU: Increased urinary output, dysuria
INTEG: Rash, urticaria, bruising, flushing, diaphoresis, pruritus
EENT: Tinnitus, blurred vision, miosis, diplopia
CV: Palpitations, bradycardia, change in B/P, dysrhythmias
RESP: Respiratory depression

Contraindications: Hypersensitivity to ASA products (some preparations), addiction (narcotic)

Precautions: Addictive personality, pregnancy (C), lactation, increased intracranial pressure, MI (acute), severe heart disease, respiratory depression, hepatic disease, renal disease, child <18 yr

Pharmacokinetics:
PO: Onset 15-30 min, peak 2-3 hr, duration 4-6 hr
REC: Onset slow; duration 4-6 hr
Metabolized by liver, excreted by kidneys (as metabolites), crosses placenta, excreted in breast milk, half-life 12 hr (metabolites)

Interactions/incompatibilities:
- Increased effects with other CNS depressants: alcohol, narcotics, sedative/hypnotics, antipsychotics, skeletal muscle relaxants

bold italic = life threatening reactions

NURSING CONSIDERATIONS
Assess:
• I&O ratio; check for decreasing output; may indicate urinary retention

Administer:
• With antiemetic if nausea, vomiting occur
• When pain is beginning to return; determine dosage interval by patient response

Perform/provide:
• Storage in light-resistant area at room temperature
• Assistance with ambulation
• Safety measures: siderails, night light, call bell within easy reach

Evaluate:
• Therapeutic response: decrease in pain
• CNS changes: dizziness, drowsiness, hallucinations, euphoria, LOC, pupil reaction
• Allergic reactions: rash, urticaria
• Respiratory dysfunction: respiratory depression, character, rate, rhythm; notify physician if respirations are <10/min
• Need for pain medication, physical dependence

Teach patient/family:
• To report any symptoms of CNS changes, allergic reactions
• That physical dependency may result when used for extended periods of time; not to exceed dose
• That withdrawal symptoms may occur: nausea, vomiting, cramps, fever, faintness, anorexia

Lab test interferences:
Increase: Amylase

Treatment of overdose: Narcan 0.2-0.8 IV, O₂, IV fluids, vasopressors

---

propranolol HCl
(proe-pran'oh-lole)
Inderal
Func. class.: Antihypertensive, antianginal
Chem. class.: β-Adrenergic blocker

Action: Nonselective beta-blocker with negative inotropic, chronotropic, dromotropic properties
Uses: Chronic stable angina pectoris, hypertension, supraventricular dysrhythmias, migraine, prophylaxis, MI, pheochromocytoma, essential tremor

Dosage and routes:
Dysrythmias
• *Adult:* PO 10-30 mg tid-qid; IV BOL 0.5-3 mg over 1 mg/min; may repeat in 2 min
Hypertension
• *Adult:* PO 40 mg bid or 80 mg qd (sus rel) initially; usual dose 120-240 mg/day bid-tid or 120-160 mg qd (sus rel)
Angina
• *Adult:* PO 80-320 mg in divided doses bid-qid or 80 mg qd (sus rel); usual dose 160 mg qd (sus rel)
MI
• *Adult:* PO 180-240 mg/day tid-qid
Pheochromocytoma
• *Adult:* PO 60 mg/day × 3 days preoperatively in divided doses or 30 mg/day in divided doses (inoperable tumor)
Migraine
• *Adult:* PO 80 mg/day (sus rel) or in divided doses; may increase to 160-240 mg/day in divided doses
Essential tremor
• *Adult:* PO 40 mg bid; usual dose 120 mg/day
Available forms include: Caps ext

---

rel 80, 120, 160 mg; tabs 10, 20, 40, 60, 80, 90 mg; inj 1 mg/ml, oral sol 4 mg, 8 mg/ml, conc oral sol 80 mg/ml, ext rel cap 60 mg

Side effects/adverse reactions:

RESP: Dyspnea, respiratory dysfunction, *bronchospasm*

*CV: Bradycardia, hypotension, **CHF,** *palpitations, AV block, peripheral vascular insufficiency, vasodilation

*HEMA: **Agranulocytosis, thrombocytopenia***

GI: Nausea, vomiting, diarrhea, colitis, constipation, cramps, dry mouth, hepatomegaly, gastric pain, acute pancreatitis

GU: Impotence, decreased libido, urinary tract infections

MS: Joint pain, arthralgia, muscle cramps, pain

MISC: Facial swelling, weight change, Raynaud's phenomena

INTEG: Rash, pruritus, fever

CNS: Depression, hallucinations, dizziness, fatigue, lethargy, paresthesias, bizarre dreams, disorientation

EENT: Sore throat, *laryngospasm,* blurred vision, dry eyes

META: Hyperglycemia, hypoglycemia

Contraindications: Hypersensitivity to this drug, cardiac failure, cardiogenic shock, 2nd or 3rd degree heart block, bronchospastic disease, sinus bradycardia, CHF

Precautions: Diabetes mellitus, pregnancy (C), renal disease, lactation, hyperthyroidism, COPD, hepatic disease, children, myasthenia gravis, peripheral vascular disease, hypotension

Pharmacokinetics:

PO: Onset 30 min, peak 1-1½ hr

IV: Onset 2 min, peak 15 min, duration 3-6 hr

Immediate rel half-life 3-5 hr; sus

rel half-life 8-11 hr; metabolized by liver, crosses placenta, blood-brain barrier, excreted in breast milk

Interactions/incompatibilities:

• AV block: digitalis, calcium channel blockers

• Increased negative inotropic effects: verapamil, disopyramide

• Increased effects of: reserpine, digitalis, neuromuscular blocking agents

• Decreased beta-blocking effects: norepinephrine, isoproterenol, barbiturates, rifampin, dopamine, dobutamine, smoking

• Increased beta-blocking effect: cimetidine

• Increased hypotension: quinidine, haloperidol, hydralazine

NURSING CONSIDERATIONS

Assess:

• B/P, pulse, respirations during beginning therapy

• Weight qd, report gain of 5 lb

• I&O ratio, CrCl if kidney damage is diagnosed

• ECG if using as antidysrhythmic

• Hepatic enzymes: AST, ALT, bilirubin

Administer:

• IV undiluted or diluted 10 ml D_5W for inj; give 1 mg or less/min; may be diluted in 50 ml NaCl and run 1 mg over 10-15 min

• With 8 oz of water on empty stomach

Evaluate:

• Pain: duration, time started, activity being performed, character

• Tolerance if taken over long period of time

• Headache, lightheadedness, decreased B/P; may indicate a need for decreased dosage

Teach patient/family:

• Not to discontinue abruptly, to take drug at same time each day

---

italics = common side effects   ***bold italic*** = life threatening reactions

- To avoid OTC drugs unless approved by physician
- To avoid hazardous activities if dizziness occurs
- Stress patient compliance with complete medical regimen
- To make position changes slowly to prevent fainting
- Decrease dosage over 2 weeks to prevent cardiac damage

Lab test interferences:

Increase: Serum potassium, serum uric acid, ALT/AST, alk phosphatase, LDH

Decrease: Blood glucose

---

propylthiouracil (PTU)

(proe-pill-thye-oh-yoor′a-sill)
Propyl-Thyracil*

Func. class.: Thyroid hormone antagonist

Chem. class.: Thioamide

Action: Blocks synthesis of T_3, T_4 (triiodothyronine, thyroxine), inhibits organification of iodine

Uses: Preparation for thyroidectomy, thyrotoxic crisis, hyperthyroidism, thyroid storm

Dosage and routes:

Thyrotoxic crisis

- *Adult and child:* PO same as hyperthyroidism with iodine and propranolol

Preparation for thyroidectomy

- *Adult:* 600-1200 mg/day
- *Child:* 10 mg/kg/day in divided doses

Hyperthyroidism

- *Adult:* PO 100 mg tid increasing to 300 mg q8h, if condition is severe; continue to euthyroid state, then 100 mg qd-tid
- *Child > 10 yr:* PO 100 mg tid, continue to euthyroid state, then 25 mg tid to 100 mg bid

- *Child 6-10 yr:* PO 50-150 mg in divided doses q8h

Available forms include: Tabs 50 mg

Side effects/adverse reactions:

INTEG: Rash, urticaria, pruritus, alopecia, hyperpigmentation, lupus-like syndrome

GU: Nephritis

CNS: Drowsiness, headache, vertigo, fever, paresthesias, neuritis

HEMA: Agranulocytosis, leukopenia, thrombocytopenia, hypothrombinemia, lymphadenopathy, bleeding, vasculitis, periarteritis

GI: Nausea, diarrhea, vomiting, jaundice, hepatits, loss of taste

MS: Myalgia, arthralgia, noctural, muscle cramps

Contraindications: Hypersensitivity, pregnancy (D), lactation

Precautions: Infection, bone marrow depression, hepatic disease

Pharmacokinetics:

PO: Onset 30-40 min, duration 2-4 hr, half-life 1-2 hr, excreted in urine, bile, breast milk, crosses placenta

Interactions/incompatibilities:

- Increased anticoagulant effect: heparin, oral anticoagulants

NURSING CONSIDERATIONS

Assess:

- Pulse, B/P, temperature
- I&O ratio; check for edema: puffy hands, feet, periorbits; indicates hypothyroidism
- Weight qd; same clothing, scale, time of day
- T_3, T_4, which is increased; serum TSH, which is decreased; free thyroxine index, which is increased if dosage is too low; discontinue drug 3-4 wk before RAIU
- Blood work: CBC for blood dyscrasias: leukopenia, thrombocytopenia, agranulocytosis; LFTs

---

*Available in Canada only

Administer:
• With meals to decrease GI upset
• At same time each day, to maintain drug level
• Lowest dose that relieves symptoms

Perform/provide:
• Storage in light-resistant container
• Fluids to 3-4 L/day, unless contraindicated

Evaluate:
• Therapeutic effect: weight gain, decreased pulse, decreased T_4, decreased B/P
• Overdose: peripheral edema, heat intolerance, diaphoresis, palpitations, dysrhythmias, severe tachycardia, increased temperature delirium, CNS irritability
• Hypersensitivity: rash, enlarged cervical lymph nodes, drug may need to be discontinued
• Hypoprothrombinemia: bleeding, petechiae, ecchymosis
• Clinical response: after 3 wk should include increased weight, pulse; decreased T_4
• Bone marrow depression: sore throat, fever, fatigue

Teach patient/family:
• To abstain from breast feeding after delivery
• To take pulse daily
• Report redness, swelling, sore throat, mouth lesions, which indicate blood dyscrasias
• To keep graph of weight, pulse, mood
• Avoid OTC products that contain iodine
• That seafood, other iodine products may be restricted
• Not to discontinue this medication abruptly; thyroid crisis may occur; stress patient response
• That response may take several months if thyroid is large

• Symptoms/signs of overdose: periorbital edema, cold intolerance, mental depression
• Symptoms of inadequate dose: tachycardia, diarrhea, fever, irritability

Lab test interferences:
Increases: Pro-time, AST/ALT, alk phosphatase

---

protamine sulfate
(proe′ta-meen)

Func. class.: Heparin antagon⁻ ˙
Chem. class.: Low m⸱˙
weight protein

Action: Binds heparin making .
effective
Uses: Heparin overdose
Dosage and routes:
• *Adult:* IV 1 mg of protamine/90-115 U heparin given, administer slowly 1-3 min; give undiluted to 1%, not to exceed 50 mg/10 min
Available forms include: Inj IV 50, 250 mg/ml
Side effects/adverse reactions:
CV: Hypotension, bradycardia
GI: Nausea, vomiting, anorexia
INTEG: Rash, dermatitis, urticaria
CNS: Lassitude
HEMA: Bleeding, ***anaphylaxis***
Contraindications: Hypersensitivity
Precautions: Pregnancy (C)
Pharmacokinetics:
IV: Onset 5 min, duration 2 hr
NURSING CONSIDERATIONS
Assess:
• Blood studies (Hct, platelets, occult blood in stools) q 3 mo
• Coagulation tests (APTT, ACT) 15 min after dose, then in several hours
• VS, B/P, pulse of 30 min; plus 3 hr after dose

---

italics = common side effects   ***bold italic*** = life threatening reactions

Administer:
• IV after diluting 50 mg/5 ml sterile bacteriostatic H_2O for inj; shake; give 20 mg or less over 1-3 min; may further dilute with equal volume of NaCl or D_5W and run over 2-3 hr
Perform/provide:
• Storage at 36°-46° F
Evaluate:
• Skin rash, urticaria, dermatitis
• Allergy to fish, use with caution in these patients

---

protriptyline HCl

(proe-trip′te-leen)
Triptil, Vivactil
Func. class.: Antidepressant—tricyclic
Chem. class.: Dibenzocycloheptene—secondary amine

Action: Blocks reuptake of norepinephrine, serotonin into nerve endings, increasing action of norepinephrine, serotonin in nerve cells
Uses: Depression
Dosage and routes:
• *Adult:* PO 15-40 mg/day in divided doses, may increase to 60 mg/day
Available forms include: Tabs 5, 10 mg
Side effects/adverse reactions:
HEMA: Agranulocytosis, thrombocytopenia, eosinophilia, leukopenia
CNS: Dizziness, drowsiness, confusion, headache, anxiety, tremors, stimulation, weakness, insomnia, nightmares, EPS (elderly), increased psychiatric symptoms, paresthesia
GI: Diarrhea, dry mouth, nausea, vomiting, *paralytic ileus,* increased appetite, cramps, epigas-

tric distress, jaundice, *hepatitis,* stomatitis
GU: Retention, acute renal failure
INTEG: Rash, urticaria, sweating, pruritus, photosensitivity
CV: Orthostatic hypotension, ECG changes, tachycardia, hypertension, palpitations
EENT: Blurred vision, tinnitus, mydriasis
Contraindications: Hypersensitivity to tricyclic antidepressants, recovery phase of myocardial infarction, convulsive disorders, prostatic hypertrophy
Precautions: Suicidal patients, severe depression, increased intraocular pressure, narrow-angle glaucoma, urinary retention, cardiac disease, hepatic disease, hyperthyroidism, electroshock therapy, elective surgery, pregnancy (C)
Pharmacokinetics:
PO: Onset 15-30 min, peak 24-30 hr, duration 4-6 hr; therapeutic effect 2-3 wk; metabolized by liver, excreted by kidneys, crosses placenta, half-life 54-98 hr
Interactions/incompatibilities:
• Decreased effects of: guanethidine, clonidine, indirect acting sympathomimetics (ephedrine)
• Increased effects of: direct acting sympathomimetics (epinephrine), alcohol, barbiturates, benzodiazepines, CNS depressants
• Hyperpyretic crisis, convulsions, hypertensive episode: MAOI (pargyline [Eutonyl])
NURSING CONSIDERATIONS
Assess:
• B/P (lying, standing), pulse q4h; if systolic B/P drops 20 mm Hg hold drug, notify physician; take vital signs q4h in patients with cardiovascular disease
• Blood studies: CBC, leukocytes, differential, cardiac enzymes if pa-

tient is receiving long-term therapy
• Hepatic studies: AST, ALT, bilirubin, creatinine
• Weight qwk, appetite may increase with drug
• ECG for flattening of T wave, bundle branch block, AV block, dysrhythmias in cardiac patients

Administer:
• Increased fluids, bulk in diet if constipation, urinary retention occur
• With food or milk for GI symptoms
• Dosage hs if over-sedation occurs during day; may take entire dose hs; elderly may not tolerate once/day dosing
• Gum, hard candy, or frequent sips of water for dry mouth

Perform/provide:
• Storage in tight, light-resistant container at room temperature
• Assistance with ambulation during beginning therapy since drowsiness/dizziness occurs
• Safety measures including siderails, primarily in elderly
• Checking to see PO medication swallowed

Evaluate:
• EPS primarily in elderly: rigidity, dystonia, akathisia
• Mental status: mood, sensorium, affect, suicidal tendencies, increase in psychiatric symptoms: depression, panic
• Urinary retention, constipation; constipation is more likely to occur in children
• Withdrawal symptoms: headache, nausea, vomiting, muscle pain, weakness; do not usually occur unless drug was discontinued abruptly
• Alcohol consumption; if alcohol is consumed, hold dose until morning

Teach patient/family:
• That therapeutic effects may take 2-3 wk
• To use caution in driving or other activities requiring alertness because of drowsiness, dizziness, blurred vision
• To avoid alcohol ingestion, other CNS depressants
• Not to discontinue medication quickly after long-term use, may cause nausea, headache, malaise
• To wear sunscreen or large hat since photosensitivity occurs

Lab test interferences:
Increase: Serum bilirubin, blood glucose, alk phosphatase
False increase: Urinary catecholamines
Decrease: VMA, 5-HIAA

Treatment of overdose: ECG monitoring, induce emesis, lavage, activated charcoal, administer anticonvulsant

---

pseudoephedrine HCl/pseudoephedrine sulfate

(soo-doe-e-fed′rin)
Besan, Cenafed, Eltor,* First Sign, Novafed, Robidrine, Sudabid, Sudafed/Afrinol Repetabs
Func. class.: Adrenergic
Chem. class.: Substituted phenylethylamine

Action: Causes increased contractility and heart rate by acting on β-receptors in heart; also, acts on α-receptors, causing vasoconstriction in blood vessels
Uses: Decongestant, nasal congestion

Dosage and routes:
• *Adult:* PO 60 mg q6h; EXT REL 60-120 mg q12h

---

italics = common side effects   **bold italic** = life threatening reactions

• *Child 6-12 yr:* PO 30 mg q6h, not to exceed 120 mg/day
• *Child 2-6 yr:* PO 15 mg q6h, not to exceed 60 mg/day
Available forms include: Caps ext rel 120 mg; sol 15 mg, 30 mg/5 ml, 7.5 mg/0.8 ml; tabs 30, 60, 120 mg

Side effects/adverse reactions:
CNS: Tremors, anxiety, insomnia, headache, dizziness, anxiety, hallucinations, SEIZURES
EENT: Dry nose, irritation of nose and throat
CV: Palpitations, tachycardia, hypertension, chest pain, *dysrhythmias*
GI: Anorexia, nausea, vomiting, dry mouth
GU: Dysuria

Contraindications: Hypersensitivity to sympathomimetics, narrow-angle glaucoma
Precautions: Pregnancy (C), cardiac disorders, hyperthyroidism, diabetes mellitus, prostatic hypertrophy
Pharmacokinetics:
PO: Onset 15-30 min, duration 4-6 hr, 8-12 hrs (extended release) metabolized in liver, excreted in feces and breast milk
Interactions/incompatibilities:
• Do not use with MAOIs or tricyclic antidepressants, hypertensive crisis may occur
• Decreased effect of this drug: methyldopa, urinary acidifiers, rauwolfia alkaloids
• Increased effect of this drug: urinary alkalizers

NURSING CONSIDERATIONS
Perform/provide:
• Storage at room temperature
Evaluate:
• Therapeutic response: Decreased nasal congestion

Teach patient/family:
• Reason for drug administration
• Not to use continuously, or more than recommended dose, or rebound congestion may occur
• To check with physician before using other drugs, as drug interactions may occur
• To avoid taking near hs; stimulation can occur
• Not to use if stimulation, restlessness, or tremors occur

---

psyllium
(sill'i-um)
Effersyllium Instant Mix, Hydrocil Instant Powder, Konsyl, L.A. Formula, Metamucil, Metamucil Instant Mix, Metamucil Sugar Free, Modance Bulk, Mucillium, Mucilose, Naturacil, Plain Hydrocil, Prodiem Plain,* Reguloid, Siblin, Syllact, V-Lax
Func. class.: Laxative, bulk
Chem. class.: Psyllium colloid

Action: Bulk-forming laxative
Uses: Chronic constipation, treatment of ulcerative colitis, irritable bowel syndrome
Dosage and routes:
• *Adult:* PO 5-10 ml in 8 oz of water bid or tid, then 8 oz of water or 1 premeasured packet in 8 oz of water bid or tid, then 8 oz of water
• *Child >6 yr:* 5-10 ml in 4 oz of water hs
Available forms include: Chew pieces 1.7 g/piece; pdr 309, 390, 430, 450, 486, 500, 600, 630, 654, 672, 791, 919, 950 mg/g, 1 g/g
Side effects/adverse reactions:
GI: Nausea, vomiting, anorexia, diarrhea, cramps
Contraindications: Hypersensitivity, intestinal obstruction, abdom-

---

*Available in Canada only

inal pain, nausea/vomiting, fecal impaction

Precautions: Pregnancy (C)

Pharmacokinetics: Excreted in feces

NURSING CONSIDERATIONS
Assess:
- Blood, urine electrolytes if drug is used often by patient
- I&O ratio to identify fluid loss

Administer:
- Alone for better absorption
- In morning or evening (oral dose)
- After mixing with water immediately prior to use

Evaluate:
- Therapeutic response: decrease in constipation or decreased diarrhea in colitis
- Cause of constipation; identify whether fluids, bulk, or exercise is missing from lifestyle
- Cramping, rectal bleeding, nausea, vomiting; if these symptoms occur, drug should be discontinued

Teach patient/family:
- To maintain adequate fluid consumption
- That normal bowel movements do not always occur daily
- Do not use in presence of abdominal pain, nausea, vomiting
- Notify physician if constipation unrelieved or if symptoms of electrolyte imbalance occur: muscle cramps, pain, weakness, dizziness, excessive thirst

---

pyrantel pamoate
(pi-ran'tel)
Antiminth, Combantrin*

Func. class.: Anthelmintic
Chem. class.: Pyrimidine derivative

Action: Causes paralysis in worm by neuroblockade, caused by stimulation of ganglionic receptors; worms are expelled by normal peristalsis

Uses: Pinworms, roundworms

Dosage and routes:
- *Adult and child >2 yr:* PO 11 mg/kg as single dose, not to exceed 1 g; repeat in 2 wk for pinworms

Available forms include: Oral susp 250 mg/5 ml

Side effects/adverse reactions:
INTEG: Rash
CNS: Dizziness, headache, drowsiness, insomnia, fever, weakness
GI: Nausea, vomiting, anorexia, diarrhea, distention

Contraindications: Hypersensitivity

Precautions: Seizure disorders, hepatic disease, dehydration, anemia, child <2 yr, pregnancy (C)

Pharmacokinetics:
PO: Peak 1-3 hr, metabolized in liver, excreted in feces, urine (unchanged/metabolites)

Interactions/incompatibilities:
- Antagonizes effect of pyrantel: piperazine

NURSING CONSIDERATIONS
Assess:
- Stools during entire treatment; specimens must be sent to lab while still warm

Administer:
- PO after meals to avoid GI symptoms
- After shaking suspension

Perform/provide:
- Storage in tight, light-resistant containers in cool environment

Evaluate:
- For therapeutic response: expulsion of worms, 3 negative stool cultures after completion of treatment
- For allergic reaction: rash
- For diarrhea during expulsion of worms

---

italics = common side effects   ***bold italic*** = life threatening reactions

Teach patient/family:
• Proper hygiene after BM including handwashing technique; tell patient to avoid putting fingers in mouth
• That infected person should sleep alone; do not shake bed linen; change bed linen qd, wash in hot water
• To clean toilet qd with disinfectant (green soap solution)
• Need for compliance with dosage schedule, duration of treatment
• To drink fruit juice to help expel worms
• To wear shoes, wash all fruits, vegetables well before eating

---

pyrazinamide

(peer-a-zin'a-mide)
Tebrazid*

Func. class.: Antitubercular
Chem. class.: Pyrazinoic acid amine/nicoturimide analog

Action: Bactericidal interference with lipid, nucleic acid biosynthesis
Uses: Tuberculosis, as an adjunct when other drugs are not feasible
Dosage and routes:
• *Adult:* PO 20-35 mg/kg/day in 3-4 divided doses, not to exceed 3 g/day
Available forms include: Tabs 500 mg
Side effects/adverse reactions:
INTEG: Photosensitivity, urticaria
CNS: Headache
*GI: **Hepatotoxicity,** abnormal liver function tests, peptic ulcer
GU: Urinary difficulty, increased uric acid
*HEMA: **Hemolytic anemia***
Contraindications: Hypersensitivity

Precautions: Pregnancy (C), child <13 yr
Pharmacokinetics:
PO: Peak 2 hr, half-life 9-10 hr; metabolized in liver, excreted in urine (metabolites/unchanged drug)
NURSING CONSIDERATIONS
Assess:
• Signs of anemia: Hct, Hgb, fatigue
• Liver studies q wk: ALT, AST, bilirubin
• Renal status before, q mo: BUN, creatinine, output, sp gr, urinalysis
Administer:
• With meals to decrease GI symptoms
• After C&S is completed; q mo to detect resistance
Evaluate:
• Hepatic status: decreased appetite, jaundice, dark urine, fatigue
Teach patient/family:
• That compliance with dosage schedule, length is necessary
• To avoid alcohol while taking this drug
Lab test interferences:
Increase: PBI
Decrease: 17-KS

---

pyrethrins/piperonyl butoxide

(peer'e-thrins)
A-200 Pyrinate, Barc, Blue, Pyrin-d, Pyrinyl, Rdc, Rid, TISIT, Triple X

Func. class.: Pediculocide
Chem. class.: Pyrethrin/piperonyl butoxide/petroleum distillate

---

Action: Causes paralysis, death of organism by acting as a contact poison
Uses: Head, body, pubic lice; nits

Dosage and routes:
• *Adult and child:* Apply undiluted to infested area; allow application to remain no longer than 10 min, wash thoroughly with warm water, soap, or shampoo; remove dead lice, eggs with fine-tooth comb; do not exceed 2 consecutive applications within 24 hr
• *Adult and child:* CREAM/LOTION wash area with soap, water; remove visible crusts, apply to skin surfaces, remove with soap, water in 8-12 hr; may reapply in 1 wk if needed; SHAMPOO using 30 ml, work into lather, rub for 5 min, rinse, dry with towel
Available forms include: Gel, liq, shampoo, cream, lotion
Side effects/adverse reactions:
INTEG: Irritation, pruritus, urticaria, eczema
Contraindications: Hypersensitivity, inflammation of skin, abrasions, or breaks in skin
Precautions: Child/infant, ragweed sensitivity, pregnancy (C)
Pharmacokinetics: Inactivated by GI tract, other data not available
NURSING CONSIDERATIONS
Administer:
• To body areas, scalp only; do not apply to face, lips, mouth, eyes, any mucous membrane, anus, or meatus; apply to neck down for body lice
• Topical corticosteroids as ordered to decrease contact dermatitis
• Lotions of menthol or phenol to control itching
• Topical antibiotics for infection
Perform/provide:
• Storage in tight container
• Isolation until areas on skin, scalp have cleared and treatment is completed
• Removal of nits by using a fine-

tooth comb rinsed in vinegar after treatment
Evaluate:
• Area of body involved, including nits
Teach patient/family:
• To discontinue use and notify physician if irritation or infection occurs
• To flush with water in case of contact with eyes
• To wash all inhabitants' clothing, bed linen using insecticide; preventative treatment may be required of all persons living in same house, using lotion or shampoo to decrease spread of infection
• That itching may continue for 4-6 wk
• That drug must be reapplied if accidently washed off or treatment will be ineffective
• To use externally only
• To treat sexual contacts simultaneously

---

pyridostigmine bromide
(peer-id-oh-stig'meen)
Mestinon, Regonol
Func. class.: Cholinergic
Chem. class.: Tertiary amine carbamate

Action: Inhibits destruction of acetylcholine, which increases concentration at sites where acetylcholine is released; this facilitates transmission of impulses across myoneural junction
Uses: Nondepolarizing muscle relaxant antagonist, myasthenia gravis
Dosage and routes:
Myasthenia gravis
• *Adult:* PO 60-180 mg bid-qid, not to exceed 1.5 g/day; IM/IV 1/30 of PO dose, sus rel 180-540 mg 1-2

× day at intervals of at least 6 hr

Tubocurare antagonist

• *Adult:* 0.6-1.2 mg IV atropine, then 10-30 mg

Available forms include: Tabs 60 mg; tabs sus rel 180 mg; syr 60 mg/5 ml; inj IM/IV 5 mg/ml

Side effects/adverse reactions:

INTEG: Rash, urticaria, flushing

CNS: Dizziness, headache, sweating, confusion, weakness, *convulsions,* incoordination, paralysis

GI: Nausea, diarrhea, vomiting, cramps

CV: Tachycardia, dysrhythmias, bradycardia, AV block, hypotension, ECG changes, *cardiac arrest*

GU: Frequency, incontinence

RESP: Respiratory depression, bronchospasm, constriction, laryngospasm, respiratory arrest

EENT: Miosis, blurred vision, lacrimation

Contraindications: Bradycardia, hypotension, obstruction of intestine, renal system

Precautions: Seizure disorders, bronchial asthma, coronary occlusion, hyperthyroidism, dysrhythmias, peptic ulcer, megacolon, poor GI motility, pregnancy (C)

Pharmacokinetics:

PO: Onset 20-30 min, duration 3-6 hr

IM/IV/SC: Onset 2-15 min, duration 2½-4 hr

Metabolized in liver, excreted in urine

Interactions/incompatibilities:

• Decreased action: gallamine, metocurine, pancuronium, tubocurarine, atropine

• Increased action: decamethonium, succinylcholine

• Decreased action of pyridostigmine: aminoglycosides, anesthetics, procainamide, quinidine, mecamylamine, polymyxin, magne-sium, corticosteroids, antidysrhythmics

NURSING CONSIDERATIONS

Assess:

• VS, respiration q8h

• I&O ratio; check for urinary retention or incontinence

Administer:

• IV undiluted, give through Y-tube or 3-way stopcock, give 0.5 mg or less/min

• Only with atropine sulfate available for cholinergic crisis

• Only after all other cholinergics have been discontinued

• Increased doses if tolerance occurs

• Larger doses after exercise or fatigue

• With food or milk to decrease GI symptoms

• On empty stomach for better absorption

Perform/provide:

• Storage at room temperature

Evaluate:

• Therapeutic response: increased muscle strength, hand grasp, improved gait, absence of labored breathing (if severe)

• Bradycardia, hypotension, bronchospasm, headache, dizziness, convulsions, respiratory depression; drug should be discontinued if toxicity occurs

Teach patient/family:

• Not to crush or chew sus rel prep

• That drug is not a cure, it only relieves symptoms

• To wear Medic Alert ID specifying myasthenia gravis, drugs taken

Treatment of overdose:

Discontinue drug, atropine 1-4 mg IV

pyridoxine HCl (vitamin B₆)

(peer-i-dox-een)

Beesix, HexaBetalin, Hexacrest

Func. class.: Vitamin B₆, water soluble

Action: Needed for fat, protein, carbohydrate metabolism; enhances glycogen release from liver and muscle tissue; needed as coenzyme for metabolic transformations of a variety of amino acids

Uses: Vitamin B₆ deficiency associated with inborn errors of metabolism, seizures, isoniazid therapy, oral contraceptives, or alcoholic polyneuritis

Dosage and routes:

Vitamin B₆ deficiency

• *Adult:* PO/IM/IV 10-20 mg qd × 3 wk, then 2-5 mg qd

• *Child:* PO/IM/IV 100 mg until desired response

Inborn errors of metabolism

• *Adult:* IM/IV/PO 600 mg or less qd, then 50 mg qd for life

• *Child:* IM/PO/IV 100 mg, then 2-10 mg IM or 10-100 mg PO qd

Deficiency caused by isoniazid

• *Adult:* PO 100 mg qd × 3 wk, then 50 mg qd

• *Child:* PO dose titrated to patient response

Prevention of deficiency caused by isoniazid

• *Adult:* PO 25-50 mg qd

• *Child:* PO 0.5-1.5 mg qd

• *Infant:* PO 0.1-0.5 mg qd

Available forms include: Tabs 10, 25, 50, 100, 200, 250, 500 mg; tabs time released 500 mg; inj IM-IV 100 mg/ml

Side effects/adverse reactions:

CNS: Paresthesia, flushing, warmth, lethargy (rare with normal renal function)

INTEG: Pain at injection site

Contraindications: Hypersensitivity

Precautions: Pregnancy (A), lactation, children, Parkinson's disease

Pharmacokinetics:

PO/INJ: Half-life 2-3 wk, metabolized in liver, excreted in urine

Interactions/incompatibilities:

• Decreased effects of: levodopa

• Decreased effects of pyridoxine: oral contraceptives, INH, cycloserine, hydralazine, penicillamine

NURSING CONSIDERATIONS

Assess:

• Pyridoxine levels throughout treatment

Administer:

• IV undiluted or added to most IV sol; give 50 mg or less/1 min if undiluted

• Z-tract to minimize pain

Perform/provide:

• Storage in tight, light-resistant container

Evaluate:

• Therapeutic response: absence of nausea, vomiting, anorexia, skin lesions, glossitis, stomatitis, edema, convulsions, restlessness, paresthesia

• Nutritional status: yeast, liver, legumes, bananas, green vegetables, whole grains

Teach patient/family:

• To avoid vitamin supplements unless directed by physician

• To keep out of children's reach

• To increase meat, bananas, potatoes, lima beans, whole grain cereals

P

---

italics = common side effects   ***bold italic*** = life threatening reactions

pyrimethamine

(peer-i-meth'a-meen)
Daraprim, Fansidar (with sulfa-
doxine)
Func. class.: Antimalarial
Chem. class.: Folic acid antagonist

Action: Inhibits folic acid metab-
olism in parasite, prevents trans-
mission by stopping growth of fer-
tilized gametes
Uses: Malaria, prophylaxis, toxo-
plasmodium vivax
Dosage and routes:
Prophylaxis of malaria
• *Adult:* PO 1 tab q wk or 2 tabs q
2 wk (Fansidar)
• *Child 9-14 yr:* PO ¾ tab q wk or
1½ tabs q 2 wk (Fansidar)
• *Child >10 yr:* PO 25 mg q wk
• *Child 4-10 yr:* PO 12.5 mg q wk
• *Child 4-8 yr:* PO ½ tab q wk or
1 tab q 2 wk (Fansidar)
• *Child <4 yr:* PO ¼ tab q wk or
½ tab q 2 wk (Fansidar)
• *Child <4 yr:* PO 6.25 mg q wk
Acute attacks of malaria
• *Adult:* PO 2-3 tabs as a single
dose (Fansidar) alone or with qui-
nine or primaquine
• *Child 9-14 yr:* 2 tabs
• *Child 4-8 yr:* 1 tab
• *Child <4 yr:* ½ tab
Toxoplasmosis
• *Adult:* PO 100 mg, then 25 mg
qd × 4-5 wk, with 1 g sulfadiazine
q6h
• *Child:* PO 1 mg/kg, then 0.25
mg/kg qd × 4-5 wk, with sulfa-
diazine 100 mg/kg/day in divided
doses q6h
Available forms include: Tabs 25
mg; combo tabs 500 mg sulfadox-
ine/25 mg pyrimethamine
Side effects/adverse reactions:
RESP: Respiratory failure

INTEG: Skin eruptions, photosensitivity
CNS: Stimulation, irritability, ***convulsions,*** tremors, ataxia, fatigue
*GI: Nausea, vomiting, cramps, an-
orexia,* diarrhea, atrophic glossitis,
gastritis
*HEMA: **Thrombocytopenia, leukopenia, pancytopenia, megaloblastic anemia,*** decreased folic acid,
agranulocytosis
Contraindications: Hypersensitivity, chloroquine-resistant malaria,
megaloblastic anemia caused by
folate deficiency
Precautions: Blood dyscrasias,
seizure disorder, pregnancy (C)
Pharmacokinetics:
PO: Peak 2 hr, half-life 111 hr; metabolized in liver, highly protein
bound, excreted in urine (metabolites)
Interactions/incompatibilities:
• Synergestic action: para-amino-
benzoic acid or folic acid
NURSING CONSIDERATIONS
Assess:
• Folic acid level, megaloblastic
anemia occurs
• Blood studies, CBC, platelets,
since blood dyscrasias occur; twice
weekly if dosage is increased
Administer:
• Leucovorin IM 3-9 mg/day × 3
days if folic acid deficiency occurs
• Before or after meals at same
time each day to maintain drug
level to decrease GI symptoms
Perform/provide:
• Storage in tight, light-resistant
containers
Evaluate:
• For toxicity: vomiting, anorexia,
seizure, blood dyscrasia, glossitis;
drug should be discontinued immediately
Teach patient/family:
• To report visual problems, fever,

---

*Available in Canada only

fatigue, bruising, bleeding; may indicate blood dyscrasias

Treatment of overdose: Gastric lavage, administer short-acting barbiturate, leucovorin, respiratory support if needed

---

quazepam
Doral

Func. class.: Sedative-hypnotic
Chem. class.: Benzodiazepine derivative

Controlled Substance Schedule IV (USA)

Action: Produces CNS depression at the limbic, thalamic, hypothalamic levels of CNS; may be mediated by neurotransmitter γ-aminobutyric acid (GABA); results are sedation, hypnosis, skeletal muscle relaxation, anticonvulsant activity, anxiolytic action

Uses: Insomnia

Dosage and routes:
Adult: PO 7.5 mg hs, may increase if needed

Available forms include: Tabs 7.5, 15 mg

Side effects/adverse reactions:
*HEMA: **Leukopenia, granulocytopenia** (rare)*
CNS: Lethargy, drowsiness, daytime sedation, dizziness, confusion, lightheadedness, headache, anxiety, irritability, weakness, tremor, depression
GI: Nausea, vomiting, diarrhea, heartburn, abdominal pain, constipation, anorexia, taste alteration
CV: Chest pain, pulse changes, palpitations, tachycardia
MISC: Joint pain, congestion, dermatitis, sweating

Contraindications: Hypersensitivity to benzodiazepines, pregnancy, lactation

Precautions: Hepatic disease, renal disease, suicidal individuals, drug abuse, elderly, psychosis, child <18 yr, lactation, depression, pulmonary insufficiency

Pharmacokinetics:
PO: Onset 15-45 min, duration 7-8 hr; metabolized by liver, excreted by kidneys (inactive/active metabolites), crosses placenta, excreted in breast milk

Interactions/incompatibilities:
• Increased effects of quazepam: cimetidine, disulfiram
• Increased CNS depression: alcohol, CNS depressants
• Decreased effect of quazepam: antacids

NURSING CONSIDERATIONS
Assess:
• Blood studies: Hct, Hgb, RBCs (if on long-term therapy)
• Hepatic studies: AST, ALT, bilirubin

Administer:
• After removal of cigarettes, to prevent fires
• After trying conservative measures for insomnia
• ½-1 hr before hs for sleeplessness
• On empty stomach for fast onset, but may be taken with food if GI symptoms occur

Perform/provide:
• Assistance with ambulation after receiving dose
• Safety measure: siderails, night light, call bell within easy reach
• Checking to see PO medication has been swallowed
• Storage in tight container in cool environment

Evaluate:
• Therapeutic response: ability to sleep at night, decreased amount of early morning awakening
• Mental status: mood, sensorium, affect, memory (long, short)

---

italics = common side effects   ***bold italic*** = life threatening reactions

• Blood dyscrasias: fever, sore throat, bruising, rash, jaundice, epistaxis (rare)
• Type of sleep problem: falling asleep, staying asleep

Teach patient/family:
• To avoid driving or other activities requiring alertness until drug is stabilized
• To avoid alcohol ingestion or CNS depressants; serious CNS depression may result
• That effects may take two nights for benefits to be noticed
• Alternate measures to improve sleep: reading, exercise several hours before hs, warm bath, warm milk, TV, self-hypnosis, deep breathing
• That hangover is common in elderly, but less common than with barbiturates

Lab test interferences:
Increase: AST/ALT, serum bilirubin
Decrease: RAI uptake

Treatment of overdose: Lavage, activated charcoal, monitor electrolytes, vital signs

---

quinacrine HCl

(kwin'a-kreen)
Atabrine

Func. class.: Anthelmintic
Chem. class.: Acridine dye derivative

Action: Causes worm scolex to detach from GI tract
Uses: Giardiasis, tapeworms (cestodiasis), malaria
Dosage and routes:
• *Adult:* PO 100 mg × 5-7 days
• *Child:* PO 7 mg/kg/day in 3 divided doses pc × 5 days, not to exceed 300 mg/day; may repeat in 2 wk if needed; administer 1-3 mo for malaria

Available forms include: Tabs 100 mg
Side effects/adverse reactions:
INTEG: Rash, dermatitis, yellow pigmentation of skin, urticaria
CNS: Dizziness, headache, insomnia, restlessness, confusion, behavioral changes, psychosis, *convulsions*
EENT: Bad taste, oral irritation, corneal deposits, retinopathy
GI: Nausea, vomiting, anorexia, diarrhea, cramps, hepatitis
HEMA: Aplastic anemia, agranulocytosis
Contraindications: Hypersensitivity, porphyria, psoriasis
Precautions: Seizure disorders, elderly, psychosis, alcoholism, hepatic disease, depression, child <12 yr, G-6-PD deficiency, pregnancy (C)
Pharmacokinetics:
PO: Peak 8 hr, metabolized by the liver (slowly), excreted primarily in urine, crosses placenta, high protein bindings
Interactions/incompatibilities:
• Increased toxicity: primaquine, hepatotoxic drugs
• Disulfiram-like reaction: alcohol

NURSING CONSIDERATIONS
Assess:
• Stools during entire treatment, collect entire stools × 48 hr, pass through sieve, check for scolex (yellow tapeworms)
• CBC, ophthalmic exam if used for long-term treatment
• Stools 2 wk after last dose for giardiasis
Administer:
• By duodenal tube for pork tapeworm; prevents vomiting, transportation of parasites into stomach
• Bland liquid diet, no fat, or no-

---

residue 24-48 hr before beginning therapy; patient should be fasting night before, given saline enemas, cleansing enema before beginning therapy (tapeworms only)

• Laxatives before treatment to cleanse bowel

• After meals with fluids for giardiasis, malaria

• In jam or honey to disguise bitter taste of pulverized tablets (children)

Perform/provide:

• Storage in tight containers

Evaluate:

• For therapeutic response: expulsion of worms, 3 negative stool cultures after completion of treatment

• For allergic reaction (rash), visual problems (halos, blurring, inability to focus)

• For infection in other family members since infection from person to person is common

• Mental status: affect, mood, behavioral changes

Teach patient/family:

• Proper hygiene after BM including handwashing technique; tell patient to avoid putting fingers in mouth

• To clean toilet qd with disinfectant (green soap solution)

• Need for compliance with dosage schedule, duration of treatment

• That skin, urine may turn deep yellow

• To report any visual changes

• Not to drink alcohol

Lab test interferences:

False positive: Adrenal function tests

Increase: 17-OHCS (Mattingly method)

Treatment of overdose: Induce vomiting

---

quinestrol

(kwin-ess′trole)

Estrovis

Func. class.: Estrogen

Chem. class.: Nonsteroidal synthetic estrogen

Action: Needed for adequate functioning of female reproductive system; affects release of pituitary gonadotropins, inhibits ovulation, promotes adequate calcium use in bone structures

Uses: Menopause, atrophic vaginitis, kraurosis vulvae, female castration, female hypogonadism, primary ovarian failure

Dosage and routes:

• *Adult:* PO 100 µg qd × 1 wk, then 100 µg q wk starting 2 wk after beginning treatment; may increase to 200 µg/wk

Available forms include: Tabs 100 µg

Side effects/adverse reactions:

CNS: Dizziness, headache, migraine, depression

CV: Hypotension, thrombophlebitis, edema, *thromboembolism, stroke, pulmonary embolism, myocardial infarction*

GI: Nausea, vomiting, diarrhea, anorexia, pancreatitis, cramps, constipation, increased appetite, increased weight, *cholestatic jaundice*

EENT: Contact lens intolerance, increased myopia, astigmatism

GU: Amenorrhea, cervical erosion, breakthrough bleeding, dysmenorrhea, vaginal candidiasis, breast changes, *gynecomastia, testicular atrophy, impotence*

INTEG: Rash, urticaria, acne, hirsutism, alopecia, oily skin, seborrhea, purpura, melasma

---

italics = common side effects   ***bold italic*** = life threatening reactions

META: Folic acid deficiency, hypercalcemia, hyperglycemia

Contraindications: Breast cancer, thromboembolic disorders, reproductive cancer, genital bleeding (abnormal, undiagnosed), pregnancy (X)

Precautions: Hypertension, asthma, blood dyscrasias, gallbladder disease, CHF, diabetes mellitus, bone disease, depression, migraine headache, convulsive disorders, hepatic disease, renal disease, family history of cancer of breast or reproductive tract

Pharmacokinetics:

PO: Degraded in liver, excreted in urine, crosses placenta, excreted in breast milk

Interactions/incompatibilities:
• Decreased action of: anticoagulants, oral hypoglycemics
• Toxicity: tricyclic antidepressants
• Decreased action of quinestrol: anticonvulsants, barbiturates, phenylbutazone, rifampin
• Increased action of: corticosteroids

NURSING CONSIDERATIONS
Assess:
• Urine glucose in patient with diabetes; increased urine glucose may occur
• Weight daily, notify physician of weekly weight gain >5 lb; if increase, diurectic may be ordered
• B/P q4h, watch for increase caused by water and sodium retention
• I&O ratio, be alert for decreasing urinary output and increasing edema
• Liver function studies, including AST, ALT, bilirubin, alk phosphatase

Administer:
• Titrated dose, use lowest effective dose

• With food or milk to decrease GI symptoms

Evaluate:
• Therapeutic response: reversal of menopause or decrease in tumor size in prostatic cancer
• Edema, hypertension, cardiac symptoms, jaundice, calcemia
• Mental status: affect mood, behavioral changes, aggression

Teach patient/family:
• To weigh weekly, report gain >5 lb
• To report breast lumps, vaginal bleeding, edema, jaundice, dark urine, clay-colored stools, dyspnea, headache, blurred vision, abdominal pain, numbness or stiffness in legs, chest pain; male to report impotence or gynecomastia

---

quinidine gluconate/ quinidine polygalacturonate/quinidine sulfate

(kwin'i-deen)

Biquin Durales,* Duraquin,* Quinaglute Dura-Tabs, Quinate, Quinatime, Quin-Release/Cardioquin, Cin-Quin, Novoquindin, Quine, Quinidex Extentabs, Quinora

Func. class.: Antidysrhythmic (Class IA)

Chem. class.: Quinine dextro isomer

Action: Increases action potential duration and effective refractory period, thus decreasing myocardial excitability

Uses: PVCs, atrial fibrillation, PAT, ventricular tachycardia, atrial dysrhythmias

Dosage and routes:

Atrial fibrillation/flutter
• *Adult:* PO 200 mg q2-3h × 5-8 doses, may increase qd until sinus

rhythm is restored, max 4 g/day given only after digitalization

Paroxysmal supraventricular tachycardia

• *Adult:* PO 400-600 mg q2-3h

All other dysrhythmias

• *Adult:* PO 50-200 mg as a test dose, then 200-400 mg q4-6h; IM 600 mg, then 400 mg q2h, after test dose (gluconate); IV INF 800 mg in 40 ml D_5W run at 16 mg/min

Available forms include: (Gluconate) tabs sus rel 324, 330 mg; inj IM gluconate 80 mg/ml (sulfate) tabs 100, 200, 300 mg; caps 200, 300 mg; tabs sus rel 300 mg; inj IV (polygalacturonate) tabs 275 mg, sulfate 200 mg/ml

Side effects/adverse reactions:

CNS: Headache, dizziness, involuntary movement, confusion, psychosis, restlessness, irritability, syncope, excitement

EENT: Tinnitus, blurred vision, hearing loss, mydriasis, disturbed color vision

GI: Nausea, vomiting, anorexia, diarrhea, *hepatotoxicity*

CV: Hypotension, bradycardia, PVCs, *heart block, cardiovascular collapse, arrest*

HEMA: Thrombocytopenia, hemolytic anemia, agranulocytosis, hypoprothrombinemia

RESP: Dyspnea, *respiratory depression*

INTEG: Rash, urticaria, angioedema, swelling, photosensitivity

Contraindications: Hypersensitivity, blood dyscrasias, severe heart block, myasthenia gravis

Precautions: Prancacy (C), lactation, children, renal disease, potassium imbalance, liver disease, CHF, respiratory depression

Pharmacokinetics:

PO: Peak 0.5-6 hr, duration 6-8 hr; half-life 6-7 hr, metabolized in liver, excreted unchanged by kidneys

Interactions/incompatibilities:

• Increased effects of: neuromuscular blockers, digoxin, coumadin

• Increased effects of quinidine: cimetidine, propranolol, thiazides, sodium bicarbonate, carbonic anhydrase inhibitors, antacids, hydroxide suspensions

• May decrease effects of quinidine: barbiturates, phenytoin, rifampin, nifedipine

• Additive vagolytic effect: anticholinergic blockers

• Additive cardiac depression: other antidysrhythmics, phenothiazines, reserpine

NURSING CONSIDERATIONS
Assess:

• ECG continuously to determine increased PR or QRS segments; if these develop, discontinue or reduce dose

• Blood levels (therapeutic level 2-6 µg/ml)

• B/P continuously for fluctuations

Administer:

• IV after diluting 800 mg/40 ml or more D_5; give 16 mg or less over 1 min as infusion; use infusion pump

• IM injection in deltoid; aspirate to avoid intravascular administration

Evaluate:

• Cinchonism: tinnitus, headache, nausea, dizziness, fever, vertigo, tremor; may lead to hearing loss

• Cardiac rate, respiration: rate, rhythm, character, continuously

• Respiratory status: rate, rhythm, lung fields for rales

• CNS effects: dizziness, confusion, psychosis, paresthesias, convulsions; drug should be discontinued

---

italics = common side effects   ***bold italic*** = life threatening reactions

• Lung fields, bilateral rales may occur in CHF patient
• Increased respiration, increased pulse; drug should be discontinued
Lab test interferences:
Increase: CPK
Treatment of overdose: O_2, artificial ventilation, ECG, administer dopamine for circulatory depression, administer diazepam or thiopental for convulsions

---

quinine sulfate

(kwye'nine)
Novoquine,* Quinamm, Quine, Quinite, Quiphile, Strema, Quin-260

Func. class.: Antimalarial
Chem. class.: Cinchoma tree alkaloid

Action: Inhibits parasite replications, transcription of DNA to RNA by forming complexes with DNA of parasite
Uses: *Plasmodium falciparum* malaria, nocturnal leg cramps
Dosage and routes:
• *Adult:* PO 650 mg q8h × 10 days, given with pyrimethamine 25 mg q12h × 3 days, with sulfadiazine 500 mg qid × 5 days
Available forms include: Caps 130, 195, 200, 300, 325 mg; tabs 260, 325 mg
Side effects/adverse reactions:
RESP: Dysuria
INTEG: Pruritus, pigmentary changes, skin eruptions, lichen planus–like eruptions, flushing, facial edema, sweating
*HEMA: **Thrombocytopenia, purpura, hypothrombinemia, hemolysis***
CNS: Headache, stimulation, fatigue, irritability, ***convulsion,*** bad dreams, dizziness, fever, confusion, anxiety
EENT: Blurred vision, corneal changes, retinal changes, difficulty focusing, tinnitus, vertigo, deafness, photophobia, diplopia, night blindness
GI: Nausea, vomiting, anorexia, diarrhea, epigastric pain
CV: Angina, dysrhythmias, tachycardia, hypotension, ***acute circulatory failure***
ENDO: Hypoglycemia
Contraindications: Hypersensitivity, G-6-PD deficiency, retinal field changes, pregnancy (X)
Precautions: Blood dyscrasias, severe GI disease, neurologic disease, severe hepatic disease, psoriasis, cardiac dysrhythmias
Pharmacokinetics:
PO: Peak 1-3 hr, metabolized in liver, excreted in urine, half-life 4-5 hr
Interactions/incompatibilities:
• Toxicity: $NaHCO_3$, acetazolamide
• Decreased absorption: magnesium or aluminum salts
• Increase levels of: digoxin, digitoxin, neuromuscular blockers, other anticoagulants
NURSING CONSIDERATIONS
Assess:
• B/P, pulse, if administered IV, watch for hypotension, tachycardia
• Liver studies weekly: ALT, AST, bilirubin
• Blood studies, CBC, since blood dyscrasias occur
Administer:
• By slow IV
• Before or after meals at same time each day to maintain drug level
Perform/provide:
• Storage in tight, light-resistant container

---

* Available in Canada only

Evaluate:
- For cinchonism: nausea, blurred vision, tinnitus, headache, difficulty focusing

Teach patient/family:
- To avoid OTC preparations: cold preparations, tonic water

Lab test interferences:
Increase: 17-KS
Interference: 17-OHCS

---

rabies immune globulin, human

Hyperab, Imogam

Func. class.: Immune serum
Chem. class.: IgG

Action: Provides passive immunity; given with HDCV; may be used regardless of time of bite, treatment

Uses: Exposure to rabies

Dosage and routes:
- *Adult and child:* IM 20 IU/kg given at same time as 1st rabies vaccine; infiltrate wound with ½ dose, then administer rest IM, 1 ml dose on each of days 3, 7, 14, 28 after 1st dose

Available forms include: Inj IM 125 IU/ml

Side effects/adverse reactions:
INTEG: Pain at injection site, rash, pruritus
MS: Arthralgia
SYST: Lymphadenopathy, **anaphylaxis**, fever
CNS: Headache, fatigue, malaise
GI: Abdominal pain

Contraindications: Hypersensitivity to equine products and thimerosal

Interactions/incompatibilities:
- Decreased action of rabies immune globulin: corticosteroids, immunosuppressants

---

NURSING CONSIDERATIONS
Administer:
- Test dose: dilute drug either with 1:100 or 1:1000 0.9% NaCl for injection, inject 0.1 ml 0.9% NaCl in other arm intradermally, check for wheal 10 mm or > after 10 min; if present, drug should not be used
- Only after epinephrine 1:1000, resuscitative equipment are available
- Only if human immune serum is not available
- As soon as possible after exposure

Perform/provide:
- Storage at 2°-8°C

Evaluate:
- Allergic reactions: dyspnea, rash, pruritus, eruptions

Teach patient/family:
- That pain, swelling, itching may occur at injection site
- To take acetaminophen to alleviate headache, fever, and pain

---

radioactive iodine (sodium iodide) ^{131}I

Func. class.: Antithyroid
Chem. class.: Radiopharmaceutical

Action: Converted to protein-bound iodine by thyroid gland for use when needed

Uses:
High dose: Thyroid cancer, hyperthyroidism
Low dose: Visualization to determine thyroid cancer, diagnostic aid in thyroid function studies

Dosage and routes:
Thyroid cancer
- *Adult:* PO 50-150 mCi, may repeat depending on clinical status
Hyperthyroidism

R

---

italics = common side effects   ***bold italic*** = life threatening reactions

• *Adult:* PO 4-10 mCi, depending on serum thyroxine level
Available forms include: Caps 1-50, 0.8-100 mCi; oral sol 7.05 mCi/ml, 3.5-150 mCi/vial
Side effects/adverse reactions:
ENDO: Hypothyroidism, **hyperthyroid adenoma,** transient thyroiditis
INTEG: Alopecia
HEMA: **Eosinophilia, lymphedema, leukemia, bone marrow depression, leukopenia,** anemia
GI: Nausea, diarrhea, vomiting
EENT: Sore throat, cough
Contraindications: Recent MI, lactation, large nodular goiter, pregnancy (X), <30 yr, vomiting/diarrhea, acute hyperthyroidism, use of thyroid drugs
Pharmacokinetics:
PO: Onset 3-6 days, excreted in urine, sweat, feces, crosses placenta, excreted in breast milk, excreted in 56 days
Interactions/incompatibilities:
• Hypothyroidism: lithium
• Decreased uptake if recent intake of stable iodine, thyroid, antithyroid drugs
NURSING CONSIDERATIONS
Assess:
• Weight qd in same clothing, scale, time of day
• Blood work, including CBC for blood dyscrasias (leukopenia, thrombocytopenia, agranulocytosis)
Administer:
• Only after discontinuing all other antithyroid agents × 5-7 days
• After NPO overnight, food delays action
• After menstruation (10 days) or during
Perform/provide:
• Limited contact with patient ½ hr/day for each person
• Adequate rest after treatment

• Fluids to 3-4 L/day for 48 hr after agent is administered to remove agent from body
Evaluate:
• Therapeutic effect: weight gain, decreased pulse, decreased T_4, B/P
• Overdose: peripheral edema, heat intolerance, diaphoresis, palpitations, dysrhythmias, severe tachycardia, increased temperature delirium, CNS irritability
• Hypersensitivity: rash, enlarged cervical lymph nodes; drug may need to be discontinued
• Hypoprothrombinemia: bleeding, petechiae, ecchymosis
• Clinical response: after 3 wk should include increased weight, pulse; decreased T_4
• Bone marrow depression: sore throat, fever, fatigue
Teach patient/family:
• To empty bladder often during treatment, avoids radiation of gonads
• Report redness, swelling, sore throat, mouth lesions; indicate blood dyscrasias
• To avoid extended contact with children or spouse for 1 week
• That bathroom may be used by entire family
• Not to take antithyroid agents but propranolol, which decreases hyperthyroid symptoms, until total effects of ^{131}I has taken effect (about 6 wk)
• Avoid coughing, expectorating for 24 hr (saliva and vomiting are highly radioactive for 6-8 hr)

---

ranitidine
(ra-nye' te-deen)
Zantac
Func. class.: H_2 histamine receptor antagonist

Action: Inhibits histamine at H_2 receptor site in parietal cells, which inhibits gastric acid secretion

Uses: Duodenal ulcer, Zollinger-Ellison syndrome, gastric ulcers, hypersecretory conditions, gastroesophageal reflux disease, stress ulcers

Dosage and routes:
• *Adult:* PO 150 mg bid, 300 mg hs; IM 50 mg q6-8h; IV BOL 50 mg diluted to 20 ml over 5 min q6-8h IV INT INF 50 mg/100 ml D₅ over 15-20 min, q6-8h

Available forms include: Tabs 150, 300 mg; inj 25 mg/ml IM, IV

Side effects/adverse reactions:
CNS: Headache, sleeplessness, dizziness, confusion, agitation, depression, hallucination
GI: Constipation, abdominal pain, diarrhea, nausea, vomiting, *hepatotoxicity*
GU: Impotence, gynecomastia
CV: Tachycardia, bradycardia, PVCs
EENT: Blurred vision, increased ocular pressure
INTEG: Urticaria, rash, fever

Contraindications: Hypersensitivity

Precautions: Pregnancy (B), lactation, child <12 yr, hepatic disease, renal disease

Pharmacokinetics:
PO: Peak 2-3 hr, duration 8-12 hr; metabolized by liver, excreted in urine, breast milk, half-life 2-3 hr

Interactions/incompatibilities:
• Increased toxicity; anticoagulants, metoprolol
• Decreased absorption of: ketoconazole
• Decreased absorption of ranitidine: antacids

NURSING CONSIDERATIONS
Assess:
• Gastric pH (>5 should be maintained)
• I&O ratio, BUN, creatinine

Administer:
• With meals for prolonged drug effect
• Antacids 1 hr before or 1 hr after ranitidine
• IV after diluting 50 mg/20 ml of compatible sol and give 50 mg or less/5 min or more; may dilute 50 mg/50-100 ml of compatible sol and give over 15-20 min

Perform/provide:
• Storage at room temperature

Evaluate:
• Mental status: confusion, dizziness, depression, anxiety, weakness, tremors, psychosis, diarrhea, abdominal discomfort, jaundice; report immediately
• GI complaints: nausea, vomiting, diarrhea, cramps

Teach patient/family:
• That gynecomastia, impotence may occur but are reversible
• To avoid driving or other hazardous activities until patient is stabilized on this medication
• To avoid black pepper, caffeine, alcohol, harsh spices, extremes in temperature of food
• That drug must be continued for prescribed time to be effective

Lab test interferences:
Increase: AST/ALT, alk phosphatase, creatinine, LDH, bilirubin
False positive: Urine protein

R

---

regular insulin

Beef Regular Iletin II, Humulin BR, Humulin R, Iletin Regular,* Novolin R, Pork Regular Iletin II, Regular Iletin I, Regular Pork Insulin, Regular purified Pork, Novolin R PenFill, Velosulin

Func. class.: Antidiabetic
Chem. class.: Exogenous unmodified insulin

Action: Decreases blood sugar, indirectly increases blood pyruvate, lactate, decreases phosphate, potassium

Uses: Adult-onset diabetes, juvenile diabetes, ketoacidosis, Type I, II, NIDDM, IDDM, hyperkalemia

Dosage and routes:

Ketoacidosis

• *Adult:* IV/IM 5-10 U, then 5-10 U/hr until desired response, then switch to SC dose; IV/INF 2-12 U (50 U/500 ml of normal saline)

• *Child:* IV/IM 0.1 U/kg

Replacement

• *Adult:* SC dosage individualized by blood, urine glucose levels, up to qid given ½ hr before meals

Available forms include: IV/IM/SC inj U 40, U 100/ml

Side effects/adverse reactions:

CNS: Headache, lethargy, tremors, weakness, fatigue, delirium, sweating

CV: Tachycardia, palpitations

EENT: Blurred vision, dry mouth

GI: Hunger, nausea

META: Hypoglycemia

INTEG: Flushing, rash, urticaria, warmth, lipodystrophy, lipohypertrophy

SYST: Anaphylaxis

Contraindications: Hypersensitivity

Precautions: Pregnancy (B)

Interactions/incompatibilities:

• Increased hypoglycemia: salicylate, alcohol, β-blockers, anabolic steroids, fenfluramine, guanethidine, oral hypoglycemics, MAOIs, tetracycline, sulfinpyrazone

• Decrease hypoglycemia: thiazides, thyroid hormones, oral contraceptives, corticosteroids, estrogens, dobutamine, epinephrine, dextrothyroxine, smoking

• Mask signs/symptoms of hypoglycemia: β-blocker

Pharmacokinetics:

SC: Onset 30-60 min, peak 2-3 hr, duration 5-7 hr

IV: Onset 10-30 min, peak 30-60 min, duration 1-2 hr, half-life 3-5 min

Metabolized by liver, muscle, kidneys, excreted in urine

NURSING CONSIDERATIONS

Assess:

• Fasting blood glucose, 2 hr PP (60-100 mg/dl normal fasting level) (70-130 mg/dl-normal 2 hr level)

• Urine ketones during illness; insulin requirements increase during times of stress, illness

Administer:

• After warming to room temperature by rotating in palms, to prevent lipodystrophy (from injecting cold insulin)

• ½ hr ac, so peak action coincides with peak sugar level

• Increased doses if tolerance occurs

• Human insulin to those allergic to beef or pork

• IV undiluted through Y-tube or 3-way stopcock, give 50 U or less/min; may be diluted in 0.9% NS or 0.45% saline for INF; run at rate ordered

Perform/provide:

• Storage at room temperature for <1 month, keep in cool area, refrigerate all other supply, do not use discolored, or cloudy solution

• Rotation of injection sites: abdomen, upper back, thighs, upper arm, buttocks; keep record of sites

Evaluate:

• Therapeutic response: decrease in polyuria, polydipsia, polyphagia, clear sensorium, absence of dizziness, stable gait

• Hypoglycemic/hyperglycemic

reaction that can occur soon after meals

Teach patient/family:

• That blurred vision occurs, not to change corrective lens until vision is stabilized 1-2 mo

• To keep insulin, equipment available at all times

• That drug does not cure diabetes, but controls symptoms

• To carry Medic Alert ID as diabetic

• Hypoglycemia reaction: headache, tremors, fatigue, weakness, sweating

• Dosage, route, mixing instructions if any diet restrictions, disease process

• To carry candy or lump sugar to treat hypoglycemia

• Symptoms of ketoacidosis: nausea, thirst, polyuria, dry mouth, decrease B/P, dry, flushed skin, acetone breath, drowsiness, Kussmaul respirations

• That a plan is necessary for diet, exercise; all food on diet should be eaten, exercise routine should not vary

• Urine glucose testing; make sure patient is able to determine glucose, acetone levels, also home blood glucose monitoring

• The pregnant patient to use glucose oxidase reagents

• To avoid OTC drugs unless directed by physician

Lab test interferences:

Increase: VMA

Decrease: Potassium, calcium

Interference: Liver function studies, thyroid function studies

Treatment of overdose: 10%-50% glucose PO if conscious or IV if comatose or 1 mg glucagon

regular insulin concentrated

Regular (concentrated) Iletin II U-500

Func. class.: Antidiabetic

Chem. class.: Exogenous unmodified insulin

Action: Decreases blood sugar, indirectly increases blood pyruvate, lactate, decreases phosphate, potassium

Uses: Treatment of diabetic patients with marked insulin resistance (>200 U/day)

Dosage and routes:

• *Adult:* SC/IM dosage individualized by blood, urine glucose qd-tid

Available forms include: Inj SC, IM 500 U/ml

Side effects/adverse reactions:

CNS: Headache, lethargy, tremors, weakness, fatigue, delirium, sweating

CV: Tachycardia, palpitations

EENT: Blurred vision

GI: Hunger, nausea, dry mouth

META: Hypoglycemia

INTEG: Flushing, rash, urticaria, warmth, lipodystrophy, lipohypertrophy

SYST: **Anaphylaxis**

MISC: Thirst, leg pain, increased urination

Contraindications: Hypersensitivity

Precautions: Pregnancy (B)

Pharmacokinetics:

SC: Onset 30-60 min, peak 2-5 hr, duration 5-7 hr

Metabolized by liver, muscle, kidneys, excreted in urine

Interactions/incompatibilities:

• Increased hypoglycemia: salicylate, alcohol, β-blockers, anabolic steroids, fenfluramine, guanethi-

R

dine, oral hypoglycemics, MAOIs, tetracycline, sulfinpyrazone
• Decreased hypoglycemia: thiazides, thyroid hormones, oral contraceptives, corticosteroids, estrogens, smoking, dextrothyroxine, dobutamine, epinephrine

NURSING CONSIDERATIONS
Assess:
• Fasting blood glucose, 2 hr PP (60-100 mg/dl normal fasting level) (70-130 mg/dl-normal 2 hr level)
• Urine ketones during times of illness; insulin requirements increase during stress, illness

Administer:
• After warming to room temperature by rotating in palms, to prevent lipodystrophy from injecting cold insulin
• ½ hr ac, so peak action coincides with peak sugar level
• Increased doses if tolerance occurs

Perform/provide:
• Storage in refrigerator, do not freeze, do not use discolored, or cloudy solution
• Rotation of injection sites: abdomen, upper back, thighs, upper arms, buttocks; keep record of sites

Evaluate:
• Therapeutic response: decrease in polyuria, polydipsia, polyphagia, clear sensorium, absence of dizziness, stable gait
• Hypoglycemic/hyperglycemic reaction that can occur soon after meals or suddenly while on therapy

Teach patient/family:
• That blurred vision occurs, not to change corrective lens until vision is stabilized 1-2 mo
• To keep insulin, equipment available at all times
• That drug does not cure diabetes, but controls symptoms

• To carry Medic Alert ID as diabetic
• Hypoglycemia reaction: headache, tremors, fatigue, weakness
• Dosage, route, mixing instructions if any diet restrictions, disease process
• To carry candy or lump sugar to treat hypoglycemia
• Symptoms of ketoacidosis: nausea, thirst, polyuria, dry mouth, decrease B/P, dry, flushed skin, acetone breath, drowsiness, Kussmaul respirations
• That a plan is necessary for diet, exercise; all food on diet should be eaten, exercise routine should not vary
• Urine glucose testing, make sure patient is able to determine glucose, acetone levels
• The pregnant patient to use glucose oxidase reagents
• To avoid OTC drugs unless directed by physician

Lab test interferences:
Increase: VMA
Decrease: Potassium, calcium
Interference: Liver function studies, thyroid function studies
Treatment of overdose: 10%-50% glucose PO if conscious or IV if comatose or 1 mg glucagon

---

reserpine

(re-ser′peen)

Broserpine, Elserpine, Hyperine, Rauserpin, Reserfia,* Serpasil, Serpate, Sertina, Tensin, Zepine

Func. class.: Antihypertensive
Chem. class.: Antiadrenergic agent

Action: Inhibits norepinephrine release, depleting norepinephrine stores in adrenergic nerve endings
Uses: Hypertension; relief in agitated psychotic states unable to tol-

erate phenothiazines or requiring antihypertensive medication

Dosage and routes:

Hypertension

• *Adult:* PO 0.25-0.5 mg qd × 1-2 wk, then 0.1-0.25 mg qd maintenance

• *Child:* PO 0.07 mg/kg or 2 mg/m² given with hydralzine IM q12-24 h

Pyschiatric disorders

• *Adult:* 0.5 mg/day (range 0.1-1 mg)

Available forms include: Tabs 0.2, 0.1, 0.25, 1 mg; caps-time rel 0.5 mg; inj 2.5 mg/ml

Side effects/adverse reactions:

CV: Bradycardia, chest pain, dysrhythmias, prolonged bleeding time, ***thrombocytopenia,*** purpura

CNS: Drowsiness, fatigue, lethargy, dizziness, depression, anxiety, headache, increased dreaming, nightmares, convulsions, Parkinsonism, EPS (high doses)

GI: Nausea, vomiting, cramps, peptic ulcer, dry mouth, increased appetite, anorexia

INTEG: Rash, purpura, alopecia, flushing, warm feeling, pruritus, ecchymosis

EENT: Lacrimation, miosis, blurred vision, ptosis, dry mouth, epistaxis

GU: Impotence, dysuria, nocturia, sodium, water retention, edema, breast engorgement, galactorrhea, gynecomastia

RESP: ***Bronchospasm,*** dyspnea, cough, rales

Contraindications: Hypersensitivity, depression/suicidal patients, active peptic ulcer disease, ulcerative colitis, pregnancy (D)

Precautions: Pregnancy, lactation, seizure disorders, renal disease

Pharmacokinetics:

PO: Peak 4 hr, duration 2-6 wk; half-life 50-100 hr, metabolized by liver, excreted in urine, feces, crosses placenta, blood-brain barrier, excreted in breast milk

Interactions/incompatibilities:

• Increased hypotension: diuretics, hypotension, β-blockers, methotrimeprazine

• Dysrhythmias: cardiac glycosides

• Increased cardiac depression: quinidine, procainamide

• Excitation, hypertension: MAOIs

• Increased CNS depression: barbiturates, alcohol, narcotics

• Increased pressor effects: epinephrine, isoproterenol, norepinephrine

• Decreased pressor effects: ephedrine, amphetamine

NURSING CONSIDERATIONS

Assess:

• Renal function studies in renal impairment (BUN, creatinine)

• Bleeding time, check for ecchymosis, thrombocytopenia, purpura

• I&O in renal disease patient

Evaluate:

• Cardiac status: B/P, pulse, watch for hypotension, bradycardia

• Edema in feet, legs daily; take weight daily

• Skin turgor, dryness of mucous membranes for hydration status

• Symptoms of CHF: edema, dyspnea, wet rales

Teach patient/family:

• To avoid driving, hazardous activities if drowsiness occurs

• Not to discontinue drug abruptly

• Not to use OTC products (cough, cold preparations) unless directed by physician

• To report bradycardia, dizziness, confusion, depression, fever, sore throat

• That impotence, gynecomastia may occur but is reversible

• To rise slowly to sitting or stand-

R

---

italics = common side effects   ***bold italic*** = life threatening reactions

ing position to minimize orthostatic hypotension
• That therapeutic effect may take 2-4 wk
Lab test interferences:
Increase: VMA excretion, 5-HIAA excretion
Interferences: 17-OHCS, 17-KS
Treatment of overdose: Lavage, IV atropine for bradycardia, supportive therapy

---

Rh₀ (D) immune globulin, human

Gamulin Rh, HypoRho-D, MICRhoGAM, Mini-Gamulin RH, RHoGAM, Win-Rho*

Func. class.: Immunizing agent
Chem. class.: IgG

Action: Supresses immune response of non-sensitized Rh_o (D or D_u)-negative patients who are exposed to Rh_o (D or D^u)-positive blood
Uses: Prevention of isoimmunization in Rh-negative women exposed to Rh positive blood, given after abortions, miscarriages, amniocentesis
Dosage and routes:
Obstetrical use
• *Adult:* IM 1 vial if fetal packed RBCs <15 ml, or 2 vials if fetal packed RBCs >15 ml; given within 72 hr of delivery or miscarriage
Transfusion error
• *Adult:* IM Give within 72 hr
Available forms include: Inj IM single dose vial
Side effects/adverse reactions:
INTEG: Irritation at injection site, fever
CNS: Lethargy
MS: Myalgia
Contraindications: Previous im-

munization with this drug, Rh_o (O)-positive/D^u-positive patient
NURSING CONSIDERATIONS
Administer:
• After sending newborn's cord blood to lab after delivery for cross match, type, infant must be Rh-positive, with Rh-negative mother
• IM only in deltoid, aspirate
• Only equal lot numbers of drug, cross-match
• Only MICRhoGAM for abortions
Evaluate:
• Allergic reaction: rash, urticaria, nausea, fever, wheezing
Perform/provide:
• Storage in refrigerator
Teach patient/family:
• How drug works, that drug does need to be given after subsequent deliveries if baby is Rh positive

---

riboflavin (vitamin B₂)

(rey'boo-flay-vin)
Riobin-50 and others
Func. class.: Vitamin B_2, water soluble

Action: Needed for respiratory reactions by catalyzing proteins and normal vision
Uses: Vitamin B_2 deficiency or polyneuritis, cheilosis adjunct with thiamine
Dosage and routes:
• *Adult and child >12 yr:* PO 5-50 mg qd
• *Child <12 yr:* PO 2-10 mg qd
Available forms include: Tabs 5, 10, 25, 50, 100 mg
Side effects/adverse reactions:
GU: Yellow discoloration of urine (large doses)
Contraindications: Child <12 yr
Precautions: Pregnancy (A)
Pharmacokinetics:
PO: Half-life 65-85 min, 60% pro-

tein-bound, unused amounts excreted in urine (unchanged)

Interactions/incompatibilities:
• Decreased action of: tetracyclines

NURSING CONSIDERATIONS
Administer:
• With food for better absorption

Perform/provide:
• Storage in tight, light-resistant container

Evaluate:
• Therapeutic response: absence of headache, GI problems, cheilosis, skin lesions, depression, burning, itchy eyes, anemia
• Nutritional status: liver, eggs, dairy products, yeast, whole grain, green vegetables

Teach patient/family:
• That urine may turn bright yellow
• On addition of needed foods that are rich in riboflavin

Lab test interferences:
• May cause false elevations of urinary catecholamines

---

rifampin

(rif'am-pin)
Rifadin, Rimactane, Rofact*

Func. class.: Antitubercular
Chem. class.: Rifamycin B derivative

Action: Inhibits DNA-dependent polymerase, decreases tubercle bacilli replication

Uses: Pulmonary tuberculosis, meningococcal carriers (prevention)

Dosage and routes:
• *Adult:* PO 600 mg/day as single dose 1 hr ac or 2 hr pc
• *Child >5 yr:* PO 10-20 mg/kg/day as single dose 1 hr ac or 2 hr pc, not to exceed 600 mg/day, with other antituberculars

Meningococcal carriers

• *Adult:* PO 600 mg bid × 2 days
• *Child >5 yr:* PO 10 mg/kg bid × 2 days, not to exceed 600 mg/dose

Available forms include: Caps 150, 300 mg

Side effects/adverse reactions:
CV: **CHF, dysrhythmias**
CNS: Headache, anxiety, drowsiness, tremors, **convulsions,** lethargy, depression, confusion, psychosis, aggression
EENT: Blurred vision, optic neuritis, photophobia
HEMA: **Hemolytic anemia, thrombocytopenia, leukopenia**

Contraindications: Hypersensitivity

Precautions: Pregnancy (C), child <13 yr

Pharmacokinetics:
PO: Peak 2-3 hr, duration >24 hr, half-life 3 hr; metabolized in liver (active/inactive metabolites), excreted in urine as free drug (30% crosses placenta), excreted in breast milk

Interactions/incompatibilities:
• Decreased action: barbiturates, clofibrate, corticosteroids, dapsone, anticoagulants, antidiabetics, hormones, digoxin, PAS, alcohol, oral contraceptives
• Hepatotoxicity: INH

NURSING CONSIDERATIONS
Assess:
• Signs of anemia: Hct, Hgb, fatigue
• Liver studies q wk: ALT, AST, bilirubin
• Renal status before, q mo: BUN, creatinine, output, sp gr, urinalysis

Administer:
• With meals to decrease GI symptoms even though absorption will be decreased

R

---

italics = common side effects   ***bold italic*** = life threatening reactions

- Antiemetic if vomiting occurs
- After C&S is completed; q mo to detect resistance

Evaluate:

- Mental status often: affect, mood, behavioral changes (psychosis may occur)
- Hepatic status: decreased appetite, jaundice, dark urine, fatigue

Teach patient/family:

- That compliance with dosage schedule, duration is necessary
- That scheduled appointments must be kept; relapse may occur
- To avoid alcohol while taking drug
- That urine, feces, saliva, sputum, sweat, tears may be colored red-orange; soft contact lenses may be permanently stained

Lab test interferences:

Interference: Folate level, vitamin B_{12}, BSP, gall bladder studies

---

ritodrine HCl

(ri′toe-dreen)

Yutopar

Func. class.: Tocolytic, uterine relaxant

Chem. class.: β_2-adrenergic agonist

Action: Reduces frequency, intensity of uterine contractions by stimulation of the β_2 receptors in uterine smooth muscle

Uses: Preterm labor

Dosage and routes:

- Adult: IV INF 150 mg/500 ml (0.3 mg/ml) given 0.1 mg/min, increased gradually by 0.05 mg/min q10 min until desired response; PO 10 mg given ½ hr before termination of IV, then 10 mg q2h × 24 hr, then 10-20 mg q4-6h, not to exceed 120 mg/day

Available forms include: Tabs 10 mg; inj 10 mg/ml

Side effects/adverse reactions:

MISC: Erythema, rash, dyspnea, hyperventilation, glycosuria, lactic acidosis

META: Hyperglycemia

CNS: Headache, restlessness, anxiety, nervousness, sweating, chills, drowsiness, tremor

GI: Nausea, vomiting, anorexia, malaise, bloating, constipation, diarrhea

CV: Altered maternal, fetal heart rate, B/P, dysrhythmias, palpitation, chest pain

Contraindications: Hypersensitivity, eclampsia, hypertension, dysrhythmias, thyrotoxicosis, before 20th wk of pregnancy, antepartum hemorrhage, intrauterine fetal death, maternal cardiac disease, pulmonary hypertension, uncontrolled diabetes

Precautions: Migraine, sulfite sensitivity, pregnancy-induced hypertension, hypertension, diabetes

Pharmacokinetics:

PO: Peak ½-1 hr

IV: Peak 1 hr, half-life 6 min, 1½-2½ hr, >10 hr, metabolized in liver, excreted in urine, crosses placenta

Interactions/incompatibilities:

- Pulmonary edema: corticosteroids
- Increased CV effects of ritodrine: magnesium sulfate, diazoxide, meperidine, potent general anesthetics
- Increased effects of: sympathomimetic amines
- Systemic hypertension: atropine
- Decreased action of ritodrine: beta-blockers

NURSING CONSIDERATIONS

Assess:

- Maternal, fetal heart tones during infusion

- Intensity, length of uterine contractions
- Fluid intake to prevent fluid overload; discontinue if this occurs
- Blood glucose in diabetics

Administer:
- Only clear solutions
- After dilutions: 150 mg/500 ml D₅W or NS, give at 0.3 mg/ml
- After infusion pump, or monitor carefully

Perform/provide:
- Positioning of patient in left lateral recumbent position to decrease hypotension, increase renal blood flow

Evaluate:
- Therapeutic response: decreased intensity, length of contraction, absence of preterm labor, decreased B/P

Teach patient/family:
- To remain in bed during infusion

Lab test interferences:
Increase: Blood glucose, free fatty acids, insulin, GTT
Decrease: Potassium

---

salicylic acid

Calicylic, Keralyt, Salacid, Salonil
Func. class.: Keratolytic

Action: Corrects abnormal keratinization and causes peeling of skin
Uses: Dandruff, seborrheic dermatitis, psoriasis, multiple superficial epitheliomatoses
Dosage and routes:
- *Adult:* TOP apply as needed, cover at night
Available forms include: Powder, cream 2%, 2.5%, 10%; gel 6%, 17%; oint 25%, 60%; plaster 40%; pledgets 0.5%; shampoo 2%, 4%; solution 0.5%, 13.6%, 17%; stick 2%; susp 2%

Side effects/adverse reactions:
INTEG: Irritation, drying
CNS: Salicylism: hearing loss, tinnitus, dizziness, confusion, headache, hyperventilation
Contraindications: Hypersensitivity
Precautions: Pregnancy (C), diabetes

NURSING CONSIDERATIONS
Assess:
- Platelets, WBC if systemic absorption occurs

Administer:
- Only to intact skin, do not use on inflamed, denuded skin
- After wetting skin, wash thoroughly each AM after treatment
- Using an occlusive dressing to increase absorption, apply more often to areas where occlusion is impossible

Evaluate:
- Therapeutic response: decrease in dandruff, size of lesions
- Salicylism: tinnitus, hearing loss, dizziness, confusion, headache, hyperventilation
- Allergic reactions: irritation, redness

Teach patient/family:
- To avoid contact with eyes, mucous membranes
- To apply lotion if drying occurs
- To avoid applying to large areas, salicylate toxicity may occur

S

---

salsalate

(sal-sa'late)
Disalcid, Mono-Gesic
Func. class.: Nonnarcotic analgesic
Chem. class.: Salicylate

Action: Blocks formation of peripheral prostaglandins, which causes pain and inflammation, an-

---

tipyretic action results from inhibition of hypothalamic heat-regulating center, does not inhibit platelet aggregation

Uses: Mild to moderate pain or fever including arthritis, juvenile rheumatoid arthritis

Dosage and routes:
• *Adult:* PO 3000 mg/day in divided doses

Available forms include: Caps 500 mg; tabs 500, 750 mg

Side effects/adverse reactions:
*HEMA: **Thrombocytopenia, agranulocytosis, leukopenia, neutropenia, hemolytic anemia,*** increased pro-time

CNS: Stimulation, drowsiness, dizziness, confusion, ***convulsions,*** headache, flushing, hallucinations, coma

GI: Nausea, vomiting, GI bleeding, diarrhea, heartburn, anorexia, ***hepatotoxicity***

INTEG: Rash, urticaria, bruising

EENT: Tinnitus, hearing loss

CV: Rapid pulse, ***pulmonary edema***

RESP: Wheezing, hyperpnea

ENDO: Hypoglycemia, hyponatremia, hypokalemia, alteration in acid-base balance

Contraindications: Hypersensitivity to salicylates, NSAIDs, GI bleeding, bleeding disorders, children < 3 yr, vitamin K deficiency

Precautions: Anemia, hepatic disease, renal disease, Hodgkin's disease, pregnancy (C), lactation

Pharmacokinetics: Metabolized by liver, excreted by kidneys, half-life 1 hr, highly protein bound, crosses blood-brain barrier and placenta slowly

Interactions/incompatibilities:
• Decreased effects of salsalate: antacids, steroids, urinary alkalizers

• Increased blood loss: alcohol, heparin, ibuprofen, warfarin
• Increased effects of: anticoagulants, insulin, methotrexate, probenecid
• Decreased effects of: spironolactone, sulfinpyrazone, sulfonylmides, loop diuretics
• Toxic effects: PABA
• Decreased blood sugar levels: salicylates

NURSING CONSIDERATIONS
Assess:
• Liver function studies: AST, ALT, bilirubin, creatinine if patient is on long-term therapy
• Renal function studies: BUN, urine creatinine if patient is on long-term therapy
• Blood studies: CBC, Hct, Hgb, pro-time if patient is on long-term therapy
• I&O ratio; decreasing output may indicate renal failure (long-term therapy)

Administer:
• To patient crushed or whole; chewable tablets may be chewed
• With food or milk to decrease gastric symptoms; give 30 min before or 2 hr after meals
• With full glass of water

Evaluate:
• Hepatotoxicity: dark urine, clay-colored stools, yellowing of skin, sclera, itching, abdominal pain, fever, diarrhea if patient is on long-term therapy
• Allergic reactions: rash, urticaria; if these occur, drug may need to be discontinued
• Renal dysfunction: decreased urine output
• Ototoxicity: tinnitus, ringing, roaring in ears; audiometric testing is needed before, after long-term therapy

---

* Available in Canada only

- Visual changes: blurring, halos, corneal and retinal damage
- Edema in feet, ankles, legs
- Prior drug history; there are many drug interactions

Teach patient/family:
- To report any symptoms of hepatotoxicity, renal toxicity, visual changes, ototoxicity, allergic reactions (long-term therapy)
- Not to exceed recommended dosage; acute poisoning may result
- To read label on other OTC drugs; many contain aspirin
- That therapeutic response takes 2 wk (arthritis)
- To avoid alcohol ingestion; GI bleeding may occur

Lab test interferences:
Increase: Coagulation studies, liver function studies, serum uric acid, amylase, CO_2, urinary protein
Decrease: Serum potassium, PBI, cholesterol
Interfere: Urine catecholamines, pregnancy test

Treatment of overdose: Lavage, activated charcoal, monitor electrolytes, VS

---

scopolamine (transdermal)

(skoe-pol'-a-meen)
Transderm-Scop

Func. class.: Antiemetic, anticholinergic
Chem. class.: Belladonna alkaloid

Action: Competitive antagonism of acetylcholine at receptor site in eye, smooth muscle, cardiac muscle, glandular cells; inhibition of vestibular input to the CNS, resulting in inhibition of vomiting reflex

Uses: Prevention of motion sickness

Dosage and routes:
- *Adult:* PATCH 1 placed behind ear 4-5 hr before travel
- Not recommended for children
Available forms include: Patch, 0.5 mg delivered in 72 hr

Side effects/adverse reactions:
INTEG: Rash, erythema
GU: Difficult urination
CNS: Dizziness, drowsiness, confusion, disorientation, memory disturbances, hallucinations
EENT: Blurred vision, altered depth perception, *dilated pupils,* photophobia, *dry mouth,* dry, itchy, red eyes, acute narrow-angle glaucoma

Contraindications: Hypersensitivity, glaucoma

Precautions: Children, elderly, pregnancy (C), pyloric, urinary, bladder neck, intestinal obstruction, liver, kidney disease

Pharmacokinetics:
PATCH: Onset 4-5 hr, duration 72 hr

Interactions/incompatibilities:
- Increased anticholinergic effects: antihistamines, antidepressants

NURSING CONSIDERATIONS
Teach patient/family:
- To avoid hazardous activities, activities requiring alertness; dizziness may occur
- To wash, dry hands before and after applying to surface behind ear
- To change patch q72h
- To apply at least 4 hr before traveling
- If blurred vision, severe dizziness, drowsiness occurs, to discontinue use, use another type of antiemetic
- To read label of all OTC medications; if any scopolamine is found in product, avoid use
- To keep out of children's reach

S

---

italics = common side effects   ***bold italic*** = life threatening reactions

scopolamine hydro-bromide

(skoe-pol′a-meen)

Func. class.: Cholinergic blocker
Chem. class.: Belladonna alkaloid

Action: Inhibits acetylcholine at receptor sites in autonomic nervous system, which controls secretions, free acids in stomach; blocks central muscarinic receptors, which decreases involuntary movements

Uses: Reduction of secretions before surgery, calm delirium, motion sickness

Dosage and routes:
Parkinson symptoms
• *Adult:* IM/SC/IV 0.3-0.6 mg tid-qid diluted using dilution provided
• *Child:* SC 0.006 mg/kg tid-qid or 0.2 mg/m^2
Preoperatively
• *Adult:* SC 0.4-0.6 mg

Available forms include: Inj 0.3, 0.4, 0.86, 1 mg/ml

Side effects/adverse reactions:
CNS: Confusion, anxiety, restlessness, irritability, delusions, hallucinations, headache, sedation, depression, incoherence, dizziness, excitement, delirium, flushing, weakness
INTEG: Urticaria
MISC: Suppression of lactation, nasal congestion, decreased sweating
EENT: Blurred vision, photophobia, dilated pupils, difficulty swallowing, mydriasis, cycloplegia
CV: Palpitations, tachycardia, postural hypotension, paradoxical bradycardia
GI: Dryness of mouth, constipation, nausea, vomiting, abdominal distress, *paralytic ileus*
GU: Hesitancy, retention

Contraindications: Hypersensitivity, narrow-angle glaucoma, myasthenia gravis, GI/GU obstruction, hypersensitivity to belladonna, barbiturates

Precautions: Pregnancy (C), elderly, lactation, prostatic hypertrophy, CHF, hypertension, dysrhythmia, children, gastric ulcer

Pharmacokinetics:
SC/IM: Peak 30-45 min, duration 7 hr
IV: Peak 10-15 min, duration 4 hr
Excreted in urine, bile, feces (unchanged)

Interactions/incompatibilities:
• Increased anticholinergic effect: alcohol, narcotics, antihistamines, phenothiazines, tricyclics
• Do not mix with diazepam, chloramphenicol, pentobarbital, sodium bicarbonate in syringe or solution

NURSING CONSIDERATIONS
Assess:
• I&O ratio; retention commonly causes decreased urinary output

Administer:
• Parenteral dose with patient recumbent to prevent postural hypotension
• Administer with or after meals for GI upset; may give with fluids other than water
• At hs to avoid daytime drowsiness in patient with parkinsonism
• Parenteral dose slowly; keep in bed for at least 1 hr after dose
• With analgesic to avoid behavioral changes when given as a preop

Perform/provide:
• Storage at room temperature in light-resistant containers
• Hard candy, frequent drinks, sugarless gum to relieve dry mouth

Evaluate:
• Parkinsonism, extrapyramidal symptoms: shuffling gait, muscle rigidity, involuntary movements
• Urinary hesitancy, retention, palpate bladder if retention occurs

---

* Available in Canada only

- Constipation; increase fluids, bulk, exercise if this occurs
- For tolerance over long-term therapy; dose may need to be increased or changed
- Mental status: affect, mood, CNS depression, worsening of mental symptoms during early therapy

Teach patient/family:
- Not to discontinue this drug abruptly; to taper off over 1 wk
- To avoid driving or other hazardous activities; drowsiness may occur
- To avoid OTC medication: cough, cold preparations with alcohol, antihistamines unless directed by physician

---

scopolamine hydrobromide (optic)

(skoe-pol′a-meen)
Isopto-Hyoscine

Func. class.: Mydriatic
Chem. class.: Synthetic alkaloid

Action: Blocks response of iris sphincter muscle, muscle of accommodation of ciliary body to cholinergic stimulation, resulting in dilation, paralysis of accommodation

Uses: Uveitis, iritis

Dosage and routes:
- *Adult:* INSTILL 1-2 gtts before refraction or 1-2 gtts qd-tid for iritis or uveitis
- *Child:* INSTILL 1 gtt bid × 2 days before refraction

Available forms include: Sol 0.25%

Side effects/adverse reactions:
CV: Tachycardia
CNS: Confusion, somnolence, flushing, fever
EENT: Blurred vision, photopho-

bia, increased intraocular pressure, irritation, edema

Contraindications: Hypersensitivity, children <6 yr, narrow-angle glaucoma, increased intraocular pressure, infants

Precautions: Children, elderly, hypertension, hyperthyroidism, diabetes, pregnancy (C)

Pharmacokinetics:
INSTILL: Peak 20-30 min, duration 3-7 days

NURSING CONSIDERATIONS
Evaluate:
- Therapeutic response: decrease in inflammation, cycloplegic refraction
- Eye pain, discontinue use

Teach patient/family:
- To report change in vision, blurring or loss of sight, trouble breathing, inhibition of sweating, flushing
- Method of instillation: pressure on lacrimal sac for 1 min, do not touch dropper to eye
- That blurred vision will decrease with repeated use of drug
- Not to engage in hazardous activities until able to see
- Wait 5 min to use other drops
- Do not blink more than usual

---

secobarbital/secobarbital sodium

(see-koe-bar′bi-tal)
Seconal/Secogen Sodium,* Seconal Sodium, Seral*

Func. class.: Sedative/hypnotic-barbiturate
Chem. class.: Barbitone (short acting)

Controlled Substance Schedule II (USA), Schedule G (Canada)

Action: Depresses activity in brain cells primarily in reticular activating system in brainstem; selectively depresses neurons in posterior hypothalamus, limbic structures; able to decrease seizure activity by inhibition of epileptic activity in CNS

Uses: Insomnia, sedation, preoperative medication, status epilepticus, acute tetanus convulsions

Dosage and routes:

Insomnia
• *Adult:* PO/IM 100-200 mg hs
• *Child:* IM 3-5 mg/kg, not to exceed 100 mg, not to inject >5 ml in one site; REC 4-5 mg/kg

Sedation/preoperatively
• *Adult:* PO 200-300 mg 1-2 hr preoperatively
• *Child:* PO 50-100 mg 1-2 hr preoperatively; REC 4-5 mg/kg 1-2 hr preoperatively

Status epilepticus
• *Adult and child:* IM/IV 250-350 mg

Acute psychotic agitation
• *Adult and child:* IM/IV 5.5 mg/kg q3-4h

Available forms include: Caps 50, 100 mg; tabs 100 mg, inj IM, IV 50 mg/ml; powder, rec supp 200 mg

Side effects/adverse reactions:

CNS: Lethargy, drowsiness, hangover, dizziness, paradoxical stimulation in the elderly and children, lightheadedness, dependence, CNS depression, mental depression, slurred speech

GI: Nausea, vomiting, diarrhea, constipation

INTEG: Rash, urticaria, pain, abscesses at injection site, angioedema, thrombophlebitis, *Stevens-Johnson syndrome*

CV: Hypotension, bradycardia

RESP: Depression, *apnea, laryngospasm, bronchospasm*

HEMA: Agranulocytosis, thrombocytopenia, megaloblastic anemia (long-term treatment)

Contraindications: Hypersensitivity to barbiturates, respiratory depression, addiction to barbiturates, severe liver impairment, porphyria, uncontrolled severe pain

Precautions: Anemia, pregnancy (D), lactation, hepatic disease, renal disease, hypertension, elderly, acute/chronic pain

Pharmacokinetics:

IM: Onset 10-15 min, duration 4-6 hr

REC: Onset slow, duration 3-6 hr Metabolized by liver, excreted by kidneys (metabolites); half-life 15-40 hr

Interactions/incompatibilities:
• Do not mix with other drugs in solution or syringe
• Increased CNS depression: alcohol, MAOIs, sedative, narcotics
• Decreased effect of: oral anticoagulants, corticosteroids, griseofulvin, quinidine
• Decreased half-life of doxycycline

NURSING CONSIDERATIONS

Assess:
• VS q30 min after parenteral route for 2 hr
• Blood studies: Hct, Hgb, RBCs, serum folate, vitamin D (if on long-term therapy); pro-time in patients receiving anticoagulants
• Hepatic studies: AST, ALT, bilirubin; if increased, the drug is usually discontinued

Administer:
• After removal of cigarettes, to prevent fires
• IM injection in deep large muscle mass to prevent tissue sloughing and abscesses
• After conservative measures have been tried for insomnia

---

*Available in Canada only

- Within 30 min of mixing with sterile water for injection, reconstitute after rotating ampule, do not shake, do not use cloudy solution, may be given directly, or indirectly
- IV only with resuscitative equipment available, administer at <100 mg/min (only by qualified personnel)
- ½-1hr before hs for sleeplessness
- On empty stomach for best absorption
- For <14 days since drug is not effective after that; tolerance develops
- Crushed or whole
- Alone, do not mix with other drugs or inject if there is precipitate
- After cleansing enema if given rectally preoperatively in children

Perform/provide:
- Assistance with ambulation after receiving dose
- Safety measure: siderails, nightlight, callbell within easy reach
- Checking to see PO medication has been swallowed
- Storage of suppositories in refrigerator; do not use aqueous solutions containing precipitate

Evaluate:
- Therapeutic response: ability to sleep at night, decreased amount of early morning awakening if taking drug for insomnia, or decrease in number, severity of seizures if taking drug for seizure disorder
- Unresolved pain, as drug may cause severe stimulation if pain is present
- Mental status: mood, sensorium, affect, memory (long, short)
- Physical dependency: more frequent requests for medication, shakes, anxiety
- Barbiturate toxicity: hypotension; pulmonary constriction; cold, clammy skin; cyanosis of lips; insomnia; nausea; vomiting; hallucinations; delirium; weakness; mild symptoms may occur in 8-12 hr without drug
- Respiratory dysfunction: respiratory depression, character, rate, rhythm; hold drug if respirations <10/min or if pupils dilated
- Blood dyscrasias: fever, sore throat, bruising, rash, jaundice, epistaxis
- Perianal irritation if rectal forms used

Teach patient/family:
- That morning hangover is common
- That drug is indicated only for short-term treatment of insomnia and is probably ineffective after 2 wk
- That physical dependency may result when used for extended periods of time (45-90 days depending on dose)
- To avoid driving or other activities requiring alertness
- To avoid alcohol ingestion or CNS depressants; serious CNS depression may result
- Not to discontinue medication quickly after long-term use; drug should be tapered over 1-2 wk
- To tell all prescribers that barbiturate is being taken
- That withdrawal insomnia may occur after short-term use; do not start using drug again, insomnia will improve in 1-3 nights, may experience increased dreaming
- That effects may take 2 nights for benefits to be noticed
- Alternate measures to improve sleep (reading, exercise several hours before hs, warm bath, warm milk, TV, self-hypnosis, deep breathing)

Lab test interferences:
False increase: Sulfobromophthalein

---

italics = common side effects   ***bold italic*** = life threatening reactions

Treatment of overdose: Lavage, activated charcoal, warming blanket, vital signs, hemodialysis, I&O ratio

---

selegiline HCl (L-Deprenyl)

(sel-ee-gill-ene)
Eldepryl

Func. class.: Antiparkinson agent
Chem. class.: Levorotatory acetylanic derivative of phenethylamine

Action: Increased dopaminergic activity by inhibition of MAO type B activity; not fully understood
Uses: Adjunct management of Parkinson's disease in patients being treated with levodopa/carbidopa who have had a poor response to therapy
Dosage and routes:
• *Adult:* PO 10 mg/day in divided doses 5 mg at breakfast and lunch, after 2-3 days begin to reduce the dose of levodopa/carbidopa 10%-30%
Available forms: Tabs 5 mg
Side effects/adverse reactions:
CNS: Increased tremors, chorea, restlessness, blepharospasm, increased bradykinesia, grimacing, tardive dyskinesia, dystonic symptoms, involuntary movements, increased apraxia, hallucinations, dizziness, mood changes, nightmares, delusions, lethargy, apathy, overstimulation, sleep disturbances, headache, migraine, numbness, muscle cramps, confusion, anxiety, tiredness, vertigo, personality change, back/leg pain
CV: Orthostatic hypotension, hypertension, dysrhythmia, palpitations, angina pectoris, hypotension, tachycardia, edema, sinus bradycardia, syncope

GI: Nausea, vomiting, constipation, weight loss, anorexia, diarrhea, heartburn, rectal bleeding, poor appetite, dysphagia
GU: Slow urination, nocturia, prostatic hypertrophy, hesitation, retention, frequency, sexual dysfunction
INTEG: Increased sweating, alopecia, hematoma, rash, photosensitivity, facial hair
RESP: Asthma, shortness of breath
EENT: Diplopia, dry mouth, blurred vision, tinnitus
Contraindications: Hypersensitivity
Precautions: Pregnancy (C), lactation, children
Pharmacokinetics:
Rapidly absorbed, peak ½-2 hr; rapidly metabolized (active metabolites: N-desmethyldeprenyl, amphetamine, methamphetamine), metabolites excreted in urine
Interactions/incompatibilities:
• Fatal interaction: opioids (especially meperidine), do not administer together
NURSING CONSIDERATIONS
Assess:
• B/P, respiration
Administer:
• Drug up until NPO before surgery
• Adjust dosage, depending on patient response
• With meals; limit protein taken with drug
• At doses <10 mg/day because of risks associated with nonselective inhibition of MAO
Perform/provide:
• Assistance with ambulation, during beginning therapy
Evaluate:
• Mental status: affect, mood behavioral changes, depression; perform suicide assessment

---

* Available in Canada only

• Therapeutic response: decrease in akathesia, increased mood
Teach patient/family:
• To change positions slowly to prevent orthostatic hypotension
• To report side effects: twitching, eye spasms; indicate overdose
• To use drug exactly as prescribed; if drug is discontinued abruptly, parkinsonian crisis may occur
• That urine, sweat may darken
Lab test interferences:
False positive: urine ketones, urine glucose
False negative: urine glucose (glucose oxidase)
False increase: uric acid, urine protein
Decrease: VMA
Treatment of overdose: IV fluids for hypotension, IV dilute pressure agent for B/P titration

---

selenium sulfide

(cee-leen'ee-um)
Exsel, Selsun, Selsen-Blue
Func. class.: Local antiseborrheic, antifungal

Action: Appears to have cytostatic effect on epidural cells and reduces corneocyte production
Uses: Dandruff, seborrhea; dermatitis of the scalp, versicolor
Dosage and routes:
• *Adult and child:* TOP wash hair with 1-2 tsp, leave on 2-3 min; rinse, repeat, use 2 applications/wk × 2 wk, then 3-4 wk or as needed
Available forms include: Shampoo lotion 1%, 2.5%
Side effects/adverse reactions:
INTEG: Oiliness of hair/scalp, alopecia, discoloration of hair
Contraindications: Hypersensitiv-

ity to sulfur preparations, inflamed skin
Precautions: Infants, pregnancy (C)
NURSING CONSIDERATIONS
Perform/provide:
• Thorough hair rinsing after use
• Storage at room temperature in tight container
Evaluate:
• Toxicity: tremors, perspiration, pain in abdomen, weakness, anorexia
• Area of body involved, including time involved, what helps or aggravates condition
Teach patient/family:
• To avoid contact with eyes, genital area
• To discontinue use if rash or irritation occurs
• That drug may damage jewelry, remove before application
• That drug is not be taken internally

---

senna

(sin'na)
Black Draught, Casafru, Senexan, Senokot, X-Prep
Func. class.: Laxative
Chem. class.: Anthraquinone

Action: Stimulates peristalsis by action on Auerbach's plexis
Uses: Constipation, bowel preparation for surgery or examination
Dosage and routes:
• *Adult:* PO 1-8 tabs (Senokot), ½ to 4 tsps. of granules added to water or juice; REC SUPP 1-2 hs; SYR 1-4 tsps. hs, 7.5-15 ml (Black Draught); ¾ oz dissolved in 2.5 oz liquid given between 2-4 PM the day before procedure (X-Prep)
• *Child >27 kg:* ½ adult dose; do not use Black Draught for children

• *Child 1 mo-1 yr:* SYR 1.25-2.5 ml (Senokot) hs
Available forms include: Supp 625 mg, 30 mg sennosides; powder 662 mg/g, 6, 15 mg sennosides/3g; tabs 8.6 sennosides, 180 mg
Side effects/adverse reactions:
GI: Nausea, vomiting, anorexia, cramps, diarrhea
META: Hypocalcemia, enteropathy, alkalosis, hypokalemia, *tetany*
Contraindications: Hypersensitivity, GI bleeding, obstruction, CHF, lactation, abdominal pain, nausea/ vomiting, appendicitis, acute surgical abdomen
Precautions: Pregnancy (C)
Pharmacokinetics:
PO: Onset 6-24 hr; metabolized by liver, excreted in feces
Interactions/incompatibilities:
• Do not use with antabuse
NURSING CONSIDERATIONS
Assess:
• Blood, urine electrolytes if drug is used often by patient
• I&O ratio to identify fluid loss
Administer:
• In morning or evening (oral dose)
Evaluate:
• Therapeutic response: decrease in constipation
• Cause of constipation; identify whether fluids, bulk, or exercise is missing from lifestyle
• Cramping, rectal bleeding, nausea, vomiting; if these symptoms occur, drug should be discontinued
Teach patient/family:
• That urine, feces may turn yellow-brown to red
• Not to use laxatives for long-term therapy; bowel tone will be lost
• That normal bowel movements do not always occur daily
• Not to use in presence of abdominal pain, nausea, vomiting
• To notify physician if constipation unrelieved or if symptoms of electrolyte imbalance occur: muscle cramps, pain, weakness, dizziness, excessive thirst

---

silver nitrate
Func. class.: Keratolytic

Action: Possesses antiinfective, astringent, caustic properties
Uses: Cauterization of lesions, warts, burns (low concentrations)
Dosage and routes:
• *Adult and child:* TOP Apply to area to be treated
Available forms include: Sticks, sol 10%, 25%, 50%
Side effects/adverse reactions:
INTEG: Skin discoloration
Contraindications: Hypersensitivity
Interactions/incompatibilities:
• Not to be used with alkalis, phosphates, thimerosol, benzalkonium chloride, halogenated acids
NURSING CONSIDERATIONS
Administer:
• After moistening stick with water
• To burns using a wet dressing (low concentrations 0.125%)
Evaluate:
• Therapeutic response: absence of lesions, healing of burned areas
Perform/provide:
• Storage in cool area
Teach patient/family:
• To avoid contact with clothing or unaffected areas, discoloration may occur

---

silver nitrate 1% (ophthalmic)
Func. class.: Antiinfective

Action: Inhibits metabolic actions in susceptible organisms

Uses: Prevention, treatment of gonorrheal ophthalmia neonatorum
Dosage and routes:
• *Neonate:* INSTILL 2 gtts of 1% solution into each eye
Available forms include: Sol
Side effects/adverse reactions:
EENT: Redness, discharge, edema, swelling
Contraindications: Hypersensitivity
Precautions: Antibiotic hypersensitivity, pregnancy (C)
NURSING CONSIDERATIONS
Administer:
• After washing hands
Perform/provide:
• Storage at room temperature, in tight, light-resistant container
Evaluate:
• Allergy: itching, lacrimation, redness, swelling

---

silver protein, mild

Argyrol S.S., Silvol, Solargentum
Func. class.: Disinfectant
Chem. class.: Silver colloidal compound

Action: Destroys gram-positive, gram-negative organisms
Uses: Eye, nose, throat, swelling, infection
Dosage and routes:
• *Adult and child:* TOP, SOL Use as needed
Available forms include: Top sol 5%, 10%, 25%; eyedrops 20%
Side effects/adverse reactions:
INTEG: Irritation, discoloration of tissue
Contraindications: Hypersensitivity
Precautions: Pregnancy (C)
NURSING CONSIDERATIONS
Administer:
• To area to be treated only; do not apply to healthy skin

Perform/provide:
• Storage in tight container
Evaluate:
• Area of body involved: irritation, rash, breaks, dryness, scales

---

silver sulfadiazine (topical)

(sul-fa-dye'a-zeen)
Flamazine, Flint SSD, Silvadene
Func. class.: Local antiinfective
Chem. class.: Sulfonamide

Action: Interferes with bacterial cell wall synthesis
Uses: Burns (2nd, 3rd degree); prevention of wound sepsis
Dosage and routes:
• *Adult and child:* TOP apply 1/16 in to affected area qd-bid
Available forms include: Cream 10 mg/g
Side effects/adverse reactions:
INTEG: Rash, urticaria, stinging, burning, itching, pain
HEMA: Reversible leukopenia
Contraindications: Hypersensitivity, child <2 mo
Precautions: Impaired renal function, pregnancy (C), impaired hepatic function, lactation
NURSING CONSIDERATIONS
Administer:
• Using aseptic technique
• Enough medication to completely cover burns, keep covered with medication at all times
• After cleansing debris before each application
• Analgesic before application if needed
Perform/provide:
• Storage at room temperature in dry place
Evaluate:
• Allergic reaction: burning, stinging, swelling, redness

S

---

italics = common side effects   ***bold italic*** = life threatening reactions

• Therapeutic response: development of granulation tissue
• Renal function studies, check for crystalluria
Teach patient/family:
• That drug may be continued until graft can be done

---

simethicone

(si-meth'-i-kone)
Gas-X, Mylicon, Ovol,* Phazyme, Silain
Func. class.: Antiflatulent

Action: Disperses, prevents gas pockets in GI system
Uses: Flatulence
Dosage and routes:
• *Adult and child >12 yr:* PO 40-100 mg pc, hs
Available forms include: Chew tabs 40, 80 mg; tabs 50, 60, 95, 125 mg; drops 40 mg/0.6 ml
Side effects/adverse reactions:
GI: Belching, rectal flatus
Contraindications: Hypersensitivity
Precautions: Pregnancy (C)
NURSING CONSIDERATIONS
Evaluate:
• Therapeutic response: absence of flatulence
Teach patient/family:
• That tablets must be chewed
• Shake suspension well before pouring

---

sodium bicarbonate

Func. class.: Alkalinizer
Chem. class.: $NaHCO_3$

Action: Orally neutralizes gastric acid, which forms water, NaCl, CO_2; increases plasma bicarbonate, which buffers H^+ ion concentration; reverses acidosis

Uses: Acidosis (metabolic), cardiac arrest, alkalinization (systemic/urinary) antacid
Dosage and routes:
Acidosis
• *Adult and child:* IV INF 2-5 mEq/kg over 4-8 hr depending on CO_2, pH
Cardiac arrest
• *Adult and child:* IV BOL 1 mEq/kg, then 0.5 mEq/kg q10 min, then doses based an ABGs
• *Infant:* IV INF not to exceed 8 mEq/kg/day based on ABGs (4.2% sol)
Alkalinization
• *Adult:* PO 325 mg-2 g qid
• *Child:* PO 12-120 mg/kg/day
Antacid
• *Adult:* PO 300 mg-2 g chewed, taken with water
Available forms include: Tabs 325, 520, 650 mg; powd; inj 4%, 4.2%, 5%, 7.5%, 8.4%
Side effects/adverse reactions:
CNS: Irritability, headache, confusion, stimulation, tremors, *twitching, hyperreflexia, tetany,* weakness, *convulsions* caused by alkalosis
CV: Irregular pulse, *cardiac arrest,* water retention, edema, weight gain
GI: Flatulence, belching, distension, *paralytic ileus*
META: Alkalosis
GU: Calculi
RESP: Shallow, slow respirations, cyanosis, *apnea*
Contraindications: Hypertension, peptic ulcer, renal disease
Precautions: CHF, cirrhosis, toxemia, renal disease, pregnancy (C)
Pharmacokinetics:
PO: Onset 2 min, duration 10 min
IV: Onset 15 min, duration 1-2 hr, excreted in urine

---

*Available in Canada only

Interactions/incompatibilities:
• Increases effects: amphetamines, mecamylamine, barbiturates, salicylates, quinine, quinidine, pseudoephedrine
• Decreases effects: lithium, chlorpropamide
• Increased sodium and decreased potassium: corticosteroids
• Do not mix solution with other drugs

NURSING CONSIDERATIONS
Assess:
• Respiratory and pulse rate, rhythm, depth, notify physician of abnormalities
• Electrolytes, blood pH, PO_2, HCO_3, during treatment
• Urine pH, urinary output, during beginning treatment
• Extravasation with IV administration (tissue sloughing, ulceration, and necrosis)
• Weight daily with initial therapy
Administer:
• IV diluted in an equal amount of compatible sol
Evaluate:
• Alkalosis: irritability, confusion, twitching, hyperreflexia stimulation, slow respirations, cyanosis, irregular pulse
• Milk-alkali syndrome: confusion, headache, nausea, vomiting, anorexia, urinary stones, hypercalcemia
Teach patient/family:
• To chew antacid tablets and drink 8 oz water
• Not to take antacid with milk, or milk-alkali syndrome may result
• Not to use antacid for more than 2 weeks
Lab tests interferences:
Increase: Urinary urobilinogen
False positive: Urinary protein, blood lactate

sodium biphosphate/ sodium phosphate
Enemeez, Fleet Enema, Phospho-Soda, Saf-tip Phosphate Enema/Sal-Hepatica
Func. class.: Laxative, saline

Action: Increases water absorption in the small intestine by osmotic action
Uses: Constipation, bowel or rectal preparation for surgery, examination
Dosage and routes:
• *Adult:* PO 5-20 ml with water; POWDER 4 g dissolved in water; SOL 20-46 ml mixed with 4 oz cold water; ENEMA 2-4.5 oz
Available forms include: Powder, sol
Side effects/adverse reactions:
GI: Nausea, cramps, diarrhea
META: Electrolyte, fluid imbalances
Contraindications: Hypersensitivity, rectal fissures, abdominal pain, nausea/vomiting, appendicitis, acute surgical abdomen, ulcerated hemorrhoids, sodium-restricted diets (Sal-Hepatica, PhosphoSoda)
Precautions: Pregnancy (C)
Pharmacokinetics: Excreted in feces
NURSING CONSIDERATIONS
Assess:
• Blood, urine electrolytes if drug is used often by patient
• I&O ratio to identify fluid loss
Administer:
• Alone for better absorption; do not take within 1 hr of other drugs
Evaluate:
• Therapeutic response: decrease in constipation
• Cause of constipation; identify whether fluids, bulk, or exercise is missing from lifestyle

italics = common side effects   ***bold italic*** = life threatening reactions

• Cramping, rectal bleeding, nausea, vomiting; if these symptoms occur, drug should be discontinued
Teach patient/family:
• Not to use laxatives for long-term therapy; bowel tone will be lost
• That normal bowel movements do not always occur daily
• Do not use in presence of abdominal pain, nausea, vomiting
• Notify physician if constipation unrelieved or if symptoms of electrolyte imbalance occur: muscle cramps, pain, weakness, dizziness, excessive thirst
• To maintain adequate fluid consumption

---

sodium chloride, hypertonic

Adsorbonac Ophthalmic Solution, Muro Ointment, Sodium Chloride Ointment

Func. class.: Miscellaneous ophthalmic agent
Chem. class.: Hyperosmolar ophthalmic

Action: Reduces corneal edema by osmosis of water through corneal epithelium which is semipermeable
Uses: Reduce corneal edema
Dosage and routes:
• *Adult:* INSTILL 1-2 gtts q3-4h or ointment hs
Available forms include: Sol 2%, 5%; oint 5%
Side effects/adverse reactions:
EENT: Stinging
Contraindications: Hypersensitivity

NURSING CONSIDERATIONS
Perform/provide:
• Storage in tight container
Teach patient/family:
• Method of instillation, including pressure on lacrimal sac for 1 min,

and not to touch dropper to eye
• That blurred vision is common with oint
• To report double vision, rapid change in vision, appearance of floating spots, acute redness of eyes

---

sodium fluoride

Fluor-A-Day,* Fluoritabs, Flura-Drops, Fluotic,* Luride Lozitabs, Karidium, Pediaflor

Func. class.: Trace elements
Chem. class.: Fluorideion

Action: Needed for hard tooth enamel, and for resistance to periodontal disease; reduces acid production by dental bacteria
Uses: Prevention of dental caries
Dosage and routes:
• *Adult and child >12 yr:* TOP 10 ml 0.2% sol qd after brushing teeth, rinse mouth for >1 min with sol
• *Child 6-12 yr:* TOP 5 ml 0.2% sol
• *Child >3 yr:* PO 1 mg qd
• *Child <3 yr:* PO 0.5 mg
Available forms include: Tabs chewable 0.25 mg; tabs 0.5, 1 mg, tab effervescent 10 mg; drops 0.125, 0.25, 0.5 mg/ml; rinse supplements 0.2 mg/ml, rinse 0.01%, 0.02%, 0.09%; gel 0.1%, 0.5%, 1.23%
Side effects/adverse reactions:
ACUTE OVERDOSE: **Black tarry stools, bloody vomit, diarrhea, decreased respiration, increased salivation, watery eyes**
CHRONIC OVERDOSE: **Hypocalcemia and tetany, respiratory arrest, sores in mouth, constipation, loss of appetite, nausea, vomiting, weight loss, discoloration of teeth** (white, black, brown)
Contraindications: Hypersensitivity, pregnancy (D)
Precautions: Child < 6 yr

Pharmacokinetics:
PO: Excreted in urine and feces, crosses placenta, breast milk
Interactions/incompatibilities:
• Avoid use with dairy products
NURSING CONSIDERATIONS
Assess:
• Use in children
Administer:
• Drops after meals with fluids or undiluted tablets, may be chewed; do not swallow whole, may be given with water or juice, avoid milk
Evaluate:
• Therapeutic response: absence of dental caries
• Nutritional status: increase fluoride content of water, decrease carbohydrate snacks, increase fish, tea, mineral water
Teach patient/family:
• To monitor children using gel or rinse, not to be swallowed
• Not to drink, eat, or rinse mouth for at least ½ hr
• Not to use during pregnancy
• To apply after brushing and flossing hs
• Store out of children's reach

---

sodium hypochlorite
Modified Dakin's Solution
Func. class.: Disinfectant

Action: Destroys microorganism
Uses: Cleansing wounds, athlete's foot
Dosage and routes:
• *Adult and child:* SOL use as needed
Available forms include: Top sol 0.5%
Side effects/adverse reactions:
INTEG: Irritation, bleeding at site
Contraindications: Hypersensitivity
Precautions: Pregnancy (C)

NURSING CONSIDERATIONS
Administer:
• New solution each time applied
• Only to skin; application to hair may result in bleaching
• To area that will not bleed, or clotting may be reduced
Evaluate:
• Area of the body involved: irritation, rash, breaks, dryness, scales

---

sodium lactate
Func. class.: Alkalinizer

Action: Removes lactate and hydrogen, which leads to alkalinization; lactate is converted to CO_2 and water
Uses: Acidosis (metabolic), alkalinization (urinary)
Dosage and routes:
Acidosis
• *Adult:* IV 1/6 molar (167 mEq lactate/L)
Alkalinization
• *Adult:* IV 30 ml of 1/6 molar sol/kg in divided doses
Available forms include: Inj IV
Side effects/adverse reactions:
CNS: Irritability, headache, confusion, stimulation, tremors, *twitching, hyperreflexia, **tetany,** weakness, **convulsions***
CV: Irregular pulse, **cardiac arrest**
GI: Flatulence, belching, distension, **paralytic ileus**
META: Alkalosis
RESP: Shallow, slow respirations, cyanosis, **apnea**
Contraindications: Hypertension, peptic ulcer
Precautions: CHF, cirrhosis, toxemia, renal disease, pregnancy (C)
Pharmacokinetics:
PO: Onset 2 min, duration 10 min
IV: Onset immediate

S

---

italics = common side effects   ***bold italic*** = life threatening reactions

Interactions/incompatibilities:
• Increased effects: amphetamines, mecamylamine, lithium, barbiturates, salicylates, quinine, quinidine, pseudoephedrine
• Do not mix solution with other drugs

NURSING CONSIDERATIONS
Assess:
• Respiratory rate, rhythm, depth, notify physician of abnormalities
• Electrolytes, blood pH, PO_2, HCO_3, during treatment
• Urine pH, urinary output, during beginning treatment

Administer:
• IV INF; dilute 5 mEq/ml added to IV solutions or TPN; run at 2-5 mEq/kg over 4-8 hr, check for extravasation

Evaluate:
• Alkalosis: irritability, confusion, twitching, hyperreflexia, stimulation, slow respirations, cyanosis, irregular pulse

Lab tests interferences:
Increase: Urinary urobilinogen
False positive: Urinary protein, blood lactate

---

sodium polystyrene sulfonate

(pol-ee-stye′-reen)
Kayexalate, SPS Suspension

Func. class.: Potassium-removing resin

Chem. class.: Cation exchange resin

Action: Removes potassium by exchanging sodium for potassium in body; occurs primarily in large intestine

Uses: Hyperkalemia in conjunction with other measures

Dosage and routes:
• *Adult:* PO 15 g qd-qid; rectal enema 30-50 g/100 ml of sorbitol warmer to body temperature q6h
• *Child:* 1 mEq of potassium exchanged/g of resin, approximate dose 1g/kg q6h

Available forms include: Susp, powd, 15 g polystyrene sulfonate, 21.5 ml sorbitol, 1.5 g (65 mEq) sodium/60 ml

Side effects/adverse reactions:
GI: Constipation, anorexia, nausea, vomiting, diarrhea (sorbitol), fecal impaction, gastric irritation
META: Hypocalcemia, hypokalemia, hypomagnesium, sodium retention

Precautions: Pregnancy (C), renal failure, CHF, severe edema, severe hypertension

Interactions/incompatibilities:
• Decreased effect of sodium polystyrene: antacids, laxatives
• Increased toxicity: cardiac glycosides

NURSING CONSIDERATIONS
Assess:
• Bowel function daily
• Hypotension: confusion, irritability, muscular pain, weakness

Administer:
• Oral dose as susp mixed with water or syrup (20-100 ml)
• Mild laxative as ordered to prevent constipation and fecal impaction
• Sorbitol as ordered to prevent constipation
• Retention enema after mixing with warm water; introduce by gravity, continue stirring, flush with 100 ml of fluid, clamp, and leave in place

Perform/provide:
• Retention of enema for at least ½-1 hr
• Irrigation of colon after enema with 1-2 qt of nonsodium solution, drain

---

• Storage of freshly prepared solution for 24 hr at room temperature
Evaluate:
• Serum potassium, calcium, magnesium, sodium, acid-base balance

---

sodium thiosalicylate

Arthrolate, Asproject, Rexolate, Tusal, Thiosal
Func. class.: Nonnarcotic analgesic
Chem. class.: Salicylate

Action: Blocks pain impulses in CNS that occur in response to inhibition of prostaglandin synthesis; antipyretic action results from inhibition of hypothalamic heat-regulating center
Uses: Mild to moderate pain (rheumatic fever, acute gout)
Dosage and routes:
Pain
• *Adult:* IM 50-100 mg qd or qod
Rheumatic fever
• *Adult:* IM 100-150 mg q4-6h for 3 days, then 100 mg bid
Arthritis
• *Adult:* IM 100 mg/day
Available forms include: Inj IM 50 mg/ml
Side effects/adverse reactions:
*HEMA: **Thrombocytopenia, agranulocytosis, leukopenia, neutropenia, hemolytic anemia,*** increased pro-time
CNS: Stimulation, drowsiness, dizziness, confusion, ***convulsions,*** headache, flushing, hallucinations, coma
GI: Nausea, vomiting, GI bleeding, diarrhea, heartburn, anorexia, **hepatitis**
INTEG: Rash, urticaria, bruising
EENT: Tinnitus, hearing loss
CV: Rapid pulse, ***pulmonary edema***

RESP: Wheezing, hyperpnea
ENDO: Hypoglycemia, hyponatremia, hypokalemia
Contraindications: Hypersensitivity to salicylates, GI bleeding, bleeding disorders, children < 3 yr, vitamin K deficiency, peptic ulcer
Precautions: Anemia, hepatic disease, renal disease, Hodgkin's disease, pregnancy (C), lactation
Pharmacokinetics:
PO: Onset 15-30 min, peak 1-2 hr, duration 4-6 hr
REC: Onset slow, duration 4-6 hr, Metabolized by liver, excreted by kidneys, crosses placenta, excreted in breast milk, half-life 1-3½ hr
Interactions/incompatibilities:
• Decreased effects of sodium thiosalicylate: antacids, steroids, urinary alkalizers
• Increased blood loss: alcohol, heparin
• Increased effects of: anticoagulants, insulin, methotrexate
• Decreased effects of: probenecid, spironolactone, sulfinpyrazone, sulfonylmides
• Toxic effects: PABA
• Decreased blood sugar levels: salicylates
NURSING CONSIDERATIONS
Assess:
• Liver function studies: ALT, AST, bilirubin, creatinine if patient is on long-term therapy
• Renal function studies: BUN, urine creatinine if patient is on long-term therapy
• Blood studies: CBC, Hct, Hgb, pro-time if patient is on long-term therapy
• I&O ratio; decreasing output may indicate renal failure (long-term therapy)
Evaluate:
• Hepatotoxicity: dark urine, clay-colored stools, yellowing of skin,

S

---

italics = common side effects   ***bold italic*** = life threatening reactions

sclera, itching, abdominal pain, fever, diarrhea if patient is on long-term therapy
• Allergic reactions: rash, urticaria; if these occur, drug may need to be discontinued
• Renal dysfunction: decreased urine output
• Ototoxicity: tinnitus, ringing, roaring in ears; audiometric testing is needed before, after long-term therapy
• Visual changes: blurring, halos, corneal, retinal damage
• Edema in feet, ankles, legs
• Prior drug history; there are many drug interactions

Teach patient/family:
• To report any symptoms of hepatotoxicity, renal toxicity, visual changes, ototoxicity, allergic reactions (long-term therapy)
• Not to exceed recommended dosage; acute poisoning may result
• To read label on other OTC drugs; many contain aspirin
• That therapeutic response takes 2 wk (arthritis)
• To avoid alcohol ingestion; GI bleeding may occur

Lab test interferences:
Increase: Coagulation studies, liver function studies, serum uric acid, amylase, CO_2, urinary protein
Decrease: Serum potassium, PBI, cholesterol
Interfere: Urine catecholamines, pregnancy test

Treatment of overdose: Lavage, activated charcoal, monitor electrolytes, VS

somatotropin (human growth hormone)

(soe-ma-toe-troe'pin)
Asellacrin, Crescormon, Humatrope*

Func. class.: Pituitary hormone
Chem. class.: Growth hormone

Action: Stimulates growth
Uses: Pituitary growth hormone deficiency (hypopituitary dwarfism)
Dosage and routes:
• *Child:* IM 2 IU 3 × /wk, less than 48 hr between doses, may give 4 IU if growth is <1 inch/6 mo
Available forms include: Inj IM, IV 2, 4, 10 IU

Side effects/adverse reactions:
GU: Hypercalciuria
INTEG: Rash, urticaria, pain, inflammation at injection site
CNS: Headache, growth of intracranial tumor
ENDO: Hyperglycemia, ketosis, hypothyroidism
SYST: Antibodies to growth hormone

Contraindications: Hypersensitivity to benzyl-alcohol, closed epiphyses, intracranial lesions
Precautions: Diabetes mellitus, hypothyroidism, pregnancy (C)
Pharmacokinetics:
Half-life 15-60 min, duration 7 days; metabolized in liver
Interactions/incompatibilities:
• Decreased growth: glucocorticosteroids
• Epiphyseal closure: androgens, thyroid hormones

NURSING CONSIDERATIONS
Assess:
• Growth hormone antibodies if patient fails to respond to therapy
• Thyroid function tests: T_3, T_4, T_7, TSH to identify hypothyroidism

---

Administer:
• IM, rotate injection site
• After reconstituting 10 IU/5 ml bacteriostatic water for injection, do not shake

Perform/provide:
• Storage in refrigerator for <1 mo if reconstituted <1 wk; do not use discolored or cloudy solutions

Evaluate:
• Allergic reaction: rash, itching, fever, nausea, wheezing
• Hypercalciuria: urinary stones, groin, flank pain, nausea, vomiting, frequency, hematuria, chills
• Growth rate of child at intervals during treatment

---

spectinomycin dihydro-chloride

(spek-ti-noe-mye′sin)
Trobicin

Func. class.: Antibiotic
Chem. class.: Aminocyclitol

Action: Inhibits bacterial synthesis by binding to 30S subunit on ribosomes

Uses: Gonorrhea

Dosage and routes:
• *Adult:* IM 2-4 g as single dose

Available forms include: Inj IM 2, 4 g

Side effects/adverse reactions:
CNS: Dizziness, chills, fever, insomnia, headache, anxiety
HEMA: Anemia
GI: Nausea, vomiting, increased BUN
GU: Decreased urine output
INTEG: Pain at injection site, urticaria, rash, pruritus, fever

Contraindications: Hypersensitivity, syphilis

Precautions: Pregnancy (B), infants, children

Pharmacokinetics:
IM: Peak 1-2 hr, duration >8 hr, half-life 1-3 hr, excreted in urine (active form)

NURSING CONSIDERATIONS
Assess:
• Gonorrhea culture after treatment
• I&O ratio; report decreased output
• Liver studies: AST, ALT, serum alk phosphatase following multiple doses
• Blood studies: Hct, Hgb, BUN if multiple diagnoses given
• Serologic test for syphilis 3 mo after treatment

Administer:
• After shaking vial
• IM in deep muscle mass
• With 20-gauge needle; no more than 5 ml per site

Perform/provide:
• Storage at room temperature; reconstituted solutions should be discarded after 24 hr
• Treatment of partner, report infection

Evaluate:
• Therapeutic response: negative gonorrhea culture after treatment
• Allergies before treatment, reaction of each medication

---

spironolactone

(speer′on-oh-lak′tone)
Aldactone

Func. class.: Potassium-sparing diuretic
Chem. class.: Aldosterone antagonist

Action: Competes with aldosterone at receptor sites in distal tubule, resulting in excretion of sodium chloride, water, retention of potassium, phosphate

Uses: Edema, hypertension, di-

S

---

italics = common side effects   ***bold italic*** = life threatening reactions

uretic-induced hypokalemia, primary hyperaldosteronism (diagnosis, short-term treatment, long-term treatment), nephrotic syndrome, cirrhosis of the liver with ascites

Dosage and routes:
Edema/hypertension
• *Adult:* PO 25-200 mg/qd in single or divided doses
• *Child:* PO 3.3 mg/kg/day in single or divided doses
Hypokalemia
• *Adult:* PO 25-100 mg/day; if PO, K supplements are unable to be used
Primary hyperaldosteronism diagnosis
• *Adult:* PO 400 mg/day × 4 days or 4 wk depending on test, then 100-400 mg/day maintenance
Available forms include: Tab 25, 50, 100 mg

Side effects/adverse reactions:
CNS: Headache, confusion, drowsiness, lethargy, ataxia
GI: Diarrhea, cramps, *bleeding,* gastritis, vomiting
INTEG: Rash, pruritus, urticaria
ENDO: Impotence, gynecomastia, irregular menses, amenorrhea, postmenopausal bleeding, hirsutism, deepening voice
HEMA: Decreased WBCs, platelets
ELECT: Hyperchloremic metabolic acidosis, hyperkalemia, hyponatremia

Contraindications: Hypersensitivity, anuria, severe renal disease, hyperkalemia, pregnancy (D)

Precautions: Dehydration, hepatic disease, lactation

Pharmacokinetics:
PO: Onset 24-48 hr, peak 48-72 hr; metabolized in liver, excreted in urine, crosses placenta

Interactions/incompatibilities:
• Increased action of: antihypertensives, digitalis, lithium

• Increased hyperkalemia: potassium sparing diuretics, potassium products, ACE inhibitors, salt substitutes
• Decreased effect of spironolactone: ASA

NURSING CONSIDERATIONS
Assess:
• Electrolytes: sodium chloride, potassium, BUN, serum creatinine, ABGs, CBC
• Weight, I&O daily to determine fluid loss; effect of drug may be decreased if used qd

Administer:
• In AM to avoid interference with sleep
• With food, if nausea occurs, absorption may be decreased slightly

Evaluate:
• Improvement in edema of feet, legs, sacral area daily if medication is being used in CHF
• Improvement in CVP q8h
• Signs of metabolic acidosis: drowsiness, restlessness
• Rashes, temperature elevation qd
• Confusion, especially in elderly, take safety precautions if needed
• Hydration: skin turgor, thirst, dry mucous membranes

Perform/provide:
• Protection from light

Teach patient/family:
• That drowsiness, ataxia, mental confusion may occur; observe caution in driving
• To notify physician of cramps, diarrhea, lethargy, thirst, headache, skin rash, menstrual abnormalities, deepening voice, breast enlargement

Lab test interferences:
Interfere: 17-OHCS, 17-KS, radioimmunoassay, digoxin assay

Treatment of overdose: Lavage if taken orally, monitor electrolytes,

---

administer IV fluids, monitor hydration, renal, CV status

---

stanozolol

(stan-oh'zoe'lole)
Winstrol

Func. class.: Androgenic anabolic steroid
Chem. class.: Halogenated testosterone derivative

Action: Increases weight by building body tissue, increases potassium, phosphorus, chloride, and nitrogen levels, increases bone development
Uses: Prevention of hereditary angioedema, aplastic anemia to increase hemoglobin
Dosage and routes:
Aplastic anemia (possibly effective)
• *Adult:* PO 2 mg tid
• *Child 6-12 yr:* PO up to 2 mg tid
• *Child <6 yr:* PO 1 mg bid
Angioedema
• *Adult:* PO 2 mg tid, then decrease q1-3 mo, down to 2 mg qd or q2 days
Available forms include: Tabs 2 mg
Side effects/adverse reactions:
INTEG: Rash, acneiform lesions, oily hair, skin, flushing, sweating, acne vulgaris, alopecia, hirsutism
CNS: Dizziness, headache, fatigue, tremors, paresthesias, flushing, sweating, anxiety, lability, insomnia
MS: Cramps, spasms
CV: Increased B/P
GU: **Hematuria,** amenorrhea, vaginitis, decreased libido, decreased breast size, clitoral hypertrophy, testicular atrophy
GI: Nausea, vomiting, constipation, weight gain, *cholestatic jaundice*
EENT: Carpal tunnel syndrome, conjunctival edema, nasal congestion
ENDO: Abnormal GTT
Contraindications: Severe renal disease, severe cardiac disease, severe hepatic disease, hypersensitivity, pregnancy (X), lactation, genital bleeding (abnormal)
Precautions: Diabetes mellitus, CV disease, MI
Pharmacokinetics:
PO: Metabolized in liver, excreted in urine, crosses placenta, excreted in breast milk
Interactions/incompatibilities:
• Increased effects of: oral antidiabetics, oxyphenbutazone
• Increased PT: anticoagulants
• Edema: ACTH, adrenal steroids
• Decreased effects of: insulin
NURSING CONSIDERATIONS
Assess:
• Weight daily, notify physician if weekly weight gain is >5 lb
• B/P q4h
• I&O ratio; be alert for decreasing urinary output, increasing edema
• Growth rate in children since growth rate may be uneven (linear/bone browth) when used for extended period
• Electrolytes: K, Na, Cl, Ca; cholesterol
• Liver function studies: ALT, AST, bilirubin
Administer:
• Titrated dose, use lowest effective dose
Perform/provide:
• Diet with increased calories and protein; decrease sodium if edema occurs
• Supportive drug of anemia
Evaluate:
• Therapeutic response: occurs in 4-6 wk in osteoporosis

---

italics = common side effects   **bold italic** = life threatening reactions

• Edema, hypertension, cardiac symptoms, jaundice
• Mental status: affect, mood, behavioral changes, aggression
• Signs of masculinization in female: increased libido, deepening of voice, breast tissue, enlarged clitoris, menstrual irregularities; male: gynecomastia, impotence, testicular atrophy
• Hypercalcemia: lethargy, polyuria, polydipsia, nausea, vomiting, constipation; drug may need to be decreased
• Hypoglycemia in diabetics, since oral anticoagulant action is decreased

Teach patient/family:
• Drug needs to be combined with complete health plan: diet, rest, exercise
• To notify physician if therapeutic response decreases
• Not to discontinue this medication abruptly
• About change in sex characteristics
• Women to report menstrual irregularities
• That 1-3 mo course is necessary for response in breast cancer
• Procedure for use of buccal tablets (requires 30-60 min to dissolve, change absorption site with each dose; do not eat, drink, chew, or smoke while tablet is in place)

Lab test interferences:
Increase: Serum cholesterol, blood glucose, urine glucose
Decrease: Serum calcium, serum potassium, T_4, T_3, thyroid ^{131}I uptake test, urine 17-OHCS

streptokinase

(strep-toe-kye'nase)
Kabikinase, Streptase
Func. class.: Thrombolytic enzyme
Chem. class.: β-Hemolytic streptococcus filtrate (purified)

Action: Activates conversion of plasminogen to plasmin (fibrinolysin): plasmin is able to break down clots (fibrin), fibrinogen, factors V, VII, occlusion of venous access lines

Uses: Deep vein thrombosis, pulmonary embolism, arterial thrombosis, arterial embolism, arteriovenous cannula occlusion, lysis of coronary artery thrombi after MI, acute evolving transmural MI

Dosage and routes:
Lysis of coronary artery thrombi
• *Adult:* CC 20,000 IU, then 2000 IU/min over 1 hr as IV INF
Arteriovenous cannula occlusion
• *Adult:* IV INF 250,000 IU/2 ml sol into occluded limb of cannula run over 1/2 hr, clamp for 2 hr, aspirate contents, flush with NaCl sol and reconnect
Thrombosis/embolism
• *Adult:* IV INF 250,000 IU over 1/2 hr, then 100,000 IU/hr for 72 hr for deep thrombosis, 100,000 IU/hr over 24-72 hr for pulmonary embolism
Acute evolving transmural MI:
• *Adult:* IV INF 1,500,000 IU diluted to a volume of 45 ml; give within 1 hr

Available forms include: Inj IV 250,000, 600,000, 750,000 IU

Side effects/adverse reactions:
*HEMA: Decreased Hct, **bleeding***
INTEG: Rash, urticaria, phlebitis at IV inf site, itching, flushing, headache

---

* Available in Canada only

CNS: Headache, fever
GI: Nausea
RESP: Altered respirations, SOB, ***bronchospasm***
MS: Low back pain
CV: Hypertension, dysrhythmias
EENT: Periorbital edema
*SYST: **GI, GU, intracranial retroperitoneal bleeding,** surface bleeding, **anaphylaxis***
Contraindications: Hypersensitivity, active bleeding, intraspinal surgery, neoplasms of the CNS, ulcerative colitis/enteritis, severe hypertension, renal disease, hepatic disease, hypocoagulation, COPD, subacute bacterial endocarditis, rheumatic valvular disease, cerebral embolism/thrombosis/hemorrhage, intraarterial diagnostic procedure or surgery (10 days), recent major surgery
Precautions: Arterial emboli from left side of heart, pregnancy (C)
Pharmacokinetics:
IV: Excreted in bile, urine, half-life <20 min
Interactions/incompatibilities:
• Bleeding potential: aspirin, indomethacin, phenylbutazone, anticoagulants

NURSING CONSIDERATIONS
Assess:
• VS, B/P, pulse, resp, neuro signs, temp at least q4h, temp >104° F or indicators of internal bleed, cardiac rhythm following intracoronary administration
• For neurologic changes that may indicate intracranial bleeding
• Retroperitoneal bleeding: back pain, leg weakness, diminished pulses
Administer:
• As soon as thrombi identified; not useful for thrombi over 1 wk old
• Cryoprecipatate or fresh, frozen plasma if bleeding occurs

• Loading dose at beginning of therapy may require increase loading doses
• Heparin after fibrinogen level is over 100 mg/dl. Heparin infusion to increase PTT to 1.5-2 × baseline for 3-7 days
• After reconstituting with 5 ml of NS or D$_5$W; do not shake, further dilute to total volume of 45 ml; may be diluted to 500 ml in 45 ml increments; may dilute vial in 15 ml NS, further dilute 750,000 IU/50 ml NS or D$_5$W; further dilute 1,500,000 IU dose/100 ml or more
• About 10% patients have high streptococcal antibody titres requiring increased loading doses
• IV therapy using 0.8 μm filter
Perform/provide:
• Bed rest during entire course of treatment
• Avoidance of venous or arterial puncture, inj, rectal temp
• Treatment of fever with acetaminophen or aspirin
• Pressure for 30 sec to minor bleeding sites; inform physician if this does not attain hemostasis; apply pressure dressing
Evaluate:
• Allergy: fever, rash, itching, chills; mild reaction may be treated with antihistamines
• For bleeding during 1st hr of treatment: hematuria, hematemesis, bleeding from mucous membranes, epistaxis, ecchymosis
• Blood studies (Hct, platelets, PTT, PT, TT, APTT) before starting therapy; PT or APTT must be less than ×2 control before starting therapy TT ot PT q3-4h during treatment
Lab test interferences:
Increase: PT, APTT, TT

S

---

italics = common side effects   ***bold italic*** = life threatening reactions

streptomycin sulfate

(strep-toe-mye'sin)

Func. class.: Antibiotic
Chem. class.: Aminoglycoside

Action: Interferes with protein synthesis in bacterial cell by binding to ribosomal subunit, causing inaccurate peptide sequence to form in protein chain, causing bacterial death

Uses: Sensitive strains of *M. tuberculosis,* nontuberculous infections caused by sensitive strains of *Y. pestus, Brucella, H. influenzae, K. pneumoniae, E. coli, E. aerogenes, S. viridans, F. tularensis*

Dosage and routes:

Tuberculosis

• *Adult:* IM 1g qd × 2-3 mo, then 1 g 2-3 times/week given with other antitubercular drugs

• *Child:* IM 20-40 mg/kg/day in divided doses given with other antitubercular drugs

Streptococcal endocarditis

• *Adult:* IM 1 g q12h × 1 wk with penicillin, then 500 mg bid for 1 wk

Enterococcal endocarditis

• *Adult:* IM 1 g q12h × 2 wk, then 500 mg q12h × 4 wk with penicillin

Available forms include: Inj IM 1, 5 g

Side effects/adverse reactions:

GU: Oliguria, hematuria, renal damage, azotemia, renal failure, nephrotoxicity

CNS: Confusion, depression, numbness, tremors, *convulsions,* muscle twitching, *neurotoxicity*

EENT: Ototoxicity, deafness, visual disturbances

HEMA: Agranulocytosis, thrombocytopenia, leukopenia, eosinophilia, anemia

GI: Nausea, vomiting, anorexia, increased ALT, AST, bilirubin, hepatomegaly, *hepatic necrosis,* splenomegaly

CV: Hypotension, myocarditis

INTEG: Rash, burning urticaria, photosensitivity, dermatitis

Contraindications: Severe renal disease, hypersensitivity

Precautions: Neonates, mild renal disease, pregnancy (B), myasthenia gravis, lactation, hearing deficits, elderly

Pharmacokinetics:

IM: Onset rapid, peak 1-2 hr; plasma half-life 5-6 hr, not metabolized, excreted unchanged in urine, crosses placental barrier

Interactions/incompatibilities:

• Increased ototoxicity, neurotoxicity, nephrotoxicity: other aminoglycosides, amphotericin B, polymyxin, vancomycin, ethacrynic acid, furosemide, mannitol, methoxyflurane, cisplatin, cephalosporins

• Decreased effects of: parenteral penicillins

• Do not mix in solution or syringe: carbenicillin, ticarcillin, amphotericin B, cephalothin, erythromycin, heparin

• Increased effects: nondepolarizing muscle relaxants

NURSING CONSIDERATIONS

Assess:

• Weight before treatment; calculation of dosage is usually done based on ideal body weight, but may be calculated on actual body weight

• I&O ratio, urinalysis daily for proteinuria, cells, casts; report sudden change in urine output

• Serum peak 60 min after IM injection, trough level drawn just before next dose; blood level should be 2-4 times bacteriostatic level

• Urine pH if drug is used for UTI; urine should be kept alkaline

Administer:

• IM injection in large muscle mass, rotate injection sites

• Drug in evenly spaced doses to maintain blood level

Perform/provide:

• Adequate fluids of 2-3 L/day unless contraindicated to prevent irritation of tubules

• Supervised ambulation, other safety measures with vestibular dysfunction

Evaluate:

• Therapeutic effect: absence of fever, draining wounds, negative C&S after treatment

• Renal impairment by securing urine for CrCl testing, BUN, serum creatinine; lower dosage should be given in renal impairment (CrCl <80 ml/min)

• Deafness by audiometric testing, ringing, roaring in ears, vertigo; assess hearing before, during, after treatment

• Dehydration: high sp gr, decrease in skin turgor, dry mucous membranes, dark urine

• Overgrowth of infection: increased temperature, malaise, redness, pain, swelling, perineal itching, diarrhea, stomatitis, change in cough, sputum

• C&S before starting treatment to identify infecting organism

• Vestibular dysfunction: nausea, vomiting, dizziness, headache; drug should be discontinued if severe

• Injection sites for redness, swelling, abscesses; use warm compresses at site

Teach patient/family:

• To report headache, dizziness, symptoms of overgrowth of infection, renal impairment

• To report loss of hearing, ringing, roaring in ears, fullness in head

Treatment of overdose: Hemodialysis, monitor serum levels of drug

---

streptozocin

(strep-toe-zoe′sin)

Zanosar

Func. class.: Antineoplastic alkylating agent

Chem. class.: Nitrosourea

Action: Alkylates DNA, RNA; inhibits enzymes that allow synthesis of amino acids in proteins; is also responsible for cross-linking DNA strands

Uses: Metastatic islet cell carcinoma of pancreas

Dosage and routes:

• *Adult:* IV 500 mg/m^2 × 5 days q6wk until desired response, alternate with 1000 mg/m^2 qwk × 2 wk, not to exceed 1500 mg/m^2 in 1 dose

Available forms include: Inj IV 1 g

Side effects/adverse reactions:

*HEMA: **Thrombocytopenia, leukopenia, pancytopenia***

CNS: Confusion, depression, lethargy

GI: Nausea, vomiting, diarrhea, weight loss, **hepatotoxicity**

*GU: **Azotemia, anuria,** hypophosphatemia, glycosuria, renal tubular acidosis, **renal toxicity***

Contraindications: Hypersensitivity

Precautions: Radiation therapy, children, lactation, pregnancy (C), hepatic disease, renal disease

Pharmacokinetics:

IV: Metabolized by liver, excreted in urine, half-life 5 min, terminal 35-40 min

S

---

italics = common side effects   ***bold italic*** = life threatening reactions

Interactions/incompatibilities:
• Increased toxicity: neurotoxic agents, other antineoplastics
• Increased action of: doxorubicin
• Decreased effect of streptozocin: phenytoin

NURSING CONSIDERATIONS
Assess:
• CBC, differential, platelet count weekly; withhold drug if WBC is <4000 or platelet count is <75,000; notify physician of results
• Renal function studies: BUN, serum uric acid, phosphate urine CrCl before, during therapy
• I&O ratio; report fall in urine output of 30 ml/hr
• Monitor temperature q4h (may indicate beginning infection)
• Liver function tests before, during therapy (bilirubin, AST, ALT, LDH) as needed or monthly

Administer:
• Antiemetic 30-60 min before giving drug to prevent vomiting
• Antibiotics for prophylaxis of infection
• IV after diluting 1 g/9.5 ml 0.9% NaCl or D₅; may be further diluted in 50-250 mg; may be given directly over 5-15 min
• Using 21-, 23-, 25-gauge needle
• Topical or systemic analgesics for pain
• Local or systemic drugs for infection

Perform/provide:
• Storage protected from light; refrigerate reconstituted solution, stable for 48 hr at room temperature
• Strict medical asepsis, protective isolation if WBC levels are low
• Special skin care
• Warm skin compresses at injection site for inflammation
• Adequate hydration that may reduce renal toxicity

Evaluate:
• Bleeding: hematuria, guaiac, bruising or petechiae, mucosa or orifices q8h
• Food preferences; list likes, dislikes
• Inflammation of mucosa, breaks in skin
• Yellowing of skin, sclera, dark urine, clay-colored stools, itchy skin, abdominal pain, fever, diarrhea
• Local irritation, pain, burning, discoloration at injection site
• Symptoms indicating severe allergic reaction: rash, urticaria, itching, flushing

Teach patient/family:
• Of protective isolation precautions
• To report signs of infection: increased temperature, sore throat, flu symptoms
• To report signs of anemia: fatigue, headache, faintness, shortness of breath, irritability
• To avoid use of razors or commercial mouthwash
• To avoid use of aspirin products or ibuprofen

---

succinylcholine chloride
(suk-sin-ill-koe'leen)
Anectine, Anectine Flo-Pack Powder, Quelicin, Brevidil 'm'* (bromide salt), Scaline*, Sucostrin*, Sux-Cert*

Func. class.: Neuromuscular blocker (depolarizing-ultra short)

Action: Inhibits transmission of nerve impulses by binding with cholinergic receptor sites, antagonizing action of acetylcholine
Uses: Facilitation of endotracheal intubation, skeletal muscle relaxa-

---

tion during orthopedic manipulations

Dosage and routes:
• *Adult:* IV 25-75 mg, then 2.5 mg/min as needed; IM 2.5 mg/kg, not to exceed 150 mg
• *Child:* IV/IM 1-2 mg/kg, not to exceed 150 mg IM
Available forms include: Inj IM, IV 20, 50, 100 mg/ml; powder for inj 100, 500 mg/vial, 1 g/vial
Side effects/adverse reactions:
CV: Bradycardia, tachycardia, increased, decreased B/P, *sinus arrest, dysrhythmias*
RESP: Prolonged apnea, bronchospasm, cyanosis, respiratory depression
EENT: Increased secretions, increased intraocular pressure
MS: Weakness, muscle pain, fasciculations, prolonged relaxation
HEMA: Myoglobulinemia
INTEG: Rash, flushing, pruritus, urticaria
Contraindications: Hypersensitivity, malignant hyperthermia, decreased plasma pseudocholinesterase
Precautions: Pregnancy (C), cardiac disease, severe burns, fractures—fasciculations may increase damage, lactation, children <2 yr, electrolyte imbalances, dehydration, neuromuscular disease, respiratory disease, collagen diseases, glaucoma, eye surgery, penetrating eye wounds, elderly or debilitated patients
Pharmacokinetics:
IV: Onset 1 min, peak 2-3 min, duration 6-10 min
IM: Onset 2-3 min
Hydrolyzed in urine (active/inactive metabolites)
Interactions/incompatibilities:
• Increased neuromuscular blockade: aminoglycosides, clindamycin, lincomycin, quinidine, local anesthetics, polymyxin antibiotics, lithium, narcotic analgesics, thiazides, enflurane, isoflurane
• Dysrhythmias: theophylline
• Do not mix with barbiturates in solution or syringe

NURSING CONSIDERATIONS
Assess:
• For electrolyte imbalances (K, Mg); may lead to increased action of this drug
• Vital signs (B/P, pulse, respirations, airway) until fully recovered; rate, depth, pattern of respirations, strength of hand grip
• I&O ratio; check for urinary retention, frequency, hesitancy
Administer:
• Using nerve stimulator by anesthesiologist to determine neuromuscular blockade
• Anticholinesterase to reverse neuromuscular blockade
• IV INF; dilute 1-2 mg/ml in compatible sol, give 0.5-10 mg/min, titrate to patient response; may be given directly over 1 min
• Deep IM, preferably high in deltoid muscle
Perform/provide:
• Storage in refrigerator, powder at room temp, close tightly
• Reassurance if communication is difficult during recovery from neuromuscular blockade, post-operative stiffness is normal, soon subsides
Evaluate:
• Therapeutic response: paralysis of jaw, eyelid, head, neck, rest of body
• Recovery: decreased paralysis of face, diaphragm, leg, arm, rest of body
• Allergic reactions: rash, fever, respiratory distress, pruritus; drug should be discontinued

S

---

italics = common side effects   ***bold italic*** = life threatening reactions

Treatment of overdose: Edrophonium or neostigmine, atropine, monitor VS; may require mechanical ventilation

---

sucralfate
(soo-kral'fate)
Carafate, Sulcrate*
Func. class.: Protectant
Chem. class.: Aluminum hydroxide/sulfated sucrose

Action: Forms a complex that adheres to ulcer site, adsorbs pepsin
Uses: Duodenal ulcer
Dosage and routes:
• *Adult:* PO 1 g qid 1 hr ac, hs
Available forms include: Tabs 1 g
Side effects/adverse reactions:
CNS: Drowsiness, dizziness
GI: Dry mouth, constipation, nausea, gastric pain, vomiting
INTEG: Urticaria, rash, pruritus
Contraindications: Hypersensitivity
Precautions: Pregnancy (B), lactation, children
Pharmacokinetics:
PO: Duration up to 5 hr
Interactions/incompatibilities:
• Decreased action of: tetracyclines, phenytoin, fat-soluble vitamins
NURSING CONSIDERATIONS
Assess:
• Gastric pH (>5 should be maintained)
Perform/provide:
• Storage at room temperature
Evaluate:
• Therapeutic response: absence of pain, or GI complaints
Teach patient/family:
• To avoid black pepper, caffeine, alcohol, harsh spices, extremes in temperature of food
• To take on empty stomach

• To take full course of therapy
• To avoid antacids within ½ hr of drug

---

sufentanil citrate
(soo-fen'ta-nil)
Sufenta
Func. class.: Narcotic analgesics
Chem. class.: Opiate, synthetic

Controlled Substance Schedule II
Action: Inhibits ascending pain pathways in CNS, increases pain threshold, alters pain perception
Uses: Primary anesthetic, adjunct to general anesthetic
Dosage and routes:
Primary anesthetic
• *Adult:* IV 8-30 µg/kg given with 100% O_2, a muscle relaxant
Adjunct
• *Adult:* IV 1-8 µg/kg given with nitrous oxide/O_2
Available forms include: Inj IV 50 µg/ml
Side effects/adverse reactions:
CNS: Drowsiness, dizziness, confusion, headache, sedation, euphoria
GI: Nausea, vomiting, anorexia, constipation, cramps
GU: Increased urinary output, dysuria, urinary retention
INTEG: Rash, urticaria, bruising, flushing, diaphoresis, pruritus
EENT: Tinnitus, blurred vision, miosis, diplopia
CV: Palpitations, bradycardia, change in B/P
RESP: Respiratory depression
Contraindications: Hypersensitivity, addiction (narcotic)
Precautions: Addictive personality, pregnancy (C), lactation, increased intracranial pressure, MI (acute), severe heart disease, re-

---

spiratory depression, hepatic disease, renal disease, child <18 yr

Pharmacokinetics:
Half-life 1-2 hr

Interactions/incompatibilities:
• Increased effects with other CNS depressants: alcohol, narcotics, sedative/hypnotics, antipsychotics, skeletal muscle relaxants

NURSING CONSIDERATIONS
Assess:
• I&O ratio; check for decreasing output (may indicate urinary retention)

Administer:
• IV undiluted over 1-2 min or give as INF
• With antiemetic if nausea, vomiting occur

Perform/provide:
• Storage in light-resistant area at room temperature
• Safety measures: siderails, night light, call bell within easy reach

Evaluate:
• Therapeutic response: maintenance of anesthesia
• CNS changes: dizziness, drowsiness, hallucinations, euphoria, LOC, pupil reaction
• Allergic reactions: rash, urticaria
• Respiratory dysfunction: respiratory depression, character, rate, rhythm; notify physician if respirations are <10/min
• Need for pain medication, physical dependence

Teach patient/family:
• To report any symptoms of CNS changes, allergic reactions

Lab test interferences:
Increase: Amylase

Treatment of overdose: Narcan 0.2-0.8 IV, O₂, IV fluids, vasopressors

sulfacetamide sodium (ophthalmic)
(sul-fa-see'ta-mide)
Bleph-10, Cetamide, Isopto Cetamide, Sodium Sulamyd, Sulf-O
Func. class.: Antibacterial

Action: Inhibits folic acid synthesis by preventing PABA use, which is necessary for bacterial growth

Uses: Conjunctivitis, superficial eye infections, corneal ulcers

Dosage and routes:
• *Adult and child:* INSTILL 1-2 gtts q2-3h; TOP apply ½-1 inch oint into conjunctival sac qid-tid and at bedtime

Available forms include: Sterile ophth sol 10%, 15%, 30%; sterile ophth oint 10%

Side effects/adverse reactions:
EENT: Burning, stinging, swelling

Contraindications: Hypersensitivity

Precautions: Antibiotic hypersensitivity, pregnancy (C)

NURSING CONSIDERATIONS
Administer:
• After washing hands, cleanse crusts or discharge from eye before application

Perform/provide:
• Storage at room temperature

Evaluate:
• Therapeutic response: absence of redness, inflammation, tearing
• Allergy: itching, lacrimation, redness, swelling

Teach patient/family:
• To use drug exactly as prescribed
• Not to use eye makeup, towels, washcloths, eye medication of others; reinfection may occur
• That drug container tip should not be touched to eye
• To report itching, increased red-

ness, burning, stinging; drug should be discontinued

• That drug may cause blurred vision when ointment is applied

---

sulfacytine
(sul-fa-sye′teen)
Renoquid

Func. class.: Antibiotic
Chem. class.: Short-acting sulfonamide

Action: Interferes with bacterial biosynthesis of proteins by competitive antagonism of PABA
Uses: Urinary tract infections
Dosage and routes:
• *Adult:* PO 500 mg, then 250 mg qid × 10 days
Available forms include: Tabs 250 mg
Side effects/adverse reactions:
SYST: Anaphylaxis
GI: Nausea, vomiting, abdominal pain, stomatitis, *hepatitis,* glossitis, pancreatitis, diarrhea, *enterocolitis*
CNS: Headache, confusion, insomnia, hallucinations, depression, vertigo, fatigue, anxiety, *convulsions,* drug fever, chills
HEMA: Leukopenia, neutropenia, thrombocytopenia, agranulocytosis, hemolytic anemia
INTEG: Rash, dermatitis, urticaria, *Stevens-Johnson syndrome,* erythema, photosensitivity
GU: Renal failure, toxic nephrosis, increased BUN, creatinine, crystalluria
CV: Allergic myocarditis
Contraindications: Hypersensitivity to sulfonamides, pregnancy at term, child <14 yr
Precautions: Pregnancy (C), lactation, impaired hepatic function, severe allergy, bronchial asthma

Pharmacokinetics:
PO: Rapidly absorbed, peak 2-3 hr; half-life 4 hr, metabolized in liver, excreted in urine (active drug), breast milk, crosses placenta, protein-binding 86%
Interactions/incompatibilities:
• Decreased effectiveness: oral contraceptives
• Increased hypoglycemic response: sulfonylurea agents
• Increased anticoagulant effects: oral anticoagulants
• Decreased renal excretion of: methotrexate
• Decreased hepatic clearance of: phenytoin
NURSING CONSIDERATIONS
Assess:
• I&O ratio; note color, character, pH of urine if drug administered for urinary tract infections; output should be 800 ml less than intake; if urine is highly acidic, alkalization may be needed
• Kidney function studies: BUN, creatinine, urinalysis if on long-term therapy
Administer:
• With full glass of water to maintain adequate hydration; increase fluids to 2000 ml/day to decrease crystallization in kidneys
• Medication after C&S; repeat C&S after full course of medication completed
• With resuscitative equipment available; severe allergic reactions may occur
Perform/provide:
• Storage in tight, light-resistant containers at room temperature
Evaluate:
• Therapeutic effectiveness: absence of pain, fever, C&S negative
• Blood dyscrasias: skin rash, fever, sore throat, bruising, bleeding, fatigue, joint pain

---

- Allergic reaction: rash, dermatitis, urticaria, pruritus, dyspnea, bronchospasm

Teach patient/family:
- To take each oral dose with full glass of water to prevent crystalluria
- To complete full course of treatment to prevent superimposed infection
- To avoid sunlight or use sunscreen to prevent burns
- To avoid OTC medications, (aspirin, vitamin C) unless directed by physician
- To use alternative contraceptive measures; decreased effectiveness of oral contraceptives may result
- To notify physician if skin rash, sore throat, fever, mouth sores, unusual bruising, bleeding occur

Lab test interferences:
False positive: Urinary glucose test (Benedict's method)

---

sulfadiazine

(sul-fa-dye′a-zeen)
Microsulfon
Func. class.: Antibiotic
Chem. class.: Sulfonamide, intermediate acting

Action: Interferes with bacterial biosynthesis of proteins by competitive antagonism of PABA

Uses: Urinary tract infections, rheumatic fever prophylaxis, adjunctive in toxoplasmosis

Dosage and routes:
Urinary tract infections
- *Adult:* PO 2-4 g, then 0.5-1 g q6h × 10 days
- *Child:* PO 75 mg/kg or 2 g/m², then 150 mg/kg/day or 4 g/m² in 4-6 divided doses

Rheumatic fever prophylaxis
- *Child >30 kg:* PO 1 g qd

- *Child <30 kg:* PO 500 mg qd

Available forms include: Tabs 500 mg

Side effects/adverse reactions:
*SYST: **Anaphylaxis***
GI: Nausea, vomiting, abdominal pain, stomatitis, ***hepatitis,*** glossitis, pancreatitis, diarrhea, ***enterocolitis***
CNS: Headache, confusion, insomnia, hallucinations, depression, vertigo, fatigue, anxiety, ***convulsions,*** drug fever, chills
*HEMA: **Leukopenia, neutropenia, thrombocytopenia, agranulocytosis, hemolytic anemia***
INTEG: Rash, dermatitis, urticaria, ***Stevens-Johnson syndrome,*** erythema, photosensitivity
*GU: **Renal failure, toxic nephrosis,*** increased BUN, creatinine, crystalluria
*CV: **Allergic myocarditis***

Contraindications: Hypersensitivity to sulfonamides, pregnancy at term

Precautions: Pregnancy (C), lactation, impaired hepatic function, severe allergy, bronchial asthma

Pharmacokinetics:
PO: Rapidly absorbed, onset ½ hr, peak 3-6 hr, 30%-50% bound to plasma proteins, half-life 8-10 hr, excreted in urine, breast milk, crosses placenta

Interactions/incompatibilities:
- Decreased absorption of: digoxin
- Decreased effectiveness: oral contraceptives
- Increased hypoglycemic response: sulfonylurea agents
- Increased anticoagulant effects: oral anticoagulants
- Decreased renal excretion of: methotrexate
- Decreased hepatic clearance of: phenytoin

---

italics = common side effects   **bold italic** = life threatening reactions

NURSING CONSIDERATIONS
Assess:
• I&O ratio; note color, character, pH of urine if drug administered for urinary tract infections; output should be 800 ml less than intake; if urine is highly acidic, alkalization may be needed
• Kidney function studies: BUN, creatinine, urinalysis if on long-term therapy
Administer:
• With full glass of water to maintain adequate hydration; increase fluids to 2000 ml/day to decrease crystallization in kidneys
• Medication after C&S; repeat C&S after full course of medication completed
• With resuscitative equipment available; severe allergic reactions may occur
Perform/provide:
• Storage in tight, light-resistant containers at room temperature
Evaluate:
• Therapeutic effectiveness: absence of pain, fever, C&S negative
• Blood dyscrasias: skin rash, fever, sore throat, bruising, bleeding, fatigue, joint pain
• Allergic reaction: rash, dermatitis, urticaria, pruritus, dyspnea, bronchospasm
Teach patient/family:
• To take each oral dose with full glass of water to prevent crystalluria
• To complete full course of treatment to prevent superimposed infection
• To avoid sunlight or use sunscreen to prevent burns
• To avoid OTC medication (aspirin, vitamin C) unless directed by physician
• To use alternative contraceptive measures; decreased effectiveness of oral contraceptives may result
• To notify physician if skin rash, sore throat, fever, mouth scores, unusual bruising, bleeding occur
Lab test interferences:
False positive: Urinary glucose test (Benedict's method)

---

sulfamethizole
(sul-fa-meth′i-zole)
Bursul, Microsul, Proklar, Sulfasol, Sulfurine, Thiosulfil, Utrasul
Func. class.: Antibiotic
Chem. class.: Sulfonamide, short acting

Action: Interferes with bacterial biosynthesis of proteins by competitive antagonism of PABA
Uses: Urinary tract infections
Dosage and routes:
• *Adult:* PO 0.5-1 g tid-qid
• *Child* >2 mo: PO 30-45 mg/kg/day in divided doses q6h
Available forms include: Tabs 250, 500 mg
Side effects/adverse reactions:
*SYST: **Anaphylaxis***
GI: Nausea, vomiting, abdominal pain, stomatitis, ***hepatitis,*** glossitis, pancreatitis, diarrhea, ***enterocolitis***
CNS: Headache, confusion, insomnia, hallucinations, depression, vertigo, fatigue, anxiety, ***convulsions,*** drug fever, chills
*HEMA: **Leukopenia, neutropenia, thrombocytopenia, agranulocytosis, hemolytic anemia***
INTEG: Rash, dermatitis, urticaria, ***Stevens-Johnson syndrome,*** erythema, photosensitivity
*GU: **Renal failure, toxic nephrosis,*** increased BUN, creatinine, crystalluria
*CV: **Allergic myocarditis***
Contraindications: Hypersensitiv-

ity to sulfonamides, pregnancy at term

Precautions: Pregnancy (C), lactation, impaired hepatic function, severe allergy, bronchial asthma

Pharmacokinetics:

PO: Rapidly absorbed, peak 2 hr, 90% bound to plasma proteins, excreted in urine, breast milk, crosses placenta

Interactions/incompatibilities:
• Decreased absorption of: digoxin
• Decreased effectiveness: oral contraceptives
• Increased hypoglycemic response: sulfonylurea agents
• Increased anticoagulant effects: oral anticoagulants
• Decreased renal excretion of: methotrexate
• Decreased hepatic clearance of: phenytoin

NURSING CONSIDERATIONS
Assess:
• I&O ratio; note color, character, pH of urine if drug administered for urinary tract infections; output should be 800 ml less than intake; if urine is highly acidic, alkalization may be needed
• Kidney function studies: BUN, creatinine, urinalysis if on long-term therapy

Administer:
• With full glass of water to maintain adequate hydration; increase fluids to 2000 ml/day to decrease crystallization in kidneys
• Medication after C&S; repeat C&S after full course of medication completed
• With resuscitative equipment available; severe allergic reactions may occur

Perform/provide:
• Storage in tight, light-resistant containers at room temperature

Evaluate:
• Therapeutic effectiveness: absence of pain, fever, C&S negative
• Blood dyscrasias: skin rash, fever, sore throat, bruising, bleeding, fatigue, joint pain
• Allergic reaction: rash, dermatitis, urticaria, pruritus, dyspnea, bronchospasm

Teach patient/family:
• To take each oral dose with full glass of water to prevent crystalluria
• To complete full course of treatment to prevent superimposed infection
• To avoid sunlight or use sunscreen to prevent burns
• To avoid OTC medication (aspirin, vitamin C) unless directed by physician
• To use alternative contraceptive measures; decreased effectiveness of oral contraceptives may result
• To notify physician if skin rash, sore throat, fever, mouth sores, unusual bruising, bleeding occur

Lab test interferences:
False positive: Urinary glucose test (Benedict's method)

sulfamethoxazole

(sul-fa-meth-ox'a-zole)
Gamazole, Gantanol, Urobak

Func. class.: Antibiotic
Chem. class.: Sulfonamide, intermediate acting

Action: Interferes with bacterial biosynthesis of proteins by competitive antagonism of PABA

Uses: Urinary tract infections, lymphogranuloma venereum, systemic infections

Dosage and routes:
• *Adult:* PO 2 g, then 1 g bid or tid for 7-10 days

- Child >2 mo: PO 50-60 mg/kg then 25-30 mg/kg bid, not to exceed 75 mg/kg/day

Lymphogranuloma venereum

- Adult: PO 1 g bid × 14 days

Available forms include: Tabs 500 mg, 1 g; oral susp 500 mg/5ml

Side effects/adverse reactions:

SYST: Anaphylaxis

GI: Nausea, vomiting, abdominal pain, stomatitis, *hepatitis,* glossitis, pancreatitis, diarrhea, *enterocolitis*

CNS: Headache, confusion, insomnia, hallucinations, depression, vertigo, fatigue, anxiety, convulsions, drug fever, chills

HEMA: Leukopenia, neutropenia, thrombocytopenia, agranulocytosis, hemolytic anemia

INTEG: Rash, dermatitis, urticaria, *Stevens-Johnson syndrome,* erythema, photosensitivity

GU: Renal failure, toxic nephrosis, increased BUN, creatinine, crystalluria

CV: Allergic myocarditis

Contraindications: Hypersensitivity to sulfonamides, pregnancy at term

Precautions: Pregnancy (C), lactation, impaired hepatic function, severe allergy, bronchial asthma

Pharmacokinetics:

PO: Poorly absorbed, peak 3-4 hr, 50%-70% bound to plasma proteins, half-life 7-12 hr, excreted in urine (unchanged 90%), breast milk, crosses placenta

Interactions/incompatibilities:

- Decreased absorption of: digoxin
- Decreased effectiveness: oral contraceptives
- Increased toxicity: phenothiazines, probenecid
- Increased hypoglycemic response: sulfonylurea agents

- Increased anticoagulant effects: oral anticoagulants
- Decreased renal excretion of: methotrexate
- Decreased hepatic clearance of: phenytoin

NURSING CONSIDERATIONS
Assess:

- I&O ratio; note color, character, pH of urine if drug administered for urinary tract infections; output should be 800 ml less than intake; if urine is highly acidic, alkalization may be needed
- Kidney function studies: BUN, creatinine, urinalysis if on long-term therapy

Administer:

- With full glass of water to maintain adequate hydration; increase fluids to 2000 ml/day to decrease crystallization in kidneys
- Medication after C&S; repeat C&S after full course of medication completed
- With resuscitative equipment available; severe allergic reactions may occur

Perform/provide:

- Storage in tight, light-resistant containers at room temperature

Evaluate:

- Therapeutic effectiveness: absence of pain, fever, C&S negative
- Blood dyscrasias: skin rash, fever, sore throat, bruising, bleeding, fatigue, joint pain
- Allergic reaction: rash, dermatitis, urticaria, pruritus, dyspnea, bronchospasm

Teach patient/family:

- To take each oral dose with full glass of water to prevent crystalluria
- To complete full course of treatment to prevent superimposed infection

- To avoid sunlight or use sunscreen to prevent burns
- To avoid OTC medication (aspirin, vitamin C) unless directed by physician
- To use alternative contraceptive measures; decreased effectiveness of oral contraceptives may result
- To notify physician if skin rash, sore throat, fever, mouth sores, unusual bruising, bleeding occur

Lab test interferences:
False positive: Urinary glucose test (Benedict's method)

---

sulfapyridine

(sul-fa-peer'i-deen)
Dagenan*
Func. class.: Antibiotic
Chem. class.: Sulfonamide, intermediate acting

Action: Interferes with bacterial biosynthesis of proteins by competitive antagonism of PABA
Uses: Dermatitis herpetiformis
Dosage and routes:
- *Adult:* PO 500 mg qid until lesions are improved, then decrease dose by 500 mg/day q3 days until maintenance dose is achieved
Available forms include: Tabs 500 mg

Side effects/adverse reactions:
SYST: Anaphylaxis
GI: Nausea, vomiting, abdominal pain, stomatitis, ***hepatitis,*** glossitis, pancreatitis, diarrhea, ***enterocolitis***
CNS: Headache, confusion, insomnia, hallucinations, depression, vertigo, fatigue, anxiety, ***convulsions,*** drug fever, chills
*HEMA: **Leukopenia, neutropenia, thrombocytopenia, agranulocytosis, hemolytic anemia***
INTEG: Rash, dermatitis, urticaria,

Stevens-Johnson syndrome, erythema, photosensitivity
*GU: **Renal failure, toxic nephrosis,*** increased BUN, creatinine, crystalluria
*CV: **Allergic myocarditis***
Contraindications: Hypersensitivity to sulfonamides, pregnancy at term, child <14 yr
Precautions: Pregnancy (C), lactation, impaired hepatic function, severe allergy, bronchial asthma
Pharmacokinetics:
PO: Slowly absorbed, peak 5-7 hr, 10%-45% bound to plasma proteins, half-life 7-12 hr, excreted in urine, breast milk, crosses placenta
Interactions/incompatibilities:
- Decreased absorption of: digoxin
- Decreased effectiveness: oral contraceptives
- Increased toxicity: phenothiazines, probenecid
- Increased hypoglycemic response: sulfonylurea agents
- Increased anticoagulant effects: oral anticoagulants
- Decreased renal excretion of: methotrexate
- Decreased hepatic clearance of: phenytoin

NURSING CONSIDERATIONS
Assess:
- I&O ratio; note color, character, pH of urine if drug administered for urinary tract infections; output should be 800 ml less than intake; if urine is highly acidic, alkalization may be needed
- Kidney function studies: BUN, creatinine, urinalysis if on long-term therapy

Administer
- With full glass of water to maintain adequate hydration; increase

S

---

italics = common side effects   ***bold italic*** = life threatening reactions

fluids to 2000 ml/day to decrease crystallization in kidneys
• Medication after C&S; repeat C&S after full course of medication completed
• With resuscitative equipment available, severe allergic reactions may occur

Perform/provide:
• Storage in tight, light-resistant containers at room temperature

Evaluate:
• Therapeutic effectiveness: absence of pain, fever, C&S negative
• Blood dyscrasias: skin rash, fever, sore throat, bruising, bleeding, fatigue, joint pain
• Allergic reaction: rash, dermatitis, urticaria, pruritus, dyspnea, bronchospasm

Teach patient/family:
• To take each oral dose with full glass of water to prevent crystalluria
• To complete full course of treatment to prevent superimposed infection
• To avoid sunlight or use sunscreen to prevent burns
• To avoid OTC medication (aspirin, vitamin C) unless directed by physician
• To use alternative contraceptive measures; decreased effectiveness of oral contraceptives may result
• To notify physician if skin rash, sore throat, fever, mouth sores, unusual bruising, bleeding occur

Lab test interferences:
False positive: Urinary glucose test (Benedict's method)

---

sulfasalazine
(sul-fa-sal′a-zeen)
Azulfidine, SAS-500, Salazopyrin*
Func. class.: Antiinflammatory
Chem. class.: Sulfonamide

Action: Drug acts as a prodrug to deliver sulfapyridine and 5-aminosalicylic acid to colon

Uses: Ulcerative colitis

Dosage and routes:
• *Adult:* PO 3-4 g/day in divided doses; maintenance 1.5-2 g/day in divided doses q6h
• *Child >2 yrs.:* PO 40-60 mg/kg/day in 3-6 divided doses, then 30 mg/kg/day in 4 doses

Available forms include: Tabs 500 mg; oral susp 250 mg/5ml; enteric-coated tabs 500 mg

Side effects/adverse reactions:
*SYST: **Anaphylaxis***
GI: Nausea, vomiting, abdominal pain, stomatitis, ***hepatitis,*** glossitis, pancreatitis, diarrhea
CNS: Headache, confusion, insomnia, hallucinations, depression, vertigo, fatigue, anxiety, ***convulsions,*** drug fever, chills
*HEMA: **Leukopenia, neutropenia, thrombocytopenia, agranulocytosis, hemolytic anemia***
INTEG: Rash, dermatitis, urticaria, ***Stevens-Johnson syndrome,*** erythema, photosensitivity
*GU: **Renal failure, toxic nephrosis,*** increased BUN, creatinine, crystalluria
*CV: **Allergic myocarditis***

Contraindications: Hypersensitivity to sulfonamides or salicylates, pregnancy at term, child <14 yr

Precautions: Pregnancy (C), lactation, impaired hepatic function, severe allergy, bronchial asthma

Pharmacokinetics:
PO: Partially absorbed, peak 1½-6 hr, half-life 5-10 hr, excreted in urine as sulfasalazine (15%), sulfapyridine (60%), 5-aminosalicylic acid and metabolites (20%-33%), breast milk, crosses placenta

Interactions/incompatibilities:
• Decreased absorption of: digoxin, folic acid

---

*Available in Canada only

• Decreased effectiveness: oral contraceptives
• Increased hypoglycemic response: sulfonylurea agents
• Increased anticoagulant effects: oral anticoagulants
• Decreased renal excretion of: methotrexate
• Decreased hepatic clearance of: phenytoin

NURSING CONSIDERATIONS
Assess:
• I&O ratio; note color, character, pH of urine if drug administered for urinary tract infections; output should be 800 ml less than intake; if urine is highly acidic, alkalization may be needed
• Kidney function studies: BUN, creatinine, urinalysis if on long-term therapy

Administer:
• With full glass of water to maintain adequate hydration; increase fluids to 2000 ml/day to decrease crystallization in kidneys
• Medication after C&S; repeat C&S after full course of medication completed
• With resuscitative equipment available; severe allergic reactions may occur
• Total daily dose in evenly spaced doses and after meals to help minimize GI intolerance

Perform/provide:
• Storage in tight, light-resistant containers at room temperature

Evaluate:
• Therapeutic effectiveness: absence of fever, mucus in stools
• Blood dyscrasias: skin rash, fever, sore throat, bruising, bleeding, fatigue, joint pain
• Allergic reaction: rash, dermatitis, urticaria, pruritus, dyspnea, bronchospasm

Teach patient family:
• To take each oral dose with full glass of water to prevent crystalluria
• To complete full course of treatment to prevent superimposed infection
• To avoid sunlight or use sunscreen to prevent burns
• To avoid OTC medication (aspirin, vitamin C) unless directed by physician
• To use alternative contraceptive measures; decreased effectiveness of oral contraceptives may result
• To notify physician if skin rash, sore throat, fever, mouth sores, unusual bruising, bleeding occur

Lab test intereferences:
False positive: Urinary glucose test

---

sulfinpyrazone
(sul-fin-peer'a-zone)
Antazone, Anturan,* Anturane, Zynol
Func. class.: Uricosuric
Chem. class.: Pyrazolone

Action: Inhibits tubular reabsorption of urates, with increased excretion of uric acid; inhibits prostaglandin synthesis which decreases platelet aggregation
Uses: Inhibition of platelet aggregation, gout

Dosage and routes:
Inhibition of platelet aggregation
• *Adult:* PO 200 mg qid
Gout/gouty arthritis
• *Adult:* PO 100-200 mg bid for 1 wk, then 200-400 mg bid, not to exceed 800 mg/day
Available forms include: Tabs 100 mg; caps 200 mg
Side effects/adverse reactions:
CNS: Dizziness, ***convulsions, coma***
EENT: Tinnitus

S

---

italics = common side effects   ***bold italic*** = life threatening reactions

GU: Renal calculi, hypoglycemia
*GI: Gastric irritation, nausea, vomiting, anorexia, **hepatic necrosis,*** GI bleeding
INTEG: Rash, dermatitis, pruritus, fever, photosensitivity
*HEMA: **Agranulocytosis*** (rare)
*RESP: **Apnea,*** irregular respirations
Contraindications: Hypersensitivity to pyrazolone derivatives, severe hepatic disease, blood dyscrasias, severe renal disease, CrCl <50 mg/min, active peptic ulcer, GI inflammation, renal calculi
Precautions: Pregnancy (C), lactation
Pharmacokinetics:
PO: Peak 1-2 hr, duration 4-6 hr, half-life 3 hr, metabolized by liver, excreted in urine
Interactions/incompatibilities:
• Increased toxicity: sulfa drugs, dapsone, clofibrate, PAS, indomethacin, rifampin, naproxen, methotrexate, pantothenic acid, tolbutamide, warfarin
• Decreased effects of sulfinpyrazone: salicylates, xanthines

NURSING CONSIDERATIONS
Assess:
• Uric acid levels (3-7 mg/dl)
• Respiratory rate, rhythm, depth; notify physician of abnormalities
• Renal function
• Bleeding tendencies, RBC and Hct
• I & O
• Electrolytes, CO_2 before, during treatment
• Urine pH, output, glucose during beginning treatment
Administer:
• With glass of milk
• With food for GI symptoms
• Increased fluids to prevent calculi; alkalinization of urine may be required

Evaluate:
• Therapeutic response: absence of pain, stiffness in joints
Lab test interferences:
Increase: PSP, aminohippuric acid
Teach patient/family:
• To avoid aspirin, alcohol, high purine diet

---

sulfisoxazole

(sul-fi-sox′a-zole)
Barazole, Gantrisin, Novosoxazole,* Rosoxol, Soxomide, Urizole
Func. class.: Antibiotic
Chem. class.: Sulfonamide, short acting

Action: Interferes with bacterial biosynthesis of proteins by competitive antagonism of PABA
Uses: Urinary tract, systemic infections; chancroid; trachoma; toxoplasmosis; acute otitis media; lymphogranuloma venerium, eye infections
Dosage and routes:
• *Adult:* PO 2-4 g loading dose, then 1-2 g qid × 7-10 days
• *Child >2 mo:* PO 75 mg/kg or 2 g/m² loading dose then 150 mg/kg/day or 4 g/m²/day in divided doses q6h, not to exceed 6 g/day
Available forms include: Tabs 500 mg; syr, pediatric susp 500 mg/5 ml; emul 1 g/5 ml
Side effects/adverse reactions:
*SYST: **Anaphylaxis***
GI: Nausea, vomiting, abdominal pain, stomatitis, ***hepatitis,*** glossitis, pancreatitis, diarrhea, ***enterocolitis***
CNS: Headache, confusion, insomnia, hallucinations, depression, vertigo, fatigue, anxiety, ***convulsions,*** drug fever, chills
*HEMA: **Leukopenia, neutropenia,***

thrombocytopenia, agranulocytosis, hemolytic anemia
INTEG: Rash, dermatitis, urticaria, **Stevens-Johnson syndrome,** erythema, photosensitivity
GU: **Renal failure, toxic nephrosis,** increased BUN, creatinine, crystalluria
CV: **Allergic myocarditis**
Contraindications: Hypersensitivity to sulfonamides, pregnancy at term
Precautions: Pregnancy (C), lactation, impaired hepatic function, severe allergy, bronchial asthma
Pharmacokinetics:
PO: Rapidly absorbed, peak 2-4 hr, 85% protein bound; half-life 4-7 hr, excreted in urine, crosses placenta
Interactions/incompatibilities:
• Decreased absorption of: digoxin, folic acid
• Decreased effectiveness: oral contraceptives
• Increased hypoglycemic response: sulfonylurea agents
• Increased anticoagulant effect: oral anticoagulants
• Decreased renal excretion of: methotrexate
• Decreased hepatic clearance of: phenytoin
NURSING CONSIDERATIONS
Assess:
• I&O ratio; note color, character, pH of urine if drug administered for urinary tract infections; output should be 800 ml less than intake; if urine is highly acidic, alkalization may be needed
• Kidney function studies: BUN, creatinine, urinalysis if on long-term therapy
Administer:
• With full glass of water to maintain adequate hydration; increase fluids to 2000 ml/day to decrease crystallization in kidneys

• Medication after C&S; repeat C&S after full course of medication completed
• With resuscitative equipment available; severe allergic reactions may occur
Perform/provide:
• Storage in tight, light-resistant containers at room temperature
Evaluate:
• Therapeutic effectiveness: absence of pain, fever, C&S negative
• Blood dyscrasias: skin rash, fever, sore throat, bruising, bleeding, fatigue, joint pain
• Allergic reaction: rash, dermatitis, urticaria, pruritus, dyspnea, bronchospasm
Teach patient/family:
• Take each oral dose with full glass of water to prevent crystalluria
• To complete full course of treatment to prevent superimposed infection
• To avoid sunlight or use sunscreen to prevent burns; avoid hazardous activities if dizziness occurs
• To avoid OTC medication (aspirin, vitamin C) unless directed by physician
• To use alternative contraceptive measures; decreased effectiveness of oral contraceptives may result
• To notify physician if skin rash, sore throat, fever, mouth sores, unusual bruising, bleeding occur
Lab test interferences:
False positive: Urinary glucose test

---

sulindac

(sul-in'dak)
Clinoril, Novosudac*
Func. class.: Nonsteroidal antiinflammatory
Chem. class.: Indeneacetic acid derivative

Action: Inhibits prostaglandin syn-

---

italics = common side effects
bold italic = life threatening reactions

thesis by decreasing an enzyme needed for biosynthesis; possesses analgesic, antiinflammatory, antipyretic properties

Uses: Mild to moderate pain, osteoarthritis, rheumatoid, gouty arthritis

Dosage and routes:
Arthritis
• *Adult:* PO 150 mg bid, may increase to 200 mg bid
Bursitis/acute arthritis
• *Adult:* PO 200 mg bid × 1-2 wk, then reduce dose
Available forms include: Tabs 150, 200 mg

Side effects/adverse reactions:
GI: Nausea, anorexia, vomiting, diarrhea, jaundice, ***cholestatic hepatitis,*** constipation, flatulence, cramps, dry mouth, peptic ulcer
CNS: Dizziness, drowsiness, fatigue, tremors, confusion, insomnia, anxiety, depression
CV: Tachycardia, peripheral edema, palpitations, dysrhythmias
INTEG: Purpura, rash, pruritus, sweating
GU: ***Nephrotoxicity: dysuria, hematuria, oliguria, azotemia***
HEMA: ***Blood dyscrasias***
EENT: Tinnitus, hearing loss, blurred vision

Contraindications: Hypersensitivity, asthma, severe renal disease, severe hepatic disease

Precautions: Pregnancy (C), lactation, children, bleeding disorders, GI disorders, cardiac disorders, hypersensitivity to other antiinflammatory agents

Pharmacokinetics:
PO: Peak 2 hr, half-life 3-3½ hr; metabolized in liver, excreted in urine (metabolites) excreted in breast milk, 93% protein binding

Interactions/incompatibilities:
• Increased action of: coumarin, phenytoin, sulfonamides when used with this drug

NURSING CONSIDERATIONS
Assess:
• Renal, liver, blood studies: BUN, creatinine, AST, ALT, HgB, before treatment, periodically thereafter
• Audiometric, ophthalmic exam before, during, after treatment
Administer:
• With food to decrease GI symptoms; best to take on empty stomach to facilitate absorption
Perform/provide:
• Storage at room temperature
Evaluate:
• Therapeutic response: decreased pain, stiffness, swelling in joints, ability to move more easily
• For eye, ear problems: blurred vision, tinnitus (may indicate toxicity)
Teach patient/family:
• To report blurred vision or ringing, roaring in ears (may indicate toxicity)
• To avoid driving or other hazardous activities if dizziness or drowsiness occurs
• To report change in urine pattern, weight increase, edema, pain increase in joints, fever, blood in urine (indicates nephrotoxicity)
• That therapeutic effects may take up to 1 mo

---

sutilains
(soo'ti-lains)
Travase
Func. class.: Topical enzyme preparation
Chem. class.: Proteolytic enzyme concentration

Action: Digests necrotic tissue, hemoglobin, exudate that impairs adequate wound healing

Uses: Debridement in decubitus ulcers, severe burns, peripheral vascular ulcers, pyogenic wounds, ulcers secondary to peripheral vascular disease

Dosage and routes:
• *Adult and child:* TOP apply to affected area, ½-inch beyond area to be debrided, cover loosely with wet dressing, reapply tid-qid

Available forms include: Top oint 82,000 casein U/g

Side effects/adverse reactions:
CNS: Pain, paresthesias
INTEG: Bleeding, dermatitis

Contraindications: Hypersensitivity, severe wounds

Precautions: Pregnancy (C)

Pharmacokinetics:
TOP: Onset 1 hr, peak 6 hr, duration 8-12 hr

Interactions/incompatibilities:
• Decreased action: benzalkonium chloride, hexachlorophene, iodine, nitrofurazone, silver nitrate, thimerosal products, detergents

NURSING CONSIDERATIONS
Administer:
• Cover with dressing (loose, wet)
• After putting on gloves to protect healthy skin, wash after application
• After covering healthy skin with protectant such as petrolatum

Perform/provide:
• Refrigeration after use
• Wear gloves
• Thorough cleansing of wound with sterile water with 0.9% NaCl
• Thorough moistening of wound area
• Changing gloves, then applying ointment in thin layer

Evaluate:
• Therapeutic response: clean, pink wound after 5-7 days (burns) or 8-12 days (ulcers)
• Area of body involved, including time involved, what helps or aggravates condition

Teach patient/family:
• To discontinue use if rash, irritation occurs
• To avoid contact with eyes

---

talbutal
(tal'byoo-tal)
Lotusate

Func. class.: Sedative/hypnotic-barbiturate (intermediate acting)
Chem. class.: Barbitone

Controlled Substance Schedule II (USA), Schedule G (Canada)

Action: Depresses activity in brain cells primarily in reticular activating system in brainstem; selectively depresses neurons in posterior hypothalamus, limbic structures

Uses: Insomnia, short-term treatment only

Dosage and routes:
• *Adult:* PO 120 mg hs

Available forms include: Tabs 120 mg

Side effects/adverse reactions:
CNS: Lethargy, drowsiness, hangover, dizziness, paradoxical stimulation in elderly and children, lightheadedness, dependence, CNS depression, mental depression, slurred speech
GI: Nausea, vomiting, diarrhea, constipation
INTEG: Rash, urticaria, pain, abscesses at injection site, angioedema, thrombophlebitis, ***Stevens-Johnson syndrome***
CV: Hypotension, bradycardia
RESP: Depression, apnea, ***laryngospasm, bronchospasm***
*HEMA: **Agranulocytosis, thrombocytopenia, megaloblastic anemia** (long-term treatment)*

Contraindications: Hypersensitiv-

ity to barbiturates, respiratory depression, addiction to barbiturates, severe liver impairment, porphyria, pregnancy (D), uncontrolled severe pain

Precautions: Anemia, lactation, hepatic disease, renal disease, hypertension, elderly, acute/chronic pain

Pharmacokinetics:
Onset 30-45 min, duration 4-6 hr; metabolized by liver, excreted by kidneys (metabolites)

Interactions/incompatibilities:

• Increased CNS depression: alcohol, MAOIs, sedative, narcotics

• Decreased effect of: oral anticoagulants, corticosteroids, griseofulvin, quinidine

• Decreased half-life of: doxycycline

NURSING CONSIDERATIONS
Assess:

• Blood studies: Hct, Hgb, RBCs, if blood dyscrasias are suspected

• Hepatic studies: AST, ALT, bilirubin, if hepatic damage has occurred

Administer:

• After removal of cigarettes, to prevent fires

• After trying conservative measures for insomnia

• ½-1 hr before hs for sleeplessness

• On empty stomach for best absorption

• For < 14 days since drug is not effective after that, tolerance develops

• Crushed or whole

Perform/provide:

• Assistance with ambulation after receiving dose

• Safety measure: siderails, night-light, call bell within easy reach

• Checking to see PO medication has been swallowed

• Storage in tight container in cool environment

Evaluate:

• Therapeutic response: ability to sleep at night, decreased amount of early morning awakening

• Mental status: mood, sensorium, affect, memory (long, short)

• Physical dependency: more frequent requests for medication, shakes, anxiety

• Barbiturate toxicity: hypotension; pupillary constriction; cold, clammy skin; cyanosis of lips; insomnia; nausea; vomiting; hallucinations; delirium; weakness; mild symptoms may occur in 8-12 hr without drug

• Respiratory dysfunction: respiratory depression, character, rate, rhythm; hold drug if respirations are < 10/min or if pupils are dilated (rare)

• Blood dyscrasias: fever, sore throat, bruising, rash, jaundice, epistaxis (rare)

Teach patient/family:

• That morning hangover is common

• That drug is indicated only for short-term treatment of insomnia and is probably ineffective after 2 wk

• That physical dependency may result when used for extended periods of time (45-90 days depending on dose)

• To avoid driving or other activities requiring alertness

• To avoid alcohol ingestion or CNS depressants; serious CNS depression may result

• To tell all prescribers that barbiturate is being taken

• That withdrawal insomnia may occur after short-term use; do not start using drug again; insomnia

will improve in 1-3 nights; may experience increased dreaming
• That effects may take 2 nights for benefits to be noticed
• Alternate measures to improve sleep (reading, exercise several hours before hs, warm bath, warm milk, TV, self-hypnosis, deep breathing)

Lab test interferences:
False increase: Sulfobromophthalein

Treatment of overdose: Lavage, activated charcoal, warming blanket, vital signs, hemodialysis, I&O ratio

---

tamoxifen citrate

(ta-mox'i-fen)
Nolvadex, Tamofen,* Tamone*
Func. class.: Antineoplastic
Chem. class.: Hormone, antiestrogen

Action: Inhibits cell division by binding to cytoplasmic receptors (estrogen receptors); resembles normal cell complex but inhibits DNA synthesis

Uses: Advanced breast carcinoma that has not responded to other therapy in estrogen receptor positive patients (usually postmenopausal)

Dosage and routes:
• *Adult:* PO 10-20 mg bid
Available forms include: Tabs 10 mg

Side effects/adverse reactions:
*HEMA: **Thrombocytopenia, leukopenia***
GI: Nausea, vomiting, altered taste (anorexia)
GU: Vaginal bleeding, pruritus vulvae
INTEG: Rash, alopecia
CV: Chest pain

CNS: Hot flashes, headache, lightheadedness, depression
META: Hypercalcemia
EENT: Ocular lesions, retinopathy, corneal opacity, blurred vision (high doses)

Contraindications: Hypersensitivity, pregnancy (D)

Precautions: Leukopenia, thrombocytopenia, lactation, cataracts

Pharmacokinetics:
PO: Peak 4-7 hr, half-life 7 days (1 wk terminal), excreted primarily in feces

NURSING CONSIDERATIONS

Assess:
• CBC, differential, platelet count weekly; withhold drug if WBC is <4000 or platelet count is <75,000; notify physician of results

Administer:
• Antacid before oral agent; give drug after evening meal, before bedtime
• Antiemetic 30-60 min before giving drug to prevent vomiting

Perform/provide:
• Liquid diet, if needed including cola, Jello; dry toast or crackers may be added if patient is not nauseated or vomiting
• Increase fluid intake to 2-3 L/day to prevent dehydration
• Nutritious diet with iron, vitamin supplements as ordered
• Storage in light-resistant container at room temperature

Evaluate:
• Bleeding: hematuria, guaiac, bruising, petechiae, mucosa or orifices q8h
• Food preferences; list likes, dislikes
• Effects of alopecia on body image; discuss feelings about body changes
• Symptoms indicating severe al-

T

---

italics = common side effects   ***bold italic*** = life threatening reactions

lergic reactions: rash, pruritus, urticaria, purpuric skin lesions, itching, flushing

Teach patient/family:
• To report any complaints, side effects to nurse or physician
• That vaginal bleeding, pruritus, hot flashes, can occur, are reversible after discontinuing treatment
• To immediately report decreased visual acuity, which may be irreversible. Stress need for routine eye exams, who should be told about tamoxifen therapy
• To report vaginal bleeding immediately
• That tumor flare may occur: increase in size of tumor, increased bone pain and will subside rapidly May take analgesics for pain. Premenopausal women need to use mechanical birth control because ovulation may be induced
• That hair may be lost during treatment; a wig or hairpiece may make patient feel better; new hair may be different in color, texture

Lab test interferences:
Increase: Serum Ca

---

temazepam

(te-maz'e-pam)
Razepam, Restoril, Temaz
Func. class.: Sedative-hypnotic
Chem. class.: Benzodiazepine

Controlled Substance Schedule IV (USA), Schedule F (Canada)
Action: Produces CNS depression at limbic, thalamic, hypothalamic levels of the CNS; may be mediated by neurotransmitter gamma aminobutyric acid (GABA); results are sedation, hypnosis, skeletal muscle relaxation, anticonvulsant activity, anxiolytic action
Uses: Insomnia

Dosage and routes:
• *Adult:* PO 15-30 mg hs
Available forms include: Caps 15, 30 mg

Side effects/adverse reactions:
HEMA: **Leukopenia, granulocytopenia** (rare)
CNS: Lethargy, drowsiness, daytime sedation, dizziness, confusion, lightheadedness, headache, anxiety, irritability
GI: Nausea, vomiting, diarrhea, heartburn, abdominal pain, constipation, anorexia
CV: Chest pain, pulse changes

Contraindications: Hypersensitivity to benzodiazepines, pregnancy (X), lactation, intermittent porphyria
Precautions: Anemia, hepatic disease, renal disease, suicidal individuals, drug abuse, elderly, psychosis, child < 15 yr, acute narrow-angle glaucoma, seizure disorders

Pharmacokinetics:
PO: Onset 30-45 min, duration 6-8 hr, half-life 10-20 hr; metabolized by liver, excreted by kidneys, crosses placenta, excreted in breast milk

Interactions/incompatibilities:
• Increased effects of: cimetidine, disulfiram
• Increased action of both drugs: alcohol, CNS depressants
• Decreased effect of: antacids

NURSING CONSIDERATIONS
Assess:
• Blood studies: Hct, Hgb, RBCs (if on long-term therapy)
• Hepatic studies: AST, ALT, bilirubin (if on long-term therapy)
Administer:
• After removal of cigarettes, to prevent fires
• After trying conservative measures for insomnia

---

* Available in Canada only

- ½-1 hr before hs for sleeplessness
- On empty stomach fast onset, but may be taken with food if GI symptoms occur

Perform/provide:
- Assistance with ambulation after receiving dose
- Safety measure: siderails, nightlight, callbell within easy reach
- Checking to see PO medication has been swallowed
- Storage in tight container in cool environment

Evaluate:
- Therapeutic response: ability to sleep at night, decreased amount of early morning awakening if taking drug for insomnia
- Mental status: mood, sensorium, affect, memory (long, short)
- Blood dyscrasias: fever, sore throat, bruising, rash, jaundice, epistaxis (rare)
- Type of sleep problem: falling asleep, staying asleep

Teach patient/family:
- To avoid driving or other activities requiring alertness until drug is stabilized
- To avoid alcohol ingestion or CNS depressants; serious CNS depression may result
- That effects may take 2 nights for benefits to be noticed
- Alternate measures to improve sleep: reading, exercise several hours before hs, warm bath, warm milk, TV, self-hypnosis, deep breathing
- That hangover is common in elderly, but less common than with barbiturates

Lab test interferences:
Increase: ALT/AST, serum bilirubin
Decrease: RAI uptake
False increase: Urinary 17-OHCS
Treatment of overdose: Lavage, activated charcoal, monitor electrolytes, vital signs

terazosin

(ter-ay'zoe-sin)
Hytrin
Func. class.: Antihypertensive, anti-adrenergic

Action: Decreases total vascular resistance, which is responsible for a decrease in B/P; this occurs by blockade of α-1 adrenoreceptors

Uses: Hypertension as a single agent or in combination with diuretics or β-blockers

Dosage and routes:
- *Adult:* PO 1 mg hs, may increase dose slowly to desired response; not to exceed 20 mg/day

Available forms include: Tabs 1, 2, 5 mg

Side effects/adverse reactions:
CV: Palpitations, orthostatic hypotension, tachycardia, edema, rebound hypertension
CNS: Dizziness, headache, drowsiness, anxiety, depression, vertigo, weakness, fatigue
GI: Nausea, vomiting, diarrhea, constipation, abdominal pain
GU: Urinary frequency, incontinence, impotence, priapism
EENT: Blurred vision, epistaxis, tinnitus, dry mouth, red sclera, nasal congestion, sinusitis
RESP: Dyspnea

Contraindications: Hypersensitivity

Precautions: Pregnancy (C), children, lactation

Pharmacokinetics:
Peak 1 hr, half-life 9-12 hr, highly bound to plasma proteins; metabolized in liver, excreted in urine, feces

Interactions/incompatibilities:

T

---

italics = common side effects   ***bold italic*** = life threatening reactions

• Increased hypotensive effects: β-blockers, nitroglycerin, verapamil, nifedipine

NURSING CONSIDERATIONS
Assess:
• B/P
• Pulse, jugular venous distention q4h
• BUN, uric acid if on long-term therapy
• Weight daily, I&O

Perform/provide:
• Storage in tight containers in cool environment

Evaluate:
• Edema in feet, legs daily
• Skin turgor, dryness of mucous membranes for hydration status
• Rales, dyspnea, orthopnea q30 min

Teach patient/family:
• That fainting occasionally occurs after first dose; do not drive or operate machinery for 4 hr after first dose or take first dose hs
• To rise slowly from sitting/lying position

---

terbutaline sulfate
(ter-byoo´te-leen)
Brethaire, Brethine, Bricanyl
Func. class.: Selective β₂-agonist
Chem. class.: Catecholamine

Action: Relaxes bronchial smooth muscle by direct action on β₂-adrenergic receptors, through accumulation of cAMP at β-adrenergic receptor sites

Uses: Bronchospasm, premature labor

Dosage and routes:
Bronchospasm
• *Adult and child >12 yr:* INH 2 puffs q1 min apart, then q4-6h; PO 2.5-5 mg q8h; SC 0.25 mg q8h
Premature Labor

• *Adult:* IV INF: 0.01 mg/min, increased by 0.005 mg q10 min, not to exceed 0.025 mg/min; SC 0.25 mg q1h; PO 5 mg q4h × 48 hr, then 5 mg q6h as maintenance for above doses

Available forms include: Tabs 2.5, 5 mg; aerosol 0.2 mg/actuation

Side effects/adverse reactions:
CNS: Tremors, anxiety, insomnia, headache, dizziness, stimulation
CV: Palpitations, tachycardia, hypertension, *cardiac arrest*
GI: Nausea, vomiting

Contraindications: Hypersensitivity to sympathomimetics, narrow-angle glaucoma, tachydysrhythmias

Precautions: Pregnancy (B), cardiac disorders, hyperthyroidism, diabetes mellitus, prostatic hypertrophy, lactation, elderly, hypertensive, glaucoma

Pharmacokinetics:
PO: Onset ½ hr, duration 4-8 hr
SC: Onset 6-15 min, duration 1½-4 hr
INH: Onset 5-30 min, duration 3-6 hr

Interactions/incompatibilities:
• Increased effects of both drugs: other sympathomimetics
• Decreased action: β-blockers
• Hypertensive crisis: MAOIs

NURSING CONSIDERATIONS
Assess:
• Respiratory function: vital capacity, forced expiratory volume, ABGs, B/P, pulse

Administer:
• IV, run 10 μg/min; may increase 5 μg q10 min, titrate to response; after ½-1 hr taper dose by 5 μg, switch to PO as soon as possible
• 2 hr before hs to avoid sleeplessness

Perform/provide:
• Storage at room temperature, do not use discolored solutions

---

*Available in Canada only

Evaluate:
• Therapeutic response: absence of dyspnea, wheezing
• Tolerance over long-term therapy, dose may need to be increased or changed

Teach patient/family:
• Not to use OTC medications; extra stimulation may occur
• Use of inhaler; review package insert with patient
• To avoid getting aerosol in eyes
• To wash inhaler in warm water and dry qd, rinse mouth after use
• On all aspects of drug; avoid smoking, smoke-filled rooms, persons with respiratory infections
• To increase fluids >2 L/day; allow 15 min between inhalation of this drug and inhaler containing steroid

Treatment of overdose: Administer an α-blocker, then norepinephrine for severe hypotension

---

terconazole

(ter-kon′-a-zole)
Terazol 7

Func. class.: Local antiinfective
Chem. class.: Antifungal

Action: Interferes with fungal DNA replication; binds sterols in fungal cell membranes, which increases permeability, leaking of nutrients

Uses: Vaginal, vulvae, vulvovaginal candidiasis (moniliasis)

Dosage and routes:
• *Adult:* Vag 5 g (1 applicator) hs × 7 days

Available forms include: Vag cream 0.4%

Side effects/adverse reactions:
GU: Vulvovaginal burning, itching, pelvic cramps

INTEG: Rash, urticaria, stinging, burning
MISC: Headache, body pain

Contraindications: Hypersensitivity

Precautions: Children <2 yr, pregnancy, lactation

NURSING CONSIDERATIONS
Administer:
• Enough medication to completely cover lesions
• After cleansing with soap, water before each application, dry well

Perform/provide:
• Storage at room temperature in dry place

Evaluate:
• Allergic reactions: burning, stinging, swelling, redness
• Therapeutic response: decrease in size, number of lesions

Teach patient/family:
• To avoid use of OTC creams, ointments, lotions unless directed by physician
• To use medical asepsis (hand washing) before, after each application
• To avoid contact with eyes

---

terfenadine

(ter-fin′-a-deen)
Seldane

Func. class.: Antihistamine
Chem. class.: Butyrophenone derivative

Action: Acts on blood vessels, GI, respiratory system by competing with histamine for H_1-receptor site; decreases allergic response by blocking histamine

Uses: Rhinitis, allergy symptoms

Dosage and routes:
• *Adult and child >12 yr:* PO 60 mg bid
• *Child <12 yr:* PO 15-30 mg bid

T

Available forms include: Tabs 60 mg

Side effects/adverse reactions:
CNS: Dizziness, poor coordination
RESP: Increased thick secretions
GI: Anorexia, increased liver function tests, dry mouth
GU: Retention

Contraindications: Hypersensitivity

Precautions: Pregnancy (C)

Pharmacokinetics:
PO: Peak 1-2 hr, 97% bound to plasma proteins, half-life is biphasic 3½ hr, 16-23 hr

NURSING CONSIDERATIONS
Assess:
• I&O ratio; be alert for urinary retention, frequency, dysuria; drug should be discontinued if these occur
• CBC during long-term therapy

Administer:
• With meals if GI symptoms occur; absorption may slightly decrease

Perform/provide:
• Hard candy, gum, frequent rinsing of mouth for dryness
• Storage in tight, light-resistant container

Evaluate:
• Therapeutic response: absence of running or congested nose or rashes
• Respiratory status: rate, rhythm, increase in bronchial secretions, wheezing, chest tightness

Teach patient/family:
• To notify physician if confusion, sedation, hypotension occurs

Lab test interferences:
False negative: Skin allergy tests

Treatment of overdose: Administer ipecac syrup or lavage, diazepam, vasopressors, barbiturates (short-acting)

---

terpin hydrate
(ter'pin)

Func. class.: Expectorant

Action: Direct action on respiratory tract, which increases fluids, allows for expectoration

Uses: Bronchial secretions

Dosage and routes:
• *Adult:* ELIX 5-10 ml q4-6h

Available forms include: Elix terpin hydrate codeine 10 mg codeine/ 85 mg terpin hydrate; elix, plain 85 mg/5 ml

Side effects/adverse reactions:
GI: Nausea, vomiting, anorexia

Contraindications: Hypersensitivity, child <12 yr

Precautions: Pregnancy (C)

NURSING CONSIDERATIONS
Administer:
• With glass of water or food to decrease GI irritation

Perform/provide:
• Storage at room temperature

Evaluate:
• Therapeutic response: absence of thick secretions
• Cough: type, frequency, character including sputum

Teach patient/family:
• To avoid driving, other hazardous activities until patient is stabilized on this medication (if combined with codeine, drowsiness occurs)
• Not to exceed recommended dosage

---

testolactone
(tess-toe-lak'tone)
Teslac

Func. class.: Antineoplastic
Chem. class.: Hormone, androgen

Action: Acts on adrenal cortex to

---

suppress activity; reduces estrone synthesis

Uses: Advanced breast carcinoma in postmenopausal women, prostatic cancer

Dosage and routes:
• *Adult:* PO 250 mg qid
Available forms include: Tabs 50 mg

Side effects/adverse reactions:
GI: Nausea, vomiting, anorexia, glossitis
GU: Urinary retention, ***renal failure***
INTEG: Rash, nail changes, facial hair growth
CV: Orthostatic hypertension, edema
CNS: Paresthesias, dizziness
EENT: Deepening voice
META: Hypercalcemia

Contraindications: Hypersensitivity, premenopausal women, carcinoma of male breast

Precautions: Renal disease, hypercalcemia, cardiac disease, pregnancy (C)

Pharmacokinetics: None known

Interactions/incompatibilities:
• Enhanced effects of: oral anticoagulants

NURSING CONSIDERATIONS
Assess:
• CA⁺ levels
• B/P q4h, tell patient to rise slowly from sitting or lying down

Administer:
• For at least 3 mo or longer for desired response

Evaluate:
• Food preferences; list likes, dislikes
• Edema in feet, joint, stomach pain, shaking
• Symptoms indicating severe allergic reaction: rash, pruritus, urticaria, purpuric skin lesions, itching, flushing

• Anorexia, nausea, vomiting, constipation, weakness, loss of muscle tone (indicating hypercalcemia)

Teach patient/family:
• To recognize and report signs of hepatotoxicity, hypercalcemia, virilization

Lab test interferences:
Increase: Urinary 17-OHCS
Decrease: Estradiol

---

testosterone

(tess-toss′ter-one)
Histerone, Malogen, Testoject
Func. class.: Androgenic anabolic steroid
Chem. class.: Halogenated testosterone derivative

Action: Increases weight by building body tissue, increases potassium, phosphorus, chloride, nitrogen levels, increases bone development

Uses: Breast engorgement, breast cancer in postmenopausal women, eunuchoidism, eunuchism, male climacteric

Dosage and routes:
Breast engorgement
• *Adult:* IM 25-50 mg/day × 3-4 days
Breast cancer
• *Adult:* IM 100 mg 3 ×/wk
Male climacteric/eunuchoidism/eunuchism
• *Adult:* IM 10-25 mg 2-5 ×/wk
Available forms include: Inj IM 25, 50, 100 mg/ml

Side effects/adverse reactions:
INTEG: Rash, acneiform lesions, oily hair, skin, flushing, sweating, acne vulgaris, alopecia, hirsutism
CNS: Dizziness, headache, fatigue, tremors, paresthesias, flushing,

T

sweating, anxiety, lability, insomnia

MS: Cramps, spasms

CV: Increased B/P

GU: Hematuria, amenorrhea, vaginitis, decreased libido, decreased breast size, clitoral hypertrophy, testicular atrophy

GI: Nausea, vomiting, constipation, weight gain, *cholestatic jaundice*

EENT: Carpal tunnel syndrome, conjunctival edema, nasal congestion

ENDO: Abnormal GTT

Contraindications: Severe renal disease, severe cardiac disease, severe hepatic disease, hypersensitivity, pregnancy (X), lactation, genital bleeding (abnormal)

Precautions: Diabetes mellitus, CV disease, MI

Pharmacokinetics:

PO: Metabolized in liver, excreted in urine, crosses placenta, excreted in breast milk

Interactions/incompatibilities:

• Increased effects of: oral antidiabetics, oxyphenbutazone
• Increased PT: anticoagulants
• Edema: ACTH, adrenal steroids
• Decreased effects of: insulin

NURSING CONSIDERATIONS

Assess:

• Weight daily, notify physician if weekly weight gain is >5 lb
• B/P q4h
• I&O ratio; be alert for decreasing urinary output, increasing edema
• Growth rate in children since growth rate may be uneven (linear/bone browth) when used for extended period
• Electrolytes: K, Na, Cl, Ca; cholesterol
• Liver function studies: ALT, AST, bilirubin

Administer:

• Titrated dose, use lowest effective dose
• IM deep into upper outer quadrant of gluteal muscle

Perform/provide:

• Diet with increased calories and protein; decrease sodium if edema occurs
• Supportive drug of anemia

Evaluate:

• Therapeutic response: occurs in 4-6 wk in osteoporosis
• Edema, hypertension, cardiac symptoms, jaundice
• Mental status: affect, mood, behavioral changes, aggression
• Signs of masculinization in female: increased libido, deepening of voice, breast tissue, enlarged clitoris, menstrual irregularities; male: gynecomastia, impotence, testicular atrophy
• Hypercalcemia: lethargy, polyuria, polydipsia, nausea, vomiting, constipation; drug may need to be decreased
• Hypoglycemia in diabetics, since oral anticoagulant action is decreased

Teach patient/family:

• Drug needs to be combined with complete health plan: diet, rest, exercise
• To notify physician if therapeutic response decreases
• Not to discontinue this medication abruptly
• About changes in sex characteristics
• Women to report menstrual irregularities
• That 1-3 mo course is necessary for response in breast cancer

Lab test interferences:

Increase: Serum cholesterol, blood glucose, urine glucose

Decrease: Serum calcium, serum

potassium, T_4, T_3, thyroid ^{131}I uptake test, urine 17-OHCS, 17-KS

testosterone cypionate/ testosterone enanthate/ testosterone propionate

Andro-Cyp, Andronate, Depotest, Dep-Test, Depo-Testosterone, Duratest/Android-T LA, Andro-LA, Andryl, Delatestryl, Everone, Malogen,* Malogex,* Testostroval-PA/Androlan, Androlin, Testex

Func. class.: Androgenic anabolic steroid

Chem. class.: Halogenated testosterone derivative

Action: Increases weight by building body tissue, increases potassium, phosphorus, chloride, nitrogen levels, increases bone development

Uses: Female breast cancer, eunuchoidism, male climacteric, oligospermia, impotence, osteoporosis

Dosage and routes:

Oligospermia

• *Adult:* IM 100-200 mg q4-6 wk (cypionate or enanthate)

Breast cancer

• *Adult:* IM 50-100 mg 3 × /wk (propionate) or 200-400 mg q2-4 wk (cypionate or enanthate)

Male climacteric/eunuchoidism/ eunuchism

• *Adult:* IM 10-25 mg 2-4 × /wk (propionate)

Available forms include: Propionate inj IM 25, 50, 100 mg/ml; enanthate inj IM 100, 200 mg/ml; cypionate inj IM 50, 100, 200 mg/ml

Side effects/adverse reactions:

INTEG: Rash, acneiform lesions, oily hair, skin, flushing, sweating, acne vulgaris, alopecia, hirsutism

CNS: Dizziness, headache, fatigue, tremors, paresthesias, flushing, sweating, anxiety, lability, insomnia

MS: Cramps, spasms

CV: Increased B/P

GU: Hematuria, amenorrhea, vaginitis, decreased libido, decreased breast size, clitoral hypertrophy, testicular atrophy

GI: Nausea, vomiting, constipation, weight gain, *cholestatic jaundice*

EENT: Carpal tunnel syndrome, conjunctional edema, nasal congestion

ENDO: Abnormal GTT

Contraindications: Severe renal disease, severe cardiac disease, severe hepatic disease, hypersensitivity, pregnancy (X), lactation, genital bleeding (abnormal)

Precautions: Diabetes mellitus, CV disease, MI

Pharmacokinetics:

PO: Metabolized in liver, excreted in urine, breast milk; crosses placenta

Interactions/incompatibilities:

• Increased effects of: oral antidiabetics, oxyphenbutazone

• Increased PT: anticoagulants

• Edema: ACTH, adrenal steroids

• Decreased effects of: insulin

NURSING CONSIDERATIONS

Assess:

• Weight daily, notify physician if weekly weight gain is >5 lb

• B/P q4h

• I&O ratio; be alert for decreasing urinary output, increasing edema

• Growth rate in children since growth rate may be uneven (linear/bone growth) used for extended periods of time

• Electrolytes: K, Na, Cl, Ca; cholesterol

T

---

italics = common side effects   ***bold italic*** = life threatening reactions

• Liver function studies: ALT, AST, bilirubin
Administer:
• Titrated dose; use lowest effective dose
• IM deep into upper outer quadrant of gluteal muscle
Perform/provide:
• Diet with increased calories, protein; decrease sodium if edema occurs
• Supportive drug of anemia
Evaluate:
• Therapeutic response: occurs in 4-6 wk in osteoporosis
• Edema, hypertension, cardiac symptoms, jaundice
• Mental status: affect, mood, behavioral changes, aggression
• Signs of masculinization in female: increased libido, deepening of voice, breast tissue, enlarge clitoris, menstrual irregularities; male: gynecomastia, impotence, testicular atrophy
• Hypercalcemia: lethargy, polyuria, polydipsia, nausea, vomiting, constipation; drug may need to be decreased
• Hypoglycemia in diabetics, since oral anticoagulant action is decreased
Teach patient/family:
• That drug needs to be combined with complete health plan: diet, rest, exercise
• To notify physician if therapeutic response decreases
• Not to discontinue this medication abruptly
• About changes in sex characteristics
• Women to report menstrual irregularities
• That 1-3 mo course is necessary for response in breast cancer
• Procedure for use of buccal tablets (requires 30-60 min to dissolve, change absorption site with each dose; do not eat, drink, chew, or smoke while tablet is in place)
Lab test interferences:
Increase: Serum cholesterol, blood glucose, urine glucose
Decrease: Serum calcium, serum potassium, T_4, T_3, thyroid ^{131}I uptake test, urine 17-OHCS, 17-KS, PBI

---

tetanus toxoid, adsorbed; tetanus toxoid
Func. class.: Toxoid

Action: Produces specific antibodies to tetanus
Uses: Tetanus toxoid: used for prophylactic treatment of wounds
Dosage and routes:
• *Adult and child:* IM 0.5 ml q4-6 wk × 2 doses, then 0.5 ml 1 yr after dose 2 (adsorbed); SC/IM 0.5 ml q4-8 wk × 3 doses, then 0.5 ml ½-1 yr after dose 3
Available forms include: Inj adsorbed IM 5, 10 LfU/0.5 ml; inj IM, SC 4, 5 LfU/0.5 ml
Side effects/adverse reactions:
GI: Nausea, vomiting, anorexia
INTEG: Skin abscess, urticaria, itching, swelling
CV: Tachycardia, hypotension
SYST: Lymphadenitis, ***anaphylaxis***
CNS: Crying, fretfulness, fever, drowsiness
MS: Osteomyelitis
Contraindications: Hypersensitivity, active infection, poliomyelitis outbreak, immunosuppression
Precautions: Pregnancy
NURSING CONSIDERATIONS
Assess:
• For skin reactions: swelling, rash, urticaria
Administer:
• At least 4 wk apart × 3 doses for children >6 wk old

---

*Available in Canada only

• Only with epinephrine 1:1000 on unit to treat laryngospasm
• IM only; not to be given SC (vastus lateralis in infants, deltoid in adults)

Evaluate:
• For history of allergies, skin conditions (eczema, psoriasis, dermatitis), reactions to vaccinations
• For anaphylaxis: inability to breathe, bronchospasm

Teach patient/family:
• That doses are given at least 4 wk apart × 3 doses; booster needed at 10 yr intervals

---

tetracaine/tetracaine HCl (topical)

(tet'-ra-cane)
Cetacaine, Pontocaine
Func. class.: Topical anesthetic

Action: Inhibits nerve impulses from sensory nerves, which produces anesthesia

Uses: Pruritus, sunburn, toothache, sore throat, cold sores, oral pain, rectal pain and irritation, control of gagging

Dosage and routes:
• *Adult and child:* TOP apply to affected area 1 oz for adult ¼ oz for child

Available forms include: Sol 2%; aero spray, liq, oint, gel

Side effects/adverse reactions:
INTEG: Rash, irritation, sensitization

Contraindications: Hypersensitivity, infants <1 yr, application to large areas, PABA allergies

Precautions: Child <6 yr, sepsis, pregnancy (C), denuded skin

NURSING CONSIDERATIONS
Administer:
• After cleansing and drying of affected area

Evaluate:
• Allergy: rash, irritation, reddening, swelling
• Therapeutic response: absence of pain, itching of affected area
• Infection: if affected area is infected, do not apply

Teach patient/family:
• To report rash, irritation, redness, swelling
• How to apply solution

---

tetracaine HCl

(tet'-ra-caine)
Pontocaine
Func. class.: Ophthalmic anesthetic
Chem. class.: Ester

Action: Decreases ion permeability by stabilizing neuronal membrane

Uses: Cataract extraction, tonometry, gonioscopy, removal of foreign objects, corneal suture removal, glaucoma surgery

Dosage and routes:
• *Adult and child:* Instill 1-2 gtts before procedure

Available forms include: Sol 0.5%; oint 0.5%

Side effects/adverse reactions:
EENT: Blurred vision, stinging, burning, lacrimation, photophobia, conjunctival redness
INTEG: Contact dermatitis

Contraindications: Hypersensitivity to paraaminobenzoic acid

Precautions: Abnormal levels of plasma esterases, allergies, hyperthyroidism, hypertension, cardiac disease, pregnancy (C)

Pharmacokinetics:
Instill: Onset 13-30 sec, duration 15-20 min

Interactions/incompatibilities:
• Decreases antibacterial action of: sulfonamides

T

---

italics = common side effects   ***bold italic*** = life threatening reactions

NURSING CONSIDERATIONS
Assess:
• Previous hypersensitivity to anesthetics
Perform/provide:
• Protective covering for eye
• Storage at room temperature in tight, light resistant container; refrigerate
Teach patient/family:
• To report change in vision, with blurring or loss of sight, trouble breathing, sweating, flushing
• Not to touch or rub eye, which may further damage eye
• That someone must drive the patient home after the appointment

---

tetracaine HCl
(tet-ra'-kane)
Pontocaine
Func. class.: Local anesthetic
Chem. class.: Ester

Action: Competes with calcium for sites in nerve membrane that control sodium transport across cell membrane; decreases rise of depolarization phase of action potential
Uses: Spinal anesthesia, epidural, peripheral nerve block, perineum, lower extremities
Dosage and routes:
Varies depending on route of anesthesia
Available forms include: Inj 0.2%, 0.3%, 1%; powder
Side effects/adverse reactions:
CNS: Anxiety, restlessness, *convulsions, loss of consciousness,* drowsiness, disorientation, tremors, shivering
CV: Myocardial depression, cardiac arrest, dysrhythmias, bradycardia, hypotension, hypertension, fetal bradycardia

GI: Nausea, vomiting
EENT: Blurred vision, tinnitus, pupil constriction
INTEG: Rash, urticaria, allergic reactions, edema, burning, skin discoloration at injection site, tissue necrosis
RESP: Status asthmaticus, respiratory arrest, anaphylaxis
Contraindications: Hypersensitivity, child <12 yr, elderly, severe liver disease
Precautions: Elderly, severe drug allergies, pregnancy (C)
Pharmacokinetics:
Onset 15 min, duration 3 hr; metabolized by liver, excreted in urine (metabolites)
Interactions/incompatibilities:
• Dysrhythmias: epinephrine, halothane, enflurane
• Hypertension: MAOIs, tricyclic antidepressants, phenothiazines
• Decreased action of tetracaine: chloroprocaine
NURSING CONSIDERATIONS
Assess:
• B/P, pulse, respiration during treatment
• Fetal heart tones if drug is used during labor
Administer:
• Only drugs that are not cloudy, do not contain precipitate
• Only with crash cart, resuscitative equipment nearby
• Only drugs without preservatives for epidural or caudal anesthesia
Perform/provide:
• Use of new solution, discard unused portions
Evaluate:
• Therapeutic response: anesthesia necessary for procedure
• Allergic reactions: rash, urticaria, itching
• Cardiac status: ECG for dys-

---

*Available in Canada only

rhythmias, pulse, B/P, during anesthesia

Treatment of overdose: Airway, O_2, vasopressor, IV fluids, anticonvulsants for seizures

---

tetracycline HCl
(tet-ra-sye'kleen)

Achromycin, Bicycline, Cefracycline,* Cycline, Cyclopar, Medicycline,* Neo-Tetrine,* Novotetra,* Panmycin, Sarocycline, Sumycin, Tetracyn, Tetralan, Tetralean,* Trexin, Tetracap

Func. class.: Broad spectrum antibiotic/antiinfective
Chem. class.: Tetracycline

Action: Inhibits protein synthesis and phosphorylation in microorganisms

Uses: Syphilis, chlamydia trachomatis, gonorrhea, lymphogranuloma venereum, uncommon gram positive/negative organisms, rickettsial infections

Dosage and routes:
• *Adult:* PO 250-500 mg q6h; IM 250 mg/day or 150 mg q12h; IV 250-500 mg q8-12h
• *Child >8 yr:* PO 25-50 mg/kg/day in divided doses q6h; IM 15-25 mg/kg/day in divided doses q8-12h; IV 10-20 mg/kg/day in divided doses q12h

Gonorrhea
• *Adult:* PO 1.5 g, then 500 mg qid for a total of 9 g × 7 days

Chlamydia trachomatis
• *Adult:* PO 500 mg qid × 7 days

Syphilis
• *Adult:* PO 2-3 g in divided doses × 10-15 days; if syphilis duration > 1 yr, must treat 30 days

Brucellosis
• *Adult:* PO 500 mg qid × 3 wk with 1 g streptomycin IM 2 ×/day

× 1 wk, and 1 ×/day the second wk

Urethral syndrome in women
• *Adult:* PO 500 mg qid × 7 days
Rape Victims
• *Adult:* PO 500 mg qid × 7 days
Acne
• *Adult:* 1 g/day in divided doses, maintenance 125-500 mg per day

Available forms include: Oral susp, caps 100, 200, 500 mg; tabs 250, 500 mg; powder for inj

Side effects/adverse reactions:
CNS: Fever, headache, paresthesia
HEMA: Eosinophilia, neutropenia, thrombocytopenia, leukocytosis, hemolytic anemia
EENT: Dysphagia, glossitis, decreased calcification of deciduous teeth, abdominal pain, oral candidiasis
GI: Nausea, vomiting, diarrhea, anorexia, enterocolitis, *hepatotoxicity,* flatulence, abdominal cramps, epigastric burning, stomatitis, *pseudomembranous colitis*
CV: Pericarditis
GU: Increased BUN, polyuria, polydipsia, *renal failure, nephrotoxicity*
INTEG: Rash, urticaria, photosensitivity, *increased pigmentation, exfoliative dermatitis,* pruritus, *angioedema*

Contraindications: Hypersensitivity to tetracyclines, children <8 yr, pregnancy (D), lactation
Precautions: Renal disease, hepatic disease, IM: cross-sensitivity to "caine-type" local anesthetics

Pharmacokinetics:
PO: Peak 2-3 hr, duration 6 hr, half-life 6-10 hr; excreted in urine, crosses placenta, excreted in breast milk, 20%-60% protein bound

Interactions/incompatibilities:
• Decreased effect of tetracycline:

---

italics = common side effects   ***bold italic*** = life threatening reactions

T

antacids, NaHCO₃, dairy products, alkali products, iron, kaolin/pectin
• Increased effect: anticoagulants
• Decreased effect: penicillins
• Nephrotoxicity: methoxyflurane
• Do not mix with other drugs

NURSING CONSIDERATIONS
Assess:
• Signs of anemia: Hct, Hgb, fatigue
• I&O ratio
• Blood studies: PT, CBC, AST, ALT, BUN, creatinine

Administer:
• IM: deep; no more than 2 ml/injection site
• IV after diluting 250 mg or less/5 ml of sterile H₂O; may be further diluted with 100 ml or more D₅W or NS; give 100 mg or less over 5 min or more
• After C&S obtained
• 2 hr before or after ferrous products; 3 hr after antacid or kaolin/pectin products

Perform/provide:
• Storage in tight, light-resistant container at room temperature

Evaluate:
• Therapeutic response: decreased temperature, absence of lesions, negative C&S
• Allergic reactions: rash, itching, pruritus, angioedema
• Nausea, vomiting, diarrhea; administer antiemetic, antacids as ordered
• Overgrowth of infection: increased temperature, malaise, redness, pain, swelling, drainage, perineal itching, diarrhea, changes in cough or sputum

Teach patient/family:
• To avoid sun exposure since burns may occur; sunscreen does not seem to decrease photosensitivity
• Of diabetic to avoid use of Clin-istix, Diastix, or Tes-Tape for urine glucose testing
• That all prescribed medication must be taken to prevent superimposed infection
• To avoid milk products, take with a full glass of water

Lab test interferences:
False negative: Urine glucose with Clinistix or Tes-Tape
False increase: Urinary catecholamines

---

tetracycline HCl (ophthalmic)

(tet-ra-sye'kleen)
Achromycin Ophthalmic
Func. class.: Antiinfective

Action: Inhibits bacterial protein synthesis
Uses: Infection of eye, ophthalmia neonatorum
Dosage and routes:
• *Adult and child:* INSTILL 1-2 gtts bid-qid as needed
Ophthalmia neonatorum
• *Neonate:* TOP 1-2 gtts into each eye immediately after delivery; SOL, 1 gtt q6-12 hr more frequently
Available forms include: Oint 1%, Susp drops 1%
Side effects/adverse reactions:
EENT: Poor corneal wound healing, overgrowth of nonsusceptible organisms
Contraindications: Hypersensitivity, pregnancy (D)
Precautions: Antibiotic hypersensitivity

NURSING CONSIDERATIONS
Administer:
• After washing hands, cleanse crusts or discharge from eye before application

---

Perform/provide:
• Storage at room temperature, in light-resistant container
Evaluate:
• Therapeutic response: absence of redness, inflammation, tearing
• Allergy: itching, lacrimation, redness, swelling
Teach patient/family:
• To use drug exactly as prescribed, shake well before using
• Not to use eye make-up, towels, washcloths, or eye medication of others, or reinfection may occur
• That drug container tip should not be touched to eye
• To report itching, increased redness, burning, stinging, swelling; drug should be discontinued
• That drug may cause blurred vision when ointment is applied

---

tetracycline HCl (topical)
(tet-ra-sye'kleen)
Achromycin
Func. class.: Local antiinfective
Chem. class.: Tetracycline

Action: Interferes with microorganism protein synthesis
Uses: Acne vulgaris, skin abrasions
Dosage and routes:
• *Adult and child >12 yr:* TOP apply to affected area bid
Available forms include: Oint 3%; sol 0.22%
Side effects/adverse reactions:
INTEG: Rash, urticaria, stinging, burning, redness, swelling, photosensitivity
Contraindications: Hypersensitivity, pregnancy (D)
Precautions: Lactation
NURSING CONSIDERATIONS
Administer:
• Enough medication to completely cover lesions

• After cleansing with soap, water before each application, dry well
Perform/provide:
• Storage at room temperature in dry place, use within 2 mo or discard
Evaluate:
• Allergic reaction: burning, stinging, swelling, redness
• Therapeutic response: decrease in size, number of lesions
Teach patient/family:
• To apply with glove to prevent further infection
• To avoid use of OTC creams, ointments, lotions unless directed by physician
• To use medical asepsis (hand washing) before, after each application, avoid eyes, nose, mouth
• To notify physician if condition worsens
• That some stinging may occur
• To avoid sunlight or ultraviolet light or burning may occur
• That staining of clothing and skin may occur

---

tetrahydrozoline HCl
(tet-ra-hi-droz-o-leen)
Murine Plus, Optigene, Soothe, Visine
Func. class.: Ophthalmic vasoconstrictor
Chem. class.: Direct sympathomimetic amine

Action: Vasoconstriction of eye arterioles; decreases eye engorgement by stimulation of α-adrenergic receptors
Uses: Ocular congestion, irritation, itching
Dosage and routes:
• *Adult and child >2 yr:* INSTILL 1-2 gtts bid or tid

T

---

italics = common side effects   ***bold italic*** = life threatening reactions

Available forms include: Sol 0.05%

Side effects/adverse reactions:

CNS: Headache, dizziness, weakness

CV: Bradycardia, hypertension, dysrhythmias, tachycardia, *CV collapse,* palpitation

EENT: Stinging, lacrimation, blurred vision, conjunctival allergy

Contraindications: Hypersensitivity, glaucoma (narrow-angle)

Precautions: Severe hypertension, diabetes, hyperthyroidism, elderly, severe arteriosclerosis, cardiac disease, infants, pregnancy (C)

Pharmacokinetics:

INSTILL: Duration 2-3 hr

Interactions/incompatibilities:

• Increased pressor effects: MAOIs, tricyclic antidepressants

NURSING CONSIDERATIONS

Assess:

• B/P, pulse, systemic absorption does occur

Perform/provide:

• Storage in tight, light-resistant container; do not use discolored solutions

Teach patient/family:

• To report change in vision, blurring, loss of sight; breathing trouble, sweating, flushing

• Method of instillation; tilt head backward, hold dropper over eye, drop medication inside lower lid, using pressure on inside corner of eye hold 1 min, do not touch dropper to eye

• That blurred vision will decrease with repeated use of drug

• To notify physician if headache, spots, redness, pain occurs; discontinue use

• To use sunglasses if photophobia occurs

• To use exactly as prescribed

tetrahydrozoline HCl

(tet-ra-hye-drozz a-leen)

Tyzine HCl, Tyzine Pediatric

Func. class.: Nasal decongestant

Chem. class.: Sympathomimetic amine

Action: Produces vasoconstriction (rapid, long-acting) of arterioles thereby decreasing fluid exudation, mucosal engorgement

Uses: Nasal congestion

Dosage and routes:

• *Adult and child >6 yr:* INSTILL 2-4 gtts or sprays q4-6h prn (0.1%)

• *Child 2-6 yr:* INSTILL 2-3 gtts q4-6h prn (0.05%)

Available forms include: Sol 0.05%, 0.1%

Side effects/adverse reactions:

GI: Nausea, vomiting, anorexia

EENT: Irritation, burning, sneezing, stinging, dryness, rebound congestion

INTEG: Contact dermatitis

CNS: Anxiety, restlessness, tremors, weakness, insomnia, dizziness, fever, headache

Contraindications: Hypersensitivity to sympathomimetic amines

Precautions: Child <6 yr, elderly, diabetes, cardiovascular disease, hypertension, hyperthyroidism, increased ICP, prostatic hypertrophy, pregnancy (C), glaucoma

Interactions/incompatibilities:

• Hypertension: MAOIs, β-adrenergic blockers

• Hypotension: methyldopa, mecamylamine, reserpine

NURSING CONSIDERATIONS

Administer:

• No more than q4h

• For <4 consecutive days

Perform/provide:

• Environmental humidification to decrease nasal congestion, dryness

• Storage in light-resistant containers; do not expose to high temperatures

Evaluate:
• Redness, swelling, pain in nasal passages

Teach patient/family:
• Stinging may occur for several applications; drying of mucosa may be decreased by environmental humidification
• To notify physician if irregular pulse, insomnia, dizziness, or tremors occur
• Proper administration to avoid systemic absorption

---

theophylline, theophylline sodium glycinate

(thee-off'i-lin)

Aquaphyllin, Bronkodyl, Elixophyllin, Slo-Phyllin, Somophyllin-T/ Accurbron, Aerolate, Aquaphyllin, Asmalix, Elixicon, Elixomin, Elixophyllin, Lanophyllin, Lixolin, Theo-Dur, Theo-24, Theo-Dur Sprinkle, Theolair, Theolixir, Theon, Theophyl, Lodrane, Slo-bid, Slo-Phyllin, Theovent, Theo-Time

Func. class.: Spasmolytic
Chem. class.: Xanthine, ethylenediamide

Action: Relaxes smooth muscle of respiratory system by blocking phosphodiesterase, which increases cyclic AMP

Uses: Bronchial asthma, bronchospasm of COPD, chronic bronchitis

Dosage and routes:
Bronchospasm, bronchial asthma
• *Adult:* PO 100-200 mg q6h, dosage must be individualized; REC 250-500 mg q8-12h
• *Child:* PO 50-100 mg q6h, not to exceed 12 mg/kg/24 hr
COPD, chronic bronchitis

• *Adult:* PO 330-660 mg q6-8h pc (sodium glycinate)
• *Child >12 yr:* PO 220-330 mg q6-8h pc (sodium glycinate)
• *Child 6-12 yr:* PO 330 mg q6-8h pc (sodium glycinate)
• *Child 3-6 yr:* PO 110-165 mg q6-8h pc (sodium glycinate)
• *Child 1-3 yr:* PO 55-110 mg q6-8h pc (sodium glycinate)

Available forms include: Caps 50, 100, 200, 250 mg; tabs 100, 125, 200, 225, 250, 300 mg; tabs timerelease 100, 200, 250, 300, 400, 500 mg; caps time-release 50, 65, 100, 125, 130, 200, 250, 260, 300, 400, 500 mg; elix 80, 11.25 mg/15 ml; sol 80 mg/15 ml; liq 80, 150, 160 mg/15 ml; susp 300 mg/15 ml

Side effects/adverse reactions:
CNS: Anxiety, restlessness, insomnia, dizziness, convulsions, headache, light-headedness, muscle twitching
CV: Palpitations, sinus tachycardia, hypotension, other dysrhythmias
GI: Nausea, vomiting, anorexia, diarrhea, bitter taste, dyspepsia, gastric distress
RESP: Increased rate
INTEG: Flushing, urticaria

Contraindications: Hypersensitivity to xanthines, tachydysrhythmias

Precautions: Elderly, CHF, cor pulmonale, hepatic disease, active peptic ulcer disease, diabetes mellitus, hyperthyroidism, hypertension, children, pregnancy (C)

Pharmacokinetics:
SOL: Peak 1 hr, metabolized in liver, excreted in urine, breast milk, crosses placenta

Interactions/incompatibilities:
• Increased action of theophylline: cimetidine, propranolol, erythromycin, troleandomycin

T

---

italics = common side effects   ***bold italic*** = life threatening reactions

- May increase effects of: anticoagulants
- Cardiotoxicity: β-blockers
- Decreased effect of: lithium

NURSING CONSIDERATIONS

Assess:

- Theophylline blood levels (therapeutic level is 10-20 μg/ml); toxicity may occur with small increase above 20 μg/ml
- Monitor I&O; diuresis occurs, dehydration may result in elderly or children
- Signs of toxicity: irritability, insomnia, restlessness, tremors, nausea, vomiting

Administer:

- PO after meals to decrease GI symptoms; absorption may be affected

Evaluate:

- Respiratory rate, rhythm, depth; auscultate lung fields bilaterally; notify physician of abnormalities
- Allergic reactions: rash, urticaria; if these occur, drug should be discontinued

Teach patient/family

- To check OTC medications, current prescription medications for ephedrine, which will increase stimulation, to avoid alcohol or caffeine
- To avoid hazardous activities; dizziness may occur
- If GI upset occurs, to take drug with 8 oz water; avoid food, absorption may be decreased
- Not to crush, dissolve, or chew slow-release products
- May sprinkle contents of bead-filled capsule over food for children's use
- To notify physician of toxicity: nausea, vomiting, anxiety, insomnia, convulsions
- To notify physician of change in smoking habit; dosage may need to be changed

---

thiabendazole

(thye-a-ben′da-zole)

Mintezol, Minzolum

Func. class.: Anthelmintic

Chem. class.: Benzimadazole derivative

Action: Inhibits anaerobic metabolism, disrupts microtubules

Uses: Pinworm, roundworm, threadworm, whipworm, trichinosis, hookworm, cutaneous larva migrans (creeping eruption)

Dosage and routes:

- *Adult and child:* PO 25 mg/kg in 2 doses qd × 2-5 days, not to exceed 3 g/day

Available forms include: Tabs, chew 500 mg; oral susp 500 mg/5 ml

Side effects/adverse reactions:

*SYST: **Anaphylaxis***

*GU: **Hematuria, nephrotoxicity,*** enuresis, abnormal smell of urine

INTEG: Rash, pruritus, fever, flushing, ***convulsions,*** behavioral changes

CNS: Dizziness, headache, drowsiness

EENT: Tinnitus, blurred vision, xanthopsia

GI: Nausea, vomiting, anorexia, diarrhea, jaundice, liver damage, epigastric distress

CV: Hypotension, bradycardia

Contraindications: Hypersensitivity

Precautions: Severe malnutrition, hepatic disease, renal disease, anemia, severe dehydration, child <14 kg, pregnancy (C)

Pharmacokinetics:

PO: Peak 1-2 hr, metabolized com-

---

pletely by liver, excreted in feces, urine

NURSING CONSIDERATIONS
Assess:
• Stools periodically during entire treatment

Administer:
• Suspension after shaking
• PO after meals to avoid GI symptoms

Perform/provide:
• Storage in tight containers

Teach patient/family:
• Proper hygiene after BM including handwashing technique; tell patient to avoid putting fingers in mouth
• That infected person should sleep alone; do not shake bed linen; change bed linen qd
• To clean toilet qd with disinfectant (green soap solution)
• Need for compliance with dosage schedule, duration of treatment
• To drink fruit juice to remove mucus that intestinal tapeworms burrow in; aids in expulsion of worms
• To avoid hazardous activities if drowsiness occurs

Treatment of overdose: Induce emesis or gastric lavage

---

thiamine HCl (vitamin B₁)

Apatate Drops, Betaline S, Betaxin,* Revitonus, Thia

Func. class.: Vitamin B₁
Chem. class.: Water soluble

Action: Needed for pyruvate metabolism

Uses: Vitamin B₁ deficiency or polyneuritis, cheilosis adjunct with thiamine beriberi, Wernicke-Korsakoff syndrome, pellagra

Dosage and routes:
Beriberi

• *Adult:* IM 10-500 mg tid × 2 wk, then 5-10 mg qd × 1 mo
• *Child:* IM 10-50 mg qd × 4-6 wk

Anemia/alcoholism/pregnancy/ pellagra
• *Adult:* PO 100 mg qd
• *Child:* PO 10-50 mg qd in divided doses

Beriberi with cardiac failure
• *Adult and child:* IV 100-500 mg

Wernicke's encephalopathy
• *Adult:* IV 500 mg or less, then 100 mg bid

Available forms include: Tabs 5, 10, 25, 50, 100, 250, 500 mg; inj IM, IV 100, 200 mg/ml

Side effects/adverse reactions:
CNS: Weakness, restlessness
GI: Hemorrhage, *nausea, diarrhea*
CV: **Collapse, pulmonary edema,** hypotension
INTEG: **Angioneurotic edema,** cyanosis, sweating, warmth
SYST: **Anaphylaxis**
EENT: Tightness of throat

Contraindications: None known
Precautions: Pregnancy (A)

Pharmacokinetics:
PO/INJ: Unused amounts excreted in urine (unchanged)

NURSING CONSIDERATIONS
Assess:
• Thiamine levels throughout treatment

Administer:
• By IM injection, rotate sites if pain and inflammation occur; do not mix with alkaline solutions; Z-track to minimize pain
• Application of cold may decrease pain

Perform/provide:
• Storage in tight, light-resistant container

Evaluate:
• Therapeutic response: absence of nausea, vomiting, anorexia, insom-

---

italics = common side effects   ***bold italic*** = life threatening reactions

nia, tachycardia, paresthesias, depression, muscle weakness
• Nutritional status: yeast, beef, liver, whole or enriched grains, legumes
Teach patient/family:
• Necessary foods to be included in diet: yeast, beef, liver, legumes, whole grain

---

thiethylperazine maleate

(thye-eth-il-per'-a-zeen)
Torecan
Func. class.: Antiemetic
Chem. class.: Phenothiazine, piperazine derivative

Action: Acts centrally by blocking chemoreceptor trigger zone, which in turn acts on vomiting center
Uses: Nausea, vomiting
Dosage and routes:
• *Adult:* PO/IM/REC 10 mg/qd-tid
Available forms include: Tabs 10 mg; supp 10 mg; inj 5 mg/ml
Side effects/adverse reactions:
GU: Urinary retention, dark urine
CNS: Euphoria, depression, restlessness, tremor, extrapyramidal symptoms, *convulsions*
GI: Nausea, vomiting, anorexia, dry mouth, diarrhea, constipation, weight loss, metallic taste, cramps
CV: Circulatory failure, tachycardia, postural hypotension, EKG changes
RESP: Respiratory depression
Contraindications: Hypersensitivity to phenothiazines, coma, seizure, encephalopathy, bone marrow depression
Precautions: Children <2 yr, pregnancy (C), elderly
Pharmacokinetics:
PO: Onset 45-60 min

REC: Onset 45-60 min, metabolized by liver, excreted by kidneys, crosses placenta, excreted in breast milk
Interactions/incompatibilities:
• Decreased effect of thiethylperazine: barbiturates, antacids
• Increased anticholinergic action: anticholinergics, antiparkinson drugs, antidepressants
• Do not mix with other drug in syringe or solution
NURSING CONSIDERATIONS
Assess:
• VS, B/P; check patients with cardiac disease more often
Administer:
• IM injection in large muscle mass; aspirate to avoid IV administration
Evaluate:
• Therapeutic response: absence of nausea, vomiting
• Respiratory status before, during, after administration of emetic; check rate, rhythm, character; respiratory depression can occur rapidly with elderly or debilitated patients
Teach patient/family:
• To avoid hazardous activities, activities requiring alertness; dizziness may occur

---

thimerosal

(thye-mer'oh-sal)
Aeroaid Thimerosal, Merthiolate
Func. class.: Disinfectant
Chem. class.: Mercurial

Action: Destroys microorganisms (bacteria, fungi)
Uses: Cleansing wounds, disinfection of skin preoperatively
Dosage and routes:
Adult and child: SOL Apply locally qd-tid

---

*Available in Canada only

Available forms include: Top sol 0.1%; tinc 0.1%

Side effects/adverse reactions:
INTEG: Irritation, contact dermatitis, erythema

Contraindications: Hypersensitivity to mercurial compounds, external ear wax removal

Precautions: Pregnancy (C)

Interactions/incompatibilities:
• Do not use with acids, heavy metals, permanganate, aluminum salts, iodine

NURSING CONSIDERATIONS
Administer:
• After cleaning wound of all debris if using tincture; do not apply dressing to wet area
Perform/provide:
• Storage in tight, light-resistant container
Evaluate:
• Area of body involved: irritation, rash, breaks, redness, dryness, itching

---

thioguanine (6-TG)

(thye-oh-gwah'neen)
TG, 6-Thioguanine, Lanvis*

Func. class.: Antineoplastic-antimetabolite
Chem. class.: Purine analog

Action: Interferes with synthesis, utilization of purine nucleotides; effect is related to substitution of ribonucleotides into DNA

Uses: Acute leukemias, chronic granulocytic leukemia, lymphomas, multiple myeloma, solid tumors

Dosage and routes:
• *Adult and child:* PO 2 mg/kg/day, then increase slowly to 3 mg/kg/day after 4 wk

Available forms include: Tabs 40 mg

Side effects/adverse reactions:
*HEMA: **Thrombocytopenia, leukopenia, myelosuppression, anemia***
*GI: Nausea, vomiting, anorexia, diarrhea, stomatitis, **hepatotoxicity,** gastritis, jaundice*
*GU: **Renal failure,** hyperuricemia, oliguria*
INTEG: Rash, dermatitis, dry skin

Contraindications: Prior drug resistance, leukopenia (<2500/mm³), thrombocytopenia (<100,000/mm³), anemia, pregnancy (D)

Precautions: Liver disease

Pharmacokinetics: Oral form absorbed only 30%, metabolized in liver, only small amounts excreted in urine (unchanged)

Interactions/incompatibilities:
• Increased toxicity: radiation, other antineoplastics

NURSING CONSIDERATIONS
Assess:
• CBC, differential, platelet count weekly; withhold drug if WBC is <3500/mm³ or platelet count is <100,000/mm³; notify physician of these results; drug should be discontinued
• Renal function studies: BUN, serum uric acid, urine CrCl, electrolytes before, during therapy
• I&O ratio; report fall in urine output to <30 ml/hr
• Monitor temperature q4h; fever may indicate beginning infection
• Liver function tests before, during therapy: bilirubin, alk phosphatase, AST, ALT
• Bleeding time, coagulation time during treatment
Administer:
• Antacid before oral agent; give drug after evening meal before bedtime
• Antiemetic 30-60 min before giving drug to prevent vomiting

---

italics = common side effects   ***bold italic*** = life threatening reactions

- Allopurinol or sodium bicarbonate to maintain uric acid levels, alkalinization of urine
- Antibiotics for prophylaxis of infection
- Topical or systemic analgesics for pain
- Transfusion for anemia

Perform/provide:
- Strict medical asepsis, protective isolation if WBC levels are low
- Liquid diet: carbonated beverage, Jello; dry toast, crackers may be added when patient is not nauseated or vomiting
- Increase fluid intake to 2-3 L/day to prevent urate deposits, calculi formation, unless contraindicated
- Diet low in purines: absence of organ meats (kidney, liver), dried beans, peas to maintain alkaline urine
- Rinsing of mouth tid-qid with water, club soda, brushing of teeth bid-tid with soft brush or cotton-tipped applicators for stomatitis; use unwaxed dental floss
- Nutritious diet with iron, vitamin supplements as ordered
- Storage in tightly closed container in cool environment

Evaluate:
- Bleeding: hematuria, guaiac, bruising, petechiae, mucosa or orifices q8h
- Food preferences; list likes, dislikes
- Hepatotoxicity: yellowing of skin, sclera, dark urine, clay-colored stools, pruritus, abdominal pain, fever, diarrhea
- Buccal cavity q8h for dryness, sores, ulceration, white patches, oral pain, bleeding, dysphagia
- Symptoms indicating severe allergic reaction: rash, urticaria, itching, flushing

Teach patient/family:
- Why protective isolation precautions are needed
- To report any complaints, side effects to nurse or physician: black tarry stools, chills, fever, sore throat, bleeding, bruising, cough, shortness of breath, dark, bloody urine
- To avoid foods with citric acid, hot or rough texture if stomatitis is present
- To report stomatitis: any bleeding, white spots, ulcerations in mouth; tell patient to examine mouth qd, report symptoms
- That contraceptive measures are recommended during therapy
- To drink 10-12 glasses of fluid/day

Lab test interferences:
Increase: Uric acid (blood, urine)

---

thiopental sodium

(thye-oh-pen′tal)
Pentothal
Func. class.: General anesthetic
Chem. class.: Barbiturate

Controlled Substance Schedule III

Action: Acts in reticular-activating system to produce anesthesia

Uses: Short general anesthesia, narcoanalysis, induction anesthesia before other anesthetics

Dosage and routes:
Induction
- *Adult:* IV 210-280 mg or 3-4 ml/kg

General anesthetic
- *Adult:* IV 50-75 mg given at 20-40 sec intervals

Narcoanalysis
- *Adult:* IV 200 mg/min, not to exceed 50 ml/min

Available forms include: Inj IV

---

*Available in Canada only

Side effects/adverse reactions:
*RESP: **Respiratory depression, bronchospasm***
CNS: Retrograde amnesia, prolonged somnolence
CV: Tachycardia, hypotension, ***myocardial depression, dysrhythmias***
EENT: Sneezing, coughing
INTEG: Chills, *shivering,* necrosis, pain at injection site
MS: Muscle irritability

Contraindications: Hypersensitivity, status asthmaticus, hepatic/intermittent porphyrias

Precautions: Severe cardiovascular disease, renal disease, hypotension, liver disease, myxedema, myasthenia gravis, asthma, increased intracranial pressure, pregnancy (C)

Pharmacokinetics:
IV: Onset 30-40 sec; half-life 11½ hr, crosses placenta

Interactions/incompatibilities:
• Increased action: CNS depressants
• Do not mix with atropine or silicone in solution or syringe

NURSING CONSIDERATIONS
Assess:
• VS q3-5 min during IV administration, after dose, q4 hr postoperatively

Administer:
• IV after diluting 500 mg/20 ml sterile H_2O for inj; give each 25 mg or less/min, titrate to response
• Only with crash cart, resuscitative equipment nearby

Evaluate:
• Therapeutic response: maintenance of anesthesia
• Extravasation, if it occurs use nitroprusside or chloroprocaine to decrease pain, increase circulation
• Dysrhythmias or myocardial depression

thioridazine HCl

(thye-or-rid' a-zeen)
Mellaril, Millazine, Novoridazine,* SK Thioridazine

Func. class.: Antipsychotic/neuroleptic
Chem. class.: Phenothiazine, piperidine

Action: Depresses cerebral cortex, hypothalamus, limbic system, which control activity, aggression; blocks neurotransmission produced by dopamine at synapse; exhibits strong α-adrenergic, anticholinergic blocking action; mechanism for antipsychotic effects is unclear

Uses: Psychotic disorders, schizophrenia, behavioral problems in children, alcohol withdrawal as adjunct, anxiety, major depressive disorders, organic brain syndrome

Dosage and routes:
Psychosis
• *Adult:* PO 25-100 mg tid, max dose 800 mg/day; dose is gradually increased to desired response, then reduced to minimum maintenance

Depression/behavioral problems/ organic brain syndrome
• *Adult:* PO 25 tid, range from 10 mg bid-qid to 50 mg tid-qid
• *Child 2-12 yr:* PO 0.5-3 mg/kg/ day in divided doses

Available forms include: Tabs 10, 15, 25, 50, 100, 150, 200, 300 mg; conc 30, 100 mg/ml; susp 25, 100 mg/5 ml

Side effects/adverse reactions:
*RESP: **Laryngospasm,** dyspnea, **respiratory depression***
*CNS: Extrapyramidal symptoms (rare): pseudoparkinsonism, akathisia, dystonia, tardive dyskinesia, **seizures,** headache*
HEMA: Anemia, ***leukopenia, leukocytosis, agranulocytosis***

T

---

italics = common side effects   ***bold italic*** = life threatening reactions

INTEG: Rash, photosensitivity, dermatitis

EENT: Blurred vision, glaucoma

GI: Dry mouth, nausea, vomiting, anorexia, constipation, diarrhea, jaundice, weight gain

GU: Urinary retention, urinary frequency, enuresis, impotence, amenorrhea, gynecomastia

CV: Orthostatic hypotension, hypertension, *cardiac arrest,* ECG changes, *tachycardia*

Contraindications: Hypersensitivity, blood dyscrasias, coma, child <2 yr, brain damage, bone marrow depression

Precautions: Pregnancy (C), lactation, seizure disorders, hypertension, hepatic disease, cardiac disease

Pharmacokinetics:

PO: Onset erratic, peak 2-4 hr; metabolized by liver, excreted in urine, crosses placenta, enters breast milk, half-life 26-36 hr

Interactions/incompatibilities:

• Oversedation: other CNS depressants, alcohol, barbiturate anesthetics

• Toxicity: epinephrine

• Decreased absorption: aluminum hydroxide or magnesium hydroxide antacids

• Decreased effects of: lithium, levodopa

• Increased effects of both drugs: β-adrenergic blockers, alcohol

• Increased anticholinergic effects: anticholinergics

NURSING CONSIDERATIONS
Assess:

• Swallowing of PO medication; check for hoarding or giving of medication to other patients

• I&O ratio; palpate bladder if low urinary output occurs

• Bilirubin, CBC, liver function studies monthly

• Urinalysis is recommended before and during prolonged therapy

Administer:

• Antiparkinsonian agent, after securing order from physician to be used if extrapyramidal symptoms occur

• Concentrate mixed in citrus juices or distilled or acidified tap water

Perform/provide:

• Decreased noise input by dimming lights, avoiding loud noises

• Supervised ambulation until stabilized on medication; do not involve in strenuous exercise program because fainting is possible; patient should not stand still for long periods of time

• Increased fluids to prevent constipation

• Sips of water, candy, gum for dry mouth

• Storage in tight, light-resistant container

Evaluate:

• Therapeutic response: decrease in emotional excitement, hallucinations, delusions, paranoia, reorganization of patterns of thought, speech

• Affect, orientation, LOC, reflexes, gait, coordination, sleep pattern disturbances

• B/P standing and lying; also include pulse and respirations q4h during initial treatment; establish baseline before starting treatment; report drops of 30 mm Hg

• Dizziness, faintness, palpitations, tachycardia on rising

• Extrapyramidal symptoms including akathisia (inability to sit still, no pattern to movements), tardive dyskinesia (bizarre movements of jaw, mouth, tongue, extremities), pseudoparkinsonism (ri-

gidity, tremors, pill rolling, shuffling gait)
• For neuroleptic malignant syndrome: altered mental status, muscle rigidity, increased CPK, hyperthermia
• Skin turgor daily
• Constipation, urinary retention daily; if these occur, increase bulk, water in diet

Teach patient/family:
• That orthostatic hypotension occurs frequently, and to rise from sitting or lying position gradually
• To remain lying down after IM injection for at least 30 min
• To avoid hot tubs, hot showers, or tub baths since hypotension may occur
• To avoid abrupt withdrawal of thioridazine or extrapyramidal symptoms may result; drugs should be withdrawn slowly
• To avoid OTC preparations (cough, hayfever, cold) unless approved by physician since serious drug interactions may occur; avoid use with alcohol or CNS depressants, increased drowsiness may occur
• To use a sunscreen during sun exposure to prevent burns
• Regarding compliance with drug regimen
• About necessity for meticulous oral hygiene since oral candidiasis may occur
• To report sore throat, malaise, fever, bleeding, mouth sores; if these occur, CBC should be drawn and drug discontinued
• In hot weather, heat stroke may occur; take extra precautions to stay cool

Lab test interferences:
Increase: Liver function tests, cardiac enzymes, cholesterol, blood glucose, prolactin, bilirubin, PBI, cholinesterase, ^{131}I
Decrease: Hormones (blood, urine)
False positive: Pregnancy tests, PKU
False negative: Urinary steroids
Treatment of overdose: Lavage if orally injested, provide an airway; do not induce vomiting

---

thiotepa

(thye-oh-tep'a)
Thiotepa, TSPA
Func. class.: Antineoplastic
Chem. class.: Alkylating agent

Action: Responsible for cross-linking DNA strands leading to cell death
Uses: Hodgkin's disease, lymphomas; breast, ovarian, lung, bladder, cancer; neoplastic effusions
Dosage and routes:
• *Adult:* IV 50.2 mg/kg × 5 days, then 0.2 mg/kg q1-3 wk
Neoplastic effusions
• *Adult:* INTRACAVITY 10-15 mg
Bladder cancer
• *Adult:* INSTILL 60 mg/60 ml water for inj in bladder once weekly × 4 wk
Available forms include: Inj 15 mg, powder for inj
Side effects/adverse reactions:
CNS: Dizziness, headache
HEMA: ***Thrombocytopenia, leukopenia, pancytopenia***
GI: Nausea, vomiting, anorexia, stomatitis
GU: Hyperuricemia, ***hematuria, amenorrhea, azoospermia***
INTEG: Rash, pruritus
Contraindications: Hypersensitivity, pregnancy (D)
Precautions: Radiation therapy,

T

---

bone marrow suppression, impaired renal or hepatic function

Pharmacokinetics:

Onset slow, metabolized in liver, excreted in urine

Interactions/incompatibilities:

• Increased apnea: succinylcholine

NURSING CONSIDERATIONS

Assess:

• CBC, differential, platelet count weekly; withhold drug if WBC is <4000 or platelet count is <75,000; notify physician of results

• Renal function studies: BUN, serum uric acid, urine CrCl before, during therapy

• I&O ratio, report fall in urine output of 30 ml/hr

• Monitor temperature q4h (may indicate beginning infection)

• Liver function tests before, during therapy (bilirubin, AST, ALT, LDH) as needed or monthly

Administer:

• IV after diluting 15 mg/1.5 ml of sterile H_2O for inj; give over 1-3 min; may be further diluted in 50-100 ml compatible sol

• Antiemetic 30-60 min before giving drug to prevent vomiting

• Allopurinol or sodium bicarbonate to maintain uric acid levels, alkalinization of urine

• Antibiotics for prophylaxis of infection

• Local or systemic drugs for infection

Perform/provide:

• Storage in light-resistant container, refrigerate

• Strict medical asepsis, protective isolation if WBC levels are low

• Special skin care

• Increase fluid intake to 2-3 L/day to prevent urate deposits, calculi formation

• Diet low in purines: organ meats (kidney, liver), dried beans, peas to maintain alkaline urine

• Rinsing of mouth tid-qid with water; brushing of teeth bid-tid with soft brush or cotton tipped applicators for stomatitis; use unwaxed dental floss

• Warm compresses at injection site for inflammation

Evaluate:

• Bleeding: hematuria, guaiac, bruising or petechiae, mucosa or orifices q8h

• Food preferences; list likes, dislikes

• Inflammation of mucosa, breaks in skin

• Yellowing of skin, sclera, dark urine, clay-colored stools, itchy skin, abdominal pain, fever, diarrhea

• Buccal cavity q8h for dryness, sores, ulceration, white patches, oral pain, bleeding, dysphagia

• Symptoms indicating severe allergic reaction: rash, pruritus, urticaria, itching, flushing

Teach patient/family:

• Of protective isolation precautions

• That azoospermia or amenorrhea can occur; reversible after discontinuing treatment

• To avoid foods with citric acid, hot or rough texture

• To report any bleeding, white spots or ulcerations in mouth to physician, tell patient to examine mouth qd

• To report signs of infection: increased temperature, sore throat, flu symptoms

• To report signs of anemia: fatigue, headache, faintness, shortness of breath, irritability

• To avoid use of razors or commercial mouthwash

---

* Available in Canada only

- To avoid use of aspirin products or ibuprofen

---

thiothixene

(thye-oh-thix'een)
Navane

Func. class.: Antipsychotic/neuroleptic
Chem. class.: Thioxanthene

Action: Depresses cerebral cortex, hypothalamus, limbic system, which control activity, aggression; blocks neurotransmission produced by dopamine at synapse; exhibits strong α-adrenergic blocking action; mechanism for antipsychotic effects is unclear

Uses: Psychotic disorders, schizophrenia, acute agitation

Dosage and routes:
- *Adult:* PO 2-5 mg bid-qid depending on severity of condition; dose is gradually increased to 15-30 mg if needed; IM 4 mg bid-qid, max dose is 30 mg qd; administer PO dose as soon as possible

Available forms include: Caps 1, 2, 5, 10, 20 mg; conc 5 mg/ml; inj IM 2 mg/ml; powder for inj 5 mg/ml

Side effects/adverse reactions:
RESP: ***Laryngospasm,*** dyspnea, ***respiratory depression***
CNS: Extrapyramidal symptoms: pseudoparkinsonism, akathisia, dystonia, tardive dyskinesia, seizures, *headache*
HEMA: Anemia, ***leukopenia, leukocytosis, agranulocytosis***
INTEG: Rash, photosensitivity, dermatitis
EENT: Blurred vision, glaucoma
GI: Dry mouth, nausea, vomiting, anorexia, constipation, diarrhea, jaundice, weight gain
GU: Urinary retention, urinary frequency, enuresis, impotence, amenorrhea, gynecomastia
CV: Orthostatic hypotension, hypertension, ***cardiac arrest,*** ECG changes, ***tachycardia***

Contraindications: Hypersensitivity, blood dyscrasias, child <12 yr, bone marrow depression, circulatory collapse, CNS depression, coma, alcoholism, CV disease, hepatic disease, Reye's syndrome

Precautions: Pregnancy (C), lactation, seizure disorders, hypertension, hepatic disease

Pharmacokinetics:
PO: Onset slow, peak 2-8 hr, duration up to 12 hr
IM: Onset 15-30 min, peak 1-6 hr, duration up to 12 hr
Metabolized by liver, excreted in urine, crosses placenta, enters breast milk, half-life 34 hr

Interactions/incompatibilities:
- Oversedation: other CNS depressants, alcohol, barbiturate anesthetics
- Toxicity: epinephrine
- Decreased absorption: aluminum hydroxide or magnesium hydroxide antacids
- Decreased effects of thiothixene: lithium, levodopa
- Increased effects of both drugs: β-adrenergic blockers, alcohol
- Increased anticholinergic effects: anticholinergics

NURSING CONSIDERATIONS
Assess:
- Swallowing of PO medication; check for hoarding or giving of medication to other patients
- I&O ratio, palpate bladder if low urinary output occurs
- Bilirubin, CBC, liver function studies monthly
- Urinalysis is recommended before and during prolonged therapy

---

italics = common side effects   ***bold italic*** = life threatening reactions

Administer:
• Antiparkinsonian agent, after securing order from physician to be used if EPS occur
• Concentrate mixed in citrus juices or distilled or acidified tap water
• IM injection into large muscle mass

Perform/provide:
• Decreased noise input by dimming lights, avoiding loud noises
• Supervised ambulation until stabilized on medication; do not involve in strenuous exercise program because fainting is possible; patient should not stand still for long periods of time
• Increased fluids to prevent constipation
• Sips of water, candy, gum for dry mouth
• Storage in tight, light-resistant container; place reconstituted solutions at room temperature for up to 48 hr

Evaluate:
• Therapeutic response: decrease in emotional excitement, hallucinations, delusions, paranoia, reorganization of patterns of thought, speech
• Affect, orientation, LOC, reflexes, gait, coordination, sleep pattern disturbances
• B/P standing and lying; also include pulse and respirations q4h during initial treatment; establish baseline before starting treatment; report drops of 30 mm Hg
• Dizziness, faintness, palpitations, tachycardia on rising
• EPS including akathisia (inability to sit still, no pattern to movements), tardive dyskinesia (bizarre movements of jaw, mouth, tongue, extremities), pseudoparkinsonism (rigidity, tremors, pill rolling, shuffling gait)
• For neuroleptic malignant syndrome: muscle rigidity, altered mental status, increased CPK, hyperthermia
• Constipation, urinary retention daily; if these occur, increase bulk, water in diet

Teach patient/family:
• That orthostatic hypotension occurs frequently, and to rise from sitting or lying position gradually
• To remain lying down after IM inj for at least 30 min
• To avoid hot tubs, hot showers, or tub baths since hypotension may occur
• To avoid abrupt withdrawal of this drug or EPS may result; drugs should be withdrawn slowly
• To avoid OTC preparations (cough, hayfever, cold) unless approved by physician since serious drug interactions may occur; avoid use with alcohol or CNS depressants, increased drowsiness may occur
• To use a sunscreen during sun exposure to prevent burns
• Regarding compliance with drug regimen
• About EPS and necessity for meticulous oral hygiene since oral candidiasis may occur
• To report sore throat, malaise, fever, bleeding, mouth sores; if these occur, CBC should be drawn and drug discontinued
• In hot weather, heat stroke may occur; take extra precautions to stay cool

Lab test interferences:
Increase: Liver function tests, cardiac enzymes, cholesterol, blood glucose, prolactin, bilirubin, PBI, cholinesterase, ^{131}I
Decrease: Uric acid

Treatment of overdose: Lavage if orally injested, provide an airway; *do not induce vomiting*

thrombin

Thrombinar, Thrombostat
Func. class.: Hemostatic
Chem. class.: Bovine thrombin

Action: Converts fibrinogen to fibrin, promotes clotting
Uses: GI hemorrhage, bleeding in dental, plastic, nasal, laryngeal surgery, skin grafting
Dosage and routes:
• *Adult:* TOP apply 100 U/1 ml sterile isotonic NaCl or distilled water in light to moderate bleeding, or 1000-2000 U/ml sterile isotonic NaCl in severe bleeding. Dry area before applying
Available forms include: Powder 1000, 5000, 10,000, 20,000, 50,000 U
Side effects/adverse reactions:
INTEG: Rash, allergic reactions
*HEMA: **Intravascular clotting when entering large blood vessels***
Contraindications: Hypersensitivity to bovine products
Precautions: Pregnancy (C)
NURSING CONSIDERATIONS
Administer:
• Only to area sponged free of blood
• After preparing with NS, isotonic saline
• After having blood available for transfusion
Perform/provide:
• Storage in refrigerator, use reconstituted solution within 3 hr, discard unused portion
Evaluate:
• For allergic reactions: fever, rash, itching, changes in VS; thrombosis formation

thyroglobulin

(thye-roe-glob'yoo-lin)
Proloid
Func. class.: Thyroid hormone
Chem. class.: Combination of natural T_4/T_3; ratio 2.5 to 1

Action: Increases metabolic rates, increases cardiac output, O_2 consumption, body temperature, blood volume, growth, development at cellular level
Uses: Hypothyroidism
Dosage and routes:
Hypothyroidism
Adult: 32 mg/day increasing q2-3 wks to desired response; maintenance 65-200 mg/day
Available forms include: Tabs 32, 65, 100, 130, 200 mg
Side effects/adverse reactions:
INTEG: Sweating, alopecia
CNS: Anxiety, insomnia, tremors, headache, heat intolerance, fever, coma, thyroid storm
CV: Tachycardia, palpitations, angina, dysrhythmias, hypertension, CHF
GI: Nausea, diarrhea, increased or decreased appetite, cramps
GU: Menstrual irregularities
Contraindications: Adrenal insufficiency, myocardial infarction, thyrotoxicosis
Precautions: Elderly, angina pectoris, hypertension, ischemia, cardiac disease, pregnancy (A), lactation
Pharmacokinetics:
PO: Peak 12-48 hr, half-life 6-7 days
Interactions/incompatibilities:
• Decreased absorption of thyroglobulin: cholestyramine
• Increased effects of: anticoagulants, sympathomimetics, tricyclic

T

---

italics = common side effects　　　　***bold italic*** = life threatening reactions

antidepressants, catecholamines
• Decreased effects of: digitalis drugs, insulin, hypoglycemics
• Decreased effects of liothyronine: estrogens

NURSING CONSIDERATIONS
Assess:
• B/P, pulse before each dose
• I&O ratio
• Weight qd in same clothing, using same scale, at same time of day
• Height, growth rate if given to a child
• T₃, T₄, which are decreased, radioimmunoassay of TSH, which is increased, radio uptake, which is decreased if patient is on too low a dose of medication
• Pro-time may require decreased anticoagulant, check for bleeding, bruising

Administer:
• In AM if possible as a single dose to decrease sleeplessness
• At same time each day to maintain drug level
• Only for hormone imbalances, not to be used for obesity, male infertility, menstrual conditions, lethargy
• Lowest dose that relieves symptoms

Perform/provide:
• Removal of medication 4 wk before RAIU test

Evaluate:
• Therapeutic response: absence of depression, increased weight loss, diuresis, pulse, appetite, absence of constipation, peripheral edema, cold intolerance, pale, cool dry skin, brittle nails, alopecia, coarse hair, menorrhagia, night blindness, paresthesias, syncope, stupor, coma, rosy cheeks
• Increased nervousness, excitability, irritability, which may indicate

too high dose of medication usually after 1-3 wk of treatment
• Cardiac status: angina, palpitation, chest pain, change in VS

Teach patient/family:
• To report excitability, irritability, anxiety, which indicate overdose
• Not to switch brands unless approved by physician
• That hypothyroid child will show almost immediate behavior/personality change
• That drug is not to be taken to reduce weight
• To avoid OTC preparations with iodine, read labels
• To avoid iodine food, salt iodinized, soy beans, tofu, turnips, some seafood, some bread

Lab test interferences:
Increase: CPK, LDH, AST, PBI, blood glucose
Decrease: TSH, ¹³¹I uptake test, uric acid, triglycerides

---

thyroid USP (desiccated)
(thye-roid)
Armour Thyroid, Cholaxin,* S-P-T, Thyrar, Thyro-Teric, Thyroid Serone, Thyroid USP Enseals

Func. class.: Thyroid hormone
Chem. class.: Active thyroid hormone in natural state and ratio

---

Action: Increases metabolic rates, increases cardiac output, O₂ consumption, body temperature, blood volume, growth, development at cellular level
Uses: Hypothyroidism, cretinism, myxedema
Dosage and routes:
Hypothyroidism
• *Adult:* PO 65 mg qd, increased by 65 mg q30 days until desired response, maintenance dose 65-195 mg qd

---

*Available in Canada only

- *Geriatric:* PO 7.5-15 mg qd, double dose q6-8 wk until desired response

Cretinism/juvenile hypothyroidism
- *Child over 1 yr:* PO up to 180 mg qd titrated to response
- *Child 4-12 mo:* PO 30-60 mg qd
- *Child 1-4 mo:* PO 15-30 mg qd, may increase q2 wk, titrated to response, maintenance dose 30-45 mg qd

Myxedema
- *Adult:* PO 16 mg qd, double dose q2 wk, maintenance 65-195 mg/ day

Available forms include: Tabs 16, 32, 65, 98, 130, 195, 260, 325 mg; tabs enteric coated 32, 65, 130 mg; sugar-coated tabs 32, 65, 130, 195 mg; caps 65, 130, 195, 325 mg

Side effects/adverse reactions:
CNS: Insomnia, tremors, headache, thyroid storm
CV: Tachycardia, palpitations, angina, dysrhythmias, hypertension, **cardiac arrest**
GI: Nausea, diarrhea, increased or decreased appetite, cramps
MISC: Menstrual irregularities, weight loss, sweating, heat intolerance, fever

Contraindications: Adrenal insufficiency, myocardial infarction, thyrotoxicosis

Precautions: Elderly, angina pectoris, hypertension, ischemia, cardiac disease, pregnancy (A), lactation

Pharmacokinetics:
PO: Peak 12-48 hr, half-life 6-7 days

Interactions/incompatibilities:
- Decreased absorption of thyroid: cholestyramine
- Increased effects of: anticoagulants, sympathomimetics, tricyclic antidepressants, catecholamines

- Decreased effects of: digitalis drugs, insulin, hypoglycemics
- Decreased effects of thyroid: estrogens

NURSING CONSIDERATIONS
Assess:
- B/P, pulse before each dose
- I&O ratio
- Weight qd in same clothing, using same scale, at same time of day
- Height, growth rate if given to a child
- T_3, T_4, which are decreased, radioimmunoassay of TSH, which is increased, radio uptake, which is decreased if patient is on too low a dose of medication
- Pro-time may require decreased anticoagulant, check for bleeding, bruising

Administer:
- In AM if possible as a single dose to decrease sleeplessness
- At same time each day to maintain drug level
- Only for hormone imbalances, not to be used for obesity, male infertility, menstrual conditions, lethargy
- Lowest dose that relieves symptoms

Perform/provide:
- Removal of medication 4 wk before RAIU test

Evaluate:
- Therapeutic response: absence of depression, increased weight loss, diuresis, pulse, appetite, absence of constipation, peripheral edema, cold intolerance, pale, cool dry skin, brittle nails, alopecia, coarse hair, menorrhagia, night blindness, paresthesias, syncope, stupor, coma, rosy cheeks
- Increased nervousness, excitability, irritability, may indicate too high dose of medication usually after 1-3 wk of treatment

T

---

italics = common side effects   ***bold italic*** = life threatening reactions

• Cardiac status: angina, palpitation, chest pain, change in VS
Teach patient/family:
• That hair loss will occur in child, is temporary
• To report excitability, irritability, anxiety; indicates overdose
• Not to switch brands unless directed by physician
• That hypothyroid child will show almost immediate behavior/personality change
• That treatment drug is not to be taken to reduce weight
• To avoid OTC preparations with iodine; read labels
• To avoid iodine food, salt-iodinized, soy beans, tofu, turnips, some seafood, some bread
Lab test interferences:
Increase: CPK, LDH, AST, PBI, blood glucose
Decrease: TSH, ^{131}I uptake test, uric acid, triglycerides

---

thyrotropin (thyroid-stimulating hormone, or TSH)

(thye-roe-troe'pin)
Thytropar
Func. class.: Thyroid hormone
Chem. class.: TSH

Action: Increases uptake of iodine by thyroid gland, increases production of thyroid hormone, increases release of thyroid hormone
Uses: Diagnosis of thyroid cancer, diagnosis of primary/secondary hypothyroidism
Dosage and routes:
Diagnosis of hypothyroidism
• *Adult:* IM/SC 10 Units qd × 1-3 days
Diagnosis of thyroid cancer
• *Adult:* IM/SC 10 IU qd × 3-7 days

Treatment of thyroid cancer
• *Adult:* IM/SC 10 Units qd × 3-8 days
Available forms include: Powder for inj 10 IU/vial
Side effects/adverse reactions:
INTEG: Urticaria
CNS: Headache, fever
CV: Tachycardia, angina, *atrial fibrillation, CHF,* hypotension
GI: Nausea, vomiting
SYST: **Anaphylactic reactions**
Contraindications: Hypersensitivity, coronary thrombosis, untreated Addison's Disease
Precautions: Angina pectoris, adrenal insufficiency, pregnancy (C), lactation, children
Pharmacokinetics:
IM/SC: Onset 8 hr, peak 24-48 hr
NURSING CONSIDERATIONS
Administer:
• After dilution with 2 ml sterile saline solution
• Three-day dose schedule for myxedema (pituitary)
• In combination with ^{131}I to treat thyroid cancer
Treatment of overdose: Discontinue drug, administer supportive care

---

ticarcillin disodium

(tye-kar-sill'in)
Ticaripen,* Ticar
Func. class.: Broad-spectrum antibiotic
Chem. class.: Extended-spectrum penicillin

Action: Interferes with cell wall replication of susceptible organisms; osmotically unstable cell wall swells, bursts from osmotic pressure.
Uses: Respiratory, soft tissue, urinary tract infections, bacterial sep-

---

ticemia; effective for gram-positive cocci *(S. aureus, S. faecalis, S. pneumoniae)*, gram-negative cocci *(N. gonorrhoeae)*, gram-positive bacilli *(C. perfringens, C. tetani)*, gram-negative bacilli *(Bacteroides, F. nucleatum, E. coli, P. mirabilis, Salmonella, M. morganii, P. rettgeri, Enterobacter, P. aeruginosa, Serratia, Peptococcus, Peptostreptococcus, Eubacterium)*

Dosage and routes:
• *Adult:* IV/IM 12-24 g/day in divided doses q3-6h, infuse over ½-2 hr
• *Child:* IV/IM 50-300 mg/kg/day in divided doses q4-8h
• *Neonates:* IV INF 75-100 mg/kg/8-12 hr
Available forms include: Inj IM, IV 1, 3, 6, 20, 30 g, IV INF 3 g

Side effects/adverse reactions:
HEMA: Anemia, increased bleeding time, ***bone marrow depression, granulocytopenia***
GI:Nausea, vomiting, diarrhea, increased AST, ALT, abdominal pain, glossitis, colitis
GU: Oliguria, proteinuria, hematuria, *vaginitis, moniliasis, **glomerulonephritis***
CNS: Lethargy, hallucinations, anxiety, depression, twitching, ***coma, convulsions***
META: Hypokalemia

Contraindications: Hypersensitivity to penicillins

Precautions: Hypersensitivity to cephalosporins, pregnancy (B)

Pharmacokinetics:
IM: Peak 1 hr, duration 4-6 hr
IV: Peak 30-45 min, duration 4 hr, Half-life 70 min, small amount metabolized in liver, excreted in urine, breast milk

Interactions/incompatibilities:
• Decreased antimicrobial effect of

ticarcillin: tetracyclines, erythromycins, aminoglycosides IV
• Increased ticarcillin concentrations: aspirin, probenecid

NURSING CONSIDERATIONS
Assess:
• I&O ratio; report hematuria, oliguria since penicillin in high doses is nephrotoxic
• Any patient with compromised renal system since drug is excreted slowly in poor renal system function; toxicity may occur rapidly
• Liver studies: AST, ALT
• Blood studies: WBC, RBC, H&H, bleeding time
• Renal studies: urinalysis, protein, blood
• C&S before drug therapy; drug may be taken as soon as culture is taken

Administer:
• IV after diluting 1 g or less/4 ml sterile H_2O for inj; dilute further with 10-20 ml or more compatible sol; give 1 g or less/5 min or more or by intermittent INF over ½-2 hr or by continuous INF
• Drug after C&S has been completed

Perform/provide:
• Adrenalin, suction, tracheostomy set, endotracheal intubation equipment
• Adequate fluid intake (2000 ml) during diarrhea episodes
• Scratch test to assess allergy, after securing order from physician; usually done when penicillin is only drug of choice
• Storage at room temperature, reconstituted solution for 72 hr at room temperature

Evaluate:
• Therapeutic effectiveness: absence of fever, purulent drainage, redness, inflammation

T

---

italics = common side effects   ***bold italic*** = life threatening reactions

• Bowel pattern before, during treatment
• Skin eruptions after administration of penicillin to 1 wk after discontinuing drug
• Respiratory status: rate, character, wheezing, tightness in chest
• Allergies before initiation of treatment, reaction of each medication; highlight allergies on chart, Kardex

Teach patient/family:
• That culture may be taken after completed course of medication
• To report sore throat, fever, fatigue (could indicate superimposed infection)
• To wear or carry Medic Alert ID if allergic to penicillins
• To notify nurse of diarrhea

Lab test interferences:
False positive: Urine glucose, urine protein

Treatment of overdose: Withdraw drug, maintain airway, administer epinephrine, aminophylline, O_2, IV corticosteroids for anaphylaxis

---

ticarcillin disodium/ clavulanate potassium
Timentin

Func. class.: Broad-spectrum antibiotic
Chem. class.: Extended-spectrum penicillin

Action: Interferes with cell wall replication of susceptible organisms; osmotically unstable cell wall swells, bursts from osmotic pressure

Uses: Respiratory, soft tissue, and urinary tract infections, bacterial septicemia; effective for gram-positive cocci (*S. aureus, S. faecalis,*

S. pneumoniae), gram-negative cocci (*N. gonorrhoeae*), gram-positive bacilli (*C. perfringens, C. tetani*), gram-negative bacilli (*Bacteroides, F. nucleatum, E. coli, P. mirabilis, Salmonella, M. morganii, P. rettgeri, Enterobacter, P. aeruginosa, Serratia, Peptococcus, Peptostreptococcus, Eubacterium*)

Dosage and routes:
• *Adult:* IV INF 1 vial containing ticarcillin 3 g, clavulanate potassium 0.1 g q4-6h, infuse over 30 min
• *Child <60 kg:* 200-300 mg ticarcillin/kg/day in divided doses q4-6h

Available forms include: Inj IM, IV 3 g ticarcillin and 0.1g clavulanate; IV INF 3 g ticarcillin and 0.1 g clavulanate

Side effects/adverse reactions:
HEMA: Anemia, increased bleeding time, **bone marrow depression, granulocytopenia**
GI: Nausea, vomiting, diarrhea, increased AST, ALT, abdominal pain, glossitis, colitis
GU: Oliguria, proteinuria, hematuria, *vaginitis, moniliasis,* **glomerulonephritis**
CNS: Lethargy, hallucinations, anxiety, depression, twitching, **coma, convulsions**
META: Hyperkalemia, hypokalemia, alkalosis, hypernatremia

Contraindications: Hypersensitivity to penicillins; neonates
Precautions: Hypersensitivity to cephalosporins, pregnancy (B)

Pharmacokinetics:
IV: Peak 30-45 min, duration 4 hr, half-life 64-68 min

Interactions/incompatibilities:
• Decreased antimicrobial effect of ticarcillin: tetracyclines, erythromycins, aminoglycosides IV

• Increased ticarcillin concentrations: aspirin, probenecid

NURSING CONSIDERATIONS
Assess:
• I&O ratio; report hematuria, oliguria since penicillin in high doses is nephrotoxic
• Any patient with compromised renal system, since drug is excreted slowly in poor renal system function; toxicity may occur rapidly
• Liver studies: AST, ALT
• Blood studies: WBC, RBC, H&H, bleeding time
• Renal studies: urinalysis, protein, blood
• C&S before drug therapy; drug may be taken as soon as culture is taken

Administer:
• IV after diluting 3.1 g or less/13 ml of sterile H₂O or NaCl, shake; may further dilute in 50-100 ml or more compatible sol and run over ½ hr
• Drug after C&S has been completed

Perform/provide:
• Adrenalin, suction, tracheostomy set, endotracheal intubation equipment
• Adequate fluid intake (2000 ml) during diarrhea episodes
• Scratch test to assess allergy, after securing order from physician; usually done when penicillin is only drug of choice
• Storage at room temperature, reconstituted solution for 12-24 hr or 3-7 days refrigerated

Evaluate:
• Therapeutic effectiveness: absence of fever, purulent drainage, redness, inflammation
• Bowel pattern before, during treatment
• Skin eruptions after administra-

tion of penicillin to 1 wk after discontinuing drug
• Respiratory status: rate, character, wheezing, and tightness in chest
• Allergies before initiation of treatment, reaction of each medication; highlight allergies on chart, Kardex

Teach patient/family:
• That culture may be taken after completed course of medication
• To report sore throat, fever, fatigue (could indicate superimposed infection)
• To wear or carry Medic Alert ID if allergic to penicillins

Lab test interferences:
False positive: Urine glucose, urine protein

Treatment of overdose: Withdraw drug, maintain airway, administer epinephrine, aminophylline, O₂, IV corticosteroids for anaphylaxis

---

timolol maleate
(tye′moe-lole)
Blocadren
Func. class.: Antihypertensive
Chem. class.: Nonselective β-blocker

Action: Competitively blocks stimulation of β-adrenergic receptor within vascular smooth muscle; produces chronotropic, inotropic activity (decreases rate of SA node discharge, increases recovery time), slows conduction of AV node, decreases heart rate, which decreases O₂ consumption in myocardium; also, decreases renin-aldosterone-angiotensin system, at high doses inhibits β-2 receptors in bronchial system
Uses: Mild to moderate hyperten-

italics = common side effects   ***bold italic*** = life threatening reactions

sion, sinus tachycardia, persistent atrial extrasystoles, tachydysrhythmias, prophylaxis of angina pectoris, reduction of mortality after MI

Dosage and routes:
Hypertension
• *Adult:* PO 10 mg bid, or 100 mg qd, may increase by 10 mg q2-3 days, not to exceed 60 mg/day
Myocardial infarction
• *Adult:* 10 mg bid
Available forms include: Tabs 5, 10, 20 mg

Side effects/adverse reactions:
CV: Hypotension, bradycardia, **CHF,** edema, chest pain, bradycardia, claudication
CNS: Insomnia, dizziness, hallucinations, anxiety
GI: Nausea, vomiting, ***ischemic colitis,*** diarrhea, *abdominal pain,* ***mesenteric arterial thrombosis***
INTEG: Rash, alopecia, pruritus, fever
HEMA: ***Agranulocytosis, thrombocytopenia, purpura***
EENT: Visual changes, sore throat, *double vision,* dry burning eyes
GU: Impotence, frequency
RESP: ***Bronchospasm,*** *dyspnea,* cough, rales
META: Hypoglycemia
MUSC: Joint pain, muscle pain

Contraindications: Hypersensitivity to β-blockers, cardiogenic shock, heart block (2nd, 3rd degree), sinus bradycardia, CHF, cardiac failure

Precautions: Major surgery, pregnancy (C), lactation, diabetes mellitus, renal disease, thyroid disease, COPD, well compensated heart failure, CAD, nonallergic bronchospasm

Pharmacokinetics:
PO: Peak 2-4 hr; half-life 3-4 hr, excreted 30%-45% unchanged, 60%-65% is metabolized by liver, excreted in breast milk

Interactions/incompatibilities:
• Increased hypotension, bradycardia: reserpine, hydralazine, methyldopa, prazosin, anticholinergics
• Decreased antihypertensive effects: idomethacin
• Increased hypoglycemic effects: insulin
• Decreased bronchodilation: theophyllines

NURSING CONSIDERATIONS
Assess:
• I&O, weight daily
• B/P during initial treatment, periodically thereafter, pulse q4h; note rate, rhythm, quality
• Apical/radial pulse before administration; notify physician of any significant changes
• Baselines in renal, liver function tests before therapy begins

Administer:
• PO ac, hs, tablet may be crushed or swallowed whole
• Reduced dosage in renal dysfunction

Perform/provide:
• Storage in dry area at room temperature, do not freeze

Evaluate:
• Therapeutic response: decreased B/P after 1-2 wk
• Edema in feet, legs daily
• Skin turgor, dryness of mucous membranes for hydration status

Teach patient/family:
• To take with or immediately after meals
• Not to discontinue drug abruptly, taper over 2 wk, may cause precipitate angina
• Not to use OTC products containing α-adrenergic stimulants (nasal decongestants, cold prepa-

rations) unless directed by physician

• To report bradycardia, dizziness, confusion, depression, fever, sore throat, shortness of breath to physician

• To take pulse at home, advise when to notify physician

• To avoid alcohol, smoking, sodium intake

• To comply with weight control, dietary adjustments, modified exercise program

• To carry Medic Alert ID to identify drug you are taking, allergies

• To avoid hazardous activities if dizziness is present

• To report symptoms of CHF: difficult breathing, especially on exertion or when lying down, night cough, swelling of extremities

• To take medication hs to maintain effect of orthostatic hypotension

• To wear support hose to minimize effects of orthostatic hypotension

Lab test interferences:
Increase: Liver function tests, renal function tests, K, uric acid
Decrease: Hct, Hgb, HDL

Treatment of overdose: Lavage, IV atropine for bradycardia, IV theophylline for bronchospasm, digitalis, O₂, diuretic for cardiac failure, hemodialysis, administer vasopressor (norepinephrine)

---

timolol maleate (optic)
(tye′moe-lole)
Timoptic Solution
Func. class.: β-Adrenergic blocker
Chem. class.: I-isomer

Action: Reduces production of aqueous humor by unknown mechanism
Uses: Ocular hypertension, chronic open-angle glaucoma, secondary glaucoma, aphakic glaucoma

Dosage and routes:
• *Adult:* INSTILL 1 gtt of 0.25% sol in affected eye(s) bid, then 1 gtt for maintenance, may increase to 1 gtt of 0.5% sol bid if needed
Available forms include: Sol 0.25%, 0.5%

Side effects/adverse reactions:
CNS: Weakness, fatigue, depression, anxiety, headache, confusion
GI: Nausea, anorexia, dyspepsia
EENT: Eye irritation, conjunctivitis, keratitis
INTEG: Rash, urticaria
CV: Bradycardia, hypotension, dysrhythmias

Contraindications: Hypersensitivity, asthma, 2nd/3rd degree heart block, right ventricular failure, congenital glaucoma (infants), COPD

Pharmacokinetics:
INSTILL: Onset 15-30 min, peak 1-2 h, duration 24 hr

Interactions/incompatibilities:
• Toxicity: β-adrenergic blockers
• Increased effect: propranolol, metoprolol

NURSING CONSIDERATIONS
Teach patient/family:
• To report change in vision, with blurring or loss of sight, trouble breathing, sweating, flushing, since systemic absorption may occur
• Method of instillation, including pressure on lacrimal sac for 1 min, and not to touch dropper to eye
• That long-term therapy may be required
• That blurred vision will decrease with continued use of drug

T

---

italics = common side effects   ***bold italic*** = life threatening reactions

tiopronin

(tye-o-pro'-nen)
Thiola
Func. class.: Orphan drug
Chem. class.: Active reducing, complexing thiol compound

Action: Prevents cystine (kidney) stone formation by increasing amount of water-soluble cystine
Uses: Prevention of kidney stone formation in patients with severe homozygous cystinuria with urinary cystine greater than 500 mg/day, who are resistant to conservative treatment
Dosage and routes:
• *Adult:* PO 800-1000 mg/day, given in divided doses tid at least 1 hr before or 2 hr after meals
• *Child:* PO 15 mg/kg/day, given in divided doses tid at least 1 hr before or 2 hr after meals
Available forms include: Tabs 100 mg
Side effects/adverse reactions:
MISC: Blunting of taste
INTEG: Erythema, maculopapular rash, wrinkling skin, lupus-like syndrome (fever, arthralgia, lymphadenopathy), pruritus
CNS: Drug fever
META: Vitamin B_6 deficiency
Contraindications: History of agranulocytosis, thrombocytopenia, aplastic anemia
Precautions: Pregnancy (C), lactation, myasthenia gravis, Goodpasture's syndrome, children <9 yr
Pharmacokinetics:
Reduction of urinary cystine of 250-500 mg on 1-2 g/day may be expected; excreted in urine 78% in 3 days
NURSING CONSIDERATIONS
Assess:
• I&O during treatment, check urine for stones, strain all urine, keep output at 2 L/day
• Diet for alkaline foods: dairy products, prevent overindulgence of sodium alkali foods since hypercalcinuria results
• Urine pH, notify physician of pH over 7
• Urinary cystine 1 mo after treatment, q3 mo thereafter
Administer:
• After adequate hydration, conservative treatment: 3 L/day of fluid, 16 oz of fluid at meals and hs
Perform/provide:
• Storage at room temperature
Evaluate:
• Therapeutic response: decrease in urinary cystine to <250 mg/L, absence of pain or hematuria
Teach patient/family:
• To watch for lupuslike syndrome: fever, joint pain, swollen lymph glands; drug may need to be discontinued

tobramycin (ophthalmic)

(toe-bra-mye'sin)
Nebcin, Tobrex
Func. class.: Antiinfective
Chem. class.: Aminoglycoside

Action: Inhibits bacterial protein synthesis
Uses: Infection of eye
Dosage and routes:
• *Adult and child:* INSTILL 1-2 gtts q1-4h depending on infection; OINT: 1 cm bid-tid
Available forms include: Oint 0.3%; sol 0.3%
Side effects/adverse reactions:
EENT: Poor corneal wound healing, visual haze, (temporary), overgrowth of nonsusceptible organisms

---

* Available in Canada only

Contraindications: Hypersensitivity

Precautions: Antibiotic hypersensitivity, pregnancy (D)

NURSING CONSIDERATIONS
Administer:
• After washing hands, cleanse crusts or discharge from eye before application
• Apply pressure on lacrimal sac for 1 min

Perform/provide:
• Storage at room temperature

Evaluate:
• Therapeutic response: absence of redness, inflammation, tearing
• Allergy: itching, lacrimation, redness, swelling

Teach patient/family:
• To use drug exactly as prescribed
• Not to use eye make-up, towels, washcloths, or eye medication of others, or reinfection may occur
• That drug container tip should not be touched to eye
• To report itching, increased redness, burning, stinging; drug should be discontinued
• That drug may cause blurred vision when ointment is applied

---

tobramycin sulfate
(toe-bra-mye′sin)
Nebcin
Func. class.: Antibiotic
Chem. class.: Aminoglycoside

Action: Interferes with protein synthesis in bacterial cell by binding to ribosomal subunit, causing inaccurate peptide sequence to form in protein chain, causing bacterial death

Uses: Severe systemic infections of CNS, respiratory, GI, urinary tract, bone, skin, soft tissues caused by *P. aeruginosa, E. coli, Enterobac-*

ter, Providencia, Citrobacter, Staphylococcus, Proteus, Klebsiella, Serratia

Dosage and routes:
• *Adult:* IM/IV 3 mg/kg/day in divided doses q8h; may give up to 5 mg/kg/day in divided doses q6-8h
• *Child:* IM/IV 6-7.5 mg/kg/day in 3-4 equally divided doses
• *Neonates <1 wk:* IM up to 4 mg/kg/day in divided doses q12h; IV up to 4 mg/kg/day in divided doses q12h diluted in 50-100 mg NS or D₅W; give over 30-60 min

Available forms include: Inj IM, IV 10, 40 mg/ml; powder for inj 1.2 g; inj 20 mg/2 ml

Side effects/adverse reactions:
GU: Oliguria, hematuria, renal damage, azotemia, renal failure, nephrotoxicity
CNS: Confusion, depression, numbness, tremors, *convulsions,* muscle twitching, *neurotoxicity*
EENT: Ototoxicity, deafness, visual disturbances
HEMA: Agranulocytosis, thrombocytopenia, leukopenia, eosinophilia, anemia
GI: Nausea, vomiting, anorexia, increased ALT, AST, bilirubin, hepatomegaly, *hepatic necrosis,* splenomegaly
CV: Hypotension, myocarditis
INTEG: Rash, burning, urticaria, photosensitivity, dermatitis

Contraindications: Severe renal disease, hypersensitivity to aminoglycosides

Precautions: Neonates, mild renal disease, pregnancy (D), myasthenia gravis, lactation, hearing deficits

Pharmacokinetics:
IM: Onset rapid, peak 1-2 hr
IV: Onset immediate, peak 1-2 hr
Plasma half-life 1-3 hr, not metabolized, excreted unchanged in urine, crosses placental barrier

---

italics = common side effects   ***bold italic*** = life threatening reactions

Interactions/incompatibilities:

• Increased ototoxicity, neurotoxicity, nephrotoxicity: other aminoglycosides, amphotericin B, polymyxin, vancomycin, ethacrynic acid, furosemide, mannitol, methoxyflurane, cisplatin, cephalosporins

• Decreased effects of: parenteral penicillins

• Do not mix in solution or syringe: carbenicillin, ticarcillin, amphotericin B, cephalothin, erythromycin, heparin

• Increased effects: nondepolarizing muscle relaxants

NURSING CONSIDERATIONS
Assess:

• Weight before treatment; calculation of dosage is usually done based on ideal body weight, but may be calculated on actual body weight

• I&O ratio, urinalysis daily for proteinuria, cells, casts; report sudden change in urine output

• VS during infusion, watch for hypotension, change in pulse

• IV site for thrombophlebitis including pain, redness, swelling q30 min, change site if needed; apply warm compresses to discontinued site

• Serum peak, drawn at 30-60 min after IV infusion or 60 min after IM injection, trough level drawn just before next dose; blood level should be 2-4 times bacteriostatic level

• Urine pH if drug is used for UTI; urine should be kept alkaline

Administer:

• IV diluted in 50-100 ml NS or D_5W (adult), infuse over 20-60 min

• IM injection in large muscle mass, rotate injection sites

• Drug in evenly spaced doses to maintain blood level

• Bicarbonate to alkalinize urine if ordered in treating UTI, as drug is most active in an alkaline environment

Perform/provide:

• Adequate fluids of 2-3 L/day unless contraindicated to prevent irritation of tubules

• Flush of IV line with NS or D_5W after infusion

• Supervised ambulation, other safety measures with vestibular dysfunction

Evaluate:

• Therapeutic effect: absence of fever, draining wounds, negative C&S after treatment

• Renal impairment by securing urine for CrCl testing, BUN, serum creatinine; lower dosage should be given in renal impairment (CrCl <80 ml/min)

• Deafness by audiometric testing, ringing, roaring in ears, vertigo; assess hearing before, during, after treatment

• Dehydration: high sp gr, decrease in skin turgor, dry mucous membranes, dark urine

• Overgrowth of infection: increased temperature, malaise, redness, pain, swelling, perineal itching, diarrhea, stomatitis, change in cough, sputum

• C&S before starting treatment to identify infecting organism

• Vestibular dysfunction: nausea, vomiting, dizziness, headache, drug should be discontinued if severe

• Injection sites for redness, swelling, abscesses; use warm compresses at site

Teach patient/family:

• To report headache, dizziness, symptoms of overgrowth of infection, renal impairment

• To report loss of hearing, ringing,

---

roaring in ears, feeling of fullness in head

Treatment of overdose: Hemodialysis, monitor serum levels of drug

---

tocainide HCl

(toe-kay′nide)
Tonocard
Func. class.: Antidysrhythmic (Class IB)
Chem. class.: Lidocaine analog

Action: Decreases sodium and potassium, resulting in decreased excitability of myocardial cells
Uses: PVCs, ventricular tachycardia
Dosage and routes:
• *Adult:* PO 400 mg q8h
Available forms include: Tabs 400, 600 mg
Side effects/adverse reactions:
CNS: Headache, dizziness, involuntary movement, confusion, psychosis, restlessness, irritability, paresthesias, tremors, *seizures*
EENT: Tinnitus, blurred vision, hearing loss
GI: Nausea, vomiting, anorexia, diarrhea, hepatitis
CV: Hypotension, bradycardia, angina, PVCs, *heart block, cardiovascular collapse, arrest, CHF,* chest pain, tachycardia
RESP: Dyspnea, *respiratory depression, pulmonary fibrosis*
INTEG: Rash, urticaria, edema, swelling
HEMA: Blood dyscrasias: leukopenia, agranulocytosis, hypoplastic anemia, thrombocytopenia
Contraindications: Hypersensitivity to amides, severe heart block
Precautions: Pregnancy (C), lactation, children, renal disease, liver disease, CHF, respiratory depression, myasthenia gravis, blood dyscrasias

Pharmacokinetics:
PO: Peak 0.5-3 hr; half-life 10-17 hr, metabolized by liver, excreted in urine
Interactions/incompatibilities:
• Increased effects: propranolol, quinidine and all other antidysrhythmics
NURSING CONSIDERATIONS
Assess:
• Chest x-ray, pulmonary function tests, liver enzymes during treatments
• CBC during beginning treatment
• I&O ratio; check for decreasing output
• Blood levels (therapeutic level 4-10 μg/ml)
• B/P continuously for fluctuations
• Lung fields, bilateral rales may occur in CHF patient
• Increased respiration, increased pulse; drug should be discontinued
Evaluate:
• Toxicity: fine tremors, dizziness
• Blood dyscrasias: fatigue, sore throat, fever, bruising, increased temperature
• Cardiac rate, respiration: rate, rhythm, character
Lab test interferences:
Increase: CPK
Positive: ANA titer
Treatment of overdose: O_2, artificial ventilation, ECG, administer dopamine for circulatory depression, administer diazepam or thiopental for convulsions

---

tolazamide

(tole-az′a-mide)
Ronase, Tolamide, Tolinase
Func. class.: Antidiabetic
Chem. class.: Sulfonylurea (1st generation)

Action: Causes functioning β-cells

in pancreas to release insulin, leading to drop in blood glucose levels; may improve binding to insulin receptors or increase the number of insulin receptors; this drug not effective if patient lacks functioning β-cells

Uses: Type II (NIDDM) diabetes mellitus

Dosage and routes:
• *Adult:* PO 100 mg/day for FBS <200 mg/dl or 250 mg/day for FBS >200 mg/dl; dose should be titrated to patient response (1 g or less/day)

Available forms include: Tabs 100, 250, 500 mg

Side effects/adverse reactions:
CNS: Headache, weakness, fatigue, lethargy, dizziness, vertigo, tinnitus

GI: Nausea, vomiting, diarrhea, constipation, gas, *hepatotoxicity, jaundice,* heartburn

HEMA: Leukopenia, thrombocytopenia, agranulocytosis, aplastic anemia, pancytopenia, hemolytic anemia

INTEG: Rash, (rare) allergic reactions, pruritus, urticaria, eczema, photo-sensitivity, erythema

ENDO: Hypoglycemia

Contraindications: Hypersensitivity to sulfonylureas, juvenile or brittle diabetes

Precautions: Pregnancy (C), elderly, cardiac disease, thyroid disease, severe hypoglycemic reactions, renal disease, hepatic disease

Pharmacokinetics:
PO: Completely absorbed by GI route; onset 4-6 hr, peak 4-8 hr, duration 12-24 hr; half-life 7 hr, metabolized in liver, excreted in urine (metabolites), breast milk, highly protein bound

Interactions/incompatibilities:
• Increased hypoglycemic reaction:

oral anticoagulants, chloramphenicol, cimetidine, MAOIs, insulin, guanethidine, methyldopa, nonsteroidal anti-inflammatories, salicylates, probenecid, sulfonamides, ranitidine
• Mask symptoms of hypoglycemia: β-blockers
• Decreased effects of both drugs: diazoxide
• Decreased action of tolazamide: calcium channel blockers, corticosteroids, oral contraceptives, thiazide diuretics, thyroid preparations, estrogens, phenothiazines, phenytoin, rifampin, isoniazide, phenobarbital, sympathomimetics
• Disulfiram-like reaction: alcohol

NURSING CONSIDERATIONS
Administer:
• Drug 30 min before meal

Perform/provide:
• Storage in tight container in cool environment

Evaluate:
• Therapeutic response: decrease in polyuria, polydipsia, polyphagia, clear sensorium, absence of dizziness, stable gait
• Hypoglycemic/hyperglycemic reaction that can occur soon after meals

Teach patient/family:
• To check for symptoms of cholestatic jaundice (dark urine, pruritus, yellow sclera); if these occur a physician should be notified
• To use a capillary blood glucose test while on this drug
• To test urine glucose levels with Chemstrip 3 × /day
• The symptoms of hypo/hyperglycemia, what to do about each
• That this drug must be continued on a daily basis; explain consequence of discontinuing drug abruptly
• To take drug in morning to pre-

vent hypoglycemic reactions at night
• To avoid OTC medications and alcohol unless prescribed by a physician
• That diabetes is a life-long illness, drug will not cure disease
• That all food included in diet plan must be eaten in order to prevent hypoglycemia
• To carry a Medic-Alert ID for emergency purposes
Treatment of overdose: 10%-50% glucose solution IV or 1 mg glucagon

tolazoline HCl

(toe-laz′a-leen)
Priscoline
Func. class.: Peripheral vasodilator
Chem. class.: Imidazoline derivative

Action: Peripheral vasodilation occurs by direct relaxation on vascular smooth muscle; also has weak α- and β-adrenergic properties
Uses: Persistent pulmonary hypertension of newborn
Dosage and routes:
• *Newborn:* IV 1-2 mg/kg via scalp vein; IV INF 1-2 mg/kg/hr
Available forms include: Inj SC, IM, IV 25 mg/ml
Side effects/adverse reactions:
CV: Orthostatic hypotension, tachycardia, dysrhythmias, hypertension, *cardiovascular collapse*
RESP: Pulmonary hemorrhage
GU: Edema, oliguria, hematuria
GI: Nausea, vomiting, diarrhea, peptic ulcer, *GI hemorrhage, hepatitis*
INTEG: Flushing, tingling, rash, chills, sweating, increased pilomotor activity

HEMA: Thrombocytopenia, leukopenia
Contraindications: Hypersensitivity, CVA, CAD
Precautions: Pregnancy (C), active peptic ulcer, lactation, mitral stenosis
Pharmacokinetics:
IM/SC: Peak 30-60 min, duration 3-4 hr, excreted in urine, half-life 3-10 hr
Interactions/incompatibilities:
• Increased effects with alcohol, β-blockers, antihypertensive
• Decrease B/P, rebound hypertension: epinephrine
• Do not mix in syringe or solution with any other drugs
NURSING CONSIDERATIONS
Assess:
• ABGs, electrolytes, VS in newborn
• B/P, pulse during treatment until stable; take B/P lying, standing; orthostatic hypotension is common
• Hepatic tests: AST, ALT, bilirubin; liver enzymes may increase
• Blood studies: CBC, platelets; watch for thrombocytopenia, agranulocytosis
Administer:
• IV undiluted, give 10 mg or less over 1 min; may be diluted in compatible sol, run over 1 hr
• Ordered analgesic if headache develops
• Intraarterial to patient in supine position
• To patient who is sitting or lying down during treatment
Perform/provide:
• Storage at room temperature, protect from light
Evaluate:
• Therapeutic response: decrease in pulmonary hypertension or pulse volume, increased temperature in

italics = common side effects   ***bold italic*** = life threatening reactions

extremities, ability to walk without pain
• Hepatic involvement: nausea, vomiting, jaundice; drug should be discontinued if this occurs
• For bleeding from GI tract: coffee grounds vomitus, increased pulse, pain in upper gastric area
• Affected areas for changes in temperature, color

Teach patient/family:
• To report jaundice, dark urine, joint pain, fatigue, malaise, bruising, easy bleeding, which may indicate blood dyscrasias
• That it is necessary to quit smoking to prevent excessive vasoconstriction if prescribed for PVD
• To avoid hazardous activities until stabilized on medication; dizziness may occur

Treatment of overdose: Administer IV fluids, head-low position

---

tolbutamide

(tole-byoo'ta-mide)
Mobenol,* Novobutamide,* Orinase, Oramide, Tolbutone*

Func. class.: Antidiabetic
Chem. class.: Sulfonylurea (1st generation)

Action: Causes functioning β-cells in pancreas to release insulin, leading to drop in blood glucose levels; may improve binding to insulin receptors or increase the number of insulin receptors; this drug is not effective if patient lacks functioning β-cells

Uses: Type II (NIDDM) diabetes mellitus

Dosage and routes:
• *Adult:* PO 1-2 g/day in divided doses, titrated to patient response
Available forms include: Tabs 250, 500 mg

Side effects/adverse reactions:
CNS: Headache, weakness, paresthesia, tinnitus, dizziness, vertigo
GI: Nausea, fullness, heartburn, *hepatotoxicity, cholestatic jaundice,* taste alteration, diarrhea
HEMA: Leukopenia, thrombocytopenia, agranulocytosis, aplastic anemia, increased AST, ALT, alk phosphatase
INTEG: Rash, allergic reactions, pruritus, urticaria, eczema, photosensitivity, erythema
ENDO: Hypoglycemia
MS: Joint pains

Contraindications: Hypersensitivity to sulfonylureas, juvenile or brittle diabetes

Precautions: Pregnancy (C), elderly, cardiac disease, thyroid disease, severe hypoglycemic reactions, renal disease, hepatic disease

Pharmacokinetics:
PO: Completely absorbed by GI route; onset 30-60 min, peak 3-5 hr, duration 6-12 hr; half-life 4-5 hr, metabolized in liver, excreted in urine (metabolites), breast milk, 90%-95% is plasma protein bound

Interactions/incompatibilities:
• Increased hypoglycemic reaction: oral anticoagulants, chloramphenicol, cimetidine, MAOIs, insulin, guanethidine, methyldopa, nonsteroidal antiinflammatories, salicylates, probenecid, sulfonamides, ranitidine
• Mask symptoms of hypoglycemia: β-blockers
• Decreased effects of both drugs: diazoxide
• Increased effects of tolbutamide: insulin, MAOIs
• Decreased action of tolbutamide: calcium channel blockers, corticosteroids, oral contraceptives, thiazide diuretics, thyroid preparations, estrogens, phenobarbital,

---

phenytoin, rifampin, phenothiazines, sympathomimetics

NURSING CONSIDERATIONS

Administer:

• Drug 30 min before meals

Perform/provide:

• Storage in tight container in cool environment

Evaluate:

• Therapeutic response: decrease in polyuria, polydipsia, polyphagia, clear sensorium, absence of dizziness, stable gait

• Hypoglycemic/hyperglycemic reaction that can occur soon after meals

Teach patient/family:

• To check for symptoms of cholestatic jaundice (dark urine, pruritus, yellow sclera); if these occur a physician should be notified

• To use a capillary blood glucose test while on this drug

• To test urine glucose levels with Chemstrip 3 × /day

• The symptoms of hypo/hyperglycemia, what to do about each

• That this drug must be continued on a daily basis; explain consequence of discontinuing drug abruptly

• To take drug in morning to prevent hypoglycemic reactions at night

• To avoid OTC medications and alcohol unless prescribed by a physician

• That diabetes is a life-long illness, drug will not cure disease

• That all food included in diet plan must be eaten in order to prevent hypoglycemia

• To carry a Medic-Alert ID for emergency purposes

Lab test interferences:

Decrease: RAIU test

Interfere: Urinary albumin

Treatment of overdose: 10%-50%

glucose solution IV or 1 mg glucagon

---

tolmetin sodium

(tole′met-in)

Tolectin, Tolectin DS

Func. class.: Nonsteroidal antiinflammatory

Chem. class.: Pyrrole acetic acid derivative

Action: Inhibits prostaglandin synthesis by decreasing an enzyme needed for biosynthesis; possesses analgesic, antiinflammatory, antipyretic properties

Uses: Mild to moderate pain, osteoarthritis, rheumatoid arthritis

Dosage and routes:

• *Adult:* PO 400 mg tid-qid, not to exceed 2 g/day

• *Child >2 yr:* PO 15-30 mg/kg/day in 3 or 4 divided doses

Available forms include: Caps 400 mg; tabs 200 mg

Side effects/adverse reactions:

GI: Nausea, anorexia, vomiting, diarrhea, jaundice, ***cholestatic hepatitis,*** constipation, flatulence, cramps, dry mouth, peptic ulcer

CNS: Dizziness, drowsiness, fatigue, tremors, confusion, insomnia, anxiety, depression

CV: Tachycardia, peripheral edema, palpitations, dysrhythmias

INTEG: Purpura, rash, pruritus, sweating

GU: ***Nephrotoxicity: dysuria, hematuria, oliguria, azotemia***

HEMA: ***Blood dyscrasias***

EENT: Tinnitus, hearing loss, blurred vision

Contraindications: Hypersensitivity, asthma, severe renal disease, severe hepatic disease

Precautions: Pregnancy (B), lac-

---

italics = common side effects   ***bold italic*** = life threatening reactions

tation, children, bleeding disorders, children, bleeding disorders, GI disorders, cardiac disorders, hypersensitivity to other antiinflammatory agents, peptic ulcer disease

Pharmacokinetics:

PO: Peak 2 hr, half-life 3-3½ hr; metabolized in liver, excreted in urine (metabolites), excreted in breast milk, 99% protein binding

Interactions/incompatibilities:

• Increased action of: coumarin, phenytoin, sulfonamides when used with this drug

NURSING CONSIDERATIONS

Assess:

• Renal, liver, blood studies: BUN, creatinine, AST, ALT, Hgb before treatment, periodically thereafter

• Audiometric, ophthalmic exam before, during, after treatment

Administer:

• With food to decrease GI symptoms; best to take on empty stomach to facilitate absorption

Perform/provide:

• Storage at room temperature

Evaluate:

• Therapeutic response: decreased pain, stiffness, swelling in joints, ability to move more easily

• For eye, ear problems: blurred vision, tinnitus (may indicate toxicity)

Teach patient/family:

• To report blurred vision or ringing, roaring in ears (may indicate toxicity)

• To avoid driving or other hazardous activities if dizziness or drowsiness occurs

• To report change in urine pattern, weight increase, edema, pain increase in joints, fever, blood in urine (indicates nephrotoxicity)

• That therapeutic effects may take up to 1 mo

tolnaftate (topical)

(tole-naf'tate)

Aftate, Footwork, Fungatin, Genaspor, NP-27, Pitrex, Tinactin, Zeasorb-AF

Func. class.: Local antiinfective
Chem. class.: Antifungal

Action: Interferes with fungal cell membrane, which increases permeability, leaking of cell nutrients

Uses: Tinea pedis, tinea cruris, tinea corporis, tinea capitis, tinea unguium, versicolor

Dosage and routes:

• *Adult and child:* TOP apply to affected area bid for 2-6 wk, rub in

Available forms include: Cream, powder, aerosol powder, aerosol liq, gel, pump spray liquid 1%

Side effects/adverse reactions:

INTEG: Rash, urticaria, stinging

Contraindications: Hypersensitivity, nail infections

Precautions: Pregnancy (C), lactation

NURSING CONSIDERATIONS

Administer:

• Aerosol powder after shaking

• Enough medication to completely cover lesions

• After cleansing with soap, water before each application, dry well

Perform/provide:

• Storage at room temperature in dry place, do not puncture or incinerate aerosol container

Evaluate:

• Allergic reaction: burning, stinging, swelling, redness

• Therapeutic response: decrease in size, number of lesions

Teach patient/family:

• To apply with glove to prevent further infection

• To avoid use of OTC creams,

ointments, lotions unless directed by physician
• To use medical asepsis (hand washing) before, after each application
• To avoid contact with eyes
• To notify physician if condition worsens or does not improve in 10 days

---

trace elements (chromium, copper, iodide, manganese, selenium, zinc)

Func. class.: Minerals

Action: Needed for adequate absorption and synthesis of amino acids
Uses: Prevention of trace element deficiency
Dosage and routes:
Chromium
• *Adult:* IV 10-15 μg qd
• *Child:* IV 0.14-0.20 μg/kg/day
Copper
• *Adult:* IV 0.5-1.5 mg/day
• *Child:* IV .05-0.2 mg/kg/day
Iodine
• *Adult:* IV 1 μg/kg/day
Manganese
• *Adult:* IV 1-3 mg/day
Selenium
• *Adult:* IV 40-120 μg/day
• *Child:* IV 3 μg/kg/day
Zinc
• *Adult:* IV 2-4 mg/day
• *Child:* IV 0.05 mg/kg/day
Available forms include: Many forms available—see particular elements
Side effects/adverse reactions:
None known
Precautions: Liver, biliary disease
NURSING CONSIDERATIONS
Assess:
• Trace element levels, notify physician if low copper 0.07-0.15 mg/ml, zinc 0.05-0.15 mg/100 ml, manganese 4-20 μg/100 ml, selenium 0.1-0.19 μg/ml
Administer:
• By IV infusion, often mixed with TPN solution
Evaluate:
• Therapeutic response: absence of element deficiency
• Trace element deficiency if patient is receiving TPN for extended periods of time

---

tranylcypromine sulfate

(tran-ill-sip'roe-meen)
Parnate
Func. class.: Antidepressant-MAOI
Chem. class.: Nonhydrazine

Action: Increases concentrations of endogenous epinephrine, norepinephrine, serotonin, dopamine in storage sites in CNS by inhibition of MAO; increased concentration reduces depression
Uses: Depression, when uncontrolled by other means
Dosage and routes:
• *Adult:* PO 10 mg bid, may increase to 30 mg/day after 2 wk
Available forms include: Tabs 10 mg
Side effects/adverse reactions:
HEMA: Anemia
CNS: Dizziness, drowsiness, confusion, headache, anxiety, tremors, stimulation, weakness, hyperreflexia, mania, insomnia, fatigue, weight gain
GI: Constipation, dry mouth, nausea, vomiting, *anorexia,* diarrhea, weight gain
GU: Change in libido, frequency
INTEG: Rash, flushing, increased perspiration

T

---

italics = common side effects   ***bold italic*** = life threatening reactions

CV: *Orthostatic hypotension, hypertension, dysrhythmias,* hypertensive crisis

EENT: Blurred vision

ENDO: **SIADH-like syndrome**

Contraindications: Hypersensitivity to MAOIs, elderly, hypertension, CHF, severe hepatic disease, pheochromocytoma, severe renal disease, severe cardiac disease

Precautions: Suicidal patients, convulsive disorders, severe depression, schizophrenia, hyperactivity, diabetes mellitus, pregnancy (C)

Pharmacokinetics:

Metabolized by liver, excreted by kidneys, crosses placenta, excreted in breast milk

Interactions/incompatibilities:

• Increased pressor effects: guanethidine, clonidine, indirect acting sympathomimetics (ephedrine)

• Increased effects of: direct acting sympathomimetics (epinephrine), alcohol, barbiturates, benzodiazepines, CNS depressants, levodopa

• Hyperpyretic crisis, convulsions, hypertensive episode: tricyclic antidepressants, meperidine

• Hypoglycemic effect increased: insulin

NURSING CONSIDERATIONS

Assess:

• B/P (lying, standing), pulse; if systolic B/P drops 20 mm Hg hold drug, notify physician

• Blood studies: CBC, leukocytes, cardiac enzymes if patient is receiving long-term therapy

• Hepatic studies: ALT, AST, bilirubin, creatinine; hepatotoxicity may occur

Administer:

• Increased fluids, bulk in diet if constipation, urinary retention occur

• With food or milk for GI symptoms

• Crushed if patient is unable to swallow medication whole

• Dosage hs if over-sedation occurs during day

• Gum, hard candy, or frequent sips of water for dry mouth

• Phentolamine for severe hypertension

Perform/provide:

• Storage in tight container in cool environment

• Assistance with ambulation during beginning therapy since drowsiness/dizziness occurs

• Safety measures including siderails

• Checking to see PO medication swallowed

Evaluate:

• Toxicity: increased headache, palpitation, discontinue drug immediately; prodromal signs of hypertensive crisis

• Mental status: mood, sensorium, affect, memory (long, short), increase in psychiatric symptoms

• Urinary retention, constipation, edema, take weight weekly

• Withdrawal symptoms: headache, nausea, vomiting, muscle pain, weakness

Teach patient/family:

• That therapeutic effects may take 1-4 wk

• To avoid driving or other activities requiring alertness

• To avoid alcohol ingestion, CNS depressants or OTC medications: cold, weight, hay fever, cough syrup

• Not to discontinue medication quickly after long-term use

• To avoid high tyramine foods: cheese (aged), sour cream, beer, wine, pickled products, liver, raisins, bananas, figs, avocados, meat

---

* Available in Canada only

tenderizers, chocolate, yogurt; increase caffeine
• Report headache, palpitation, neck stiffness
Treatment of overdose: Lavage, activated charcoal, monitor electrolytes, vital signs, diazepam IV, NaHCO₃

trazodone HCl
(tray'zoe-done)
Desyrel
Func. class.: Antidepressant—tricyclic-like
Chem. class.: Triazolopyridine

Action: Selectively inhibits serotonin uptake by brain, potentiates behavorial changes
Uses: Depression
Dosage and routes:
• *Adult:* PO 150 mg/day in divided doses, may be increase by 50 mg/day q3-4d, not to exceed 600 mg/day
Available forms include: Tabs 50, 100, 150, 300 mg
Side effects/adverse reactions:
*HEMA: **Agranulocytosis, thrombocytopenia, eosinophilia, leukopenia***
CNS: Dizziness, drowsiness, confusion, headache, anxiety, tremors, stimulation, weakness, insomnia, nightmares, EPS (elderly), increase in psychiatric symptoms
GI: Diarrhea, dry mouth, nausea, vomiting, ***paralytic ileus,*** increased appetite, cramps, epigastric distress, jaundice, ***hepatitis,*** stomatitis
*GU: Retention, **acute renal failure, priapism***
INTEG: Rash, urticaria, sweating, pruritus, photosensitivity
*CV: Orthostatic hypotension, ECG changes, tachycardia, **hypertension,*** palpitations
EENT: Blurred vision, tinnitus, mydriasis
Contraindications: Hypersensitivity to tricyclic antidepressants, recovery phase of myocardial infarction, convulsive disorders, prostatic hypertrophy
Precautions: Suicidal patients, severe depression, increased intraocular pressure, narrow-angle glaucoma, urinary retention, cardiac disease, hepatic disease, hyperthyroidism, electroshock therapy, elective surgery, pregnancy (C)
Pharmacokinetics:
Metabolized by liver, excreted by kidneys, feces; half-life 4.4-7.5 hr
Interactions/incompatibilities:
• Decreased effects of: guanethidine, clonidine, indirect acting sympathomimetics (ephedrine)
• Increased effects of: direct acting sympathomimetics (epinephrine), alcohol, barbiturates, benzodiazepines, CNS depressants
• Hyperpyretic crisis, convulsions, hypertensive episode: MAOI (pargyline [Eutonyl])
NURSING CONSIDERATIONS
Assess:
• B/P (lying, standing), pulse q4h; if systolic B/P drops 20 mm Hg hold drug, notify physician; take vital signs q4h in patients with cardiovascular disease
• Blood studies: CBC, leukocytes, differential, cardiac enzymes if patient is receiving long-term therapy
• Hepatic studies: AST, ALT, bilirubin, creatinine
• Weight qwk, appetite may increase with drug
• ECG for flattening of T wave, bundle branch block, AV block, dysrhythmias in cardiac patients

italics = common side effects   ***bold italic*** = life threatening reactions

Administer:
• Increased fluids, bulk in diet if constipation, urinary retention occur
• With food or milk for GI symptoms
• Dosage hs if over-sedation occurs during day; may take entire dose hs; elderly may not tolerate once/day dosing
• Gum, hard candy, or frequent sips of water for dry mouth

Perform/provide:
• Storage in tight, light-resistant container at room temperature
• Assistance with ambulation during beginning therapy since drowsiness/dizziness occurs
• Safety measures including side-rails, primarily in elderly
• Checking to see PO medication swallowed

Evaluate:
• EPS primarily in elderly: rigidity, dystonia, akathisia
• Mental status: mood, sensorium, affect, suicidal tendencies, increase in psychiatric symptoms: depression, panic
• Urinary retention, constipation; constipation is more likely to occur in children
• Withdrawal symptoms: headache, nausea, vomiting, muscle pain, weakness; do not usually occur unless drug was discontinued abruptly
• Alcohol consumption; if alcohol is consumed, hold dose until morning

Teach patient/family:
• That therapeutic effects may take 2-3 wk
• To use caution in driving or other activities requiring alertness because of drowsiness, dizziness, blurred vision
• To avoid alcohol ingestion, other CNS depressants
• Not to discontinue medication quickly after long-term use, may cause nausea, headache, malaise
• To wear sunscreen or large hat since photosensitivity occurs

Lab test interferences:
Increase: Serum bilirubin, blood glucose, alk phosphatase
False increase: Urinary catecholamines
Decrease: VMA, 5-HIAA

Treatment of overdose: ECG monitoring, induce emesis, lavage, activated charcoal, administer anticonvulsant

---

tretinoin (vitamin A acid, retinoic acid)

(tret'i-noyn)
Retin-A, Stievaa*

Func. class.: Vitamin A acid/acne product
Chem. class.: Tretinoin derivative

Action: Decreases cohesiveness of follicular epithelium, decreases microcomedone formation

Uses: Acne vulgaris (grades 1-3); unlabeled use: skin cancer

Dosage and routes:
• *Adult and child:* TOP cleanse area, apply hs; cover lightly

Available forms include: Top cream 0.1%, 0.05%; top gel 0.025%, 0.01%; top liq 0.05%

Side effects/adverse reactions:
INTEG: Rash, stinging, warmth, redness, erythema, blistering, crusting, peeling, contact dermatitis, hypo/hyperpigmentation

Contraindications: Hypersensitivity

Precautions: Pregnancy (B), lactation, eczema, sunburn

Pharmacokinetics:

TOP: Poor absorption, excreted in urine

Interactions/incompatibilities:

• Increase peeling: medication containing agents such as sulfur, benzoyl peroxide, resorcinol, salicylic acid

• Use with caution medicated or abrasive soaps or cleansers that have drying effect, products with high concentrations of alcohol astringents

NURSING CONSIDERATIONS

Administer:

• Once daily before hs; cover area lightly using gauze

Perform/provide:

• Storage at room temperature

• Washing of hands after application

Evaluate:

• Therapeutic response: decrease in size and number of lesions

• Area of body involved, including time involved, what helps or aggravates condition

Teach patient/family:

• To avoid application on normal skin or getting cream in eyes, nose, or other mucous membranes

• To avoid sunlight or sunlamps

• Treatment may cause warmth, stinging; dryness, peeling will occur

• Cosmetics may be used over drug, do not use shaving lotions

• That rash may occur during first 1-3 wk of therapy

• That drug does not cure condition, only relieves symptoms

triamcinolone/triamcinolone acetonide/triamcinolone diacetate/triamcinolone hexacetonide

(trye-am-sin'oh-lone)

Aristocort, Kenacort, Azmacort, Kenalog/Amcort/Cenocort Forte, Triam-Forte, Trisoject/Aristospan

Func. class.: Corticosteroid

Chem. class.: Glucocorticoid, intermediate-acting

Action: Decreases inflammation by suppression of migration of polymorphonuclear leukocytes, fibroblasts, reversal to increase capillary permeability and lysosomal stabilization

Uses: Severe inflammation, immunosuppresion, neoplasms, asthma (steroid dependent), collagen, respiratory, dermatologic disorders

Dosage and routes:

• *Adult:* PO 4-48 mg/day in divided doses qd-qid; IM 40 mg q wk (acetonide, or diacetate), 5-48 mg into neoplasms (diacetate, acetonide), 2-40 mg into joint or soft tissue (diacetate, acetonide), 0.5 mg/sq in of affected intralesional skin (hexacetonide), 2-20 mg into joint or soft tissue (hexacetonide)

Asthma

• *Adult:* INH 2 tid-qid, not to exceed 16 INH/day

• *Child 6-12 yr:* INH 1-2 tid-qid, not to exceed 12 INH/day

Available forms include: Tabs 1, 2, 4, 8, 16 mg; syr 2 mg/5 ml, 4.85 mg/5 ml; inj 25, 40 mg/ml diacetate; inj 3, 10, 40 mg/ml acetonide; inj 20, 5 mg/ml hexacetonide

T

---

italics = common side effects   ***bold italic*** = life threatening reactions

Side effects/adverse reactions:

INTEG: Acne, poor wound healing, ecchymosis, petechiae

CNS: Depression, flushing, sweating, headache, mood changes

*CV: Hypertension, **circulatory collapse, thrombophlebitis, embolism,** tachycardia, edema*

*HEMA: **Thrombocytopenia***

MS: Fractures, osteoporosis, weakness

*GI: Diarrhea, nausea, abdominal distention, **GI hemorrhage,** increased appetite, **pancreatitis***

EENT: Fungal infections, increased intraocular pressure, blurred vision

Contraindications: Psychosis, hypersensitivity, idiopathic thrombocytopenia, acute glomerulonephritis, amebiasis, fungal infections, nonasthmatic bronchial disease, child <2 yr, AIDS, TB

Precautions: Pregnancy (C), diabetes mellitus, glaucoma, osteoporosis, seizure disorders, ulcerative colitis, CHF, myasthenia gravis, renal disease, esophagitis, peptic ulcer

Pharmacokinetics:

PO/IM: Peak 1-2 hr, 2 days, 1-6 wk (IM), half-life 2-5 hr

Interactions/incompatibilities:

• Decreased action of triamcinolone: cholestyramine, colestipol, barbiturates, rifampin, ephedrine, phenytoin, theophylline

• Decreased effects of: anticoagulants, anticonvulsants, antidiabetics, ambenonium, neostigmine, isoniazid, toxoids, vaccines

• Increased side effects: alcohol, salicylates, indomethacin, amphotericin B, digitalis preparations

• Increased action of triamcinolone: salicylates, estrogens, indomethacin

NURSING CONSIDERATIONS

Assess:

• Potassium, blood sugar, urine glucose while on long-term therapy; hypokalemia and hyperglycemia

• Weight daily, notify physician if weekly gain >5 lb

• B/P q4h, pulse, notify physician if chest pain occurs

• I&O ratio, be alert for decreasing urinary output and increasing edema

• Plasma cortisol levels during long-term therapy (normal level: 138-635 nmol/L SI units when drawn at 8 AM)

Administer:

• After shaking suspension (parenteral)

• Titrated dose, use lowest effective dose

• IM injection deeply in large mass, rotate sites, avoid deltoid, use 21G needle

• In one dose in AM to prevent adrenal suppression, avoid SC administration, damage may be done to tissue

• With food or milk to decrease GI symptoms

Perform/provide:

• Assistance with ambulation in patient with bone tissue disease to prevent fractures

Evaluate:

• Therapeutic response: ease of respirations, decreased inflammation

• Infection: increased temperature, WBC, even after withdrawal of medication. Drug masks infections symptoms

• Potassium depletion: paresthesias, fatigue, nausea, vomiting, depression, polyuria, dysrhythmias, weakness

• Edema, hypertension, cardiac symptoms

• Mental status: affect, mood, behavioral changes, aggression

Teach patient/family:
• That ID as steroid user should be carried
• To notify physician if therapeutic response decreases; dosage adjustment may be needed
• Not to discontinue this medication abruptly or adrenal crisis can result
• To avoid OTC products: salicylates, alcohol in cough products, cold preparations unless directed by physician
• About cushingoid symptoms
• Symptoms of adrenal insufficiency: nausea, anorexia, fatigue, dizziness, dyspnea, weakness, joint pain

Lab test interferences:
Increase: Cholesterol, sodium, blood glucose, uric acid, calcium, urine glucose
Decrease: Calcium, potassium, T$_4$, T$_3$, thyroid ^{131}I uptake test, urine 17-OHCS, 17-KS, PBI
False negative: Skin allergy tests

---

triamcinolone acetonide

(trye-am-sin'oh-lone)
Acetospan, Azmacort, Aristocort, Cenocort A$_2$, Kenalog, Tramacort, Triami-A, Triamonide, Tri-kort, Trilog
Func. class.: Topical corticosteroid
Chem. class.: Synthetic fluorinated agent, group II potency (0.5%), group III potency (0.1%), group IV potency (0.025%)

Action: Possesses antipruritic, antiinflammatory actions
Uses: Psoriasis, eczema, contact dermatitis, pruritus
Dosage and routes:
• *Adult and child:* Apply to affected area bid-qid
Available forms include: Oint

0.025%, 0.1%, 0.5%; cream 0.025%, 0.1%, 0.5%; lotion 0.025%, 0.1%; aerosol 0.2 mg/2 sec; paste 0.1%

Side effects/adverse reactions:
INTEG: Burning, dryness, itching, irritation, acne, folliculitis, hypertrichosis, perioral dermatitis, hypopigmentation, atrophy, striae, miliaria, allergic contact dermatitis, secondary infection

Contraindications: Hypersensitivity to corticosteroids, fungal infections
Precautions: Pregnancy (C), lactation, viral infections, bacterial infections

NURSING CONSIDERATIONS
Assess:
• Temperature; if fever develops, drug should be discontinued
Administer:
• Only to affected areas; do not get in eyes
• Medication, then cover with occlusive dressing (only if prescribed), seal to normal skin, change q12h; use occlusive dressing with extreme caution (group II potency), systemic absorption may occur
• Only to dermatoses; do not use on weeping, denuded, or infected area
Perform/provide:
• Cleansing before application of drug; apply to slightly moist skin; use gloves and a cotton-tipped applicator
• Treatment for a few days after area has cleared
• Storage at room temperature
Evaluate:
• Therapeutic response: absence of severe itching, patches on skin, flaking
• For systemic absorption: in-

---

italics = common side effects

bold italic = life threatening reactions

creased temperature, inflammation, irritation
Teach patient/family:
• To avoid sunlight on affected area; burns may occur

---

triamcinolone acetonide (topical-oral)

(trye-am-sin'oh-lone)
Kenalog in Orabase
Func. class.: Topical anesthetic
Chem. class.: Synthetic fluorinated adrenal corticosteroid

Action: Inhibits nerve impulses from sensory nerves
Uses: Oral pain
Dosage and routes:
• *Adult and child:* TOP press ¼ inch into affected area until film appears, repeat bid-tid
Available forms include: Paste 0.1%
Side effects/adverse reactions:
INTEG: Rash, irritation, sensitization
Contraindications: Hypersensitivity, infants <1 yr, application to large areas, presence of fungal, viral, or bacterial infections of mouth or throat
Precautions: Child <6 yr, sepsis, pregnancy (C), denuded skin
NURSING CONSIDERATIONS
Administer:
• After cleansing oral cavity
Evaluate:
• Allergy: rash, irritation, reddening, swelling
• Therapeutic response: absence of pain in affected area
• Infection: if affected area is infected, do not apply
Teach patient/family:
• To report rash, irritation, redness, swelling
• How to apply paste

---

triamterene

(trye-am'ter-een)
Dyrenium
Func. class.: Potassium-sparing diuretic
Chem. class.: Pteridine derivative

Action: Acts on distal tubule to inhibit reabsorption of sodium, chloride
Uses: Edema; may be used with other diuretics, hypertension
Dosage and routes:
• *Adults:* PO 100 mg bid pc, not to exceed 300 mg
Available forms include: Cap 50, 100 mg
Side effects/adverse reactions:
GI: Nausea, diarrhea, vomiting, dry mouth, jaundice, liver disease
ELECT: Hyperkalemia, hyponatremia, hypochloremia
CNS: Weakness, headache, dizziness
INTEG: Photosensitivity, rash
*HEMA: **Thrombocytopenia, megaloblastic anemia,** low folic acid levels*
*GU: **Azotemia, interstitial nephritis,** increased BUN, creatinine, renal stones*
Contraindications: Hypersensitivity, anuria, severe renal disease, severe hepatic disease, hyperkalemia, pregnancy (D)
Precautions: Dehydration, hepatic disease, lactation, CHF, renal disease, cirrhosis
Pharmacokinetics:
PO: Onset 2 hr, peak 6-8 hr, duration 12-16 hr; half-life 3 hr; metabolized in liver, excreted in bile and urine
Interactions/incompatibilities:
• Nephrotoxicity: indomethacin
• Enhanced action of: antihypertensives, lithium, amantadine

• Increased hyperkalemia: other potassium sparing diuretics, potassium products, ACE inhibitors, salt substitutes

NURSING CONSIDERATIONS
Assess:
• Weight, I&O daily to determine fluid loss; effect of drug may be decreased if used qd
• Electrolytes: potassium, sodium, chloride; include BUN, blood sugar, CBC, serum creatinine, blood pH, ABGs, liver function tests

Administer:
• In AM to avoid interference with sleep
• With food if nausea occurs; absorption may be decreased slightly

Evaluate:
• Improvement in edema of feet, legs, sacral area daily if medication is being used in CHF
• Improvement in CVP q8h
• Signs of metabolic acidosis: drowsiness, restlessness
• Rashes, temperature elevation qd
• Confusion, especially in elderly, take safety precautions if needed
• Hydration: skin turgor, thirst, dry mucous membranes

Teach patient/family:
• To take medication after meals for GI upset
• To avoid prolonged exposure to sunlight since photosensitivity may occur
• To notify physician if weakness, headache, nausea, vomiting, dry mouth, fever, sore throat, mouth sores, unusual bleeding or bruising occurs
• That drug must be tapered to prevent excessive rebound K excretion

Lab test interferences:
Interfere: quinidine serum levels, LDH

Treatment of overdose: Lavage if taken orally, monitor electrolytes, administer IV fluids, dialysis, monitor hydration, CV, renal status

---

triazolam

(trye-ay′zoe-lam)
Halcion
Func. class.: Sedative-hypnotic
Chem. class.: Benzodiazepine

Controlled Substance Schedule IV (USA), Schedule F (Canada)
Action: Produces CNS depression at limbic, thalamic, hypothalamic levels of CNS; may be mediated by neurotransmitter gamma aminobutyric acid (GABA); results are sedation, hypnosis, skeletal muscle relaxation, anticonvulsant activity, anxiolytic action
Uses: Insomnia
Dosage and routes:
• *Adult:* PO 0.125-0.5 mg hs
• *Elderly:* PO 0.125-0.25 mg hs
Available forms include: Tabs 0.125, 0.25, 0.5 mg
Side effects/adverse reactions:
HEMA: **Leukopenia, granulocytopenia** (rare)
CNS: Headache, lethargy, drowsiness, daytime sedation, dizziness, confusion, lightheadedness, anxiety, irritability, amnesia, poor coordination
GI: Nausea, vomiting, diarrhea, heartburn, abdominal pain, constipation
CV: Chest pain, pulse changes
Contraindications: Hypersensitivity to benzodiazepines, pregnancy (X), lactation, intermittent porphyria
Precautions: Anemia, hepatic disease, renal disease, suicidal individuals, drug abuse, elderly, psychosis, child < 15 yr, acute nar-

T

---

italics = common side effects   **bold italic** = life threatening reactions

row-angle glaucoma, seizure disorders

Pharmacokinetics:
PO: Onset 30-45 min, duration 6-8 hr; metabolized by liver, excreted by kidneys (inactive metabolites), crosses placenta, excreted in breast milk; half-life 2-3 hr

Interactions/incompatibilities:
• Increased effects of: cimetidine, disulfiram, erythromycin
• Increased action of both drugs: alcohol, CNS depressants
• Decreased effect of: antacids

NURSING CONSIDERATIONS
Assess:
• Blood studies: Hct, Hgb, RBCs, if blood dyscrasias are suspected (rare)
• Hepatic studies: AST, ALT, bilirubin if liver damage has occurred

Administer:
• After removal of cigarettes, to prevent fires
• After trying conservative measures for insomnia
• ½-1 hr before hs for sleeplessness
• On empty stomach fast onset, but may be taken with food if GI symptoms occur

Perform/provide:
• Assistance with ambulation after receiving dose
• Safety measure: siderails, night-light, callbell within easy reach
• Checking to see PO medication has been swallowed
• Storage in tight container in cool environment

Evaluate:
• Therapeutic response: ability to sleep at night, decreased amount of early morning awakening if taking drug for insomnia
• Mental status: mood, sensorium, affect, memory (long, short)
• Blood dyscrasias: fever, sore throat, bruising, rash, jaundice, epistaxis (rare)
• Type of sleep problem: falling asleep, staying asleep

Teach patient/family:
• That dependence is possible after long-term use
• To avoid driving or other activities requiring alertness until drug is stabilized
• To avoid alcohol ingestion or CNS depressants; serious CNS depression may result
• That effects may take 2 nights for benefits to be noticed
• Alternate measures to improve sleep: reading, exercise several hours before hs, warm bath, warm milk, TV, self-hypnosis, deep breathing
• That hangover is common in elderly, but less common than with barbiturates, rebound insomnia may occur for 1-2 nights after discontinuing drug

Lab test interferences:
Increase: ALT, AST, serum bilirubin
Decrease: RAI uptake
False increase: Urinary 17-OHCS

Treatment of overdose: Lavage, activated charcoal, monitor electrolytes, vital signs

---

trientine HCl
(trye-in'-teen)
Cuprid

Func. class.: Heavy metal antagonist

Chem. class.: Chelating agent (thiol compound)

Action: Binds with ions of lead, mercury, copper, iron, zinc to form a water-soluble complex excreted by kidneys

Uses: Wilson's disease

---

*Available in Canada only

Dosage and routes:
• *Adult:* PO 750-2000 mg in divided doses bid-qid
• *Child:* PO 500-1500 mg in divided doses bid-qid
Available forms include: Caps 125, 250 mg; tabs 250 mg
Side effects/adverse reactions:
HEMA: Anemia, *iron deficiency*
INTEG: Urticaria, fever
SYST: Hypersensitivity
GI: Epigastric distress, anorexia, heartburn
Contraindications: Hypersensitivity
Precautions: Pregnancy (C)
Pharmacokinetics:
PO: Peak 1 hr, metabolized in liver, excreted in urine
Interactions/incompatibilities:
• Decreased action: mineral supplements
NURSING CONSIDERATIONS
Assess:
• Monitor hepatic, renal studies: ALT/AST, alk phosphatase, BUN, creatinine, serum copper level
• Monitor I&O
• For anemia: fatigue, Hct, Hgb
Administer:
• On an empty stomach, ½-1 hr before meals or 2 hr after meals
• B₆ daily; depleted when this drug is used
Evaluate:
• Therapeutic response: improvement in neurologic, psychiatric symptoms
• Allergic reactions (rash, urticaria); if these occur, drug should be discontinued
Teach patient/family:
• That therapeutic effect may take 1-3 mo or longer
• To report urticaria, fever, fatigue

trifluoperazine HCl

(trye-floo-oh-per'a-zeen)
Novoflurazine,* Solazine,* Suprazine, Stelazine, Terfluzine,* Triflurin*

Func. class.: Antipsychotic/neuroleptic
Chem. class.: Phenothiazine, piperazine

Action: Depresses cerebral cortex, hypothalamus, limbic system, which control activity, aggression; blocks neurotransmission produced by dopamine at synapse; exhibits strong α-adrenergic, anticholinergic blocking action; mechanism for antipsychotic effects is unclear
Uses: Psychotic disorders, nonpsychotic anxiety, schizophrenia
Dosage and routes:
Psychotic disorders
• *Adult:* PO 2-5 mg bid, usual range 15-20 mg/day, may require 40 mg/day or more; IM 1-2 mg q4-6h
• *Child >6 yr:* PO 1 mg qd or bid; IM *not recommended for children,* but 1 mg may be given qd or bid
Nonpsychotic anxiety
• *Adult:* PO 1-2 mg bid, not to exceed 5 mg/day; do not give longer than 12 wk
Available forms include: Tabs 1, 2, 5, 10, 20 mg; conc 10 mg/ml; inj IM 2 mg/ml
Side effects/adverse reactions:
RESP: **Laryngospasm**, dyspnea, **respiratory depression**
CNS: Extrapyramidal symptoms: pseudoparkinsonism, akathisia, dystonia, tardive dyskinesia, seizures, *headache*
HEMA: Anemia, **leukopenia, leukocytosis, agranulocytosis**
INTEG: **Rash**, photosensitivity, dermatitis

T

---

italics = common side effects   ***bold italic*** = life threatening reactions

EENT: Blurred vision, glaucoma

GI: Dry mouth, nausea, vomiting, anorexia, constipation, diarrhea, jaundice, weight gain

GU: Urinary retention, urinary frequency, enuresis, impotence, amenorrhea, gynecomastia

CV: Orthostatic hypotension, hypertension, *cardiac arrest,* ECG changes, *tachycardia*

Contraindications: Hypersensitivity, cardiovascular disease, coma, blood dyscrasias, severe hepatic disease, child <6 yr

Precautions: Breast cancer, seizure disorders, pregnancy (C), lactation

Pharmacokinetics:

PO: Onset rapid, peak 2-3 hr, duration 12 hr

IM: Onset immediate, peak 1 hr, duration 12 hr

Metabolized by liver, excreted in urine, crosses placenta, enters breast milk

Interactions/incompatibilities:

• Oversedation: other CNS depressants, alcohol, barbiturate anesthetics

• Toxicity: epinephrine

• Decreased absorption: aluminum hydroxide or magnesium hydroxide antacids

• Decreased effects of: lithium, levodopa

• Increased effects of both drugs: β-adrenergic blockers, alcohol

• Increased anticholinergic effects: anticholinergics

NURSING CONSIDERATIONS

Assess:

• Swallowing of PO medication; check for hoarding or giving of medication to other patients

• I&O ratio; palpate bladder if low urinary output occurs

• Bilirubin, CBC, liver function studies monthly

• Urinalysis is recommended before and during prolonged therapy

Administer:

• Antiparkinsonian agent, after securing order from physician to be used if EPS occur

• Conc in 120 ml of tomato or fruit juice, milk, orange, carbonated beverage, coffee, tea, water, or semisolid foods (soup, pudding)

Perform/provide:

• Decreased noise input by dimming lights, avoiding loud noises

• Supervised ambulation until stabilized on medication; do not involve in strenuous exercise program because fainting is possible; patient should not stand still for long periods of time

• Increased fluids to prevent constipation

• Sips of water, candy, gum for dry mouth

• Storage in tight, light-resistant container, oral solutions in amber bottles; slight yellowing of inj or conc is common, does not affect potency.

Evaluate:

• Therapeutic response: decrease in emotional excitement, hallucinations, delusions, paranoia, reorganization of patterns of thought, speech

• Affect, orientation, LOC, reflexes, gait, coordination, sleep pattern disturbances

• B/P standing and lying; also include pulse, respirations q4h during initial treatment; establish baseline before starting treatment; report drops of 30 mm Hg

• Dizziness, faintness, palpitations, tachycardia on rising

• EPS including akathisia (inability to sit still, no pattern to movements), tardive dyskinesia (bizarre movements of jaw, mouth, tongue,

---

* Available in Canada only

extremities), pseudoparkinsonism (rigidity, tremors, pill rolling, shuffling gait)

• Skin turgor daily

• Constipation, urinary retention daily; if these occur increase bulk, water in diet

Teach patient/family:

• That orthostatic hypotension occurs frequently, and to rise from sitting or lying position gradually

• To remain lying down after IM injection for at least 30 min

• To avoid hot tubs, hot showers, or tub baths since hypotension may occur

• To avoid abrupt withdrawal of this drug or EPS may result; drugs should be withdrawn slowly

• To avoid OTC preparations (cough, hayfever, cold) unless approved by physician since serious drug interactions may occur; avoid use with alcohol or CNS depressants, increased drowsiness may occur

• To use a sunscreen during sun exposure to prevent burns

• Regarding compliance with drug regimen

• About necessity for meticulous oral hygiene since oral candidiasis may occur

• To report sore throat, malaise, fever, bleeding, mouth sores; if these occur, CBC should be drawn and drug discontinued

• In hot weather, that heat stroke may occur; take extra precautions to stay cool

Lab test interferences:

Increase: Liver function tests, cardiac enzymes, cholesterol, blood glucose, prolactin, bilirubin, PBI, cholinesterase, ^{131}I

Decrease: Hormones (blood and urine)

False positive: Pregnancy tests, PKU

False negative: Urinary steroids, 17-OHCS

Treatment of overdose: Lavage if orally ingested, provide an airway; *do not induce vomiting*

---

triflupromazine HCl

(trye-floo-proe′ma-zeen)
Vesprin

Func. class.: Antipsychotic/neuroleptic

Chem. class.: Phenothiazine, aliphatic

Action: Depresses cerebral cortex, hypothalamus, limbic system, which control activity, aggression; blocks neurotransmission produced by dopamine at synapse; exhibits strong α-adrenergic, anticholinergic blocking action; mechanism for antipsychotic effects is unclear

Uses: Psychotic disorders, schizophrenia, acute agitation, nausea, vomiting

Dosage and routes:

Psychosis

• *Adult:* PO 10-50 mg bid-tid depending on severity of condition; dose is gradually increased to desired dose; IM 60 mg; not to exceed 150 mg/day

• *Child >2 yr:* PO 0.5-2 mg/kg/day in 3 divided doses; may increase to 10 mg if needed; IM 0.2 to 0.25 mg/kg to a maximum total dose of 10 mg/day

Nausea/vomiting

• *Adult:* PO 20-30 mg qd; IV 1-3 mg; IM 5-15 mg, q4h, max 60 mg qd

• *Child >2 yr:* PO/IM 0.2 mg/kg, max 10 mg qd

Acute agitation

• *Adult:* IM 60-150 mg/qd in 3 divided doses

• *Child >2 yr:* IM 0.2-0.25 mg/kg/day in divided doses, max 10 mg/qd

Available forms include: Tabs 10, 25, 50 mg (Canada only); inj IM, IV 10, 20 mg/ml

Side effects/adverse reactions:

RESP: Laryngospasm, dyspnea, *respiratory depression*

CNS: Extrapyramidal symptoms: pseudoparkinsonism, akathisia, dystonia, tardive dyskinesia, drowsiness, headache, seizures

HEMA: Anemia, *leukopenia, leukocytosis, agranulocytosis*

INTEG: Rash, photosensitivity, dermatitis

EENT: Blurred vision, glaucoma

GI: Dry mouth, nausea, vomiting, anorexia, constipation, diarrhea, jaundice, weight gain

GU: Urinary retention, urinary frequency, enuresis, impotence, amenorrhea, gynecomastia

CV: Orthostatic hypotension, hypertension, *cardiac arrest,* ECG changes, *tachycardia*

Contraindications: Hypersensitivity, blood dyscrasias, coma, child <2½ yr, brain damage, bone marrow depression

Precautions: Pregnancy (C), lactation, seizure disorders, hypertension, hepatic disease, cardiac disease

Pharmacokinetics:

PO: Onset erratic, peak 2-4 hr, duration 4-6 hr

IM: Onset 15-30 min, peak 15-20 min, duration 4-6 hr

Metabolized by liver, excreted in urine and feces, crosses placenta, enters breast milk

Interactions/incompatibilities:

• Oversedation: other CNS depressants, alcohol, barbiturate anesthetics

• Toxicity: epinephrine

• Decreased absorption: aluminum hydroxide or magnesium hydroxide antacids

• Decreased effects of: lithium, levodopa

• Increased effects of both drugs: β-adrenergic blockers, alcohol

• Increased anticholinergic effects: anticholinergics

NURSING CONSIDERATIONS

Assess:

• Swallowing of PO medication; check for hoarding or giving of medication to other patients

• I&O ratio; palpate bladder if low urinary output occurs

• Bilirubin, CBC, liver function studies monthly

• Urinalysis is recommended before and during prolonged therapy

Administer:

• IV after diluting 10 mg/9 ml of NS; give 1 mg or less/2 min

• Antiparkinsonian agent, after securing order from physician to be used if extrapyramidal symptoms occur

• IM injection into large muscle mass

Perform/provide:

• Decreased noise input by dimming lights, avoiding loud noises

• Supervised ambulation until stabilized on medication; do not involve in strenuous exercise program because fainting is possible; patient should not stand still for long periods of time

• Increased fluids to prevent constipation

• Sips of water, candy, gum for dry mouth

• Storage in tight, light-resistant container

*Available in Canada only

Evaluate:

• Therapeutic response: decrease in emotional excitement, hallucinations, delusions, paranoia, reorganization of patterns of thought, speech

• Affect, orientation, LOC, reflexes, gait, coordination, sleep pattern disturbances

• B/P standing and lying; also include pulse, respirations q4h during initial treatment; establish baseline before starting treatment; report drops of 30 mm Hg

• For neuroleptic malignant syndrome: altered mental status, muscle rigidity, increased CPK, hyperthermia

• Dizziness, faintness, palpitations, tachycardia on rising

• Extrapyramidal symptoms including akathisia (inability to sit still, no pattern to movements), tardive dyskinesia (bizarre movements of jaw, mouth, tongue, extremities), pseudoparkinsonism (rigidity, tremors, pill rolling, shuffling gait)

• Constipation, urinary retention daily; if these occur increase bulk, water in the diet

Teach patient/family:

• That orthostatic hypotension occurs frequently, and to rise from sitting or lying position gradually

• To remain lying down after IM injection for at least 30 min

• To avoid hot tubs, hot showers, or tub baths since hypotension may occur

• To avoid abrupt withdrawal of this drug or extrapyramidal symptoms may result; drugs should be withdrawn slowly

• To avoid OTC preparations (cough, hayfever, cold) unless approved by physician since serious drug interactions may occur; avoid use with alcohol or CNS depressants, increased drowsiness may occur

• To use sunscreen during sun exposure to prevent burns

• Regarding compliance with drug regimen

• About necessity for meticulous oral hygiene since oral candidiasis may occur

• To report sore throat, malaise, fever, bleeding, mouth sores; if these occur, CBC should be drawn and drug discontinued

• In hot weather, heat stroke may occur; take extra precautions to stay cool

Lab test interferences:

Increase: Liver function tests, cardiac enzymes, cholesterol, blood glucose, prolactin, bilirubin, PBI, cholinesterase, ^{131}I

Decrease: Hormones (blood and urine)

False positive: Pregnancy tests, PKU

False negative: Urinary steroids

Treatment of overdose: Lavage if orally ingested, provide an airway; *do not induce vomiting*

---

trifluridine (ophthalmic)
(trye-flure′i-deen)
Viroptic Ophthalmic Solution
Func. class.: Antiviral
Chem. class.: Pyrimidine nucleoside

Action: Inhibits viral DNA synthesis and replication

Uses: Primary keratoconjunctivitis, recurring epithelial keratitis

Dosage and routes:

• *Adult and child:* INSTILL 1 gtt q2h, not to exceed 9 gtts/day, until corneal epithelium is regrown, then 1 gtt q4h × 1 wk

Available forms include: Sol 1%

Side effects/adverse reactions:
EENT: Burning, stinging, swelling, photophobia
Contraindications: Hypersensitivity
Precautions: Antibiotic hypersensitivity, pregnancy (C)
NURSING CONSIDERATIONS
Administer:
• After washing hands, cleanse crusts or discharge from eye before application
Perform/provide:
• Storage in refrigerator
Evaluate:
• Therapeutic response: absence of redness, inflammation, tearing
• Allergy: itching, lacrimation, redness, swelling
Teach patient/family:
• To use drug exactly as prescribed
• Not to use eye make-up, towels, washcloths, or eye medication of others, or reinfection may occur
• That drug container tip should not be touched to eye
• To report itching, increased redness, burning, stinging; drug should be discontinued

---

trihexyphenidyl HCl
(trye-hex-ee-fen'i-dill)
Aparkane,* Aphen, Artane, Hexaphen, Novohexidyl,* T.H.P., Trihexane, Trihexidyl, Trihexy
Func. class.: Cholinergic blocker
Chem. class.: Synthetic tertiary amine

Action: Blocks central muscarinic receptors, which decreases involuntary movements
Uses: Parkinson symptoms
Dosage and routes:
Parkinson symptoms
• *Adult:* PO 1 mg, increased by 2 mg q3-5 days to a total of 6-10 mg/day
Drug-induced extrapyramidal symptoms
• *Adult:* PO 1 mg/day; usual dose 5-15 mg/day
Available forms include: Tabs 2, 5 mg; caps sus-rel 5 mg; elix 2 mg/5 ml
Side effects/adverse reactions:
CNS: Confusion, anxiety, restlessness, irritability, delusions, hallucinations, headache, sedation, depression, incoherence, dizziness, flushing, weakness
EENT: Blurred vision, photophobia, dilated pupils, difficulty swallowing
CV: Palpitations, tachycardia, postural hypotension
INTEG: Urticaria, rash
MISC: Suppression of lactation, nasal congestion, decreased sweating, increased temperature
MS: Weakness, cramping
GI: Dryness of mouth, constipation, nausea, vomiting, abdominal distress, *paralytic ileus*
GU: Hesitancy, retention
Contraindications: Hypersensitivity, narrow-angle glaucoma, myasthenia gravis, GI/GU obstruction, tachycardia, myocardial ischemia, unstable CV disease
Precautions: Pregnancy (C), elderly, lactation, tachycardia, prostatic hypertrophy, abdominal obstruction, infection, children, gastric ulcer
Pharmacokinetics:
PO: Onset 1 hr, peak 2-3 hr, duration 6-12 hr, excreted in urine
Interactions/incompatibilities:
• Increased anticholinergic effects: antihistamines, phenothiazines, amantadine
NURSING CONSIDERATIONS
Assess:
• I&O ratio; retention commonly

---

causes decreased urinary output
• B/P, pulse frequently while dose is being determined
Administer:
• With or after meals for GI upset; may give with fluids other than water
• At hs to avoid daytime drowsiness in patient with parkinsonism
Perform/provide:
• Storage at room temperature in light resistant containers
• Hard candy, frequent drinks, sugarless gum to relieve dry mouth
Evaluate:
• Parkinsonism: shuffling gait, muscle rigidity, involuntary movements
• Urinary hesitancy, retention; palpate bladder if retention occurs
• Constipation; increase fluids, bulk, exercise if this occurs
• For tolerance over long-term therapy; dose may need to be increased or changed
• Mental status: affect, mood, CNS depression, worsening of mental symptoms during early therapy
Teach patient/family:
• Not to discontinue this drug abruptly; to taper off over 1 wk
• To avoid driving or other hazardous activities; drowsiness may occur
• To avoid OTC medications: cough, cold preparations with alcohol, antihistamines unless directed by physician
• To avoid sudden position changes
• To avoid hot climates, overheating may occur

---

trilostane
(trye-loss-tane)
Modrastane
Func. class.: Antineoplastic
Chem. class.: Hormone, adrenal steroid inhibitor

Action: Inhibits DNA, RNA, protein synthesis; derived from *Streptomyces verticillus;* replication is decreased by binding to DNA, which causes strand splitting; drug is phase specific in G_2, M phases
Uses: Metastatic breast cancer, adrenal cancer, suppression of adrenal function in Cushing's syndrome
Dosage and routes:
• *Adult:* PO 30 mg qid, may increase q3-4d up to 480 mg/day
Available forms include: Caps 30, 60 mg
Side effects/adverse reactions:
HEMA: ***Thrombocytopenia, leukopenia, myelosuppression, anemia***
GI: Nausea, vomiting, anorexia, ***hepatotoxicity***
GU: Hirsutism
INTEG: Rash, pruritus
CV: Hypotension, tachycardia
CNS: Dizziness, headache
Contraindications: Hypersensitivity, hypothyroidism, pregnancy (X)
Precautions: Renal disease, hepatic disease, respiratory disease
Pharmacokinetics: Half-life 13 hr, metabolized in liver, excreted in urine, crosses placenta
NURSING CONSIDERATIONS
Assess:
• CBC, differential, platelet count weekly; withhold drug if WBC is <4000 or platelet count is <75,000; notify physician of results
• Renal function studies: BUN, serum uric acid, urine CrCl, electrolytes before, during therapy
• I&O ratio; report fall in urine output of 30 ml/hr
• Monitor temperature q4h (may indicate beginning infection)
• Liver function tests before, during therapy (bilirubin, AST, ALT, LDH) as needed or monthly
• RBC, Hct, Hgb since these may be decreased

T

italics = common side effects   ***bold italic*** = life threatening reactions

Administer:
• Medications by oral route; if possible avoid IM, SC, IV routes to prevent infections
• Antacid before oral agent, give last dose of drug after evening meal, before bedtime
• Antiemetic 30-60 min before giving drug to prevent vomiting
• Local or systemic drugs for infection

Perform/provide:
• Nutritious diet with iron, vitamin supplements as ordered

Evaluate:
• Bleeding: hematuria, guaiac, bruising, petechiae, mucosa or orifices q8h
• Food preferences; list likes, dislikes
• Inflammation of mucosa, breaks in skin
• Yellowing of skin, sclera, dark urine, clay-colored stools, itchy skin, abdominal pain, fever, diarrhea
• Symptoms indicating severe allergic reactions: rash, pruritus, urticaria, purpuric skin lesions, itching, flushing

Teach patient/family:
• To report any complaints, side effects to nurse or physician
• That masculinization can occur, is reversible after discontinuing treatment

---

trimeprazine tartrate
(trye-mep′ra-zeerı)
Panectyl,* Temaril

Func. class.: Antihistamine
Chem. class.: Phenothiazine analog, H_1-receptor antagonist

Action: Acts on blood vessels, GI, respiratory system by competing with histamine for H_1-receptor site; decreases allergic response by blocking histamine

Uses: Pruritus

Dosage and routes:
• *Adult:* PO 2.5 mg qid; TIME-REL 5 mg bid
• *Child 3-12 yr:* PO 2.5 mg tid or hs
• *Child 6 mo-1 yr:* PO 1.25 mg tid or hs

Available forms include: Tabs 2.5 mg; spans 5 mg; syr 2.5 mg/5 ml

Side effects/adverse reactions:
CNS: Dizziness, drowsiness, poor condition, fatigue, anxiety, euphoria, confusion, paresthesia, neuritis
CV: Hypotension, palpitations, tachycardia
RESP: Increased thick secretions, wheezing, chest tightness
*HEMA: **Thrombocytopenia, agranulocytosis, hemolytic anemia***
GI: Dry mouth, nausea, vomiting, anorexia, constipation, diarrhea
INTEG: Rash, urticaria, photosensitivity
GU: Retention, dysuria, frequency
EENT: Blurred vision, dilated pupils, tinnitus, nasal stuffiness, dry nose, throat, mouth

Contraindications: Hypersensitivity to H_1-receptor antagonist, acute asthma attack, lower respiratory tract disease

Precautions: Increased intraocular pressure, renal disease, cardiac disease, hypertension, bronchial asthma, seizure disorder, stenosed peptic ulcers, hyperthyroidism, prostatic hypertrophy, bladder neck obstruction, pregnancy (C)

Interactions/incompatibilities:
• Increased CNS depression: barbiturates, narcotics, hypnotics, tricyclic antidepressants, alcohol
• Decreased effect of: oral anticoagulants, heparin

• Increased effect of trimeprazine: MAOIs

NURSING CONSIDERATIONS
Assess:
• I&O ratio; be alert for urinary retention, frequency, dysuria; drug should be discontinued if these occur
• CBC during long-term therapy
Administer:
• Coffee, tea, cola (caffeine) to decrease drowsiness
• With meals if GI symptoms occur; absorption may slightly decrease
• Sustained-release formulation only to adults
Perform/provide:
• Hard candy, gum, frequent rinsing of mouth for dryness
• Storage in tight container at room temperature
Evaluate:
• Therapeutic response: decreased itching associated with pruritus
• Respiratory status: rate, rhythm, increase in bronchial secretions, wheezing, chest tightness
• Cardiac status: palpitations, increased pulse, hypotension
Teach patient/family:
• To notify physician if confusion, sedation, hypotension occurs
• To avoid driving or other hazardous activity if drowsiness occurs
• To avoid concurrent use of alcohol or other CNS depressants
Lab test interferences:
False negative: Skin allergy tests
Treatment of overdose: Administer ipecac syrup or lavage, diazepam, vasopressors, barbiturates (short-acting)

trimethadione
(trye-meth-a-dye'one)
Tridione
Func. class.: Anticonvulsant
Chem. class.: Oxazolidinedione

Action: Decreases seizures in cortex, basal ganglia; decreases synaptic stimulation to low-frequency impulses
Uses: Refractory absence (petit mal) seizures
Dosage and routes:
• *Adult:* PO 300 mg tid, may increase by 300 mg/wk, not to exceed 600 mg qid
• *Child:* PO 20-50 mg/kg/day, may increase by 150-300 mg/wk
Available forms include: Caps 300 mg; chew tabs 150 mg; sol 200 mg/ 5 ml; oral sol 40 mg/ml
Side effects/adverse reactions:
*HEMA: **Thrombocytopenia, agranulocytosis, leukopenia, neutropenia, hemolytic anemia,*** increased pro-time, *eosinophilia, **aplastic anemia***
CNS: Drowsiness, dizziness, fatigue, paresthesia, irritability, headache, insomnia
GU: Vaginal bleeding, albuminuria, nephrosis, abdominal pain, weight loss
GI: Nausea, vomiting, bleeding gums, abnormal liver function tests
*INTEG: **Exfoliative dermatitis,*** rash, alopecia, petechiae, erythema
EENT: Photophobia, diplopia, epistaxis, retinal hemorrhage
CV: Hypertension, hypotension
Contraindications: Hypersensitivity, blood dyscrasias, pregnancy (D)
Precautions: Hepatic disease, renal disease
Pharmacokinetics:
PO: Peak 30 min-2 hr, excreted by kidneys, half-life 6-13 days

T

---

italics = common side effects   ***bold italic*** = life threatening reactions

NURSING CONSIDERATIONS
Assess:
- Blood studies: Hct, Hgb, RBCs, serum folate, vitamin D; hepatic studies: AST, ALT, bilirubin, creatinine; drug should be stopped if neutrophil count falls below 2500/mm^3 if on long-term therapy

Administer:
- After diluting oral solution with water, give slowly through lavage needle
- Oral with juice or milk to cover taste/smell; decreases GI symptoms

Perform/provide:
- Ventilation of room

Evaluate:
- Mental status: mood, sensorium, affect, memory (long, short)
- Rash, alopecia, convulsions; discontinue drug if these occur

Teach patient/family:
- To notify physician if skin rash, alopecia, sore throat, fever, bruising, epistaxis occur
- That physical dependency may result when used for extended periods
- To avoid driving, other activities that require alertness
- Not to discontinue medication quickly after long-term use; convulsions may result

---

trimethaphan camsylate
(trye-meth'a-fan)
Arfonad

Func. class.: Antihypertensive
Chem. class.: Ganglionic blocker

Action: Occupies receptor site, prevents acetylcholine from attaching to postsynaptic nerve endings in sympathetic, parasympathetic ganglia

Uses: Hypertensive emergencies, production of controlled hypotension during surgery

Dosage and routes:
- *Adult:* IV INF dilute 500 mg in 500 ml of 5% dextrose injection, run at 3-4 mg/min, adjust to maintain B/P at desired rate; range 0.3-6.0 mg/min
- *Child:* 50-150 μg/kg/min

Available forms include: Inj IV 50 mg/ml

Side effects/adverse reactions:
CV: Orthostatic hypotension, angina, tachycardia, edema
GI: Nausea, vomiting, anorexia, dry mouth, diarrhea, constipation
CNS: Headache, agitation, weakness, restlessness
INTEG: Rash, urticaria, pruritus
*RESP: **Respiratory arrest***
EENT: Blurred vision, diplopia, pupillary dilation
GU: Urinary retention

Contraindications: Uncorrected respiratory insufficiency, hypersensitivity, pregnancy (C), hypovolemic shock, glaucoma, uncorrected anemia

Precautions: Elderly, debilitated, allergic individuals, cardiac disease, degenerative CNS disease, hepatic disease, renal disease, diabetes mellitus, Addison's disease, children

Pharmacokinetics:
IV: Onset 1-2 min, duration up to 30 min; excreted in urine, crosses placenta

Interactions/incompatibilities:
- Increased effects of diuretics, antihypertensives, anesthetics
- Do not mix with any drug in syringe or solution

NURSING CONSIDERATIONS
Assess:
- Electrolytes: K, Na, Cl, CO_2
- Renal function studies: BUN, creatinine

- B/P during initial treatment, periodically thereafter
- Weight daily, I&O
- ECG throughout treatment if there is a history of cardiac problems

Administer:
- IV infusion by microdrip regulator
- Diluted solution only (500 mg of drug/500 ml or more of D₅W)

Perform/provide:
- Artificial ventilation equipment nearby
- Use of only freshly prepared solution
- Elevate patient's head to control B/P

Evaluate:
- Therapeutic effect: decreased B/P, primarily systolic B/P
- Nausea, vomiting, diarrhea
- Edema in feet, legs daily
- Skin turgor, dryness of mucous membranes for hydration status
- Constipation: number of stools, consistency, give stool softener as ordered or increase bulk in diet if constipation occurs, or antidiarrheal for diarrhea
- Respiratory dysfunction: bronchospasm, wheezing, tachypnea, respiratory arrest
- Signs of peripheral vascular collapse

Teach patient/family:
- That lying in bed is needed during infusion

Treatment of overdose: Administer vasopressors, phenylephrine, mephentermine

trimethobenzamide

(trye-meth-oh-ben'za-mide)
Spengan, Ticon, Tigan
Func. class.: Antiemetic, anticholinergic
Chem. class.: Ethanolamine derivative

Action: Acts centrally by blocking chemoreceptor trigger zone, which in turn acts on vomiting center

Uses: Nausea, vomiting, prevention of postoperative vomiting

Dosage and routes:
Postoperative vomiting
- *Adult:* IM/REC 200 mg before or during surgery; may repeat 3 hr after

Discontinuing anesthesia
- *Child 13-40 kg:* PO/REC 100-200 mg tid-qid
- *Child <13 kg:* PO/REC 100 mg tid-qid

Nausea/vomiting
- *Adult:* PO 250 mg tid-qid; IM/REC 200 mg tid-qid

Available forms include: Caps 100, 250 mg; supp 100, 200 mg; inj IM 100 mg/ml

Side effects/adverse reactions:
CNS: Drowsiness, restlessness, headache, dizziness, insomnia, confusion, nervousness, tingling, vertigo, extrapyramidal symptoms
GI: Nausea, anorexia, diarrhea, vomiting, constipation
CV: Hypertension, hypotension, palpitation
INTEG: Rash, urticaria, fever, chills, flushing
EENT: Dry mouth, blurred vision, diplopia, nasal congestion, photosensitivity

Contraindications: Hypersensitivity to narcotics, shock, children (parenterally)

---

italics = common side effects   ***bold italic*** = life threatening reactions

Precautions: Children, cardiac dysrhythmias, elderly, asthma, pregnancy (C), prostatic hypertrophy, bladder-neck obstruction, narrow-angle glaucoma, stenosing peptic ulcer, pyloroduodenal obstruction

Pharmacokinetics:
PO: Onset 20-40 min, duration 3-4 hr
IM: Onset 15 min, duration 2-3 hr, metabolized by liver, excreted by kidneys

Interactions/incompatibilities:
• Increased effect: CNS depressants
• May mask ototoxic symptoms associated with antibiotics

NURSING CONSIDERATIONS
Assess:
• VS, B/P; check patients with cardiac disease more often

Administer:
• IM injection in large muscle mass; aspirate to avoid IV administration
• Tablets may be swallowed whole, chewed, allowed to dissolve

Evaluate:
• Signs of toxicity of other drugs or masking of symptoms of disease: brain tumor, intestinal obstruction
• Observe for drowsiness, dizziness

Teach patient/family:
• To avoid hazardous activities, activities requiring alertness; dizziness may occur; instruct patient to request assistance with ambulation
• To avoid alcohol, other depressants
• To keep out of children's reach

---

trimethoprim
(trye-meth'oh-prim)
Proloprim, Trimpex
Func. class.: Urinary antiinfective
Chem. class.: Folate antagonist

Action: Prevents bacterial synthesis by blocking enzyme reduction of dihyodrofolic acid

Uses: *E.coli, P. mirabilis, Klebsiella, Enterobacter* urinary tract infections

Dosage and routes:
• *Adult:* PO 100 mg q12h
Available forms include: Tabs 100, 200 mg

Side effects/adverse reactions:
*INTEG: **Exfoliative dermatitis**,* pruritus, rash
*HEMA: **Thrombocytopenia, leukopenia, neutropenia, megaloblastic anemia*** (rare)
GI: Nausea, vomiting, abdominal pain, abnormal taste, increased AST, ALT, bilirubin, creatinine
CNS: Fever

Contraindications: Hypersensitivity, CrCl <15 ml/min, renal disease, hepatic disease, megaloblastic anemia

Precautions: Folate deficiency, pregnancy (C), lactation, fragile X chromosome, children <12 yr old

Pharmacokinetics:
PO: Peak 1-4 hr, half-life 8-11 hr, metabolized in liver, excreted in urine (unchanged 60%), breast milk, crosses placenta

Interactions/incompatabilities:
• Decreased action of: phenytoin

NURSING CONSIDERATIONS
Assess:
• Nocturia; may indicate drug resistance
• Signs of infection, anemia
• AST/ALT, BUN, bilirubin, creatinine, urine cultures
• C&S before drug therapy; drug may be taken as soon as culture is obtained

Administer:
• With full glass of water

Perform/provide:
• Storage in tight, light-resistant container

---

*Available in Canada only

- Adequate intake of fluids (2000 ml) to decrease bacteria in bladder

Evaluate:
- Therapeutic response: absence of pain in bladder area, negative C&S
- Skin eruptions

Teach patient/family:
- Aspects of drug therapy: need to complete entire course of medication to ensure organism death (10-14 days); culture may be taken after completed course of medication
- That drug must be taken in equal intervals around clock to maintain blood levels
- To notify nurse of nausea, vomiting

---

trimipramine maleate

(tri-mip'ra-meen)
Surmontil
Func. class.: Antidepressant—tricyclic
Chem. class.: Tertiary amine

Action: Selectively inhibits serotonin uptake by brain; potentiates behavioral changes

Uses: Depression, enuresis in children

Dosage and routes:
- *Adult:* PO 75 mg/day in divided doses, may be increased to 200 mg/day
- *Child >6 yr:* 25 mg hs, may increase to 50 mg in children <12 yr or 75 mg in children >12 yr

Available forms include: Caps 25, 50, 100 mg

Side effects/adverse reactions:
*HEMA: **Agranulocytosis, thrombocytopenia, eosinophilia, leukopenia***
CNS: Dizziness, drowsiness, confusion, headache, anxiety, tremors, stimulation, weakness, insomnia,

nightmares, EPS (elderly), increase in psychiatric symptoms
GI: Diarrhea, dry mouth, nausea, vomiting, ***paralytic ileus,*** increased appetite, cramps, epigastric distress, jaundice, ***hepatitis,*** stomatitis
*GU: Retention, **acute renal failure***
INTEG: Rash, urticaria, sweating, pruritus, photosensitivity
*CV: Orthostatic hypotension, ECG changes, tachycardia, **hypertension,*** palpitations
EENT: Blurred vision, tinnitus, mydriasis

Contraindications: Hypersensitivity to tricyclic antidepressants, recovery phase of myocardial infarction, convulsive disorders, prostatic hypertrophy

Precautions: Suicidal patients, severe depression, increased intraocular pressure, narrow-angle glaucoma, urinary retention, cardiac disease, hepatic disease, hyperthyroidism, electroshock therapy, elective surgery, pregnancy (C)

Pharmacokinetics:
Metabolized by liver, excreted by kidneys, steady state 2-6 days; half-life 7-30 hr

Interactions/incompatibilities:
- Decreased effects of: guanethidine, clonidine, indirect acting sympathomimetics (ephedrine)
- Increased effects of: direct acting sympathomimetics (epinephrine), alcohol, barbiturates, benzodiazepines, CNS depressants
- Hyperpyretic crisis, convulsions, hypertensive episode: MAOI (pargyline [Eutonyl])

NURSING CONSIDERATIONS
Assess:
- B/P (lying, standing), pulse q4h; if systolic B/P drops 20 mm Hg hold drug, notify physician; take

T

---

italics = common side effects   ***bold italic*** = life threatening reactions

vital signs q4h in patients with cardiovascular disease
• Blood studies: CBC, leukocytes, differential, cardiac enzymes if patient is receiving long-term therapy
• Hepatic studies: AST, ALT, bilirubin, creatinine
• Weight qwk, appetite may increase with drug
• ECG for flattening of T wave, bundle branch block, AV block, dysrhythmias in cardiac patients

Administer:
• Increased fluids, bulk in diet if constipation, urinary retention occur
• With food or milk for GI symptoms
• Dosage hs if over-sedation occurs during day; may take entire dose hs; elderly may not tolerate once/day dosing
• Gum, hard candy, or frequent sips of water for dry mouth

Perform/provide:
• Storage in tight, light-resistant container at room temperature
• Assistance with ambulation during beginning therapy since drowsiness/dizziness occurs
• Safety measures, including siderails primarily in elderly
• Checking to see PO medication swallowed

Evaluate:
• EPS primarily in elderly: rigidity, dystonia, akathisia
• Mental status: mood, sensorium, affect, suicidal tendencies, increase in psychiatric symptoms: depression, panic
• Urinary retention, constipation; constipation is more likely to occur in children
• Withdrawal symptoms: headache, nausea, vomiting, muscle pain, weakness; do not usually occur unless drug was discontinued abruptly
• Alcohol consumption; if alcohol is consumed, hold dose until morning

Teach patient/family:
• That therapeutic effects may take 2-3 wk
• To use caution in driving or other activities requiring alertness because of drowsiness, dizziness, blurred vision
• To avoid alcohol ingestion, other CNS depressants
• Not to discontinue medication quickly after long-term use, may cause nausea, headache, malaise
• To wear sunscreen or large hat since photosensitivity occurs

Lab test interferences:
Increase: Serum bilirubin, blood glucose, alk phosphatase
False increase: Urinary catecholamines
Decrease: VMA, 5-HIAA

Treatment of overdose: ECG monitoring, induce emesis, lavage, activated charcoal, administer anticonvulsant

---

tripelennamine HCl

(tri-pel-een'a-meen)
PBZ-SR, Pelamine, Pyribenzamine, Ro-Hist

Func. class.: Antihistamine
Chem. class.: Ethylenediamine derivative

Action: Acts on blood vessels, GI, respiratory system, by competing with histamine for H_1-receptor site; decreases allergic response by blocking histamine
Uses: Rhinitis, allergy symptoms
Dosage and routes:
• *Adult:* PO 25-50 mg q4-6h, not to exceed 600 mg/day; TIME-REL

---

* Available in Canada only

100 mg bid-tid, not to exceed 600 mg/day
• *Child >5 yr:* TIME-REL 50 mg q8-12hr, not to exceed 300 mg/day
• *Child <5 yr:* PO 5 mg/kg/day in 4-6 divided doses, not to exceed 300 mg/day
Available forms include: Tab 25, 50 mg; time-rel tab 100 mg; elix 37.5 mg/5 ml
Side effects/adverse reactions:
CNS: Dizziness, drowsiness, poor coordination, fatigue, anxiety, euphoria, confusion, paresthesia, neuritis
CV: Hypotension, palpitations, tachycardia
RESP: Increased thick secretions, wheezing, chest tightness
*HEMA: **Thrombocytopenia, agranulocytosis, hemolytic anemia***
GI: Constipation, dry mouth, nausea, vomiting, anorexia, diarrhea
INTEG: Rash, urticaria, photosensitivity
GU: Retention, dysuria, frequency
EENT: Blurred vision, dilated pupils, tinnitus, nasal stuffiness, dry nose, throat, mouth
Contraindications: Hypersensitivity to H₁-receptor antagonist, acute asthma attack, lower respiratory tract disease
Precautions: Increased intraocular pressure, renal disease, cardiac disease, hypertension, bronchial asthma, seizure disorder, stenosed peptic ulcers, hyperthyroidism, prostatic hypertrophy, bladder neck obstruction, pregnancy (C)
Pharmacokinetics:
PO: Onset 15-30 min, duration 4-6 hr, detoxified in liver, excreted by kidneys
Interactions/incompatibilities:
• Increased CNS depressants: barbiturates, narcotics, hypnotics, tricyclic antidepressants, alcohol

• Decreased effect of: oral anticoagulants, heparin
• Increased effect of tripelennamine: MAOIs
NURSING CONSIDERATIONS
Assess:
• I&O ratio; be alert for urinary retention, frequency, dysuria; drug should be discontinued if these occur
• CBC during long-term therapy
Administer:
• With meals if GI symptoms occur; absorption may slightly decrease
• Time-release formulation to adults only
Perform/provide:
• Hard candy, gum, frequent rinsing of mouth for dryness
• Storage in tight container at room temperature
Evaluate:
• Therapeutic response: decrease itching associated with pruritus
• Respiratory status: rate, rhythm, increase in bronchial secretions, wheezing, chest tightness
• Cardiac status: palpitations, increased pulse, hypotension
Teach patient/family:
• All aspects of drug use; to notify physician if confusion, sedation, hypotension occurs
• To avoid driving or other hazardous activity if drowsiness occurs
• To avoid concurrent use of alcohol or other CNS depressants
Lab test interferences:
False negative: Skin allergy test
False positive: Urine pregnancy tests
Treatment of overdose: Administer ipecac syrup or lavage, diazepam, vasopressors, barbiturates (short-acting)

italics = common side effects   ***bold italic*** = life threatening reactions

triprolidine HCl

(trye-proe'li-deen)
Actifed,* Actidil, Bayidyl
Func. class.: Antihistamine
Chem. class.: Alkylamine, H₁-receptor antagonist

Action: Acts on blood vessels, GI, respiratory system, by competing with histamine for H₁-receptor site; decreases allergic response by blocking histamine

Uses: Rhinitis, allergy symptoms

Dosage and routes:
• *Adult:* PO 2.5 mg tid-qid
• *Child >6 yr:* PO 1.25 mg tid-qid
• *Child 4-6 yr:* PO 0.9 mg tid-qid
• *Child 2-4 yr:* PO 0.6 mg tid-qid
• *Child 4 mo-2 yr:* 0.3 mg tid-qid
Available forms include: Tab 2.5 mg; syr 1.25 mg/5 ml

Side effects/adverse reactions:
CNS: Dizziness, drowsiness, poor coordination, fatigue, anxiety, euphoria, confusion, paresthesia, neuritis
CV: Hypotension, palpitations, tachycardia
RESP: Increased thick secretions, wheezing, chest tightness
HEMA: Thrombocytopenia, agranulocytosis, hemolytic anemia
GI: Constipation, dry mouth, nausea, vomiting, anorexia, diarrhea
INTEG: Rash, urticaria, photosensitivity
GU: Retention, dysuria, frequency
EENT: Blurred vision, dilated pupils, tinnitus, nasal stuffiness, dry nose, throat, mouth

Contraindications: Hypersensitivity to H₁-receptor antagonist, acute asthma attack, lower respiratory tract disease

Precautions: Increased intraocular pressure, renal disease, cardiac disease, hypertension, bronchial asthma, seizure disorder, stenosed peptic ulcers, hyperthyroidism, prostatic hypertrophy, bladder neck obstruction, pregnancy (C)

Pharmacokinetics:
PO: Onset 20-60 min, duration 8-12 hr, detoxified in liver, excreted by kidneys (metabolites/free drug), half-life 20-24 hr

Interactions/incompatibilities:
• Increased CNS depressants: barbiturates, narcotics, hypnotics, tricyclic antidepressants, alcohol
• Decreased effect of: oral anticoagulants, heparin
• Increased effect of triprolidine: MAOIs

NURSING CONSIDERATIONS
Assess:
• I&O ratio; be alert for urinary retention, frequency, dysuria; drug should be discontinued if these occur
• CBC during long-term therapy

Administer:
• With meals if GI symptoms occur; absorption may slightly decrease
• Time-release formulation to adults only

Perform/provide:
• Hard candy, gum, frequent rinsing of mouth for dryness
• Storage in tight container at room temperature

Evaluate:
• Therapeutic response: decreased itching associated with pruritus
• Respiratory status: rate, rhythm, increase in bronchial secretions, wheezing, chest tightness
• Cardiac status: palpitations, increased pulse, hypotension

Teach patient/family:
• All aspects of drug use; to notify

---

physician if confusion, sedation, hypotension occurs
• To avoid driving or other hazardous activity if drowsiness occurs
• To avoid concurrent use of alcohol or other CNS depressants while taking this drug

Lab test interferences:
False negative: Skin allergy tests
Treatment of overdose: Administer ipecac syrup or lavage, diazepam, vasopressors, barbiturates (short-acting)

---

troleandomycin

(troe-lee-an-doe-mye′sin)
TAO
Func. class.: Antibacterial, macrolide
Chem. class.: Oleandomycin derivative

Action: Inhibits cell wall bacterial synthesis by binding to 50S subunit of ribosome
Uses: *P. pneumonia* or group A β-hemolytic streptococcal respiratory infections
Dosage and routes:
• *Adult:* PO 250-500 mg q6h
• *Child:* PO 6.6-11 mg/kg q6h
Available forms include: Caps 250 mg
Side effects/adverse reactions:
*SYST: **Anaphylaxis***
INTEG: Urticaria, rash
GI: Nausea, vomiting, rectal burning, esophagitis, *abdominal cramps, **cholangiolytic hepatitis***
Contraindications: Hypersensitivity, minor infections
Precautions: Hepatic disease, pregnancy, lactation
Pharmacokinetics:
PO: Peak 2 hr, duration >12 hr, metabolized in liver, excreted in urine (active drug 25%) and bile

Interactions/incompatibilities:
• Increased ischemic reactions: ergotamine preparations
• Increased theophylline levels: theophylline
• Increased action of: carbamazepine, corticosteroids
• Cholestatic jaundice: oral contraceptives

NURSING CONSIDERATIONS
Assess:
• Liver studies: AST, ALT
• C&S before drug therapy; drug may be taken as soon as culture is taken; C&S may be taken after treatment
Perform/provide:
• Storage at room temperature
• Adrenalin, suction, tracheostomy set, endotracheal intubation equipment on unit
Evaluate:
• Jaundice, fever, nausea, vomiting, right upper quadrant pain indicating cholestatic hepatitis; drug should be discontinued
Teach patient/family:
• To take oral drug on empty stomach with full glass of water
• Aspects of drug therapy: need to complete entire course of medication to ensure organism death (10 days); culture may be taken after completed course of medication
• To report sore throat, fever, fatigue; could indicate superimposed infection
• That drug must be taken in equal intervals around clock to maintain blood levels
Lab test interferences:
False increase: Urinary 17-KS, 17-OHCS

T

---

tromethamine

(troe-meth′a-meen)
Tham, Tham-E
Func. class.: Alkalinizer
Chem. class.: Amine

Action: Proton acceptor which corrects acidosis by combining with hydrogen ions to form bicarbonate and buffer; acts as diuretic (osmotic)

Uses: Acidosis (metabolic) associated with cardiac disease or COPD

Dosage and routes:
• *Adult:* 0.3 M required = kg of weight × HCO_3 deficit (mEq/L)
• *Child:* Same as above given over 3-6 hr, not to exceed 40 ml/kg

Available forms include: Inj IV 36 mg/ml, powd for inj IV 36 g

Side effects/adverse reactions:
CV: Irregular pulse, **cardiac arrest**
META: Alkalosis, hypoglycemia, hyperkalemia
RESP: Shallow, slow respirations, cyanosis, **apnea**
GI: **Hepatic necrosis**
INTEG: Infection at injection site, extravasation

Contraindications: Hypersensitivity, anuria, uremia

Precautions: Severe respiratory disease/respiratory depression, pregnancy (C), cardiac edema, renal disease, infants

Pharmacokinetics:
IV: Excreted in urine

NURSING CONSIDERATIONS
Assess:
• Respiratory rate, rhythm, depth, notify physician of abnormalities that may indicate acidosis
• Electrolytes, blood glucose, chloride CO_2, before, during treatment
• Urine pH, urinary output, urine glucose during beginning treatment
• I&O ratio, report large increase or decrease
• IV site for extravasation, phlebitis, thrombosis
• For signs of K^+ depletion

Administer:
• IV slowly to avoid pain at infusion site and toxicity
• IV undiluted as INF or added to priming fluid or ACD blood; give 5 ml or less/min

Teach patient/family:
• To increase K + in diet: bananas, oranges, cantaloupe, honeydew, spinach, potatoes, dried fruit

tropicamide (optic)

(troe-pik′a-mide)
Mydriacyl
Func. class.: Mydriatic, cycloplegia, anticholinergic
Chem. class.: Belladonna alkaloid

Action: Blocks response of sphincter muscle of iris and ciliary body dilatation and paralysis of accommodation

Uses: Fundus exam, cycloplegic refraction

Dosage and routes:
• *Adult and child:* INSTILL 1-2 gtts of 1% sol, repeat in 5 min (refraction) or 1-2 gtts of 0.5% sol 15-20 min before exam (fundus examination)

Available forms include: Sol 0.5%, 1%

Side effects/adverse reactions:
SYST: Tachycardia, confusion, hallucinations, emotional changes in children, fever, flushing, dry skin, dry mouth, abdominal discomfort (infants: bladder distention, irregular pulse, **respiratory depression**)

Contraindications: Hypersensitiv-

ity, infants <3 mo, glaucoma, conjunctivitis

Precautions: Pregnancy (C)

Pharmacokinetics:

INSTILL: Peak 20-40 min, (mydriasis), 20-35 min, (cycloplegia)

NURSING CONSIDERATIONS
Evaluate:
• Eye pain, discontinue use
Teach patient/family:
• To report change in vision, with blurring or loss of sight, trouble breathing, flushing
• Method of instillation, including pressure on lacrimal sac for 1 min, and not to touch dropper to eye
• That blurred vision will decrease with repeated use of drug
• Not to engage in hazardous activities until able to see
• To wait 5 min to use other drops
• Not to blink more than usual
• That dark glasses may be worn if photophobia occurs

---

tubocurarine chloride

(too-boe-kyoo-ar'een)
Tubarine*

Func. class.: Neuromuscular blockers

Chem. class.: Curare alkaloid

Action: Inhibits transmission of nerve impulses by binding with cholinergic receptor sites, antagonizing action of acetylcholine

Uses: Facilitation of endotracheal intubation, skeletal muscle relaxation during mechanical ventilation, surgery, or general anesthesia

Dosage and routes:
• *Adult:* IV BOL 0.4-0.5 mg/kg, then 0.08-0.10 mg/kg 20-45 min after 1st dose if needed for prolonged procedures

Available forms include: Inj IV 3 mg/ml, 20 U/ml

Side effects/adverse reactions:

CV: Bradycardia, tachycardia, increased, decreased B/P

RESP: **Prolonged apnea, bronchospasm, cyanosis, respiratory depression**

EENT: Increased secretions

INTEG: Rash, flushing, pruritus, urticaria

Contraindications: Hypersensitivity

Precautions: Pregnancy (C), cardiac disease, lactation, children <2 yr, electrolyte imbalances, dehydration, neuromuscular disease, respiratory disease

Pharmacokinetics:

IV: Onset 15 sec, peak 2-3 min, duration ½-1½ hr; half-life 1-3 hr, degraded in liver, kidney (minimally), excreted in urine (unchanged) crosses placenta

Interactions/incompatibilities:
• Increased neuromuscular blockade: aminoglycosides, clindamycin, lincomycin, quinidine, local anesthetics, polymyxin antibiotics, lithium, narcotic analgesics, thiazides, enflurane, isoflurane
• Dysrhythmias: theophylline
• Do not mix with barbiturates in solution or syringe

NURSING CONSIDERATIONS
Assess:
• For electrolyte imbalances (K, Mg); may lead to increased action of this drug
• Vital signs (B/P, pulse, respirations, airway) q15 min until fully recovered; rate, depth, pattern of respirations, strength of hand grip
• I&O ratio; check for urinary retention, frequency, hesitancy

Administer:
• With diazepam, or morphine when used for therapeutic paralysis; this drug provides no sedation alone

---

italics = common side effects   **bold italic** = life threatening reactions

• Using nerve stimulator by anesthesiologist to determine neuromuscular blockade
• Anticholinesterase to reverse neuromuscular blockade
• IV undiluted 3 mg/ml; give single dose over 1-1½ sec by qualified person

Perform/provide:
• Storage in light-resistant area; use only fresh solution
• Reassurance if communication is difficult during recovery from neuromuscular blockade

Evaluate:
• Therapeutic response: paralysis of jaw, eyelid, head, neck, rest of body
• Recovery: decreased paralysis of face, diaphragm, leg, arm, rest of body; allow to fully recover before completing a neuro assessment
• Allergic reactions: rash, fever, respiratory distress, pruritus; drug should be discontinued

Treatment of overdose: Edrophonium or neostigmine, atropine, monitor VS; may require mechanical ventilation

---

undecylenic acid (topical)

(un-dek'-sye-lin-ik)
Cruex, Desenex, NP-27, Ting, Unde-Jen

Func. class.: Local antiinfective
Chem. class.: Antifungal, antibacterial

Action: Interferes with fungal cell membrane permeability
Uses: Tinea cruris, pedis, diaper rash, minor skin irritations
Dosage and routes:
• *Adult and child:* TOP apply to affected areas bid

Available forms include: Powder, oint, cream, liq, foam, soap
Side effects/adverse reactions:
INTEG: Rash, urticaria, stinging, burning
Contraindications: Hypersensitivity
Precautions: Pregnancy (C), lactation, impaired circulation, diabetes mellitus

NURSING CONSIDERATIONS
Administer:
• Enough medication to completely cover lesions
• After cleansing with soap, water before each application, dry well
Perform/provide:
• Storage at room temperature in dry place
Evaluate for:
• Allergic reaction: burning, stinging, swelling, redness
• Therapeutic response: decrease in size, number of lesions
Teach patient/family:
• To apply with glove to prevent further infection
• To avoid use of OTC creams, ointments, lotions unless directed by physician
• To use medical asepsis (hand washing) before, after each application
• To avoid inhaling and contact with eyes or other mucous membranes

---

uracil mustard

(yoor'a-sill)

Func. class.: Antineoplastic alkylating agent
Chem. class.: Nitrogen mustard

Action: Responsible for cross-linking DNA strands leading to cell death
Uses: Hodgkin's disease, lympho-

---

mas; cervix, ovarian, lung cancer; chronic lymphocytic, myelocytic leukemia; reticulum cell sarcoma, mycosis fungoides; polycythemia vera

Dosage and routes:
• *Adult:* PO 1-2 mg/day × 3 mo or desired response, then 1 mg/day for 3 out of 4 wk until desired response or 3-5 mg × 7 days, not to exceed total dose of 0.5 mg/kg then 1 mg/day until desired response, then 1 mg/day 3 out of 4 wk

Available forms include: Caps 1 mg

Side effects/adverse reactions:
*HEMA: **Thrombocytopenia, leukopenia,** anemia*
*GI: Nausea, vomiting, diarrhea, **hepatotoxicity***
GU: Amenorrhea, azoospermia
INTEG: Alopecia, dermatitis, pruritus, rash

Contraindications: Severe thrombocytopenia/leukopenia, hypersensitivity, pregnancy (X)

Precautions: Radiation therapy

Pharmacokinetics:
Excreted unchanged in urine

Interactions/incompatibilities:
• Increased toxicity: antineoplastics, radiation

NURSING CONSIDERATIONS
Assess:
• CBC, differential, platelet count weekly; withhold drug if WBC is <4000 or platelet count is <75,000; notify physician of results
• Renal function studies: BUN, serum uric acid, urine CrCl before, during therapy
• I&O ratio; report fall in urine output of 30 ml/hr
• Monitor temperature q4h (may indicate beginning infection)
• Liver function tests before, during therapy (bilirubin, AST, ALT, LDH) as needed or monthly

Administer:
• Medications by oral route if possible; avoid IM, SC, IV routes to prevent infections
• Antacid before oral agent; give drug after evening meal, before bedtime
• Antiemetic 30-60 min before giving drug to prevent vomiting
• Antibiotics for prophylaxis of infection
• Topical or systemic analgesics for pain
• Local or systemic drugs for infection

Perform/provide:
• Storage in tight container at room temperature
• Strict medical asepsis, protective isolation if WBC levels are low
• Special skin care
• Liquid diet, including cola, Jello; dry toast or crackers may be added if patient is not nauseated or vomiting
• Increase fluid intake to 2-3 L/day to prevent urate deposits, calculi formation

Evaluate:
• Bleeding: hematuria, guaiac, bruising or petechiae, mucosa or orifices q8h
• Food preferences; list likes, dislikes
• Yellowing of skin, sclera, dark urine, clay-colored stools, itchy skin, abdominal pain, fever, diarrhea
• Effects of alopecia on body image; discuss feelings about body changes
• Inflammation of mucosa, breaks in skin
• Symptoms indicating severe allergic reaction: rash, pruritus, urticaria, itching
• Check for tartrazine dye allergy

U

---

italics = common side effects   ***bold italic*** = life threatening reactions

Teach patient/family:
• Of protective isolation precautions
• To report signs of infection: increased temperature, sore throat, flu symptoms
• To report signs of anemia: fatigue, headache, faintness, shortness of breath, irritability
• To avoid use of razors or commercial mouthwash
• To avoid use of aspirin products or ibuprofen
• That azoospermia, amenorrhea can occur; are reversible after discontinuing treatment
• That hair may be lost during treatment; a wig or hairpiece may make patient feel better; new hair may be different in color, texture
• To avoid foods with citric acid, hot or rough texture

---

urea

(yoor-ee'a)
Ureaphil, Carbamex*
Func. class.: Diuretic, osmotic
Chem. class.: Carbonic acid diamide salt

Action: Elevates plasma osmolality increasing flow of water into the extracellular compartment
Uses: To decrease intracranial pressure, intraocular pressure
Dosage and routes:
• *Adult:* IV 1-1.5 g/kg of a 30% sol over 1-3 hr
• *Child >2 yr:* IV 0.5-1.5 g/kg, not to exceed 4 ml/min
• *Child <2 yr:* IV 0.1 g/kg, not to exceed 4 ml/min
Available forms include: Inj IV 40 g/150 ml
Side effects/adverse reactions:
CNS: Dizziness, headache, disorientation, fever, syncope, headache
GI: Nausea, vomiting
INTEG: Venous thrombosis, phlebitis, extravasation
CV: Postural hypotension
Contraindications: Severe renal disease, active intracranial bleeding, marked dehydration, liver failure
Precautions: Hepatic disease, renal disease, pregnancy (C), electrolyte imbalances, lactation
Pharmacokinetics:
IV: Onset ½-1 hr, peak 1 hr, duration 3-10 hr, (diuresis) 5-6 hr (intraocular pressure); half-life 1 hr, excreted in urine, crosses placenta, excreted in breast milk
Interactions/incompatibilities:
• Incompatible with whole blood, in solution or syringe with any other drug or solution
• Increased renal excretion of: lithium

NURSING CONSIDERATIONS
Assess:
• Weight, I&O daily to determine fluid loss; effect of drug may be decreased if used qd
• Rate, depth, rhythm of respiration, effect of exertion
• B/P lying, standing, postural hypotension may occur
• Electrolytes: potassium, sodium, chloride; include BUN, blood sugar, CBC, serum creatinine, blood pH, ABGs, liver function tests
Administer:
• IV after diluting 30 g/100 ml diluent with D_5, D_{10}; run 30% sol over 1-2 hr; check for extravasation; do not exceed 4 ml/min; use IV filter
• Within minutes of reconstitution. Solution becomes ammonia on standing
Evaluate:
• Improvement in edema of feet,

---

legs, sacral area daily if medication is being used in CHF
• Improvement in CVP q8h
• Signs of metabolic acidosis: drowsiness, restlessness
• Signs of hypokalemia: postural hypotension, malaise, fatigue, tachycardia, leg cramps, weakness
• Temperature elevation, signs of extravasation qd
• Confusion, especially in elderly, take safety precautions if needed
• Hydration: skin turgor, thirst, dry mucous membranes

Teach patient/family:
• That drug will cause diuresis in ½ hr

Treatment of overdose: Lavage if taken orally, monitor electrolytes, administer IV fluids, monitor BUN, hydration, CV status

---

urofollitropin

(yoor-oo-foll′aa-tropin)
Metrodin

Func. class.: Ovulation stimulant
Chem. class.: Gonadotropin

Action: Stimulates ovarian follicular growth in primary ovarian failure

Uses: Induction of ovulation in polycystic ovarian disease in those who have elevated LH/FSH ratios and have failed to respond to other treatment

Dosage and routes:
• *Adult:* IM 75 IU/day × 7-12 days, then 5000-10,000 U HCG 1 day after last urofollitropin, if pregnancy does not occur; may repeat for 2 courses before increasing dose to 150 IU/day 7-12 days then 5000-10,000 U HCG 1 day after last urofollitropin; may repeat for 2 more courses

Available forms include: Powder

for injection 0.83 mg (76 IU FSH)/ amp

Side effects/adverse reactions:
CNS: Malaise
GI: Nausea, vomiting, constipation, increased appetite, abdominal pain
INTEG: Rash, dermatitis, urticaria, alopecia
GU: Polyuria, frequency, **birth defects, spontaneous abortions,** multiple ovulation, breast pain

Contraindications: Hypersensitivity, pregnancy, undiagnosed vaginal bleeding, intracranial lesion, ovarian cyst not caused by polycystic ovarian disease

Precautions: Lactation, arterial thromboembolism

Pharmacokinetics:
Detoxified in liver, excreted in feces, stored in fat

NURSING CONSIDERATIONS
Assess:
• At same time qd to maintain drug level

Teach patient/family:
• Multiple births are common after taking this drug
• To notify physician if low abdominal pain occurs; may indicate ovarian cyst, cyst rupture
• Method of taking, recording basal body temperature to determine whether ovulation has occurred
• If ovulation can be determined (there is a slight decrease then a sharp increase for ovulation) to attempt coitus 3 days before and qod until after ovulation
• If pregnancy is suspected, physician must be notified immediately

U

---

italics = common side effects   ***bold italic*** = life threatening reactions

urokinase

(yoor-oh-kin'ase)
Abbokinase, Win-Kinase
Func. class.: Thrombolytic enzyme
Chem. class.: β-Hemolytic streptococcus filtrate (purified)

Action: Promotes thrombolysis by enhancing the change of plasminogen to plasmin

Uses: Venous thrombosis, pulmonary embolism, arterial thrombosis, arterial embolism, arteriovenous cannula occlusion, lysis of coronary artery thrombi after myocardial infarction

Dosage and routes:
Lysis of pulmonary emboli
• *Adult:* IV 4400 IU/kg/hr × 12-24 hr not to exceed 200 ml; then IV heparin, then anticoagulants

Coronary artery thrombosis
• *Adult:* INSTILL 6000 IU/min into occluded artery for 1-2 hr after giving IV bol of heparin 2500-10,000 U

Venous catheter occlusion
• *Adult:* INSTILL 5000 IU into line, wait 5 min, then aspirate, repeat aspiration attempts q5min × ½ hr; if occlusion has not been removed, then cap line and wait ½-1 hr then aspirate; may need 2nd dose if still occluded

Available forms include: Inj

Side effects/adverse reactions:
*HEMA: Decreased Hct, **bleeding***
INTEG: Rash, urticaria, phlebitis at IV infusion site, itching, flushing, headache
CNS: Headache, fever,
GI: Nausea
RESP: Altered respirations, SOB, ***bronchospasm***
MS: Low back pain

CV: Hypertension, dysrhythmias
EENT: Periorbital edema
*SYST: **GI, GU, intracranial, retroperitoneal bleeding,** surface bleeding, **anaphylaxis***
Contraindications: Hypersensitivity, active bleeding, intraspinal surgery, neoplasms of CNS, ulcerative colitis/enteritis, severe hypertension, renal disease, hepatic disease, hypocoagulation, COPD, subacute bacterial endocarditis, rheumatic valvular disease, cerebral embolism/thrombosis/hemorrhage, intraarterial diagnostic procedure or surgery (10 days), recent major surgery
Precautions: Arterial emboli from left side of heart, pregnancy (B)
Pharmacokinetics:
IV: Half-life 10-20 min, small amounts excreted in urine
Interactions/incompatibilities:
• Bleeding potential: aspirin, indomethacin, phenylbutazone, anticoagulants

NURSING CONSIDERATIONS
Assess:
• VS, B/P, pulse, resp, neuro signs, temp at least q4h, temp >104° F or indicators of internal bleed, cardiac rhythm following intracoronary administration
• For neurologic changes that may indicate intracranial bleeding
• Retroperitoneal bleeding: back pain, leg weakness, diminished pulses
Administer:
• Using infusion pump, terminal filter (0.45 μm or smaller)
• IV reconstitute only with 5.2 ml sterile water for injection (not bacteriostatic water), and roll (not shake) to enhance reconstitution; further dilute with 190 ml; give as intermittent INF or give to clear cannula by using 1 ml of diluted

drug; inject into cannula slowly, clamp 5 min, aspirate clot

• As soon as thrombi identified; not useful for thrombi over 1 wk old

• Cryoprecipitate or fresh, frozen plasma if bleeding occurs

• Loading dose at beginning of therapy may require increased loading doses

• Heparin therapy after thrombolytic therapy is discontinued, TT or APTT less than 2 times control (about 3-4 hr)

• About 10% patients have high streptococcal antibody titres, requiring increased loading doses

• Store in refrigerator; use immediately after reconstitution

Perform/provide:

• Bed rest during entire course of treatment

• Avoidance of venous or arterial puncture procedures: inj, rectal temp

• Treatment of fever with acetaminophen or aspirin

• Pressure for 30 sec to minor bleeding sites; inform physician if hemostasis not attained, apply pressure dressing

Evaluate:

• Allergy: fever, rash, itching, chills; mild reaction may be treated with antihistamines

• Bleeding during 1st hr of treatment (hematuria, hematemesis, bleeding from mucous membranes, epistaxis, ecchymosis)

• Blood studies (Hct, platelets, PTT, PT, TT, APTT) before starting therapy; PT or APTT must be less than 2 × control before starting therapy TT ot PT q3-4h during treatment

Lab test interferences:

Increase: PT, APTT, TT

ursodiol
(your-soo'-dee-ol)

Actigall

Func. class.: Gallstone solubilizing agent

Chem. class.: Ursodeoxycholic acid

Action: Suppresses hepatic synthesis, secretion of cholesterol; inhibits intestinal absorption of cholesterol

Uses: Dissolution of radiolucent, noncalcified gallbladder stones (less than 20 mm in diameter) in which surgery is not indicated

Dosage and routes:

• *Adult:* PO 8-10 mg/kg/day in 2-3 divided doses using gallbladder ultrasound q6 mo; determine if stones have dissolved, if so continue therapy, repeat ultrasound within 1-3 mo

Available forms include: Caps 300 mg

Side effects/adverse reactions:

GI: Diarrhea, nausea, vomiting, abdominal pain, constipation, stomatitis, flatulence, dyspepsia, biliary pain

INTEG: Pruritus, rash, urticaria, dry skin, sweating, alopecia

CNS: Headache, anxiety, depression, insomnia, fatigue

MS: Arthralgia, myalgia, back pain

OTHER: Cough, rhinitis

Contraindications: Calcified cholesterol stones, radiopaque stones, radiolucent bile pigment stones, chronic liver disease, hypersensitivity

Precautions: Pregnancy (B), lactation, children

Pharmacokinetics: 80% excreted in feces, 20% metabolized, excreted into bile, lost in feces

U

---

italics = common side effects   **bold italic** = life threatening reactions

Interactions/incompatibilities:

• Reduced action of ursodiol: cholestyramine, colestipol, aluminum-based antacids

NURSING CONSIDERATIONS
Assess:

• GI status: diarrhea, abdominal pain, nausea, vomiting; drug may have to be discontinued if side effects are severe

• Skin for pruritus, rash, urticaria, dry skin; provide soothing lotion to lesions

• Muscular/skeletal status: aches or stiffness in joints

Administer:

• For up to 9-12 mo; if no improvement is seen, discontinue drug

Evaluate:

• Therapeutic response: decreasing size of stones on ultrasound

Teach patient/family:

• That anxiety, depression, insomnia are side effects and are reversible after discontinuing drug

---

valproate sodium/valproate sodium—valproic acid/valproic acid
(val-proe′ate)

Depakene Syrup, Myproic Acid Syrup/Depakote/Depakene, Myproic Acid

Func. class.: Anticonvulsant
Chem. class.: Carboxylic acid derivative

Action: Increases levels of gamma-aminobutyric acid (GABA) in brain

Uses: Simple, complex (petit mal) absence, mixed, tonic-clonic (grand mal) seizures

Dosage and routes:

• *Adult and child:* PO 15 mg/kg/day divided in 2-3 doses, may increase by 5-10 mg/kg/day q wk,

not to exceed 30 mg/kg/day in 2-3 divided doses

Available forms include: Caps 250 mg; tabs 125, 250, 500 mg; syr 250 mg/5 ml

Side effects/adverse reactions:

HEMA: Thrombocytopenia, leukopenia, lymphocytosis, increased pro-time

CNS: Sedation, drowsiness, dizziness, headache, incoordination, paresthesia, depression, hallucinations, behavioral changes, tremors, aggression, weakness

GI: Nausea, vomiting, constipation, diarrhea, heartburn, anorexia, cramps, *hepatic failure, pancreatitis, toxic hepatitis,* stomatitis

INTEG: Rash, alopecia, bruising

GU: Enuresis, irregular menses

Contraindications: Hypersensitivity

Precautions: MI (recovery phase), hepatic disease, renal disease, Addison's disease, pregnancy (D), lactation

Pharmacokinetics:

PO: Onset 15-30 min, peak 1-4 hr, duration 4-6 hr

REC: Onset slow, duration 4-6 hr

Metabolized by liver, excreted by kidneys, feces, crosses placenta, excreted in breast milk, half-life 6-16 hr

Interactions/incompatibilities:

• Increased effects: CNS depressants

• Increased toxicity: salicylates, warfarin, sulfinpyrazone

NURSING CONSIDERATIONS
Assess:

• Blood studies: Hct, Hgb, RBCs, serum folate, pro-time vitamin D if on long-term therapy

• Hepatic studies: AST, ALT, bilirubin, creatinine, failure

---

* Available in Canada only

- Blood levels: therapeutic level 50-100 µg/ml

Administer:

- Tablets or capsules whole
- Elixir alone; do not dilute with carbonated beverage; do not give syrup to patients on sodium restriction
- Give with food or milk to decrease GI symptoms

Evaluate:

- Mental status: mood, sensorium, affect, memory (long, short)
- Respiratory dysfunction: respiratory depression, character, rate, rhythm; hold drug if respirations are <12/min or if pupils are dilated

Teach patient/family:

- That physical dependency may result when used for extended periods
- To avoid driving, other activities that require alertness
- Not to discontinue medication quickly after long-term use; convulsions may result

Lab test interferences:

False-positive: Ketones

---

vancomycin HCl

(van-koe-mye'sin)
Vancocin

Func. class.: Antibacterial
Chem. class.: Tricyclic glucopeptide

Action: Inhibits bacterial cell wall synthesis

Uses: Resistant staphylococcal infections, pseudomembranous colitis, staphylococcal enterocolitis, endocarditis prophylaxis for dental procedures

Dosage and routes:
Serious staphylococcal infections
- *Adult:* IV 500 mg q6h or 1 g q12h

- *Child:* IV 40 mg/kg/day divided q6h
- *Neonates:* IV 15 mg/kg initially followed by 10 mg/kg q8-12h

Pseudomembranous/staphylococcal enterocolitis
- *Adult:* PO 500 mg -2 g/day in 3-4 divided doses for 7-10 days
- *Child:* PO 40 mg/kg/day divided q6h, not to exceed 2 g/day

Endocarditis prophylaxis
- *Adult:* IV 1 g over 1 hr, 1 hr before dental procedure

Available forms include: Pulvules 125, 250 mg; powder for oral sol 1, 10 g; powder for inj IV 500 mg

Side effects/adverse reactions:

*CV: **Cardiac arrest, vascular collapse***

*EENT: **Ototoxicity, permanent deafness,** tinnitus*

*HEMA: **Leukopenia, eosinophilia, neutropenia***

*GI: **Nausea***

RESP: Wheezing, dyspnea

*SYST: **Anaphylaxis***

*GU: **Nephrotoxicity,** increased BUN, creatinine, albumin, **fatal uremia***

INTEG: Chills, fever, rash, thrombophlebitis at injection site, urticaria, pruritus, necrosis

Contradindications: Hypersensitivity, decreased hearing

Precautions: Renal disease, pregnancy (C), lactation, elderly, neonates

Pharmacokinetics:
Peak 5 min IV trough 12 hr, half-life 4-8 hr, excreted in urine (active form), crosses placenta

Interactions/incompatibilities:
- Ototoxicity or nephrotoxicity: aminoglycosides, cephalosporins, colistin, polymyxin, bacitracin, cisplatin, amphotericin B
- Do not mix in solution or syringe

V

with alkaline solutions; check product information

NURSING CONSIDERATIONS
Assess:
• I&O ratio; report hematuria, oliguria since nephrotoxicity may occur
• Any patient with compromised renal system; drug is excreted slowly in poor renal system function; toxicity may occur rapidly
• Blood studies: WBC
• C&S before drug therapy; drug may be taken as soon as culture is taken
• Auditory function during, after treatment
• B/P during administration; sudden drop may indicate Redman's syndrome
• Signs of infection

Administer:
• After reconstitution with 10 ml sterile water for injection 500 mg/100 ml; further dilution is needed for IV
• Infuse over 60 min; avoid extravasation

Perform/provide:
• Storage at room temperature for up to 2 wk after reconstitution
• Adrenalin, suction, tracheostomy set, endotracheal intubation equipment on unit; anaphylaxis may occur
• Adequate intake of fluids (2000 ml) to prevent nephrotoxicity

Evaluate:
• Therapeutic response: absence of fever, sore throat
• Hearing loss, ringing, roaring in ears; drug should be discontinued
• Skin eruptions
• Respiratory status: rate, character, wheezing, tightness in chest
• Allergies before treatment, reaction of each medication; place allergies on chart, Kardex in bright red letters; notify all people giving drugs

Teach patient/family:
• Aspects of drug therapy: need to complete entire course of medication to ensure organism death (7-10 days); culture may be taken after completed course of medication
• To report sore throat, fever, fatigue; could indicate superimposed infection
• That drug must be taken in equal intervals around clock to maintain blood levels

---

vasopressin (antidiuretic hormone)/vasopressin tannate

(vay-soe-press'in)
Pitressin Synthetic/Pitressin Tannate

Func. class.: Pituitary hormone
Chem. class.: Lysine vasopressin

Action: Promotes reabsorption of water by action on renal tubular epithelium; causes vasoconstriction
Uses: Diabetes insipidus (nonnephrogenic/nonpsychogenic), abdominal distention postoperatively, bleeding esophageal varices
Dosage and routes:
Diabetes insipidus
• *Adult:* IM/SC 5-10 units bid-qid as needed; IM/SC 2.5-5 units q2-3 days (Pitressin Tannate) for chronic therapy
• *Child:* IM/SC 2.5-10 units bid-qid as needed; IM/SC 1.25-2.5 units q2-3 days (Pitressin Tannate) for chronic therapy
Abdominal distention
• *Adult:* IM 5 units, then q3-4h, increasing to 10 units if needed (aqueous)
Available forms include: Inj IM,

SC 20, 5 U/ml (tannate), spray, cotton pledgets

Side effects/adverse reactions:

EENT: Nasal irritation, congestion, rhinitis

CNS: Drowsiness, headache, lethargy, flushing

GU: Vulval pain

GI: Nausea, heartburn, cramps

CV: Increased B/P

MISC: Tremor, sweating, vertigo, urticaria, bronchial constriction

Contraindications: Hypersensitivity, chronic nephritis

Precautions: CAD, pregnancy (C)

Pharmacokinetics:

NASAL: Onset 1 hr, duration 3-8 hr, half-life 15 min; metabolized in liver, kidneys, excreted in urine

NURSING CONSIDERATIONS

Assess:

• Pulse, B/P, when giving drug IV or IM

• I&O ratio, weight daily, check for edema in extremities, if water retention is severe, diuretic may be prescribed

Evaluate:

• Therapeutic response: absence of severe thirst, decreased urine output, osmolality

• Water intoxication: lethargy, behavioral changes, disorientation, neuromuscular excitability

---

vecuronium bromide

(vek-yoo-roe′nee-um)

Norcuron

Func. class.: Neuromuscular blocker

Action: Inhibits transmission of nerve impulses by binding with cholinergic receptor sites, antagonizing action of acetylcholine

Uses: Facilitation of endotracheal intubation, skeletal muscle relaxation during mechanical ventilation, surgery, or general anesthesia

Dosage and routes:

• *Adult and child >9 yr:* IV BOL 0.08-0.10 mg/kg, then 0.010-0.015 mg/kg for prolonged procedures

Available forms include: IV 10 mg/5 ml

Side effects/adverse reactions:

CNS: Skeletal muscle weakness or paralysis, rarely

*RESP: **Prolonged apnea, possible respiratory paralysis***

Contraindications: Hypersensitivity

Precautions: Pregnancy (C), cardiac disease, lactation, children <2 yr, electrolyte imbalances, dehydration, neuromuscular disease, respiratory disease

Pharmacokinetics:

IV: Onset 15 min, peak 3-5 min, duration 45-60 min; half-life 65-75 min, not metabolized, excreted in feces, crosses placenta

Interactions/incompatibilities:

• Increased neuromuscular blockade: aminoglycosides, clindamycin, lincomycin, quinidine, local anesthetics, polymyxin antibiotics, lithium, narcotic analgesics, thiazides, enflurane, isoflurane

• Dysrhythmias: theophylline

• Do not mix with barbiturates in solution or syringe

NURSING CONSIDERATIONS

Assess:

• For electrolyte imbalances (K, Mg); may lead to increased action of this drug

• Vital signs (B/P, pulse, respirations, airway) q15 min until fully recovered; rate, depth, pattern of respirations, strength of hand grip

• I&O ratio; check for urinary retention, frequency, hesitancy

Administer:

• With diazepam or morphine

V

---

when used for therapeutic paralysis; this drug provides no sedation alone
• Using nerve stimulator by anesthesiologist to determine neuromuscular blockade
• Anticholinesterase to reverse neuromuscular blockade
• IV after diluting with diluent provided; further dilute each dose/5-10 ml; may give as continuous INF 10-20 mg/100 ml, titrate to patient response (only by qualified person)

Perform/provide:
• Storage in refrigerator, discard in 24 hr
• Reassurance if communication is difficult during recovery from neuromuscular blockade

Evaluate:
• Therapeutic response: paralysis of jaw, eyelid, head, neck, rest of body
• Recovery: decreased paralysis of face, diaphragm, leg, arm, rest of body; allow to recover fully before completing a neuro assessment
• Allergic reactions: rash, fever, respiratory distress, pruritus; drug should be discontinued

Treatment of overdose: Edrophonium or neostigmine, atropine, monitor VS; may require mechanical ventilation

---

verapamil HCl
(ver-ap'-a-mill)
Calan, Isoptin
Func. class.: Calcium channel blocker
Chem. class.: Phenylalkylamine

Action: Inhibits calcium ion influx across cell membrane during cardiac depolarization; produces relaxation of coronary vascular smooth muscle, dilates coronary arteries, decreases SA/AV node conduction, dilates peripheral arteries

Uses: Chronic stable angina pectoris, vasospastic angina, dysrhythmias, hypertension

Dosage and routes:
• *Adult:* PO 80 mg tid or qid, increase gwk; IV BOL 5-10 mg > 2 min, repeat if necessary in 30 min
• *Child 0-1 yr:* IV BOL 0.1-0.2 mg/kg > 2 min with ECG monitoring, repeat if necessary in 30 min
• *Child 1-15 yr:* IV BOL 0.1-0.3 mg/kg over > 2 min, repeat in 30 min, not to exceed 10 mg in a single dose

Available forms include: Tabs 40, 80, 120; sus rel tabs, 240 mg; inj 2.5 mg/ml

Side effects/adverse reactions:
CV: Edema, CHF, bradycardia, hypotension, palpitations, AV block
GI: Nausea, diarrhea, gastric upset, constipation, increased liver function studies
GU: Nocturia, polyuria
CNS: Headache, drowsiness, dizziness, anxiety, depression, weakness, insomnia, confusion, lightheadedness

Contraindications: Sick sinus syndrome, 2nd or 3rd degree heart block, hypotension less than 90 mm Hg systolic, cardiogenic shock, severe CHF

Precautions: CHF, hypotension, hepatic injury, pregnancy (C), lactation, children, renal disease, concomitant β-blocker therapy

Pharmacokinetics:
IV: Onset 3 min, peak 3-5 min, duration 10-20 min
PO: Onset variable, peak 3-4 hr, duration 17-24 hr, half-life (biphasic) 4 min, 3-7 hr (terminal)
Metabolized by liver, excreted in urine (96% as metabolites)

---

* Available in Canada only

Interactions/incompatibilities:
- Increased hypotension: prazosin, quinidine
- Increased effects: β-blockers, antihypertensives, cimetidine
- Decreased effects of: lithium
- Increased levels of: digoxin, theophylline, cyclosporine, carbamazepine, nondepolarizing muscle relaxants

NURSING CONSIDERATIONS
Administer:
- IV undiluted through Y-tube or 3-way stopcock of compatible sol; give over 2 min, or 3 min elderly
- Before meals, hs, sus rel give with food

Evaluate:
- Therapeutic response: decreased anginal pain, decreased B/P, dysrhythmias
- Cardiac status: B/P, pulse, respiration, ECG intervals (PR, QRS, QT)

Teach patient/family:
- How to take pulse before taking drug; record or graph should be kept
- To avoid hazardous activities until stabilized on drug, dizziness is no longer a problem
- To limit caffeine consumption
- To avoid OTC drugs unless directed by a physician
- Stress patient compliance to all areas of medical regimen: diet, exercise, stress reduction, drug therapy

Lab test interferences:
Increase: Liver function tests
Treatment of overdose: Defibrillation, atropine for AV block, vasopressor for hypotension

vidarabine (ophthalmic)
(vye-dare'a-been)
Vira-A Ophthalmic
Func. class.: Antiviral
Chem. class.: Purine nucleoside

Action: Inhibits viral DNA synthesis by blocking DNA polymerase
Uses: Herpes simplex, cytomegalovirus, varicella zoster
Dosage and routes:
- *Adult and child:* TOP ½ inch oint into conjunctival sac q3h, 5 times daily
Available forms include: Oint 3%
Side effects/adverse reactions:
EENT: Burning, stinging, photophobia, pain, temporary visual haze
Contraindications: Hypersensitivity
Precautions: Antibiotic hypersensitivity, pregnancy (C)

NURSING CONSIDERATIONS
Administer:
- After washing hands, cleanse crusts or discharge from eye before application
Perform/provide:
- Storage at room temperature
Evaluate:
- Therapeutic response: absence of redness, inflammation, tearing
- Allergy: itching, lacrimation, redness, swelling
Teach patient/family:
- To use drug exactly as prescribed
- Not to use eye makeup, towels, washcloths, or eye medication of others, or reinfection may occur
- That drug container tip should not be touched to eye
- To report itching, increased redness, burning, stinging, photophobia, drug should be discontinued
- That drug may cause blurred vision when ointment is applied

italics = common side effects **bold italic** = life threatening reactions

• To use sunglasses to prevent photophobia

---

vidarabine

(vye-dare′a-been)
Vira-A

Func. class.: Antibacterial, antiviral
Chem. class.: Purine nucleoside

Action: Inhibits bacterial/viral replication by preventing DNA synthesis

Uses: Herpes simplex virus encephalitis, varicella-zoster encephalomyelitis

Dosage and routes:
• *Adult and child:* IV INF 15 mg/kg/day × 10 days; infuse over 12-24 hr

Available forms include: Inj IV 200 mg/ml

Side effects/adverse reactions:
CNS: Psychosis, hallucinations, dizziness, weakness, tremors, *fatal metabolic encephalopathy,* confusion, malaise
GU: SIADH
HEMA: Anemia, thrombocytopenia, neutropenia
GI: Nausea, vomiting, anorexia, diarrhea, weight loss
INTEG: Pain, thrombophlebitis at injection site

Contraindications: Hypersensitivity

Precautions: Renal disease, liver disease, lactation, pregnancy (C)

Pharmacokinetics: Crosses blood-brain barrier, excreted by kidneys (metabolites), crosses placenta, half-life 1½-3 hr

Interactions/incompatibilities:
• Increased neurologic side effects: allopurinol

NURSING CONSIDERATIONS
Assess:
• Liver studies: AST, ALT

• Blood studies: WBC, diff, RBC, Hct, Hgb, platelets
• Renal studies: urinalysis, protein, blood
• C&S before drug therapy; drug may be taken as soon as culture is taken; C&S may be taken after therapy

Administer:
• Shake solution; dilute to 450 mg/L IV; give fluid at constant rate over 12-24 hr, using in-line filter with mean pore diameter of 0.45 mm or less

Evaluate:
• Therapeutic response: decreased amount of lesion, itching
• Bowel pattern before, during treatment
• Fluid overload; drug requires large volume to stay in solutions
• Weakness, tremors, confusion, dizziness, psychosis; if these occur, drug might need to be decreased or discontinued

---

vinblastine sulfate (VLB)

(vin-blast′een)
Velban, Velbe*

Func. class.: Antineoplastic
Chem. class.: Vinca rosea alkaloid

Action: Inhibits mitotic activity, arrests cell cycle at metaphase; inhibits RNA synthesis, blocks cellular use of glutamic acid needed for purine synthesis; a vesicant

Uses: Breast, testicular cancer, lymphomas, neuroblastoma, Hodgkin's non-Hodgkin's lymphomas, mycosis fungoides, histiocytosis, Kaposi's sarcoma

Dosage and routes:
• *Adult and child:* IV 0.1 mg/kg or 3.7 mg/m² q wk or q2 wk, not to exceed 0.5 mg/kg or 18.5 mg/m² q wk in adults

---

Available forms include: Inj IV, powder 10 mg for 10 ml IV inj

Side effects/adverse reactions:

HEMA: **Thrombocytopenia, leukopenia, myelosupppression**

GI: *Nausea, vomiting,* ileus, *anorexia, stomatitis,* constipation, abdominal pain, GI, rectal bleeding, **hepatotoxicity,** pharyngitis, stomatitis

GU: Urinary retention, **renal failure**

INTEG: *Rash,* alopecia, photosensitivity

RESP: **Fibrosis, pulmonary infiltrate**

CV: Tachycardia, orthostatic hypotension

CNS: Paresthesias, peripheral neuropathy, depression, headache, **convulsions**

META: SIADH

Contraindications: Hypersensitivity, infants, pregnancy (D)

Precautions: Renal disease, hepatic disease

Pharmacokinetics: Half-life (triphasic) 35 min, 53 min, 19 hr, metabolized in liver, excreted in urine, feces, crosses blood-brain barrier

Interactions/incompatibilities:
- Increased action of: methotrexate
- Do not use with radiation
- Synergism: bleomycin
- Decreased phenytoin level: phenytoin
- Bronchospasm: mitomycin

NURSING CONSIDERATIONS

Assess:
- CBC, differential, platelet count weekly, withhold drug if WBC is <4000 or platelet count is <75,000; notify physician of results
- Pulmonary function tests, chest X-ray studies before, during therapy; chest X-ray film should be obtained q2 wk during treatment
- Neurologic status: sensory-vibratory evaluation if side effects occur
- Renal function studies: BUN, serum uric acid, urine CrCl, electrolytes before, during therapy
- I&O ratio, report fall in urine output of 30 ml/hr
- Monitor temperature q4h; may indicate beginning infection
- Liver function tests before, during therapy (bilirubin, AST, ALT, LDH) as needed or monthly
- RBC, Hct, Hgb since these may be decreased

Administer:
- IV after diluting 10 mg/10 ml NaCl; give through Y-tube or 3-way stopcock or directly over 1 min
- Hyaluronidase 150 U/ml in 1 ml NaCl, warm compress for extravasation
- Antacid before oral agent; give drug after evening meal before bedtime
- Antiemetic 30-60 min before giving drug and prn to prevent vomiting
- Local or systemic drugs for infection
- Transfusion for anemia
- Antispasmodic for GI symptoms

Perform/provide:
- Deep-breathing exercises with patient 3-4 × day; place in semi-Fowler's position
- Liquid diet: cola, Jell-O; dry toast or crackers may be added if patient is not nauseated or vomiting
- Increase fluid intake to 2-3 L/day to prevent urate deposits, calculi formation
- Rinsing of mouth 3-4 × day with water
- Brushing of teeth 2-3 × day with soft brush or cotton-tipped applicators for stomatitis; use unwaxed dental floss

italics = common side effects   **bold italic** = life threatening reactions

- Nutritious diet with iron, vitamin supplements
- HOB increased to facilitate breathing

Evaluate:
- Bleeding: hematuria, guaiac, bruising or petechiae, mucosa of orifices q8h
- Dyspnea, rales, unproductive cough, chest pain, tachypnea, fatigue, increased pulse, pallor, lethargy
- Food preferences; list likes, dislikes
- Effects of alopecia on body image; discuss feelings about body changes
- Sensitivity of feet/hands, which precedes neuropathy
- Inflammation of mucosa, breaks in skin
- Yellowing of skin and sclera, dark urine, clay-colored stools, itchy skin, abdominal pain, fever, diarrhea
- Buccal cavity q8h for dryness, sores or ulceration, white patches, oral pain, bleeding, dysphagia
- Local irritation, pain, burning, discoloration at injection site
- Symptoms indicating severe allergic reaction: rash, pruritus, urticaria, purpuric skin lesions, itching, flushing
- Frequency of stools and characteristics: cramping, acidosis; signs of dehydration: rapid respirations, poor skin turgor, decreased urine output, dry skin, restlessness, weakness

Teach patient/family:
- To report any complaints or side effects to the nurse or physician
- To report any changes in breathing or coughing
- That hair may be lost during treatment, a wig or hairpiece may make patient feel better; tell patient that

new hair may be different in color, texture
- To report change in gait or numbness in extremities; may indicate neuropathy
- To avoid foods with citric acid, hot or rough texture
- To report any bleeding, white spots or ulcerations in mouth to physician; tell patient to examine mouth qd

---

vincristine sulfate (VCR)

(vin-kris'teen)
Oncovin
Func. class.: Antineoplastic
Chem. class.: Vinca alkaloid

Action: Inhibits mitotic activity, arrests cell cycle at metaphase; inhibits RNA synthesis, blocks cellular use of glutamic acid needed for purine synthesis; a vesicant

Uses: Breast, lung cancer, lymphomas, neuroblastoma, Hodgkin's disease, acute lymphoblastic and other leukemias, rhabdomyosarcoma, Wilm's tumor, osteogenic and other sarcomas

Dosage and routes:
- *Adult:* IV 1-2 mg/m^2/wk, not to exceed 2 mg
- *Child:* IV 1.5-2 mg/m^2/wk, not to exceed 2 mg

Available forms include: Inj IV 1 mg/ml

Side effects/adverse reactions:
INTEG: Alopecia
HEMA: **Thrombocytopenia, leukopenia, myelosuppression, anemia**
GI: Nausea, vomiting, anorexia, stomatitis, constipation, **paralytic ileus**, abdominal pain, **hepatotoxicity**
CV: Orthostatic hypotension
CNS: Decreased reflexes, numbness, weakness, motor difficulties,

CNS depression, cranial nerve paralysis, *seizures*

Contraindications: Hypersensitivity, infants, pregnancy (D)

Precautions: Renal disease, hepatic disease, hypertension, neuromuscular disease

Pharmacokinetics: Half-life (triphasic) 0.85 min, 7.4 min, 164 min, metabolized in liver, excreted in bile, feces, crosses placental barrier, crosses blood-brain barrier

Interactions/incompatibilities:

• Increased action of: methotrexate
• Do not use with radiation
• Neurotoxicity: peripheral nervous system drugs
• Decreased digoxin level: digoxin
• Decreased action of vincristine: L-asparaginase
• Acute pulmonary reactions: Mitomycin-c

NURSING CONSIDERATIONS
Assess:

• CBC, differential, platelet count weekly; withhold drug if WBC is <4000 or platelet count is <75,000; notify physician of results
• Renal function studies: BUN, serum uric acid, urine CrCl, electrolytes before, during therapy
• I&O ratio, report fall in urine output of 30 ml/hr
• Monitor temperature q4h; may indicate beginning infection
• Liver function tests before, during therapy (bilirubin, AST, ALT, LDH) as needed or monthly
• RBC, Hct, Hgb since these may be decreased
• Deep tendon reflexes; drug is neurotoxic

Administer:

• Agents to prevent constipation
• Antiemetic 30-60 min before giving drug and prn to prevent vomiting

• IV after diluting with diluent provided or 1 mg/10 ml of sterile H_2O or NaCl; give through Y-tube or 3-way stopcock or directly over 1 min
• Hyaluronidase 150 U/ml in 1 ml NaCl, apply warm compress for extravasation
• Transfusion for anemia
• Antispasmodic for GI symptoms

Perform/provide:

• Liquid diet: cola, Jell-O; dry toast or crackers may be added if patient is not nauseated or vomiting
• Rinsing of mouth 3-4 × day with water
• Brushing of teeth 2-3 × day with soft brush or cotton-tipped applicators for stomatitis; use unwaxed dental floss
• Nutritious diet with iron, vitamin supplements

Evaluate:

• Sensitivity of feet/hands, which precedes neuropathy
• Bleeding: hematuria, guaiac, bruising or petechiae, mucosa of orifices q8h
• Food preferences; list likes, dislikes
• Effects of alopecia on body image, discuss feelings about body changes
• Inflammation of mucosa, breaks in skin
• Yellowing of skin and sclera, dark urine, clay-colored stools, itchy skin, abdominal pain, fever, diarrhea
• Buccal cavity q8h for dryness, sores or ulceration, white patches, oral pain, bleeding, dysphagia
• Symptoms indicating severe allergic reaction: rash, pruritus, urticaria, purpuric skin lesions, itching, flushing
• Frequency of stools, characteristics: cramping, acidosis; signs of dehydration: rapid respirations,

V

---

italics = common side effects   ***bold italic*** = life threatening reactions

poor skin turgor, decreased urine output, dry skin, restlessness, weakness

Teach patient/family:
• To report change in gait or numbness in extremities; may indicate neuropathy
• To report any complaints or side effects to nurse or physician
• To report any bleeding, white spots or ulcerations in mouth to physician; tell patient to examine mouth qd

---

vitamin A
Acon, Afaxin, Aquasol A, Natola

Func. class.: Vitamin, fat soluble
Chem. class.: Retinol

Action: Needed for normal bone and teeth development, visual dark adaptation, skin disease, mucosa tissue repair, assists in production of adrenal steroids, cholesterol, RNA

Uses: Vitamin A deficiency

Dosage and routes:
• *Adult and child >8 yr:* PO 100,000-500,000 IU qd 3 days, then 50,000 qd × 2 wk; dose based on severity of deficiency; maintenance 10,000-20,000 IU for 2 mo
• *Child 1-8 yr:* IM 17,500-35,000 IU qd × 10 days
• *Infants <1 yr:* IM 7500-15,000 IU × 10 days
Maintenance
• Child 4-8 yr: IM 15,000 IU qd × 2 mo
• Child <4 yr: IM 10,000 IU qd × 2 mo
Available forms include: Caps 10,000, 25,000, 50,000 IU; drops 5,000 IU; inj 50,000 IU/ml

Side effects/adverse reactions:
GI: Nausea, vomiting, anorexia, abdominal pain, *jaundice*

CNS: Headache, increased intracranial pressure, intracranial hypertension, lethargy, malaise
EENT: Gingivitis, papillaedema, exophthalmos, inflammation of tongue and lips
INTEG: Drying of skin, pruritus, increased pigmentation, night sweats, alopecia
MS: Arthraglia, retarded growth, hard areas on bone
META: Hypomenorrhea, hypercalcemia

Contraindications: Hypersensitivity to vitamin A, malabsorption syndrome (PO)

Precautions: Lactation, impaired renal function, pregnancy (A)

Pharmacokinetics:
PO/INJ: Stored in liver, kidneys, fat; excreted (metabolites) in urine, feces

Interactions/incompatibilities:
• Decreased absorption of vitamin A: mineral oil
• Increased levels of vitamin A: corticosteroids

NURSING CONSIDERATIONS
Administer:
• With food (PO) for better absorption

Perform/provide:
• Storage in tight, light-resistant container

Evaluate:
• Nutritional status: yellow and dark green vegetables, yellow/orange fruits, vitamin A fortified foods, liver, egg yolks
• Vitamin A deficiency: decreased growth, night blindness, dry, brittle nails, hair loss, urinary stones, increased infection, hyperkeratosis of skin, drying of cornea
• Therapeutic response: increased growth rate, weight; absence of dry skin and mucous membranes, night blindness

---

* Available in Canada only

Teach patient/family:
• Not to use mineral oil while taking this drug
• To notify a physician of nausea, vomiting, lip cracking, loss of hair, headache
• Not to take more than the prescribed amount

Lab test interferences:
False increase: Bilirubin, serum cholesterol

Treatment of overdose: Discontinue drug

---

vitamin D (cholecalciferol, vitamin D₃ or ergocalciferol, vitamin D₂)

Calciferol, Deltalin, Drisdol, Hytakerol, Radiostol,* Radiostol Forte*

Func. class.: Vitamin D
Chem. class.: Fat soluble

Action: Needed for regulation of calcium, phosphate levels, normal bone development, parathyroid activity, neuromuscular functioning

Uses: Vitamin D deficiency, rickets, renal osteodystrophy, hypoparathyroidism, hypophosphatemia, psoriasis, rheumatoid arthritis

Dosage and routes:
• *Adult:* PO/IM 12,000 IU qd, then increased to 500,000 IU/day
• *Child:* PO/IM 1500/5000 IU qd × 2-4 wk, may repeat after 2 wk or 600,000 IU as single dose

Hypoparathyroidism
• *Adult and child:* PO/IM 200,000 IU given with 4 g calcium tab

Available forms include: Tabs 400, 1000, 50,000 IU; caps 25,000, 50,000; liq 8000 IU/ml; inj 500,000 IU/ml, 500,000 IU/5 ml IM

Side effects/adverse reactions:
GI: Nausea, vomiting, anorexia, cramps, diarrhea, constipation, metallic taste, dry mouth, decreased libido
CNS: Fatigue, weakness, drowsiness, convulsions, headache, psychosis
GU: Polyuria, nocturia, ***hematuria, albuminuria, renal failure***
CV: Hypertension, dysrhythmias
MS: Decreased bone growth, early joint pain, early muscle pain
INTEG: Pruritus, photophobia

Contraindications: Hypersensitivity, hypercalcemia, renal dysfunction, hyperphosphatemia

Precautions: Cardiovascular disease, renal calculi, pregnancy (A)

Pharmacokinetics:
PO/INJ: Half-life 7-12 hr, stored in liver, duration 2 mo, excreted in bile (metabolites) and urine

Interactions/incompatibilities:
• Decreased effects of vitamin D: cholestyramine, colestipol, phenobarbital, phenytoin
• Increased toxicity: diuretics (thiazides), antacids, verapamil

NURSING CONSIDERATIONS
Assess:
• Vitamin D levels q2 wk during treatment
• Ca, PO₄, Mg, BUN, alk phosphatase, urine Ca, creatinine

Administer:
• IM injection in deep muscle mass, administer slowly

Evaluate:
• Therapeutic response: absence of rickets/osteomalacia, adequate calcium/phosphate levels, decrease in bone pain
• Nutritional status: egg yolk, fortified dairy products, cod, halibut, salmon, sardines

Teach patient/family:
• Necessary foods to be included in diet

V

---

italics = common side effects   ***bold italic*** = life threatening reactions

• To avoid vitamin supplements unless directed by physician
• To keep doctor's appointments since line between therapeutic and toxic doses is narrow
• To report weakness, lethargy, headache, anorexia, loss of weight
• Nausea, vomiting, abdominal cramps, diarrhea, constipation, excessive thirst, polyuria, muscle and bone pain
• To decrease intake of antacids containing magnesium

---

vitamin E

Alfacol, Aquasol E, Daltose,* E-Ferol, Eprolin, Hy-E-Plex, Kell-E, Lethopherol, Maxi-E, Pertropin, Tocopher-Caps, Tocopherol

Func. class.: Vitamin E
Chem. class.: Fat soluble

Action: Needed for digestion and metabolism of polyunsaturated fats, decreased platelet aggregation, decreases blood clot formation, promotes normal growth, and development of muscle tissue, prostaglandin synthesis

Uses: Vitamin E deficiency, impaired fat absorption, hemolytic anemia in premature neonates, prevention of retrolental fibroplasia, sickle cell anemia, supplement in malabsorption syndrome

Dosage and routes:
• *Adult:* PO/IM 60-75 IU qd, not to exceed 300 IU/day
• *Child:* PO/IM 1 mg/0.6 g of dietary fat

Available forms include: Caps 50, 100, 200, 400, 500, 600, 1000 IU; 74, 165, 294, 331 mg; tabs 200, 400 IU; 331 mg; drops 50 mg/ml

Side effects/adverse reactions:
META: Altered metabolism of hor-

mones, thyroid, pituitary, adrenal, altered immunity
MS: Weakness
CNS: Headache, fatigue
GI: Nausea, cramps, diarrhea
GU: Gonadal dysfunction
CV: Increased risk thrombophlebitis
EENT: Blurred vision
INTEG: Sterile abscess, contact dermatitis

Contraindications: None significant

Precautions: Pregnancy (A)

Pharmacokinetics:
PO: Metabolized in liver, excreted in bile

Interactions/incompatibilities:
• Increased action of: oral anticoagulants

NURSING CONSIDERATIONS

Assess:
• BUN, creatinine
• Vitamin E levels during treatment
• CBC; hemolytic anemia may occur

Administer:
• Topically to moisturize dry skin

Perform/provide:
• Storage in tight, light-resistant container

Evaluate:
• Therapeutic response: absence of hemolytic anemia, adequate vitamin E levels, improvement in skin lesions, decreased edema
• Nutritional status: wheat germ, dark green leafy vegetables, nuts, eggs, liver, vegetable oils, dairy products, cereals

Teach patient/family:
• Necessary foods to be included in diet
• To avoid vitamin supplements unless directed by physician

---

warfarin sodium

(war′far-in)

Coumadin, Panwarfin, Sofarin, Carfin, Warfilone Sodium,* Warnerin*

Func. class.: Anticoagulant

Action: Interferes with blood clotting by indirect means; depresses hepatic synthesis of vitamin K-dependent coagulation factors (II, VII, IX, X)

Uses: Pulmonary emboli, deep vein thrombosis, myocardial infarction, atrial dysrhythmias

Dosage and routes:
• *Adult:* PO 10-15 mg × 3 days, then titrated to PT qd or 40-60 mg for 1 day, then 2-10 mg qd titrated to PT level

Available forms include: Tabs 1 mg, 2, 2.5, 5, 7.5, 10 mg; inj 50 mg/2 ml

Side effects/adverse reactions:

GI: Diarrhea, nausea, vomiting, anorexia, stomatitis, cramps, *hepatitis*

GU: Hematuria

INTEG: Rash, dermatitis, urticaria, alopecia, pruritus

CNS: Fever

HEMA: Hemorrhage, agranulocytosis, leukopenia, eosinophilia

Contraindications: Hypersensitivity, hemophilia, leukemia with bleeding, peptic ulcer disease, thrombocytopenic purpura, hepatic disease (severe), severe hypertension, subacute bacterial endocarditis, acute nephritis, blood dyscrasias, pregnancy (D), eclampsia, preeclampsia

Precautions: Alcoholism, elderly

Pharmacokinetics:

PO: Onset 12-24 hr, peak 1½-3 days, duration 3-5 days, half-life 1½-2½ days; metabolized in liver, excreted in urine/feces (active/inactive metabolites), crosses placenta 99% bound to plasma proteins

Interactions/incompatibilities:
• Increased action of warfarin: allopurinol, chloramphenicol, clofibrate, amiodarone, diflunisal, heparin, steroids, cimetidine, disulfiram, thyroid, glucagon, metronidazole, quinidine, sulindac, sulfinpyrazone, sulfonamides, clofibrate, cholestyramine, salicylates, ethacrynic acids, indomethacin, mefenamic acid, oxyphenbutazones, phenylbutazone
• Decreased action of warfarin: barbiturates, griseofulvin, haloperidol, ethchlorvynol, carbamazepine, rifampin, oral contraceptives, phenytoin, estrogens, vitamin K
• Increased toxicity: oral sulfonylureas, phenytoin

NURSING CONSIDERATIONS

Assess:
• Blood studies (Hct, platelets, occult blood in stools) q 3 mo
• Prothrombin time, which should be 1½-2 × control, PT; often done qd initially
• B/P, watch for increasing signs of hypertension

Administer:
• At same time each day to maintain steady blood levels
• Avoiding all IM injections that may cause bleeding

Perform/provide:
• Storage in tight container

Evaluate:
• Therapeutic response: decrease of deep vein thrombosis
• Bleeding gums, petechiae, ecchymosis, black tarry stools, hematuria
• Fever, skin rash, urticaria

---

italics = common side effects   ***bold italic*** = life threatening reactions

• Needed dosage change q 1-2 wk; when stable, PT q 3 wk
Teach patient/family:
• To avoid OTC preparations that may cause serious drug interactions unless directed by physician
• To use soft-bristle toothbrush to avoid bleeding gums, electric razor
• To carry a Medic-Alert ID identifying drug taken
• Stress patient compliance
• To report any signs of bleeding: gums, under skin, urine, stools
• To avoid hazardous activities (football, hockey, skiing) or dangerous work
Lab test interferences:
Increase: T_3 uptake
Decrease: Uric acid
Treatment of overdose: Administer vitamin K

---

xylometazoline HCl (nasal)

(xye-loe-met-az'oh-leen)
Neo-Synephrine II, Otrivin, Sine-Off Nasal Spray, Sinex-LA
Func. class.: Nasal decongestant
Chem. class.: Sympathomimetic amine

Action: Dilates arterioles of nasal membrane, which decreases congestion
Uses: Nasal congestion
Dosage and routes:
• *Adult and child >12 yr:* INSTILL 2-3 gtts or 2 sprays q8-10h (0.1%)
• *Child <12 yr:* INSTILL 2-3 gtts or 1% spray q8-10h (0.05%)
Available forms include: Sol 0.05%, 0.1%
Side effects/adverse reactions:
EENT: Irritation, burning, sneezing, stinging, dryness, rebound congestion

INTEG: Contact dermatitis
Contraindications: Hypersensitivity to sympathomimetic amines
Precautions: Pregnancy (C), glaucoma
Pharmacokinetics:
INSTILL: Onset 5-10 min, duration 5-6 hr

NURSING CONSIDERATIONS
Administer:
• No more than q4h
• For <4 consecutive days
Perform/provide:
• Environmental humidification to decrease nasal congestion, dryness
• Storage in light-resistant containers; do not expose to high temperatures
Evaluate:
• Redness, swelling, pain in nasal passages
Teach patient/family:
• To avoid contamination of container
• Stinging may occur for a few applications; drying of mucosa may be decreased by environmental humidification
• To notify physician if irregular pulse, insomnia, dizziness, or tremors occur
• Proper administration to avoid systemic absorption

---

zidovudine (formerly azidothymidine or AZT)

(zid-oo'-vue-dine)
Retrovir
Func. class.: Antiviral
Chem. class.: Thymidine analog

Action: Inhibits replication of HIV virus by interfering with transcription of RNA and DNA
Uses: Symptomatic HIV infections (AIDS, ARC), confirmed *P. carinii*

---

*Available in Canada only

pneumonia, or absolute CD4 lymphocytes of $<200/mm_3$

Dosage and routes:
• *Adult:* PO 200 mg q4h, may need to stop treatment if severe bone marrow depression occurs, and restart after bone marrow recovery

Available forms include: Caps 100 mg

Side effects/adverse reactions:
*HEMA: **Granulocytopenia, anemia***
CNS: Fever, headache, malaise, diaphoresis, dizziness, insomnia, paresthesia, somnolence, chills, tremor, twitching, anxiety, confusion, depression, lability, vertigo, loss of mental acuity
GI: Nausea, vomiting, diarrhea, anorexia, cramps, dyspepsia, constipation, dysphagia, flatulence, rectal bleeding, mouth ulcer
RESP: Dyspnea
EENT: Taste change, hearing loss, photophobia
INTEG: Rash, acne, pruritus, urticaria
MS: Myalgia, arthralgia, muscle spasm
GU: Dysuria, polyuria, frequency, hesitancy

Contraindications: Hypersensitivity

Precautions: Granulocyte count $<1000/mm_3$ or Hgb <9.5 g/dl, pregnancy (C), lactation, children, severe renal disease, severe hepatic function

Pharmacokinetics:
PO: Rapidly absorbed from GI tract, peak ½-1½ hr, metabolized in liver (inactive metabolites), excreted by kidneys

Interactions/incompatibilities:
• Toxicity: amphotericin B, dapsone, flucytosine, adriamycin, interferon vincristine, vinblastine, pentamidine, probenecid, experimental nucleoside analogues, benzodiazepines, cimetidine, morphine, sulfonamides
• Granulocytopenia: acetaminophen, aspirin, indomethacin

NURSING CONSIDERATIONS
Assess:
• Blood counts q2 wk, watch for decreasing granulocytes, Hgb; if low, therapy may need to be discontinued and restarted after hematologic recovery; blood transfusions may be required

Administer:
• By mouth, capsules should be swallowed whole
• Trimethoprim-sulfamethoxazole, pyrimethamine, or acyclovir as ordered to prevent opportunistic infections; if these drugs are given, watch for neurotoxicity

Perform/provide:
• Storage in cool environment, protect from light

Evaluate:
• Blood dyscrasias (anemia, granulocytopenia): bruising, fatigue, bleeding, poor healing

Teach patient/family:
• Drug is not cure for AIDS, but will control symptoms
• To call physician if sore throat, swollen lymph nodes, malaise, fever occur since other infections may occur
• That even with drug administration, patient is still infective and may pass AIDS virus on to others
• That follow-up visits must be continued since serious toxicity may occur, blood counts must be done q2 wk
• That drug must be taken q4h around clock even during night
• That serious drug interactions may occur if OTC products are ingested, check with physician first if taking aspirin, acetaminophen, indomethacin

Y

Z

italics = common side effects   ***bold italic*** = life threatening reactions

• That other drugs may be necessary to prevent other infections
• That drug may cause fainting or dizziness

---

zinc sulfate

Eye-Sed Ophthalmic, Op-Thal-Zin
Func. class.: Ophthalmic vasoconstrictor
Chem. class.: Zinc product

Action: Vasoconstriction occurs by action on conjunctiva
Uses: Ocular congestion, irritation, itching
Dosage and routes:
• *Adult and child >2 yr:* INSTILL 1-2 gtts bid or tid
Available forms include: Sol 0.217%, 0.25%
Side effects/adverse reactions:
EENT: Eye irritation, burning
Contraindications: Hypersensitivity
Precautions: Narrow-angle glaucoma, pregnancy (C)
NURSING CONSIDERATIONS
Perform/provide:
• Storage in tight container
Teach patient/family:
• To report change in vision, or irritation
• Method of instillation; tilt head backward, hold dropper over eye, drop medication inside lower lid, using pressure on inside corner of eye hold 1 min, do not touch dropper to eye

---

zinc sulfate

Orazinc
Func. class.: Trace element

Action: Needed for adequate healing, bone and joint development (23% zinc)
Uses: Prevention of zinc deficiency, adjunct to vitamin A therapy
Dosage and routes:
• *Adult:* PO 200-220 mg tid
• *Child:* PO 0.3 mg/kg/day
Available forms include: Tabs 110, 200, 220 mg; caps 110, 220 mg
Side effects/adverse reactions:
GI: Nausea, vomiting, cramps, heartburn, ulcer formation
OVERDOSE: Diarrhea, rash, dehydration, restlessness
Precautions: Pregnancy (A)
Interactions/incompatibilities:
• Decreased absorption of: other covalent cations
NURSING CONSIDERATIONS
Assess:
• Zinc levels during treatment
Administer:
• With meals to decrease gastric upset; avoid dairy products
Evaluate:
• Therapeutic response: absence of zinc deficiency
Teach patient/family:
• That element will need to be taken for 2 mo to be effective
• To immediately report nausea, diarrhea, rash, severe vomiting, restlessness

---

*Available in Canada only

Appendix a

Abbreviations

ā	before	ASHD	arteriosclerotic heart disease
aa	of each	AV	atrioventricular
AB	abortion	BAL	blood alcohol level
abd	abdomen	bid	twice a day
ABGs	arterial blood gases	BM	bowel movement
ac	before meals	BMR	basal metabolism rate
ACE	angiotensin-converting enzyme	B/P	blood pressure
ad lib	as desired	BPH	benign prostatic hypertrophy
ADA	American Diabetes Association	bpm	beats per minute
ADH	antidiuretic hormone	BS	blood sugar
AKA	also known as	BSP	bromsulphalein
ALT	alanine aminotransferase, serum	BUN	blood urea nitrogen
AMA	against medical advice	Bx	biopsy
		c̄	with
amb	ambulation	cap	capsules
ANA	antinuclear antibodies	C	Celsius (centigrade)
ant	anterior	Ca	cancer
AP	anterior-posterior	CAD	coronary artery disease
APTT	activated partial thromboplastin time	cath	catheterization or catheterize
AROM	active range of motion	CC	chief complaint
ASA	acetylsalicylic acid, aspirin	cc	cubic centimeter
ASAP	as soon as possible	CBC	complete blood count
AST	aspartate aminotransferase, serum	CHF	congestive heart failure

cm	centimeter	elix	elixir
CNS	central nervous system	EPS	extrapyrimidal symptoms
CO_2	carbon dioxide	ESR	erythrocyte sedimentation rate
c/o	complains of	F	Farenheit
COPD	chronic obstructive pulmonary disease	FBS	fasting blood sugar
CPAP	continuous positive airway pressure	FHT	fetal heart tones
CPK	creatinine phosphokinase	FIo_2	inspired oxygen concentration
CPR	cardiopulmonary resuscitation	FSH	follicle-stimulating hormone
CrCl	creatinine clearance	fx	fracture
C section	cesarean section	g	gram
C&S	culture and sensiturty	gal	gallon
CSF	cerebrospinal fluid	gr	grain
CV	cardiovascular	GTT	glucose tolerance test
CVA	cerebrovascular accident	gtt	drop
CVP	central venous pressure	GI	gastrointestinal
		GU	genitourinary
D&C	dilatation and curettage	Gyn	gynecology
DM	diabetes mellitus	H	hypodermically
DOA	dead on arrival	H & H	hematocrit and hemoglobin
DOB	date of birth	Hct	hematocrit
dr	dram	HCG	human chorionic gonadotropin
dsg	dressing	HDCV	human diploid cell rabies vaccine
D_5W	5% glucose in distilled water	Hgb	hemoglobin
dx	diagnosis	5-HIAA	5-hydroxyindole-acetic acid
ECG	electrocardiogram (EKG)	H_2O	water
EDTA	ethylenediaminetetraacetic acid	HOB	head of bed
EEG	electroencephalogram	HR	heart rate
		hr	hour
EENT	ear, eye, nose, and throat	hs	at bedtime
		Hx	history
		IgG	immunoglobulin G

IM	intramuscular
INH	inhalation
inj	injection
IPPB	intermittent positive pressure breathing
I&O	intake and output
ITP	idiopathic thrombocytopenic purpura
IUD	intrauterine contraceptive device
IV	intravenous
IVAC	intravenous controller
IVP	intravenous pyelogram
IVPB	intravenous piggyback
K	potassium
Kg	kilogram
L or l	left
L	liter
lat	lateral
lb	pound
LDH	lactic dehydrogenase
LE	lupus erythematosus
LH	luteinizing hormone
liq	liquid
LLQ	left lower quadrant
LMP	last menstrual period
LOC	loss of consciousness
LR	lactated Ringer's solution
LUQ	left upper quadrant
M	meter
m	minim
m^2	square meter
MAOI	monoamine oxidase inhibitor

MCA	motorcycle accident
mEq	milliequivalent
mg	milligram
μg	microgram
MI	myocardial infarction
min	minute
mixt	mixture
ml	milliliter
mm	millimeter
mo	month
MRC	medical research council
MVA	motorvehicle accident
Na	sodium
NC	nasal cannula
neg	negative
NKA	no known allergies
noc	night
NPO	nothing by mouth (Lat. *nulla per os*)
NS	normal saline
NV	neurovascular
O$_2$	oxygen
OBS	organic brain syndrome
OD	right eye
OOB	out of bed
OR	operating room
ORIF	open reduction, internal fixation
OS	left eye
os	mouth
OTC	over the counter
OU	each eye
oz	ounce
p̄	after
p	pulse

P56	plasma-lyte 56	**qod**	every other day
Pa$_{CO_2}$	arterial carbon dioxide tension (pressure)	**qPM**	every night
		qs	quantity sufficient
		qt	quart
Pa$_{O_2}$	arterial oxygen tension (pressure)	**q2h**	every 2 hours
PBI	protein-bound iodine	**q3h**	every 3 hours
PAT	paroxysmal atrial tachycardia	**q4h**	every 4 hours
		q6h	every 6 hours
PCN	penicillin	**q12h**	every 12 hours
PCWP	pulmonary capillary wedge pressure	**R**	respirations, rectal
		r	right
PE	physical examination	**RAIU**	radioactive iodine uptake
PEEP	positive end expiratory pressure	**RBC(s)**	red blood count or cell(s)
PERRLA	pupils equal, round, react to light and accommodation	**REM**	rapid eye movement
		RLQ	right lower quadrant
		R/O	rule out
pH	hydrogen ion concentration	**ROM**	range of motion
		RUQ	right upper quadrant
PO	by mouth	**Rx**	therapy, treatment, or prescription
postop	postoperatively		
PP	post prandial	**s̄**	without
PPD	purified protein derivative	**SAN**	sinoatrial node
		SC	subcutaneous
preop	preoperatively	**sig**	label
prep	preparation	**SIMV**	synchronous intermittent mandatory ventilation
prn	as needed		
pro-time, PT	prothrombin time		
		SL	sublingual
PTT	partial thromboplastin time	**SOB**	short of breath
		sol	solution
PVC	premature ventricular contraction	**ss**	one half
		stat	at once
q	every	**surg**	surgical
qAM	every morning	**Sx**	symptoms
qd	every day	**supp**	suppository
qh	every hour	**syr**	syrup
qid	four times a day	**T**	temperature

T&A	tonsillectomy and adenoidectomy		**VD**	veneral disease
tab	tablet		**VMA**	vanillylmandelic acid
TAH	total abdominal hysterectomy		**VO**	verbal order
tbsp	tablespoon		**vol**	volume
temp	temperature		**VS**	vital signs
tid	three times daily		**WBC**	white blood count
tinc	tincture		**wk**	week
TPN	total parenteral nutrition		**WNL**	within normal limits
TPR	temperature, pulse, respirations		**wt**	weight
top	topical		**yr**	year
TSH	thyroid-stimulating hormone		$>$	greater than
tsp	teaspoon		$<$	less than
TT	thrombin time		$=$	equal
U	unit		$\neq$	not equal
UA	urinalysis		$\uparrow$	increase
UV	ultraviolet		$\downarrow$	decrease
vag	vaginal		$2°$	secondary
			$°$	degree
			%	percent
			@	at

Appendix b

Commonly used antibiotics in adults and children

amoxicillin
  Adult: PO 750 mg-1.5 g qd in divided doses q8h
  Child: PO 20-40 mg/kg/day in divided doses q8h
ampicillin
  Adult: PO 1-2 g qd in divided doses q6h
       IM/IV 2-8 g qd in divided doses q4-6h
  Child: PO 50-100 mg/kg/day in divided doses q6h
       IM/IV 100-200 mg/kg/day in divided doses q6h
cefaclor
  Adult: PO 250-500 mg q8h
  Child: PO 24-40 mg/kg/day in divided doses q8h
cephalexin
  Adult: PO 250-500 mg q6h
  Child: PO 25-50 mg/kg/day in 4 equal doses
chloramphenicol
  Adult and child >3 mo: 50-100 mg/kg/day in divided doses q6h
clindamycin
  Adult: PO 150-450 mg q6h
       IM/IV 300 mg q6-12h
  Child >1 mo: PO 8-25 mg/kg/day in divided doses q6-8h
            IM/IV 15-40 mg/kg/day in divided doses q6-8h
erythromycin
  Adult: 250 mg-500 mg q6h
  Child: 30-50 mg/kg/day in divided doses q6h
gentamicin
  Adult: IV INF 3-5 mg/kg/day in divided doses q8h
  Child: IV/IM 2-2.5 mg/kg q8h
  Neonates and infants: IV/IM 2.5 mg/kg q8h
kanamycin
  Adult and child: IV INF/IM 15 mg/kg/day in divided doses
               q8-12h
methicillin
  Adult: IM/IV 4-12 g/day in divided doses q4-6h
  Child: IM/IV 50-300 mg/kg/day in divided doses q4-12h
       PO 25-50 mg/kg/day in divided doses q6h
  Neonates: IM 10 mg/kg q12h

nafcillin
Adult: PO/IM/IV 2-6 g/day in divided doses q4-6h
Child: IM 25 mg/kg q12h

oxacillin
Adult: PO 2-6 g/day in divided doses q4-6h
IM/IV 2-12 g/day in divided doses q4-6h
Child: PO/IM/IV 50-100 mg/kg/day in divided doses q6h

penicillin G benzathine
Adult: IM 1.2 million U

penicillin G potassium
Adult: PO 400,000-500,000 U q6-8h
Child <12 yr: PO 25,000-90,000 U/kg/day in 3-6 divided doses

penicillin G procaine
Adult and child: IM 600,000-1.2 million U in 1-2 doses/day
Newborn: IM 50,000 U/kg qd

nitrofurantoin
Adult and child >12 yr: PO 50-100 mg qid pc

sulfisoxazole
Adult: PO 2-4 g loading dose, then 1-2 g qid
Child >2 mo: PO 75 mg/kg or 2 g/m² loading dose then 150 mg/kg/day or 4 g/m² day in divided doses q6h

ticarcillin
Adult: IV/IM 12-24 g/day in divided doses q3-6h
Child: IV/IM 50-300 mg/kg/day in divided doses q4-8h
Neonates: IV INF 75-100 mg/kg q8-12h

Appendix c

Nomogram for calculation of body surface area

Place a straight edge from the patient's height in the left column to his weight in the right column. The point of intersection on the body surface area column indicates the body surface area (BSA). Reproduced from Behrman, R.E., and Vaughn, V.C. (editors): Nelson's textbook of pediatrics, ed. 12, Philadelphia, 1983, W.B. Saunders Co.

Appendix d

How to prepare a medication card

Medication cards are easy to develop from Mosby's Nursing Drug Reference because all the information can be easily found in each individual drug monograph. The key is to use only the most essential information in the monograph since space on the medication card is more limited.

First, locate the generic drug (1) and trade name (2) in the drug monograph and place them, as well as the functional classification (3), on the card. If you are unfamiliar with how to pronounce the generic name, you should also include the pronunciation (4) in the upper right-hand corner of the card. The action (5) should be simplified so you will be able to explain the basic physiologic response of the drug. Identify the reason your patient is receiving this particular drug and place that use (6) first, with all other uses listed afterward.

Next, dosage and routes (7) should be copied exactly as given in the drug monograph; identify the dosage and route your patient is receiving. Side effects/adverse reactions (8) should be listed by body system. Only include the most common *(italicized)* and life-threatening *(bold italic);* you can refer to the others in the drug handbook, if needed. Contraindications and precautions (9) can be grouped together and checked before giving the medication. Also, copy the pharmacokinetics (10) so you can refer to this information after you administer the drug. Important drug interactions and incompatibilities (11) should be listed on the card and carefully checked before administering the drug.

Nursing considerations (12), which are grouped under the headings of assess, administer, perform/provide, evaluate, and teach patient/family, can be placed on the back of the card for easy reference. These nursing considerations can be simplified to save space. For example, the following assessment criteria from the drug monograph can be abbreviated as shown below:

Assess:
• I&O, report hematuria, oliguria since penicillin in high doses is neurotoxic
• Culture, sensitivity before drug therapy; drug may be taken as soon as culture is taken

Assess:
• I&O, report hematuria, oliguria
• C&S—begin drug after culture is taken

Example of medication card

FRONT

(1) Generic drug:	(4) Pronunciation:
(2) Trade name:	
(3) Classification:	

(5) Action:

(6) Uses:

(7) Dosage and routes:

(8) Side effects/adverse reactions:

(9) Contraindications/precautions:

(10) Pharmacokinetics:

(11) Interactions/incompatibilities:

BACK

(12) Nursing considerations

Assess:

Administer:

Perform/provide:

Evaluate:

Teach patient/family:

Appendix e

Controlled substance chart

Drugs	United States	Canada
Heroin, LSD, peyote, marijuana, mescaline	Schedule I	Schedule H
Opium (morphine, meperidine), amphetamines, cocaine, short-acting barbiturates (secobarbital)	Schedule II	Schedule F
Glutethimide, paregoric, phendimetrazine	Schedule III	Schedule F
Chloral hydrate, chlordiazepoxide, diazepam, mazindol, meprobamate, phenobarbital	Schedule IV	Schedule F
Antidiarrheals with opium, antitussives	Schedule V	

Appendix f

FDA pregnancy categories

A No risk demonstrated to the fetus in any trimester

B No adverse effects in animals, no human studies available

C Only given after risks to the fetus are considered; animal studies have shown adverse reactions, no human studies available

D Definite fetal risks, may be given in spite of risks if needed in life-threatening conditions

X Absolute fetal abnormalities; not to be used anytime in pregnancy

Appendix g
Bibliography

Clark JB, Queener SF, Karb VB: Pharmacological basis of nursing practice, ed 3, St Louis, 1990, Mosby–Year Book, Inc.

Drug Information 90: Bethesda, 1990, American Hospital Formulary Service.

Facts and Comparisons: Philadelphia, updated monthly, JB Lippincott Co.

Gahart BL: Intravenous medications, ed 7, St Louis, 1991, Mosby–Year Book, Inc.

Goodman A, and others: Goodman and Gilman's The pharmacological basis of therapeutics, ed 7, New York, 1985, Macmillan Publishing Co.

McKenry LM and Salerno E: Mosby's pharmacology in nursing, ed 17, St Louis, 1989, Mosby–Year Book, Inc.

Mediphor Editorial Group: Drug interaction facts, Philadelphia, updated quarterly, JB Lippincott Co.

Appendix h

Combination products

Aceta with Codeine, Empracet
with Codeine Phosphate 30 mg
No. 3, Tylenol with Codeine
No. 3: acetaminophen 300 mg
with codeine phosphate 30 mg
Achromycin Intramuscular:
tetracycline HCl 100 mg with
procaine HCl 40 mg
Achromycin Intramuscular:
tetracycline HCl 250 mg with
procaine HCl 40 mg
Aethralgen: salicylamide 250
mg with acetaminophen 250 mg
Alazide, Spironazide, Spiro-
zide: spironolactone 25 mg with
hydrochlorothiazide 25 mg
Aldactazide 25/25: spironolactone 25 mg with hydrochlorothiazide 25 mg
Aldactazide 50/50: spironolactone 50 mg with hydrochlorothiazide 50 mg
Aldoclor-15: methyldopa 250
mg with chlorothiazide 15 mg
Aldoclor-150: methyldopa
250 mg with chlorothiazide
150 mg
Aldoclor-250: methyldopa
250 mg with chlorothiazide
250 mg
Aldoril-15, Methyldopa and Hydrochlorothiazide Tablets 250
mg/15 mg: methyldopa 250 mg
with hydrochlorothiazide 15 mg
Aldoril-25, Methyldopa and Hydrochlorothiazide Tablets 250
mg/25 mg: methyldopa 250 mg
with hydrochlorothiazide 25 mg

Aldoril D30, Alodopa-H-30,
Methyldopa and Hydrochlorothiazide Tablets 500 mg/30 mg:
methyldopa 500 mg with hydrochlorothiazide 30 mg
Aldoril D50, Alodopa-H-50,
Methyldopa and Hydrochlorothiazide Tablets 500 mg/50 mg:
methyldopa 500 mg with hydrochlorothiazide 50 mg
Amaphen with Codeine No. 3:
acetaminophen 325 mg with butalbital 50 mg, caffeine 40 mg,
codeine phosphate 30 mg
Ambenyl: diphenhydramine HCl
12.5 mg/5 ml with codeine phosphate 10 mg/5 ml
Anacin: aspirin 400 mg with caffeine 32 mg
Anexsia: hydrocodone bitartrate
7.5 mg with acetaminophen
650 mg
Anexsia with Codeine, Empirin
with Codeine 30 mg No. 3: codeine 30 mg with aspirin 325 mg
Anodynos-DHC, DIA-Gesic:
acetaminophen 150 mg with aspirin 230 mg, caffeine 30 mg, hydrocodone bitartrate 5 mg
Antrocol: atropine sulfate 0.195
mg with phenobarbital 16 mg
Antrocol Elixir: atropine sulfate
0.039 mg/ml with phenobarbital
3 mg/ml
A.P.C. with Codeine No. 3
Tabloid: aspirin 227 mg with caffeine 32 mg, codeine phosphate
30 mg, phenacetin 162 mg

COMBINATION PRODUCTS

A.P.C. with Codeine No. 4
Tabloid: aspirin 227 mg with caffeine 32 mg, codeine phosphate 60 mg, phenobarbital 162 mg
Apresazide 25/25, Aprozide 25/25, Hydralazine 25/25, Hydralazine-Thiazide 25/25: hydralazine HCl 25 mg with hydrochlorothiazide 25 mg
Apresazide 50/50, Aprozide 50/50, Hydralazine 50/50, Hydralazine-Thiazide 50/50: hydralazine HCl 50 mg with hydrochlorothiazide 50 mg
Apresazide 100/50, Aprozide 100/50, Hydralazine 100/50, Hydralazine-Thiazide 100/50: hydralazine HCl 100 mg with hydrochlorothiazide 50 mg
Apresodex, Apresoline-Esidrix, Hydralazine-Thiazide: hydralazine HCl 25 mg with hydrochlorothiazide 15 mg
Aralen Phosphate with Primaquine Phosphate: chloroquine phosphate 300 mg (of chloroquine) with primaquine phosphate 45 mg (of primaquine)
A.S.A. and Codeine Compound No. 3 Pulvules: codeine 30 mg with aspirin 380 mg, caffeine 30 mg
Ascriptin with Codeine No. 2: aspirin 325 mg with codeine phosphate 15 mg, buffers
Ascriptin with Codeine No. 3: aspirin 325 mg with codeine phosphate 30 mg, buffers
Atropine, Demerol Injection: meperidine HCl 50 mg/ml with atropine sulfate 0.4 mg/ml
Atropine, Demerol Injection: meperidine HCl 75 mg/ml with atropine sulfate 0.4 mg/ml
Axotal: aspirin 650 mg with butalbital 50 mg
Azo-Gamazole, Azo Gantanol, Azo-Sulfamethoxazole: sulfamethoxazole 500 mg with phenazopyridine HCl 100 mg
Azo-Gantrisin, Azo-Gulfasin, Azo-Sulfisocon, Azo-Sulfamethoxazole: sulfisoxazole 500 mg with phenazopyridine HCl 50 mg
B-A-C: aspirin 650 mg with butalbital 50 mg, caffeine 40 mg, buffers
B-A-C No. 3: aspirin 325 mg with butalbital 50 mg, caffeine 40 mg, codeine phosphate 30 mg, buffers
Bancap: acetaminophen 325 mg with butalbital 50 mg
Bancap HC, Dolacet, Hydrocet, Vicoden: hydrocodone bitartrate 5 mg with acetaminophen 500 mg
Barbidonna: belladonna alkaloids, atropine sulfate 0.025 mg, hyoscyamine sulfate 0.1286 mg, phenobarbital 16 mg, scopolamine hydrobromide 0.0074 mg
Barbidonna Elixir: belladonna alkaloids, atropine sulfate 0.034 mg/5 ml, hyoscyamine sulfate 0.0174 mg/5 ml, phenobarbital 21.6 mg/ml, scopolamine hydrobromide 0.01 mg/5 ml
Barbidonna No. 2: belladonna alkaloids, atropine sulfate 0.025 mg, hyoscyamine sulfate 0.1286 mg, phenobarbital 32 mg, scopolamine hydrobromide 0.0074 mg
Bayer Children's Cold Medicine, St. Joseph's Cold Tablets for Children: phenylpropanolamine HCl 3.125 mg with aspirin 81 mg
Bayer Cold Syrup for Children: dextromethorphan hydrobromide 7.5 mg/5 ml with phenylpropanolamine HCl 9 mg/5 ml
BC Powder: aspirin 650 mg with caffeine 32 mg, salicylamide 195 mg
Belap, Pheno-Bella: belladonna

extract 10.8 mg (0.135 mg of alkaloids of belladonna leaf) with phenobarbital 16.2 mg

Belladenal-S: levorotatory belladonna alkaloids malates 0.25 mg (of levorotatory belladonna alkaloids) with phenobarbital 50 mg

Bellalphen, Donnatal, Hyosophen: belladonna alkaloids atropine sulfate 0.0194 mg, hyoscyamine sulfate 0.1037 mg, phenobarbital 16.2 mg, scopolamine hydrobromide 0.0065 mg

Bellergal: ergotamine tartrate 0.3 mg with levorotatory belladonna alkaloids malates 0.1 mg (of levorotatory belladonna alkaloids), phenobarbital 20 mg

Bellergal-S: ergotamine tartrate 0.6 mg with levorotatory belladonna alkaloids malates 0.2 mg (of lavorotatory belladonna alkaloids 40 mg)

Benadryl: diphenhydramine HCl 25 mg with pseudoephedrine HCl 60 mg

Benylin: diphenhydramine HCl 12.5 mg/5 ml with pseudoephedrine HCl 30 mg/5 ml

Benylin DM: dextromethorphan hydrobromide 5 mg/5 ml with guaifenesin 100 mg/5 ml

Bexophene, Darvon Compound-65 Pulvules, Dolene Compound-65, Doxaphene Compound, Propoxyphene-AC, Propoxyphene Compound-65, SK-65: propoxyphene HCl 65 mg with aspirin 389 mg, caffeine 32.4 mg

Bicillin C-R: 150,000 units (of penicillin G) per ml with penicillin G benzathine 150,000 units (of penicillin G) per ml

Bicillin C-R: penicillin G procaine 300,000 units (of penicillin G) per ml with penicillin G benzathine 300,000 units (of penicillin G) per ml

Bicillin C-R 900/300: penicillin G procaine 150,000 units (of penicillin G) per ml with penicillin G benzathine 450,000 units (of penicillin G) per ml

B&O Supprettes No. 15A: powdered opium 30 mg with belladonna extract 16.2 mg (equivalent to belladonna alkaloids 0.21 mg)

B&O Supprettes No. 16A: powdered opium 60 mg with belladonna extract 16.2 mg (equivalent to belladonna alkaloids 0.21 mg)

Bromo-seltzer Granules: acetaminophen 325 mg/capful measure with citric acid 2.224 g/capful measure, sodium bicarbonate 2.871 g/capful measure

Butibel: belladonna extract 15 mg (0.187 mg of alkaloids of belladonna leaf) with butabarbital sodium 15 mg

Butibel Elixir: belladonna extract 15 mg (0.187 mg of alkaloids of belladonna leaf) with butabarbital sodium 15 mg

Cafatine, Cafergot, Caffeien-Ergotamine, Ercaf, Lanatrate: ergotamine tartrate 1 mg with caffeine 100 mg

Cafatine PB, Cafergot, Caferate-PB, Ergo-Caff with Phenobarbital, Migergot PB: ergotamine tartrate 2 mg with caffeine 100 mg, levorotatory belladonna alkaloids malates 0.25 mg (of levorotatory belladonna alkaloids), phenobarbital 60 mg

Cafergot: ergotamine tartrate 1 mg with caffeine 100 mg, levorotatory alkaloids malates 0.125 mg (of levorotatory belladonna alkaloids), phenobarbital sodium 30 mg

Cafergot, Wigraine: ergotamine

COMBINATION PRODUCTS

tartrate 2 mg with caffeine 100 mg

Caladryl: diphenhydramine HCl 1% with calamine 8%, camphor 0.1%

Calcidrine Syrup: codeine 8.4 mg/5 ml with calcium iodide anhydrous 152 mg/5 ml

Cantri, Vagilia: sulfisoxazole 10% with allantoin 2%, aminacrine HCl 0.2%

Capital and Codeine: codeine 30 mg with acetaminophen 325 mg

Capital with Codeine: acetaminophen 120 mg/5 ml with codeine 12 mg/5 ml

Capozide 25/15: captopril 25 mg with hydrochlorothiazide 15 mg

Capozide 25/25: captopril 25 mg with hydrochlorothiazide 25 mg

Capozide 50/15: captopril 50 mg with hydrochlorothiazide 15 mg

Capozide 50/25: captopril 50 mg with hydrochlorothiazide 25 mg

Carisoprodol Compound, Soprodol Compound, Soma Compound, Soprodol Compound: risoprodol 200 mg with aspirin 325 mg

CDP Plus, Clindex, Clinoxide, Clipoxide, Librax, Lidox, Lidoxide: clidinium bromide 2.5 mg with chlordiazepoxide HCl 5 mg

Chardonna-2: belladonna extract 15 mg (0.187 mg of alkaloids of belladonna leaf) with phenobarbital 15 mg

Cherapas, Hydroserpine Plus, Ser-A-Gen, Ser-Ap-Es, Serathide, Serpazide, Tri-Hydroserpine, Unipres: reserpine 0.1 mg with hydralazine HCl 25 mg, hydrochlothiazide 15 mg

Children's Hold 4 Hour: dextromethorphan hydrobromide 3.75 mg with phenylpropanolamine HCl 6.25 mg

Chlorofon-F, Chlorzone Forte, Paracet Forte, Parafon Forte, Zoxaphen: chlorzoxazone 250 mg with acetaminophen 300 mg

Chloroserp-250, Chloroserpine-250, Diupres-250: reserpine 0.125 mg with chlorothiazide 250 mg

Chloroserp-500, Chloropserpine-500, Diupres-500: reserpine 0.125 mg with chlorothiazide 500 mg

Clindex, Clinoxide, Clipoxide, Librax, Lidox: chlordiazepoxide HCl 5 mg with clidinium bromide 2.5 mg

Co-Gesic, Damacet-P, Duradyne, Hy-Phen, Norcet, Vicodin: hydrocodone bitartrate 5 mg with acetaminophen 500 mg

Codalan No. 1: acetaminophen 500 mg with caffeine 30 mg, codeine phosphate 8 mg

Codalan No. 2: acetaminophen 500 mg with caffeine 30 mg, codeine phosphate 15 mg

Codalan No. 3: acetaminophen 500 mg with caffeine 30 mg, codeine phosphate 30 mg

Codxym, Percodan, Roxiprin: oxycodone HCl 4.5 mg, oxycodone terephthalate 0.38 mg with aspirin 325 mg

Combipres 0.1 mg: clonidine HCl 0.1 mg with chlorthalidone 15 mg

Combipres 0.2 mg: clonidine HCl 0.2 mg with chlorthalidone 15 mg

Combipres 0.3 mg: clonidine HCl 0.3 mg with chlorthalidone 15 mg

Comtrex: dextromethorphan hydrobromide 10 mg with acetaminophen 325 mg, chlorpheniramine maleate 2 mg, phenylpropanolamine hydrochloride 12.5 mg

Comtrex: dextromethorphan hydrobromide 3.3 mg/5 ml with acetaminophen 108.3 mg/5 ml, chlorpheniramine maleate 0.67 mg/5 ml, phenylpropanolamine HCl 4.2 mg/5 ml

Conar Expectorant: dextromethorphan hydrobromide 15 mg/5 ml with guaifenesin 100 mg/5 ml, phenylephrine HCl 10 mg/5 ml

Conar: dextromethorphan hydrobromide 15 mg with acetaminophen 300 mg, guaifenesin 100 mg, phenylephrine HCl 10 mg

Conar Syrup: dextromethorphan hydrobromide 15 mg/5 ml with phenylephrine HCl 10 mg/5 ml

Congespirin: phenylpropanolamine HCl 6.25 mg/5 ml with acetaminophen 130 mg/5 ml

Congespirin, Aspirin-Free: acetaminophen 81 mg with phenylephrine HCl 81 mg

Contac Jr.: dextromethorphan hydrobromide 5 mg/5 ml with acetaminophen 160 mg/5 ml, pseudoephedrine HCl 15 mg/5 ml

Contac Severe Cold Formula, Nyquil Nighttime Cold Medicine, Nytime Cold Medicine, Quiet Nite: dextromethorphan hydrobromide 5 mg/5 ml with acetaminophen 167 mg/5 ml, doxylamine succinate 1.25 mg/5 ml, pseudoephedrine HCl 10 mg/5 ml

Copavin Pulvules: codeine sulfate 15 mg with papaverine HCl 15 mg

Corzide 40/5: bendroflumethiazide 5 mg with nadolol 4 mg

Corzide 80/5: bendroflumethiazide 5 mg with nadolol 40 mg

CoTylenol: dextromethorphan hydrobromide 5 mg/5 ml with acetaminophen 108.3 mg/5 ml, chlorpheniramine maleate 0.67 mg/5 ml, pseudoephedrine HCl 10 mg/5 ml

CoTylenol Cold Medication Tablets: dextromethorphan hydrobromide 15 mg with acetaminophen 325 mg, chlorpheniramine maleate 2 mg, pseudoephedrine HCl 30 mg

Cremacoat 3: dextromethorphan hydrobromide 6.7 mg/5 ml with guaifenesin 66.7 mg/5 ml, phenylpropanolamine HCl 12.5 mg/5 ml

Cremacoat 4: dextromethorphan hydrobromide 6.7 mg/5 ml with doxylamine succinate 2.5 mg/5 ml, phenylpropanolamine HCl 12.5 mg/5 ml

Damason-P: hydrocodone bitartrate 5 mg with aspirin 224 mg, caffeine 32 mg

Darvocet-N 50, Propoxyphene Napsylate with Acetaminophen Tablets: acetaminophen 325 mg with propoxyphene napsylate 50 mg

Darvocet-N 100, Doxapap-N, Propacet 100: propoxyphene napsylate 100 mg with acetaminophen 650 mg

Darvon Compound Pulvules: aspirin 389 mg with caffeine 32.4 mg propoxyphene HCl 32 mg

Darvon Compound-65 Pulvules, Dolene Compound-65, SK-65-Compound: aspirin 389 mg with caffeine 32.4 mg, propoxyphene HCl 65 mg

Darvon with A.S.A. Pulvules: aspirin 325 mg with propoxyphene HCl 65 mg

Darvon-N and A.S.A.: aspirin 325 mg with propoxyphene napsylate 100 mg

Deconex: phenylpropanolamine HCl 18 mg with acetaminophen 325 mg

Demerol APAP: acetaminophen 300 mg with meperidine HCl 50 mg

Demi-Regroton: chlorthalidone 25 mg with reserpine 0.125 mg

Deprol: meprobamate 400 mg with benactyzine HCl 1 mg

Dihydrocodeine Compound Modified, Synalgos: aspirin 356.4 mg with caffeine 30 mg and dihydrocodeine bitartrate 16 mg

Dilantin with Phenobarbital Kapseals: Phenytoin Sodium 100 mg with Phenobarbital 32 mg

Dilantin with Phenobarbital Kapseals: phenobarbital 16 mg with phenytoin sodium 100 mg

Dimetane-DX Cough Syrup: dextromethorphan hydrobromide 10 mg/5 ml with brompheniramine maleate 2 mg/5 ml, pseudoephedrine HCl 30 mg/5 ml

Diurese, Matatensin No. 4, Trichlormethiazide with Reserpine Tablets, Trichlortensin: trichlormethiazide 4 mg with reserpine 0.1 mg

Diutensen: methyclothiazide 2.5 mg with cryptenamine tannates 2 mg (of cryptenamine)

Diutensen: reserpine 0.1 mg with methyclothiazide 2.5 mg

Diutensin-R: methyclothiazide 25 mg with reserpine 0.1 mg

Diutrim: phenylpropanolamine HCl 75 mg with benzocaine 9 mg, carboxymethylcellulose 75 mg

Dolene AP-65: acetaminophen 650 mg with propoxyphene HCl 65 mg

Donnatal: belladonna alkaloids atropine sulfate 0.0194 mg, hyoscyamine sulfate 0.1037 mg, phenobarbital 32.4 mg, scopolamine hydrobromide 0.0065 mg

Donnatal Elixir, Hyosophen Elixir: belladonna alkaloids atropine sulfate 0.0194 mg/5 ml, hyoscyamine sulfate 0.1037 mg/5 ml, phenobarbital 16.2 mg/5 ml, scopolamine hydrobromide 0.0065/5 ml

Donnatal Extentabs: belladonna alkaloids atropine sulfate 0.0582 mg, hyoscyamine sulfate 0.3111 mg, phenobarbital 48.6 mg, scopolamine hydrobromide 0.0195 mg

Donnatal, Hyosophen: belladonna alkaloids atropine sulfate 0.0194 mg, hyoscyamine sulfate 0.1037 mg, phenobarbital 16.2 mg, scopolamine hydrobromide 0.0065 mg

Dorcol Children's Cough Syrup: dextromethorphan hydrobromide 5 mg/5 ml with guaifenesin 50 mg/5 ml, pseudoephedrine HCl 15 mg/5 ml

DUO-Medihaler: isoproterenol HCl 160 μg/metered spray with phenylephrine bitartrate 240 μg/metered spray

Dyazide: hydrochlorothiazide 25 mg with triamterene 50 mg

Ebdecon, Phenapap No. 2: acetaminophen 325 mg with phenylpropanolamine HCl 25 mg

Empirin with Codeine 15 mg No. 2: codeine 15 mg with aspirin 325 mg

Empirin with Codeine 60 mg No. 4: aspirin 325 mg with codeine phosphate 60 mg

Empracet with Codeine Phosphate 60 mg No. 4, Tylenol

with Codeine No. 4: acetaminophen 300 mg with codeine phosphate 60 mg

Endecon, Phenapap No. 2: phenylpropanolamine HCl 25 mg with acetaminophen 325 mg

Enduronyl, Eserdine Forte, Methyclothiazide and Deserpidine Tablets 5 mg/0.5 mg, Methy-Deserpidine Forte, Methy-Deserpidine Strong: methyclothiazide 5 mg with deserpidine 0.5 mg

Enduronyl, Eserdine, Methyclothiazide, Deserpidine Tablets 5 mg/0.25 mg: deserpidine 0.25 mg with methychlothiazide 5 mg

Entex: guaifenesin 200 mg with phenylephrine HCl 5 mg with phenylpropanolamine HCl 45 mg

Entex LA: guaifenesin 400 mg with phenylpropanolamine HCl 75 mg

Epromate, Equagesic, Equazine-M, Hepto-M, Mepro Compound, Meprogesic, Micranin: meprobamate 200 mg with aspirin 325 mg

Equagesic, Equazine-M, Mepro-Analgesic, Mepor Compound, Micrainin: aspirin 325 mg with meprobamate 200 mg

Esgic, Fioricet: acetaminophen 325 mg with butalbital 50 mg, caffeine 40 mg

Esimil: guanethidine monosulfate 10 mg (equivalent to guanethidine sulfate 8.4 mg) with hydrochlorothiazide 25 mg

Eutron Filmtab: pargyline HCl 25 mg with methyclothiazide 5 mg

Excedrin: acetaminophen 194 mg with aspirin 227 mg, caffeine 33 mg, buffers

Excedrin: aspirin 250 mg with acetaminophen 250 mg, caffeine 65 mg

Excedrin P.M.: acetaminophen 500 mg with diphenhydramine citrate 38 mg

Femguard, Sulfa-Gyn, Sultrin, Sulfa, Trysul: miscellaneous sulfonamide-sulfonamide sulfabenzamide 3.7%, sulfacetamide 2.85%, sulfisoxazole 3.42%, and urea 0.64%

Fiorinal: aspirin 325 mg with butalbital 50 mg, caffeine 40 mg

Fiorinal with Codeine No. 1: aspirin 325 mg with butalbital 50 mg, caffeine 40 mg, codeine phosphate 7.5 mg

Fiorinal with Codeine No. 2: aspirin 325 mg with butalbital 50 mg, caffeine 40 mg, and codeine phosphate 15 mg

Fiorinal with Codeine No. 3: aspirin 325 mg with butalbital 50 mg, caffeine 40 mg, codeine phosphate 30 mg

Firgesic, Ursinus Inlay Tablets: aspirin 325 mg with pseudoephedrine HCl 30 mg

G-1: acetaminophen 500 mg with butalbital 50 mg, caffeine 40 mg

G-2: acetaminophen 500 mg with butalbital 50 mg, codeine phosphate 15 mg

G-3, Sedapap No. 3: codeine 30 mg with acetaminophen 500 mg, butalbital 50 mg

G-3: acetaminophen 500 mg with butalbital 50 mg, codeine phosphate 30 mg

Gemnisyn: acetaminophen 325 mg with aspirin 325 mg

Goody's Headache Powder: acetaminophen 260 mg with aspirin 520 mg, caffeine 32.5 mg

Hybephen: belladonna alkaloids atropine sulfate 0.0233 mg, hyoscyamine sulfate 0.1277 mg, phenobarbital 15 mg,

COMBINATION PRODUCTS

scopolamine hydrobromide 0.0094 mg

Hydro-Fluserpine No 1, Hydropine, Salazide-Demi, Salutensin-Demi: reserpine 0.125 mg with hydroflumethiazide 25 mg

Hydro-Fluserpine No. 2, Hydropine H.P., Salazide, Salutensin: hydroflumethiazide 50 mg with reserpine 0.125 mg

Hydrogesic: hydrocodone bitartrate 7.5 mg with acetaminophen 650 mg

Hydromox R: quinethazone 50 mg with reserpine 0.125 mg

Hydropres-25, Hydro-Reserpine-25, Hydroserp, Hydroserpine No. 1, Hydrosine 25 mg, Mallopress: reserpine 0.125 mg with hydrochlorothiazide 25 mg

Hydropres-50, Hydro-Reserpine-50, Hydroserp, Hydroserpine No. 2, Hydrosine 50 mg, Hydrotensin, Hydroserpalan: reserpine 0.125 mg with hydrochlorothiazide 50 mg

Inderide 40/25, Propranolol HCl, Hydrochlorothiazide Tablets 40/25: propranolol HCl 40 mg with hydrochlorothiazide 25 mg

Inderide 80/25, Propranolol HCl, Hydrochlorothiazide Tablets 80/25: propranolol HCl 80 mg with hydrochlorothiazide 25 mg

Inderide LA 80/50: propranolol HCl 80 mg with hydrochlorothiazide 50 mg

Inderide LA 120/50: propranolol HCl 120 mg with hydrochlorothiazide 50 mg

Inderide LA 160/50: propranolol HCl 160 mg with hydrochlorothiazide 50 mg

INH: isoniazid 1 tablet, isoniazid 300 mg

Iophen DM, Tussi-Organidin

DM: dextromethorphan hydrobromide 10 mg/5 ml with iodinated glycerol 30 mg/5 ml

Kinesed: belladonna alkaloids atropine sulfate 0.02 mg, hyoscyamine sulfate 0.12 mg, phenobarbital 16 mg, scopolamine hydrobromide 0.007 mg

Levsin with Phenobarbital Tablets, Anaspaz: hyoscyamine sulfate 0.125 mg with phenobarbital

Levsinex with Phenobarbital Elixir: hyoscyamine sulfate 0.125 mg/5 ml with phenobarbital 15 mg/5 ml

Levsinex with Phenobarbital Time-caps: hyoscyamine sulfate 0.375 mg with phenobarbital 45 mg

Levsin-PB: hyoscyamine sulfate 0.125 mg/ml with phenobarbital 15 mg/ml

Lopressor HCT 50/25: metoprolol tartrate 50 mg with hydrochlorothiazide 25 mg

Lopressor HCT 100/25: metoprolol tartrate 100 mg with hydrochlorothiazide 25 mg

Lopressor HCT 100/50: metoprolol tartrate 100 mg with hydrochlorothiazide 50 mg

Maximum Strength Anacin: aspirin 500 mg with caffeine 32 mg

Maximum Strength Midol for Cramps: aspirin 500 mg with caffeine 32.4 mg, cinnamedrine HCl 14.9 mg

Maxzide: hydrochlorothiazide 50 mg with triamterene 75 mg

Mediqueall: dextromethorphan hydrobromide 15 mg with pseudoephedrine HCl 30 mg

Menrium 5-2: chlordiazepoxide 5 mg with esterified estrogens 0.2 mg

Menrium 5-4: chlordiazepoxide 5 mg with esterified estrogens 0.4 mg

Menrium 10-4: chlordiazepoxide 10 mg with esterified estrogens 0.4 mg

Mepergan: meperidine HCl 25 mg/ml with promethazine HCl 25 mg/ml

Mepergan Fortis: meperidine HCl 50 mg with promethazine HCl 25 mg

Metatensin No. 2: reserpine 0.1 mg with trichlormethiazide 2 mg

Midol Caplets: aspirin 454 mg with caffeine 32.4 mg, cinnamedrine HCl 14.9 mg

Midol PMS Caplets: acetaminophen 500 mg with pamabrom 25 mg, pyrilamine maleate 15 mg

Milprem-200, PMB 200: meprobamate 200 mg with conjugated estrogens 0.45 mg

Milprem-400, PMB 400: meprobamate 400 mg with conjugated estrogens 0.45 mg

Minizide 1: prazosin HCl 1 mg (of prazosin) with polythiazide 0.5 mg

Minizide 2: prazosin HCl 2 mg (of prazosin) with polythiazide 0.5 mg

Minizide 5: prazosin HCl 5 mg (of prazosin) with polythiazide 0.5 mg

Morphine, Atropine Sulfate Injection: morphine sulfate 16 mg/ml with atropine sulfate 0.4 mg/ml

Myapap with Codeine, Tylenol with Codeine: acetaminophen 120 mg/5 ml with codeine phosphate 12 mg/5 ml

Mysteclin F: amphotericin B 25 mg/5 ml with tetracycline equivalent to tetracycline HCl 25 mg/5 ml

Mysteclin-F: amphotericin B 50 mg with tetracycline equivalent to tetracycline HCl 250 mg

Mysteclin-F: tetracycline equivalent to 125 mg tetracycline HCl per 5 ml with amphotericin B 25 mg/5 ml

Mysteclin-F: tetracycline equivalent to 350 mg tetracycline HCl with amphotericin B 50 mg/5 ml

Mysteclin-F Syrup: tetracycline equivalent to 125 mg tetracycline HCl per 5 ml with amphotericin B 25 mg/5 ml

Naldecon-DX Adult: dextromethorphan hydrobromide 15 mg/5 ml with guaifenesin 200 mg/5 ml, phenylpropanolamine HCl 18 mg/5 ml

Naldecon-DX Children's Syrup: dextromethorphan hydrobromide 7.5 mg/5 ml with guaifenesin 100 mg/5 ml, phenylpropanolamine HCl 9 mg/5 ml

Naldegisic: acetaminophen 325 mg with pseudoephedrine HCl 15 mg

Naturetin with K 5 mg: bendroflumethiazide 5 mg with potassium chloride 500 mg

Neosporin G.U. Irrigant: polymyxin B sulfate 200,000 units (of polymyxin B)

Norgesic: orphenadrine citrate 25 mg with aspirin 385 mg, caffeine 30 mg

Norgesic Forte: orphenadrine citrate 50 mg with aspirin 770 mg, caffeine 60 mg

Novahistine Cough and Cold Formula: dextromethorphan hydrobromide 10 mg/5 ml with chlorpheniramine maleate 2 mg/5 ml, pseudoephedrine HCl 30 mg/5 ml

Opium and Belladonna: powdered opium 60 mg with belladonna extract 15 mg (equivalent to belladonna alkaloids 0.2 mg)

Oreticyl 25: deserpidine 0.125

COMBINATION PRODUCTS

mg with hydrochlorothiazide 25 mg

Oreticyl 50: deserpidine 0.125 mg with hydrochlorothiazide 50 mg

Oreticyl Forte: deserpidine 0.25 mg with hydrochlorothiazide 50 mg

Ornex: phenylpropanolamine HCl 12.5 mg with acetaminophen 325 mg

Orthoxicol Cough Syrup: dextromethorphan hydrobromide 10 mg/5 ml with methoxyphenamine HCl 17 mg/5 ml

Oxymycin, Terramycin Intramuscular Solution: oxytetracycline 50 mg/ml with lidocaine 2%

Pamprin: acetaminophen 325 mg with pamabrom 25 mg, pyrilamine maleate 12.5 mg

Pamprin Maximum Cramp Relief: acetaminophen 500 mg with pamabrom 25 mg, pyrilamine maleate 15 mg

Pathibamate-200: meprobamate 200 mg with tridihexethyl chloride 25 mg

Pathibamate-400: meprobamate 400 mg with tridihexethyl chloride 25 mg

Pediacare 3: dextromethorphan hydrobromide 5 mg/5 ml with chlorpheniramine maleate 1 mg/5 ml, pseudoephedrine HCl 15 mg/5 ml

Pediacare 3 Chewable Tablets: dextromethorphan hydrobromide 2.5 mg with chlorpheniramine maleate 0.5 mg, pseudophedrine HCl 7.5 mg

Pediazole: erythromycin ethlysuccinate 200 mg (of erythromycin) per 5 ml with sulfisoxazole acetyl 600 mg (of sulfisoxazole) per 5 ml

Penntuss: codeine polistirex

equivalent to codeine 10 mg/5 ml with chlorpheniramine polistirex equivalent to chlorpheniramine maleate 4 mg/5 ml

Percodan-Demi: aspirin 325 mg with oxycodone HCl 2.25 mg, oxycodone terephthalate 0.19 mg

Percogesic: acetaminophen 325 mg with phenyltoloxamine citrate 30 mg

Peri-Colace: docusate sodium 100 mg with cusanthranol 30 mg

Persistin: salsalate 487.5 mg with aspirin 162.5 mg

Phenaphen with Codeine No. 2: acetaminophen 325 mg with codeine phosphate 15 mg

Phenaphen with Codeine No. 2, Proval No. 3: codeine 30 mg with acetaminophen 325 mg

Phenaphen with Codeine No. 3, Proval No. 2: acetaminophen 325 mg with codeine phosphate 30 mg

Phenaphen with Codeine No. 4: acetaminophen 325 mg with codeine phosphate 60 mg

Phenaphen-650 with Codeine: acetaminophen 650 mg with codeine phosphate 30 mg

Phenergan: promethazine HCl 6.25 mg/5 ml with phenylephrine HCl 5 mg/5 ml

Phenergan-D: promethazine HCl 6.25 mg with pseudoephedrine HCl 60 mg

Phenergan VC Syrup, Promethazine HCl VC: promethazine HCl 6.25 mg/5 ml with phenylephrine HCl 5 mg/5 ml

Phenergan with Dextromethorphan: dextromethorphan hydrobromide 15 mg/5 ml with promethazine HCl 6.35 mg/5 ml

Phrenilin: acetaminophen 325 mg with butalbital 50 mg, caffeine 40 mg

Phrenilin Forte: acetaminophen 650 mg with butalbital 50 mg
Phrenilin with Codeine No. 3: acetaminophen 325 mg with butalbital 50 mg, codeine phosphate 30 mg
Propoxyphene HCl/65, Wygesic: acetaminophen 650 mg with propoxyphene HCl 65 mg
Prunicodeine: terpin hydrate 29 mg/5 ml with codeine sulfate 10 mg/5 ml
Rautrax: rauwolfia 50 mg with flumethiazide 400 mg, potassium chloride 400 mg
Rautrax-N: bendroflumethiazide 4 mg with rauwolfia serpentina 50 mg, potassium chloride 400 mg
Rauzide: bendroflumethiazide 4 mg with rauwolfia serpentina 50 mg
Regroton: reserpine 0.25 mg with chlorthalidone 50 mg
Renese: reserpine 0.25 mg with polythiazide 2 mg
Rifamate: isoniazid 150 mg with rifampin 300 mg
Rimactane: isoniazid 2 capsules, rifampin 300 mg
Rimactane: rifampin 1 tablet, isoniazid 300 mg
Rimactane: rifampin 2 capsules, rifampin 300 mg
Robaxisal, Robomol/ASA: methocarbamol 400 mg with aspirin 325 mg
Robitussin-DM: dextromethorphan hydrobromide 15 mg/5 ml with guaifenesin 100 mg/5 ml
Roxicet: oxycodone HCl 5 mg/5 ml with acetaminophen 325 mg/5 ml
S-A-C: salicylamide 230 mg with acetaminophen 150 mg, caffeine 30 mg
Salimeth Forte: salicylamide 600 mg with acetaminophen 250 mg

S.B.P.: secobarbital sodium 50 mg with butabarbital sodium 30 mg, phenobarbital 15 mg
Serpasil-Apresoline HCl No. 1: hydralazine HCl 25 mg with reserpine 0.1 mg
Serpasil-Apresoline HCl No. 2: hydralazine HCl 25 mg with reserpine 0.2 mg
Serpasil-Esidrix No. 1: reserpine 0.1 mg with hydrochlorothiazide 25 mg
Serpasil-Esidrix No. 2: reserpine 0.1 mg with hydrochlorothiazide 50 mg
Sine-Aid: acetaminophen 325 mg with pseudoephedrine HCl 30 mg
Sine-Aid Extra Strength Caplets, Tylenol Sinus Maximum Strength Caplets: acetaminophen 500 mg with pseudoephedrine HCl 30 mg
Sine-Off Extra Strength, Sinutab: acetaminophen 500 mg with pseudoephedrine HCl 30 mg
Sinubid: acetaminophen 600 mg with phenylpropanolamine HCl 100 mg, phenyltoloxamine citrate 66 mg
Sinutab Maximum Nighttime: acetaminophen 167 mg/5 ml with diphenhydramine HCl 8.3 mg/5 ml, pseudoephedrine HCl 10 mg/5 ml
Sinutab II Maximum, Tylenol maximum strength sinus: acetaminophen 500 mg with pseudoephedrine HCl 30 mg
SK-APAP with Codeine, Tylenol with Codeine No. 2: codeine 5 mg with acetaminophen 300 mg
Soma Compound with Codeine: codeine 16 mg with aspirin 325 mg, carisoprodol 200 mg
Somines Pain Relief: acetaminophen 500 mg with diphenhydramine HCl 25 mg

COMBINATION PRODUCTS

Spec-T: Phenylpropanolamine 10.5 mg with Benzocaine 10 mg, Phenylephrine HCl 5 mg

Spec-T Sore Throat Cough Suppressant: dextromethorphan hydrobromide 10 mg with benzocaine 10 mg

Sudafed Cough Syrup: dextromethorphan hydrobromide 5 mg/ 5 ml with guaifenesin 100 mg/5 ml, pseudoephedrine HCl 15 mg/ 5 ml

Sultrin: miscellaneous sulfonamide-sulfonamide sulfabenzamide 184 mg, sulfacetamide 143.75 mg, sulfathiazole 172.5 mg, urea 31.83 mg

Talacen: pentazocine HCl 25 mg (of pentazocine) with acetaminophen 650 mg

Talwin Compound Caplets: aspirin 325 mg with pentazocine HCl 12.5 mg (of pentazocine)

Tenoretic 50: atenolol 50 mg with chlorthalidone 25 mg

Tenoretic 100: atenolol 100 mg with chlorthalidone 25 mg

Terpin Hydrate and Codeine: terpin hydrate 85 mg/5 ml with dextromethorphan hydrobromide 10 mg/5 ml (with alcohol 39%-44%)

Terramycin Intramuscular Solution: oxytetracycline 125 mg/ml with lidocaine 2%

T-Gesic: hydrocodone bitartrate 5 mg with acetaminophen 325 mg, butalbital 30 mg, caffeine 40 mg

Timolide 10/25: timolol maleate 10 mg with hydrochlorothiazide 25 mg

Trendar: acetaminophen 325 mg with pamabrom 25 mg

Triaminic-DM Cough Formula: dextromethorphan hydrobromide 10 mg/5 ml with phenylpropanolamine HCl 12.5 mg/5 ml

Triaminicol: dextromethorphan

hydrobromide 10 mg/5 ml with chlorpheniramine maleate 2 mg/5 ml, phenylpropanolamine HCl 12.5 mg/5 ml

Trigesic: aspirin 230 mg with acetaminophen 125 mg, caffeine 30 mg

Tuinal 50 mg Pulvules: secobarbital sodium 25 mg with amobarbital sodium 25 mg

Tuinal 100 mg Pulvules: secobarbital sodium 50 mg with amobarbital sodium 50 mg

Tuinal 200 mg Pulvules: secobarbital sodium 100 mg with amobarbital sodium 100 mg

Tylenol with Codeine No. 1: acetaminophen 300 mg with codeine phosphate 7.5 mg

Tylenol with Codeine No. 2: acetaminophen 300 mg with codeine phosphate 15 mg

Tylenol with Codeine No. 3: acetaminophen 300 mg with codeine phosphate 30 mg

Tylenol with Codeine No. 4: acetaminophen 300 mg with codeine phosphate 60 mg

Tylox: acetaminophen 500 mg with oxycodone HCl 5 mg

Urobiotic-250: oxytetracycline HCl 250 mg (of oxytetracycline) with phenazopyridine HCl 50 mg, sulfamethizole 250 mg

Vanquish Caplets: aspirin 227 mg with acetaminophen 194 mg, caffeine 30 mg, buffers

Vaseretic 10-25: enalapril maleate 10 mg with hydrochlorothiazide 25 mg

Vicks Childrens Cough Syrup: dextromethorphan hydrobromide 3.5 mg/5 ml with guaifenesin 25 mg/5 ml

Vicks Cough Silencers: dextromethorphan hydrobromide 2.5 mg with benzocaine 1 mg

Vicks Daycare: dextromethorphan hydrobromide 10 mg with acetaminophen 325 mg, guaifenesin 100 mg, pseudoephedrine HCl 30 mg

Vicks Daycare: dextromethorphan hydrobromide 3.3 mg/5 ml with acetaminophen 108.3 mg/5 ml, guaifenesin 33.3 mg/5 ml, pseudoephedrine HCl 10 mg/5 ml

Vicks Formula 44 Cough Control Discs: dextromethorphan hydrobromide 5 mg with benzocaine 1.25 mg

Vicks Formula 44 Cough Mixture: dextromethorphan hydrobromide 15 mg/ 5 ml with doxylamine succinate 3.75 mg/5 ml

Vicks Formula 44D: dextromethorphan hydrobromide 10 mg/5 ml with guaifenesin 66.7 mg/5 ml, pseudoephedrine HCl 20 mg/ 5 ml

Vicks Formula 44M: dextromethorphan hydrobromide 7.4 mg/5 ml with acetaminophen 125 mg/5 ml, guaifenesin 50 mg/5 ml, pseudoephedrine HCl 15 mg/ 5 ml

Westrim-1: phenylpropanolamine HCl 25 mg with benzocaine 5 mg, methylcellulose 300 mg

Wyanoids: belladonna extract 15 mg (0.19 mg of alkaloids of belladonna leaf) with ephedrine 3 mg

Ziradyl: diphenhydramine HCl 2% with zinc oxide 2%

COMBINATION PRODUCTS

Index

Entries can be identified as follows: generic name, Trade Name, DRUG CATEGORY, *Combination Product.*

Entries can be identified as follows: generic name, Trade Name, DRUG CATEGORY, *Combination Product.*

Entries can be identified as follows: generic name, Trade Name, DRUG CATEGORY, *Combination Product.*

Entries can be identified as follows: generic name, Trade Name, DRUG CATEGORY, *Combination Product*.

Entries can be identified as follows: generic name, Trade Name, DRUG CATEGORY, *Combination Product.*

Entries can be identified as follows: generic name, Trade Name, DRUG CATEGORY, *Combination Product*.

Entries can be identified as follows: generic name, Trade Name, DRUG CATEGORY, *Combination Product.*

Entries can be identified as follows: generic name, Trade Name, DRUG CATEGORY, *Combination Product*.

Entries can be identified as follows: generic name, Trade Name, DRUG CATEGORY, *Combination Product.*

INDEX

Entries can be identified as follows: generic name, Trade Name, DRUG CATEGORY,
Combination Product.

Entries can be identified as follows: generic name, Trade Name, DRUG CATEGORY, *Combination Product*.

Entries can be identified as follows: generic name, Trade Name, DRUG CATEGORY, *Combination Product.*

Entries can be identified as follows: generic name, Trade Name, DRUG CATEGORY, *Combination Product.*

Entries can be identified as follows: generic name, Trade Name, DRUG CATEGORY, *Combination Product.*

Entries can be identified as follows: generic name, Trade Name, DRUG CATEGORY, *Combination Product.*

Entries can be identified as follows: generic name, Trade Name, DRUG CATEGORY, *Combination Product.*

Entries can be identified as follows: generic name, Trade Name, DRUG CATEGORY, *Combination Product.*

Entries can be identified as follows: generic name, Trade Name, DRUG CATEGORY, *Combination Product*.

Entries can be identified as follows: generic name, Trade Name, DRUG CATEGORY, *Combination Product.*

Entries can be identified as follows: generic name, Trade Name, DRUG CATEGORY,
Combination Product.

Entries can be identified as follows: generic name, Trade Name, DRUG CATEGORY, *Combination Product.*

Entries can be identified as follows: generic name, Trade Name, DRUG CATEGORY, *Combination Product.*

Entries can be identified as follows: generic name, Trade Name, DRUG CATEGORY, *Combination Product.*

Entries can be identified as follows: generic name, Trade Name, DRUG CATEGORY, *Combination Product*.

Entries can be identified as follows: generic name, Trade Name, DRUG CATEGORY, *Combination Product.*

Entries can be identified as follows: generic name, Trade Name, DRUG CATEGORY, *Combination Product.*

Entries can be identified as follows: generic name, Trade Name, DRUG CATEGORY, *Combination Product.*

Entries can be identified as follows: generic name, Trade Name, DRUG CATEGORY, *Combination Product*.

Entries can be identified as follows: generic name, Trade Name, DRUG CATEGORY, *Combination Product.*

Entries can be identified as follows: generic name, Trade Name, DRUG CATEGORY, *Combination Product.*

Entries can be identified as follows: generic name, Trade Name, DRUG CATEGORY, *Combination Product.*

Entries can be identified as follows: generic name, Trade Name, DRUG CATEGORY, *Combination Product.*

Entries can be identified as follows: generic name, Trade Name, DRUG CATEGORY,
Combination Product.

Entries can be identified as follows: generic name, Trade Name, DRUG CATEGORY, *Combination Product.*

Entries can be identified as follows: generic name, Trade Name, DRUG CATEGORY, *Combination Product.*

Entries can be identified as follows: generic name, Trade Name, DRUG CATEGORY, *Combination Product*.

Entries can be identified as follows: generic name, Trade Name, DRUG CATEGORY, *Combination Product.*

Entries can be identified as follows: generic name, Trade Name, DRUG CATEGORY, *Combination Product.*

Entries can be identified as follows: generic name, Trade Name, DRUG CATEGORY, *Combination Product*.

Entries can be identified as follows: generic name, Trade Name, DRUG CATEGORY, *Combination Product.*

Entries can be identified as follows: generic name, Trade Name, DRUG CATEGORY, *Combination Product.*

INDEX

Entries can be identified as follows: generic name, Trade Name, DRUG CATEGORY,
Combination Product.

Notes

Notes

Notes

Notes

Notes

Compatibility Chart

	Atropine	Butorphanol	Chlordiazepoxide	Chlorpromazine	Codeine	Diazepam	Dimenhydrinate	Diphenhydramine	Droperidol	Fentanyl	Glycopyrrolate
Atropine		C	I	C		I	C	C	C	C	C
Butorphanol	C		I	C		I	I	C	C	C	
Chlordiazepoxide	I	I		I	I	I	I	I	I	I	I
Chlorpromazine	C	C	I			I	I	C	C	C	C
Codeine			I			I					
Diazepam	I	I	I	I	I		I	I	I	I	I
Dimenhydrinate	C	I	I	I		I		C	C	C	I
Diphenhydramine	C	C	I	C		I	C		C	C	C
Droperidol	C	C	I	C		I	C	C		C	C
Fentanyl	C	C	I	C		I	C	C	C		C
Glycopyrrolate	C		I	C		I	I	C	C	C	
Hydroxyzine	C	C	I	C		I	I	C	C	C	C
Innovar	C	C	I	C		I	C	C	C	C	C
Lorazepam	I	I	I	I	I	I	I	I	I	I	I
Meperidine	C	C	I	C		I	C	C	C	C	C
Metoclopramide	C	C	I	C		I	C	C	C	C	
Morphine	C	C	I	C		I	C	C	C	C	C
Nalbuphine	C		I			I		C			
Pentazocine	C	C	I	C		I	C	C	C	C	I
Pentobarbital	C	I	I	I	I	I	I	I	I	I	I
Perphenazine	C	C	I	C		I	C	C	C	C	
Prochlorperazine	C	C	I	C		I	I	C	C	C	C
Promazine	C		I	C		I	I	C	C	C	C
Promethazine	C	C	I	C		I	I	C	C	C	C
Scopolamine Hbr	C	C	I	C		I	C	C	C	C	C
Secobarbital	I	I	I	I	I	I	I	I	I	I	I
Thiethylperazine		C	I			I					
Trimethobenzamide			I			I					C

Developed by Providence Memorial Hospital, El Paso, Texas.
NOTE: Give within 15 minutes of mixing. C, compatible; I, incompatible; □, no documented information